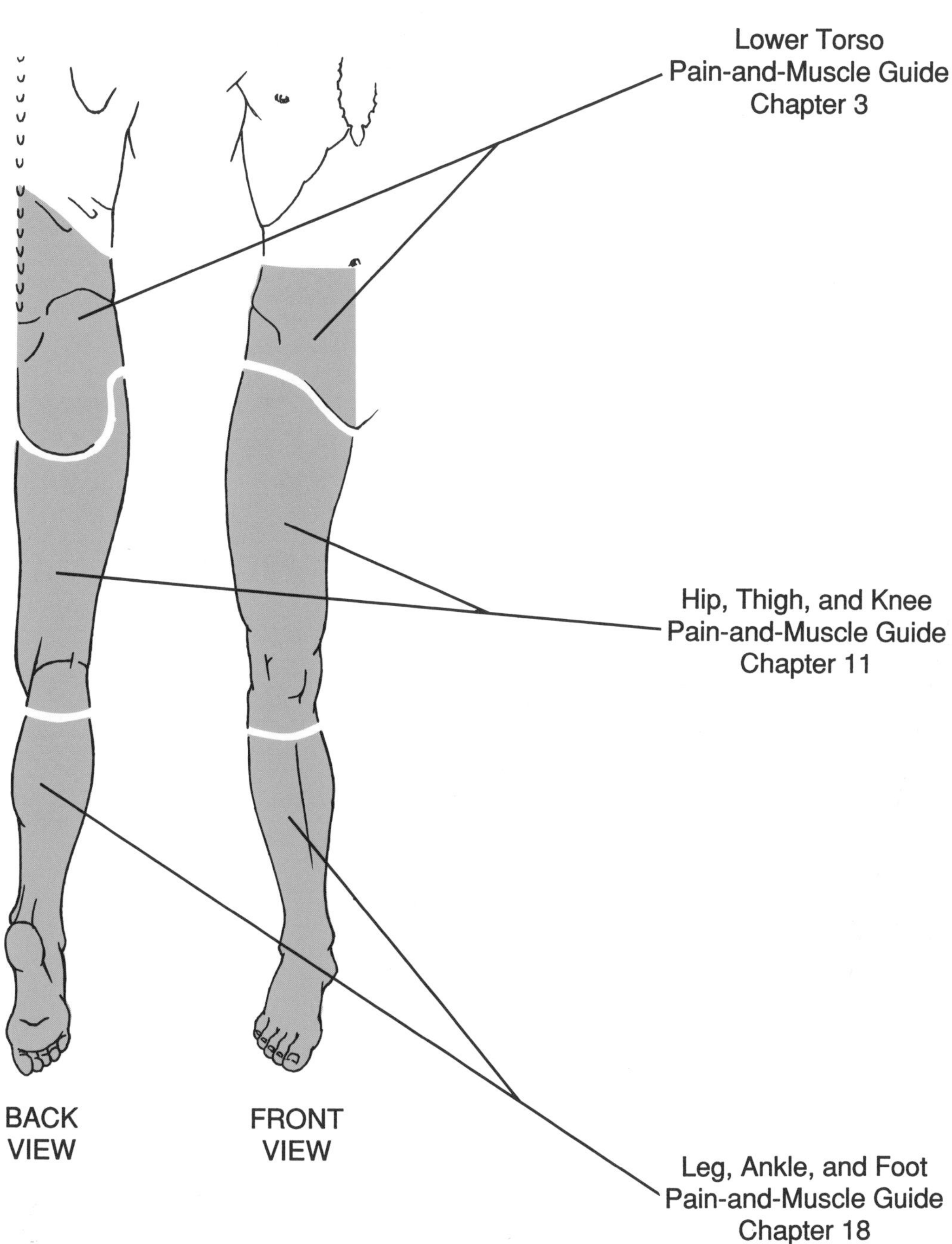

Pictorial index. The muscles that are likely to refer pain to an illustrated region of the body are listed in the Pain-and-Muscle Guide to the corresponding Part of the *Manual*. A Guide is found at the beginning of each Part, which is marked by red thumb tabs.

VOLUME 2

Myofascial Pain and Dysfunction

The Trigger Point Manual

THE LOWER EXTREMITIES

This is the second of two volumes, and contains information relating to the "lower half" of the body. Volume 1 deals with the "upper half" of the body. The contents and indices for both volumes are included in this book for the reader's convenience.

VOLUME 2

Myofascial Pain and Dysfunction

The Trigger Point Manual

THE LOWER EXTREMITIES

JANET G. TRAVELL, M.D.
Honorary Clinical Professor of Medicine
The George Washington University School of Medicine
Washington, D.C.

DAVID G. SIMONS, M.D.
Clincial Professor
Department of Physical Medicine and Rehabilitation
University of California, Irvine
Irvine, California

Illustrations by Barbara D. Cummings

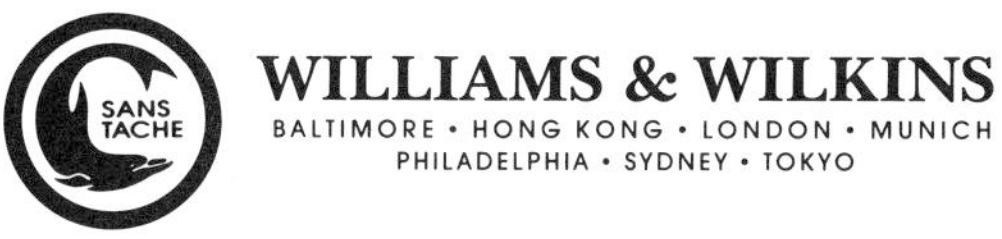
WILLIAMS & WILKINS
BALTIMORE • HONG KONG • LONDON • MUNICH
PHILADELPHIA • SYDNEY • TOKYO

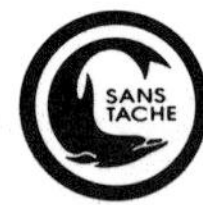

Editor: John P. Butler
Managing Editor: Linda Napora
Copy Editor: Shelley Potler
Designer: JoAnne Janowiak
Illustration Planner: Wayne Hubbel
Production Coordinator: Charles E. Zeller

Williams & Wilkins
Rose Tree Corporate Center, Building II
1400 North Providence Road, Suite 5025
Media, PA 19063-2043 USA

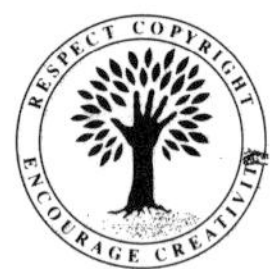

Accurate indications, adverse reactions, and dosage schedules for drugs are provided in this book, but it is possible that they may change. The reader is urged to review the package information data of the manufacturers of the medications mentioned.

Made in the United States of America

Library of Congress Cataloging-in-Publication Data
(Revised for volume 2)

Travell, Janet, 1901–
Myofascial pain and dysfunction.
Includes bibliographies and indexes.
1. Myalgia—Handbooks, manuals, etc. 2. Muscles—Diseases—Handbooks, manuals, etc. 3. Fasciae (Anatomy)—Diseases—Handbooks, manuals, etc. 4. Myofascial pain syndrome. 5. Muscles. I. Simons, David G. II. Trigger point manual. III. Title.
RC925.5.T7 1983 616.7′4 82-8555
ISBN 0-683-08366-X (v. 1)
ISBN 0-683-08367-8 (v. 2)

ISBN 0-683-08367-8

99 00 01
9 10 11 12

TO

Lois Statham Simons

whose contributions enriched this book

and

with whom it became a rewarding way of life

Foreword

John V. Basmajian

Superlatives come easily in considering what Drs. Travell and Simons have done in rounding out their epoch-making and highly successful *Trigger Point Manual* with this *Volume 2*. Many must have thought that producing the excellent Volume 1 was so exhausting that the authors were not going to be able to produce a fitting sequel. Such fans will be as delighted as I (who was impatient, not pessimistic). The pessimists were completely wrong.

I believe this volume is even better than the other because it reflects an enormous new recharging of energy that further experience, interaction, and thought have stimulated. Thus, *Volume 2* has become much more than it originally promised to be; i.e., it was to be a rounding out of practical considerations in the anatomical sense of dealing with the lower half of the body. *Volume 1*, indeed, dealt with the upper half of the body, but it also laid out the important principles of the myofascial pain syndromes (MPS) and hands-on techniques that were state-of-the-art then. This new volume has the distinction of going considerably beyond those areas to discuss rationale, new principles arising from a ground-swell of experience, and the unique place of MPS in the spectrum of musculoskeletal disorders. No book, not even Volume 1, has attempted this broad view before, and probably no other authors now could do it as well–if at all.

Myofascial trigger points and their significance in painful conditions are no longer the rather controversial subject they were before Volume 1 appeared, nor are the treatment methods taught by Drs. Travell and Simons. These are firmly established and are increasingly being validated by once skeptical clinical investigators. This volume goes beyond and opens up new ground in sensitizing clinicians to the important interfaces between myofascial pain syndromes and articular (somatic) dysfunctions on the one hand and fibromyalgia (fibrositis) on the other hand. I applaud the wise manner in which these issues are addressed, assessed, and integrated.

When I first began to learn that *Fluori-Methane* spray had a deleterious effect on the ozone layer, I was dismayed and disheartened for both my two friends and the many patients who would be denied the spray-and-stretch treatments. It is so heartwarming and exciting to see these innovators fully recognizing the environmental risks and acting with firmness. Instead of making excuses and persisting in the use of fluorocarbons, they have found adequate alternative techniques and are actively seeking adequate substitutes. My instincts assure me that they will succeed. Meanwhile, it is important that the chemical coolants are only the means to an end that can be achieved by following the lessons to be learned in *Volume 2*.

There are a multitude of clinically valuable gems throughout this volume. Some are boldly displayed (e.g., postisometric relaxation and cautions for patients with hypermobility); others are scattered liberally throughout the text and may be overlooked by the inexperienced reader.

Of course, on seeing the eloquent illustrations, casual browsers will be deeply impressed. I predict that they will soon be at risk of becoming serious and devoted readers. The drawings are not approximate renderings by a clever artist of what the authors "want." They are *exactly* what the authors require, carefully integrated with the text by a close author-artist relationship. Rarely have I seen such a perfect match.

The chapters on individual muscles "below the waist" were, of course, supposed to be the reason for ***Volume 2***. Alone, they could make the book an important aid for clinicians. But once again, they go far beyond the "How To" approach implied by the title ***Manual***. They embody the state-of-the-art of dealing with pain in and around the individual muscles in a way that I have never before seen for those muscles. Morphology, function, and common-sense approaches are melded with great style and clarity.

In short, I am greatly honored and pleased to have had the opportunity to write this Foreword. It is a volume that has set a very high mark for all authors in this field to try to reach. It is ***the*** book for its time, and an instant ***classic*** for many years to come.

John V. Basmajian, M.D., FRCPC, FACA, FACRM (Australia), FSBM, FABMR
Professor Emeritus, McMaster University
Hamilton, Ontario
Canada

Preface

Volume 2 of *The Trigger Point Manual* concerns the muscles of the lower half of the body as Volume 1 dealt with the muscles of the upper half of the body. This volume follows the same format with the same careful attention to detail found in Volume 1 and, again, reflects the close collaboration and interdependence of the coauthors who bring to it, respectively, their clinical expertise and insatiable curiosity as to how and why.

Preparation of this volume has been spurred by the broad acceptance of Volume 1. The first volume has now sold over 50,000 copies, partly because practitioners who have learned to use it have brought relief to their patients, and partly because practitioners became aware of it through the slides of all of its figures, economically supplied by the illustrator, Barbara D. Cummings. Volume 1 has been printed in English, Russian, and Italian and is scheduled to appear in German, French, and Japanese. Patients suffering from myofascial pain will benefit greatly as the recognition and management of myofascial pain syndromes are incorporated into the curricula of medical schools and physical therapy schools.

The reader will notice several differences between Volume 1 and Volume 2. This volume includes frequent references to related manual medicine diagnoses and treatment. The therapy sections describe alternative treatment techniques that do not require vapocoolant spray, techniques that will serve as a substitute until an environmentally safe vapocoolant is available. These other treatment techniques are summarized in Chapter 2.

Paragraphs set in smaller type indicate material that may not be essential to the management of patients' symptoms; however, this material cites the details and references on which summary statements are based. The supplementary references at the end of each anatomy section are provided primarily for the benefit of teachers and advanced students.

This volume includes unique features and reviews of special topics that are not available elsewhere. The chapter on the quadratus lumborum muscle contains an extensive review of the causes of functional scoliosis and how to identify them clinically. It puts lower limb-length inequality (often called a short leg) in perspective and examines in detail radiographic techniques for measuring it accurately. Chapter 6, Pelvic Floor Muscles, provides an unprecedented description of how to examine intrapelvic muscles for trigger points. A practical three-tone topographical guide (Fig. 8.5) simplifies distinguishing the three gluteal muscles and the piriformis muscle when palpating trigger points. The piriformis chapter, Chapter 10, presents a new understanding of the muscular origin of pain in sciatic, gluteal, and perineal distributions. The adductor chapter (Chapter 15) examines the remarkable complexity of the adductor magnus muscle, which helps explain why its importance is easily overlooked. The amply illustrated review of the recognition and correction of the Morton foot structure appears in Chapter 20 on the peroneal muscles. Chapter 21 reviews thoroughly the subject of nocturnal calf cramps and their close relation to trigger points in the gastrocnemius muscle.

Chapter 22 on the soleus and plantaris muscles summarizes the current literature on shin splints in relation to trigger points. The subject of postexercise muscle soreness is reviewed in the Appendix. The review shows that this phenomenon is now well understood. In summary, it is unlikely that either condition is closely associated with trigger points.

The last chapter (Chapter 28), Management of Chronic Myofascial Pain Syndrome, concerns the care of patients who have developed multiple myofascial syndromes and who fail to respond to the therapeutic measures that are usually so effective in single-muscle myofascial syndromes. This chapter distinguishes between the chronic myofascial pain syndrome and fibromyalgia.

Health professionals, when first exposed to this subject, often ask, "What does it take to become proficient?" The answer is threefold: *(a)* develop an appreciation of the ubiquity and characteristics of referred pain, *(b)* become intimately familiar with muscle anatomy, and *(c)* learn to palpate taut bands, locate trigger points, and elicit local twitch responses. To achieve the first, listen to and believe the patient. For the second, keep *The Trigger Point Manual* in the examining room to show a patient the illustration of the muscle most likely to be causing the pain (while the examiner reviews its anatomy). The third requires a motor skill that must be learned, like any other motor skill, by diligent practice.

During this volume's 8 years of gestation, many individuals have contributed to the final product in many helpful ways. The heavy burden was frequently made bearable by the enthusiasm expressed by practitioners for the value of Volume 1 to their patients and by their insistent need for Volume 2.

Through most, if not all, of this period, five individuals formed the essential team: the coauthors; the artist, Barbara D. Cummings, whose steadfast dedication and blossoming skills account for all of the original illustrations; the second author's wife, Lois Statham Simons, P.T., whose spirited discussions helped keep the manuscript on course and whose meticulous editing of every chapter polished it and ensured that it was correct and made sense; and the second author's faithful secretary, Barbara Zastrow, who typed and processed the seven (or more) drafts of each chapter and never lost her sense of humor.

Michael D. Reynolds, M.D., a rheumatologist, deserves outstanding recognition for the meticulous care and understanding with which he reviewed every chapter. He is a master of grammatic precision, concise expression, and the resolution of fuzzy statements. Any redundancy in this volume surely crept in *following* his review!

We owe a deep debt of gratitude to Robert Gerwin, M.D. for screening most of the chapters with a keen appreciation of the interface between neurology and myofascial trigger-point phenomena. Mary Maloney, P.T., enriched many chapters with her comments based on years of combining manual medicine skills with a thorough clinical knowledge of myofascial trigger points. Dannie Smith, P.T., and Ann Anderson, P.T., contributed knowledgeable reviews and suggestions for several chapters. Jay Goldstein, M.D., critically reviewed Chapter 6 on the pelvic floor muscles, based on extensive experience with patients whose pain came from intrapelvic muscles that harbored trigger points. The authors are grateful to A.J. Nielsen, P.T., for his enthusiastic support, which included willing participation as the subject in pictures from which many of the drawings were made and for access to the Physical Therapy Anatomy Laboratory.

Stimulating discussions with Prof. MUDr. Karel Lewit of Czechoslovakia greatly enriched the second author's understanding of the importance of the interactions between articular dysfunctions and myofascial trigger points.

Herbert Kent, M.D., as Chief, Rehabilitation Medicine Service at the Veterans Medical Center, Long Beach, California, and Professors Jerome Tobis, M.D., and Jen Yu, M.D., as successive Chairmen of the Department of Physical Medicine and Rehabilitation at the University of California, Irvine, have been most supportive, for which we are deeply grateful. Earle Davis, M.D., enthusiastically extended privileges for anatomical dissections at the same University and contributed helpful discussions. The second author's friend and colleague, Chang-Zern (John) Hong, M.D., has provided an ongoing opportunity for fruitful discussions of myofascial pain problems based on his outstanding clinical competence and extensive research experience.

The librarians who provided the second author with the many references used in this volume were of inestimable help. They include Karen Vogel and Ute M. Schultz in the earlier years and, later, Susan Russell, director of the Medical Center Library of the University of California, Irvine; Marge Linton, also of that library; Linda Lau Murphy, who helped make Melvyl Medline available on the second author's home computer through the library; and the interlibrary loan librarians, Chris Ashen, Jody Hammond Oppelt, and Linda Weinberger, who obtained working copies of references. The references on the piriformis syndrome collected by LeRoy P. W. Froetscher, M.D., when he was a resident helped greatly in the preparation of Chapter 10.

John Butler, our Executive Editor at Williams & Wilkins, has earned our deep gratitude for his persistent support, patience, and understanding.

Last but not least, we express appreciation to inquiring medical students and residents and to our determined critics and skeptics, who keep asking difficult and stimulating questions.

David G. Simons, M.D.
Janet G. Travell, M.D.

Acknowledgment

To my coauthor, David G. Simons, I extend my deepest appreciation for his untiring and pioneering effort in the writing of *Volume 2* of our text, *Myofascial Pain and Dysfunction: The Trigger Point Manual*. I wish to acknowledge that he has made the major contribution to the authorship of this *Volume 2*.

I am proud to have had the privilege of working with Dr. Simons for about thirty years in order to elucidate the basic neurophysiologic mechanisms of the regional myofascial pain syndromes, and to develop effective clinical methods of treatment and management for these common complex pain problems.

Janet G. Travell, M.D.

Contents for Volume 1

PART 3

PART 4

Contents to Volume 2

PART 3

CHAPTER 1
Glossary

The glossary comes first to assure that the reader knows what a term means as it is used in this manual, and to help the reader become acquainted with unfamiliar terms. The glossary is in front to encourage frequent reference to it, whenever needed. Comments concerning a definition appear in *italics*.

Abduction: Movement away from the midline. For the **toes**, it is movement away from the midline of the second toe. For the **foot**, it is movement of the forefoot horizontally outward toward the fibular side of the leg. For the **thigh**, it is movement away from the midline of the body. *Abduction is the opposite of adduction.*

Action: The actions of a muscle, as described in this volume, are the anatomical movements produced by contraction of that muscle. *To be distinguished from function.*

Active Range of Motion: The extent of movement (usually expressed in degrees) of an anatomical segment at a joint. The movement should be caused only by voluntary effort to move the body part being tested.

Active Myofascial Trigger Point: A focus of hyperirritability in a muscle or its fascia that is symptomatic with respect to pain; it causes a pattern of referred pain at rest and/or on motion that is specific for that muscle. An active trigger point is tender, prevents full lengthening of the muscle, weakens the muscle, usually refers pain on direct compression, mediates a local twitch response of its taut muscle fibers when adequately stimulated, causes tenderness in the pain reference zone, and often produces specific referred autonomic phenomena, generally in its pain reference zone. *To be distinguished from a latent myofascial trigger point.*

Acute: Of recent onset (hours, days, or a few weeks).

Adduction: Movement toward the midline. For the **toes**, it is movement toward the midline of the second digit. For the **foot**, it is movement of the forefoot horizontally inward toward the tibial side of the leg. At the **hip**, adduction is movement of the thigh toward the midline of the body. *Adduction is the opposite of abduction.*

Agonists: Muscles, or portions of muscles, so attached anatomically that when they contract, they develop forces that reinforce each other.

Anatomical Position: The erect position of the body with the face directed forward, each arm at the side and the palms of the hands facing forward, feet together with the toes directed forward. *The terms posterior, anterior, lateral, medial, etc., are applied to the body parts as they relate to each other and to the axis of the body when in this anatomical position.*[16]

Antagonists: Muscles, or portions of muscles, so attached anatomically that when they contract, they develop forces that oppose each other.

Antalgic Gait: A gait resulting from pain on weight bearing. Characteristically, the stance phase of gait is shortened on the affected side.[4]

Anterior Tilt (of the pelvis): Anterior tilt rocks the cephalad portion of the pelvis (crest of the ilium) anteriorly, tending to increase lumbar lordosis.

Associated Myofascial Trigger Point: A myofascial trigger point in one muscle that develops in response to compensatory overload, shortened position, or referred phenomena caused by trigger-point activity in another muscle. *Satellite and secondary trigger points are types of associated trigger points.*

Chronic: Long-standing (months or years), but **NOT** necessarily irreversible. *Symptoms may be mild or severe.*

ck: creatine kinase

Composite Pain Pattern: Total pain pattern referred from trigger points in two or more closely adjacent muscles. *No distinction is made between the referred pain patterns of the individual muscles.*

Concentric (contraction): Contraction as the muscle shortens.

Contracture: Sustained intrinsic activation of the contractile mechanism of muscle fibers. With contracture, muscle shortening occurs in the absence of motor unit action potentials. *This physiological definition, as used in this manual, must be differentiated from the clinical definition, which is shortening due to fibrosis. Contracture also must be distinguished from spasm.*

Coronal Plane: A frontal (vertical) plane that divides the body into anterior and posterior portions.[15]

Dorsiflexion: Turning of the foot or the toes upward.[2]

Eccentric (contraction): Contraction as the muscle lengthens.

EMG: Electromyographic.

Essential Pain Zone (Area): The region of referred pain (indicated by solid red areas in pain-pattern figures) that is present in nearly every patient when the trigger point is active. *To be distinguished from a spillover pain zone.*

Eversion: Eversion of the foot is outward (lateral) turning of the entire foot on the talus and of the forefoot on the hindfoot at the transverse tarsal joint. *The movements are complex. The term eversion is sometimes used as synonymous with pronation.*[26] *To be distinguished from inversion.*

Extrinsic Foot Muscles: Muscles that originate outside the foot and attach onto structures in the foot.

Fibromyalgia: Fibromyalgia is identified by widespread pain of at least 3 months' duration in combination with tenderness at 11 or more of the 18 specified tender point sites.[34]

Fibrositis: A term with multiple meanings. In publications prior to 1977, it was often used to identify a condition with palpable taut bands strongly suggestive of myofascial trigger points. Subsequently,[30] fibrositis is frequently used as essentially synonymous with the condition now known as fibromyalgia.[34]

First Ray: The first ray of the foot includes the first metatarsal bone and the bones (two phalanges) of the great toe. The second, third, fourth, and fifth rays comprise the corresponding sequential bones (metatarsal and phalangeal) across the foot.

Flat Palpation: Examination by finger pressure that proceeds across the muscle fibers at a right angle to their length, while compressing them against a firm underlying structure, such as bone. *It is used to detect taut bands and trigger points. To be distinguished from pincer palpation and snapping palpation.*

Forefoot: The forefoot is that part of the foot anterior to the transverse tarsal joint. The location of the transverse tarsal joint is between the navicular and the cuboid in front, and the talus and the calcaneus behind.[25]

Function: The function of a muscle, as used in this volume, concerns when and how the muscle contributes to the posture and activities of the individual. *To be distinguished from action.*

Gait Cycle: The gait cycle during ambulation is the entire period from heel-strike of one foot to the next heel-strike of the same foot.

Greater Pelvis (Pelvis Major, Large Pelvis, False Pelvis): The expanded portion of the pelvis above the brim.[12,27] *To be distinguished from the lesser pelvis.*

Groin: The groin, as used in this volume, includes the inguinal region, not just the anterior crease at the junction of the thigh with the trunk.[5]

h: Hour, a unit of time.

Hallux Valgus: Deviation of the first toe toward the lesser four toes.[6]

Hallux Varus: Deviation of the first toe away from the lesser four toes.[6]

Hammer Toe: Persistent flexion at the interphalangeal joint of the great toe,[22] or persistent flexion of the proximal interphalangeal joint with extension of the distal interphalangeal joint of one of the four lesser toes.

Hindfoot: The hindfoot is that part of the foot posterior to the transverse tarsal joint; it includes the calcaneus and the talus.

in: Inch, a unit of distance; approximately 2.54 centimeters.

Innominate Upslip: An innominate upslip (shear) dysfunction[28] is characterized by upward displacement of an innominate bone in relation to the sacrum.[29]

Intrinsic Foot Muscles: Both ends of an intrinsic foot muscle attach within the foot.

Inversion: Inversion of the foot is inward (medial) turning of the foot, including movement of the entire foot about the talus and movement of the forefoot on the hindfoot at the transverse tarsal joint. *The term inversion is sometimes used as synonymous with supination.*[26] *To be distinguished from eversion.*

Involved Muscle: A muscle that has developed one or more active or latent trigger points.

IP Joint: Interphalangeal joint.

Ischemic Compression: (also Acupressure, Myotherapy, Shiatzu, "Thumb" Therapy): Application of progressively stronger, painful pressure on a trigger point for the purpose of eliminating the trigger point's tenderness and hyperirritability. *This action blanches the compressed tissues, which usually become hyperemic (flushed) on release of the pressure.*

Jump Sign: A general involuntary pain response of the patient, who winces, may cry out, and may withdraw in response to pressure applied on a trigger point. *At one time, we erroneously used this term to describe the local twitch response of muscle fibers to trigger-point stimulation.*

kg: Kilogram, a unit of weight equal to 1,000 grams; approximately 2.2 pounds.

kg/cm²: Kilogram per square centimeter, a unit of weight or force per unit area.

LaSègue's Sign: Pain or muscle spasm in the posterior thigh when the patient lies supine with the hip flexed and knee extended, and the ankle is passively dorsiflexed. *Considered indicative of lumbar root or sciatic nerve irritation,*[20] *or of gastrocnemius muscle tightness.*

Latent Myofascial Trigger Point: A focus of hyperirritability in muscle or its fascia that is clinically quiescent with respect to spontaneous pain: it is painful only when palpated. *A latent trigger point may have all the other clinical characteristics of an active trigger point, from which it is to be distinguished.*

Lateral Rotation (External Rotation, Rotation Outward): Lateral rotation of the **thigh** at the hip or of the **leg** at the knee is rotation of the anterior surface outward from the midsagittal plane of the body. *To be distinguished from medial rotation.*

Lateral Tilt: Lateral tilt of the pelvis inclines the pelvis toward the lower side in a frontal (coronal) plane.

Leg: In this volume, the leg includes only that part of the lower limb between the knee and the ankle, not the entire lower limb.

Lesser Pelvis (Pelvis Minor, Small Pelvis, True Pelvis): The cavity of the pelvis below the brim or superior aperture.[13] *To be distinguished from the greater pelvis.*

Lewit Technique: At stretch-length of the muscle, postisometric relaxation combined with reflex potentiation of relaxation using coordinated respiration and eye movements, as described in Chapter 2, pages 10–11, of this volume.

LLLI: lower limb-length inequality.

Local Twitch Response: Transient contraction of the group of muscle fibers (usually a palpable band) that contains a trigger point. The contraction of the fibers is in response to stimulation (usually by snapping palpation or needling) of the trigger point, or sometimes of a nearby trigger point. *The local twitch response erroneously has been called a jump sign.*

Long Sitting Position: Sitting upright with the hips flexed and the knees straight (extended).

Lordosis: Lumbar lordosis is an anteroposterior curvature of the spine that places the lumbar spine in extension with the convexity of the curve facing anteriorly.

Lotus Position: An erect sitting posture with the legs crossed, so that each foot, sole upturned, rests on the upper part of the thigh of the opposite leg.[32]

Lumbago: Pain in the mid and lower back; *a descriptive term not specifying cause.*[7]

m: Meter, a defined measure of distance; *equivalent to approximately 39 inches.*

Medial Rotation (Internal Rotation, Rotation Inward): Rotation of the **thigh** at the hip or of the **leg** at the knee with the anterior surface turned inward toward the midsagittal plane of the body. *To be distinguished from lateral rotation.*

mm: Millimeter, a measure of distance equal to 1/1,000th of a meter or 1/10th of a centimeter; *approximately 1/25th of an inch.*

MP (MTP) Joint: Metatarsophalangeal joint.

mrad: Millirad, a measure of ionizing radiation: 0.001 rad.

Muscular Rheumatism (*Muskel Rheumatismus*): Muscular pain and tenderness attributed to "rheumatic" causes (especially exposure to cold), as distinguished from articular rheumatism. *Often used as synonymous with myofascial trigger-point syndromes.*

Myalgia: Pain in a muscle or muscles.[8] *Myalgia is used in two ways, to signify: (1) diffusely aching muscles due to systemic disease, such as a viral infection; and (2) the spot tenderness of a muscle or muscles as in myofascial trigger points. The reader must distinguish which use an author has in mind.*

Myofascial Pain Syndrome: Synonymous with Myofascial Syndrome and with Myofascitis. *Often a significant component of somatic dysfunction. To be distinguished from fibromyalgia.*

Myofascial Syndrome: Pain, tenderness, and autonomic phenomena referred from active myofascial trigger points, with associated dysfunction. *The specific muscle or muscle group that causes the symptoms should be identified.*

Myofascial Trigger Point: A hyperirritable spot, usually within a taut band of skeletal muscle or in the muscle's fascia. The spot is painful on compression and can give rise to characteristic referred pain, tenderness, and autonomic phenomena. *A myofascial trigger point is to be distinguished from cutaneous, ligamentous, periosteal, and nonmuscular fascial trigger points. Types include active, latent, primary, associated, satellite, and secondary.*

Myofascitis: (Myofasciitis, Myositis Fibrosa, Interstitial Myositis): As used in this text, myofascitis is the syndrome of pain, tenderness, other referred phenomena, and the dysfunction attributed to myofascial trigger points.[9,10]

Myogelosis: Circumscribed firmness and tenderness to palpation in a muscle or muscles. *The name is derived from the concept that the regions of circumscribed firmness were due to localized gelling of muscle proteins. This concept predates our understanding of sliding filaments as the basis for muscle contraction. Focal tenderness and palpable taut muscle fibers are also characteristic of myofascial trigger points. Most patients diagnosed as having myogelosis would also be diagnosed as having myofascial trigger points.*

Myotatic Unit: A group of agonist and antagonist muscles, which function together as a unit because they share common spinal reflex responses. *The agonist muscles may act together in series, or in parallel.*

Ober's Test: With the patient lying on the left side and with the left leg and thigh flexed, the examiner holds the patient's right lower limb abducted and extended. If, on the sudden withdrawal of the examiner's support, the right lower limb stays up instead of dropping down, there is contraction of the tensor fasciae femoris[1] *or shortening of the tensor fasciae latae muscle.*

Orthosis: An orthopaedic appliance intended to correct a deformity[11] *or structural inadequacy.*

Palpable Band (Taut Band, or Nodule): The group of taut muscle fibers that is associated with a myofascial trigger point and is identifiable by tactile examination of the muscle. *An evoked contraction of the muscle fibers in this band produces the local twitch response.*

Passive Range of Motion: The extent of movement (usually tested in a given plane) of an anatomical segment at a joint when movement is produced by an outside force without voluntary assistance or resistance by the subject. *The subject must relax the muscles crossing the joint.*

Pes Anserinus: The tendinous expansion and attachment of the sartorius, gracilis, and semitendinosus muscles at the medial border of the tuberosity of the tibia.[14]

Pincer Palpation: Examination of a part by holding it in a pincer grasp between the thumb and fingers. *Groups of muscle fibers are rolled between the tips of the digits to detect taut bands of fibers, to identify trigger points in the muscle, and to elicit local twitch responses. To be distinguished from flat palpation and snapping palpation.*

Plantar Flexion: Turning the foot or toes downward.[3]

Posterior Tilt: Posterior tilt of the pelvis rocks the cephalad portion of the pelvis (crest of the ilium) posteriorly, tending to flatten the lumbar spine (decrease the lumbar lordosis).

Primary Myofascial Trigger Point: A hyperirritable focus within a taut band of skeletal muscle. The hyperirritability was activated by acute or chronic overload (mechanical strain) of the muscle in which it occurs, and was not activated as the result of trigger-point activity in another muscle of the body. *To be distinguished from secondary and satellite trigger points.*

Pronation: Pronation of the foot consists of eversion and abduction of the foot, causing a lowering of its medial edge.[17]

Reactive Cramp: See **Shortening Activation**.

Rearfoot: See **Hindfoot**. *Term hindfoot is preferable.*

Reference Zone: See **Zone of Reference**

Referred Autonomic Phenomena: Vasoconstriction (blanching), coldness, sweating, pilomotor response, vasodilatation, and hypersecretion caused by activity of a trigger point but occurring in a region separate from the trigger point. The phenomena usually appear in the general area to which that trigger point refers pain.

Referred (Trigger-Point) Pain: Pain that arises in a trigger point, but is felt at a distance, often entirely remote from its source. The pattern of referred pain is reproducibly related to its site of origin. *The distribution of referred trigger-point pain rarely coincides with the entire distribution of a peripheral nerve or dermatomal segment.*

Referred (Trigger-Point) Phenomena: Sensory, motor, and autonomic phenomena, such as pain, tenderness, increased motor unit activity (spasm), vasoconstriction, vasodilatation, and hypersecretion caused by a trigger point, which usually occur at a distance from the trigger point.

Rotation, Pelvic: Rotation of the pelvis occurs in the transverse plane around the long axis of the body. Rotation of the pelvis toward the right moves the anterior part of the pelvis toward the right and the posterior part toward the left.

Sagittal Plane: A vertical anteroposterior plane that divides the body into right and left parts, or any plane parallel to it. *To be distinguished from the unique midsagittal plane, which divides the body into right and left halves.*

Satellite Myofascial Trigger Point: A focus of hyperirritability in a muscle or its fascia that became active because the muscle was located within the zone of reference of another active trigger point. *To be distinguished from a secondary trigger point.*

Sciatica: Pain in the lower back and hip radiating down the back of the thigh into the calf, cause not specified.[18]

Scoliosis: Lateral curvature of the spine.[19]

Screening Palpation: Digital examination of a muscle to determine the absence, or presence, of palpable bands and tender trigger points using flat and/or pincer palpation.

Secondary Myofascial Trigger Point: A hyperirritable spot in a muscle or its fascia that became active because its muscle was overloaded as a synergist substituting for, or as an antagonist countering the forces of, the muscle that contained the primary trigger point. *To be distinguished from a satellite trigger point.*

Shortening Activation: Activation of latent myofascial trigger points by unaccustomed sudden shortening of the muscle during stretch therapy of its antagonist. *The activated latent trigger points increase tension in the shortened muscle and can cause severe referred pain.*

SI: Sacroiliac (joint).

Snapping Palpation: A fingertip is placed on the tender spot in a taut band of muscle at right angles to the direction of the band and suddenly presses down while drawing the finger back so as to roll the underlying fibers transversely under the finger. *The motion is similar to that used to pluck a guitar string, except that firm contact with the surface is maintained. To most effectively elicit a local twitch response, the band is palpated and snapped transversely at the trigger point, with the muscle at a neutral length or slightly longer. To be distinguished from flat palpation and pincer palpation.*

Spasm: Increased tension with or without shortening of a muscle due to nonvoluntary motor unit action potentials. Spasm cannot be stopped by voluntary relaxation. *Spasm should be distinguished from contracture. Tightness of a muscle may or may not be caused by spasm.*

Spillover Pain Zone (Area): The region beyond the essential pain zone where some, but not all, patients experience referred pain from an active trigger point. *The spillover zone is indicated by red stippling in the pain-pattern figures. To be distinguished from an essential pain zone.*

Square Brackets [ ]: In this volume, square brackets set off comments or interpretations by the authors.

Stance Phase: The stance phase of gait is that portion of the gait cycle during which the foot is in contact with the ground.

Stripping Massage (Deep-stroking Massage): As described on pages 26 and 88 in Volume 1[31] and on page 9 in Chapter 2 of this volume.

Supination: Supination of the foot consists of inversion and adduction of the foot, causing an elevation of its medial edge.

Swing Phase: The swing phase is that period of the gait cycle during which the foot is not in contact with the ground.

Synergistic Muscles: In this volume, synergistic muscles are defined as muscles that assist each other in an action when they contract.

Toe (of shoe): That part of the shoe that covers the toes.

Triceps Surae: The gastrocnemius and soleus muscles considered together.

Trigger Point (Trigger Zone, Trigger Spot, Trigger Area): A focus of hyperirritability in a tissue that, when compressed, is locally tender and, if sufficiently hypersensitive, gives rise to referred pain and tenderness, and sometimes to referred autonomic phenomena and distortion of proprioception. Types include myofascial, cutaneous, fascial, ligamentous, and periosteal trigger points.

TrP: Trigger point.

TrPs: Trigger points.

Upslip: See **Innominate Upslip**.

μV: Microvolt, a measure of electrical potential: 10^{-6} volt, or 0.000001 volt.

Valgus: Used in this volume in accordance with accepted orthopaedic usage, the part distal to the structure named is bent or twisted outward: genu valgum (knock-kneed)[23] or talipes valgus (foot below the talus is turned outward).[21]

Vamp: The vamp is that part of a boot or shoe that covers the instep and toes of the foot.[33]

Varus: Used in this volume in accordance with accepted orthopedic usage, the part distal to the structure named is bent or twisted inward: genu varum (bowlegged)[24] or talipes varus (foot below the talus is turned inward).[21]

Zone of Reference: The specific region of the body at a distance from a trigger point, where the referred phenomena (sensory, motor, autonomic) that it causes are observed.

References

1. Agnew LRC, *et al.*: *Dorland's Illustrated Medical Dictionary*, 24th Ed. W.B. Saunders, Philadelphia, 1965 (p. 1546).
2. Basmajian JV, *et al.*: *Stedman's Medical Dictionary*, 24th Ed. Williams & Wilkins, Baltimore, 1982 (p. 421).
3. *Ibid.* (p. 540).
4. *Ibid.* (p. 569).
5. *Ibid.* (p. 608).
6. *Ibid.* (p. 618).
7. *Ibid.* (p. 811).
8. *Ibid.* (p. 913).
9. *Ibid.* (p. 920).
10. *Ibid.* (p. 922).
11. *Ibid.* (p. 997).
12. *Ibid.* (p. 1046).
13. *Ibid.* (p. 1047).
14. *Ibid.* (p. 1062).
15. *Ibid.* (p. 1093).
16. *Ibid.* (p. 1126).
17. *Ibid.* (p. 1148).
18. *Ibid.* (p. 1262).
19. *Ibid.* (p. 1265).
20. *Ibid.* (p. 1288).
21. *Ibid.* (p. 1408).
22. *Ibid.* (p. 1458).
23. *Ibid.* (p. 1530).
24. *Ibid.* (p. 1534).
25. Basmajian JV, Slonecker CE: *Grant's Method of Anatomy*, 11th Ed. Williams & Wilkins, Baltimore, 1989 (pp. 316–317).
26. *Ibid.* (p. 332).
27. Clemente CD: *Gray's Anatomy of the Human Body*, American Ed. 30. Lea & Febiger, Philadelphia, l985 (pp. 270–271).
28. Greenman PE: Innominate shear dysfunction in the sacroiliac syndrome. *Manual Medicine 2*:114–121, 1986.
29. Greenman PE: *Principles of Manual Medicine*. Williams & Wilkins, Baltimore, 1989 (pp. 234, 236, 246).
30. Smythe HA, Moldofsky H: Two contributions to understanding of the "fibrositis" syndrome. *Bull Rheum Dis 28*:928–931, 1977.
31. Travell JG, Simons DG: *Myofascial Pain and Dysfunction: The Trigger Point Manual*. Williams & Wilkins, Baltimore, 1983.
32. Webster N, McKechnie JL: *Webster's Unabridged Dictionary*, 2nd Ed. Dorset & Baber/New World Dictionaries/Simon and Schuster, New York, 1979 (p. 1069).
33. *Ibid.* (p. 2018).
34. Wolfe F, Smythe HA, Yunus MB, *et al.*: American College of Rheumatology 1990 criteria for the classification of fibromyalgia: report of the multicenter criteria committee. *Arth Rheum 33*: 160–172, 1990.

CHAPTER 2
General Issues

OUTLINE OF CHAPTER

This introductory chapter is not intended to cover the material previously presented in the introductory chapters (Chapters 2–4) of Volume 1.[93] It addresses new issues or issues that represent major progress in previously discussed areas. It omits a number of updates, including new prevalence data and new understanding of the neurophysiology of referred pain, which will be covered in the forthcoming revision of Volume 1. Only updates of clinical issues of immediate concern are included here.

Five topics that are new to *The Trigger Point Manual* are addressed in this chapter: the hazard posed by Fluori-Methane spray to the upper atmosphere ozone layer; alternative treatment techniques; the Lewit technique; new methods of measurement applicable to myofascial trigger points (TrPs); and current terminology of muscle pain disorders. Another section deals with sacroiliac (SI) joint mobilization. Four additional sections enlarge on topics previously addressed:[93] the hypermobility syndrome; shortening activation; injection technique; and the head-forward posture.

1. FLUORI-METHANE SPRAY: THE PROBLEM

The fact that the ozone layer of the upper atmosphere is being destroyed by environmental contaminants including the chlorofluorocarbons is widely known. Since it may be a decade or more until we can fully assess the damage that will be done by chlorofluorocarbons already released, it is of utmost importance that their release into the atmosphere be terminated quickly. Then we will have time to determine the extent of the damage already inflicted and the recovery rate of the atmosphere.

Vallentyne and Vallentyne have expressed the opinion that the use of Fluori-Methane, a mixture of chlorofluorocarbons, should be stopped.[98] Although medical use of chlorofluorocarbons releases minuscule amounts of fluorocarbon compared to those released by the refrigeration industry, we agree that everyone should cooperate fully in the elimination of this hazard to our atmosphere.[84,85]

Fortunately, alternative techniques can substitute for the method of spray and stretch using Fluori-Methane.[65,72,84,85] Meanwhile, a major research effort is underway to find a suitable replacement for Fluori-Methane, but that may take several years. The intermittent cold effect of the vapocoolant can be obtained in other ways and for that reason, in this volume, the term *spray and stretch* has been replaced by the term *intermittent cold with stretch*. Some stretching techniques used alone, without intermittent cold, also can be effective.

2. ALTERNATIVE TREATMENT TECHNIQUES

Intermittent Cold

The sensory and reflex effects of a jet stream of vapocoolant spray (such as Fluori-Methane) can also be obtained to a considerable degree by stroking with ice. Water frozen in a plastic or paper cup is a convenient form of ice. A stirring stick inserted in the cup before freezing the water provides a convenient handle to hold the ice. The ice is exposed by tearing back part of the cup and is then covered with thin plastic to prevent melting ice from making direct contact and wetting the skin. An edge of the plastic-covered ice is applied in unidirectional parallel strokes, which follow the spray patterns presented in each muscle chapter. The stroking movements progress slowly, at the same rate as the spray: 10 cm (4 in)/sec. This application of the sharp, dry edge of ice simulates the jet stream of vapocoolant spray. The skin must remain dry, because dampness reduces the rate of the change in skin temperature produced by the ice-stroking. Wetness also prolongs and diffuses the cooling effect, which delays rewarming of the skin. The clinician must avoid cooling the underlying muscle when stroking with ice, just as when applying vapocoolant spray.[65,76,93]

Although some health professionals still use ethyl chloride spray, we do not recommend its use as a vapocoolant for several reasons (*see* Volume 1[94]). It is too cold as usually applied, it is a rapidly acting general anesthetic with a very narrow safety margin, and it has been responsible for accidental death. It is flammable, and potentially explosive when the vapor is mixed with air. It is not safe to give to patients for home use.

Other Methods With Stretching

Any procedure for inactivating myofascial TrPs is facilitated if the muscle is passively lengthened to the point of resistance during the procedure, and if, following the procedure, it is actively and slowly moved from the fully shortened to the fully lengthened position (if muscle mechanics and anatomy permit). Distraction of the joint or joints crossed by the muscle while it is being stretched can also facilitate release of tension due to myofascial TrPs.

The combination of techniques employed by Karel Lewit for release of muscle tension is particularly effective and is described in detail in Section 3 of this chapter.

Ischemic compression consists of the application of sustained digital pressure to a TrP for a period of about 20 seconds to a minute. Pressure is gradually increased as the sensitivity of the TrP wanes and the tension in its taut band fades. Pressure is released when the clinician feels the TrP tension subside or when the TrP is no longer tender to pressure. This technique is illustrated on pages 26 and 87–88 of Volume 1,[93] and numerous examples are presented throughout the book. Sustained pressure should not be applied to blood vessels or a nerve; it may induce numbness and tingling. Ischemic compression should be followed by lengthening of the muscle, except when stretching is contraindicated, as in hypermobility.

Deep-stroking massage is another effective technique for muscles that are sufficiently superficial to be accessible. This procedure is described as **stripping massage** on page 88 of Volume 1.[93] (The term deep-friction massage refers to other techniques, not exactly the method discussed here.) We call it stripping massage because of the milking effect it produces. Stripping massage is performed by lubricating the skin and/or hands and applying firm pressure progressively along the length of the taut band, through the region of the TrP. Danneskiold-Samsøe and co-workers[10,11] found that application of this technique to the tender "nodules" of "fibrositis" or "myofascial pain" relieved the signs and symptoms of most patients after 10 massage sessions. Those responding had a transient elevation of serum myoglobin levels following the initial therapy sessions, but not after the final sessions when symptoms had been relieved.

Contract-relax, as taught by Voss and associates,[99] is recommended for patients presenting with marked limitation of the range of passive motion and with no active motion available in the agonistic pattern. Contract-relax employs contraction and then relaxation of the tight antagonists to permit active shortening of the weak agonist. This same technique can be used to inactivate myofascial TrPs, and to augment relaxation for the purpose of stretching the involved antagonist. In this case, the emphasis is on trying to lengthen the tight antagonist by having the patient perform an isometric contraction of the tight muscle and then allow it to relax and lengthen, only incidentally shortening the agonist. As originally described,[99] the patient is instructed to make a maximum contraction effort of the tight antagonist muscle and then relax it. (In contrast, Lewit recommends for his postisometric relaxation technique that the contraction phase be limited to a *mild* voluntary contraction of between 10% and 25% of maximum effort.[58])

Reciprocal inhibition is a well-established neurophysiological principle that can be used to assist a muscle-stretching procedure. To invoke reciprocal inhibition, the *agonist* (muscle not being stretched) is voluntarily activated *during* the period of stretch of the involved antagonist muscle (when it needs to be relaxed).

Relaxation during exhalation, described in the next section as part of the Lewit technique, can be useful by itself. By breathing deeply and slowly, and concentrating on relaxation during exhalation, the patient may reduce TrP irritability and release associated muscular tension. The muscle should be lengthened to the point of taking up all slack (to the onset of resistance) especially before and also during each cycle of this procedure.

Percussion and stretch starts with the muscle lengthened to the point of onset of passive resistance. The clinician or patient uses a hard rubber mallet or reflex hammer to hit the TrP at precisely the same place about 10 times. This should be done at a slow rate of no more than one impact per second but, at least, one impact every 5 seconds; the slower rates are likely to be more effective. This procedure may enhance or substitute for intermittent cold with stretch. The senior author considers it particularly applicable to the quadratus lumborum (self-applied), brachioradialis, long finger extensors, and to the peroneus longus and brevis. It is *not* applied to anterior or posterior compartment leg muscles because of a possible compartment syndrome, if it caused bleeding there.

Muscle energy technique involves voluntary muscle contractions by the patient against a specific counterforce provided by a clinician, whereby the patient, not the clinician, provides the corrective force. This technique has been applied to joint mobilization and can be used to lengthen a tense muscle and stretch its fasciae as well.[37,69]

Myofascial release is a combined technique using some principles from soft tissue technique, from muscle energy technique, and from inherent force craniosacral technique. It combines soft tissue changes, faulty body mechanics, and altered reflex mechanisms in both diagnosis and treatment.[37]

The use of **ultrasound** for the inactivation of TrPs was discussed on pages 89 and 90 of Volume 1.[93] This method is especially useful for deeply placed muscles that are not accessible to manual therapy.

Examples of **the use of high voltage pulsed galvanic stimulation** appear in Section 12 of Chapter 6, Pelvic Muscles.

3. LEWIT TECHNIQUE

The concept of applying postisometric relaxation in the treatment of myofascial pain was presented for the first time in a North American journal in 1984.[58] Combining this technique with reflex augmentation of relaxation[55,57] greatly enhances its effectiveness. Enhancements include the use of gravity to take up the slack in the muscle and the use of coordinated respiration and eye movements.

For this technique to be effective, the patient must be relaxed and the body well supported. The muscle is passively and gently lengthened to the point of taking up the slack (reaching the barrier or the point of initial resistance). If this initial positioning causes pain, either the extent of the movement has been excessive or the patient has actively resisted the movement.

Postisometric Relaxation

The process of postisometric relaxation is to contract the tense muscle isometrically against resistance and then to encourage it to lengthen during a period of complete voluntary relaxation. Gravity is an effective force to "encourage" release of the muscle tension.

Postisometric relaxation begins by having the patient perform an isometric contraction of the tense muscle at its initial tolerated length, while the clinician stabilizes that part of the body to prevent muscle shortening. Contraction should be slight (10–25% of maximum voluntary contraction). After holding this contraction for 3–10 sec., the patient is instructed to "let go" and to relax the body completely. During this relaxation phase, the clinician gently takes up any slack that develops in the muscle, noting the increase in range of motion. Care is taken to maintain the stretched length of the muscle and not to return it to the neutral position during subsequent cycles of isometric contraction and relaxation.[55]

Respiration

The effectiveness of postisometric relaxation is augmented by combining it with phased respiration. Since inhalation encourages contraction of most muscles and exhalation encourages their relaxation, the contraction-relaxation cycle is coordinated with these phases of respiration. The patient slowly inhales during the isometric contraction phase and then slowly exhales during the relaxation phase. These breaths should be deep. Patients who have difficulty using such a slow respiratory pattern are helped by pausing, breathing naturally several times, and relaxing between each cycle.

For the torso, inhalation facilitates moving toward the neutral erect position. Leaning forward is naturally associated with exhalation and relaxation. From the forward-flexed position, standing or sitting up straight is associated with inhalation. Similarly, when one is in a retroflexed (bent-back) position, inhalation again facilitates straightening up toward the erect position; exhalation facilitates further backward extension.

The jaw elevator muscles have a respiratory reflex response opposite to that of most muscles. The elevators are reflexly relaxed during the inhalation associated with a yawn. Since yawning requires activation of jaw depressors, this may be an example of overriding reciprocal inhibition. For these jaw elevators, the isometric contraction phase is coordinated with exhalation, and the relaxation (stretch) phase is coordinated with inhalation (the patient is instructed to yawn or imagine yawning).

Eye Movements

In general, eye movements facilitate the movement of the head and trunk in the direction of the patient's gaze and inhibit movement in the opposite direction. This holds true for lifting the head and torso as well as for stooping and rotation. Eye movement (gaze) does not facilitate side bending, however. Looking up does facilitate straightening up from the side-bent position. These eye movements should not be exaggerated, because a maximum-effort movement may have an inhibitory effect.[55,57]

4. NEW MEASUREMENT TECHNIQUES

This section will consider new developments in algometry, tissue compliance measurement, thermography, and magnetic resonance spectroscopy as they relate to an understanding of myofascial TrPs.

Algometry, tissue compliance measurement, and thermography are valuable for substantiating clinical observations and as research tools. By themselves they cannot be used for diagnosing myofascial TrPs.

Algometry

There are two types of algometers, a mechanical spring-operated force gauge and an electrical strain gauge.

Spring-operated Algometers

Pressure algometry is not new,[66] but devices specifically designed to measure pressure threshold, pressure tolerance, and tissue compliance in relation to myofascial TrPs are new.[29]

The pressure threshold is that pressure which is first perceived as painful by the subject as increasing pressure is applied. Fischer[28,29] described a spring-operated pressure threshold meter that records forces up to 11 kg. This force gauge has a 1-cm^2 circular rubber tip. The scale reads the pressure applied to the TrP directly in kg/cm^2. This device is usually sensitive enough at the low end of the scale to identify differences in sensitivity between active TrPs, yet remains on scale when measuring the higher pressure threshold of normal muscles.[20,23,29]

The companion pressure tolerance meter[29] measures the maximum pressure a subject can tolerate over muscles and bones, up to 17 kg. Normally, pressure tolerance is greater over muscle than over bone. Reversal of this relative sensitivity suggests the presence of a generalized myopathy.[22] The reason for having two similar instruments is that the threshold meter often goes off scale if one attempts to use it to measure tolerance, and the tolerance meter is too insensitive to resolve accurately the differences in the sensitivity of active TrPs.

Tunks and associates[97] developed a spring-operated algometer that was adapted from the Preston pinch gauge. The hemispheric tip of the instrument has an area of contact of 2 cm^2. The unit was designed to simulate the pressure applied by the thumb when examining a patient for the tender points of fibromyalgia.

Strain Gauge Algometers

The user can rapidly rescale the sensitivity of an electronic strain gauge algometer to perform both pressure threshold measurements and pressure tolerance measurements. Strain gauge algometers also permit direct recording and computer input.

Ohrbach and Gale[71] designed a strain gauge pressure tolerance meter for testing tender spots in masticatory muscles. It had a tip area of only 0.5 cm^2. Jensen and associates[44] developed a strain gauge pressure algometer for measurement of sensitivity in the temporal region to study patients with headache. Schiffman and co-workers[78] developed a strain gauge pressure algometer especially designed to transmit the feeling that one has when palpating a taut band. Its bluntly pointed plastic tip simulates the shape of a fingertip. Inter-rater reliability of their pressure algometer for 14 muscles of the head and neck was consistently higher than the reliability of palpation.

Applications

Using the Fischer pressure threshold meter,[20,23] comparison of normal values with those obtained at corresponding TrP sites showed that a difference between right and left sides in excess of 2 kg/cm^2 represents abnormal sensitivity. Moreover, any pressure threshold at a muscle site in excess of 3 kg/cm^2 was considered abnormal.[20,23] The muscles of females were more sensitive to pressure than were those of males in two studies using different instruments.[23,78]

List and associates[59] found the Fischer algometer reliable and valid for measuring sensitivity (tenderness) in the masseter muscle. A well-controlled study by Reeves and co-workers[77] demonstrated that the same meter provided a reliable measure of myofascial TrP sensitivity in five masticatory and neck muscles. They also found significantly increased sensitivity at the TrP compared with that of the muscle 2 cm away from the clinically determined spot of maximum tenderness. Jaeger and Reeves[41] demonstrated that myofascial TrP sensitivity decreases in response to passive stretch. Fischer[28] gave examples of the change in sensitivity observed following different therapies.

Applying the Jensen instrument to the study of migraine patients, investigators[45] concluded that myofascial TrPs appear to be a significant factor in migraine headache, contributing particularly to interval headaches between migraine attacks.

Thomas and Aidinis[89] objectively and quantitatively measured the threshold for grimacing and movement responses by pressure algometry in a patient with musculoskeletal pain syndrome during light Pentothal anesthesia.

A pressure threshold meter provides an objective measure of the effectiveness of treatment.[20,27,29] The meter itself does not identify the cause of the tenderness being measured.

Tissue Compliance Measurement

Fischer[24,29] described and illustrated a tissue compliance meter that measures the relative hardness of the subcutaneous tissue by the distance a particular pressure indents the skin. He concluded that a difference of more than 2 mm of penetration at corresponding bilateral sites indicates the presence of local muscle spasm, the taut band of a TrP, normal tendon or aponeurosis, or scar tissue.[25] He later reported clinical applications of the meter.[26]

Jansen and associates[43] evaluated the reliability of this meter by measuring normal paraspinal tissue compliance. They were unable to reproduce results at 26% of the sites after a 10-minute interval. Moreover, 85% of these normal subjects displayed at least one right vs. left side difference large enough to qualify as pathological by Fischer's criteria. On the other hand, Airaksinen and Pöntinen[1] found that correlations for within-experimenter and between-experimenter reliabilities for this same meter ranged from 0.63–0.98 at different force levels.

Of the instruments mentioned above, to our knowledge, only the Fischer devices are commercially available at this time. (They are obtainable from Pain Diagnostics and Thermography, 17 Wooley Lane East, Great Neck, New York 11021.)

The algometers described in this section afford an opportunity to do quantitative studies of myofascial TrP phenomena that have only begun to be explored. Their reliable use requires training and skill.

Thermography

Thermograms can be recorded by electronic radiometry or with films of liquid crystal. Recent advances in infrared radiation (electronic) thermography with computer analysis provide a powerful new tool for the rapid visualization of skin temperature changes. This technique can demonstrate cutaneous reflex phenomena characteristic of myofascial TrPs. The less expensive contact sheets of liquid crystal have limitations that make reliable interpretation of the findings considerably more difficult than with electronic radiometry.

Each of these thermographic techniques measures the skin surface temperature to a depth of only a few millimeters. The temperature changes correspond to changes in the circulation within, but not beneath, the skin. The endogenous cause of these temperature changes is usually sympathetic nervous system activity. The thermogram, therefore, is comparable in meaning to changes in skin resistance or changes in sweat production. However, electronic infrared thermography is superior to these other measures in convenience and in spatial as well as temporal resolution.

At this time, thermography alone is *NOT* sufficient to establish the diagnosis of myofascial TrPs. However, it can help to substantiate the presence of myofascial TrPs that have previously been identified by history and physical examination. It also offers a wealth of experimental opportunities.

Early thermographic studies of myofascial pain demonstrated circular hot spots 5–10 cm in diameter located over the TrP.[17] Diakow[12] studied a TrP (identified by physical examination) in the upper trapezius muscle of one patient and a TrP in the supraspinatus muscle of another. In each case, the specific TrP area had a hot spot approximately 2 cm in diameter overlying it. In both cases, an area within the expected referred pain zone also exhibited increased warmth, but of less intensity than at the TrP.

Whether the increased heat radiation observed was over a referred pain zone or over a TrP is unclear in most of the studies to date. Two papers[18,21] asserted that a reduced pressure threshold reading at the hot spot proved it to be a TrP. We question that firm conclusion since the observed tenderness at the hot spot could represent referred tenderness and not tenderness of the TrP itself. To date, the presence of a TrP can be established conclusively only by palpating a taut band and eliciting the characteristic referred pain pattern by the application of digital pressure on the spot of maximum tenderness in that band or by eliciting a local twitch response.

Other papers specifically related the hot spots of myofascial pain to the areas in which pain is felt.[17,19] The painful area is *usually* the pain reference zone, *not the location of the TrP*. The referred pain zone has been variously described as hot,[12,19] hot or cold,[17] and cold.[93] Failure to differentiate clearly whether the observed thermal changes are present over the TrP itself or in its referred pain zone is a potential source of confusion for the interpretation of thermographic findings.

The literature to date fails to address a number of critical questions concerning thermographic changes associated with TrPs. Was the TrP active or latent? Was the patient having pain at the time of examination? If so, where? Is the thermogram different when the patient is not having pain? What happens to the thermal pattern while the TrP is palpated to augment referred pain? Would a controlled study comparing the hot spots observed in normal subjects differ significantly from a study of the hot spots observed in myofascial pain patients? Are the tender points in fibromyalgia patients associated with similar hot spots?

The question may arise whether increased skin temperature is due to underlying muscle spasm. This question can be answered by needle electromyography. Spontaneous electrical activity of a relaxed muscle indicates muscle spasm, and a muscle that is electrically silent is not in spasm.

Magnetic Resonance Spectroscopy

^{31}P magnetic resonance spectroscopy can measure the relative concentration of phosphorus-containing metabolites within a selected volume of muscle. These metabolites reflect sequential steps of muscle energy metabolism. This technique can identify the relative concentration of sugar phosphates, inorganic phosphate, phosphocreatine, and three forms of adenine triphosphate (ATP).[14]

Kushmerick,[50] in an extensive review of the relation between ^{31}P magnetic resonance spectroscopy measurements and muscle metabolism, noted that the relative concentrations of these metabolites were measurable with an error of less than 10%. This new technique has provided simple and useful criteria for distinguishing muscle enzyme deficiencies,[14] has revealed abnormal changes in metabolite distribution following repeated lengthening contractions designed to result in mild muscle injury,[64] and has demonstrated characteristic changes due to muscle fatigue.[67,68]

Kushmerick[50] concluded that such a dynamic stress test is needed to reveal metabolic abnormalities in muscles of fibromyalgia patients. Two magnetic resonance spectroscopy studies did report several abnormal changes in metabolite distribution with exercise in some of the fibromyalgia patients studied.[46,63]

If ^{31}P nuclear magnetic resonance studies can demonstrate diffuse metabolic abnormalities in some forms of fibromyalgia, it seems likely that metabolic abnormalities should be demonstrable in the immediate vicinity of a myofascial TrP, if the area for examination can be adequately localized.

5. CURRENT TERMINOLOGY OF MUSCLE PAIN DISORDERS

The following terms are in current use and appear to relate in various ways to myofascial pain caused by TrPs. In many cases, this relation is not made clear by the respective authors or is controversial. The result can be confusion as much as enlightenment. The terms are arranged alphabetically and a reference is cited for each term.

This list is by no means complete, but represents a sample of the many terms currently in vogue. Terms that were used in the past appear on pages 9–11 of Volume 1,[93] and additional terms have been noted.[81]

Lumping several confusing and controversial diagnostic terms under a new umbrella usually adds only nosological complexity and confusion to the field of muscle pain. It is our opinion that *splitting* existing diagnoses into more clearly defined component syndromes is more likely to clarify our understanding.

Chronic Fatigue (Syndrome):[34,39,101] Chronic fatigue is now generally considered a close relative of fibromyalgia, or a partial expression of it. Since myofascial pain syndromes typically cause localized weakness rather than general fatigue, patients with chronic fatigue are more likely to have fibromyalgia than myofascial pain.

Chronic Myalgia:[51] The cited description of chronic myalgia emphasized muscle pain related to static load during repetitive assembly work, which would also be likely to activate TrPs. As defined by Larsson *et al.*, chronic myalgia also included findings characteristic of fibromyalgia. Since the patients studied were not specifically examined for myofascial syndromes, what contribution active TrPs made to the patients' conditions is not known.

Chronic Myofascial Pain:[73] The cited authors characterize patients with chronic myofascial pain as having "localized sites of deep myofascial tenderness (i.e., trigger points) with normal joint examination and negative serological screen." There is no indication that the patients were examined for signs that would distinguish myofascial TrPs from the tender points of fibromyalgia. For that reason, one cannot assume that this term was used by these authors in the same sense in which we use it.

In an effort to prevent confusion, we define the terms *chronic myofascial pain*[83] and *chronic regional myofascial pain syndrome*[81] in Chapter 28 of this volume and distinguish them from acute myofascial pain and fibromyalgia.

Fibromyalgia:[103] As currently defined, fibromyalgia is a widespread, painful condition of at least 3 months' duration that is identified by finding at least 11 tender points at 18 prescribed locations on the body. Since the diagnostic distinction between chronic regional myofascial pain syndrome and fibromyalgia can be difficult, the relation between the two conditions has recently been the subject of a major international symposium.[30] Distinguishing features of the two conditions were discussed in detail by Simons[81] and by Bennett.[5] By definition, all active TrPs at these prescribed tender point sites are also tender points, but not all tender points are TrPs.

Generalized tendomyopathy: This condition, known in German as *Generalisierte tendomyopathie*,[52,70] is frequently equated with fibromyalgia, but is described as usually beginning at a single site and developing into generalized pain over months or years. The physical examination recommended for this condition does not specifically include criteria that would identify myofascial TrPs. Therefore, like fibromyalgia, it could readily include patients with chronic regional myofascial pain syndromes.

Neuromyelopathic Pain Syndrome:[61] Patients with the neuromyelopathic pain syndrome characteristically have chronic pain that is refractory to ordinary therapy, and mild but often widespread neurological deficits. They frequently also have TrPs. Many of the characteristics of these patients are similar to those of patients whom we identify as having post-traumatic hyperirritability syndrome,[82] which is described in Chapter 28 of this volume.

Nonarticular Rheumatism:[6] The author of the cited article defines nonarticular rheumatism as including myofascial pain syndrome, fibromyalgia syndrome, tendinitis, and bursitis. This diagnostic term is often equated with the German *Weichteilrheumatismus* (*see* below).

Osteochondrosis:[74] Popelianskii reviewed the history of this term and the concepts that it encompasses, which include both myofascial pain syndromes and entrapment syndromes of spinal nerves. An extensive Russian literature employs this term.

Overuse Syndrome:[2,32,33] This syndrome was found to be particularly common among industrial workers who perform stressful repetitive activities, musicians, and athletes. Since these patients complained of weakness rather than fatigue, and reported initiating factors that are commonly associated with myofascial TrPs, we suspect that many of them may have had myofascial TrPs as one cause of their symptoms. Since the cited reports did not indicate that the muscles of the patients were examined for signs of myofascial TrPs, the role of TrPs in the overuse syndrome remains an open question.

Regional Myofascial Pain:[79] Sheon[79] uses the term *regional myofascial pain* in essentially the same way that we use the term *chronic myofascial pain syndrome*. It is a condition caused by myofascial TrPs, which needs to be distinguished from fibrositis (fibromyalgia). Chronic regional myofascial pain syndromes have three distinct phases (degrees of severity), as described by the senior author.[92]

Repetitive Strain Injury:[40,80] Repetitive strain injury is similar to the overuse syndrome and also has characteristics suggestive of the myofascial pain syndrome. The patients may have suffered from myofascial pain syndromes that went unrecognized, since there was no indication that their muscles were examined for that condition.

Tension Myalgia:[86,88,90] This term originated in the Physical Medicine Department of the Mayo Clinic and was first used in 1977 to describe painful tension of the muscles of the pelvic floor.[86] The probable relation of tension myalgia of the pelvic floor to myofascial TrPs is discussed in detail in Chapter 6 of this volume. The 1990 publication from the Mayo Clinic on this subject[90] lumps the diagnoses of myofascial pain syndrome, fibrositis, and fibromyalgia into one term, tension myalgia, which now has expanded to include muscles throughout the body.

Weichteilrheumatismus:[62] Literally meaning "soft-tissue rheumatism," this term is generally translated as "nonarticular rheumatism." Since it refers to all soft-tissue structures that may become painful, some authors[62] suggest that the proper translation is "reactive myotendopathy." It clearly encompasses myofascial pain syndromes along with numerous other conditions.

6. MOBILIZATION OF THE SACROILIAC JOINT
(Fig. 2.1)

Despite earlier controversy, it is now well established that the sacroiliac (SI) joint normally has mobility that decreases with advancing age.[36] Mobility is less in males than in females and the joint usually becomes ankylosed in elderly men.[36,100] Frigerio and associates[31] demonstrated several centimeters of rotational movement of the innominate bones relative to the sacrum. However, Weisl[100] pointed out that the concept of an axis of rotation in the SI joint is meaningless; the two opposing surfaces of the SI joint are so uneven that there is much scatter in the location of the most likely centers of rotation in the frontal and sagittal planes. For this reason, and because of the energy that would be needed to separate the joint surfaces as they are held together by the surrounding ligaments, Wilder and associates[102] concluded that the SI joint functions primarily as a shock absorber.

According to Lewit,[56] the SI joint is one of three joints in the body for which movement can neither be caused by, nor opposed by, muscles. However, abnormal muscle tension can help to hold the joint in a displaced position. (The other two such joints are the acromioclavicular and the tibiofibular.[56]) Porterfield[75] presents an outstanding description, with illustrations, of the examination of a patient for pelvic articular dysfunction in relation to muscle function. Egund and associates[15] described the diagnostic value of stereoscopic visualization of the pelvic bones for the identification of SI joint displacements.

Diagnosis and treatment of dysfunction of the SI joint have been described by numerous authors.[8,13,37,38,53,60,69,75] The following sections on diagnosis and treatment describe a method that the senior author has employed successfully.

Diagnosis

The patient has experienced a sudden or a gradual onset of pain in the region of one or, occasionally, both SI joints. The pain may be felt at both SI joints even when only one is displaced, but is usually worse on the side of the affected joint. Onset commonly is related to a simple motion that combines bending forward, tilting the pelvis, and twisting the trunk, such as a short golf swing, shoveling snow, stooping and reaching sideways to pick up an object on the floor, or getting up sideways out of a soft chair. The pain may also be initiated by a slight fall, pregnancy, or improper positioning during general anesthesia. Occasionally, severe pain in a sciatic distribution may be the chief symptom of SI joint dysfunction and may so predominate that the patient makes no mention of pain in the back. Some degree of pain radiation to the lower limb is common. The variable pattern of pain referred from the SI joint may include the lumbar region, the lateral aspect of the thigh, the gluteal region, the sacrum, the iliac crest, and a sciatic nerve distribution.[95,96] Limitation of mobility is variable and may be wholly incapacitating or trivial. Pain may be aggravated by bending forward, putting on shoes, crossing one thigh over the other, rising from a chair, and turning over in bed.

Steinbrocker and associates[87] injected 0.2–0.5 ml of 6% sodium chloride solution into the SI

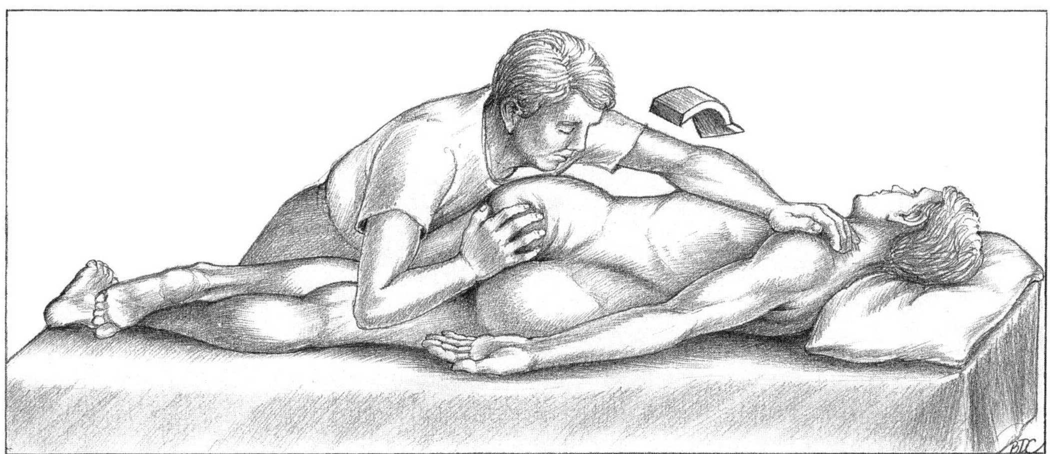

Figure 2.1. Technique for manipulation of the right sacroiliac joint. The patient lies on the affected side. The right hand exerts a smooth forceful thrust against the sacrum with a corkscrew motion upward and forward, to produce a rotary movement of the sacrum on the lowermost ilium, which is stabilized by the patient's weight. With the other hand, the operator exerts counter pressure against the upper thorax. (After Travell and Travell,[95] p. 224.)

joint and observed pain that radiated both upward and downward to the knee.

Tenderness to pressure is always present directly over the superior or inferior posterior iliac spine on the affected side. The diagnosis of SI joint dysfunction is in doubt if this tenderness is not present. In addition, muscles in the SI region develop TrP tenderness, including the lower end of the erector spinae, the quadratus lumborum, the three glutei, and the piriformis muscle. These muscles may be more tender than the posterior margin of the joint itself; this finding can be a source of confusion and misdiagnosis.

Routine X-ray films of the pelvis and lumbar spine rarely show malalignment of the SI joints.

On examination, straight-leg raising is usually limited. In more severe cases, limitation of flexion of the thigh against the abdomen is often present on the affected side. The lumbar curve is usually flattened and the pelvis is tilted upward on the affected side, causing a prominence of the hip on that side. When pain is severe, the patient walks with a distinct stoop and limps, sparing the limb on the side of the displaced SI joint.[95,96]

The left SI joint is tested for restriction by having the patient lie supine with the examiner facing the right side of the body. The right thigh is placed in full abduction and external rotation with the knee bent, foot beside the other knee, as illustrated in Figure 15.14. The right knee is gently moved up and down, using the thigh as a lever to rock the left SI joint, which is where the patient usually feels discomfort if that joint is abnormal. Sometimes pain is also induced in the SI joint on the same side as the limb being moved. If this test is not positive, SI joint dysfunction is unlikely to be present.[95,96]

Treatment

The first author of this manual has described[91] how she learned from her physician father the value of, and a technique for, manipulation of the SI joint. A 1942 photograph of her father[95] shows him demonstrating this technique, which was later used by Bierman[7] and designated "the Travell maneuver."

Before manipulating the SI joint, it is important to treat first any lumbar spinal joint dysfunction that is present. One should also ensure that any TrPs that cause shortening of the quadratus lumborum muscle have been inactivated; tension of this muscle can hold the SI joint in a malaligned position.

For manipulation of the SI joint, as illustrated in Figure 2.1, the patient lies on the affected (right) side with the right lower limb extended at the hip and the knee straight. The uppermost lower limb is allowed to fall into a natural position with the knee slightly bent and the foot hooked loosely over the ankle underneath. The arm beneath is drawn forward out of the way at a right angle with the body. The uppermost arm hangs loosely behind the back.

The operator stands in front of the patient with one hand cupping the caudal end of the sacrum. The other hand grasps the front of the patient's upper torso. Simultaneously, the operator pushes the upper torso backward and the sacrum forward and upward so that the hand on the sacrum travels along a spiral or corkscrewlike curve. This maneuver produces lordosis of the lumbar spine, a tilting forward of the upper part of the sacrum, and a twisting of the trunk; it results in a forward rotation of the sacrum on the lowermost ilium, which is stabilized by the weight of the patient's body.[95]

Force is applied smoothly and steadily (without jerks) to produce a gradual stretching movement. When maximum rotation of the trunk is obtained, a quick final thrust is provided; usually, a click is heard in the SI joint. A large reserve of strength is required in order to perform the manipulation smoothly and to sustain the effort for sufficient time to overcome muscular resistance, ordinarily from 15–30 seconds, sometimes longer.[95,96]

After the procedure, the tests described above are repeated and usually show marked improvement.

7. HYPERMOBILITY SYNDROME

Treatment with a stretching technique is *contraindicated* across joints that are truly hypermobile. When there are TrPs in muscles that cross hypermobile joints, these TrPs should be inactivated using techniques that do not extend the muscles to maximum length. Such alternative therapies include ischemic compression, TrP injection, deep stripping massage, low voltage galvanic stimulation, and ultrasound. The muscles of these patients require strengthening, not overall lengthening. However, these patients may benefit from inactivation of TrPs and release of taut bands by use of some of the methods listed.

Although there is no established standard of how much ligamentous laxity is diagnostic of the hypermobility syndrome, the Beighton criteria[35] are generally accepted. These tests have been well described and illustrated.[4,42] Between four and six of the nine possible points are required by most investigators to make a diagnosis of hypermobility. Another sign of hypermobilty is the ability of the patient to insert a tier of four knuckles, instead of the usual three, of the non-dominant hand between the incisor teeth (*see* Three-knuckle Test, pages 226–227 in Volume 1[93]). If the examiner pays attention only to the symptomatic region, an apparently normal range of motion at a joint may not be recognized as a restricted range in a hypermobile patient.

Hypermobility is not rare. Up to 5% of the adult population may be affected.[35,47] It is frequently overlooked because clinicians are trained to look for *reduced*, not *increased*, range of motion. Hypermobility normally decreases markedly throughout childhood and then more slowly during adult life.[35,54] Women generally have greater range of joint motion than men, Asians greater range than Blacks, and Blacks greater range than Caucasians.[35] Since ligamentous laxity is usually associated with weakness of postural muscles, hypermobile individuals are less able to adapt to the now common occupations in which static positions are maintained for much of the day.

The hypermobility syndrome has been associated with mitral valve prolapse, weakness of the musculotendinous support of the abdomen and pelvic floor, and hyperextensible skin that is thin, soft, and prone to develop striae. The syndrome has a dominant mode of inheritance, with sex-influenced phenotypic manifestations in most cases.[35] It may be related to rarer and more serious hereditary disorders that include Marfan syndrome, Ehlers-Danlos syndrome, and osteogenesis imperfecta.[35]

Many individuals have this condition but do not seek medical assistance. Those who do often complain of foot symptoms related to their mobile flat feet and of knee problems related to patellar hypermobility.[16]

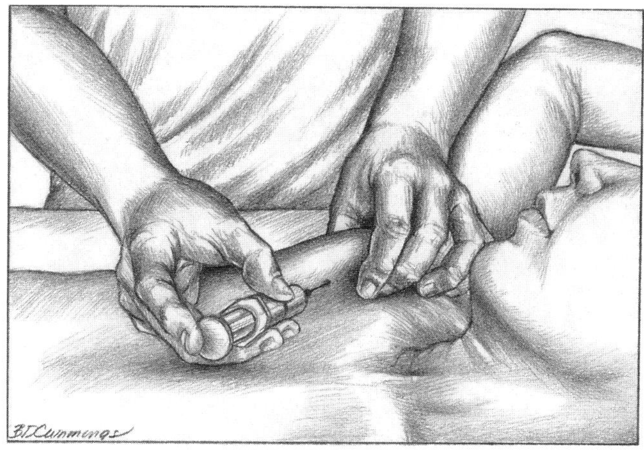

Figure 2.2. Injection of trigger points using a technique for holding the syringe that minimizes the danger of accidentally inserting the needle farther than intended if the patient makes a sudden unexpected movement. Drawn from an original photograph courtesy of John Hong, M.D., who suggested this method and who uses it successfully.

Lewit[54] identifies a group of hypermobile patients with a tendency to general instability and a lack of motor coordination that is characteristic of minimal brain dysfunction as recognized by pediatric neurologists. These hypermobile adults appear to be unable to learn motor coordination even when the patient and a competent therapist do their utmost. This group of hypermobile patients also has difficulty coping with the problems of daily life. They are likely to have difficulty working as dentists, telephone operators, or computer operators, and whenever they spend long hours bent over a desk.[54]

8. SHORTENING ACTIVATION

When a tight muscle (e.g., rectus femoris) is suddenly released, shortening activation (reactive cramp) may occur in an antagonist muscle (e.g., a hamstring muscle). As the tight muscle (rectus femoris) is lengthened well beyond its accustomed limit by inactivating its active TrPs, the antagonist (hamstring muscle) is simultaneously shortened to less than its accustomed minimum length. If the antagonist harbors latent (or mildly active) TrPs, they may be suddenly and strongly activated by being placed in this unaccustomed shorter position. The patient can then experience severe cramplike referred pain from the TrPs in this muscle that is an antagonist to the previously tight muscle. The problem is resolved if the TrPs in the antagonist muscle are inactivated by applying intermittent cold with stretch or another specific myofascial therapy. Shortening activation can be prevented by releasing the antagonist muscle before treating the tight muscle that is the source of the initial pain complaint. The peroneus longus muscle and the tibialis anterior comprise another example of functionally opposed muscles in the lower limb subject to this phenomenon. Shortening activation is discussed on pages 73–74, 360, and 589 in Volume 1.[93]

9. INJECTION TECHNIQUE

The basic principles and techniques of TrP injection are presented in Chapter 3 of Volume 1[93] and should be thoroughly studied before undertaking this procedure.

When one injects TrPs in locations that pose a hazard should the patient make a sudden unexpected movement—such as a startle reaction, sneeze, or cough—it is desirable to hold the syringe in such a manner that the syringe and needle will move with the patient. The hand that is holding the syringe should be firmly supported by the patient's body. This can be accomplished as illustrated in Figure 2.2. The syringe is held between the thumb and lesser fingers, and the plunger is depressed with the index finger while the hand rests firmly against the patient's body. This technique is particularly valuable when injecting over the lung or when the needle is directed toward major arteries or nerves.

Examples of steadying the injecting hand against the patient's body when employing the common injection technique shown in the illustrations of this manual can be found in Figures 13.5, 19.7, and 20.11 of Volume 1.[93]

10. HEAD-FORWARD POSTURE

Several muscle groups are prone to develop TrPs when an individual stands and sits with the head, neck, and/or shoulders bent forward excessively, placing the upper half of the body in a round-shouldered, slumped position. The pectoral and posterior cervical muscles are particularly likely to develop TrPs. Even temporomandibular problems can be influenced by an excessive head-forward posture. This subject is emphasized here because musculoskeletal problems in the lower half of the body can contribute strongly to this undesirable upper body posture. Anything that flattens the normal lumbar lordotic curve during sitting or standing encourages the stressful head-forward posture. Several authors emphasize the importance of recognizing this posture and improving it, especially if the patient has related symptoms.[9,49,53] As noted by Joseph,[48] posture varies markedly among apparently healthy, normal individuals; however, if the muscles are causing pain, postural strain must be identified and resolved.

The almost universal lack of adequate lumbar support by chairs and sofas encourages this unbalanced posture, because the flattened lumbar spine levers the head forward. The importance of correcting for this deficiency in seating design by providing an adequate lumbar support is illustrated in Figure 42.9*E* (p. 592) of Volume 1.[93]

Alexander[3] taught that trying to adopt a new posture that requires continuous mental and physical effort provides no lasting improvement; it only contributes to physical and mental fatigue and frustration. He recommends repositioning the head upward and letting the body follow to establish a more balanced, effortless posture.

References

1. Airaksinen O, Pöntinen PJ: The reliability of a tissue compliance meter (TCM) in the evaluation of muscle tension in healthy subjects. *Pain*, Suppl 5, 1990.
2. Ames DL: Overuse syndrome. *J Fla Med Assoc 73*:607–608, 1986.
3. Barker S: *The Alexander Technique*. Bantam Books, New York, 1978.
4. Beighton P, Grahame R, Bird H: *Hypermobility of Joints*, Ed. 2. Springer-Verlag, New York, 1989.
5. Bennett RM: Myofascial pain syndromes and the fibromyalgia syndrome: a comparative analysis, Chapter 2. In *Myofascial Pain and Fibromyalgia*, edited by J.R. Fricton, E. Awad. Raven Press, New York, 1990 (pp. 43–65).
6. Bennett RM: Nonarticular rheumatism and spondyloarthropathies. *Postgrad Med 87*:97–104, 1990.
7. Bierman W: *Physical Medicine in General Practice*. Paul B. Hoeber (Harper and Row), New York, 1944 (pp. 442–443, Fig. 265).
8. Bourdillon JF, Day EA: *Spinal Manipulation*, Ed. 4. William Heinemann Medical Books, London, 1987.
9. Brügger A: *Die Erkrankungen des Bewegungsapparates und seines Nervensystems*. Gustav Fischer Verlag, Stuttgart, New York, 1980.
10. Danneskiold-Samsøe B, Christiansen E, Andersen RB: Myofascial pain and the role of myoglobin. *Scand J Rheumatol 15*:174–178, 1986.
11. Danneskiold-Samsøe B, Christiansen E, Lund B *et al*: Regional muscle tension and pain ("fibrositis"). *Scand J Rehab 15*:17–20, 1983.
12. Diakow PRP: Thermographic imaging of myofascial trigger points. *J Manipulative Physiol Ther 11*:114–117, 1988.
13. DonTigny RL: Dysfunction of the sacroiliac joint and its treatment. *J Orthop Sports Phys Ther 1*:23–35, 1979.
14. Duboc D, Jehenson P, Dinh ST, *et al.*: Phosphorus NMR spectroscopy study of muscular enzyme deficiencies involving glycogenolysis and glycolysis. *Neurology 37*:663–671, 1987.
15. Egund N, Olsson TH, Schmid H, *et al.*: Movements in the sacroiliac joints demonstrated with roentgen stereophotogrammetry. *Acta Radiol Diagn 19*:833–846, 1978.
16. Finsterbush A, Pogrund H: The hypermobility syndrome: Musculoskeletal complaints in 100 consecutive cases of generalized joint hypermobility. *Clin Orthop 168*:124–127, 1982.
17. Fischer AA: Diagnosis and management of chronic pain in physical medicine and rehabilitation, Chapter 8. In *Current Therapy in Physiatry*, edited by A.P. Ruskin. W.B. Saunders, Philadelphia, 1984 (pp. 123–154).
18. Fischer AA: The present status of neuromuscular thermography. Academy of Neuro-muscular Thermography: Clinical Proceedings. *Postgrad Med*: Custom Communications, pp. 26–33, 1986.
19. Fischer AA: Correlation between site of pain and "hot spots" on thermogram in lower body. Academy of Neuro-muscular Thermography: Clinical Proceedings, *Postgrad Med*: Custom Communications, p. 99, 1986.
20. Fischer AA: Pressure threshold meter: its use for quantification of tender spots. *Arch Phys Med Rehabil* 67:836–838, 1986.
21. Fischer AA, Chang CH: Temperature and pressure threshold measurements in trigger points. *Thermology 1*:212–215, 1986.
22. Fischer AA: Pressure tolerance over muscles and bones in normal subjects. *Arch Phys Med Rehabil 67*:406–409, 1986.
23. Fischer AA: Pressure algometry over normal muscles. Standard values, validity and reproducibility of pressure threshold. *Pain 30*:115–126, 1987.

24. Fischer AA: Tissue compliance meter for objective, quantitative documentation of soft tissue consistency and pathology. *Arch Phys Med Rehabil 68*:122–125, 1987.
25. Fischer AA: Muscle tone in normal persons measured by tissue compliance. *J Neurol Orthop Med Surg 8*:227–233, 1987.
26. Fischer AA: Clinical use of tissue compliance meter for documentation of soft tissue pathology. *Clin J Pain 3:*23–30, 1987.
27. Fischer AA: Letter to the Editor. *Pain 28*:411–414, 1987.
28. Fischer AA: Pressure threshold measurement for diagnosis of myofascial pain and evaluation of treatment results. *Clin J Pain 2*:207–214, 1987.
29. Fischer AA: Documentation of myofascial trigger points. *Arch Phys Med Rehabil 69*:286–291, 1988.
30. Fricton JR, Awad E (eds): *Myofascial Pain and Fibromyalgia*. Raven Press, New York, 1990.
31. Frigerio NA, Stowe RR, Howe JW: Movement of the sacroiliac joint. *Clin Orthop 100*:370–377, 1974.
32. Fry HJH: Overuse syndrome, alias tenosynovitis/tendinitis: the terminological hoax. *Plast Reconstr Surg 78*:414–417, 1986.
33. Fry HJH: Prevalence of overuse (injury) syndrome in Australian music schools. *Br J Ind Med 44*:35–40, 1987.
34. Goldenberg DL, Simms RW, Geiger A, *et al.*: High frequency of fibromyalgia in patients with chronic fatigue seen in a primary care practice. *Arthritis Rheum 33*:381–387, 1990.
35. Grahame R: 'The hypermobility syndrome.' *Ann Rheum Dis 49*:197–198, 1990.
36. Gray H: Sacro-iliac joint pain: II. Mobility and axes of rotation. *Int Clin 11*:65–76, 1938 (*see* pp. 68 & 69).
37. Greenman PE. *Principles of Manual Medicine*. Williams & Wilkins, Baltimore, 1989.
38. Haldeman S (ed): *Modern Developments in the Principles and Practice of Chiropractic*. Appleton-Century-Crofts, New York, 1980.
39. Holmes GP, Kaplan JE, Gantz NM, *et al.*: Chronic fatigue syndrome: a working case definition. *Ann Intern Med 108*:387–389, 1988.
40. Ireland DCR: Repetitive strain injury. *Aust Fam Physician 15*:415–416, 1986.
41. Jaeger B, Reeves JL: Quantification of changes in myofascial trigger point sensitivity with the pressure algometer following passive stretch. *Pain 27*:203–210, 1986.
42. Janda V: *Muscle Function Testing*. Butterworths, London, 1983 (pp. 244–250).
43. Jansen RD, Nansel DD, Slosberg M: Normal paraspinal tissue compliance: the reliability of a new clinical and experimental instrument. *J Manipulative Physiol Ther 13*:243–246, 1990.
44. Jensen K, Andersen HØ, Olesen J, *et al*: Pressure-pain threshold in human temporal region. Evaluation of a new pressure algometer. *Pain 25*:313–323, 1986.
45. Jensen K, Tuxen C, Olesen J: Pericranial muscle tenderness and pressure-pain threshold in the temporal region during common migraine. *Pain 35*:65–70, 1988.
46. Jensen KE, Jacobsen S, Thomsen C, *et al.*: Paper presented to the Society of Magnetic Resonance in Medicine, San Francisco, August 22–26, 1988.
47. Jessee EF, Owen DS Jr, Sagar KB: The benign hypermobile joint syndrome. *Arthritis Rheum 23*:1053–1056, 1980.
48. Joseph J: *Man's Posture*. Charles C Thomas, Springfield, 1960.
49. Kendall HO, Kendall FP, Boynton DA: *Posture and Pain*. Williams & Wilkins, Baltimore, 1952. Reprinted by Robert E. Krieger, Melbourne, FL, 1971.
50. Kushmerick MJ: Muscle energy metabolism, nuclear magnetic resonance spectroscopy and their potential in the study of fibromyalgia. *J Rheumatol (Suppl 19) 16*:40–46, 1989.
51. Larsson S-E, Bengtsson A, Bodegård L, *et al.*: Muscle changes in work-related chronic myalgia. *Acta Orthop Scand 59*:552–556, 1988.
52. Lautenschläger J, Brückle W, Schnorrenberger CC, *et al.*: Die Messung von Druckschmerzen im Bereich von Sehnen und Muskeln bei Gesunden und Patienten mit generalisierter Tendomyopathie (Fibromyalgie-Syndrom). *Z Rheumatol 47*:397–404, 1988.
53. Lewit K: *Manipulative Therapy in Rehabilitation of the Motor System*. Butterworths, London, 1985.
54. *Ibid.* (pp. 38–39).
55. *Ibid.* (pp. 192–196, 256–257).
56. Lewit K: The muscular and articular factor in movement restriction. *Manual Med 1*:83–85, 1985.
57. Lewit K: Postisometric relaxation in combination with other methods of muscular facilitation and inhibition. *Manual Med 2*:101–104, 1986.
58. Lewit K, Simons DG: Myofascial pain: relief by post-isometric relaxation. *Arch Phys Med Rehabil 65*:452–456, 1984.
59. List T, Helkimo M, Falk G: Reliability and validity of a pressure threshold meter in recording tenderness in the masseter muscle and the anterior temporalis muscle. *J Craniomandibular Practice 7*:223–229, 1989.
60. Maigne R: *Orthopedic Medicine. A New Approach to Vertebral Manipulations*. (edited and translated by W.T. Liberson). Charles C Thomas, Springfield, 1972.
61. Margoles MS: Stress neuromyelopathic pain syndrome (SNPS): Report of 333 patients. *J Neurol Orthop Surg 4*:317–322, 1983.
62. Mathies H: Gedanken zur Nomenklatur des "Weichteilrheumatismus." *Z Rheumatol 47*: 432–433, 1988.
63. Mathur AK, Gatter RA, Bank WJ, *et al.*: Abnormal ^{31}P-NMR spectroscopy of painful muscles of patients with fibromyalgia. *Arthritis Rheum 31 (4) (suppl)*:S23, 1988.
64. McCully KK, Argov Z, Boden BA, *et al.*: Detection of muscle injury in humans with 31–P magnetic resonance spectroscopy. *Muscle Nerve 11*:212–216, 1988.
65. Mennell JM: The therapeutic use of cold. *J Am Osteopath Assoc 74*:1146–1157, 1975.
66. Merskey H, Spear FG: The reliability of the pressure algometer. *Br J Soc Clin Psychol 3*:130–136, 1964.

67. Miller RG, Boska MD, Moussavi RS, *et al.*: ^{31}P nuclear magnetic resonance studies of high energy phosphates and pH in human muscle fatigue: comparison of aerobic and anaerobic exercise. *J Clin Invest 81*:1190–1196, 1988.
68. Miller RG, Giannini D, Milner-Brown HS, *et al.*: Effects of fatiguing exercise on high-energy phosphates, force, and EMG: evidence for three phases of recovery. *Muscle Nerve 10*:810–821, 1987.
69. Mitchell FL, Moran PS, Pruzzo NA: *An Evaluation and Treatment Manual of Osteopathic Manipulative Procedures*. Mitchell, Moran, and Pruzzo Associates, Valley Park, MO, 1979.
70. Müller W, Lautenschläger J: Die generalisierte Tendomyopathie (GTM): Teil I: Klinik, Verlauf und Differentialdiagnose. *Z Rheumatol 49*:11–21, 1990.
71. Ohrbach R, Gale EN: Pressure pain thresholds, clinical assessment, and differential diagnosis: reliability and validity in patients with myogenic pain. *Pain 39*:157–169, 1989.
72. Parker R, Anderson B, Parker P: Environmentally conscious PTs. *Clinical Management 10*:11–13, 1990.
73. Perry F, Heller PH, Kamiya J, *et al.*: Altered autonomic function in patients with arthritis or with chronic myofascial pain. *Pain 39*:77–84, 1989.
74. Popelianskii Ya.Yu.: Soviet vertebroneurology: successes and problems. *Revmatologikila 4*:13–19, 1987.
75. Porterfield JA: The sacroiliac joint, Chapter 23. In *Orthopaedic and Sports Physical Therapy*, edited by J.A. Gould III and G.J. Davies, Vol. II. C.V. Mosby, St. Louis, 1985 (pp. 550–580).
76. Price R, Lehmann JF: Influence of muscle cooling on the viscoelastic response of the human ankle to sinusoidal displacements. *Arch Phys Med Rehabil 71*:745–748, 1990.
77. Reeves JL, Jaeger B, Graff-Radford SB: Reliability of the pressure algometer as a measure of myofascial trigger point sensitivity. *Pain 24*: 313–321, 1986.
78. Schiffman E, Fricton J, Haley D, Tylka D: A pressure algometer for myofascial pain syndrome: reliability and validity testing, Chapter 46. In *Proceedings of the Vth World Congress on Pain*, edited by R. Dubner, G.F. Gebhart, M.R. Bond, Vol. 3. Elsevier Science Publishers, BV, New York, 1988 (pp. 407–413).
79. Sheon RP: Regional myofascial pain and the fibrositis syndrome (fibromyalgia). *Compr Ther 12*:42–52, 1986.
80. Sikorski JM: The orthopaedic basis for repetitive strain injury. *Aust Fam Physician 17*:81–83, 1988.
81. Simons D: Muscular Pain Syndromes, Chapter 1. In *Myofascial Pain and Fibromyalgia*, edited by J.R. Fricton and E.A. Awad. Raven Press, New York, 1990 (pp. 1–41, *see* p. 31).
82. Simons DG: Myofascial pain syndrome due to trigger points, Chapter 45. In *Rehabilitation Medicine*, edited by Joseph Goodgold. C. V. Mosby Co., St. Louis, 1988 (pp. 686–723).
83. Simons DG, Simons LS: Chronic myofascial pain syndrome, Chapter 42. In *Handbook of Chronic Pain Management*, edited by C. David Tollison. Williams & Wilkins, Baltimore, 1989 (pp. 509–529).
84. Simons DG, Travell JG, Simons LS: Suggestions: alternate spray; alternative treatments. *Progress Report, Am Phys Therap Assoc 18*:2, March 1989.
85. Simons DG, Travell JG, Simons LS: Protecting the ozone layer. *Arch Phys Med Rehabil 71*:64, 1990.
86. Sinaki M, Merritt JL, Stillwell GK: Tension myalgia of the pelvic floor. *Mayo Clin Proc 52*:717–722, 1977.
87. Steinbrocker O, Isenberg SA, Silver M, *et al.*: Observations on pain produced by injection of hypertonic saline into muscles and other supportive tissues. *J Clin Invest 32*:1045–1051, 1953.
88. Stonnington HH: Tension myalgia: *Mayo Clin Proc 52*:750, 1977.
89. Thomas D, Aidinis S: Objective documentation of musculoskeletal pain syndrome by pressure algometry during thiopentone sodium (Pentothal) anesthesia. *Clin J Pain 5*:343–350, 1989.
90. Thompson JM: Tension myalgia as a diagnosis at the Mayo Clinic and its relationship to fibrositis, fibromyalgia, and myofascial pain syndrome. *Mayo Clin Proc 65*:1237–1248, 1990.
91. Travell J: *Office Hours: Day and Night*. The World Publishing Company, New York, 1968 (pp. 289–291).
92. Travell JG: Chronic myofascial pain syndromes. Mysteries of the history, Chapter 6. In *Myofascial Pain and Fibromyalgia*, edited by J.R. Fricton and E.A. Awad. Raven Press, New York, 1990 (pp. 129–137).
93. Travell JG, Simons DG: *Myofascial Pain and Dysfunction: The Trigger Point Manual*. Williams & Wilkins, Baltimore, 1983.
94. *Ibid.* (p. 67).
95. Travell W, Travell J: Technique for reduction and ambulatory treatment of sacroiliac displacement. *Arch Phys Ther 23*:222–246, 1942 (p. 224).
96. Travell J, Travell W: Therapy of low back pain by manipulation and of referred pain in the lower extremity by procaine infiltration. *Arch Phys Ther 27*:537–547, 1946.
97. Tunks E, Crook J, Norman G, Kalaher S: Tender points in fibromyalgia. *Pain 34*:11–19, 1988.
98. Vallentyne SW, Vallentyne JR: The case of the missing ozone: are physiatrists to blame? *Arch Phys Med Rehabil 69*:992–993, 1988.
99. Voss DE, Ionta MK, Myers BJ: *Proprioceptive Neuromuscular Facilitation*, Ed 3. Harper & Row, Philadelphia, 1985 (p. 304).
100. Weisl H: The movements of the sacroiliac joint. *Acta Anat 23*:80–91, 1955.
101. Wigley RD: Chronic fatigue syndrome, ME and fibromyalgia. *N Z Med J 103*:378, 1990.
102. Wilder DG, Pope MH, Frymoyer JW: The functional topography of the sacroiliac joint. *Spine 5*:575–579, 1980.
103. Wolfe F, Smythe HA, Yunus MB, *et al.*: American College of Rheumatology 1990 Criteria for the Classification of Fibromyalgia: Report of the Multicenter Criteria Committee. *Arthritis Rheum 33*:160–172, 1990.

PART 1

CHAPTER 3
Lower Torso Pain-and-Muscle Guide

INTRODUCTION TO PART 1

This first part of THE TRIGGER POINT MANUAL, Volume 2, covers muscles of three regions: lumbar muscles of the torso that were not included in Volume 1,[9] muscles of the buttock, and muscles of the pelvis. The lumbar muscles in this Part 1 are the quadratus lumborum and iliopsoas; the abdominal and paraspinal muscles were presented in Part 4 of Volume 1.[9] The gluteal muscles covered in this part are the gluteus maximus, gluteus medius, and gluteus minimus. The pelvic muscles discussed here are the intrapelvic muscles that are accessible to palpation, including the piriformis muscle. Part 1 includes the other deep lateral rotators of the thigh that connect the pelvis with the greater trochanter of the femur. This chapter also considers referred pain arising from zygapophysial (facet) joints of the lumbar spine.

Differential diagnosis of an individual muscle's referred pain pattern is considered under Section 6, Symptoms, in each muscle chapter.

PAIN GUIDE TO INVOLVED MUSCLES

This guide lists the muscles that may be responsible for referred pain in each of the areas shown in Figure 3.1. These areas, which identify where patients may complain of pain, are listed alphabetically. The muscles most likely to refer pain to a designated area are listed under the heading for that area. One uses this chart by locating the name of the area that hurts and then by looking under that heading for the muscles that are likely to cause the pain there. Then, reference should be made to the pain patterns of individual muscles; the figure and page numbers for each pattern follow in parentheses. The pain patterns of muscles that are found in Volume 1[9] are listed with a reference number. The patterns for muscles that are described in this volume are listed without a reference.

In a general way, the muscle listings follow the order of frequency in which they are likely to cause pain in that area. This order is only an approximation; the selection process by which patients reach an examiner greatly influences which of their muscles are most likely to be symptomatic. **Bold face** type indicates that the muscle refers an essential pain pattern to that pain area. Normal type indicates that the muscle may refer a spillover pattern to that pain area. TrP means trigger point.

PAIN GUIDE

ABDOMINAL PAIN

Rectus abdominis (49.2*B*, p. 664)[9]
Obliquus externus abdominis (49.1*C*, p. 662)[9]
Iliocostalis thoracis (48.1*B*, p. 638)[9]
Multifidi (48.2*B*, p. 639)[9]
Quadratus lumborum (4.1*A*, p. 30)
Pyramidalis (49.2*D*, p. 664)[9]

BUTTOCK PAIN

Gluteus medius (8.1 TrP_1 and TrP_2, p. 151)
Quadratus lumborum (4.1*A* and 4.1*B*, p. 30)
Gluteus maximus (7.1*A*, *B*, and *C*, p. 133)
Iliocostalis lumborum (48.1*C*, p. 638)[9]
Longissimus thoracis (48.1*D*, p. 638)[9]
Semitendinosus and semimembranosus (16.1*A*, p. 317)
Piriformis (10.1, p. 188)
Gluteus minimus (9.1, p. 169 and 9.2, p. 169)
Rectus abdominis (49.2*A*, p. 664)[9]
Soleus (22.1 TrP_3, p. 429)

ILIOSACRAL PAIN

Levator ani and coccygeus (6.1*A*, p. 112)
Gluteus medius (8.1 TrP_1 and TrP_3, p. 151)
Quadratus lumborum (4.1*B*, p. 30)
Gluteus maximus (7.1*B*, p. 133)
Multifidi (48.2*A* and 48.2*B*, p. 639)[9]
Rectus abdominis (49.2*A*, p. 664)[9]
Soleus (22.1 TrP_3, p. 429)

LUMBAR PAIN

Gluteus medius (8.1 TrP_1 and TrP_3, p. 151)
Multifidi (48.2*B*, p. 639)[9]
Iliopsoas (5.1, p. 90)
Longissimus thoracis (48.1*D*, p. 638)[9]
Rectus abdominis (49.2*A*, p. 664)[9]
Iliocostalis thoracis (48.1*B*, p. 638)[9]
Iliocostalis lumborum (48.1*C*, p. 638)[9]

PELVIC PAIN

Coccygeus (6.1*A*, p. 112)
Levator ani (6.1*A*, p. 112)
Obturator internus (6.1*B*, p. 112)
Adductor magnus (15.2*B*, p. 292)
Piriformis (10.1, p. 188)
Obliquus internus abdominis (p. 661)[9]

PAIN REFERRED FROM ZYGAPOPHYSIAL JOINTS

The zygapophysial (apophysial or facet) joints are probably the most carefully studied synovial joints of the body for specific referred pain patterns. The cervical zygapophysial joints have been identified as a source of head, neck, and shoulder pain;[2] the lumbar zygapophysial joints refer pain downward only, and rarely, if ever, upward.[4] This section examines the diagnosis of pain arising from zygapophysial joints. Although referred pain from this source is often unrecognized, it is diagnosable with specific techniques and it is treatable. Referred pain patterns from cervical and lumbar zygapophysial joints are clearly established. Unfortunately, as with trigger points, the cause of the referred pain and tenderness has not been firmly established.

1. DIAGNOSIS

Unambiguous identification of a zygapophysial joint as the cause of the patient's pain requires an exacting technique. Bogduk and Marsland[2] describe two ways of performing a diagnostic block of a zygapophysial joint. One way is to block the medial branch of the dorsal ramus of the spinal nerve above and below the joint, proximal to the origin of the articular branches of the nerve. The other way is direct intra-articular injection of anesthetic under image-intensifier control.[2] One of these joints can accommodate only about 1 mL or less of fluid. A greater volume infiltrates adjacent tissues.[1]

Other investigators, in addition to inserting the hypodermic needle between the articular facets under fluoroscopic control,[7] injected contrast dye to outline the joint space and confirm the needle location.[6,7] Injection of a long-acting local anesthetic, such as bupivacaine, relieves the symptoms arising from that joint, usually temporarily, but sometimes for months or years.

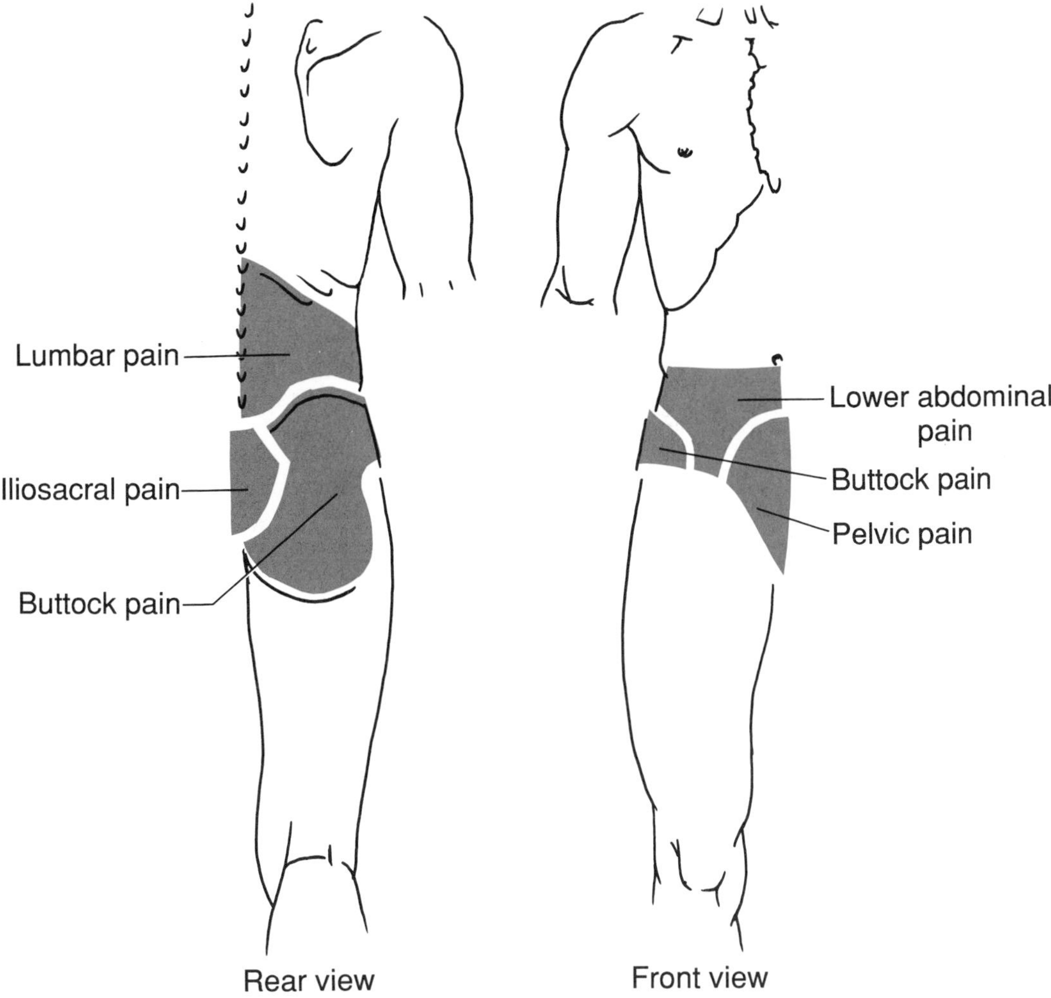

Figure 3.1. Designated areas *(red)* within the lower torso region where patients may describe myofascial pain. The pain may be referred to each designated area from the muscles that are listed in the PAIN GUIDE on the facing page.

Of 25 patients, the 14 who obtained relief from facet injection (responders) were distinguished in a number of ways from the others who did not obtain relief (non-responders).[4] Responders had a history of acute onset of pain usually associated with movement, such as bending or twisting. Non-responders experienced an insidious onset. Pain in responders was exacerbated by sitting and relieved by walking, whereas in non-responders the opposite was the case: pain was relieved by sitting and increased by walking. Pain was much more likely to extend beyond the thigh to the leg in non-responders. Also in non-responders, the Straight-leg Raising Test was more likely to produce pain below the gluteal fold. Responders complained of pain on forward flexion of the spine and they had a significantly greater average anterior-posterior diameter of the spinal canal than non-responders.

The point of maximum tenderness alone does not reliably locate the involved zygapophysial joint.[1,4] However, additional palpation to detect loss of joint mobility in the cervical spine was completely reliable in expert hands.[5] This conclusion was based on a sophisticated independent evaluation of zygapophysial joint involvement.

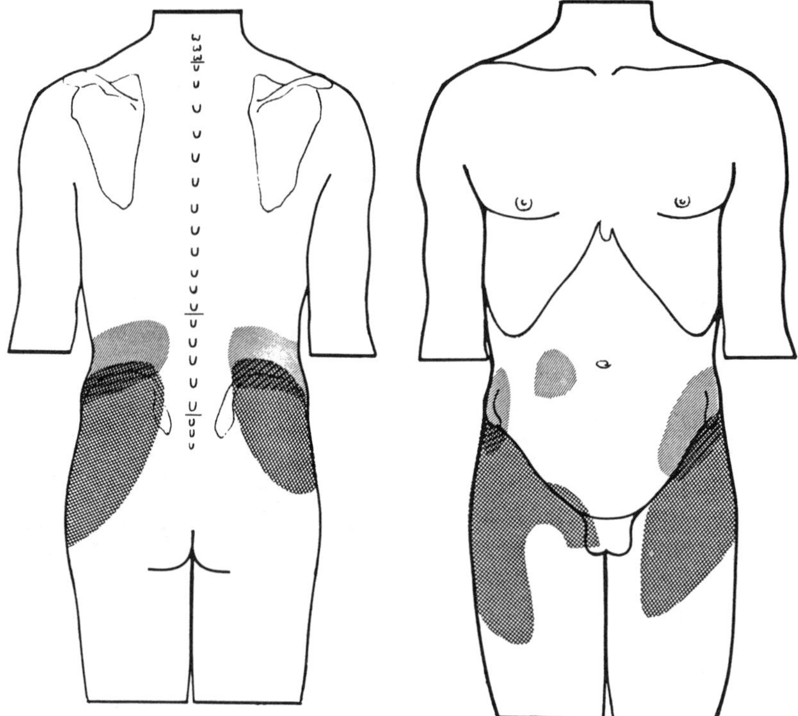

Figure 3.2. Composite referred pain patterns induced in six normal subjects by injection of hypertonic saline solution into the zygapophysial joints at L_{1-2} (*diagonal lines, superior pattern*) and at L_{4-5} (*cross-hatched, inferior pattern*). Despite the difference of three segmental levels between the stimulus injections, the referred pain patterns overlap. Reproduced by permission.[6]

2. REFERRED PHENOMENA FROM ZYGAPOPHYSIAL JOINTS

Referred Pain

The medial branch of the posterior primary ramus of each spinal nerve supplies two zygapophysial joints, one above and one below its course.[3] This branch also supplies the lumbar dorsal fasciae, the deep paraspinal muscles, the fibrous capsule of the synovial apophysial joints, and the longitudinal flaval and interspinous ligaments. It does not innervate the articular cartilage or synovium of the zygapophysial joint.[6]

Among the 14 patients noted previously who were responders to injection of a local anesthetic into the zygapophysial joint,[4] all initially had complained of pain in the sacroiliac joint or lumbosacral region; ten reported pain in part or all of the gluteal area; five reported thigh pain; four reported pain below the knee; and two reported groin pain. This indicates the relative frequency with which pain from zygapophysial joints is likely to be referred to various areas. The pattern of pain referred by lumbar zygapophysial joints corresponds to, or overlaps, pain referred by TrPs in the multifidi, quadratus lumborum, obturator internus, all three gluteal, and the piriformis muscles.

Referred pain induced by the injection of 0.4 mL of 6% sodium chloride solution into the zygapophysial joint at the L_{1-2} and the L_{4-5} levels in six normal subjects is illustrated in Figure 3.2. Clearly, the referral of pain and tenderness is not restricted to the segment stimulated. The patterns overlap despite a difference of three segmental levels. These patterns generally match well those seen in patients.[6] Similar patterns were induced by injecting hypertonic saline outside the joint capsule rather than inside it.[6] Injecting larger amounts of saline, Mooney and Robertson[7] observed more extensive referred pain patterns that sometimes reached the ankles in patients with symptoms. They observed that increasing the dose of injected saline produced more extensive referred pain patterns.

Electrical stimulation of the medial branch of the dorsal ramus of spinal nerves L_4 and L_5 in a patient presenting with low back pain reproduced the patient's pain.[1] Electrical stimulation bilaterally of the L_4 medial branch reproduced her bilateral groin pain, anterior right thigh pain, and lumbosacral pain. Bilateral stimulation of the L_5 dorsal ramus reproduced her pain in the left buttock, in the right posterior thigh, and in the right anterior leg. Bupivacaine (0.5% solution) injected in the zygapophysial joint spaces completely relieved her symptoms for 10 hours.[1]

Other Referred Phenomena

Stimulation of the posterior ramus induced electrical activity in the hamstring muscles of cats in which the rostral spinal cord had been blocked.[1] Mooney and Robertson[7] found that in patients the injection of hypertonic saline into the L_{4-5} and L_5-S_1 zygapophysial joints induced marked electromyographic activity in the hamstring muscles and limitation of straight-leg raising to less than 70°. In addition, they noted that relief of pain by injecting the zygapophysial joint with local anesthetic restored to normal values straight-leg raising that had been restricted to less than 70°. McCall *et al.*[6] reported occasional paraspinal muscle spasm observed clinically in response to intracapsular and extracapsular injection of hypertonic saline.

Mooney and Robertson[7] reported that, compared to tendon jerk responses before treatment, depressed reflexes were restored to normal in three patients following local anesthetic injection of the zygapophysial joints.

3. TREATMENT

When local anesthetic and/or steroid injection into the apophysial joint have not provided sustained relief of the pain, surgical ablative procedures have been performed on the medial branches of the posterior primary rami of spinal nerves supplying the affected joint.[1,8]

References

1. Bogduk N: Lumbar dorsal ramus syndrome. *Med J Aust 2*:537–541, 1980.
2. Bogduk N, Marsland A: The cervical zygapophysial joints as a source of neck pain. *Spine 13*: 610–617, 1988.
3. Bogduk N, Twomey LT: *Clinical Anatomy of the Lumbar Spine*. Churchill Livingstone, New York, 1987 (pp. 98–99).
4. Fairbank JCT, Park WM, McCall IW, *et al.*: Apophyseal injection of local anesthetic as a diagnostic aid in primary low-back pain syndromes. *Spine 6*:598–605, 1981.
5. Jull G, Bogduk N, Marsland A: The accuracy of manual diagnosis for cervical zygapophysial joint pain syndromes. *Med J Aust 148*:233–236, 1988.
6. McCall IW, Park WM, O'Brien JP: Induced pain referral from posterior lumbar elements in normal subjects. *Spine 4*:441–446, 1979.
7. Mooney V, Robertson J: The facet syndrome. *Clin Orthop 115*:149–156, 1976.
8. Shealy CN: Facet denervation in the management of back and sciatic pain. *Clin Orthop 115*: 157–164, 1976.
9. Travell JG, Simons DG: *Myofascial Pain and Dysfunction: The Trigger Point Manual*. Williams & Wilkins, Baltimore, 1983.

CHAPTER 4
Quadratus Lumborum Muscle

"Joker of Low Back Pain"

HIGHLIGHTS: **REFERRED PAIN** from trigger points (TrPs) in the quadratus lumborum muscle is projected posteriorly to the region of the sacroiliac (SI) joint and the lower buttock, sometimes anteriorly along the crest of the ilium to the adjacent lower quadrant of the abdomen and the groin, and to the greater trochanter. Severe referred tenderness of the greater trochanter may disrupt sleep. **ANATOMICAL ATTACHMENTS** of this muscle to three structures result in three distinct fiber groups and directions. The *iliocostal* fibers that attach, below, to the crest of the ilium and iliolumbar ligament and, above, to the 12th rib are nearly vertical. The less numerous *iliolumbar* fibers that course between the same iliac attachment, below, and the transverse processes of the upper four lumbar vertebrae, above, are directed diagonally across and extend medial to the iliocostal fibers. The *lumbocostal* fibers that span the space between the second to fourth or fifth lumbar transverse processes, below, and the 12th rib, above, are the fewest in number and lie diagonally in a direction that forms a criss-cross pattern with the iliolumbar fibers. **INNERVATION** of this muscle arises from adjacent thoracolumbar spinal nerves. Unilaterally, the quadratus lumborum can **FUNCTION** as a stabilizer of the lumbar spine and can act as a hip hiker and as a lateral flexor of the lumbar spine. Acting bilaterally, the muscle extends the lumbar spine and assists forced exhalation, as when coughing. The bilaterally paired muscles form a **FUNCTIONAL UNIT** by working together synergistically or as antagonists, depending on the function being performed. Among the **SYMPTOMS** characteristic of quadratus lumborum TrPs, low back pain is the most troublesome. The patient may be barely able to turn over in bed and unable to bear the pain of standing upright or walking. Unloading the lumbar spine of upper body weight provides much relief. Coughing or sneezing can be frightfully painful. This myofascial pain is easily mistaken for radicular pain of lumbar origin. **ACTIVATION** of TrPs in this muscle often involves simultaneously bending over and reaching to one side to pull or lift something, or a major body trauma, as in a fall or motor vehicle accident. Mechanical **PERPETUATION** of quadratus lumborum TrPs may depend on skeletal asymmetries, particularly inequality in length of lower limbs, a small hemipelvis, and/or short upper arms. **PATIENT EXAMINATION** reveals muscle guarding and restriction of trunk mobility, exhibited while rolling over on the examining table or assuming the upright posture. Lower limb-length inequalities (LLLI) and other skeletal asymmetries that cause a compensatory scoliosis are of prime importance and can be simple or confusing and difficult to estimate clinically; these asymmetries are measured most reliably by weight-bearing radiography. Short upper arms are important and easily recognized. **TRIGGER POINT EXAMINATION** of the quadratus lumborum requires positioning that separates the 12th rib from the iliac crest to make the muscle accessible to palpation and place it under gentle tension. Usually, only the most caudal iliocostal fibers can be examined by flat palpation, the rest indirectly by deep palpation of tenderness. **ASSOCIATED TRIGGER POINTS** may develop in the gluteus minimus muscle as satellites in the referred pain zone of the quadratus lumborum TrPs and project pain down the thigh in a sciatic distribution. **INTERMITTENT COLD WITH STRETCH** of this muscle is unlikely to be effective therapy unless the patient is positioned to elongate each of the three fiber groups. If stretch by side bending alone is inadequate, one or both rotary components must be added. A side lying position encourages more complete relaxation of the patient. **INJECTION AND STRETCH** of the deep quadratus lumborum TrPs require careful positioning of the patient, meticulous localization of TrP tenderness, an appropriate approach, and a needle that reaches the TrPs. **CORRECTIVE ACTIONS** for management of a compensatory lumbar scoliosis include a full-correction shoe lift for LLLI and an ischial (butt) lift for a small hemipelvis. A chair with sloped armrests or padding added to the usual horizontal armrests corrects for short upper arms. The patient must avoid angling sideways when reaching forward and down. A home program of self-stretch exercises specific for the quadratus lumborum muscle is essential.

The quadratus lumborum muscle is one of the most commonly overlooked muscular sources of low back pain and is often responsible, through satellite gluteus minimus trigger points (TrPs), for the "pseudo-disc syndrome" and the "failed surgical back syndrome."

Low back pain centered in the lumbar region, commonly called lumbago,[90] is more often of muscular origin than is generally realized. Myofascial TrP pain arising in the quadratus lumborum muscle may be paralyzingly severe, rendering weight bearing in the upright posture intolerable.

Low back pain exacts an enormous toll of misery and disability.[73] In any one year, an estimated 10–15% of adults have some work disability caused by back pain.[73] Those patients with low back pain who receive compensation are estimated to cost the country $2.7 billion per year; the Liberty Mutual Insurance Company alone paid nearly $1 million per working day in 1981.[130] How much more low back pain suffering and dysfunction remain unreported or uncompensated because no organic cause was found for the pain!

The quadratus lumborum is considered the most frequent muscular cause of low back pain among practitioners who have learned to recognize its TrPs by examination.[51,128,133] Good[51] reported the quadratus lumborum to be the muscle most commonly involved (32% of 500) in army troops with musculoskeletal pain complaints.

1. REFERRED PAIN
(Fig. 4.1)

An acute, severe onset of the quadratus lumborum myofascial pain syndrome poses a devastatingly urgent problem when the pain strikes as one is getting out of bed in the morning with a full bladder and no one to assist. The situation appears desperate until the patient discovers that the trip to the bathroom can be made on hands and knees. This posture requires no stabilization of the lumbar spine by the quadratus lumborum muscle.

The pain referred from quadratus lumborum TrPs becomes persistent when its perpetuating factors are unrecognized or neglected.

Four locations in the muscle commonly refer distinctive unilateral pain patterns (Fig. 4.1). The pain is usually deep and aching, but may be lancinating during movement. A composite of these separate patterns has been published.[126,129] Two TrP locations are superficial (lateral) and two are deep (medial); each of the pairs has a cephalad and a caudal TrP area. The superficial (lateral) TrPs refer pain more laterally and anteriorly than do the deep TrPs. Caudal TrPs tend to refer pain more distally.

TrPs in the cephalad superficial location (labeled *1*, Fig. 4.1*A*) are likely to refer pain along the crest of the ilium and sometimes to the adjacent lower quadrant of the abdomen. The pain may extend to the outer upper aspect of the groin. The more caudal superficial TrPs (location number *2*, Fig. 4.1*A*) may refer pain to the greater trochanter and outer aspect of the upper thigh. The greater trochanter can be so "sore" (tender to pressure) that the patient cannot tolerate lying on that side and pain may prevent weight bearing by the lower limb on the involved side.

The more cephalad of the deep TrPs (Fig. 4.1*B*) refer pain strongly to the area of the sacroiliac (SI) joint; bilaterally, these TrPs frequently may refer pain that extends across the upper sacral region. The caudal deep TrPs refer pain to the lower buttock.

These pain reference zones also exhibit referred tenderness,[147] especially in the SI joint area and over the greater trochanter. This tenderness is often incorrectly thought to indicate local pathology.

A few patients have described a lightning bolt (or jolt) of pain referred from deep quadratus lumborum TrPs to the front of the thigh extending from the anterior superior iliac spine to the lateral side

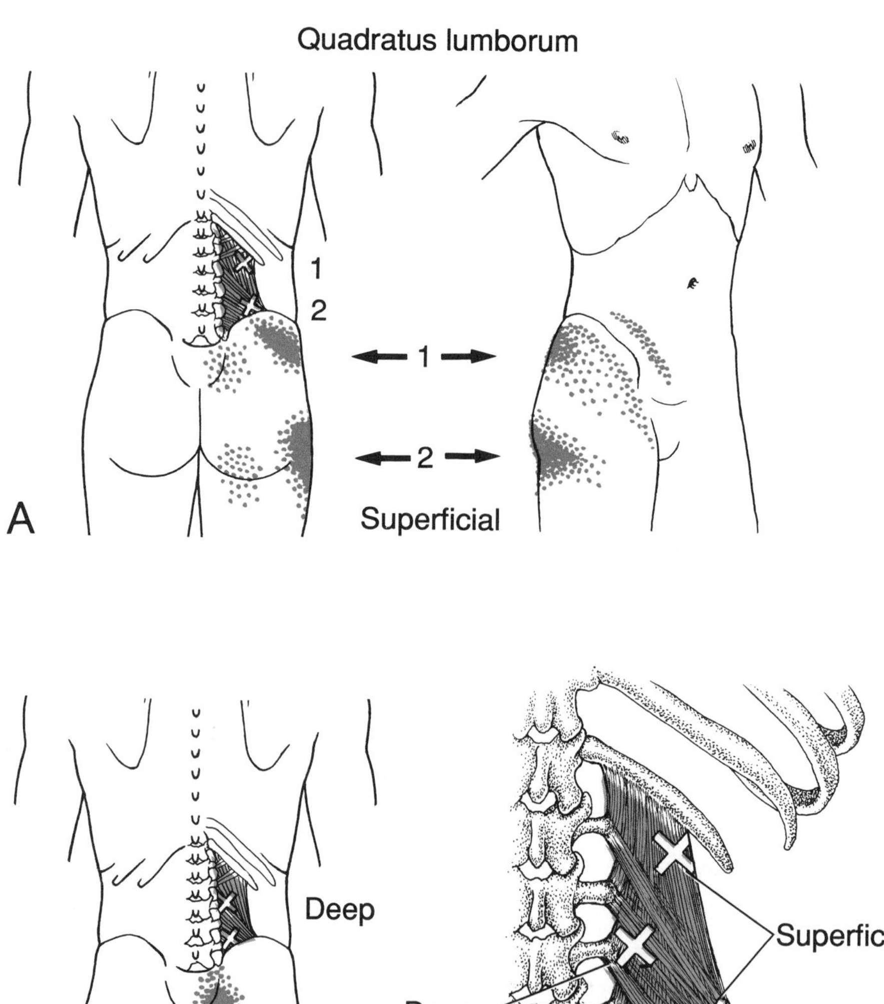

Figure 4.1. Referred pain patterns (*bright red*) of trigger points (**X**s) in the quadratus lumborum muscle (*red*). *Solid bright red* denotes an essential pain pattern, and *stippled red*, a spillover pattern. *A*, pain patterns of superficial (lateral) trigger points that are palpable *(1)* below and close to the 12th rib, and *(2)* just above the iliac crest. *B*, pain patterns of deep (more medial) trigger points close to the transverse processes of the lumbar vertebrae. The more cephalad deep trigger points refer pain to the sacroiliac joint; more caudal trigger points refer pain low in the buttock. *C*, examples of locations of trigger points in the quadratus lumborum muscle. (By permission from Postgraduate Medicine.[128])

of the upper part of the patella in a narrow band about the width of a finger. The sensation is likened to that felt when a finger is placed in an electric light socket. It has no motor component.

Vigorous contraction of the muscle to stabilize the rib cage during coughing or sneezing can cause brief but overwhelmingly severe referred pain.

Authors have identified the quadratus lumborum muscle as a source of lumbago,[52,83,98] backache,[62,111,132,134,167] and lumbar myalgia.[52] More specifically, they have identified the quadratus lumborum

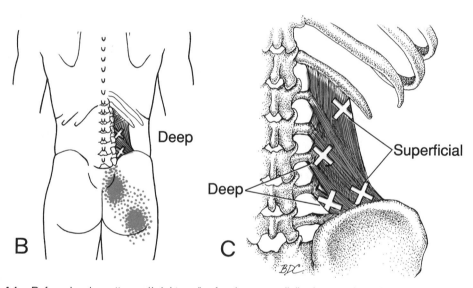

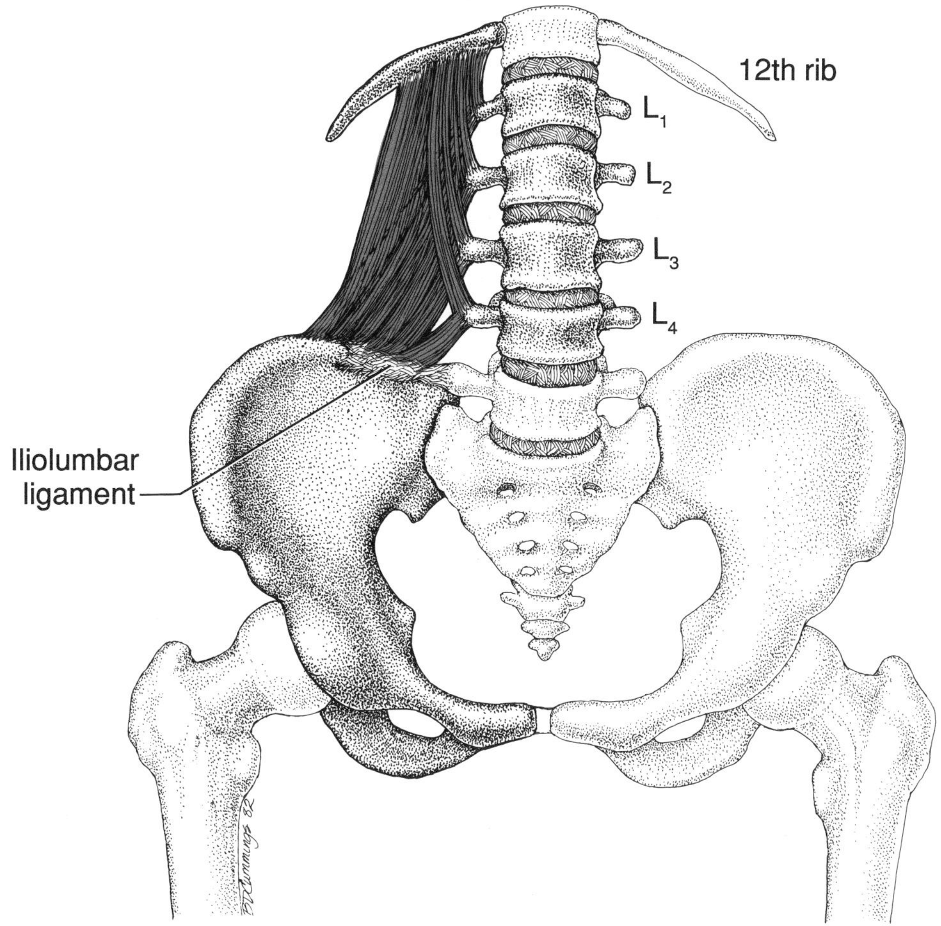

Figure 4.2. Attachments of the quadratus lumborum muscle (*red*) as seen from the front. The iliolumbar ligament is uncolored.

as referring pain to the SI region,[128,133,147] to the hip or buttock,[51,128,133,147] to the greater trochanter,[128,147] to the abdomen,[71,76,132,133,134] and to the groin.[128,147] Additional areas of pain referral from the quadratus lumborum were reported in the anterior thigh[134] and in the testicle and scrotum.[62]

2. ANATOMICAL CONSIDERATIONS AND ATTACHMENTS
(Figs. 4.2–4.4)

Fiber Arrangement

The groups of quadratus lumborum fibers are oriented in three directions (Fig. 4.2): nearly vertical iliocostal fibers, diagonal iliolumbar fibers, and diagonal lumbocostal fibers; the latter two intersect cross-wise. This means that anatomically, functionally, and when stretching the muscle, one should think of it as three muscles.

The nearly vertical fibers are always present and form the most obvious lateral portion of the muscle. These fibers slant medially as they travel cephalad, and below they tend to curve out laterally at their pelvic attachment. These iliocostal fibers attach ***above*** to approximately the medial half of the short 12th rib. ***Below*** they attach to the uppermost posterior crest of the ilium and often, also, to the iliolumbar ligament (Figs. 4.2 and 4.4). This strong ligament anchors the tip of the fifth lumbar transverse process to the crest of the ilium. Quadratus lumborum fibers interdigitate extensively with fibers of the iliolumbar ligament.

The two sets of more variable diagonal bundles of fibers attach on, and in the adjacent area close to, the tips of the transverse processes of the upper four lumbar vertebrae. These processes project laterally and in a slightly posterior direction from the *posterior* portion of the lateral surface of each vertebra and nearly at right angles to the vertical axis of the vertebra at the level of the junction between the upper and middle thirds of the vertebra. The tip of each lumbar transverse process extends well beyond the lateral edge of the vertebral body. The *iliolumbar* diagonal fibers connect ***above*** to the ends of the first three or four (L_1–L_4) transverse processes and ***below*** to the crest of the ilium and often, also, to the iliolumbar ligament. The *lumbocostal* diagonal fibers, when present, attach ***above*** to the 12th rib, and ***below*** to most, sometimes all, of the lumbar transverse processes (Figs. 4.2 and 4.3).

Both sets of diagonal fibers of the quadratus lumborum may be thought of as guy ropes that provide segmental control of lateral flexion and curvature of the lumbar spine. The iliocostal fibers provide overall lumbar curvature control.

The iliolumbar diagonal fibers are consistently shown in dorsal views.[23,55,84,99,145] They are sometimes described[25] and illustrated[168] as also forming an intermediate layer. The lumbocostal diagonal fibers are the most variable and, when present, are usually described[17,169] or illustrated[23,145] as lying anterior to the bulky lateral iliocostal fibers. These lumbocostal diagonal fibers have been described[25] and illustrated[115] as interdigitating with the other two groups of fibers. Eisler[25] draws a medial-lateral distinction that is apparent in detailed dorsal views. The diagonal iliolumbar and lumbocostal fibers comprise the medial border of the muscle and the more nearly vertical iliocostal fibers form the lateral border, with increasing overlap and interdigitation as fibers approach their iliac and costal attachments.

The diagonal fibers frequently interdigitate between layers of the more lateral longitudinal (vertical) fibers and are most apparent from the posterior view. For more detail and variations, see Eisler's classic description.

Classic Description
(Figs. 4.3 and 4.4)

By far the most complete description of the quadratus lumborum muscle is that by Eisler, published in German in 1912.[25] Because of the importance of this muscle, and because variability of some characteristics has led to inconsistencies in its description in anatomy books, the following translation is presented. Included are two illustrations (Figs. 4.3 and 4.4) of three variations as drawn by Eisler, the artist-anatomist-author.[25]

This flat, strong, moderately long, four-sided muscle extends from the dorsal part of the iliac crest to the last rib and attaches by individual serrations of its medial border to the transverse processes of the lumbar vertebrae. The lateral border is smooth and free. The two flat surfaces of the muscle face ventrally and dorsally.

The structure of the muscle is, as a rule, complicated. However, a first glance at only the lateral border gives the impression of a single compact fleshy mass (Fig. 4.4, *right side of subject*). Medially, one can usually distinguish at least two layers, between which one or more fiber layers frequently are inserted. Seen from the dorsal view (Fig. 4.3), the muscle originates for a distance of 6 cm along the iliac crest, reaching laterally 3–4 cm across its dorsal bend. This insertion on the crest is almost completely fleshy, except for a small tendinous triangle at the lateral corner. From the lateral half or lateral two thirds of the origin, the nearly parallel muscle bundles head cephalad and slightly medialward. These fibers insert on the caudal edge of the 12th rib, through a flat tendon medially. Occasionally, this main body of the muscle is anchored extensively to the lumbodorsal fascia.

Along the medial side of the muscle, the fiber bundles form divergent flat serrations, which, when completely developed, attach as tendons to the tips and adjacent parts of the caudal borders of the first four lumbar transverse processes (Fig. 4.3). The serrations increase in mass caudally and occasionally, but by no means always, overlap each other. Ventrally, they extend under the large lateral bulk of the muscle (Fig. 4.4, *right side*). The attachments of these serrations to the lumbar transverse processes are bordered on their medial side by the intertransversarii lateralis muscles.

Seen from the ventral view (Fig. 4.4), the muscle shows a marked broadening cranially [as it approaches its attachments to the transverse processes and to the 12th rib]. The origin on the crest of the ilium, on casual observation, seems to be entirely ligamentous [rather than osseous]. Here,

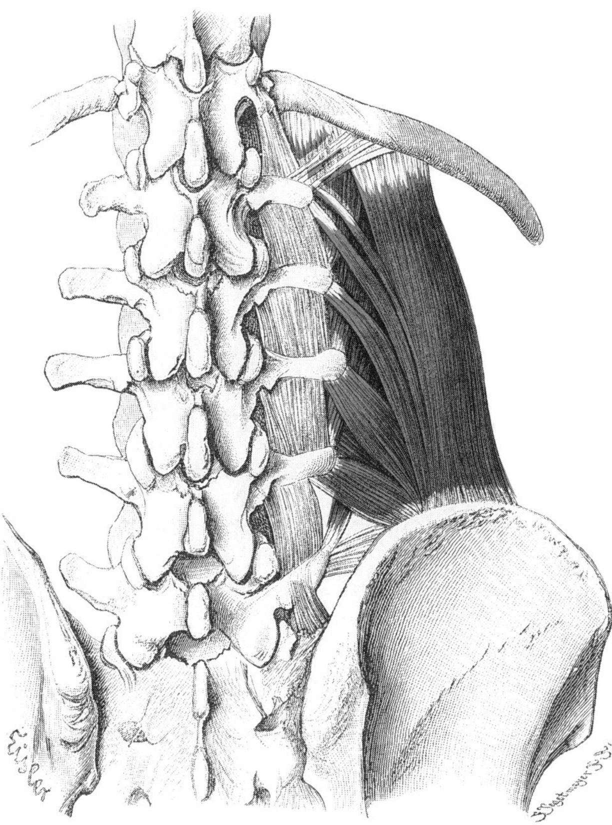

Figure 4.3. Quadratus lumborum (*red*) and intertransversarii laterales muscles (*uncolored*), dorsal view. (From Eisler,[23] *color added*.)

the bundles of fibers to the transverse processes interdigitate with the system of taut fibers belonging to the iliolumbar ligament. Near the lateral border of the muscle, the flat tendons of origin penetrate 4–5 cm cranialward into the muscle belly. Medially, fibers overlap in an alternating manner as they originate from the iliolumbar ligament and from the transverse process of the fifth lumbar vertebra. Fibers attaching to the fifth transverse process frequently form a serration that is isolated from the main origin of the muscle (Figs. 4.3 and Fig. 4.4, *configuration shown on right side of subjects*). In the most outstanding examples, that bundle represents the most caudal member of a series of such serrations. Each serration is attached by tendon to the tip and the neighboring part of the cranial border of a transverse process starting from the second lumbar vertebra. Of these serrations, as a rule, only the most caudal one is located in the ventral surface layer; the rest of them extend onto the dorsal surface.

On the whole, the bundles of the ventral layer (Fig. 4.4) are directed cranially with a somewhat stronger medial slant than those of the dorsal layer (Figs. 4.3 and 4.4). The lateral bundles arise from tendinous slips that penetrate into the muscle and spread cranially by fanning out in a pennate fashion. The medial fibers of the ventral layer run parallel to the lateral fibers just mentioned (Fig. 4.4). Laterally, the insertion along the 12th rib appears fleshy for a short distance. More medially, the insertion is tendinous as it attaches along the caudal margin of the ventral surface of the 12th rib to the area of its head. From the ventral view, some serrations may insert by narrow tendinous slips to the body of the 12th dorsal vertebra along its lateral aspect, and/or to the first lumbar vertebra, and sometimes [to the T_{12}–L_1 disc] between the vertebrae (Fig. 4.4). More rarely, serrations attach to the caudal margin or the ventral surface of the first lumbar transverse process. A part of these ventral surface fibers regularly ends in tendinous attachments to the lateral lumbocostal arch, which is a fibrous arch between the first lumbar vertebra and the 12th rib that serves as half of the lumbar origin of the diaphragm. The length of this tendinous insertion rapidly increases medially. The tendinous portion usually extends at least to the area between the quadratus arch of the diaphragm and the 12th rib.

The intermediate layer of the quadratus lumborum varies in its development from case to case

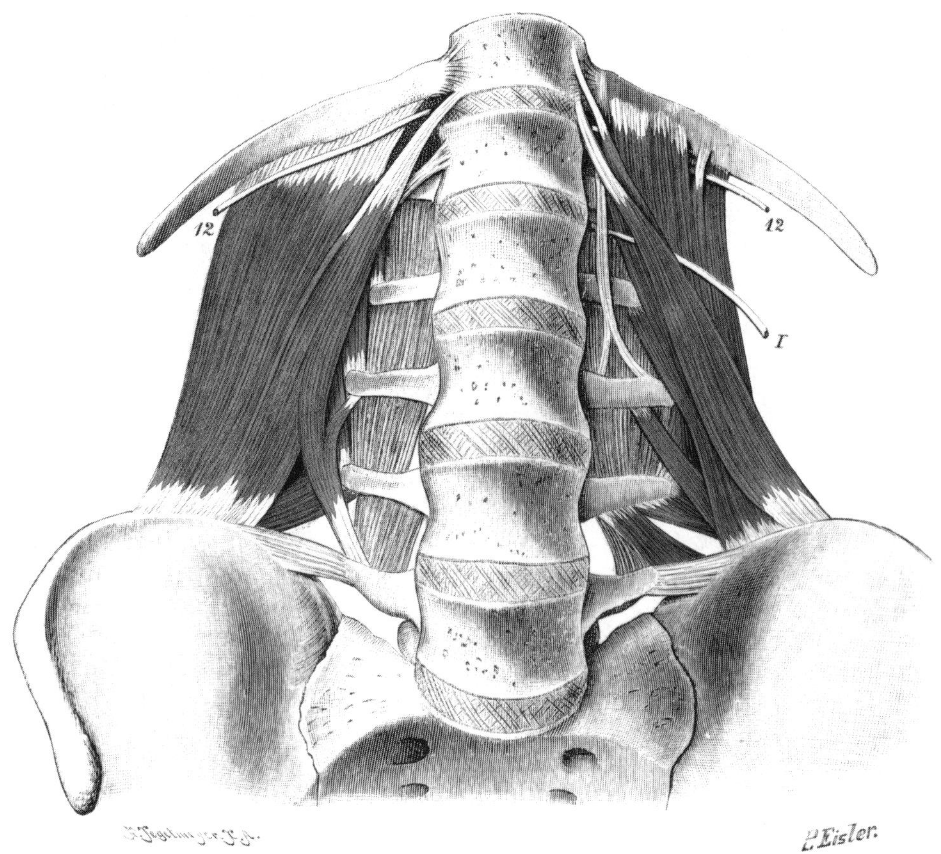

Figure 4.4. Quadratus lumborum (*red*) and intertransversarii laterales (*uncolored*) muscles, ventral view. The two halves of the figure are drawn from two different persons. *12*, 12th thoracic nerve; *I*, first lumbar nerve. (From Eisler,[24] *color added*.)

in a highly unpredictable manner. The key fact is the attachment of the intermediate-layer fibers to the long transverse process of the third lumbar vertebra. Part fleshy and part strongly tendinous, this muscular layer originates from the tip and the cranial edge of the L_3 transverse process. It has a fan-shaped distribution to the caudal edge of the ventral surface of the medial part of the 12th rib.[25]

Iliolumbar Ligament

The iliolumbar ligament develops from immature fibers of the quadratus lumborum muscle during the first two decades of life and is present only in species that assume the erect posture.[89,100] The ligament often shows degenerative changes from the fourth decade onward. It consists of two bands that connect the L_5 transverse process to the crest and inner surface of the ilium. The anterior band travels laterally in the coronal plane and serves as an attachment for the quadratus lumborum. The other band runs more obliquely and posteriorly.[89]

Loading tests in cadavers showed that the anterior band of the iliolumbar ligament chiefly restricts side bending and that the posterior band restricts mainly forward flexion of the spine. These posterior bands also appeared to prevent anterior slipping of the L_5 vertebra over the sacrum. This ligament markedly restricts movement that would otherwise be induced at the L_5–S_1 junction by activity of the quadratus lumborum muscle.

Supplemental References

There is general agreement that the quadratus lumborum muscle is anatomically complex and that its fibers usually follow three directions.[3,25,74,106,168] The variability in the extensiveness and in the dorsal or ventral location of its diagonal fibers leads to different descriptions of the muscle.

The muscle is illustrated in cross section,[15,31,56,108,135] in the ventral view showing diagonal fibers,[24,30,69,74,104,109,114] and in ventral view without diagonal fibers.[26,29,54,136,146] It is shown in dorsal view with diagonal fibers[17,23,27,55,107,115,145] and in dorsal view without diagonal fibers.[84]

3. INNERVATION

The quadratus lumborum muscle is supplied by branches of the lumbar plexus arising from spinal nerves T_{12} and either L_1–L_3[25,74,99] or L_1–L_4.[17,28]

4. FUNCTION (Figs. 4.5 and 4.6)

In an upright subject, the quadratus lumborum functions to control or "brake" side bending to the opposite side by a lengthening contraction. Stabilization of the lumbar spine on the pelvis by the quadratus lumborum is so important that, according to Knapp,[81] complete bilateral paralysis of this muscle makes walking impossible, even with braces. This muscle is also thought to stabilize the last rib for inhalation and forced exhalation.

Unilaterally, with the pelvis fixed, the quadratus lumborum muscle acts primarily as a lateral flexor of the spine to the same side (concavity toward the contracting muscle),[3,13,17,21,69,74,78,85,88,99,106,114,118,144,169] as illustrated in Figure 4.5*A* and *B*. With the spine fixed, unilateral contraction elevates (hikes) the ipsilateral hip. The quadratus lumborum assists lateral bending to the same side against resistance;[77] in so doing, it produces a scoliosis, primarily in the lumbar region. Acting bilaterally, the quadratus lumborum extends the lumbar spine.

Actions

When the subject is recumbent and the muscle is fixed at the thoracic end, it pulls the ipsilateral side of the pelvis cephalad (hikes the hip).[68,69,74,133]

Both quadratus lumborum muscles acting together were recognized as extensors of the lumbar spine by most authors,[3,69,77,106,117,144] but were reported to have a flexor action by others.[71,147] In a computer analysis[117] of the lever arms and cross-sectional areas of the regional muscles in two cadavers, the quadratus lumborum was calculated as producing approximately 9% of the muscular force exerted in lateral flexion of the spine, and 13% (in one cadaver) or 22% (in the other cadaver) of the extension power of the lumbar spine. This study confirms the extension function deduced from Figure 4.5*C*, *D*, and *E* in all positions of the lumbar spine from full flexion to full extension. In spinal rotation to the contralateral side, it was calculated as contributing 9% or 13% of the power.[117]

Based on its anatomical relations, bilateral activity of the quadratus lumborum muscles is widely identified as assisting normal inhalation by helping to stabilize the attachment of the diaphragm along the 12th rib.[69,85,88,99,106,169] It is also identified as fixing the last rib, or two, in forced exhalation.[4,17,78,114,118]

Knapp[80] concluded from clinical observations that, without apparent gluteal weakness, dropping of the pelvis on the swing side when walking in place may be caused by weakness of the oblique fibers of the quadratus lumborum on the opposite side.

The functions of the quadratus lumborum are usually described as if it had only the nearly vertical iliocostal fibers. In 1951, Knapp[80] proposed that the diagonal iliolumbar and lumbocostal fibers of the quadratus lumborum opposed the action of its own longitudinal iliocostal fibers. He aptly employed the analogy of a multi-jointed telephone pole (the spine) with cross arms (the transverse processes) through each segment. In Knapp's analogy, the iliolumbar bundles of muscle fibers corresponded to guy ropes running diagonally from the ground (iliac crest and iliolumbar ligament) to the end of each cross arm (transverse process). The iliolumbar ligament served to anchor the transverse processes of the foundation segment L_5 on S_1.

To explore the validity of this concept, the second author made tracings of anteroposterior (Fig. 4.5*A* and *B*) and lateral (Fig. 4.5*C*, *D*, and *E*) radiographs of the lumbar spine. The iliocostal muscle fibers were superimposed in Figure 4.5*A* and the diagonal fibers in Figure 4.5*B*. It appears that *IF* the upper end of the lumbar spine at T_{12} is free to move, all three divisions of the muscle flex the spine laterally with its concavity toward the active muscle (Figs. 4.5*A* and *B*, and 4.6*A*).

However, the diagonal iliolumbar fibers may have the opposite effect (Fig. 4.6*B*). According to Knapp's model, the diagonal fibers can assist flexion of the lumbar spine with the concavity *away* from those fibers, *IF* the contralateral longitudinal iliocostal fibers are simultaneously pulling the 12th rib and T_{12} vertebra to produce lateral flexion of the entire lumbar spine toward the contralateral side. This assumes that these vertical iliocostal fibers are producing a pull that balances their contralateral diagonal fibers. The diagonal lumbocostal fibers should have the same effect as the diagonal iliolumbar fibers on the same side.

PART 1

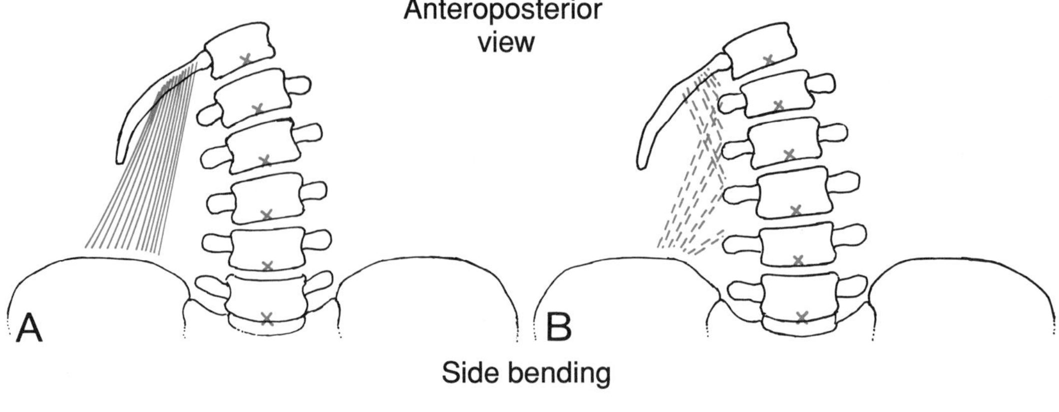

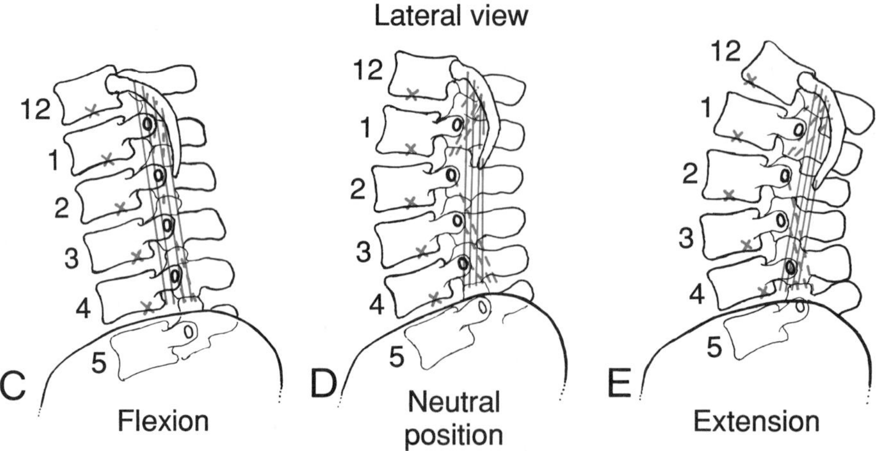

Figure 4.5. Tracings of lumbar radiographs (*black*) with quadratus lumborum fibers (*red lines*) added to show their attachments and directions. *A* and *B*, anteroposterior view; *C*, *D*, and *E*, lateral view. An **X** locates the center of rotation between two vertebrae; an *open circle* locates the tip of a transverse process. *Solid red lines* mark the longitudinal iliocostal fibers; *dashed red lines* indicate the diagonal iliolumbar and lumbocostal fibers. *A*, superficial lateral iliocostal fibers that bend the lumbar spine toward the same side. *B*, medial, deep diagonal iliolumbar and lumbocostal fibers produce the same effect. *C*, *D*, and *E* show that all fibers extend the lumbar spine when the subject stands with the lumbar spine in the flexed, neutral, or extended posture, respectively.

Functions

Implanted fine-wire electrodes recorded electromyographic (EMG) activity in the quadratus lumborum muscle during five movements:[123] lateral flexion of the spine, hip-hiking (elevation of the pelvis on the same side) when standing or sitting, extension of the lumbar spine, *forced* expiration,[4,123] and trunk rotation to the same side when the pelvis was fixed.[123] In one study,[123] activation of the quadratus lumborum was not associated with quiet respiration, but only with maneuvers that increased intra-abdominal pressure, for example, during a Valsalva maneuver (forced expiration against a closed glottis), during a vigorous verbal exclamation, or on coughing. When the standing subject bends forward, the quadratus lumborum as an extensor of the lumbar spine serves to check the forward movement against gravity, which explains why this movement aggravates TrPs in this muscle.

Waters and Morris[165] reported EMG activity in the quadratus lumborum muscle during walking. All recordings were made from the right side of the body. A burst of EMG activity in the right quadratus lumborum muscle occurred in all subjects at moderate and fast walking speeds, preceding and through right and left heel contact.[165]

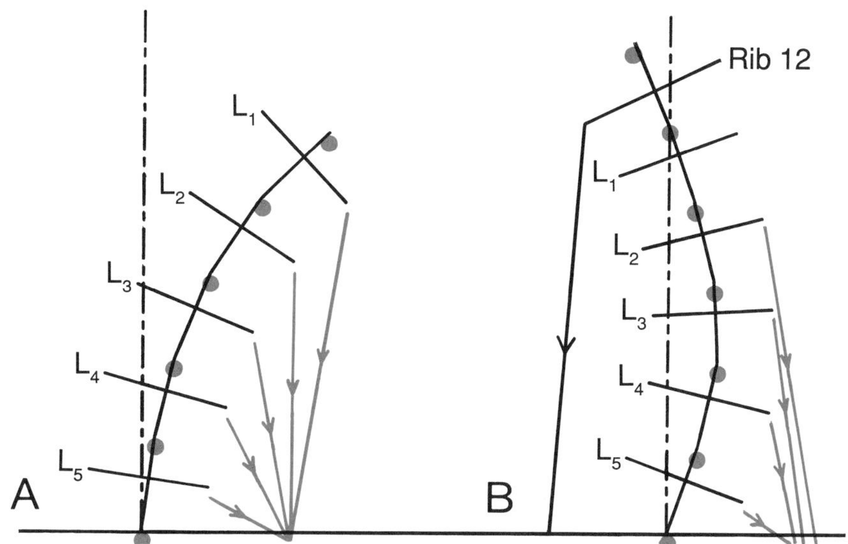

Figure 4.6. Exaggerated schematic drawing of symbolic articulated telephone pole (spine) with cross-arms (transverse processes) proposed by Knapp[80] to demonstrate two possible effects of the contraction of **diagonal** quadratus lumborum fibers on side bending of the lumbar spine. *Red arrows* indicate the direction of contractile force of the iliolumbar fibers, and the *black arrow*, of the contralateral iliocostal fibers. *Red solid circles* locate the centers of rotation between vertebrae. The *black cross-arms* represent transverse processes. *A*, the upper end of the lumbar spine is free to move producing **concavity** toward the contracting **iliolumbar** fibers. Contraction of ipsilateral iliocostal fibers (not shown) would assist this movement. *B*, in Knapp's model, the upper end of the lumbar spine is pulled to the opposite side by contraction of the contralateral iliocostal fibers (*black arrow*), presumably producing some **convexity** toward the contracting **iliolumbar** fibers. Iliolumbar (and also lumbocostal) fibers would now contribute to the convexity. Mobility of the L_5-S_1 articulation is exaggerated and action of any L_5 iliolumbar fibers present would be severely limited by the contralateral iliolumbar ligament.

5. FUNCTIONAL (MYOTATIC) UNIT

Muscles in addition to the quadratus lumborum that contribute to lateral bending of the trunk toward the same side are, in the order of their relative calculated effectiveness,[117] the external and internal abdominal obliques, the psoas, erector spinae, rectus abdominis, and the rotatores. The latissimus dorsi also can contribute significantly.[77]

The quadratus lumborum is assisted in extension by the erector spinae, multifidi, rotatores, and serratus posterior inferior muscles. The quadratus lumborum is assisted in spinal rotation to the contralateral side by the external abdominal oblique.[117]

The primary antagonist to one quadratus lumborum is the corresponding muscle on the opposite side. Therefore, TrPs and fiber shortening in one quadratus lumborum muscle frequently lead to secondary involvement of the contralateral quadratus through overload.

6. SYMPTOMS
(Fig. 4.7)

Low back pain is frequently caused by TrPs in the quadratus lumborum muscle, but this source is commonly overlooked. Acute low back pain of myofascial origin that is uncomplicated by perpetuating factors (*see* Sections 7 and 8) responds remarkably well to myofascial therapy specific to this muscle (*see* Sections 12 and 13). However, perpetuating factors are usually responsible when the low back pain has persisted for months or years, responds only temporarily to specific myofascial TrP therapy, or both. The additional stress imposed by these factors has converted the acute single-muscle syndrome into a chronic myofascial pain syndrome[127] that may include asymmetrical loading of the muscles[75] and articular dysfunction.[96]

Patient Complaints

Our patients consistently report a persistent, deep, aching pain at rest,[128] often severe in any body position but excruciating in the unsupported upright position and in sitting or standing that increases weight bearing or requires stabilization of the lumbar spine. A minimal movement of the lower part of the torso may precipitate a burst of sharp pain with a knifelike cutting quality, as also reported by Sola and Kuitert.[133] The severity of the pain from quadratus lumborum TrPs may be totally immobilizing, and its persistence emotionally depressing.

The TrPs in the quadratus lumborum restrict forward bending; the pain can functionally immobilize the lumbar spine. Patients describe difficulty in turning or leaning to the opposite side and find climbing stairs painful. Rolling onto either side from the supine position is painful and difficult. On awakening, the patient may be forced to creep on hands and knees to the bathroom. Coughing or sneezing can be agony. Arising from the supine position or getting up out of a chair may be difficult or impossible without help from the upper limbs.

In addition to back pain distributed in the primary referred patterns of this muscle (Fig. 4.1), pain may extend to the groin, testis, and scrotum, or in a sciatic distribution.[62] We attribute the latter to satellite TrPs that develop in paraspinal muscles[162] or in the posterior section of the gluteus minimus (*see* Fig. 9.2).

Patients with chronic pain due to active quadratus lumborum TrPs report loss of vitality and endurance because of the energy required to suppress the pain consciously and subconsciously and remain active in spite of it. In these cases, improvement can be judged by increased energy and activity.[133] Patients also have reported heaviness of the hips, cramping of the calves, and burning sensations in the legs and feet.[133]

Pain Relief
(Fig. 4.7)

Patients seek relief by lying supine or on the side. They find that the angle of forward or backward tilt of the hips with regard to the lumbar spine is critical. In severe cases, only creeping on all fours may provide locomotion for the sufferer.

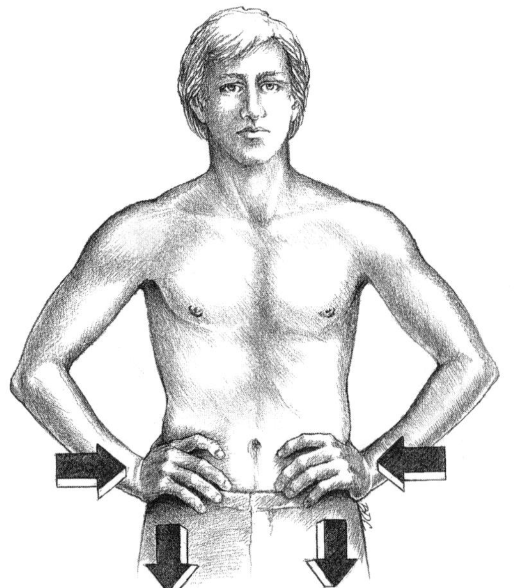

Figure 4.7. Pressure-relief technique to take sufficient load off the quadratus lumborum muscles to permit the patient to walk short distances slowly and carefully, when referred pain from an active quadratus lumborum trigger point is otherwise so severe that it prevents walking. Inward pressure holds the palms firmly on the iliac crests. The downward pressure transfers a significant portion of upper body weight directly to the hips, bypassing the lumbar spine.

Sitting and standing may be made more tolerable in severe cases by unloading some of the weight of the upper half of the body from the lumbar spine. The patient pushes down with the upper limbs against the arms of a chair or places the hands on the hips and presses downward for temporary relief (Fig. 4.7). Direct compression of the skin or pinching the skin over the quadratus lumborum may provide temporary relief (in much the same way that squeezing the skin over the sternocleidomastoid muscle can block the throat pain during swallowing due to active sternocleidomastoid TrPs).[156]

A lumbosacral support may be helpful in acute cases. If properly applied, it can reduce the workload on the quadratus lumborum by helping to stabilize the lumbar spine. After the acute stage, however, continuous use of the support can increase the irritability of quadratus lumborum TrPs by causing prolonged immobilization of the muscle. Immobilization lasting for weeks will eventually weaken the muscle, increasing its vulnerability to TrPs.

Differential Diagnosis

TrPs in other back muscles, such as the longissimus thoracis and multifidi, can also project pain to the buttock and SI joint.[158] Iliopsoas TrPs[128] refer low back pain that patients describe as radiating unilaterally up and down along the lumbosacral spine rather than horizontally across the back. The TrPs in the lower rectus abdominis[160] refer bilateral low back pain, which is described as traveling horizontally at the level of the SI joints. Pain from these other TrPs must be distinguished from quadratus lumborum TrP pain by the history, pain pattern, motions that are restricted, and by physical examination of the muscles.

Pain and tenderness referred by quadratus lumborum TrPs to the region of the greater trochanter can easily be mistaken for trochanteric bursitis.

Pain produced by satellite TrPs that refer pain in the sciatic distribution may be more annoying than the pain caused by primary quadratus lumborum TrPs.[62] This form of sciatica or "pseudo-disc syndrome"[147] is easily mistaken for an S_1 radiculopathy. This sciatic pattern of pain can be ascribed to satellite gluteus minimus TrPs when the following criteria are present: *(a)* The sciatic distribution of the patient's pain is reproduced by pressing on either the quadratus lumborum TrPs or the gluteus minimus TrPs. *(b)* The "sciatica" component can be eliminated by inactivating the gluteus minimus TrPs without treating the quadratus lumborum TrPs, but quickly recurs. *(c)* Inactivation of the quadratus lumborum TrPs immediately eliminates both the low back and sciatic pain patterns.

Radiculopathy is identified by neurological signs of motor and sensory deficits and by EMG evidence of motor root compression or sensory evoked potentials indicative of sensory root compression.

A finding of osteoarthritic spurs and/or some narrowing of lumbar disc spaces does not, by itself, establish the source of low back pain, since many people with moderate degenerative joint disease have no pain.[159] Furthermore, many patients with moderate osteoarthritis are completely relieved of low back pain when concomitant myofascial TrPs in the quadratus lumborum are inactivated.

Using an innovative dynamic radiographic technique, Friberg[39] demonstrated that the severity and frequency of low back pain correlated significantly with the amount of translatory movement between lumbar vertebrae, but did not correlate with the degree of maximal spondylo- or retrolisthetic movement. This translatory movement is an easily overlooked cause of low back pain.

Local pain from SI joint dysfunction is mimicked by pain referred from TrPs in the quadratus lumborum;[119] it is distinguished from the TrPs by testing such as that described in Chapter 2, page 17. One form of SI joint dysfunction is upslip, or innominate shear dysfunction[58] (upward displacement of an innominate bone in relation to the sacrum); it is recognized as an important source of low back and groin pain. Among 63 patients in a private orthopaedic medicine practice who were examined because of pain and found to have an innominate upslip dysfunction, the most common site of the chief pain complaint was the low back and groin (50%).[79]

Lumbar pain due to fracture of a lumbar transverse process has a sharp, knifelike, stabbing quality not characteristic of TrPs, is very localized, and matches no known pattern of referred myofascial pain. The muscles do not feel tight. The fracture is confirmed by radiography.

Distinguishing quadratus lumborum TrPs that are secondary to thoracolumbar articular dysfunction from TrPs that arise primarily from quadratus lumborum overload can be difficult. The two conditions interact strongly. Thoracolumbar articular dysfunction characteristically causes asymmetrical restriction of rotation, side bending, flexion, or sometimes extension of the thoracolumbar region. Involvement of the quadratus lumborum alone can restrict primarily side bending away from the involved side, as well as rotation and flexion of the lumbar spine.

Additional diagnoses to be considered include spinal tumors, myasthenia gravis,

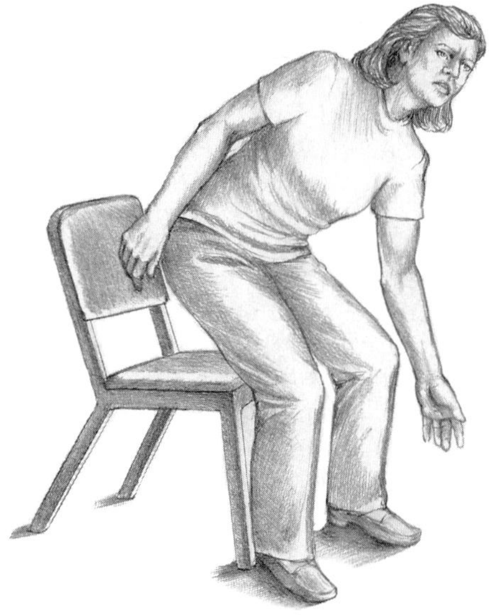

Figure 4.8. Quadratus lumborum muscle strain caused by a combined bending and twisting movement as a person gets up from a chair or picks up an object from the floor.

gallstones and liver disease, kidney stones and other urinary tract problems, intra-abdominal infections, intestinal parasites and diverticulitis, aortic aneurysm, and multiple sclerosis.

7. ACTIVATION AND PERPETUATION OF TRIGGER POINTS
(Fig. 4.8)

Activation

Myofascial TrPs in the quadratus lumborum muscle are activated acutely by awkward movements and by obvious sudden trauma, such as a motor vehicle accident.[1]

Quadratus lumborum TrPs can be activated acutely by awkward lifting of an unusually heavy load like a TV set, a child or a large dog, or by a quick stooping movement when the torso is twisted or turned somewhat to one side, often to reach for an object on the floor.[147] Another version of the latter stress is that of angling sideways while bending forward to rise from a deep-seated chair (Fig. 4.8), a low bed, or a car seat. Many patients report the onset of pain when putting on pants while standing half stooped and leaning sideways, or after losing balance as the feet became entangled in the clothing. The muscular strain of a near fall is avoided by sitting down to put on socks, pantyhose, skirt or trousers, etc., or by leaning against a wall or furniture so that balance is assured.

The quadratus lumborum muscle often develops TrPs due to an auto accident. Baker[1] investigated the occurrence of myofascial TrPs in 34 muscles of 100 occupants (drivers and passengers) who sustained a single motor vehicle impact. The quadratus lumborum was involved more frequently than any other muscle in impacts from the driver's side (81% of subjects) and in impacts from behind (79% of subjects). It was the second most commonly injured muscle (81%) when the impact was from the front and the third most common (63%) when the impact was on the passenger's side. In this study,[1] no distinction could be made between pre-existing, latent TrPs that were activated by the accident and TrPs that were initiated by this gross trauma.

Quadratus lumborum TrPs can also be activated by obscure, sustained, or repetitive strain (microtrauma) from activities such as gardening, scrubbing the floor, lifting cement blocks,[111] or by walking or jogging on a slanted surface, as on a beach or along a crowned road. In addition, when one quadratus lumborum becomes involved, the shortening of that muscle at rest tends to overload its contralateral mate and usually results in the development of TrPs in this antagonist, but with pain of less intensity.

The *sudden* introduction of a half inch difference in lower limb lengths by the application of a walking cast can activate the quadratus lumborum TrP syndrome, as has been demonstrated experimentally.[71] When quadratus lumborum pain appears immediately after an ankle fracture that required application of a walking cast, the TrP was probably activated by the strain of the fall that also caused the fracture; whereas, if the muscle pain appears a week or two after application of the cast, the chronic strain of the newly imposed limb-length inequality most likely activated latent TrPs. This pain is relieved (or prevented) by wearing on the other foot a shoe with sufficient lift to match the length of the casted lower limb.

Sola and Kuitert[133] reported the onset of quadratus lumborum myofasciitis associated with fatigue, immunization, medicinal injections, upper respiratory infections, and a twisting movement of the torso.

Perpetuation

Mechanical factors that predispose to the activation of quadratus lumborum TrPs or that perpetuate those TrPs are: a lower limb-length inequality (LLLI);[147] a small hemipelvis;[147] short upper arms;[151] a soft bed with a hammocklike sag; leaning forward with poor elbow support over a desk (frequently caused by wearing eyeglasses with too short a focal length); standing and leaning over a low sink or work surface; and deconditioned or weak abdominal muscles. Identification of the first three factors is discussed in Section 8 of this chapter; the others are discussed in Volume 1.[148]

The relative importance of LLLI and of a small hemipelvis as perpetuating factors in low back pain of quadratus lumborum origin is often revealed by a patient's relative tolerance to standing vs. sitting, and by the way he or she stands. When the patient stands with one foot forward, weight on the other foot (shorter side), or stands with feet wide apart and the pelvis shifted to one side (shorter side), and has pain when standing and walking, the problem is probably LLLI. When only sitting aggravates the pain, either short upper arms or a small hemipelvis is more likely to be the culprit. When symptoms are present in both positions, a patient is likely to have both a small hemipelvis and a shorter lower limb on the same side; that is, one side of the body is smaller.

After activation of quadratus lumborum TrPs by a sudden overload, we find that a difference in lower limb length as small as 3 mm (⅛ in) may perpetuate quadratus lumborum TrPs, and a difference of 6 mm (¼ in) commonly does so.

Gould[53] pointed out that carrying a wallet in a long back pocket where it elevates one side of the pelvis during sitting can perpetuate "back pocket sciatica" that is relieved by removing the wallet.

Important systemic factors that can perpetuate quadratus lumborum TrPs include vitamin and other nutritional deficiencies, metabolic disorders, especially thyroid inadequacies, chronic infections and infestations, and emotional stress.[147,151]

Any factor that causes chilling of the body perpetuates myofascial TrPs and must be managed. Body warmth must be maintained, especially at night, to prevent impaired sleep.

PART 1

8. PATIENT EXAMINATION
(Figs. 4.9–4.20)

OUTLINE OF SECTION 8.

This section first presents the findings on physical examination and by new imaging techniques in patients with quadratus lumborum TrPs. It then discusses how to assess three important mechanical perpetuating factors, a small hemipelvis, short upper arms, and lower limb-length inequality (LLLI).

The review of the techniques for assessing LLLI is unusually thorough because of the complexity of the topic and its critical role in quadratus lumborum TrPs. The review summarizes the clinical role of LLLI, the relation of LLLI to compensatory (functional) lumbar scoliosis, and considers in detail the radiographic assessment of LLLI and compensatory lumbar scoliosis.

Examination for Quadratus Lumborum Involvement

Physical Examination

The patient with active quadratus lumborum TrPs exhibits muscle guarding that restricts movement between the lumbar vertebrae and the sacrum during walking, lying down, turning over in bed, getting up from bed, or when arising from a chair. A vigorous cough may evoke the characteristic pain distribution.

When the patient with active quadratus lumborum TrPs is standing, the pelvis is likely to tilt downward on the side opposite to the affected muscle. The lumbar spine usually exhibits a functional lumbar scoliosis that is convex away from the side of the involved quadratus lumborum.[83] (Other configurations may appear for different reasons that are discussed later.) The normal lumbar lordosis is likely to appear flattened due to the vertebral rotation that accompanies the scoliosis, despite the fact that the quadratus lumborum is an extensor of the spine. Flexion and extension of the lumbar spine are restricted and sometimes abolished. Side bending is restricted toward the pain-free side and sometimes bilaterally.

Testing for restriction of side bending caused by tightness of the quadratus lumborum can be performed with the patient sitting, prone using two examiners as described by Jull and Janda,[75] or side lying by raising the shoulders up from the examining table.[75,93] Seated or standing, rotation of the thoracolumbar spine is usually most restricted toward the side of the involved muscle when its iliocostal fibers are afflicted.

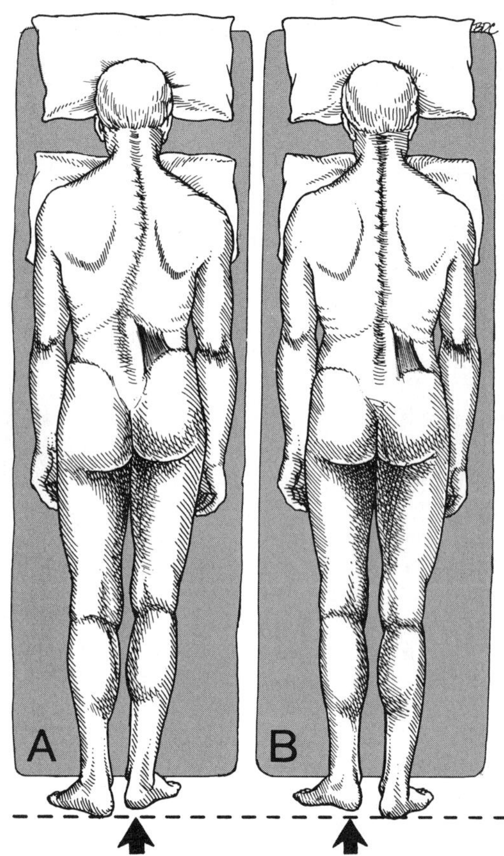

Figure 4.9. Distortion of apparent inequality in lower limb length due to a taut quadratus lumborum muscle. *A*, at the medial malleolus in the prone patient, the right lower limb appears shorter than the left due to trigger-point activity and tension in the shortened right quadratus lumborum muscle (*dark red*). *B*, true disparity in leg length becomes apparent when the trigger-point activity of the right quadratus lumborum is eliminated and the muscle returns to its normal resting length (*light red*). The S-curve functional scoliosis of the spine, seen in *A*, is also eliminated.

In recumbency, active TrPs shorten the muscle and can thus distort pelvic alignment, elevating the pelvis on the side of the tense muscle (Fig. 4.9).

Flank tenderness to deep palpation may be marked, but is easily missed because the patient's position usually closes the space between the 10th rib and the crest of the ilium,[128] and because most of the quadratus lumborum is covered pos-

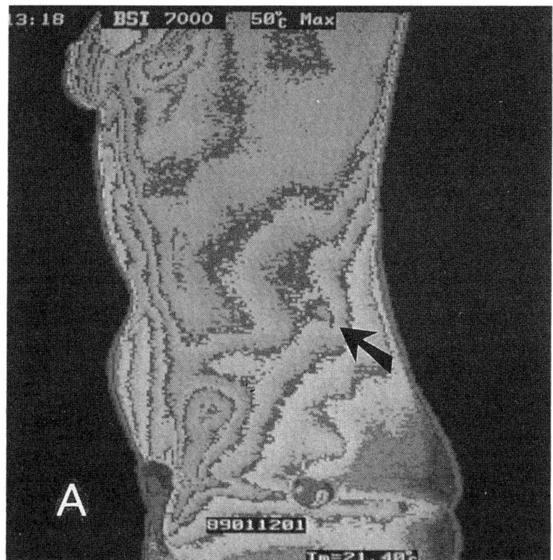

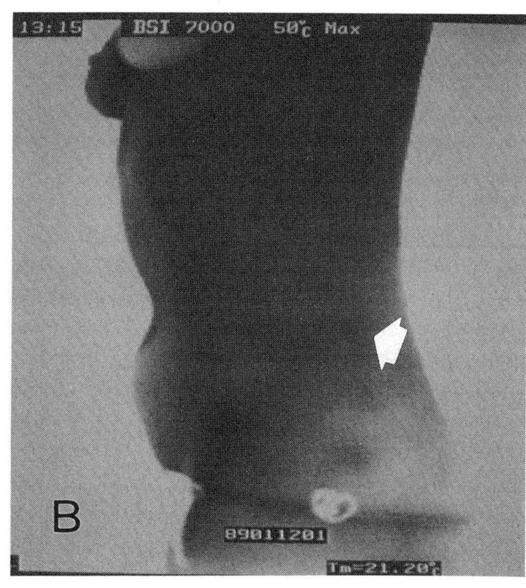

Figure 4.10. Thermogram of patient with a left quadratus lumborum trigger point shows a "hot spot" (*arrows*) of at least 0.5° C overlying the left quadratus lumborum muscle. Thermogram was obtained with a Bales Scientific MCT 7000 Medical Thermography System. *A*, color mode analysis, temperature range 23.75–30.5° C at 0.20°/L. Note the small island of increased temperature marked by the *black arrow*. *B*, corresponding gray scale recorded at resolution of 0.1°/L. "Hot spot" is identified by the small dark area marked by the *white arrow*. (Thermograms by courtesy of Bernard E. Filner, M.D., Thermographic Imaging Center of Rockville, Maryland 20850.)

teriorly by the thick mass of paraspinal muscles (*see* Fig. 4.23).

Strength of only the quadratus lumborum muscle is difficult to assess because of the parallel force generated by the lateral portions of the external and internal abdominal oblique muscles. Strength is tested during lateral flexion of the trunk and during hip hiking. Lateral flexion of the trunk is tested by having the subject lie on the opposite side with a pillow between the knees and lift the shoulders up from the examining table, while the legs are anchored. Hip hiking by this muscle is tested with the patient either prone[77] or supine.[74] He or she abducts the lower limb 20–30° and elevates the hip toward the ribs against resistance supplied by the examiner, who pulls down on the ankle on the same (affected) side.

When weakness or inhibition of the quadratus lumborum is caused by active myofascial TrPs, function may be temporarily restored while pinching the skin overlying the TrPs. A similar phenomenon is described in Volume 1 as the Sternocleidomastoid Compression Test.[156]

Examination for LLLI with the patient supine can give the impression of a shorter limb on the side of an involved quadratus lumborum muscle (Fig. 4.9*A*). This effect may more than compensate for a longer limb on that side (Fig. 4.9*B*).

Three imaging techniques (discussed in more detail in Chapter 2) hold promise for substantiating the presence of TrPs: thermography, ultrasound, and magnetic resonance spectroscopy. Zohn published thermograms of a hot spot over a quadratus lumborum TrP.[170] Figure 4.10 shows another investigator's thermograms of a 50-year-old female patient who was injured at work 5½ years earlier.

The quadratus lumborum is usually visualized on sonograms,[14] but may occasionally be sonolucent for unknown reasons. It can also be distinguished by magnetic resonance imaging. Whether either modality is capable of imaging TrPs has not, to our knowledge, been critically examined, but both measures appear to have the potential for doing so.

Examination for Small Hemipelvis (Figs. 4.11 and 4.12)

When the skeletal asymmetry of an LLLI is present, there is likely also to be a smaller hemipelvis, smaller face, and shorter upper limb on the side of the shorter lower limb. The small hemipelvis may cause symptoms in both the sitting and supine positions. Inglemark and Lindström[72] found a strong correlation (+0.78) between limb length and hemipelvis size. Therefore, LLLI can be a useful preliminary guide. Many key points on diagnosis in the seated patient and on management of a small hemipelvis are covered in Volume 1.[152] That material includes the laterally tilted pelvis during sitting, the seated examination, and determining the proper size for an ischial (butt) lift.

When Seated

The skeletal effects of a small hemipelvis during sitting, with and without correction, are illustrated in Figure 48.10 of Volume 1.[148] The figure also includes the compensatory effect of crossing the thigh of the small side over the knee on the side of the larger hemipelvis, which is also noted and illustrated by Northup.[112] A compensatory lumbar scoliosis caused by skeletal asymmetries is maintained primarily by the quadratus lumborum muscle.

If the patient has symptoms (pain) when seated, a small hemipelvis is suspect. The ischial tuberosities, on which weight is borne during sitting, are only 10–12 cm (4–5 in) apart; any difference in the size of the two sides of the pelvis is magnified farther up the torso because the spine is much longer than the distance between the ischial tuberosities.

The effect of a small hemipelvis on lumbar scoliosis is greater than that of an equal difference in leg length. Because the distance between the ischial tuberosities is approximately half the distance between the femoral heads, the effect of an asymmetrical pelvis during sitting would be greater than that of an LLLI of the same magnitude during standing. It is not unusual, however, for a patient to require approximately the same thickness of ischial (butt) lift as that required for a shoe lift.

An example of the clinical picture seen when a patient with a small hemipelvis is examined in the sitting position is illustrated in Figure 4.11*A*. It shows the pelvis tilted down on the small side, a compensatory "S" curve scoliosis, and a corresponding tilt of the shoulder-girdle axis.

Figure 4.11*B* demonstrates the restoration of skeletal symmetry by providing an appropriate lift under the ischial tuberosity on the small side. The size of the ischial lift must be adjusted for the softness and the shape of the seat.

When Supine

Some patients also experience pain when supine due to a small hemipelvis in the anteroposterior direction. Uncorrected, this asymmetry can be a significant perpetuating factor for quadratus lumborum TrPs. The patient who needs this correction fails to find relief from pain when sleeping supine at night. The pelvis on the small side tilts down toward the bed, as in Figure 4.12*A*. This asymmetry tends to aggravate and perpetuate TrPs in the quadratus lumborum muscle and ~~is~~ corrected by an appropriate lift placed under the pelvis on the small side (Fig. 4.12*B*). Counter-correction usually intensifies discomfort (Fig. 4.12*C*).

Examination for Short Upper Arms (Fig. 4.13)

This common perpetuating factor for myofascial pain is presented in Volume 1[154] and is especially important to the quadratus lumborum muscle. Short upper arms are a frequent structural variant in Caucasians, Native Americans, Polynesians, and some Orientals.

The patient with upper arms that are short in relation to torso height is most readily identified when seated upright in the standard armchair (Fig. 4.13*A*). The elbows do not reach the armrests. When the person stands, the elbows do not reach the iliac crests (Fig. 4.13*B*) as they would in persons with upper arms of the usual length (Fig. 4.13*C*).

When seated, this individual either leans to one side to rest one elbow on an armrest, which can strain the quadratus lumborum and lateral cervical muscles (Fig. 4.13*D*), or slumps forward to rest both elbows on the armrests, which can strain the posterior cervical and paraspinal muscles (Fig. 4.13*E*).

The corrective actions needed to manage this important perpetuating factor are discussed in Section 14.

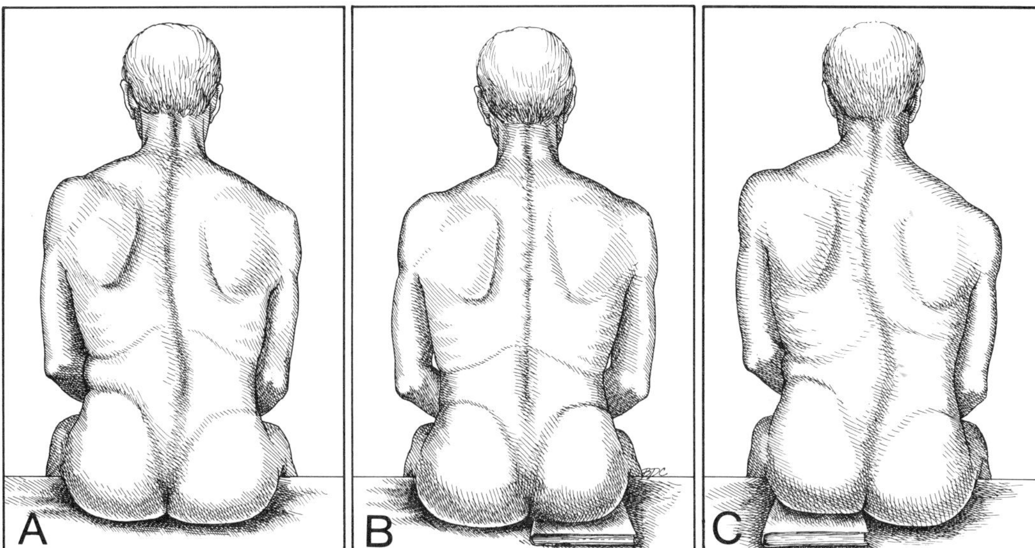

Figure 4.11. Examination of a seated subject with a small right hemipelvis. *A*, uncorrected asymmetry causes lateral tilt of the pelvis, an S-shaped functional scoliosis of the spine and tilt of the shoulder-girdle axis. *B*, correction by leveling the pelvis with an ischial (butt) lift resolves the postural distortions. *C*, counter-correction with same lift under the wrong (larger left) side. Patients immediately feel discomfort and strain from this increased asymmetry, which makes them aware of the importance of using an appropriate ischial correction whenever seated.

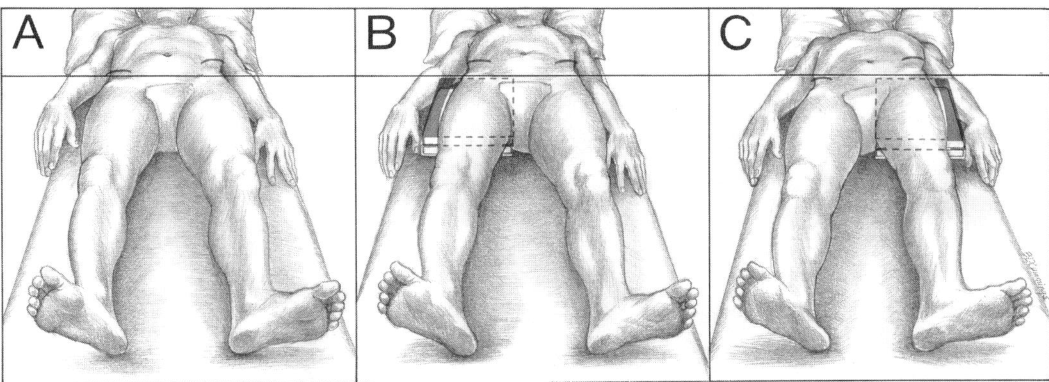

Figure 4.12. *A*, Examination of the patient with a small right hemipelvis in the anteroposterior dimension, supine position. The iliac crests are marked in *red*. The *solid black line* is level. The *red dashed lines* outline a lift under one side of the pelvis. *A*, uncorrected. The pelvis tilts, causing the right anterior superior iliac spine to sink toward the bed as compared with the left. *B*, corrected. The lift (*red book*) under the small right hemipelvis levels the anterior superior iliac spines. *C*, counter-corrected. The pelvic lift added to the wrong (large left) side exaggerates the postural distortion.

Examination for Postural Asymmetries (Figs. 4.14–4.16)

The most useful clinical technique for identifying postural asymmetries that will respond to a heel lift is described in detail on pages 107–108 and 650–653 of Volume 1.[148] Since LLLI is probably the most common source of compensatory lumbar scoliosis that overloads the quadratus lumborum muscle, this simple procedure clearly identifies an LLLI and establishes the necessary correction if no additional spinal, pelvic, or lower limb asymmetries or articular dysfunctions complicate the situation. Figures 4.14 and

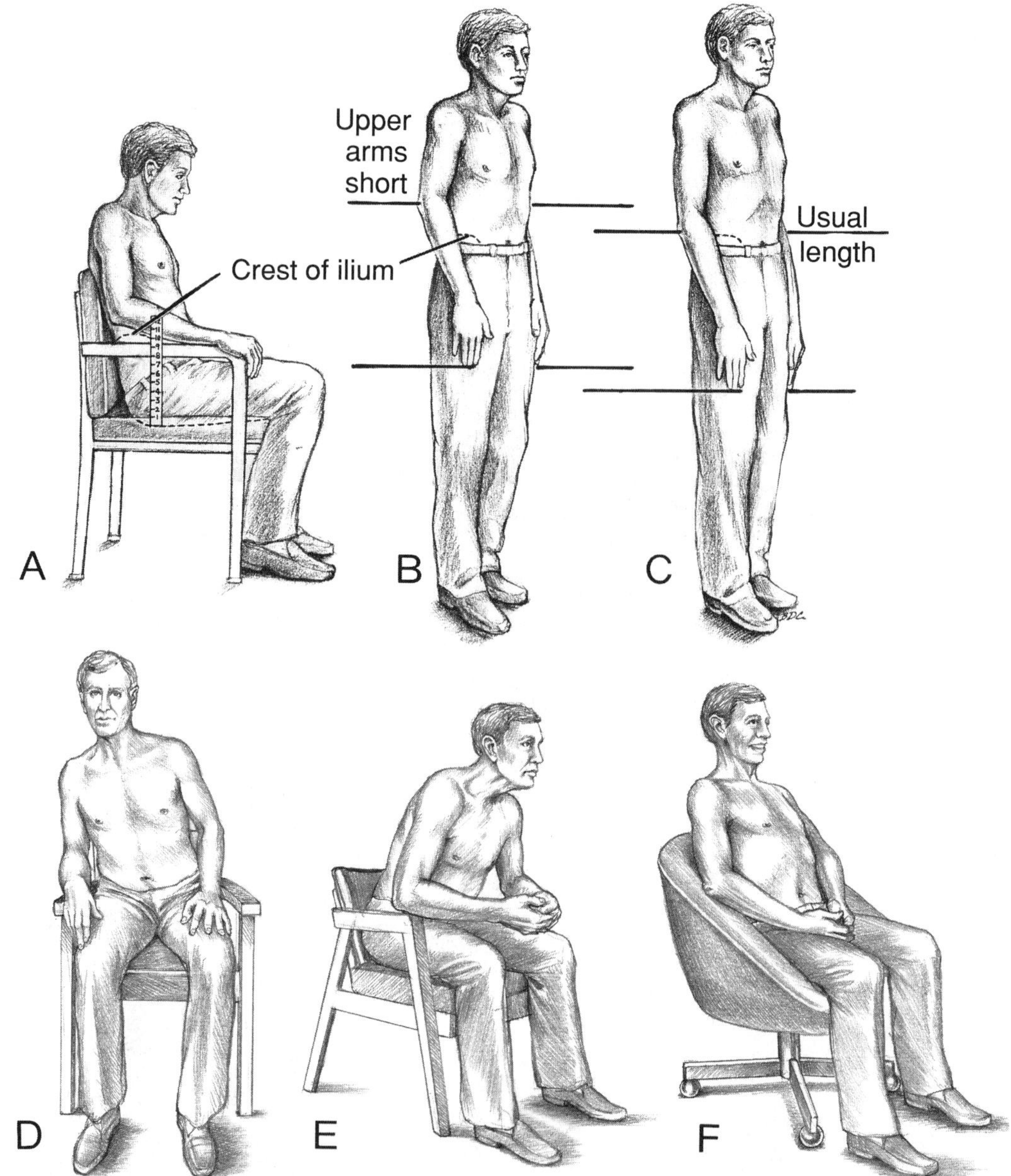

Figure 4.13. Perpetuation of quadratus lumborum trigger points because of upper arms that are short in relation to torso height. *Dashed lines* show the level of the iliac crest. *A*, failure of elbows to reach the chair armrests, which, when 9 inches above the depressed seat bottom, fit about 90% of the American population. *B*, in the relaxed standing posture, elbows of short upper arms are at a level well above the top of the iliac crest and tips of fingers are above midthigh. *C*, position of elbow and hand for the average length of the upper arms in relation to torso height in this country. *D*, compensatory seated posture: leaning sideways in an attempt to find support for the shoulder-girdle. This position strains the lumbar and cervical musculature. The quadratus lumborum and scalene muscles are particularly vulnerable. *E*, strain of paraspinal back and neck muscles caused by leaning forward to find elbow support. *F*, armchair with sloping armrests that solve this problem by providing elbow support for arms of various lengths.

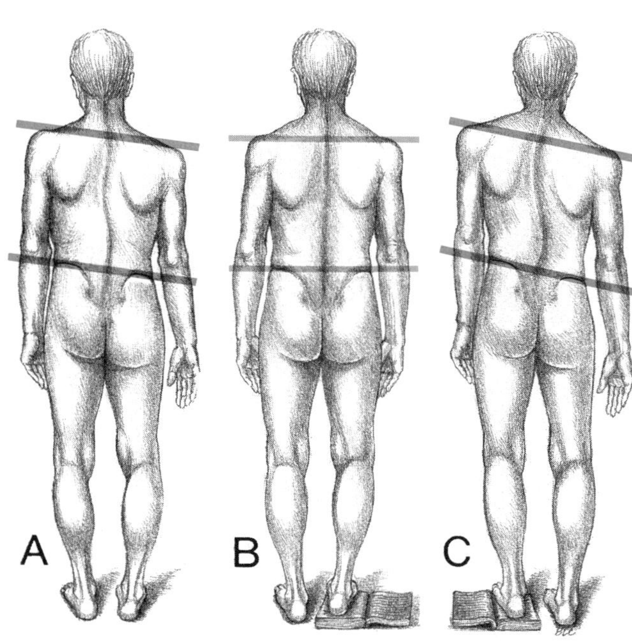

Figure 4.14. Examination of a standing patient with a shorter right lower limb, S-curve scoliosis and sagging right shoulder. *Black lines* show level iliac crests and shoulder girdles when the limb length inequality is corrected by a foot lift. *Red lines* show the angles of the pelvic and shoulder-girdle axes when tilted. *A*, uncorrected. Right hip is lower than the left hip, as is indicated by the asymmetrical outline of the waist, and by the lowered right iliac crest, right posterior superior iliac spine (*dimple*), and right buttock. The resultant functional scoliosis also tips the shoulders, usually downward on the same side when there is a large discrepancy of 10 mm (3/8 in) or more in lower limb length. Hip sway toward the left causes the right hand to hang farther away from the thigh than does the left hand. *B*, corrected. Lift under the right foot levels the pelvis and corrects the asymmetry shown in *A*. The shoulder-girdle axis and iliac crests are now level (*black lines*) and the spine is straight. *C*, counter-corrected. Placing the lift under the foot on the longer left side exaggerates the asymmetry seen in *A*. This exaggeration of the lower limb-length inequality causes immediate uncomfortable overload of postural muscles, convinces the patient that *B* is preferable to *C*, and impresses the patient with the need for correction.

PART 1

4.15 illustrate the principle. Initial assessment of the standing patient employs the clues discussed below that indicate postural asymmetry.

By adding small increments of shoe lift under the apparently short limb, an attempt is made to maximize postural symmetry and minimize postural stress felt by the patient. Then, the correction is removed from under the shorter limb and placed under the longer limb. The patient is asked how this position compares to the other. Most patients find this distinctly unpleasant, if not painful. By moving the lift from one foot to the other, the examiner confirms which is the shorter limb[49] and demonstrates to the patient the importance of maintaining the correction. If patients can see themselves in a full-length mirror, they are impressed by the visible change in symmetry and appreciate the need for correction.

This technique does not determine what additional contributing asymmetries are present, but patients help to adjust for them by selecting the correction that minimizes strain on their muscles. Correctable pelvic asymmetries should be identified and treated before modifying footwear.

Figure 4.16 shows one way of recognizing a fixed (structural) lumbar scoliosis, which is more likely to be seen in elderly males. In this case, addition of a shoe lift under the shorter leg increases body asymmetry instead of correcting it. On the other hand, adding the lift to the long leg does not help either.

The first author has noted that if the patient is asked to stand first on one foot

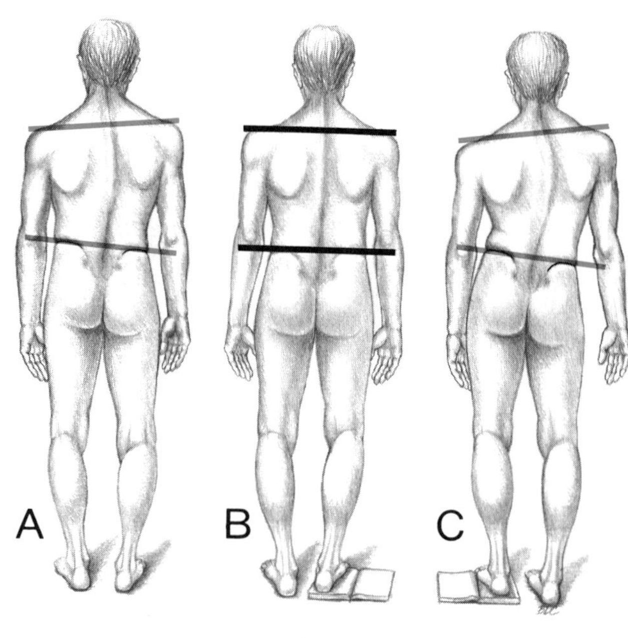

Figure 4.15. Testing a standing patient with a C-curve scoliosis and sagging left shoulder due to a shorter right lower limb. *Black lines* show level iliac crests and shoulder girdles when limb length inequality is corrected by a right foot lift. *Red lines* show the angles of the pelvic and shoulder girdle axes when tilted. *A*, uncorrected. Right hip, iliac crest, posterior superior iliac spine (*dimple*) and buttock are lower than on the left side. The angulation of the shoulder girdle and the hip sway cause the right arm to hang away from the body. This functional scoliosis tips the left shoulder-girdle axis downward on the long side; the left scapula is lower. *B*, corrected. The lift required to level the pelvis and shoulder-girdle axes and to correct the body asymmetry is more likely to measure 6 mm (1/4 inch) or less when the scoliotic curve is of this type. *C*, counter-corrected. The same foot lift placed under the longer left limb exaggerates the postural distortions of *A*. This increased asymmetry uncomfortably stresses the muscles at once so that the patient clearly prefers *B* to *C*. The difference impresses the patient with the importance of correction.

and then on the other, leveling of the pelvis and stance symmetry improve when he or she is standing on the longer limb, whereas standing on the shorter limb increases the malalignment. This becomes even more apparent when the patient stands on one foot and swings the free foot back and forth as if walking. The shorter limb swings freely, but swinging the longer limb requires marked torso tilt toward the side of the shorter limb in order to allow the foot of the longer limb to clear the floor.

By asking the patient to walk in place, Hallin[64] observed and palpated the ilia while observing the phenomenon previously described, but from the point of view of the longer limb. He detected a drop in the contralateral pelvis and a shift of the upper trunk toward the high (longer limb) side as weight was transferred to the longer limb. He described the pattern as similar to that seen when limb length is equal, but the hip abductors are weak on one side. The patient with LLLI may exhibit this same limp during walking.[67]

Evidence of Body Asymmetry (Fig. 4.17)

A number of observations help identify the presence and direction of an LLLI in the standing subject. None are completely reliable alone, but their consistency or inconsistency helps one to recognize a simple or complex condition. The examination includes checking the standing patient for stance asymmetries (including all lower limb segments), lumbar scoliosis, iliac crest height, shoulder-girdle tilt, and related body asymmetries.

Stance asymmetries provide sensitive indicators of skeletal asymmetry that can be harmful to the muscles. In the presence of LLLI, standing is a stressful condition because postural compensation induces a continuous muscular effort. The individual may try in several ways to level the pelvis and straighten the spine. One way is by shifting the foot of the

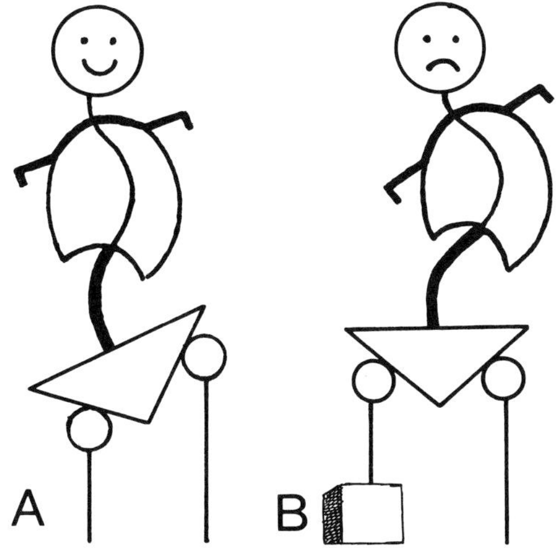

Figure 4.16. Aggravation of spinal curvature by correction of a difference in length of the lower limbs when the lumbar scoliosis is fixed (structural), not compensatory (functional). The *heavy spinal line* in the lumbar region indicates fixed scoliosis; the *thin spinal line* in the thoracic and cervical regions represents compensatory scoliosis. *A*, scoliosis with tilted pelvis and no correction of limb-length difference. *B*, aggravation of the functional scoliosis of the thoracic spine by correction of the limb-length inequality. Although a simple compensatory scoliosis due to a limb length difference may be correctable by a shoe lift, a fixed scoliosis, as seen here, may be aggravated by such a lift.

longer limb in front or to one side, thus placing more weight on the shorter limb.[67] This is readily apparent by simply observing the standing patient.

Uneven distribution of weight on the two limbs can be measured by instructing the patient to put "equal weight on both feet" while he or she stands on a pair of matching scales.[92,97] If one limb consistently registers at least 5 kg (2.3 lb) more than the other limb, the stance is abnormally asymmetrical.[97] This much difference in the scale readings can also be caused by articular dysfunction of the craniocervical junction.[97]

Functional **lumbar scoliosis** usually develops when there is LLLI. This is the most important asymmetry causing quadratus lumborum overload. Unfortunately, during examination, the true lumbar curvature may be obscured or exaggerated by the rotation of lumbar vertebrae that accompanies lateral flexion. The spinous processes can appear and feel as if they are in a straight line, while the spinal column is, in fact, scoliotic ("concave side rotation" described by Steindler in 1929).[137] The opposite situation, in which rotation of the vertebrae exaggerates the clinical appearance of scoliosis, also occurs. A radiograph reveals the true nature of this situation, as demonstrated in Figure 4.17*B* and *C*. This phenomenon has been well described and illustrated by Friberg[36,38] and by Grice.[59]

Comparison of the relative **heights of the iliac crests** (and anterior or posterior superior iliac spines) is one of the most convenient and commonly used indicators of LLLI. It is often assumed that relative crest height and LLLI relate directly to tilt of the sacral base and the L_5 vertebra, which is the factor that is most important to the quadratus lumborum muscle.[41] Unfortunately, measurement of relative iliac crest height is *not reliably* related to either LLLI or levelness of the sacral base. Tilted iliac crests indicate only an asymmetry of some kind.

If the quadratus lumborum is involved and one iliac crest is unmistakably higher than the other, one should examine for the presence of an innominate shear dysfunction;[58] this dysfunction can create evidence of LLLI when there is none.

Among 50 patients with an LLLI of at least 10 mm (3/8 in) determined radiographically, the levels of the iliac crests did not correspond to the LLLI in 12 patients (24%).[16] Fisk and Baigent[33] noted a similar lack of reliability in 26% of 31 patients who had an LLLI. Inglemark and Lindström[72] found, in 370 patients with back disorders who were studied radiographically, that 72% had a shorter limb and smaller hemipelvis on the same side. In these cases, determination based on iliac crest height could lead to an overestimation of the true LLLI. These authors[72] concluded that clinical estimation of LLLI using the relative height of the iliac crests must be considered unsatisfactory because of poor reliability.

After studying the relative positions of the anterior and posterior superior iliac spines in both the standing and seated positions, Fisk and Baigent[33] came to the same conclusion that clinical assessment of lower limb length using these pelvic landmarks is unreliable.

Gofton[49] compared these static clinical criteria with radiographic measurements and concluded that three observations

PART 1

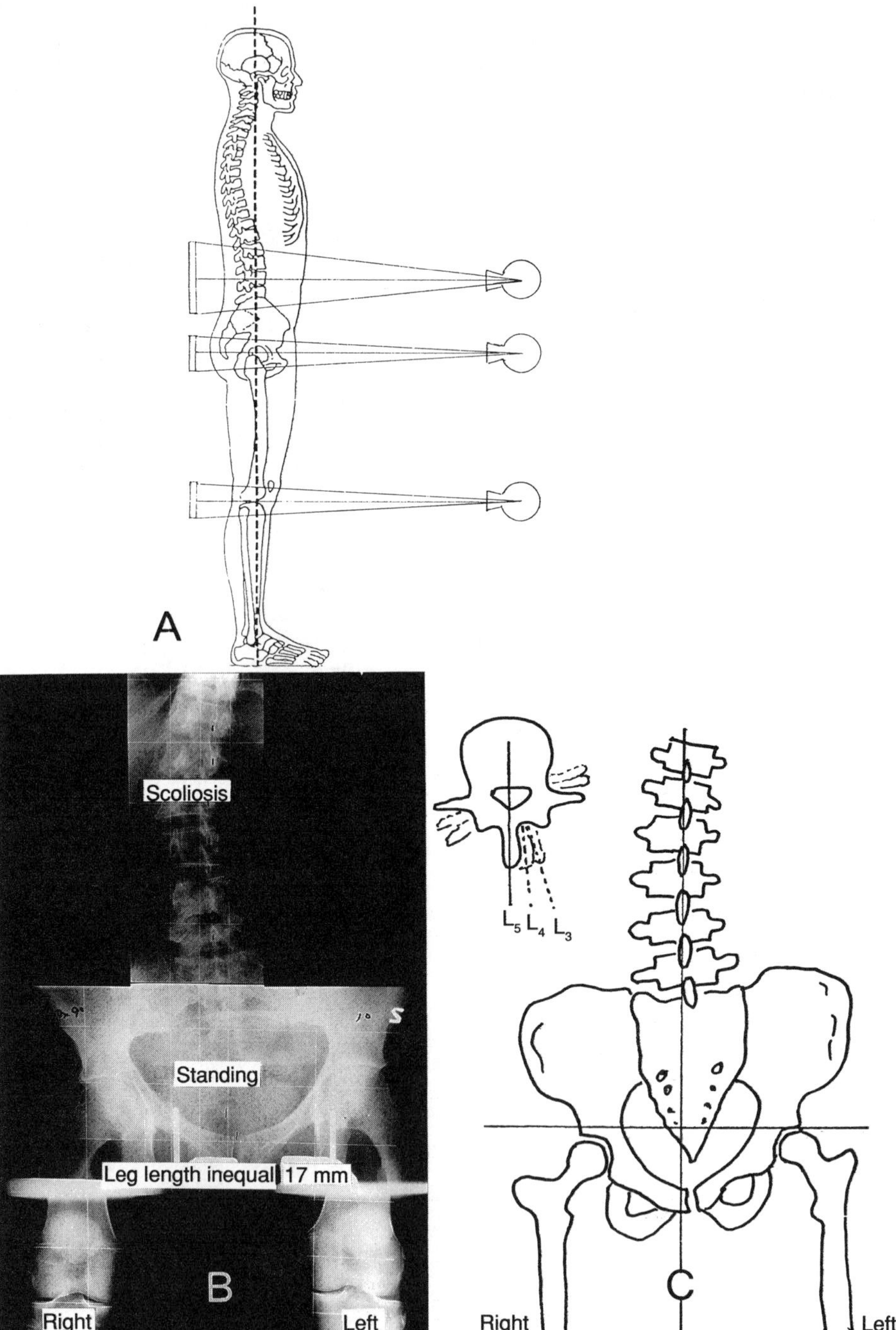

Figure 4.17. Standing radiography technique and results. *A*, Orthoradiographic method of sequential coned exposures for obtaining a film of the lumbar spine and of the hip and knee joints with minimum radiographic exposure of the patient. *B*, Example of orthoradiographic film demonstrating a postural lumbar scoliosis of 20° associated with a lower limb-length inequality of 17 mm (5⁄8 in), right side shorter. The compensatory lumbar scoliosis is convex to the right (marked *Dx*), but the lumbar spinous processes appear to have straight vertical alignment because of coupled axial rotation of the lumbar vertebrae. The two columns of mercury extend upward toward the heads of the femurs from the lower edge of the pelvic (center) exposure. The offset of the two *short vertical lines* marking the centers of the pubis and sacrum is used to measure pelvic rotation. The *Dx 9°* indicates that the right foot (short limb side) was turned out 9° and *1°S* that the left foot was turned out 1°. *C*, schematic drawing of a radiograph demonstrating how the axial rotation of lumbar vertebrae coupled with lateral bending may obscure, on clinical examination of the standing patient, the presence of scoliosis by restoring the spinous processes to nearly straight alignment. [(A) by permission of Friberg and Clinical Biomechanics;[38] (B) and (C) courtesy of Ora Friberg, M.D.]

must *all* be present in standing patients to identify significant LLLI: *(a)* protrusion laterally of the upper thigh of the long limb, *(b)* appearance of scoliosis, and *(c)* palpation of a difference in height at the top of the iliac crests. One must remember, however, that the first two of these criteria can be produced by the muscle shortening associated with TrPs of the quadratus lumborum muscle on the side of spinal concavity (Fig. 4.9). Therefore, inactivation of quadratus lumborum TrPs should precede evaluation of asymmetry.

The **relative height of the greater trochanters** in the standing position is sometimes used to estimate LLLI. Hoskins[70] was impressed by how frequently uneven angulation of the femoral necks (unilateral coxa vara or coxa valga) would cause error using this method.

A number of common clinical methods for measuring LLLI used to determine corrections for relieving quadratus lumborum and postural strain are seriously inaccurate and, when conducted with the patient recumbent, likely to be irrelevant. The following is a brief update of this literature.

Frequently used clinical methods for determining inequality in the length of the lower limbs have proven to be not only inaccurate, with observer error of ±10 mm (3/8 in) or more,[16,105,110] but sometimes misleading.[33,34,43,164] Averaged values of supine tape measurements of anterior superior iliac spine to medial malleolus distance may look useful,[7] but can be used only as a general guide because of individual variations in pelvic structure. As reviewed in Volume 1,[150] observations for LLLI made with the subject in a non-weight-bearing recumbent position are often irrelevant to quadratus lumborum strain, if not grossly misleading.[120] False and misleading values are equally likely when using the hip-to-ankle tape measure technique[16,110] and when comparing the medial malleolar levels bilaterally.[5,164] Five clinicians examined patients who were standing.[43] When compared with reliable radiological methods, over half (53%) of 196 clinical estimates of LLLI in 21 low back pain patients were wrong by more than 5 mm (3/16 in). In 13% of observations, the *wrong* limb was determined to be short.

From the foregoing, it is clear that none of the above (tilted iliac crests, tilted anterior or posterior iliac spines, or the relative height of the greater trochanters) is satisfactory as a definitive criterion of skeletal asymmetry, but each contributes to the total picture. When in doubt, a standing radiograph helps to resolve ambiguities.

If the LLLI is of interest *per se*, one can examine the **component asymmetries** that may contribute to it. Foot posture and malleolar height can be compared bilaterally in the standing subject. When the subject is lying supine with the heels approaching the buttocks, knee height (shank length) differences become apparent.[166] In the seated position, with the buttocks square against the back of the seat, differences in thigh lengths can be seen at the knees.

A number of **related asymmetries** are also useful clues to an asymmetrical pelvis and difference in lower limb length. One side of the face is also often smaller; this is most easily seen as a shorter distance between the outer corners of the eye and mouth. A tilted pelvis frequently results in a tilted shoulder-girdle axis that is detected with least ambiguity by palpating bilateral bony landmarks, such as the acromioclavicular joints or the inferior angles of the scapulae. Appearance can be deceiving if one upper trapezius muscle is tense and shortened or if a tight serratus anterior or pectoralis minor muscle has rotated or protracted one scapula. The patient may have been told that one sleeve or one pant leg needs to be shortened, or a woman patient may have been told that her skirt hangs unevenly. The foot of the shorter lower limb is likely to be smaller than its mate. The patient often has learned to test the size of new shoes on the larger foot and knows the misery that can ensue by failing to do so.

Compensatory Lumbar Scoliosis (Figs. 4.18 and 4.19)

Myofascial TrPs in the quadratus lumborum can be perpetuated by any skeletal asymmetry that tilts the base of the lumbar spine, because it is primarily the quadratus lumborum that produces the compensatory lumbar scoliosis. Maintaining this lumbar curvature needed for balance often overloads this muscle. Examples of compensatory scoliosis with radiographic illustrations are instructive.[16,22,37,38,40,43,45,46,57,63,67,105,142]

Skeletal asymmetries that can tilt the base of the lumbar spine can occur in the lower lumbar spine itself, in the pelvis, or

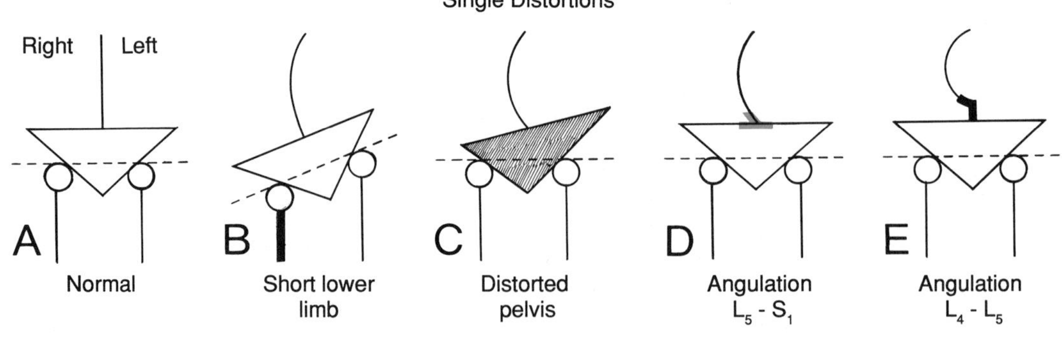

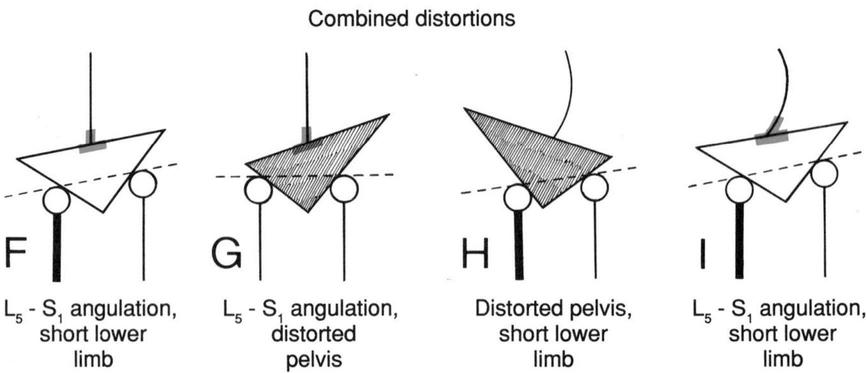

Figure 4.18. Single and combined distortions (skeletal asymmetries) of the lower limb, pelvis, and lumbar spine observed on radiographic examination. These asymmetries are usually structural where highlighted in *red*, but are likely to be compensatory (functional) and correctable where highlighted in *black*. The figures are facing the viewer. *A*, normal symmetrical lower limbs and pelvis with a straight vertical lumbar spine. *B*, shorter right lower limb, symmetrical pelvis, and compensatory spinal curvature. *C*, equal length of lower limbs, asymmetrical pelvis, and compensatory spinal curvature. *D*, equal length of lower limbs, symmetrical pelvis, angulation of L_5 to the right on a level sacral base, and compensatory spinal curvature. *E*, equal length of lower limbs, symmetrical pelvis, angulation to the right of L_4 on L_5 (may be of muscular origin) with compensatory curvature of the lumbar spine. *F*, combination of shorter right lower limb, symmetrical pelvis, and angulation to the left of L_5 on S_1. Since the two asymmetries neutralize each other, no compensatory spinal curvature results. *G*, lower limbs of equal length supporting an asymmetrical pelvis with neutralizing L_5-S_1 angulation to the left, which, similar to *F*, requires no compensatory spinal curvature. *H*, Strange combinations are sometimes seen. Here, the effect of a shorter right lower limb is overcorrected by an asymmetrical pelvis that tilts the sacral base to the left, which requires a compensatory spinal curvature. *I*, a surprisingly common combination is the shorter right lower limb supporting a symmetrical pelvis with an exaggerated deviation to the left of L_5 on S_1. This structural angulation produces a compensatory curvature of the spine that is opposite in direction to that produced by the limb-length inequality alone.

Each asymmetry illustrated occurs with nearly equal frequency on the opposite side of the body.

in the lower limbs. Spinal and pelvic asymmetries may be either structural or functional. Functional (compensatory) adaptations are reversible. Structural (fixed) asymmetries usually are correctable only with surgery. The most obvious, and apparently the most frequent, cause for a tilted sacral base is an LLLI. The severity of lumbar scoliosis is conveniently measured radiographically as the angle found between the plane of the sacral base and that of the endplate of the most inclined lumbar vertebra.[41]

Figure 4.18 illustrates common asymmetries separately and in combinations. Fixed asymmetries, such as idiopathic scoliosis of childhood and damage due to local trauma,[47] can be seen on recumbent radiographs. However, functional asymmetries are unlikely to appear in non-weight-bearing, recumbent X-ray films; standing radiographs are required to detect them. (Methods for obtaining suitable standing radiographs are presented later in this section.) In the standing position, an LLLI tilts the pelvis and sacral base downward on the side of the shorter limb (Fig. 4.18*B*), causing the lower lumbar spine to deviate toward that side. The compensatory lumbar scoliosis is convex toward the side of the shorter lower limb and restores equilibrium.

Northup[112] showed radiographically that if the foot of the long limb is not moved aside, but simply rests vertically on the ground while most of the weight is on the short limb, the compensating lumbar scoliosis becomes maximum. Bearing weight equally on both legs reduces the scoliosis. Standing with weight mainly on the long limb further reduces the scoliosis, but is uncomfortable because now the long limb must carry a major part of the weight of the short limb in addition to the rest of the body weight.

Edinger and Biedermann[22] illustrated radiographically the marked alternating lumbar scoliosis produced in normal subjects by placing a lift first under one foot and then under the other.

A tilted sacral base can also result from displaced intrapelvic articulations, for example sacroiliac (SI) joint displacement (Fig. 4.18*C*). Examination for this cause of asymmetry is covered in Chapter 2, page 17. Examination for other pelvic asymmetries is described elsewhere.[11,48,141] On the other hand, Friberg[38] found angulation of the sacral base without LLLI to be unusual among low back pain patients; it occurred in only 4 of 236 subjects.

Even with a level sacral base, a lumbar scoliosis can be caused by angulation of the spine at L_5-S_1 (Fig. 4.18*D*) or at L_4-L_5 (Fig. 4.18*E*).

Without radiographic analysis, combined asymmetries can be very confusing clinically. For example, a fixed angulation at the base of the lumbar spine can compensate for LLLI (Fig. 4.18*F*) or for a tilted sacral base caused by intrapelvic articular dysfunction (Fig. 4.18*G*) so that there is no scoliosis. However, if the fixed angulation at the base of the spine were directed toward the low side of the sacrum, it would exaggerate the effects of the pelvic or lower limb asymmetry rather than compensate for them.

Interpretation of the clinical examination becomes even more difficult when one asymmetry *overcorrects* for another. In Figure 4.18*H*, the LLLI on one side is overcorrected by pelvic asymmetry; and in Figure 4.18*I*, the LLLI is overcorrected by a fixed angulation at the base of the spine.

All of these combinations have actually been seen on radiographs of low back pain patients. A long-term study of 50 persons from childhood into adult life[63] showed a great variety of such patterns. The expected downward tilt of the sacral base on the same side as the shorter lower limb (Fig. 4.18*B*) was seen in 72% of subjects, four times as often as a sacral tilt down toward the longer lower limb (Fig. 4.18*H*), which was seen in 18% of subjects. The LLLI alone is not a very reliable indicator of the tilt of the sacral base in an *unselected* population. In one-third of the subjects, the pattern of spinal curvature changed between childhood and adulthood.[63]

A clear understanding of the nature of the skeletal configuration in patients with multiple asymmetries can be critical for the effective management of associated muscular imbalances.

Compensation for a Tilted Sacral Base

When the sacral base is tilted to one side and the spine no longer is vertical, the torso and head tilt to that side, throwing the body off balance as shown in Figure 4.19*A* and *E*. In response, one of two compensatory curvatures of the spine is commonly seen, the "S" curve of Figure 4.19*C* and *D* or the "C" curve of Figure 4.19*F* and *G*. These curves restore the head to an erect position over the center of gravity of the body, reestablish equilibrium, and level the eyes (Fig. 4.19*D* and *G*). The difference between the two curves is determined by which muscles produce them.

In the case of the **"S" curve**, the force required to produce the functional lumbar scoliosis is provided by *Force 1* of Figure 4.19*B*, *C*, and *D*, primarily by the quadratus lumborum muscle assisted by the iliocostalis. The internal and external abdomi-

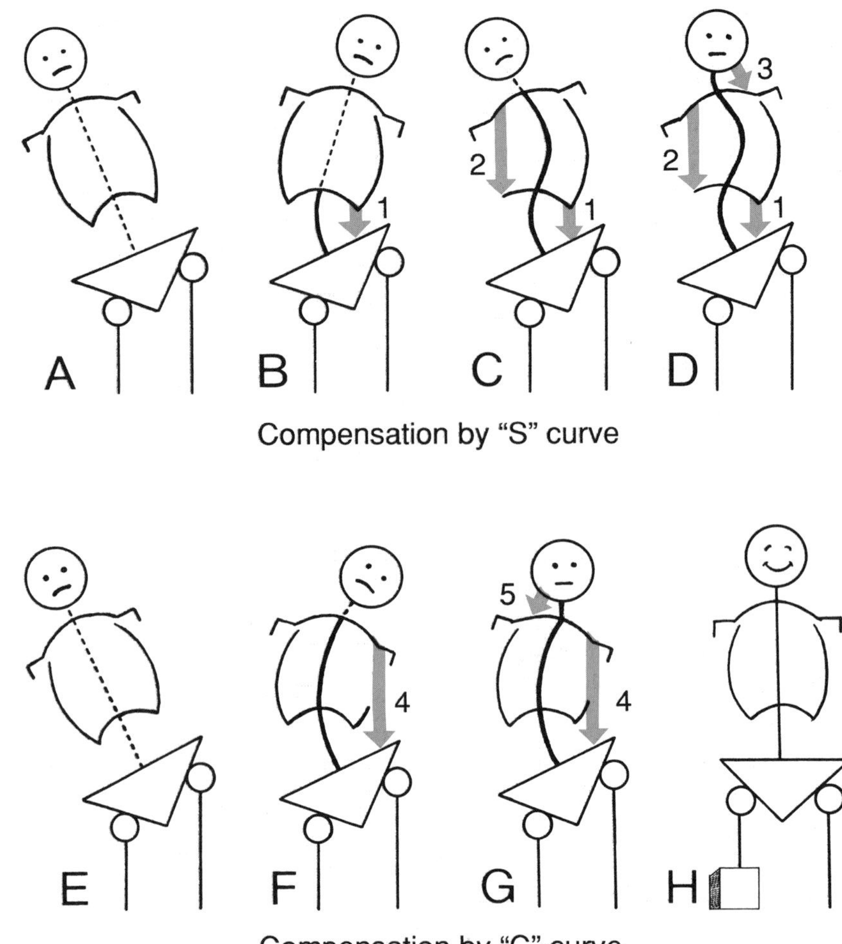

Figure 4.19. Muscular actions that produce either an "S" curve or a "C" curve functional scoliosis to compensate for a laterally tilted sacral base that is due to a lower limb-length inequality. *A* and *E* illustrate the instability and loss of equilibrium that would result if the effect of the tilted sacral base were not compensated for by muscular effort. *B*, compensation in the lumbar spine by the quadratus lumborum muscle. Force *1* brings the 12th rib and crest of the ilium closer together on the high side. The base of the thoracic spine is now tilted in the opposite direction from the tilt of the pelvis. *C*, compensation in the thoracic spine by lateral chest muscles. Force *2* pulls the shoulder girdle down on one side toward the lower thorax. The base of the cervical spine is now tilted in the opposite direction from the base of the thoracic spine, producing an "S" curve scoliosis. *D*, compensation in the cervical spine by lateral neck muscles. Force *3* places the head over the body's center of gravity, reestablishing equilibrium and leveling the eyes. *F*, compensation in the thoracolumbar spine by lateral torso musculature exerting Force *4* on the high side of the iliac crest, possibly assisted by the ipsilateral quadratus lumborum. This muscular action approximates the shoulder girdle and iliac crest on the high side. The base of the cervical spine is now tilted in the opposite direction from the tilt of the pelvis. *G*, final compensation by the lateral cervical muscles exerting Force *5* (similar to the compensation in *D* by the lateral cervical muscles, Force *3* above, but toward the other side of the body). *H*, elimination of need for compensatory scoliosis by correcting the lower limb-length inequality with a foot lift.

nal oblique muscles may also contribute to this force.

Force 2 of Figure 4.19*C* and *D* returns the spine to midline and could use the costal fibers of the pectoralis major and the lower fibers of the serratus anterior, both of which pull the shoulder girdle down. Again, the iliocostalis paraspinal muscle may assist, but with considerably less leverage.

Finally, *Force 3* in Figure 4.19*D* restores the head to the midline by action of such muscles as the scaleni, upper trapezius, levator scapulae, and splenius capitis.

In the case of the "C" **curve**, the initial correction is made more directly by Force *4* in Figure 4.19*F* and *G* using the anterior fibers of the latissimus dorsi, which extend with excellent leverage from the humerus to the crest of the ilium. The iliocostalis could assist, but with less mechanical advantage.

Force 5 of Figure 4.19*G* is essentially the same correction as Force *3* of Figure 4.19*D*, but on the other side of the neck.

It becomes obvious that a tilted sacral base is a potent source of chronic overload for many muscles and this explains why time spent to understand the cause of the tilt and correct it is well worth the effort.

Lower Limb-length Inequality

This topic of LLLI was previously reviewed in Volume 1[150] under the heading Short Leg. Little of that material is repeated here. Instead, this analysis presents a further development of those concepts.

If LLLI is the only cause of the spinal curvature that overloads the quadratus lumborum and paraspinal muscles, its recognition and correction can be a simple process. The fact that asymmetries are often complex and difficult to assess should not lead one to miss the simple, easily correctable situations.

In terms of the compensatory load imposed on the quadratus lumborum muscle, it makes little difference why the sacral base is tilted. The postural overload demanded of the muscle to keep the head erect and the eyes level over the body's center of gravity will perpetuate its TrPs regardless of the cause. Since LLLI is considered the most common cause of functional lumbar scoliosis and is certainly the one most commonly discussed in the literature, this section reviews that extensive literature. Correcting a functional lumbar scoliosis plays an essential part in the successful management of quadratus lumborum TrPs.

LLLI is quite common. About 10% of normal individuals have a 10-mm (⅜-in) difference in leg length. Uncorrected, it can contribute to osteoarthritis of the hip. To the muscles, however, LLLI is a perpetuating factor that generally causes no symptoms until quadratus lumborum TrPs are activated by a traumatic event. Then the LLLI aggravates and perpetuates the pain caused by the active TrPs. Backache correlates strongly with LLLI when the difference is measured radiographically, but it correlates poorly, if at all, when it is determined only by clinical tests. The inequality is significant during standing, walking, and jumping, but apparently is not a source of postural stress among runners, who never have both feet on the ground at the same time during running.

With careful technique, repeated LLLI determinations on the same subject by radiograms are reproducible with a maximum error of 2–5 mm (1/32–⅛ in).

The considerations required for safe and accurate standing radiographic measurement of LLLI are summarized here and presented in detail below. Gonadal exposure to ionizing radiation is minimized for male and female subjects by a "T"-shaped lead shield[45] that can be attached with Velcro to the restraining band used to prevent pelvic rotation without obscuring essential landmarks. The film should record either, or preferably both, a vertical and horizontal reference. A plumb bob hung on a fine-link jewelry chain in front of the subject facing the radiation source and a "U" tube filled with mercury attached below the arms of the gonadal shield to the restraining band in front of the patient serve this purpose. The patient should be positioned on a level surface with the feet separated by 15 cm (6 in) between medial malleoli, with the feet pointed straight forward, with body weight distributed evenly on both feet, with hips not rotated, and facing the central X-ray beam squarely. With this technique, hip sway introduces little error. Pelvic rotation up to 8° in either direction usually causes no more than a 1-mm (1/25-in) error in LLLI measurement.

The slit scanography form of standing orthoradiography permits direct comparison of the heights of the knee joints and the heads of the femurs and includes the articulations and configuration of the lumbar spine in one film. A second film taken with the heel lift that would be expected to correct the lumbar scoliosis exactly helps confirm the source of tilt of the sacral base and the extent to which the scoliosis is functional or fixed.

Table 4.1.
Incidence of Nearly 10-mm (⅜-in) Lower Limb-length Inequality (LLLI) Determined by Radiography in Patients with Low Back Pain and in Control Groups

		No. of Subjects			Incidence of LLLI	
	Investigators	With low back pain	Control group	Lower limb discrepancy (mm)	% Of patients	% Of controls
1946	Rush and Steiner[120]	1000	100	⩾11	15	4
1959	Stoddard[138]	100	50	⩾12.5	17	8
1970	Bengert[8]	324[a]		⩾10	58	
1974	Henrard, *et al.*[66]		50	⩾10		8
1979	Giles[44]	300		⩾10	13	
1983	Friberg[36]	653	359	⩾10	30	14
	Average weighted for number of subjects in each study				25%	11%

[a]Subjects also had lumbar scoliosis.

A difference in lower limb length will be considered as to prevalence and causes, its clinical importance, and the necessity, in difficult cases, for radiographic measurements rather than relying solely on clinical assessment.

Historically, one of the earliest references to LLLI comes from the Holy Bible, "The legs of the lame are not equal."[116] The classic work on the subject of limb-length difference is the German-language book by Taillard and Morscher in 1965.[142] Currently, the most informative source is the continuing series of papers by Friberg.[35–38,40,42,43] Lawrence[87] recently completed a review of literature on LLLI.

From the point of view of the lumbar spine and the musculature that controls its configuration, it makes little difference why the spine is tilted. The spinal asymmetry, regardless of cause, must be counteracted to maintain the head erect and eyes level over the body's center of gravity. Of the asymmetries described previously that can tilt the base of the spine, LLLI is considered to be the most frequent, and certainly is the one most commonly discussed in the literature.

Prevalence

Prevalence data were previously reviewed in Volume 1.[150] Additional studies include that of Friberg,[36] who examined 359 symptom-free conscript soldiers and found that 56% had LLLI of 0–4 mm (0 to less than 3⁄16 in), 30% had an LLLI of 5–9 mm (3⁄16 to nearly ⅜ in), and 14% had LLLI of 10 mm (⅜ in) or greater. Table 4.1 summarizes data from six studies. Approximately 10% of a normal population has an LLLI of 10 mm (⅜ in). This could mean that one in 10 of us is likely to develop chronic low back pain whenever a quadratus lumborum TrP is activated and then is perpetuated by this much LLLI.

One study of 50 freshmen college students[86] found that 46% had LLLI of at least 5 mm, while another study[19] of 361 male professional students reported that 48% had LLLI of more than 5 mm (3⁄16 in).

To identify the causes of LLLI in a general medical practice, Heufelder[67] examined 315 of his patients with evidence of LLLI by radiography and found that most of the true discrepancies were developmental or idiopathic. Morscher[105] listed seven categories of possible causes of LLLI.

Effects of Lower Limb-length Inequality

LLLI contributes to low back pain by imposing chronic muscular strain and overload as diagrammed in Figure 4.19. It contributes to myofascial pain syndromes only if the chronic strain activates TrPs in the overloaded muscles, or if it perpetuates TrPs that were initially activated by an acute overload. This explains why many people can have uncorrected LLLI for a lifetime without myofascial pain symptoms, whereas others have chronic pain that is relieved by the correction of the LLLI with a shoe (heel) lift. An LLLI stresses the lumbar musculature during walking but apparently not during running.

Other effects of LLLI are noteworthy. It appears to contribute significantly to the development of degenerative osteoarthritis in the hip on the side of the longer lower limb. The scoliotic spine also tends to develop osteoarthritic changes. This may be a blessing in disguise by converting the functional scoliosis that requires muscular force to maintain it into a fixed scoliosis that imposes no muscular burden. Pelvic torsion is also associated with LLLI.

Lower Limb-length Inequality and Low Back Pain. The correlation between LLLI and low back pain is usually strong when the LLLI is determined radiographically, but has been negligible when the LLLI is determined by clinical examination.[61] Table 4.1 shows that, when determined radiographically, twice as many patients with low back pain (25%) have an LLLI of at least 10 mm (3/8 in) as compared with normal control subjects (11%).

Using a careful radiographic technique, Friberg[36] found that only 25% of a group of 653 patients with chronic low back pain had less than 4 mm (3/16 in) of LLLI, whereas 57% of a control group of 359 conscript soldiers had this small an LLLI. At the other end of the scale, 12% of the patients had a 15-mm (5/8-in) or more LLLI, while only 2% of the control group had such a large difference ($p<0.001$).

Chronic pain in the low back (as well as in the hip and knee) correlated significantly with the lateral asymmetry caused by incorrect length of a prosthesis worn by veterans with amputations.[37] The 28% of amputees who had severe low back pain that was frequent or constant had a mean inequality of 22 mm (7/8 in) between the uninvolved lower limb and the amputated limb with its prosthesis applied. The 22% who had occasional and mild low back pain had a mean inequality of 6 mm (1/4 in), independent of the side of amputation. Unilateral sciatica and hip pain occurred more frequently (60%) on the side of the longer lower limb.

An orthopaedist, Bengert[8] examined radiographically 1139 of his patients who had back pain. Of this group, 324 had low back pain with lumbar scoliosis. Of this subgroup of 324 patients, 58% had at least a 1-cm (3/8-in) LLLI and 5% had more than a 5-cm (2-in) LLLI. In one recent study[61] that found no correlation between LLLI and back pain, the LLLI was measured with tape aided by a mechanical jig, not by radiography.

Lower Limb-length Inequality and Muscle Imbalance. Both asymmetry of muscle activity, as seen on EMG recordings, and increased tenderness of myofascial structures are observed in patients with LLLI.

When **standing**, if the individual with LLLI simply places the feet in the normal position, a few inches apart, the resultant tilted pelvis produces a compensatory spinal scoliosis.[22] To level the pelvis and avoid the muscle-straining scoliosis, the subject can place the longer limb forward or to one side, and stand chiefly on the shorter limb. It is also possible to stand with the feet spread wide apart and shift the pelvis toward the shorter limb, leveling the pelvic axis. (This principle is shown in Fig. 4.21*B*). The individual variations in the standing EMG[140] suggest that the mode of compensation is a highly individual matter.

In an extensive study reported in 1965, Taillard and Morscher[142] examined differences in EMG activity in standing subjects with and without LLLI. Lower limb-length discrepancy was determined initially by radiography. Subjects with a limb length difference of 2 cm (3/4 in) showed marked unilateral EMG activity in the erector spinae and gluteus maximus muscles and some increase in the triceps surae (calf) muscles on the shorter side when standing, whether the difference was structural or artificially produced by a heel lift. If the difference was only 1 cm (3/8 in) or less, no EMG asymmetry was observed.

A few years later, Strong and associates,[140] using surface electrodes, reported EMG activity in eight bilateral pairs of muscles, including paraspinal, hip, and thigh muscles. LLLI was determined by standing radiography. When the LLLI exceeded 5 mm (3/16 in), these authors observed increased EMG activity in the postural muscles of the standing subjects on the side of the longer lower limb; the activity was marked in the gluteus maximus in some subjects. Using the same instrumentation in another study, Strong and Thomas[139] reported that the combination of two asymmetrical structures that tend to neutralize each other's effects also normalizes the balance of muscular activity. They also noted that when lumbar spine convexity was associated with an asymmetrical pattern of muscle activity, the greatest activity was on the side of the concavity. This corresponds with Force *1* in Figure 4.19*B*.

Bopp[9] observed that patients with LLLI of more than 5 mm (3/16 in) always had tenderness and sometimes pain at the greater trochanter of the longer leg, and they were likely to have tenderness on the side of the longer leg at the attachment of the iliopsoas muscle on the lesser trochanter, at the transverse processes of the lumbar vertebrae, and at the attachment of the hip adductors on the os pubis. Morscher[105] corroborated these observations in his own patients. Heufelder[67] associated increased muscle tension and muscle tenderness with LLLI that was demonstrated radiographically.

Mahar and associates[101] examined the effect of simulated LLLI on postural sway as measured with a center-of-pressure force plate. They found that lifts of as little as 1-cm (3/8-in) shifted the mean center of pressure toward the longer lower limb to a significant degree. Increasing the LLLI did not increase this effect proportionately. Postural sway in a mediolateral direction, likewise, increased significantly with a 1-cm (3/8-in) LLLI, and this effect continued to increase in proportion to the magnitude of the difference in lower limb length. The author concluded that LLLI of as little as 1-cm (3/8-in) may be biomechanically important.

Lower Limb-length Inequality and Arthritic Changes. The most serious orthopaedic complication of LLLI is osteoarthritis of the hip. Arthritic changes of the spine and of the knee have also been implicated.

Wiberg's angle as illustrated in references[36,37,82,105] relates to the size of the load-bearing articular surface of the hip joint. This angle is smaller on the side of the longer limb. The resultant increase of pressure per unit area of load-bearing surface apparently promotes chondral damage and unilateral arthrosis of the hip.[82]

Gofton and Trueman[50] found that in 81% of 36 cases of degenerative osteoarthritis of the hip, the lower limb on the diseased side was longer than the limb on the healthy side. The LLLI appeared to act in concert with other conditions to cause unilateral degenerative osteoarthritis of the hip.[49]

Turula and associates[163] concluded that LLLI warrants investigation as a cause of aseptic loosening of the prosthesis and unexplained pain following hip arthroplasty.

Several authors[38,46,105] have reported development of osteophytes on lumbar vertebrae on the side of the concavity produced by LLLI, and Giles and Taylor[46] illustrated wedging of the lumbar vertebrae in a manner that would represent the conversion of a functional scoliosis to a fixed scoliosis.

Dixon and Campbell-Smith[20] demonstrated with six case histories that LLLI of 2.5 cm (1 in) or greater can produce knee damage: destruction of the lateral tibiofemoral compartment, valgus deformity, and osteoarthrosis on the side of the longer limb.

Kinesiologic Effects of Lower Limb-length Inequality. When **walking**, the person with LLLI has the option of several kinds of compensations. The individual can maintain the pelvis level at the expense of forceful plantar flexion and possible overload of the gluteal and lower limb muscles by using these muscles to vault up to the height of the longer limb, as demonstrated electromyographically.[142] Children are prone to circumduct a longer limb. Increased knee flexion during stance phase of the longer limb is not easily seen, but the increased incidence of osteoarthritis in the knee of the longer limb may relate to this means of compensation. If the patient simply allows the pelvis to drop on the side of the shorter limb, the lumbar musculature must coordinate a compensatory scoliosis with each gait cycle.

Delacerda and Wikoff[18] studied one patient with a large LLLI of 32 mm (1¼ in) and found that it caused temporal asymmetries in the phases of gait. Equalization of lower limb length by means of a shoe lift eliminated the asymmetry and decreased the kinetic energy requirement (as measured by oxygen consumption).

Botte[10] examined 25 hospital patients with low back pain for foot abnormalities. Eight patients had LLLI of more than 5 mm by X-ray. For seven of these eight patients, the longer limb showed a compensatory ankle and foot pronation in the stance position. This contributed to medial rotation of that entire limb and distorted the normal gait pattern.

By recording both EMG activity and timing of the gait cycle, Taillard and Morscher[142] found that an experimental LLLI of 2 cm (¾ in) or more seriously disrupted the timing and the relative intensity of activity of the erector spinae, gluteus maximus and medius, and triceps surae muscles. An LLLI of 1 cm (3/8 in) was not disruptive in this way.

In **runners**, Gross[60] was not able to find any evidence of consistent benefits from the use of corrective lifts in marathon runners with LLLI of 5–25 mm (3/16–1 in). When running, both feet are never on the ground at the same time; apparently no compensatory lumbar scoliosis is needed.

A force-plate study[122] of persons with LLLI demonstrated an increase in lateral force on the foot of the shorter limb (associated with supination) that disappeared with the addition of a compensatory heel lift. This force would account for the increased wear observed on the lateral side of the heel and sole of the shoe worn on the shorter limb and may represent a subconscious effort to increase limb length.

Pelvic torsion is associated with LLLI. Bourdillon and Day[11] state that "in patients with leg inequality there is a natural tendency for the pelvis to adopt the twisted position which most nearly levels the anterior superior surface of the sacrum." They illustrate how *posterior* rotation of one innominate bone lowers the sacrum on the same side. Fisk[32] illustrates how the *anterior* rotation of an innominate bone elevates that side of the sacrum. Thus, they associate compensatory anterior rotation of the innominate bone with a short lower limb and compensatory posterior rotation with a long lower limb. One would expect this functional compensation to become increasingly fixed over a period of time.

Denslow *et al.*[19] also note the likelihood of a compensatory horizontal rotation of the pelvis toward the longer limb.

Radiographic Assessment of Lumbar Scoliosis caused by Lower Limb-length Inequality (Figs. 4.20 and 4.21)

This portion concerning radiographic measurements of LLLI includes indications for radiography, patient protection from ionizing radiation, accuracy of measurement, patient positioning errors, tube positioning errors, reading, and then interpreting the films.

Indications for Radiography

Radiographs are indicated when simple corrective measures have not been sufficiently effective in relieving symptoms, after correctable lower limb dysfunction has been alleviated, after any noted pelvic torsion has been corrected, after any lumbar dysfunction has been relieved, and after TrPs causing shortening and splinting of the quadratus lumborum have been inactivated.

Greenman[57] notes the importance of first normalizing lumbopelvic mechanics; the radiographs are then useful as guidelines for corrective lift therapy. Lewit[91] illustrated the use of standing radiography in the frontal and sagittal planes to determine the cause of inclination of the base of the spinal column and to establish the optimum correction of lower limb length.

Patient Protection

Exposure of the patient to ionizing radiation can be reduced in two ways. First, the radiation field can be coned down or collimated to include only regions of concern: the tops of the femoral heads in the acetabula, the sacral base, and the lumbar spine.[42,45] Second, the subject can be fitted with a gonadal shield.

Giles and Taylor[45] in 1981 described a "T"-shaped gonadal lead shield that was suitable for men or women and could be attached by Velcro to a restraining band used to prevent pelvic rotation. In 1985, Friberg *et al.*[42] measured the radiation dose in 10 male subjects when the film for the femoral heads was taken with a lead gonadal shield measuring 12 cm (4¾ in) × 20 cm (7⅞ in) × 1.8 mm (1/16+ in) in place. This shield reduced the mean exposure to 11.4 mrad to the gonads, 989 mrad to the skin in the primary field, and 13.6 mrad to the bone marrow. The mean ovarian dose in women was calculated to be 123 mrad without a shield and 30 mrad using the same shield over the lower abdomen. Friberg *et al.* employed this shield in subsequent studies.[43]

Accuracy of Measurement

Studies show that LLLI can be measured radiographically with a maximum error of 2–5 mm (1/16–3/16 in) with an average error of about 1 mm (1/25 in).[36,38,44,50,66]

Gofton and Trueman[50] did repeat studies on 108 subjects, 66 of whom had osteoarthritis of the hip, and in 92 subjects they found no more than a 1.5 mm (1/16 in) difference in measurement as compared to the first study; in 13 subjects, differences up to 3.0 mm (⅛ in) occurred in the second study; in only three subjects did the repeat study differ as much as 5 mm (3/16 in). In the 1983 accuracy study by Friberg,[36] measurements were repeated on 25 subjects after 1–30 months, and on another 25 by adding a lift for the second measurement that equalled the LLLI recorded in the first measurement. The mean error was 0.6 mm (<1/32 in) and the maximum error was 2.0 mm (<⅛ in). Radiography is clearly the standard against which to judge the accuracy of clinical estimates.

Level and Centerline on Film

A horizontal reference must be established in order to read a film for LLLI. Using the margin of the film leads to inaccuracy. Horizontal reference points or horizontal lines, and a vertical plumb line can be recorded on the film.

Although the bottom edge of the film has been used as the horizontal reference,[10] this use assumes that: *(a)* the bottom of the Bucky tray is horizontal, or at least is parallel to the surface on which the patient is standing; *(b)* the cassette was placed squarely in the Bucky tray; and *(c)* the film was placed squarely in the cassette.[57] This approach is not considered adequate by most authors because it provides no simple way of checking that all of these conditions have been met. Often they are not.

The simplest and probably most foolproof horizontal reference is a closed loop of plastic tubing half filled with mercury and attached to either the vertical Bucky table or to the patient. Oscillations of the mercury damp out quickly, and the top of the mercury column (the meniscus) shows clearly on the X-ray film (Fig. 4.20). If the meniscus of the mercury column is close to the roof of the acetabulum on each side, the two menisci provide a convenient and reliable horizontal reference line.[12,37,42] In the second author's experience, other radio-opaque fluids based on water or oil-soluble iodine compounds tend to dry out and crystallize, produce fuzzy menisci, and are so viscous that they reach a stable position too slowly.

In addition to this highly reliable horizontal reference, Friberg attached to the cassette holder an accurately leveled acrylic plate on which were mounted 0.3-mm (0.0181-in) thick copper wires. The shadows of these wires provided horizontal reference lines and a midline vertical line on the film to facilitate subsequent analysis.[36,38]

Whenever vertical alignment and side sway are of interest, the true vertical can be established independently with a plumb bob suspended by a radio-opaque line (or fine chain) in the plane of the midpoint between the heels. This line also serves as an independent cross-check on the horizontal level. Finding a suspension wire for the plumb bob that is thick enough to register clearly on the film, but is not so stiff that it hangs crooked, can be a problem. The second author found that several lengths of a thin, small-link silver necklace chain were relatively inexpensive, always hung true, and were clearly visible on the film.

Several authors[16,33,50] place the plumb line so that it hangs freely between the patient and the X-ray tube; others[45] place it between the patient and the cassette. The latter location introduces difficulties. The patient is likely to displace the line by leaning against it. If the line is taped in position, its accuracy depends on the care that was taken to avoid displacement of the line while or after it was taped in place.

Patient Positioning Errors

The patient should be positioned on a level surface with the feet separated and aligned straight forward, the heels even and solidly on the floor, the knees straight, body weight distributed evenly on both feet, the hips not rotated, and facing the central X-ray beam squarely. Figure 4.20 summarizes a good technique.

To obtain an accurate standing radiograph for measurement of LLLI, the surface on which the patient stands must be level.[6,50] This should be tested with a spirit level; floors are not always level. A level base is assured by having the patient stand on a steel plate that is levelled using spirit levels that are welded onto the plate at a right angle to each other.[45]

Foot Positioning. The patient must keep both heels flat on the floor, in order to avoid plantar flexion of one foot to equalize weight, and must place the heels at equal distances from the cassette stand to prevent one foot being placed in front of the other.

To eliminate errors in measuring LLLI caused by side sway of the pelvis, each heel should be under its corresponding femoral head to establish a parallelogram. To achieve this, most authors separate the malleoli or inner borders of the feet by 15 cm (6 in).[6,16,33,37,38,45,57,164]

Unless pelvic side sway is extreme, an error in foot separation of a few centimeters (an inch or so) will not make any practical difference. Some authors simply mark the floor with footprints on which the subject stands; others use plates with a block between and behind the feet, or heel cups, to position the feet.

If the subject places the feet considerably closer together or farther apart than the distance between the femoral heads, side sway of the pelvis can introduce significant error in the measurement of LLLI (Fig 4.21).[12,22,50,164] Even when the feet are placed beneath the femoral heads to form a perfect parallelogram, side sway of the pelvis can still produce some distortion caused by asymmetrical projection of the X-ray beams. This generally is an insignificant error[45] that, if desired, can be identified and corrected by calculations,[113] or can be prevented by holding the hips firmly centered in front of the Bucky with a compression band.[45] However, this restraint is likely to distort the patient's lumbopelvic posture, which affects the muscles and should be recorded without distortion.

Knees Straight. Making sure that the subject keeps *both* knees straight, or equally extended, avoids the error that is inherent when one knee is flexed more than the other.[6,36,38,43,50]

Equal Weight. The instruction to "place the weight equally on both feet" or "equally through both heels" reduces the temptation for the patient to lift one heel from the floor or to bend one knee slightly in an unconscious attempt to level the pelvis and to straighten the spine.[16,45,50,63,164] The additional instruction, "relax and let your weight

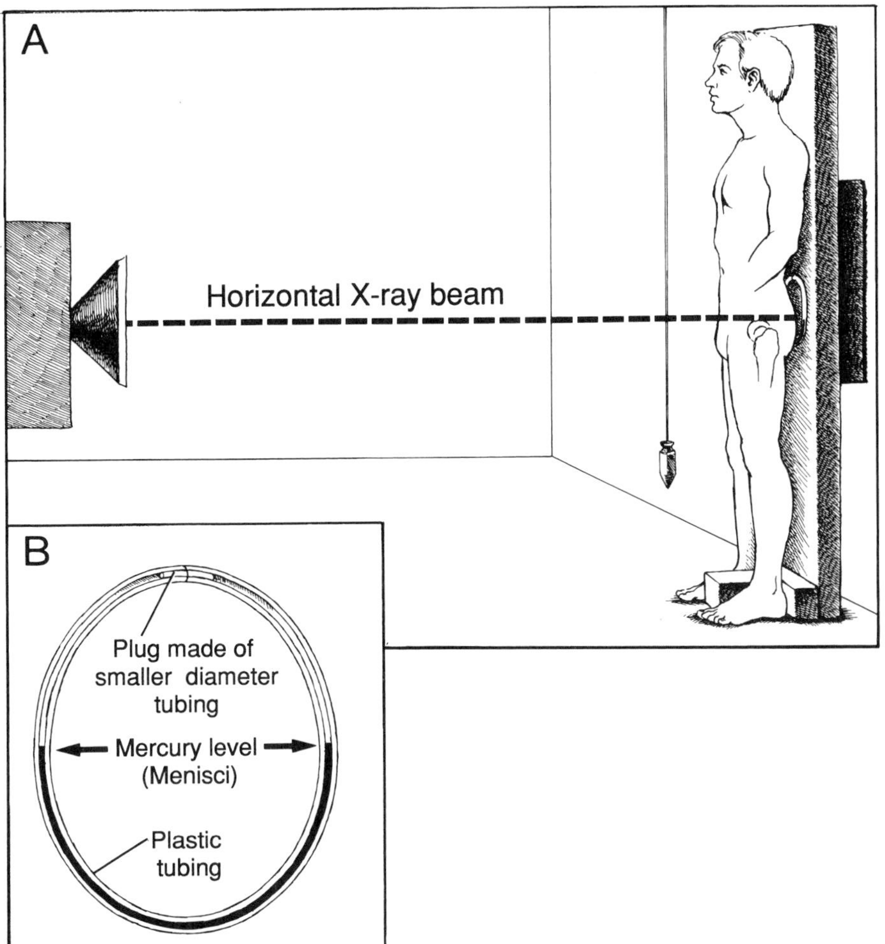

Figure 4.20. Schematic of technique for taking standing radiographs to evaluate lower body asymmetries including lower limb-length inequality. *A*, arrangement and patient positioning. The tube focus should be at least 100 cm (39 in) from the film, preferably a distance of 150 cm (5 ft) or more. A mercury level gauge is taped to the cassette holder with the menisci at the ends of the mercury column close to the level of the tops of the femoral heads. A radio-opaque plumb line is suspended in front of the patient's spine to make a vertical line on the film. The X-ray tube is adjusted so that the horizontal beam passes close to the tops of the femoral heads, the level of which is usually about halfway between the pubic tubercle and the anterior superior iliac spine. The lower edge of the film should be just below the ischial tuberosities to record the obturator foramina and the vertical dimension of each hemipelvis; this placement allows the upper edge of the film to include as much of the lumbar spine as possible. The patient stands on a level surface with a block 15 cm (6 in) wide between the feet with a backstop to position the heels. The patient is instructed to stand relaxed with equal weight on both feet held flat on the floor with knees straight, and to lean back gently against the cassette holder. *B*, level gauge, made with a plastic "O" tube half-filled with mercury. A horizontal line is determined by the two mercury menisci, which show clearly on the radiograph. The open ends of the plastic tube are connected by inserting into them a short piece of glass tubing and sealing the joints with silicone glue. The glass tubing can be protected from breakage by taping short wooden splints around it.

***settle** on your feet*," helps to reveal skeletal asymmetries.

Pelvic Rotation. The projection error caused by pelvic rotation is minimized if the X-ray beam is horizontal at the level of the top of the femoral heads.[45] Gofton and Trueman[50] considered pelvic rotation up to 8° acceptable and to be readily identifiable on the film when in excess of that.[50] The instruction for the subject to lean both buttocks back gently against the cassette holder[6,37] also helps reduce rotation error (and to keep the patient as close to the film as possible to reduce pro-

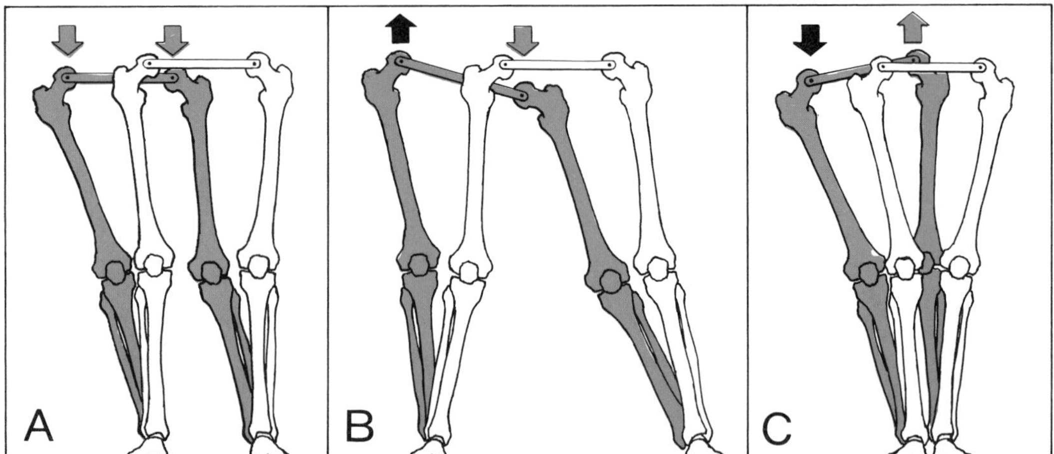

Figure 4.21. Equal-length lower limbs which demonstrate two errors that should be avoided when using standing radiography to measure lower limb-length inequality. The errors are caused by side sway of the pelvis, if the feet are not spaced properly. *A*, ankles spaced at the same distance as that between the femoral heads. **No error** in limb-length discrepancy. The limbs appear equally shortened because they form a parallelogram with the pelvis. *B*, feet spread wide apart. Lower limb on the side toward which the pelvis is shifted appears **lengthened**. *C*, feet close together. The limb on the side toward which the pelvis is shifted appears **shortened**.

jection errors). Clarke[16] found experimentally on a skeleton and on living subjects that 15° of pelvic rotation at a focal distance of 100 cm (39 in) introduced an error of less than 3 mm. Denslow and associates[19] found no rotation in 39% of 342 subjects.

Tube Positioning

Two aspects of tube positioning need to be considered: the focal distance between tube and film, and the level on the subject at which the horizontal rays are directed.

An increase in the focal distance reduces projection distortion without increasing patient exposure, but requires more tube current or a longer exposure. Most authors employed a distance of 100 cm or 1 meter (39 in).[16,22,57,72] One paper[45] reported 102 cm (40 in). A few used 150 cm (5 ft).[33,164]

For determination of LLLI, most authors attempted to direct the horizontal rays of the beam at the tops of the femoral heads.[6,37,45,50,164] There was considerable diversity of opinion as to what target best served that purpose. Recommended levels for the center of the beam included the symphysis pubis,[37] the anterior superior iliac spine,[164] and 1–2 cm (⅜–¾ in) below the anterior superior iliac spine.[38] The vertical distance between the anterior superior iliac spine or the symphysis pubis and the roof of the acetabulum depends on the degree of forward tilt of the pelvis. Therefore, the most reliable level probably is 1–2 cm (⅜–¾ in) above the upper border of the greater trochanter.

The slit scanography form of standing orthoradiography[19] (Fig. 4.17) records on one film the knee joints, the femoral heads, and a view of the articulations and configuration of the lumbar spine.

Reading and Interpreting Radiographs for Asymmetries

In addition to LLLI, radiographs can reveal the levelness of the sacral base, the degree of lumbar scoliosis, and other skeletal asymmetries of the pelvis and lumbar spine.

This review of examination of films for skeletal asymmetries addresses LLLI, levelness of the sacral base, pelvic rotation, spinal angulation, and functional vs. fixed scoliosis.

Lower Limb-length Inequality. Measurement of LLLI on a properly executed film requires only the extension of a horizontal line from the upper border of one femoral head to that of the other femoral head. The distance between that line and the top of the other femoral head is the LLLI. The film reproduced in Figure 4.17*B* shows an LLLI of 17 mm (⅝ in). The postural scoliosis of 20° is associated with a marked axial rotation that results in the clinical appearance of a straight lumbar spine, which is portrayed schematically in Figure 4.17*C*. This rotation illustrates one major difficulty in assessing lumbar scoliosis by clinical examination only.

Plane of the Sacral Base. An LLLI is important to the lumbar spine to the extent that the LLLI causes a corresponding tilt of the sacral base. Unfortunately, the plane of the sacral base is often difficult to delineate in routine standing anteroposterior or posteroanterior views of the pelvis.

Greenman[57] establishes the plane of the sacral base on a radiograph by any of the following lines, in order of preference: a line through the most posterior aspects of the sacral promontory, one through corresponding points on the sulci of the sacral ala, or one through the medial corners of the sacral articular pillars as they attach to the body of the sacrum. Heilig[65] prefers either a line through corresponding points at the lateral extensions of the L_5-S_1 disc space, or one through corresponding points on superior facets of the sacrum; if these cannot be identified, he uses a line drawn through the sulcus that lies between the body of the sacrum and the sacral ala on each side.

If a separate film is taken to better visualize the lumbosacral junction and sacroiliac joints, Greenman[57] recommends a 30° cephalic angle study of the pelvis. He pictured the pelvis with the patient supine, but the films should be more informative if taken with the subject standing.

If the curvature of the lumbar spine and the tilt of the sacral base do not correspond, the distortion may be caused by pelvic asymmetry.

Rotation of Pelvis. In standing anteroposterior X-ray films, if the pelvis is rotated, the symphysis pubis appears deviated toward the direction of rotation as compared to the position of the median sacral crest (sacral spinous processes), the obturator foramen on the side toward the direction of rotation appears narrowed, and the ischial spine appears enlarged on that side.[19] Friberg[38] found that the symphysis pubis was rotated toward the long limb in 76% of 236 cases of low back pain with LLLI. Rotation of the lumbar spine and pelvis together should be distinguished from rotation of the pelvis in relation to the non-rotated spine.

Pelvic rotation of as much as 8° is not likely to distort the LLLI measurement of a standing film more than a millimeter or two.[50] Rotation may affect muscle dynamics and postural distortions, but no study of such effects was found.

Angulation Between Vertebrae. Marked angulation between vertebrae, specifically between L_4 and L_5 or between L_5 and S_1, theoretically can be either fixed or caused by asymmetrical muscle tension. Side bending, however, is much more restricted at the lumbosacral junction than it is throughout the rest of the lumbar spine. Tanz[143] found that between the ages of 35 and 65 years, individuals without back pain had an average of 6–8° of lateral bending between each pair of lumbar vertebrae except between L_5 and S_1, where motion of only 1° or 2° was available. This means that any appreciable angulation at the lumbosacral junction is likely to be fixed and not a compensatory response under muscular control. However, lateral angulation between L_4 and L_5 can be either fixed or compensatory. The tilt can be in either the opposite direction (corrective) or the same direction, which adds to the angulation of the sacral base.

Scoliosis. If a lumbar scoliosis is observed, two questions need to be answered. The first is, what skeletal asymmetries are responsible? To answer this question, the films are examined with respect to the possibilities summarized in Figure 4.18.[57,65,105] The second question, whether the curvature is functional or fixed, can be answered by comparing films made with and without a correction, such as a shoe lift. Compensatory curves usually are modified by the correction; fixed curves are not. However, a tense quadratus lumborum can hold a compensatory curve immobile, so that it appears to be a fixed curvature.

A functional (compensatory) scoliosis that induces muscular strain can be characterized as the maximum displacement of the spine from the midline and as the maximum angle of curvature. The distance the vertebrae are displaced from the weight-bearing midline determines the total magnitude of the corrective problem confronting the muscles. Moreover, the greater the angle of curvature of the scoliosis, the more concentrated must be the corrective forces, because they must act over a shorter distance.

9. TRIGGER POINT EXAMINATION (Figs. 4.22–4.25)

The lateral border of the quadratus lumborum between the crest of the ilium and the 12th rib slopes upward and medially. As it approaches the 12th rib, the muscle passes beneath the lateral border of the iliocostalis muscle, which slopes laterally (*see* Fig. 4.25). The lower lateral portion of the quadratus lumborum lies subcuta-

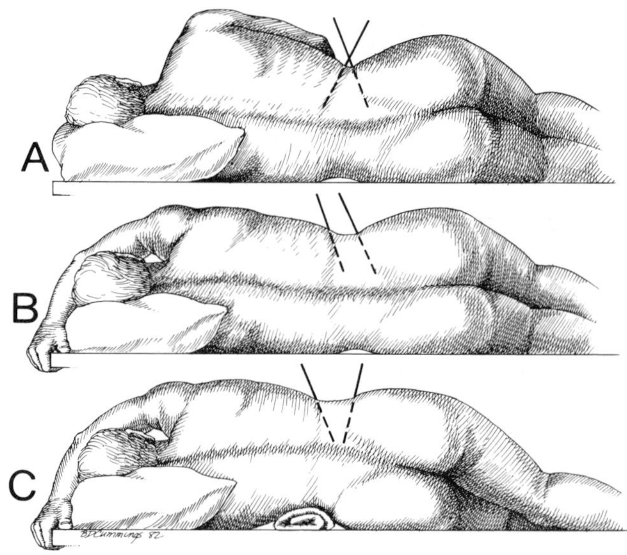

Figure 4.22. Patient positioning for examination of the quadratus lumborum muscle. *A*, the position often assumed by a patient when simply asked to lie on the side. The lines emphasize closure of the space that allows access to the muscle between the 10th or 11th rib and the crest of the ilium. *B*, partial opening of that space by having the patient reach overhead with the arm to elevate the rib cage. *C*, full opening of the space by providing a supporting lumbar roll or pillow and also by pulling the pelvis distally as the patient rests the uppermost knee behind the other knee on the examining table. This wider opening permits palpation of the quadratus lumborum muscle.

neous except for whatever portion of the latissimus dorsi muscle extends that far. The upper lateral attachment of the quadratus lumborum to the rib cage usually lies deep to both latissimus dorsi and iliocostalis fibers (*see* Fig. 4.23). When palpating the lateral border of the quadratus lumborum, it helps to remember that its fibers occasionally extend to the 11th rib.[3]

For examination of TrPs in the quadratus lumborum muscle, positioning is extremely important. Unless the patient is properly positioned lying on the uninvolved side, the TrPs in this muscle are very difficult to find.[124,125,171] The position that the patient ordinarily assumes, however (Fig. 4.22*A*), does not permit adequate palpation for deep tenderness of the quadratus lumborum muscle because of inadequate space between the 10th rib and the crest of the ilium.

Raising the arm of the side to be examined onto the top of the table behind the head elevates the thoracic cage (Fig. 4.22*B*). Dropping the knee of that side onto the examining table behind the other knee, pulls that side of the pelvis distally and lowers the iliac crest. This position creates adequate space for examining the muscle (Fig. 4.22*C*), adding the tension necessary for palpation.

However, when quadratus lumborum TrPs are very active and the muscle is especially tight and tender, this position places the quadratus lumborum muscle under painful tension. The pelvis cannot pull away from the rib cage and the knee on the side being examined does not reach the table. The leg needs support, such as the patient's other ankle.

Before starting to palpate for these TrPs, it is most important for the clinician to cut the nails very short on the digits used for palpation. This avoids unnecessary skin pain that distresses the patient and, on deep palpation, may be mistaken for TrP tenderness.

One reason why TrPs in the quadratus lumborum muscle are so easily overlooked is because almost all of this muscle lies anterior to the paraspinal muscle mass and is inaccessible from the posterior approach (Fig. 4.23) of a routine back examination. Examination for quadratus lumborum TrPs begins by palpating for the lateral edge of the paraspinal mass, the 12th rib, and the crest of the ilium. In many patients, the only part of the latissimus dorsi muscle that overlies the quadratus lumborum is its aponeurosis, which presents little obstruction to palpation. In some, however, a thick column of overlying fibers of the latissimus dorsi muscle extends to the crest of the ilium (Fig. 4.23).

Three regions in this muscle are examined for TrPs. The **first region** is deep and in the angle where the crest of the ilium and paraspinal muscle mass meet (Figs.

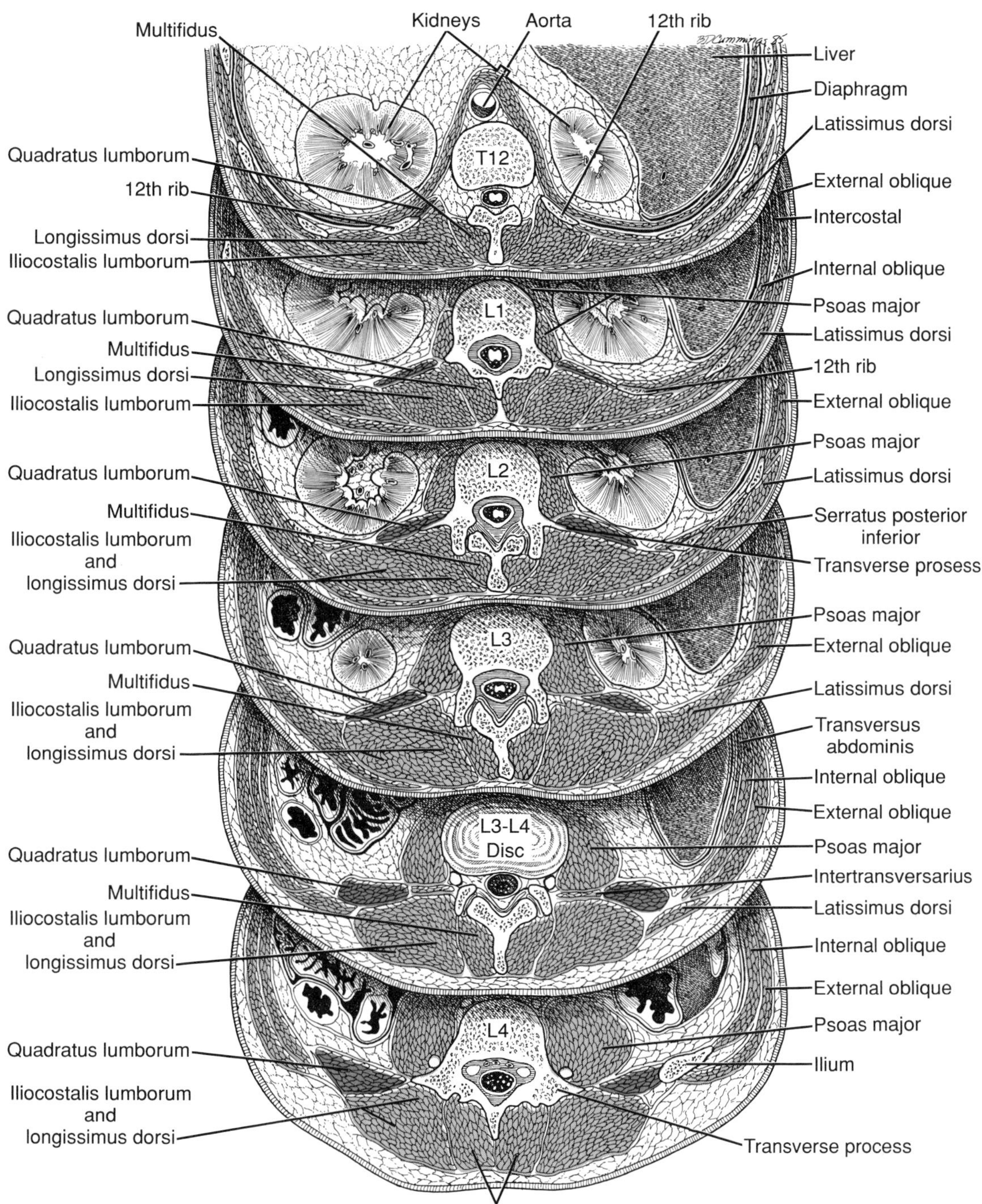

Figure 4.23. Serial cross sections of the quadratus lumborum muscle (*dark red*); other muscles, *light red*. Attachment of the muscle to the 12th rib is seen in the T_{12} and L_1 sections; attachment to a transverse process is seen in the L_2 section, and attachment to the ilium is seen in the L_4 section. The next lower section (not included) would show only the iliolumbar ligament, and no quadratus lumborum muscle. The latissimus dorsi is one muscle usually interposed between the palpating finger and the quadratus lumborum muscle. Only at the L_4 level is the muscle directly palpable beneath the skin. Adapted from Carter *et al.*[15]

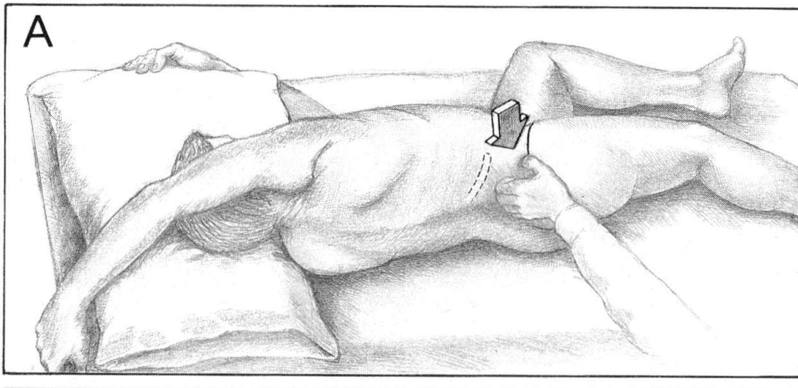

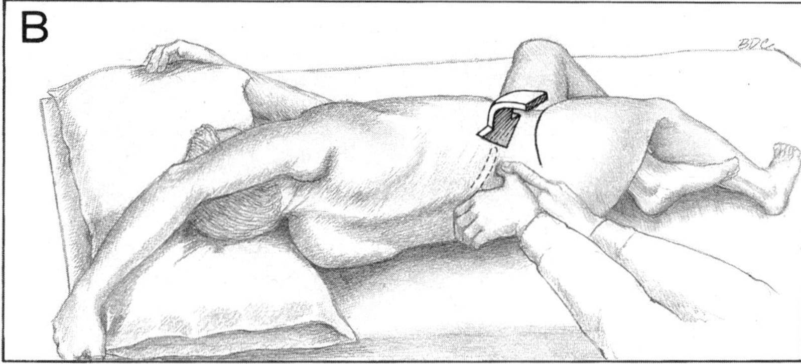

Figure 4.24. Examination for two of four trigger point locations in the right quadratus lumborum muscle. The chest is elevated by the patient's reaching upward with the uppermost arm behind the head to grasp the end of the examining table. *Dashed lines* outline the 12th rib and the *solid line* marks the crest of the ilium. The *arrows* indicate the direction in which pressure is applied to elicit spot tenderness. *A*, if the muscle is only moderately tight and sensitive to stretch, the uppermost ilium is lowered by resting the knee of the uppermost limb on the examining table behind the other knee. To locate spot tenderness at the superficial caudad trigger points, downward pressure is exerted with the thumb just above (adjacent to) the crest of the ilium and anterior to the long paraspinal muscle mass. *B*, if the muscle is very tight, that knee is placed on the ankle of the other limb to avoid excessive painful stretch of the muscle. To locate the deep, more cephalad trigger points, deep pressure is applied just caudal to the 12th rib and again anterior to the paraspinal muscles.

4.24*A* and 4.25). As seen in Figures 4.23 and 4.25, this is the thickest part of the quadratus lumborum muscle, near the level of the L_4 transverse process. This location is just cephalad to the point where many vertical iliocostal fibers and diagonal iliolumbar fibers anchor by intertwining with fibers of the iliolumbar ligament. As shown in Figure 4.24, the muscle is examined for tenderness by applying deep pressure superior to the crest of the ilium and anterior to the paraspinal muscles. The pressure is directed toward the tips of lumbar transverse processes. One must press gently at first, because remarkably little pressure on these TrPs can be exquisitely painful. Here, pressure is applied primarily to the diagonal lower iliolumbar fibers of the quadratus lumborum. These fibers are too deep for one to feel their taut bands or to elicit local twitch responses manually.

The **second region** examined for quadratus lumborum TrPs extends along the inner crest of the ilium where many of the iliocostal fibers attach. The tip of the finger is applied across the direction of the fibers shown in Figure 4.25. This flat palpation locates taut bands with tender spots in those fibers. Local twitch responses are rarely visible, unless the individual is thin and has few latissimus dorsi fibers extending this far.

If one progresses too far laterally, the fingers encounter the lateral border of the external abdominal oblique muscle; these

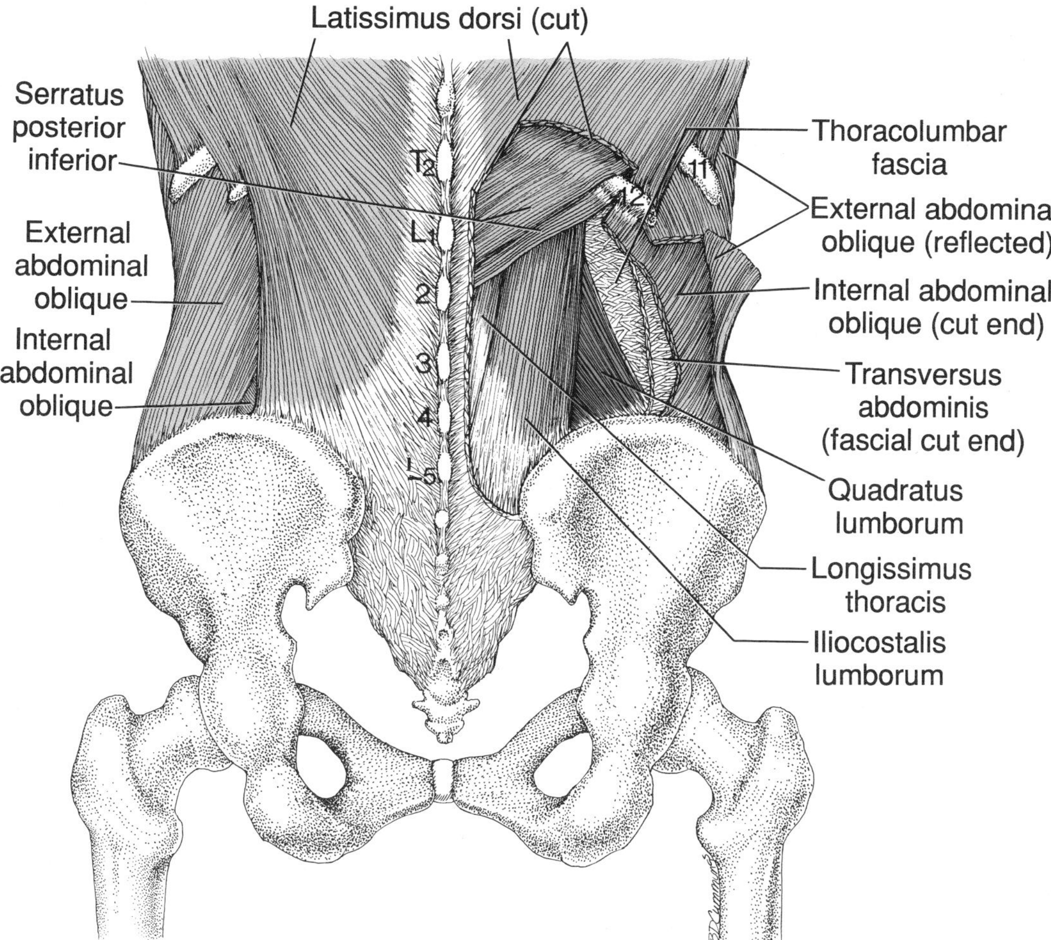

Figure 4.25. Regional anatomy of the right quadratus lumborum muscle (*dark red*). Neighboring muscles are *light red*. The thoracolumbar fascia, which lies anterior to (deep to) the quadratus lumborum muscle, is seen between the quadratus lumborum and the cut edge of the transversus abdominis. The transverse abdominal muscle, the latissimus dorsi, and the internal abdominal oblique muscles have been cut and portions removed. The external abdominal oblique has also been cut and a portion reflected.

fibers run nearly parallel to the lateral iliocostal fibers of the quadratus lumborum. The external abdominal oblique fibers may have taut bands and TrPs that can easily be mistakenly ascribed to the quadratus lumborum (Fig. 4.25). Taut bands of the external abdominal oblique muscle angle from the *tip* of the 12th rib down and forward to the *anterior* aspect of the crest of the ilium (*see* Fig. 49.3A on p. 666 of Volume 1[148]). The adjacent quadratus lumborum fibers are nearly parallel, but usually angle from the *middle* and posterior portions of the 12th rib to the *posterior* aspect of the crest of the ilium.

The **third region** lies in the angle where the paraspinal mass and the 12th rib meet (Fig. 4.24*B*). As seen in Figures 4.2, 4.23, and 4.25, deep fingertip pressure applied in the direction of the L_1-L_2 transverse processes transmits pressure to the cephalad attachment of the iliocostal and lumbocostal fibers of the quadratus lumborum. In some patients, the attachments of the iliocostal fibers extend laterally far enough along the 12th rib to be felt by flat palpation in a manner similar to that described for the second region, above. With the patient in the position shown in Figure 4.24, one can also apply pressure caudad to L_2 seeking tenderness over the L_3 transverse process between regions one and three. Only tenderness is elicited since these fibers are too deep to permit palpation of taut bands.

With sustained pressure on any one of these TrPs, one may elicit its pattern of referred pain, although penetration of the TrP with a needle is a more reliable way of eliciting pain referred by TrPs in this muscle.

In 1931, Lange[83] illustrated myogelosis of the quadratus lumborum muscle in the first region just described. He noted that when the muscle was extremely sore and tense, indurations within the muscle were not distinguishable. However, as the muscle became less tense with successive massage treatments, the palpable changes became identifiable. Following additional treatment, the muscle became less tender and abnormal muscle tension disappeared.

Other authors also located quadratus lumborum tender spots, some of which were specifically identified as TrPs, along the outer margin of the muscle,[62,132,134] near its attachments to the tips of the transverse processes of the first three lumbar vertebrae,[132,134] and along its attachment to the 12th rib.[134]

10. ENTRAPMENTS

No nerve entrapments by the quadratus lumborum muscle are known to have been identified.

11. ASSOCIATED TRIGGER POINTS

Myofascial TrPs associated with the quadratus lumborum may develop secondarily in other muscles of the functional unit, or as satellite TrPs in its pain reference zones. The quadratus lumborum TrPs may also be associated with articular dysfunction. These associated manifestations may be present simultaneously.

Secondary Trigger Points

Clinically, the muscles most likely to develop functional *secondary* myofascial TrPs due to TrPs in the quadratus lumborum are the contralateral quadratus lumborum, the ipsilateral iliopsoas, the iliocostalis between T_{11} and L_3, not infrequently the external abdominal oblique, and, occasionally, the latissimus dorsi muscle.

The two quadratus lumborum muscles work as a team bilaterally, which explains why TrPs on one side are frequently associated with less active TrPs in the quadratus muscle on the opposite side. The psoas major and lumbar paraspinal muscles help the quadratus lumborum to stabilize the lumbar spine. Both the quadratus lumborum and the lumbar paraspinal muscles are spinal extensors. The posterior fibers of the external abdominal oblique are nearly parallel to the iliocostal quadratus lumborum fibers, and have similar attachments to the rib cage and pelvis and also are likely to harbor TrPs if the quadratus lumborum does.

Satellite Trigger Points

The gluteus medius and gluteus minimus muscles commonly develop satellite TrPs since they lie in the referred pain zones of the quadratus lumborum. Patients sometimes report pain in the reference zones of the gluteus medius and minimus muscles in response to pressure on quadratus lumborum TrPs. With inactivation of the satellite gluteal TrPs, pressure on the quadratus TrP then refers pain only to its characteristic gluteal and pelvic distribution. This is not an unusual situation and, therefore, it is important to examine the quadratus lumborum muscle in patients with "sciatica."

Sola[132] observed that activity of gluteus medius TrPs often was associated with TrPs in the quadratus lumborum muscle.

Other Associations

Conversely, TrPs can develop in the quadratus lumborum as a consequence of TrPs in other muscles. Jull and Janda[75] noted that the quadratus lumborum is subject to overload when used to substitute for weak hip abductors in walking. Active TrPs in the gluteus medius and gluteus minimus muscles are one of many causes of such weakness.

Lewit[96] related blockage of motion at the thoracolumbar junction to TrPs in the iliopsoas, erector spinae, quadratus lumborum, and abdominal muscles. The importance of articular dysfunction as a perpetuating factor for TrPs in these muscles is relatively unexplored and promises to be a fertile area for investigation. On the other hand, TrP tension in these muscles can reinforce

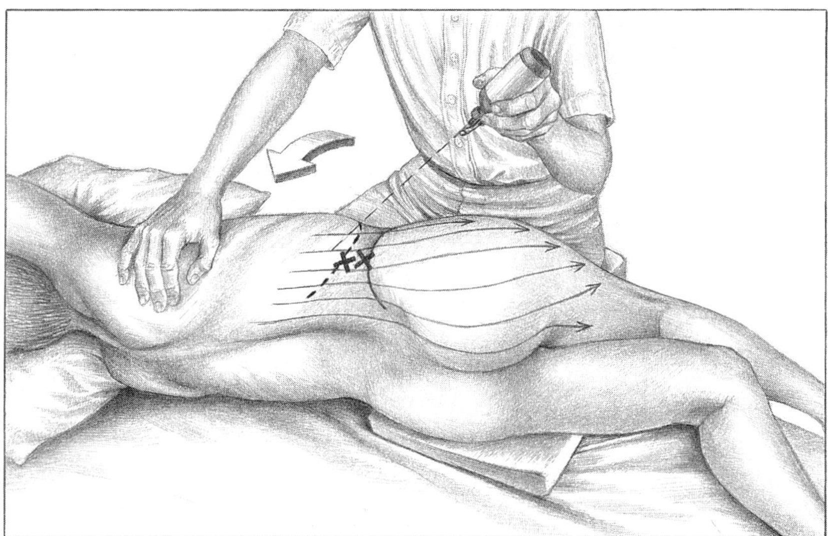

Figure 4.26. Intermittent cold with stretch of the right quadratus lumborum muscle, clinician seated. The uppermost lower limb (treated side) is swung forward. The *dashed line* marks the lower margin of the rib cage and the curved *solid line*, the crest of the ilium. Frequent sites of trigger points in this muscle are marked by **X**s. Parallel sweeps of the ice or vapocoolant spray (*thin arrows*) cover the muscle and its pain reference zones. The patient allows the uppermost thigh and leg to hang free in response to the pull of gravity, which takes up the slack as tension in the muscle releases. The operator exerts gentle pressure upward and backward against the chest (*thick arrow*) to adjust tension on the muscle and produce passive stretch. The ice or spray is also applied over all gluteal muscles, not only because the quadratus lumborum pain pattern overlaps the gluteal patterns, but also because the gluteal muscles often harbor satellite trigger points and are also stretched in this position. The foam rubber pad was added under the hip to relieve pressure on this patient's tender left greater trochanter. Positioning is better with a pillow placed as shown in Figure 4.28.

blockage of vertebral mobility at the thoracolumbar junction.

12. INTERMITTENT COLD WITH STRETCH
(Figs. 4.26–4.28)

This section first considers the use of intermittent cold with stretch for the inactivation of TrPs in the quadratus lumborum muscle. It then notes some other noninvasive methods that may be effective. Regardless of which technique is employed, the therapist should also consider the possibility of, and treat, joint dysfunction present in the thoracolumbar junction, the lumbar spine, and the pelvis. Tightness of the quadratus lumborum may also be associated with tightness of intercostal muscles that restricts excursion of the 12th rib.

The use of ice for applying intermittent cold with stretch is explained on page 9 of this volume and the use of vapocoolant with stretch is detailed on pages 67–74 of Volume 1.[148] Techniques that augment relaxation and stretch are reviewed on page 11 of this volume.

Release of myofascial TrPs in the quadratus lumborum muscle is complicated by its three different fiber directions and attachments. All fibers are stretched to some extent by the separation of the iliac crest from the 12th rib in the examination position (Fig. 4.24). The longitudinal iliocostal fibers and the diagonal deep iliolumbar fibers are most effectively elongated when this position is modified by placing the lower limb on the involved side forward while the torso on that side rotates backward (Fig. 4.26). When this position is used, the icing or spray pattern includes the gluteal muscles as well (Fig. 4.26), since they may have developed satellite TrPs and are also being passively stretched.

The lumbocostal fibers pass diagonally across the iliolumbar fibers and for elongation require trunk rotation in the oppo-

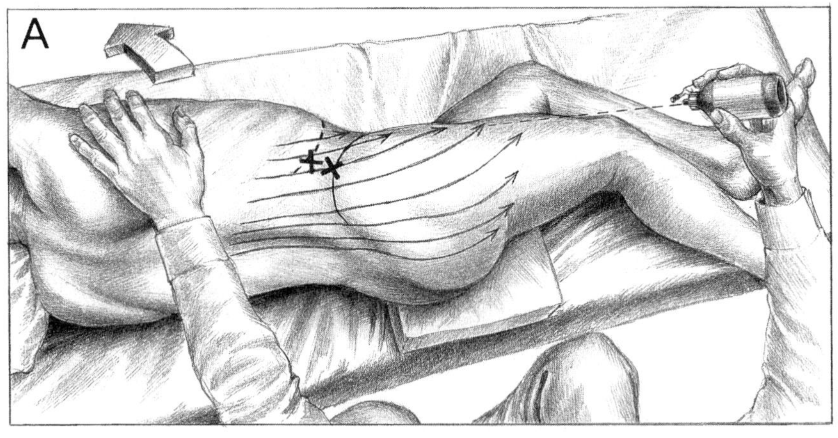

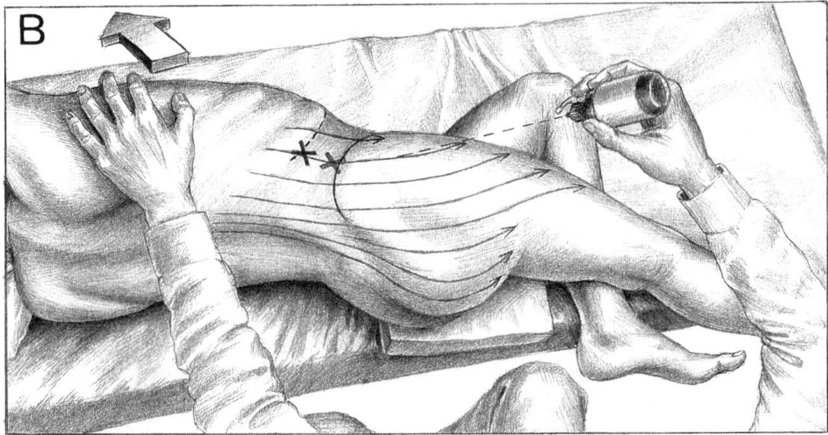

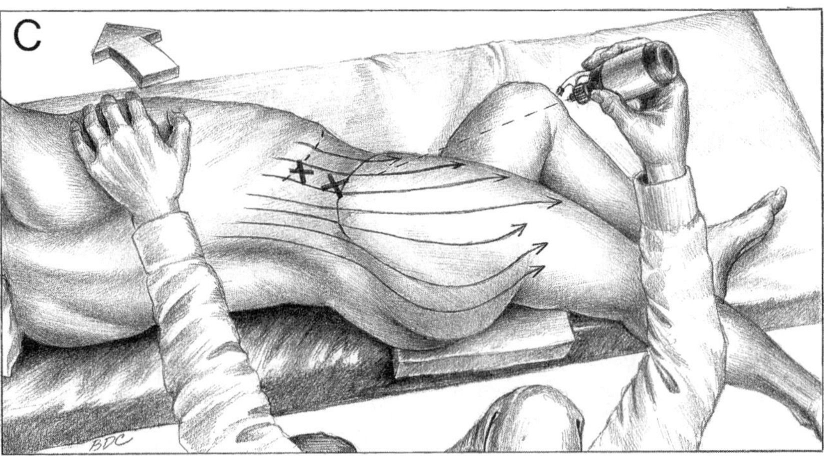

Figure 4.27. Intermittent cold with stretch of the right quadratus lumborum muscle, clinician seated. The uppermost lower limb (involved right side) is placed behind the other limb. Ice or spray patterns (*thin arrows*) cover the muscle and the distribution of pain referred from its trigger points (***X**s*). Three progressive stretch positions are shown. In all positions, the operator exerts pressure on the chest upward and forward, as indicated by the *thick arrows*. *A*, starting position in patients with severe involvement of the muscle. The right knee and leg (treatment side) rest on the table, and the uppermost arm is elevated in front of the head. *B*, increased stretch with the right thigh resting on the left leg to increase adduction at the hip and to enhance the downward pull on the pelvis. *C*, full stretch with no support under the right knee. The clinician hand pressure elevates the rib cage and increases the stretch on the quadratus lumborum muscle. If there is no hip dysfunction, the right lower limb hanging over the edge of the table may be pressed gently distalward to ensure taking up all the slack by further pulling the pelvis away from the 12th rib on that side. An intermittent cold pattern not shown here, *see* Figure 4.28*B*, also covers the skin representation of the iliopsoas muscle next to the midline over the abdomen. The foam rubber pad was placed under the hip to relieve pressure on the patient's tender greater trochanter. Positioning is better with a pillow placed as shown in Figure 4.28.

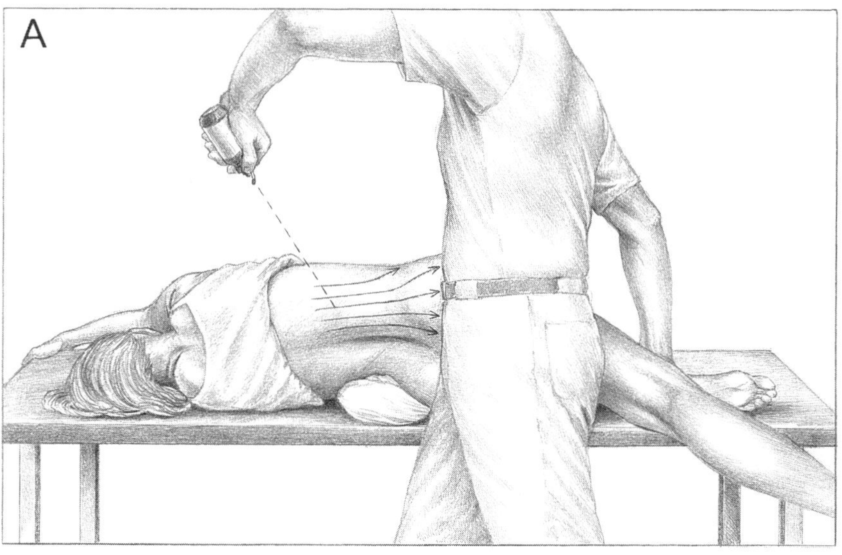

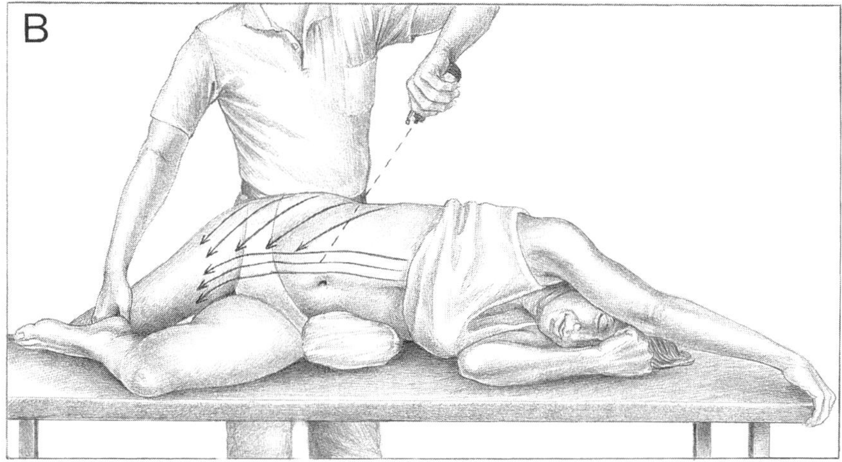

Figure 4.28. Intermittent cold with stretch of the right quadratus lumborum muscle, clinician standing. The lower limb on the involved right side is uppermost and extends behind the left lower limb. Ice or spray is applied in unidirectional parallel sweeps as indicated by the *arrows*. The patient anchors the rib cage in an elevated position by raising the arm and grasping the head of the treatment table. The pillow underneath the lumbar region helps position the muscle properly. *A*, rear view. The clinician at first holds the weight of the lower limb on the involved side to prevent painful stretch of the taut quadratus lumborum muscle. The hips of the clinician block the patient's buttocks from rolling backward over the edge of the table. *B*, front view. After a few initial applications of intermittent cold, the thigh is gradually lowered until the operator releases it to the pull of gravity. The diagonal sweeps of ice or spray extend over the lateral abdomen, hip, and groin to cover the quadratus lumborum referred pain zones. This view also shows the downward parallel sweeps applied next to the midline of the abdomen to cover the iliopsoas muscle's skin representation, which is not the same as its referred pain pattern.

site direction. To obtain rotation, the uppermost lower limb is placed behind the other limb (Figs. 4.27 and 4.28), rotating the hip on the involved side backward, while the shoulder on that side is rotated forward. This position also lengthens the iliopsoas muscle; therefore, the intermittent icing or spray pattern should include its skin representation over the abdomen (Fig. 4.28*B*).

To ensure the inactivation of TrPs in all three portions of the muscle, the patient should be treated in both positions, lower limb forward and lower limb back.

Care must be taken *not* to cause pain by forcibly stretching the muscle, but only to take up slack that has developed in response to the application of intermittent cold (and other release procedures, such as postisometric relaxation).

If the patient experiences pain when reaching overhead to grasp the head of the table, the problem is often caused by TrPs in the latissimus dorsi muscle. In this case, the restricting latissimus dorsi TrPs must be inactivated and the muscular tension released. Often this can be achieved by simply applying several parallel sweeps of ice or spray from the crest of the ilium to the upper arm along the course of the muscle fibers, while the arm is fully flexed at the shoulder. Further details on how to perform this spray-and-stretch procedure, or how to inject TrPs in the latissimus dorsi muscle, are covered in Volume 1.[157] A few sweeps of ice or vapocoolant spray combined with gentle passive stretch of the latissimus dorsi (*see* Fig. 24.4, page 399, Volume 1[148]) are useful to minimize the likelihood of recurrence, since the latissimus dorsi is part of the same functional unit as the quadratus lumborum.

The clinician can perform intermittent cold with stretch while seated, if the treatment table is low enough, or while standing, when the treatment table is the usual height. The dynamics of exerting pressure to take up the slack in the muscle is different in these two approaches.

When the clinician is seated, as in Figures 4.26 and 4.27, one end of the quadratus lumborum is anchored by having the uppermost lower limb (the limb on the side of the involved muscle) positioned as far forward (Fig. 4.26) or as far back (Fig. 4.27) as necessary to take up slack in the muscle. When the limb-forward position of the patient is used, the patient lies close to the edge of the table facing the clinician. The clinician then exerts pressure on the thorax to elevate it and rotate the chest cage away from the hip far enough to take up any additional slack that develops in response to treatment. As the muscle lengthens, excessive twisting of the trunk is avoided by successively repositioning the uppermost foot to hang farther over the edge of the table for the lower-limb-forward position (Fig. 4.26) or as shown in Figure 4.27*A*, *B*, and *C* for the lower-limb-behind position. With each repositioning, the torso is reset to a neutral position.

When the clinician is standing, the reverse strategy is used. The quadratus lumborum is anchored by having the patient reach overhead and grasp the head of the table (Fig. 4.28); slack is taken up by moving the crest of the uppermost ilium away from the 12th rib. At first, the clinician holds the thigh of that lower limb while carrying most of its weight, and then gradually lowers the limb until it can comfortably hang free against the pull of gravity. (This positioning for spraying and stretching the quadratus lumborum was described in detail by Nielsen.[111])

When the clinician stands, it is important to use the body at all times to block the patient from rolling off the table and to provide support that encourages full relaxation. When the lower limb is in the posterior position, it is helpful to use body contact against the patient's uppermost hip to control extension of the spine, which is sometimes painful. At the same time, gentle traction can be applied on the ilium, pulling it down away from the thorax. This helps lengthen the quadratus lumborum muscle.

The following two-person technique for applying intermittent cold with stretch has been found to be very effective clinically.[102]

The patient sits on the edge of the plinth with full thigh on the table and with the feet supported on a stool. *(a)* The therapist stands behind the patient, places a towel around the patient's body at the anterior superior iliac spine level, and uses the towel to support the patient. The therapist uses ice or vapocoolant for intermittent cold of the skin over the entire erector spinae as well as the quadratus lumborum. *(b)* While the assistant stands in front of the patient and gradually helps the patient bend forward, the patient uses the breathing technique with long slow exhalation to allow as much *forward bending* as possible. *(c)* The assistant then sits beside the patient and places his or her adjacent leg over the patient's thigh to stabilize the pelvis. A towel is placed around the patient's body at the anterior superior iliac spine level; the assistant uses the towel to hold the patient's weight as the therapist *side bends* the patient away from the assistant. The patient again slowly exhales to improve relaxation and passive stretch. The patient places the arm overhead when side bending in order to elevate the ribs for a full stretch of the muscle. *(d)* The side-bending stretch is repeated with a *slight turn* backward then forward in order to stretch multifidi, iliocostalis, and diagonal quadratus lumborum fibers. *(e)* The other side is then treated as in steps *(c)* and *(d)*. *(f)* The assistant stands in front of the patient and stabilizes the patient's pelvis at the anterior superior iliac spines. The therapist stands behind the patient and assists the patient in *trunk rotation* with the hips stabilized. This trunk rotation can be accomplished at various levels (thoracic and lumbar) by changing therapist hand placement for stabilization.

Following intermittent cold with stretch, the supine patient should perform a full active range of motion by alternate hip hiking (*see* Fig. 4.34). This is followed promptly by application of a moist heating pad or hot pack on the cooled skin over the quadratus lumborum muscle.

The paired quadratus lumborum muscles work as a team to control lateral angulation of the lumbar spine. Therefore, after the quadratus lumborum on one side is released, the pain is likely to shift to the other side, days or months later, because untreated latent TrPs in the contralateral muscle have now become active TrP sources of pain. For that reason, it is wise to inactivate bilateral quadratus lumborum TrPs routinely. If this is not done, at least the patient should be warned that pain may develop on the other (untreated) side.

When treatment of the quadratus lumborum has been completed, the operator should have the patient lie supine on the examining table and examine the femoral triangle for iliopsoas tenderness. If found, more complete and lasting pain relief will be ensured if that muscle is also released by intermittent cold with stretch, as described in the next chapter, page 102.

Other Non-invasive Treatments

Lange[83] reported the successful treatment of pain-producing, tender, hard places (*Myogeloses*) in the quadratus lumborum muscles of several patients by repeated forceful **massage** treatments continuing for as long as 6 weeks.

The first author has, on many occasions, inactivated quadratus lumborum TrPs by striking the area of tenderness with a **percussion hammer**, using approximately the same force ordinarily used in testing a tendon jerk. Eight to ten taps are administered to each tender area at the rate of no more than one per second. It is important that the patient is positioned so that the muscle is relaxed, but has no slack. This can be done with the patient seated, and leaning sideways away from the muscle to be stretched, while the body weight is supported on an armrest so that the muscle is not contracting against gravity. This apparently simple technique can be remarkably effective.

Postisometric relaxation with reflex augmentation is especially effective for this muscle. The procedure, described and illustrated by Lewit,[94,96] has the patient stand with feet apart, bending sideways away from the muscle to be released. The patient looks up with the eyes only, and takes in a full slow breath. During inhalation, the quadratus lumborum automatically contracts, slightly raising the trunk. Then while breathing out slowly and looking down, the patient concentrates on relaxing the tight muscles in the waist area as the pull of gravity increases the degree of side bending by gently taking up the slack.

The second author finds that the component part of the quadratus lumborum muscle being stretched by the Lewit technique is highly dependent on the combination of forward bending and side bending employed. All restricted directions must be released. It is important to have the patient concentrate on allowing the arms to hang loosely in order to achieve maximum relaxation. Before performing this procedure, the patient should have practiced successfully a method of returning to the upright posture that does not strain the extensor muscles of the low back. This may be done by holding a nearby table for support, by pushing up with the hands against the knees and thighs to straighten the trunk, or by bending the knees while straightening the

PART 1

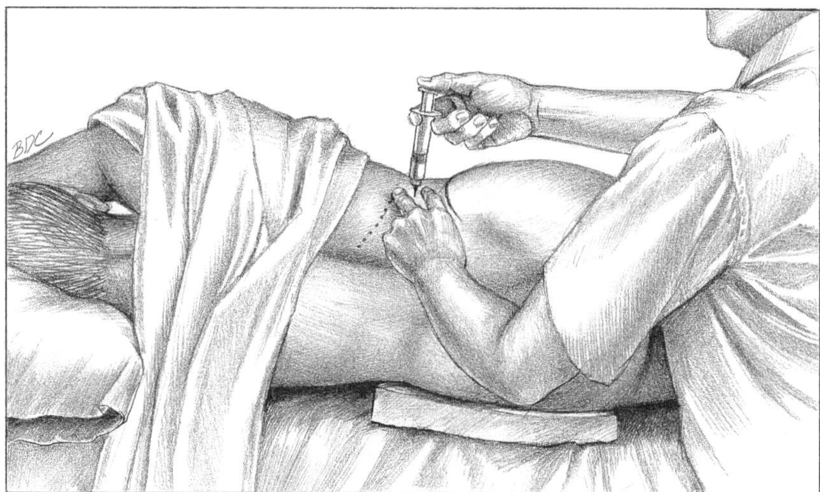

Figure 4.29. Injection of a deep trigger point high in the right quadratus lumborum muscle. The patient's legs are positioned as illustrated in Figure 4.22*C* to take up any slack in the muscle. The *solid line locates* the iliac crest; the *dotted line* marks the lower edge of the 12th rib. The needle is inserted just caudal to the 12th rib and anterior to the paraspinal muscle mass; it is directed parallel to the plane of the back (in the frontal plane) toward the L_2 and L_3 transverse processes. Caution: One must not direct the needle cephalad beyond the L_1 transverse process, since it could then penetrate the diaphragm and pleura and cause a pneumothorax, a serious complication. The foam rubber pad was added under the patient's hip to relieve pressure on a tender greater trochanter. Positioning is better with a lumbar pillow placed as illustrated in Figures 4.22*C* and 4.28.

trunk, and then, after the trunk is erect, straightening the knees. This last maneuver initially swings the hips down under the lumbar spine rather than using the lumbar extensors to lift the trunk over the hips, as occurs when one simply straightens up from a stooped position.

The "**chair twist**," described by Saudek[121] can be used as a seated lengthening technique for the quadratus lumborum. The subject leans forward at the hips and rotates the spine in a controlled movement, stretching the lateral musculature of the lumbar spine. The stretch is held 30–60 seconds on each side.

13. INJECTION AND STRETCH
(Figs. 4.29 and 4.30)

The procedure for TrP injection and stretch of any muscle appears in Volume 1.[149] Injection of TrPs in the quadratus lumborum muscle is performed with the patient in the same position that is used for examination (Fig. 4.22). Injection of TrPs in different portions of the muscle requires two different techniques, one for TrPs in those iliocostal fibers that are superficial, and another for the remaining deep TrPs.

When TrPs are localized by flat palpation in a palpable taut band of the more anterior fibers of the iliocostal portion of the quadratus lumborum (second region described previously in Section 9), near the crest of the ilium, they are injected in the same manner as other superficial TrPs, under palpatory control.[149]

When injecting the deeper TrPs that are identifiable only by deep pressure (as described previously for regions one and three in Section 9), the plane of the back in the lumbar region should be perpendicular to the treatment table. The direction of pressure that elicits pain characteristic of TrPs must be noted carefully.

The essentials of this deep injection procedure for TrPs in the quadratus lumborum muscle are illustrated in Figures 4.29 and 4.30. The lateral edge of the iliocostalis, which marks the edge of the paraspinal muscle mass, is identified and the direction to approach the spots of tenderness is confirmed. Two fingers of the examining hand span the area where pressure localized the deep tenderness, and the skin is cleansed with antiseptic.

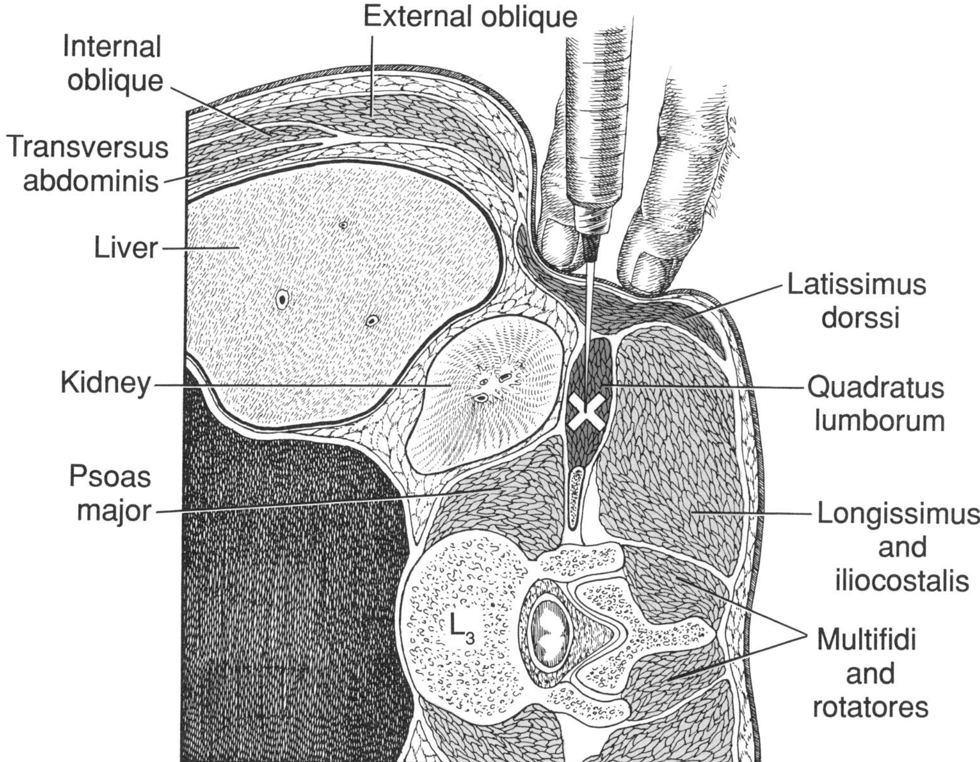

Figure 4.30. Technique for injection of a trigger point (***X***) in the quadratus lumborum muscle (*dark red*) as seen in cross section (patient side lying). The compressed latissimus dorsi muscle, through which the needle usually must pass, is *medium red*, and the other neighboring muscles are *light red*. The cross section passes through the body of the L_3 vertebra.

Pressure is applied to depress the skin over the quadratus lumborum muscle. A 62-mm to 87-mm (2½- to 3½-in) 22-gauge hypodermic needle is aimed essentially straight downward toward the tender spot, in the direction of a transverse process, and 0.5–1.0 mL of 0.5% procaine solution is injected when the patient reports pain. Often, increased resistance to needle penetration is felt at the time of the patient's pain reaction.

Penetration of a TrP in this muscle usually elicits a strong pain response (jump sign) of the patient. Local twitch responses are difficult to detect in these deep fibers. The muscle is explored with the needle for TrP tenderness by successive partial withdrawals and reinsertions, probing down to the transverse processes. Inserting the needle at the iliolumbar angle (first region described previously in Section 9) permits injection near the attachments of the muscle to the L_4 transverse process and along the iliolumbar ligament. Insertion of the needle at the lumbocostal angle (third region described previously in Section 9) permits injection near the L_2 and L_3 transverse processes. Injection cephalad of the L_1 transverse process should be avoided, but, if attempted, must be undertaken with *great care*. The quadratus lumborum and diaphragm both attach to the 12th rib,[13] and a pneumothorax will develop if the needle penetrates the diaphragm and pleura.

Injection is followed by full active range of motion of the muscle and application of a moist hot pack or heating pad over the muscle. The patient should be warned of possible postinjection soreness on the following day or two and should avoid any demanding muscular activities for at least 24 hours.

The needle must be long enough to reach to the tip of a transverse process, since the TrPs in this muscle are found at that depth. Some of the needle shaft must always be left extending *outside the skin*.

Otherwise, if the needle is inserted fully to its hub and the patient sneezes or lateral pressure is accidentally exerted on the syringe, the needle could snap at the hub and disappear under the skin with no way of recovering it short of a challenging surgical procedure.

When a needle encounters a transverse process, the tip of the needle may be bent, producing a fishhook effect. To avoid injury to the muscle, if any "scratchiness" is felt as the needle is moved in and out through the muscle, the needle should immediately be withdrawn and replaced.

Sola[134] recommended injection of quadratus lumborum TrPs along the lateral border of the muscle and at the attachments of the iliolumbar fibers to the transverse processes of the lumbar vertebrae. Baker[2] reported a patient with back pain for 4 years that was unresponsive to chymopapain injection and who required a TENS unit for pain control. Injection of quadratus lumborum TrPs provided pain relief and restored function.

When there is a poor response or no response of the TrPs to injection therapy, or if the TrPs soon recur, the clinician should look for uncorrected mechanical factors described in Section 8. The patient may also have systemic perpetuating factors, such as vitamin and other nutritional inadequacies, metabolic disorders, chronic infection, active allergies with a high histamine level, and overwhelming emotional stress.[147,151]

14. CORRECTIVE ACTIONS
(Figs. 4.31–4.34)

This section first reviews the correction of skeletal inadequacies, such as an LLLI, small hemipelvis, and short upper arms. It then identifies correctable postural errors, especially those present during sleep, and presents a summary of corrective activities. Finally, it presents corrective exercises helpful in restoring normal quadratus lumborum function.

When major weight-bearing and postural muscles develop TrPs, the patients' understanding of muscles can determine the outcome. They must learn to use, but not abuse, their muscles. It often is not possible to continue the habits and activities of one's youth. The challenge is to learn how to do what one needs and wants to do, in new ways that do not exceed the tolerance or stamina of the muscles.

Corrective Body Mechanics

This subsection considers the mechanical perpetuating factors that are particularly important to the quadratus lumborum muscle. (Systemic factors may be just as important or more so; they are covered in Chapter 4 of Volume 1.[155]) Initially, this subsection deals with skeletal asymmetries or variations that can cause quadratus lumborum overload. Emphasis is placed on LLLI, a small hemipelvis, and short upper arms.

Any problem in foot mechanics, such as pronation of the foot and ankle, that produces an asymmetrical gait may contribute to selective muscular overload,[10] including overuse of the quadratus lumborum. Appropriate corrective shoes are indicated.

Asymmetries that produce a painful functional (compensatory) scoliosis which depends on muscular contraction to maintain it, should be corrected in patients with a persistent quadratus lumborum myofascial syndrome. If appropriate examination has identified a pelvic asymmetry (*see* Section 8), an effort should be made to level the sacral base. A technique for correcting sacroiliac displacement is described in Chapter 2.

Any existing lower limb dysfunction, as well as any pelvic torsion and lumbar joint dysfunction, must be corrected to ensure that treatment of quadratus lumborum TrPs will be lasting.

Lower Limb-length Inequality

The correction of LLLI is summarized in Volume 1.[153] Here we review briefly when and why to correct LLLI, how much to correct, the influence of age on the response to correction, and how to make the correction.

The question is often asked, "Why can some people have a difference in leg length without symptoms while others with the same difference have pain and require correction?" By itself, the LLLI simply makes selected muscles work harder to compensate for the asymmetry.

When the muscles are free of TrPs, the additional stress imposed on them by the LLLI is within their tolerance. However, when the person experiences a sudden overload that initiates TrPs in the quadratus lumborum, the LLLI then becomes a perpetuating factor for those TrPs; the LLLI has taken on a totally new significance and requires correction.

When and Why to Correct. From the point of view of a myofascial pain syndrome, LLLI requires correction if two conditions are met. First, the LLLI must produce an asymmetry that requires sustained or unbalanced muscular effort to correct it. Second, the overloaded muscle must harbor TrPs, or be especially vulnerable to developing them. For reasons reviewed in Section 8, the quadratus lumborum is the muscle most likely to be overloaded by LLLI. Several authors have specifically recommended correction of LLLI for sustained relief of quadratus lumborum TrPs.[105,111,147] Correction of the LLLI often makes the difference between lasting relief and chronic suffering for patients with low back pain caused by TrPs in the quadratus lumborum muscle. (Another reason for correcting large length differences is to reduce the likelihood of developing osteoarthritis of the hip joint on the side of the longer limb,[32,40,50,142] and of the lumbar spine.[38,40,46]) However, as a rule, one must avoid making LLLI corrections that exaggerate existing spinal asymmetry and that increase the load on the muscles.[32,67,105]

In a simple situation where inclination of the sacral base corresponds to the LLLI and the lumbar spine is convex toward the shorter limb (Fig. 4.18*B*), a shoe lift that corrects the limb length inequality straightens the spine and unloads lumbar muscular strain.[38,57,67,105] However, when the lumbar scoliosis is fixed and not compensatory, the same correction displaces the upper lumbar spine (base of the thoracic spine) farther away from the midline and aggravates the asymmetry (Fig. 4.16).

If a fixed angulation at the lumbosacral junction compensates for LLLI (Fig. 4.18*F*) and straightens the spine, correction of the LLLI with a lift should not be made because it induces a compensatory lumbar scoliosis that substitutes one asymmetry for another and may cause more muscle strain, not less. Lower limb dysfunction and lumbopelvic mechanics must be normalized *prior* to adding a lift.

How Much LLLI is Significant. In our experience and that of Friberg,[38] corrections of as little as 3 mm (⅛ in) can be of significant benefit to patients with low back or hip pain and quadratus lumborum TrPs. Many studies indicate that a difference of 10 mm (⅜ in) is functionally significant.

Heufelder[67] recommended correction only if the difference is at least 10 mm (⅜ in); this value has often been used as the criterion of a clinically significant difference by those measuring LLLI radiographically (Table 4.1). If an insensitive or unreliable clinical measurement technique is employed, it is not possible to evaluate this small a difference in limb length.

Response to Correction. Several authors have made the clinical observation in older patients that what appeared to have started as a compensatory scoliosis had become fixed, and the spine showed osteoarthritic changes. Does this mean that older patients may be less responsive to (and therefore receive less benefit from) lift therapy? It would appear that there is a large individual difference with regard to this response among older patients and that they warrant a therapeutic trial of lift therapy.

In a study of 50 patients, Giles and Taylor[45] found the spinal columns of younger patients much more responsive to lift therapy than those of older patients. Scoliosis of patients in their third decade decreased 6°; in the 4th and 5th decades, it decreased 4°; in those patients over 50 years of age, scoliosis decreased only 1°. However, in a study of 288 consecutive low back pain patients ranging in age from 14–76 years (mean 45.6 years), Friberg[38] found that patients with large LLLI improved with lift therapy, despite a relatively large number of older patients.

How to Correct. We recommend full correction of LLLI. The amount of correction needed is most accurately determined by standing radiography, which was discussed in detail in Section 8 of this chapter. The clinical evaluation is described in detail on pages 107–108, Volume 1[148] and is summarized and illustrated on pages 45–51 of this chapter. The

PART 1

appropriate correction is that number of pages of a magazine or a calibrated lift,[142] which, adjusted by trial and error, eliminates asymmetry and muscle strain. Figures 4.14 and 4.15 illustrate the effects of correction on an "S" curve and a "C" curve scoliosis, respectively. Figure 4.19 diagrams the muscular implications of these two curves. The patient's feeling or sensation of symmetry and balance is an invaluable source of information. When asked, many patients can identify a 1-mm (<1/16-in) overcorrection as feeling unnatural or strained, as compared with an exact correction. Therefore, with a heel lift, special care is taken to avoid overcorrection.

The maximum amount of correction that should be attempted is not known. Delacerda and Wikoff[18] found that despite the weight imbalance imposed by a 32-mm (1⅓-in) lift, the restoration of skeletal symmetry improved kinetics of ambulation and reduced oxygen consumption.

For a small correction, a heel lift can be added as a felt-pad inserted inside the shoe of the shorter limb, or a shoe repairman can add the lift to the bottom of the heel of the shoe on the short side. Large heel inserts tend to push the patient's heel out of the shoe and felt inserts become compacted in time, losing their effectiveness. Even with only a moderate-sized correction, the result is better if half the correction is added to the heel of the shoe on the shorter side and a like amount removed from the shoe heel on the longer side.[65] We agree with others[65] that generally a heel lift of 13 mm (½ in) or more requires addition of a full *sole* lift as well. Adding the sole lift for lesser corrections adds an unnecessary asymmetrical weight that tends to alter balance.

Patient education is an essential part of this corrective therapy. If the patient is not *convinced* that there is LLLI and that its correction makes a difference, compliance will be poor. Placing the correction under the longer limb (Figs. 4.14*C* and 4.15*C*) regularly evokes an unequivocal negative reaction of the patient and emphasizes to both the patient and the clinician the importance of correcting the LLLI. By having patients observe in a mirror the difference in asymmetry without correction, with correction, and with a counter-correction under the long limb, they can see and feel for themselves the importance of the correct lift.

Even when patients thoroughly understand the need for the correction and have their footwear corrected, they are likely to forget to correct a new pair of shoes, especially after they have been symptom-free for a considerable period of time. When their symptoms return, they must be reminded to correct their new shoes and to report in a week or two whether that solves the problem.

When riding horseback, persons with LLLI are likely to have learned for themselves that they can improve balance and feel more comfortable by shortening the stirrup on the side of their shorter lower limb.

Small Hemipelvis and Short Upper Arms

The correction of a hemipelvis that is small in the *vertical* direction is described in Volume 1.[152] Essentially the same procedure as that described previously for LLLI correction is applied to patients while they are seated on a firm flat surface. A correction that is adequate on a hard unyielding surface must be increased (may need to be doubled) on a soft cushioned seat to provide the same amount of correction for elimination of pelvic tilt, scoliosis, and muscle strain. Patients learn to carry a small magazine or covered plastic foam sponge wherever they go to place under the buttock (ischial tuberosity) on the small side. A similar correction is obtained by sliding the small side of the pelvis toward the upcurved edge of a bucket seat or toward the center of a domed seat. The patient must learn to discriminate correct and incorrect positions of the pelvis by becoming aware of the way the muscles feel in each position.

A small hemipelvis in the *anteroposterior* direction is similarly corrected with the patient supine, by a lift inserted under the buttock on the small side to level the pelvis. When the examiner is in doubt about this effect, moving the correction from the small side to the large side (Fig. 4.12*C*) accentuates the asymmetry, usually increases the pain, and leaves no doubt as to which side is smaller.

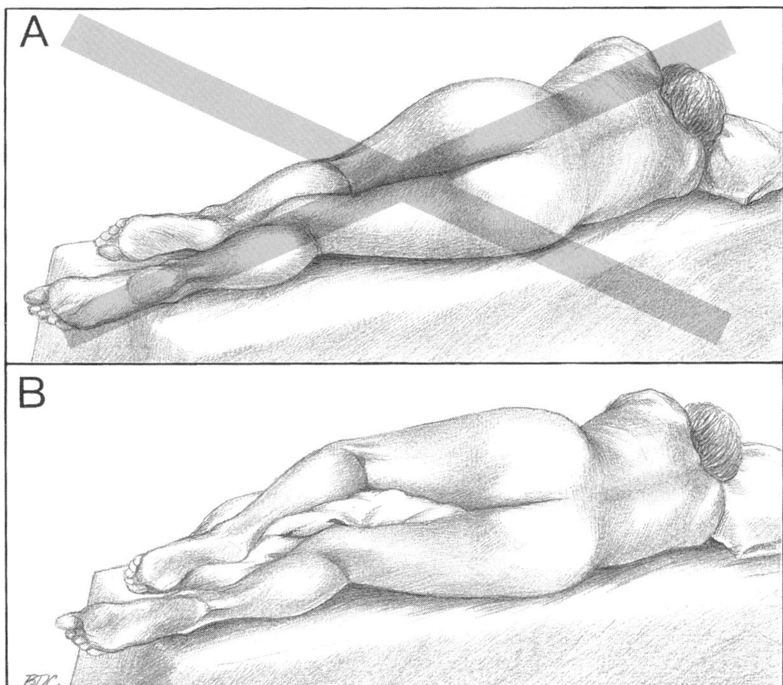

Figure 4.31. Correct side-lying posture during sleep is important to reduce irritability of quadratus lumborum trigger points. *A*, trouble-making posture (*red* ***X***) with the uppermost knee resting on the bed, causing downward tilt and forward rotation of the pelvis. This position is likely to place enough tension on the already taut quadratus lumborum fibers to evoke referred pain from their trigger points. *B*, desirable posture with uppermost hip partially flexed and the uppermost knee and leg supported on a pillow to hold the thigh horizontal. This position eliminates the troublesome pelvic and lumbar displacement.

The management of a chronic myofascial pain problem in the patient with short upper arms in relation to torso height is also covered in Volume 1.[154] When a person has short upper arms, the quadratus lumborum is placed in a shortened cramped position as the individual leans to one side to reach the armrest for elbow support (Fig. 4.13*D*). This lack of elbow support can be corrected by use of a chair with sloping armrests to provide support for arms of any length (Fig. 4.13*F*). Another approach is to adapt the chair to fit the patient by building up low flat armrests with covered plastic sponges. The armrest height to be added depends on the body structure of the patient. It can vary from 1–6 inches and must be sufficient to provide comfortable elbow support when the patient sits upright with the upper arms vertical and shoulders relaxed. When support for the arms is provided, sitting becomes a welcome new experience to people with this structural problem.

Corrective Posture and Activities (Figs. 4.31 and 4.32)

Corrective Posture

Sleeping conditions can have a profound influence on quadratus lumborum TrPs. A sagging hammocklike mattress puts the quadratus lumborum muscle in the shortened position when one lies on the opposite side. This source of aggravation is corrected by using a firm flat mattress or by placing several wooden boards ¾ inch thick longitudinally under the mattress. Each board should be 4–6 inches wide and extend nearly the length of the bed from head to foot, about 4 inches shorter than the bed at each end. The boards are readily transportable. One or two sheets of plywood cut to nearly cover the bed springs are simple and effective if portability is not an issue.

Sleeping flat on the back with knees straight places the quadratus lumborum in a relatively shortened position by causing the pelvis to tilt forward and lumbar lordosis to increase. This position can be avoided by placing a small pillow or other support under the knees, or by sleeping on one side. However, this flexed and rotated position on the side can cause the opposite problem by placing additional tension on the already taut quadratus lumborum (Fig. 4.31*A*) and can encourage further disc derangement if that already is a contributory factor.[103] A semifetal position can also cause uncomfortable tension on an irritable SI joint. These complications are avoided by placing a pillow between the knees and legs to support the uppermost lower limb, avoiding excessive flexion of the lower hip, as in Figure 4.31*B*. With a pillow appropriately placed, the lumbar spine can retain its normal curvature, protecting both the quadratus lumborum and the disc. (If the patient's problem is one of a posterior disc derangement, the preferred position is prone.)

Waterbeds tend to produce a hammock-like configuration that does not provide needed support and, therefore, may not be helpful to those who have problems with quadratus lumborum TrPs. Some recent waterbed designs employ tubes that correct this problem.

Corrective Activities

The combined flexion-rotation movement of bending forward and sideways to lift or pull something *must* be scrupulously avoided. This is a hazardous maneuver for anyone, but especially for the person with quadratus lumborum TrPs. One must turn the entire body to face the task squarely and then to perform a pure flexion-extension movement without twisting the trunk. When turning to reach behind, the patient must learn to keep the back erect, avoiding any trunk flexion during rotation. The use of an upright vacuum cleaner, rather than the low floor type, should be encouraged; the floor type favors bending over with a twisting pull to bring the unit to a new position. The worker should keep the back erect and face the vacuum cleaner, preferably with two hands on the handle, moving it straight in front and not holding it at one side.

Sustained flexion and forceful extension of the spine should be avoided. If the lower limb muscles and knees are free of problems, one can lift objects from the floor by bending the knees while keeping the torso erect. Unfortunately, people find this hard to do; not only does it require additional effort to lift the entire torso and hip regions instead of only the head, neck, and shoulders, but it also throws the load on the quadriceps femoris muscles, which, in this position, are at a mechanical disadvantage.[131] Squatting dorsiflexes the ankles and may thus be limited by a tight soleus muscle; in this case, an alternate method of reaching to the floor is illustrated in Figure 22.16.

Learning to avoid unnecessary stooping can play a critical role. The importance may not be so much in what is done, but in how it is done. One learns to make up a low bed while kneeling, rather than standing and stooping over to reach the bed. One can make up the bed by literally "walking" on the knees around it. Brushing the teeth is done while standing up straight and avoiding leaning over the sink, except to clear the mouth, while then supporting body weight with the free hand.

The muscular strain of a near fall, or injury from a fall is avoided by sitting down to put on socks, pantyhose, skirt or trousers, etc., or by leaning against a wall or heavy furniture so that balance is assured.

A common example of unnecessary forward leaning is the usual way of rising from a chair without arm support (Fig. 4.32*A*). When rising with the buttocks at the rear of the chair seat, the body is pitched forward in a stooped position to place the center of gravity over the feet. This heavily loads the extensor muscles of the back as the person straightens up.

The correct manner of rising from a chair in order to spare the back muscles is shown in Figure 4.32*B*. The buttocks are first slid forward to the front of the seat; then the body is turned sideways and one foot is placed under the front edge of the seat and under the center of gravity of the body. The body is then lifted with the torso *held erect* so that the load is placed mainly on the quadriceps femoris muscles. A push by the hands against the thighs assists the lift if the quadriceps muscles are weak.

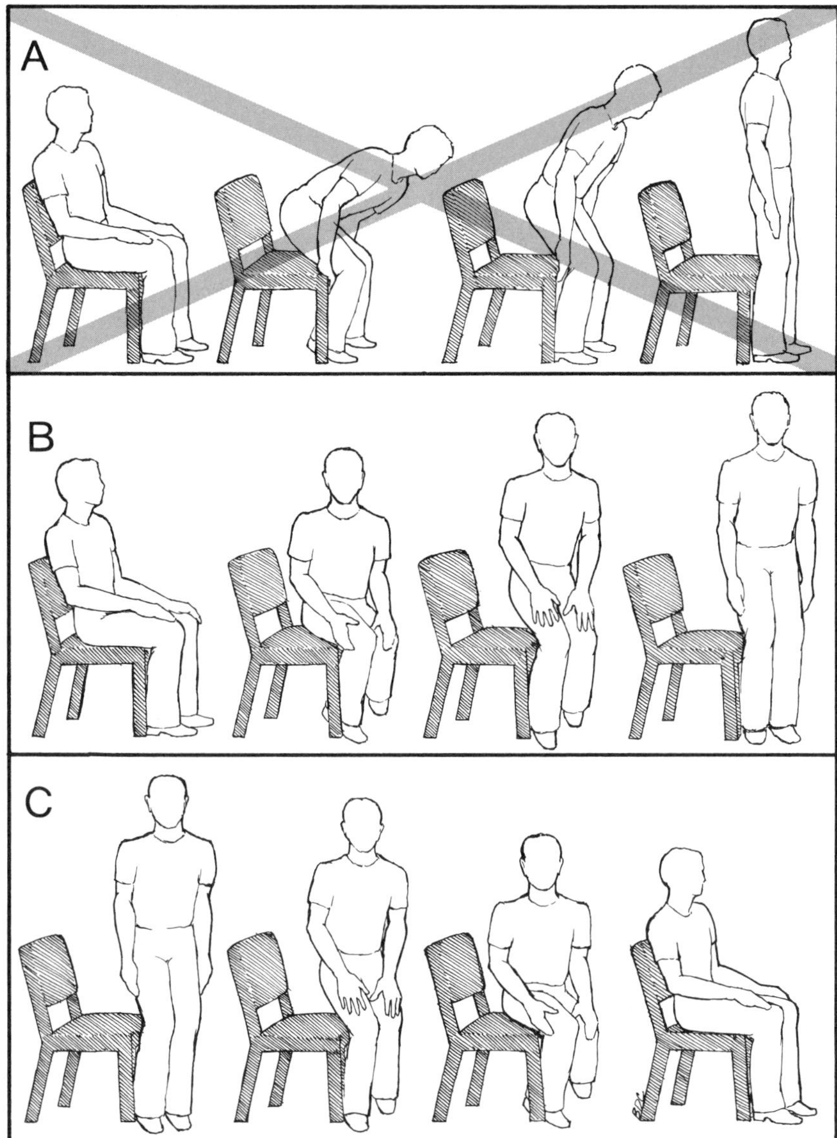

Figure 4.32. The Sit-to-stand and Stand-to-sit Techniques (reading from left to right) minimize strain on the neck and back muscles and on the intervertebral fibrocartilaginous discs while rising up from, or sitting down in a chair. *A*, back-threatening way (*red* **X**) of getting up from a chair by starting to rise with the buttocks at the rear of the seat. This sequence places the back in a strained "leaning-over" posture, with strain of the quadratus lumborum muscle. *B*, Sit-to-stand Technique with buttocks moved to the front of the seat and the body rotated at a 45° angle. This positioning permits one to keep the spine erect and with a normal lumbar lordosis throughout, between sitting and standing; it loads the hip and knee extensors instead of the thoracolumbar and cervical paraspinal and other extensor muscles. *C*, the reverse, Stand-to-sit Technique, is accomplished by first turning the body, by keeping the trunk erect while sitting down on the front of the seat, and then by sliding the buttocks backward, still keeping the spine erect.

Figure 4.32*C* shows the reverse sequence for sitting down in a way that spares the back muscles. The feet are positioned and the body angled 45° before lowering the body with the spine straight and with help from the hands on the thighs, if needed. After resting the body weight on the front of the chair seat, the person slides back in the chair to a normal sitting position.

The same principle applies to walking up stairs or climbing a ladder. If the body is turned 45° to one side, it is much easier to keep the back straight while ascending or descending.

Patients who enjoy gardening activities should sit on a low box or other seat that is 8–10 inches high while transplanting and weeding. This low seated position helps them to avoid bending over. In the house, small objects need to be placed on a chair or table rather than on the floor.

For persons who are good at horsemanship, horseback riding can be a desirable form of exercise even if they have a quadratus lumborum pain syndrome with pelvic asymmetry and/or LLLI. A small hemipelvis is compensated by sitting to one side of the sloped saddle to level the pelvis. The LLLI is compensated by shortening the stirrup on the side of the shorter limb.

For patients with LLLI, vacationing at the beach is a double hazard. The patient is likely to spend much time standing and walking with bare feet and LLLI uncorrected. Walking along a sloping shore in one direction exaggerates the LLLI; walking in the other direction may overcorrect it.

The patient with a persistent quadratus lumborum problem needs to learn how to slide and roll the hips rather than to lift them when turning over in bed at night.

Corrective Exercises
(Figs. 4.33 and 4.34)

The quadratus lumborum Supine Self-stretch Exercise (Fig. 4.33) is most effective for the diagonal iliolumbar fibers of that muscle. The exercise begins in the supine position with the hips and knees flexed (Fig. 4.33*A*). The thigh on the side of the quadratus lumborum to be stretched is adducted to the point of taking up all the slack in the muscle and the other leg is crossed over the thigh to provide resistance (Fig. 4.33*B*). The patient then relaxes and lets the pelvis on the involved side drop caudally. While the patient inhales slowly, the quadratus lumborum contracts isometrically when the patient gently and briefly attempts to abduct the thigh on the side to be stretched, against resistance provided by the other limb. During slow exhalation, the patient concentrates on relaxing ("letting go") the muscles to be elongated and uses the opposite limb to help pull the pelvis caudally by further adducting the thigh on the treatment side to take up all slack that develops (Fig. 4.33*C*). Contraction and relaxation are repeated slowly several times until no additional range of motion is achieved. Then, the patient slips the uppermost, assisting limb off the treated limb to help in pushing the latter back to the neutral position (Fig. 4.33*D*). This maneuver avoids overloading the elongated muscles while still under full stretch (a weak position). The stretch should be followed by active range of motion (hiking and lowering the hip several times).

Zohn[170] illustrates and describes four self-stretch exercises that the patient can use for the quadratus lumborum muscle. All of them primarily stretch the iliocostal fibers and not the diagonal fibers of the muscle. One stretch entails side bending while seated, another while standing. The third is performed with the patient lying on the affected side, resting on the elbow to elevate the shoulders and stretch the muscle on the underside. For the fourth stretch, the patient starts on hands and knees on the floor, hips rocked back on the heels, face down, arms stretched out overhead, and then adds side bending of the trunk.

Lewit[94–96] describes and illustrates a standing self-stretch for the quadratus lumborum with respiration augmentation, as summarized previously in Section 12 under Other Non-invasive Treatments.

The chair twist described by Saudek,[121] mentioned previously in Section 12, can be used as a seated quadratus lumborum self-stretch for the home or workplace.

Hip lowering and trunk flexion exercises are needed to maintain range of motion for the quadratus lumborum, which is a hip hiker and an extensor of the spine. The Hip-hike Exercise (Fig. 4.34) is most effective for the iliocostal fibers of the quadratus lumborum and is done initially in the supine position with the hips and knees straight. The exercise is performed alternately by first lowering one hip away from the shoulder while elevat-

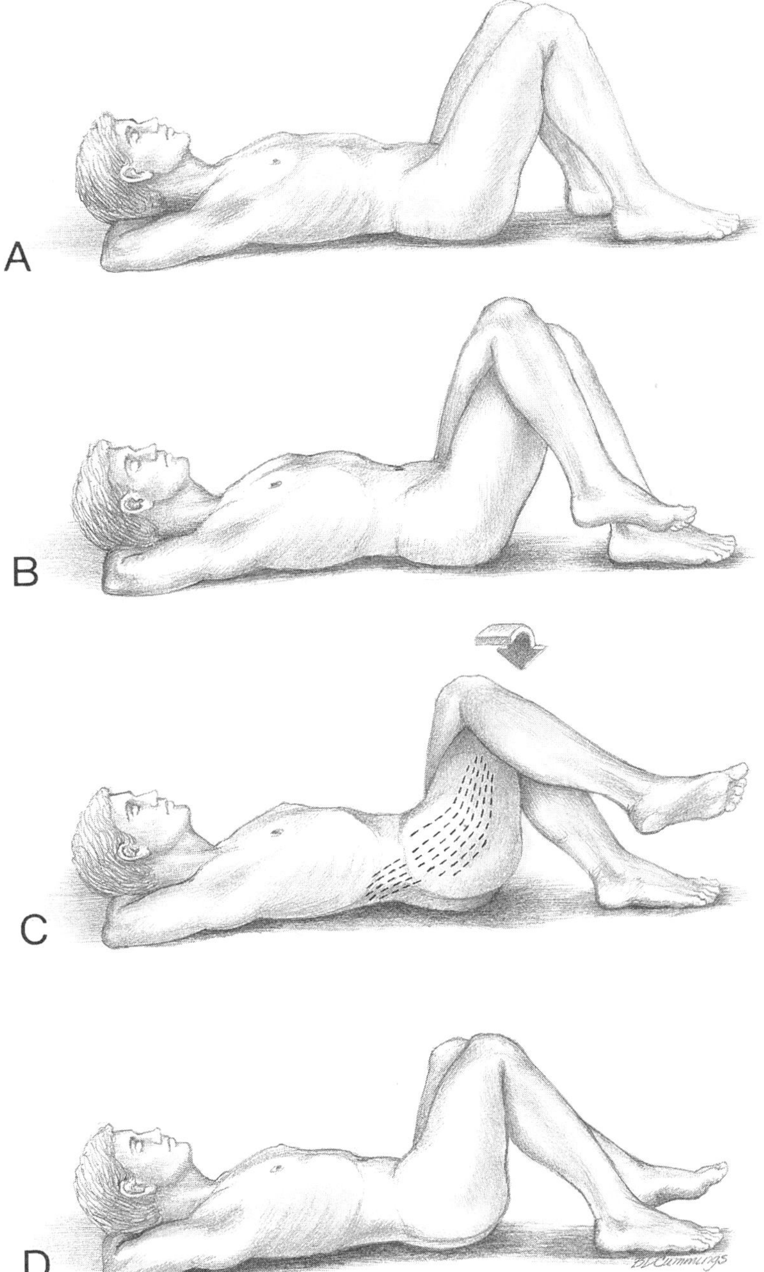

Figure 4.33. Supine Self-stretch Exercise for the right quadratus lumborum muscle. *A*, starting position, supine with the hips and knees bent. The hands are placed behind the head to elevate the rib cage. *B*, preparatory position with the controlling left leg crossed over the right thigh, the side to be stretched. After the right thigh has been adducted as far as it will go without resistance, during slow deep inhalation, the left leg is used to resist a gentle isometric abductive effort of the right thigh. *C*, as the patient slowly exhales and relaxes the right side, the left leg gently pulls the right thigh medially and downward, which rotates and pulls the right half of the pelvis caudad; this takes up slack in the quadratus lumborum and abductor fibers of the gluteal muscles (*dashed lines*). *Large arrow* indicates the direction of applied pressure. Steps *B* and *C* may be repeated until no further increase in range of motion is achieved. *D*, release of stretch by slipping the controlling (left) leg off the right knee, releasing tension and at the same time supporting the treated side. Hips and knees are then returned to the relaxed position, as in *A*.

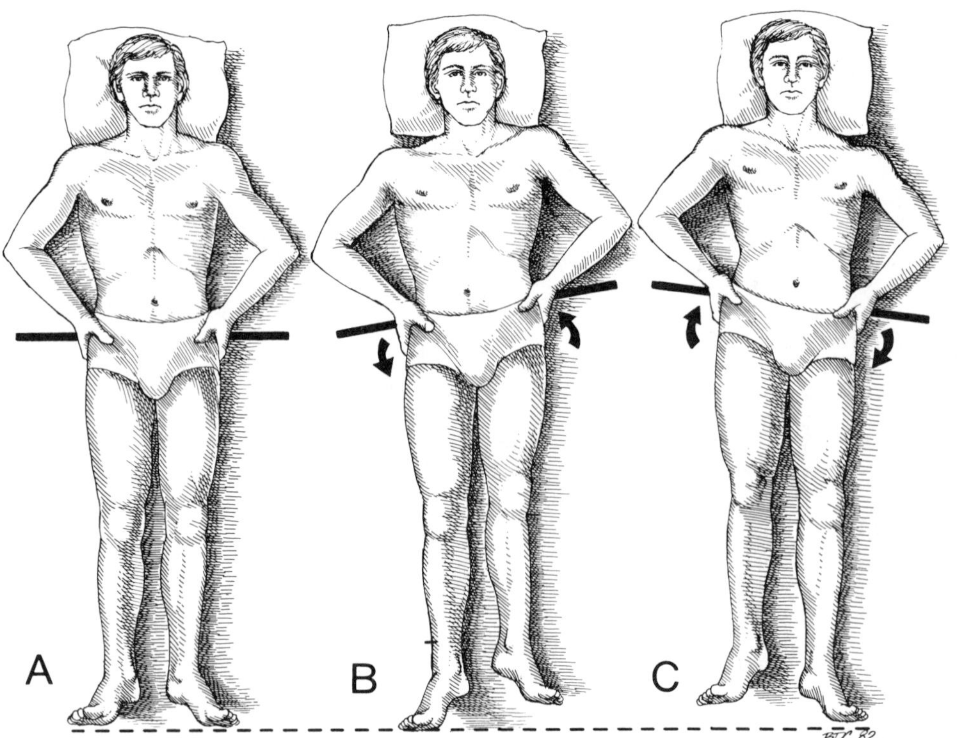

Figure 4.34. Hip-hike Exercise in the supine position to maintain active range of motion of the quadratus lumborum muscles. *A*, resting position. *B*, left hip-hike position, stretching the right quadratus lumborum. *C*, right hip-hike position, stretching the left quadratus lumborum. The patient then pauses, breathes, relaxes, and repeats the series.

ing the hip on the other side toward that shoulder, and then reversing sides. This tilting motion of the pelvis alternately stretches the quadratus lumborum on one side and then on the other side. This is more effective if done synchronously with slow respiration, breathing in while elevating the hip on the involved side and breathing out while lowering it. Additional active stretch of the quadratus lumborum occurs if the hips and knees are flexed as this exercise is performed.

A popular flexion exercise is the sit-up. However, patients frequently have weak abdominal muscles that require consideration. Since muscles exert more force with less effort during lengthening contractions than during shortening contractions, one starts with sit-backs, proceeds to abdominal curls, and finally to partial sit-ups with the knees bent to unload the iliopsoas muscle if it, too, is involved. These exercises are described and illustrated in Figure 49.11 of Volume 1.[161] One should follow a flexion exercise such as the sit-up with extension to protect the intervertebral disc.[103]

References

1. Baker BA: The muscle trigger: evidence of overload injury. *J Neurol Orthop Med Surg 7*:35–44, 1986.
2. Baker BA: Myofascial pain syndromes: Ten single muscle cases. *J Neurol Orthop Med Surg* 10:129–131, 1989.
3. Bardeen CR: The musculature, Sect. 5. In *Morris's Human Anatomy*, edited by C. M. Jackson, Ed. 6. Blakiston's Son & Co., Philadelphia, 1921 (p. 469).
4. Basmajian JV, Deluca CJ: *Muscles Alive*, Ed. 5. Williams & Wilkins, Baltimore, 1985 (pp. 385–387, 423).
5. Beal MC: A review of the short-leg problem. *J Am Osteopath Assoc 50*:109–121, 1950.
6. Beal MC: The short-leg problem. *J Am Osteopath Assoc 76*:745–751, 1977.
7. Beattie P, Isaacson K, Riddle DL, *et al*.: Validity of derived measurements of leg-length differences obtained by use of a tape measure. *Phys Ther 70*:150–157, 1990.
8. Bengert O: über die Bedeutung der Beinlängendifferenz. *Z Orthop 108*:435–445, 1970.

9. Bopp HM: Periarthrosis coxae oder Trochanterschmerz bei Beinlängedifferenzen? *Orthop Praxis 10*:261–263, 1971.
10. Botte RR: An interpretation of the pronation syndrome and foot types of patients with low back pain. *J Am Podiatr Assoc 71*:243–253, 1981.
11. Bourdillon JF, Day EA: *Spinal Manipulation*, Ed. 4. Appleton & Lange, Norwalk, 1987 (pp. 18–19, Fig. 2.2).
12. *Ibid.* (pp. 50, 52–53, Fig. 3.12).
13. Brash JC, Jamieson EB: *Cunningham's Manual of Practical Anatomy*, Ed. 10, Vol. 2. Oxford University Press, New York, 1942 (p. 389).
14. Callen PW, Filly RA, Marks WM: The quadratus lumborum muscle: a possible source of confusion in sonographic evaluation of the retroperitoneum. *J Clin Ultrasound 7*:349–52, 1979.
15. Carter BL, Morehead J, Wolpert SM, *et al.*: *Cross-Sectional Anatomy*. Appleton-Century-Crofts, New York, 1977 (Sections 29, 31–34).
16. Clarke GR: Unequal leg length: an accurate method of detection and some clinical results. *Rheum Phys Med 11*:385–390, 1972.
17. Clemente CD: *Gray's Anatomy of the Human Body*, American Ed. 30. Lea & Febiger, Philadelphia, 1985 (Fig. 6–19, p. 498).
18. Delacerda FG, Wikoff OD: Effect of lower extremity asymmetry on the kinematics of gait. *J Orthop Sports Phys Ther 3*:105–107, 1982.
19. Denslow JS, Chace JA, Gardner DL, Banner KB: Mechanical stresses in the human lumbar spine and pelvis. *J Am Osteopath Assoc 61*:705–712, 1962.
20. Dixon A St J, Campbell-Smith S: Long leg arthropathy. *Ann Rheum Dis 28*:359–365, 1969.
21. Duchenne GB: *Physiology of Motion*, translated by E.B. Kaplan. J. B. Lippincott, Philadelphia, 1949 (p. 504).
22. Edinger Von A, Biedermann F: Kurzes Bein—schiefes Becken. *Forschr Röntgenstr 86*:754–762, 1957.
23. Eisler P: *Die Muskeln des Stammes*. Gustav Fischer, Jena, 1912 (Fig. 105, p. 654).
24. *Ibid.* (Fig. 106, p. 655).
25. *Ibid.* (pp. 653–656).
26. Elze C: *Hermann Braus Anatomie des Menschen*, Ed. 3, Vol. 1, Springer-Verlag, Berlin, 1954 (Fig. 100, p. 165).
27. *Ibid.* (Fig. 274, p. 522).
28. Ferner H, Staubesand J: *Sobotta Atlas of Human Anatomy*, Ed. 10, Vol. 2. Urban & Schwarzenberg, Baltimore, 1983 (Fig. 102).
29. *Ibid.* (Fig. 136).
30. *Ibid.* (p. 137).
31. *Ibid.* (Fig. 351).
32. Fisk JW: *Medical Treatment of Neck and Back Pain*. Charles C Thomas, Springfield, 1987.
33. Fisk JW, Baigent ML: Clinical and radiological assessment of leg length. *NZ Med J 81*:477–480, 1975.
34. Ford LT, Goodman FG: X-ray studies of the lumbosacral spine. *South Med J 59*:1123–1128, 1966.
35. Friberg O: Leg length asymmetry in stress fractures. *J Sports Med 22*:485–488, 1982.
36. Friberg O: Clinical symptoms and biomechanics of lumbar spine and hip joint in leg length inequality. *Spine 8*:643–651, 1983.
37. Friberg O: Biomechanical significance of the correct length of lower limb prostheses: a clinical and radiological study. *Prosthet Orthot Int 8*: 124–129, 1984.
38. Friberg O: The statics of postural pelvic tilt scoliosis; a radiographic study on 288 consecutive chronic LBP patients. *Clin Biomechanics 2*: 211–219, 1987.
39. Friberg O: Lumbar instability: a dynamic approach by traction–compression radiography. *Spine 12*:119–129, 1987.
40. Friberg O: Hip-spine syndrome. *Manual Med 3*: 144–147, 1988.
41. Friberg O: Personal communication, 1989.
42. Friberg O, Koivisto E, Wegelius C: A radiographic method for measurement of leg length inequality. *Diagn Imag Clin Med 54*:78–81, 1985.
43. Friberg O, Nurminen M, Korhonen K, *et al.*: Accuracy and precision of clinical estimation of leg length inequality and lumbar scoliosis: comparison of clinical and radiological measurements. *International Disability Studies 10*:49–53, 1988.
44. Giles LGF: Leg length inequality: Its measurement, prevalence and its effects on the lumbar spine. *Master's preliminary thesis*. Department of Anatomy, University of Western Australia, 1979.
45. Giles LGF, Taylor JR: Low-back pain associated with leg length inequality. *Spine 6*:510–521, 1981.
46. Giles LGF, Taylor JR: Lumbar spine structural changes associated with leg length inequality. *Spine 7*:159–162, 1982.
47. Gilsanz V, Miranda J, Cleveland R, *et al.*: Scoliosis secondary to fractures of the transverse processes of lumbar vertebrae. *Radiology 134*: 627–629, 1980.
48. Gitelman R: A chiropractic approach to biomechanical disorders of the lumbar spine and pelvis, Chapter 14. In *Modern Developments in the Principles and Practice of Chiropractic*, edited by S. Haldeman. Appleton-Century-Crofts, New York, 1980 (pp. 297–330, see pp. 299–306).
49. Gofton JP: Studies in osteoarthritis of the hip: Part IV. Biomechanics and clinical considerations. *Can Med Assoc J 104*:1007–1011, 1971.
50. Gofton JP, Trueman GE: Studies in osteoarthritis of the hip: Part II. Osteoarthritis of the hip and leg-length disparity. *Can Med Assoc J 104*: 791–799, 1971.
51. Good MG: Diagnosis and treatment of sciatic pain. *Lancet 2*:597–598, 1942.
52. Good MG: What is "fibrositis"? *Rheumatism 5*: 117–123, 1949.
53. Gould N: Back-pocket sciatica. *N Engl J Med 290*:633, 1974.
54. Grant JCB: *An Atlas of Human Anatomy*, Ed. 7. Williams & Wilkins, Baltimore, 1978 (Fig. 2-119).
55. *Ibid.* (Fig. 5-28).
56. *Ibid.* (Fig. 5-29).
57. Greenman PE: Lift therapy: use and abuse. *J Am Osteopath Assoc 79*:238–250, 1979.

PART 1

58. Greenman PE: *Principles of Manual Medicine*. Williams & Wilkins, Baltimore, 1989 (p. 234, 236).
59. Grice AS: Radiographic, biomechanical and clinical factors in lumbar lateral flexion: Part I. *J Manipulative Physiol Ther* 2:26–34, 1979.
60. Gross RH: Leg length discrepancy in marathon runners. *Am J Sports Med 11*:121–124, 1983.
61. Grundy PF, Roberts CJ: Does unequal leg length cause back pain? *Lancet* 2:256–258, 1984.
62. Gutstein-Good M: Idiopathic myalgia simulating visceral and other diseases. *Lancet* 2:326–328, 1940.
63. Hagen DP: A continuing roentgenographic study of rural school children over a 15-year period. *J Am Osteopath Assoc 63*:546–557, 1964.
64. Hallin RP: Sciatic pain and the piriformis muscle. *Postgrad Med 74*:69–72, 1983.
65. Heilig D: Principles of lift therapy. *J Am Osteopath Assoc 77*:466–472, 1978.
66. Henrard J-Cl, Bismuth V, deMolmont C, Gaux J-C: Unequal length of the lower limbs: Measurement by a simple radiological method: Application to epidemiological studies. *Rev Rheum Mal Osteoartic 41*:773–779, 1974.
67. Heufelder P: Die Beinlängendifferenz aus der Sicht des Allgemeinarztes. *Z Orthop 118*:345–354, 1979.
68. Hollinshead WH: *Functional Anatomy of the Limbs and Back*, Ed. 4. W.B. Saunders, Philadelphia, 1976 (p. 400).
69. Hollinshead WH: *Anatomy for Surgeons*, Ed. 3. Vol. 3, The Back and Limbs. Harper & Row, New York, 1982 (pp. 164–165, Fig. 2-74).
70. Hoskins ER: The development of posture and its importance: III Short leg. *J Am Osteopath Assoc 34*:125–6, 1934.
71. Hudson OC, Hettesheimer CA, Robin PA: Causalgic backache. *Am J Surg 52*:297–303, 1941.
72. Inglemark BE, Lindström J: Asymmetries of the lower extremities and pelvis and their relations to lumbar scoliosis. *Acta Morphol Neerl Scand 5*:221–234, 1963.
73. Institute of Medicine: *Pain and Disability: Clinical, Behavioral, and Public Policy Perspectives*. Washington, D.C., National Academy Press, May 1987.
74. Janda J: The pelvis, Chapter 6. In *Muscle Function Testing*. Butterworths, London, 1983 (pp. 41–43).
75. Jull GA, Janda V: Muscles and motor control in low back pain: assessment and management, Chapter 10. In *Physical Therapy of the Low Back*, edited by L.T. Twomey and J.R. Taylor. Churchill Livingstone, New York, 1987 (pp. 253–278).
76. Kelly M: Some rules for the employment of local analgesic in the treatment of somatic pain. *Med J Austral 1*:235–239, 1947 (p. 236).
77. Kendall FP, McCreary EK: *Muscles, Testing and Function*, Ed. 3. Williams & Wilkins, Baltimore, 1983 (pp. 222, 230).
78. *Ibid*. (p. 227).
79. Kidd R: Pain localization with the innominate upslip dysfunction. *Manual Med* 3:103–105, 1988.
80. Knapp ME: Function of the quadratus lumborum. *Arch Phys Med Rehabil 32*:505–507, 1951.
81. Knapp ME: Exercises for lower motor neuron lesions, Chap 16. In *Therapeutic Exercise*, edited by J. V. Basmajian, Ed. 3. Williams & Wilkins, Baltimore, 1978 (p. 369).
82. Krakovits G: Über die Auswirkung einer Beinverkürzung auf die Statik und Dynamik des Hüftgelenkes. *Z Orthop 102*:418–423, 1967.
83. Lange M: *Die Muskelhärten (Myogelosen)*. J.F. Lehmanns, München, 1931 (pp. 90, 91 [Fig. 31], 92 [Case 2], 113 [Case 10] 118 [Case 13]).
84. Langman J, Woerdeman MW: *Atlas of Medical Anatomy*. W.B. Saunders, Philadelphia, 1978 (p. 143, A, B & C).
85. Last RJ: *Anatomy, Regional and Applied*, Ed. 5. Williams & Wilkins, Baltimore, 1972 (pp. 331–332).
86. Lawrence D, Pugh J, Tasharski C, Heinze W: Evaluation of a radiographic method determining short leg mensuration. *ACA J Chiropractic 18*:57–59, 1984.
87. Lawrence DJ: Chiropractic concepts of the short leg: a critical review. *J Manipulative Physiol Ther* 8:157–161, 1985.
88. Leeson CR, Leeson TS: *Human Structure*. W.B. Saunders, Philadelphia, 1972 (p. 269).
89. Leong JCY, Luk KDK, Chow DHK, Woo CW: The biomechanical functions of the iliolumbar ligament in maintaining stability of the lumbosacral junction. *Spine 12*:669–674, 1987.
90. Lewinnek GE: Management of low back pain and sciatica. *Int Anesthesiol Clin 21*:61–78, 1983.
91. Lewit K: Röntgenologische Kriterien statischer Störungen der Wirbelsäule. *Manuelle Med* 20: 26–35, 1982.
92. Lewit K: *Manipulative Therapy in Rehabilitation of the Motor System*. Butterworths, London, 1985 (p. 106, Fig. 4.1; pp. 167–8, Fig. 4.65; p. 291).
93. *Ibid*. (pp. 154–5, Fig. 4.44)
94. *Ibid*. (pp. 275–6, Fig. 6.94)
95. Lewit K: Postisometric relaxation in combination with other methods of muscular facilitation and inhibition. *Manual Med* 2:101–104, 1986.
96. Lewit K: Muscular pattern in thoraco-lumbar lesions. *Manual Med* 2:105–107, 1986.
97. Lewit K: Disturbed balance due to lesions of the cranio-cervical junction. *J Orthop Med*:58–59, (No. 3) 1988.
98. Llewellyn LJ, Jones AB: *Fibrositis*. Rebman, New York, 1915 (Fig. 53 facing p. 280).
99. Lockhart RD, Hamilton GF, Fyfe FW: *Anatomy of the Human Body*, Ed. 2. J.B. Lippincott, Philadelphia, 1969 (p. 181).
100. Luk KDK, Ho HC, Leong JCY: The iliolumbar ligament. *J Bone Joint Surg [Br] 68*:197–200, 1986.
101. Mahar RK, Kirby RL, MacLeod DA: Simulated leg-length discrepancy: its effect on mean center-of-pressure position and postural sway. *Arch Phys Med Rehabil 66*:822, 1985.
102. Maloney M, PT: Personal communication, 1990.

103. McKenzie RA: *The Lumbar Spine: Mechanical Diagnosis and Therapy*. Spinal Publications, Ltd., New Zealand, 1981.
104. McMinn RMH, Hutchings RT: *Color Atlas of Human Anatomy*. Year Book Medical Publishers, Chicago, 1977 (p. 243B–6).
105. Morscher E: Etiology and pathophysiology of leg length discrepancies. *Progr Orthop Surg 1*: 9–19, 1977.
106. Mortensen OA, Pettersen JC: The musculature, Section VI. In *Morris' Human Anatomy*, edited by B.J. Anson, Ed. 12. McGraw-Hill, New York, 1966 (p. 542).
107. Netter FH: *The Ciba Collection of Medical Illustrations*, Vol. 8, Musculoskeletal System. Part I: Anatomy, Physiology and Metabolic Disorders. Ciba-Geigy Corporation, Summit, 1987 (p. 4).
108. *Ibid*. (p. 5).
109. *Ibid*. (p. 77).
110. Nichols PJR, Bailey NTJ: The accuracy of measuring leg-length differences. *Br Med J 2*:1247–1248, 1955.
111. Nielsen AJ: Spray and stretch for myofascial pain. *Phys Ther 58*:567–569, 1978.
112. Northup GW: Osteopathic lesions. *J Am Osteopath Assoc 71*:854–865, 1972.
113. Norton JL: Pelvic side shift in standing roentgenologic postural studies. *J Am Osteopath Assoc 51*:482–484, 1952.
114. Pansky B: *Review of Gross Anatomy*, Ed. 4. Macmillan Publishing Co., Inc., New York, 1979 (pp. 306, 316–317).
115. *Ibid*. (p. 355).
116. Proverbs, Chapter 26, Verse 7. *Holy Bible*, New Testament.
117. Rab GT, Chao EYS, Stauffer RN: Muscle force analysis of the lumbar spine. *Orthop Clin North Am 8*:193–199, 1977.
118. Rasch PJ, Burke RK: *Kinesiology and Applied Anatomy*, Ed. 6. Lea & Febiger, Philadelphia, 1978 (p. 228).
119. Reynolds MD: Myofascial trigger point syndromes in the practice of rheumatology. *Arch Phys Med Rehabil 62*:111–114, 1981 (Table 1, p. 112).
120. Rush WA, Steiner HA: A study of lower extremity length inequality. *Am J Roentgen Rad Ther 56*:616–623, 1946.
121. Saudek C: C'mon let's twist. *Orthop Phys Ther Prac 1*:24–27, 1989.
122. Schuit D, Adrian M, Pidcoe P: Effect of heel lifts on ground reaction force patterns in subjects with structural leg-length discrepancies. *Phys Ther* 69:663–670, 1989.
123. Simons DG: Functions of the quadratus lumborum muscle and relation of its myofascial trigger points to low back pain. *Pain Abstracts*, Vol. 1. Second World Congress on Pain, International Assn for the Study of Pain, Montreal, Canada, August 27-September 1, 1978 (p. 245).
124. Simons DG: Myofascial pain syndromes due to trigger points: 2. Treatment and single-muscle syndromes. *Manual Med 1*:72–77, 1985.
125. Simons DG: Muskulofasziale Schmerzsyndrome infolge Triggerpunkten. *Manuelle Med 23*:134–142, 1985.
126. Simons DG: Myofascial pain syndrome due to trigger points, Chapter 45. In *Rehabilitation Medicine*, edited by J.Goodgold. C.V. Mosby Co., St. Louis, 1988 (pp. 686–723).
127. Simons DG, Simons LS: Chronic myofascial pain syndrome, Chapter 42. In *Handbook of Chronic Pain Management*, edited by C. David Tollison. Williams & Wilkins, Baltimore, 1989 (pp. 509–529).
128. Simons DG, Travell JG: Myofascial origins of low back pain. 2. Torso muscles. *Postgrad Med 73*:81–92, 1983.
129. Simons DG, Travell JG: Myofascial pain syndromes, Chapter 25. In *Textbook of Pain*, edited by P.D. Wall and R. Melzack, Ed 2. Churchill Livingstone, London, 1989 (pp. 368–385).
130. Snook SH, Jensen RC: Cost, Chapter 5. In *Occupational Low Back Pain*, edited by M.H. Pope, J.W. Frymoyer and G. Andersson. Praeger, New York, 1984 (pp. 115–121, see p. 116).
131. Snook SH, White AH: Education and training, Chapter 12. In *Occupational Low Back Pain*, edited by M.H. Pope, J.W. Frymoyer and G.Andersson. Praeger, New York, 1984 (p. 234).
132. Sola AE: Trigger point therapy, Chapter 47. In *Clinical Procedures in Emergency Medicine*, edited by J.R. Roberts and J.R. Hedges. W.B. Saunders, Philadelphia, 1985 (pp. 674–686, see pp. 682, 684).
133. Sola AE, Kuitert JH: Quadratus lumborum myofasciitis. *Northwest Med 53*:1003–1005, 1954.
134. Sola AE, Williams RL: Myofascial pain syndromes. *Neurology 6*:91–95, 1956.
135. Spalteholz W: *Handatlas der Anatomie des Menschen*, Ed. 11, Vol. 2. S. Hirzel, Leipzig, 1922 (p. 306).
136. *Ibid*. (p. 344).
137. Steindler A: *Diseases of Spine and Thorax*. C.V. Mosby, St. Louis, 1929.
138. Stoddard A: *Manual of Osteopathic Technique*. Hutchinson Medical Publications, London, 1959 (p. 212).
139. Strong R, Thomas PE: Patterns of muscle activity in the leg, hip, and torso associated with anomalous fifth lumbar conditions. *J Am Osteopath Assoc 67*:1039–1041, 1968.
140. Strong R, Thomas PE, Earl WD: Patterns of muscle activity in leg, hip, and torso during quiet standing. *J Am Osteopath Assoc 66*:1035–1038, 1967.
141. Sutton SE: Postural imbalance: examination and treatment utilizing flexion tests. *J Am Osteopath Assoc 77*:456–465, 1978.
142. Taillard W, Morscher E: *Die Beinlängenunterschiede*. S. Karger, Basel, New York, 1965 (pp. 26–42).
143. Tanz SS: Motion of the lumbar spine, a roentgenologic study. *AJR 69*:399–412, 1953 (see Fig. 6).
144. Thompson CW: *Manual of Structural Kinesiology*, Ed. 9. C.V. Mosby, St. Louis, 1981 (p. 110).
145. Toldt C: *An Atlas of Human Anatomy*, translated by M.E. Paul, Ed. 2, Vol. 1. Macmillan, New York, 1919 (p. 339).
146. *Ibid*. (p. 344).
147. Travell JG: The quadratus lumborum muscle: an overlooked cause of low back pain. *Arch Phys Med Rehabil 57*:566, 1976.

148. Travell JG, Simons DG: *Myofascial Pain and Dysfunction: The Trigger Point Manual*. Williams & Wilkins, Baltimore, 1983.
149. *Ibid.* (pp. 82–85).
150. *Ibid.* (pp. 104–109).
151. *Ibid.* (pp. 104–156).
152. *Ibid.* (pp. 106–110, 651–653, Fig. 48.10*A*).
153. *Ibid.* (pp. 108–109).
154. *Ibid.* (pp. 112–190, 196–197, Fig. 6.10).
155. *Ibid.* (pp. 114–156).
156. *Ibid.* (p. 209).
157. *Ibid.* (pp. 398–491).
158. *Ibid.* (pp. 638, 639).
159. *Ibid.* (p. 645).
160. *Ibid.* (p. 664).
161. *Ibid.* (pp. 680–681).
162. *Ibid.* (Chapter 48).
163. Turula KB, Friberg O, Lindholm TS, *et al.*: Leg length inequality after total hip arthroplasty. *Clin Orthop 202*:163–168, 1986.
164. Venn EK, Wakefield KA, Thompson PR: A comparative study of leg-length checks. *Eur J Chiropractic 31*:68–80, 1983.
165. Waters RL, Morris JM: Electrical activity of muscles of the trunk during walking. *J Anat 111*:191–199, 1972.
166. West HG Jr: Physical and spinal examination procedures utilized in the practice of chiropractic, Chapter 13. In *Modern Developments in the Principles and Practice of Chiropractic*, edited by S. Haldeman. Appleton-Century-Crofts, New York, 1980 (Fig. 13, p. 294).
167. Winter Z: Referred pain in fibrositis. *Med Rec 157*:34–37, 1944.
168. Woerdeman MW: *Atlas of Human Anatomy*, Vol. 1. Williams & Wilkins, Baltimore, 1948 (Fig. 345).
169. Woodburne RT: *Essentials of Human Anatomy*, Ed. 4. Oxford University Press, London, 1969 (p. 369).
170. Zohn DA: The quadratus lumborum: an unrecognized source of back pain, clinical and thermographic aspects. *Orthop Rev 14*:163–168, 1985.
171. Zohn DA: *Musculoskeletal Pain: Diagnosis and Physical Treatment*, Ed. 2. Little, Brown and Company, Boston, 1988 (pp. 204, 206).

CHAPTER 5
Iliopsoas Muscle

"Hidden Prankster"

HIGHLIGHTS: The iliopsoas is a "hidden prankster" in the sense that it serves many critically important functions, often causes pain, and is relatively inaccessible. Unidentified iliopsoas and/or quadratus lumborum trigger points (TrPs) are frequently responsible for a failed low back postsurgical syndrome. **REFERRED PAIN** from myofascial TrPs in the psoas major muscle extends along the spine ipsilaterally from the thoracic region to the sacroiliac area, and sometimes to the upper buttock. Pain is referred similarly from the iliacus and often also to the anterior thigh and groin. **ANATOMICAL ATTACHMENTS** of the psoas major, above, are along the sides of the lumbar vertebrae and intervertebral discs. Below, its tendon anchors to the lesser trochanter of the femur. The iliacus muscle attaches, above, to the upper two-thirds of the iliac fossa. Below, it joins the psoas major tendon and, in addition, some fibers attach directly to the femur near the lesser trochanter. The primary **FUNCTION** of the iliacus and psoas major muscles is flexion of the thigh at the hip. The psoas can assist extension of the lumbar spine (increase lumbar lordosis) when one is standing with a normal lordosis, and it plays a significant role in maintaining upright posture. Both the iliacus and psoas may assist abduction of the thigh and probably contribute slightly to lateral rotation. The psoas and sometimes the iliacus are active during sitting and standing. Both may be continuously active during ambulation. During jogging, running, or sprinting, the iliacus is active while the thigh is being flexed at the hip. It is vigorously active through the last 60° of a sit-up. The painful **SYMPTOMS** from iliopsoas TrPS are aggravated by weight-bearing activities and relieved by recumbency; relief is greater when the hip is flexed. The psoas minor syndrome is easily mistaken for appendicitis. Hemorrhage within the psoas muscle, spontaneous or associated with anticoagulation therapy, can cause a painful compression syndrome of the femoral nerve. **ACTIVATION** of iliopsoas TrPs can result from acute overload stress or from prolonged sitting with the hips acutely flexed, although they are usually activated secondarily to TrPs in other muscles of the functional unit. **PATIENT EXAMINATION** for a tight iliopsoas muscle entails tests for restriction of extension of the thigh at the hip. **TRIGGER POINT EXAMINATION** of the iliopsoas muscle requires examination at three locations. *(a)* Digital pressure exerted deep on the lateral border of the femoral triangle over the lesser trochanter elicits tenderness of distal iliacus fibers and usually from psoas musculotendinous junctions at that level. *(b)* Palpation over the inner border of the ilium behind the anterior superior iliac spine permits examination of taut bands and TrPs in the uppermost iliacus fibers. *(c)* Pressure exerted first downward on the abdomen lateral to the rectus abdominis muscle and then beneath the rectus abdominis, medially, elicits tenderness of the psoas muscles by compression against the lumbar spine. **ENTRAPMENTS** of the femoral, lateral femoral cutaneous, and the femoral branch of the genitofemoral nerves may occur in the lacuna musculorum beneath the inguinal ligament, as the nerves exit the pelvis through a narrow lacuna in the company of the iliopsoas muscle. The genitofemoral nerve regularly penetrates, and the iliohypogastric and ilioinguinal nerves occasionally penetrate the psoas major muscle as they emerge from the lumbar plexus. For **INTERMITTENT COLD WITH STRETCH** of the iliopsoas muscle, the patient lies on the opposite side, and the ice or vapocoolant is applied in downward parallel sweeps over the abdomen and anterior upper part of the thigh as the thigh is extended. Finally, parallel, distalward sweeps of intermittent cold cover the referred pain pattern on the back and buttock. Intermittent cold with stretch is followed by rewarming with moist heat and by full active range of motion. **INJECTION AND STRETCH** begin by injecting iliopsoas TrPs in the femoral triangle, while carefully avoiding the adjacent femoral nerve and artery. One can inject proximal iliacus fibers inside the iliac fossa just below the crest of the ilium through the lower abdominal wall. After application of a moist heating pad, the patient actively moves the iliopsoas through its full range of motion several times. **CORRECTIVE ACTIONS** start with inactivation of associated TrPs and correction of systemic perpetuating factors. Restricted or locked thoracolumbar, lumbosacral, or sacroiliac articulations can prevent lasting relief and need to be treated. Other mechanical approaches include correcting a lower limb-length inequality; avoiding sitting immobile for long periods, especially with an acute angle at the hip joints; normalizing paradoxical breathing; and maintaining proper positioning during sleep. An optimal management program begins with appropriate gentle hip extension exercise followed by a balanced, progressive rectus abdominis-iliopsoas strengthening program.

1. REFERRED PAIN

(Fig. 5.1)

Pain referred from trigger points (TrPs) in the iliopsoas muscle forms a distinctive **vertical** pattern ipsilaterally along the lumbar spine. It extends downward to the sacroiliac region and may spill over to include the sacrum and proximal medial buttock (Fig. 5.1).[81] The referred pain pattern usually also includes the groin and upper anteromedial aspect of the thigh on the same side. Pressure applied by abdominal palpation of either psoas or iliacus TrPs causes pain referred chiefly to the back. Palpation of TrPs near the attachment of the iliopsoas muscle (mostly iliacus fibers) on the lesser trochanter of the femur may refer pain both to the back and anteriorly to the thigh.

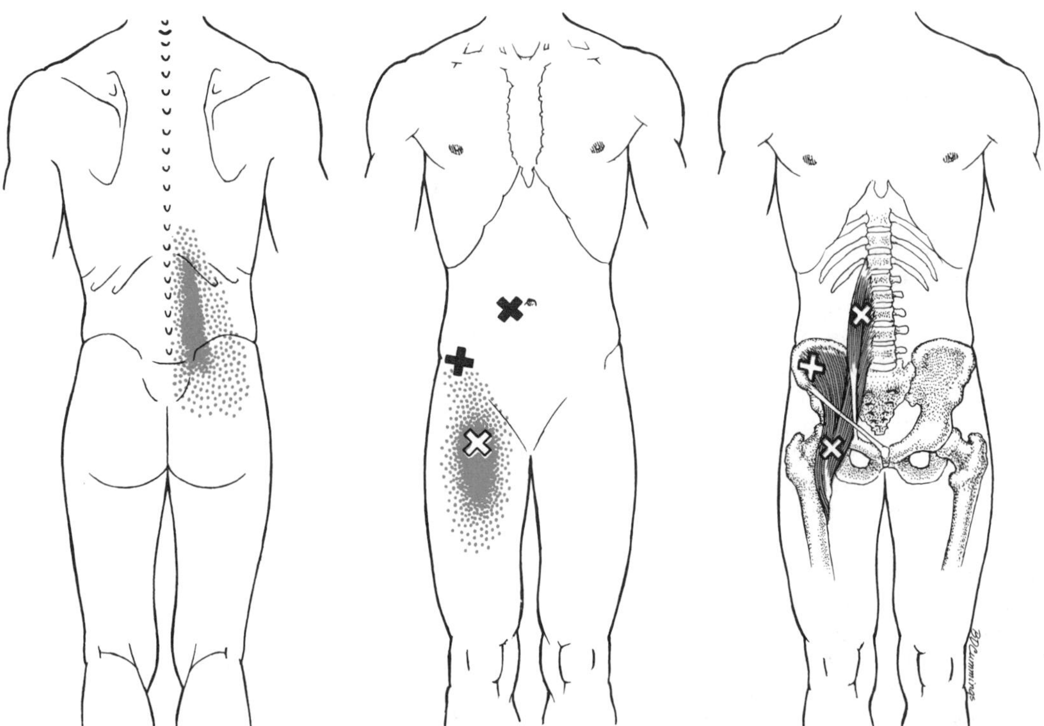

Figure 5.1. Pattern of pain (*bright red*) referred from palpable myofascial trigger points (**X**s) in the right iliopsoas muscle (*darker red*). The essential pain reference zone is *solid red*; the spill-over pattern is *stippled*.

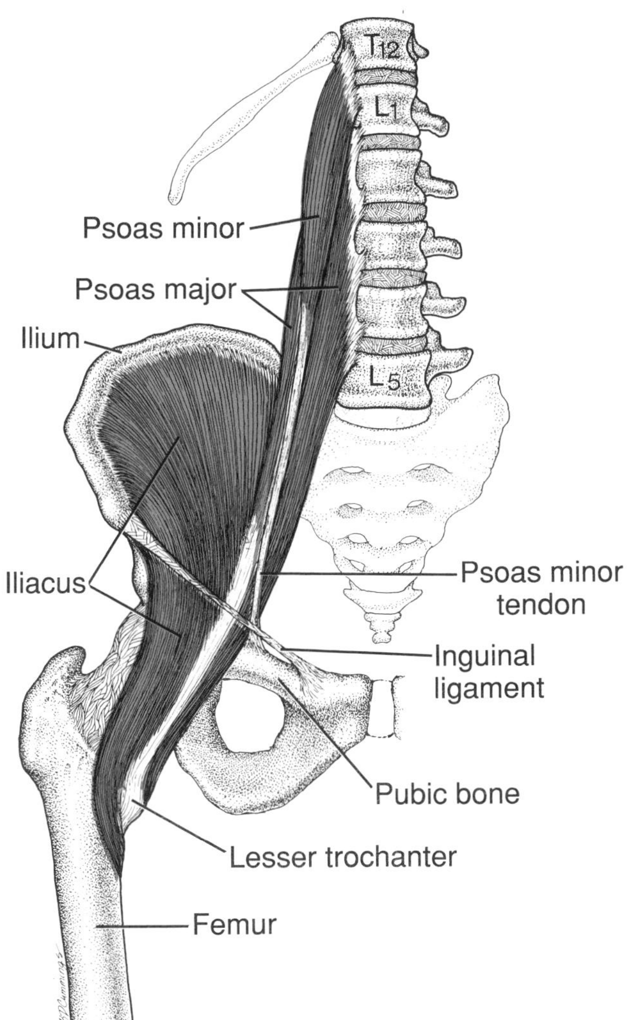

Figure 5.2. Attachments of the right psoas major, psoas minor and iliacus muscles (*red*). The psoas major crosses many articulations including those of the lumbar spine and the lumbosacral, sacroiliac, and hip joints. The psoas minor does the same, except that it does *not* cross the hip joint. The iliacus, on the other hand, crosses only the hip joint.

The senior author observed a patient who had severe pain in the hip joint and anterior thigh when walking, but could walk without pain as long as she hyperextended her lumbar spine and pressed down against the greater trochanter on the painful side.

Pain in the scrotum has been intensified by stretching the iliopsoas muscle.[47] Psoas muscle pain in the back has been reported to extend as high as the interscapular region.[24]

2. ANATOMICAL ATTACHMENTS AND CONSIDERATIONS
(Fig. 5.2)

The psoas major muscle (Fig. 5.2) attaches ***above*** by thick fasciculi to the sides of the 12th thoracic and all lumbar vertebral bodies, to the corresponding intervertebral discs, and by more slender fasciculi to the anterior surfaces and lower borders of the lumbar transverse processes.[7,17] This muscle occupies the space beside the vertebral bodies anterior to the transverse processes along the lower lumbar spine.[2] The psoas lies adjacent, anterior, and medial to the quadratus lumborum muscle in the lumbar region.[28] More distally, the psoas major passes anterior to the sacroiliac joint, then follows the border of the pelvic brim and proceeds anteriorly in front of the roof of the hip joint.[29] Inside the pelvis, it is joined by the iliacus muscle to become the iliopsoas. The psoas portion becomes largely tendinous as it passes deep to the inguinal ligament and exits the pelvis (Fig. 5.2). There it helps to form the lateral floor of the femoral triangle. The iliopsoas tendon anchors ***below*** to the lesser trochanter on the posteromedial aspect of the femur.[17]

The psoas minor muscle is variable and is absent bilaterally in from 41%[7] to over 50%[17] of bodies. When present, it lies anterior to the psoas major in the lumbar region. It attaches ***above*** to the anterolateral aspect of the 12th thoracic and one or two of the upper lumbar vertebrae. The psoas minor attaches ***below*** to the pectineal line on the superior ramus of the pubic bone, to the iliopectineal eminence, and to the iliac fascia.[17]

The iliacus muscle attaches ***above*** to the upper two-thirds of the inner surface of the iliac fossa, completely lining the lateral wall of the greater pelvis. It also anchors to the internal lip of the iliac crest. ***Below***, many of the iliacus fibers join the psoas major tendon; the remainder attach directly to the lesser trochanter anteriorly and to the adjacent femur.[17,77]

The psoas major crosses the lumbar intervertebral, lumbosacral, sacroiliac, and hip joints; the psoas minor crosses all of these *except* the hip joint. The iliacus crosses only the hip joint.

The iliacus muscle and iliopsoas tendon exit the pelvis through the lacuna musculorum in company with the femoral nerve[17] and often together with the lateral femoral cutaneous nerve. This lacuna is a firmly constricted space bounded anteriorly by the inguinal ligament, posteriorly and laterally by the pelvic bone, and medially by a thickened band of fascia, the iliopectineal arch. This restricted outlet creates a potential for nerve entrapment caused by an enlarged or shortened (thickened) iliopsoas muscle. (This entrapment is comparable to that of the sciatic and accompanying nerves by the piriformis muscle as they pass through the greater sciatic foramen, *see* Chapter 10.)

The large iliopectineal bursa[34] lies between the iliopsoas muscle anteriorly, and the capsule of the hip joint and the iliopectineal eminence of the pubis on the other side, posteriorly. This bursa may communicate with the synovial cavity of the hip joint.[17] The small, subtendinous iliac bursa[18] separates the iliopsoas tendon from the femur at its attachment to the lesser trochanter.

At each segmental level, the psoas major attaches to the medial half or so of the anterior surface of the transverse process, to the intervertebral disc, to the margins of the vertebral bodies adjacent to the disc, and to a fibrous arch that connects the upper and lower margins of each lumbar vertebral body. The fibers of this muscle are systematically overlapped by fibers from the above attachments at successively higher segmental levels. As a result, the muscle is layered, with fibers from the higher levels forming the outer surface of the muscle and those from lower levels buried sequentially more deeply within its substance.[12] Since all fibers of a muscle are nearly the same length, this structure is reflected in the distribution of distal myotendinous junctions (Fig. 5.2).

In an X-ray computed tomography study of 44 men and 52 women ranging in age from 9 to 86 years,[46] the psoas major muscle reached maximum cross-sectional area in men at age 30, declined rapidly to about two-thirds of that value by age 40, and was only one-half as large by age 60. Women showed only a slight decline in the size of this muscle with age. In both sexes, the relative density gradually declined by about 25% between the ages of 20 and 80 years.

Supplemental References

All three muscles, the psoas major, psoas minor, and iliacus, are depicted from in front with vessels or nerves removed.[28,77] The three muscles relate to nerves in the abdomen[1,27,30] and the iliopsoas muscle relates to nerves and vessels in the femoral triangle.[3,72]

Markings on the bones identify attachments of the iliacus muscle.[4,35,69]

Cross sections show all three muscles throughout their length,[14] the psoas muscle at the L_2-L_3 level,[2] the psoas muscle at a lower lumbar level,[31] and the iliopsoas just above its femoral attachment.[71] All three muscles appear in side view in a sagittal section,[32] and the iliopsoas in a frontal section through the hip joint that shows its relationship to the pelvic fascia.[29]

Illustrations portray the locations of the iliopectineal bursa[34] and the subtendinous iliac bursa.[18]

3. INNERVATION

Branches of the lumbar plexus, which contain fibers from spinal nerves L_2, L_3, and L_4, innervate the psoas major muscle. A branch of the first lumbar spinal nerve innervates the psoas minor. Spinal nerves L_2 and L_3 supply the iliacus muscle.[17]

4. FUNCTION

All allusions to the psoas muscle apply to the psoas major muscle unless otherwise stated.

Actions

Without question, the primary action of the iliacus and psoas major muscles is flexion at the hip.[7,9,17,22,37] Beyond that, there has been little general agreement through the years.[9] It now appears that the psoas major extends the lumbar spine when the individual is standing with normal lumbar lordosis but assists flexion of the lumbar spine when one bends forward.[9] The small effect that the iliopsoas exerts on rotation of the thigh is usually to assist lateral rotation.[9,11,22] The iliopsoas sometimes assists abduction at the hip but not adduction.[39] The optimal stretch position is extension of the thigh at the hip with medial or neutral rotation of the thigh and with neutral positioning or adduction of the thigh.[39]

Flexion at the Hip. Hip flexion activated the iliacus and psoas muscles regardless of position and in proportion to the effort expended. Both muscles were inactive during hip extension effort.[8,9] Electrical stimulation of the iliopsoas muscle or of only the iliacus produced primarily hip flexion.[22] Extension effort only at the knee recruited the iliacus as a **stabilizing** muscle.[37] The iliopsoas is primarily a hip flexor that requires extension at the hip to lengthen it.

Flexion or Extension of the Spine and Pelvis. The direct effect of the psoas muscle on flexion or extension of the lumbar spine is not immediately obvious anatomically.

Sophisticated analysis of mechanical moments about the L_4-L_5 interspace led to the conclusion that the psoas contributes to extension of the spine in the low lumbar region but adds only 4% to the total extension force; the erector spinae, rotatores, and quadratus lumborum, in that order, provide the primary extensor force.[75] As would be expected and as confirmed experimentally,[68] contraction of the psoas increases loading on the intervertebral discs. This muscle passes anterior to the axes of movement of the sacroiliac (SI) joint and, therefore, should exert a marked flexion force between the ilium and the sacrum.

In the standing subject, strong attempts to increase lumbar lordosis (to extend the lumbar spine) generally recruited the psoas muscle; efforts to straighten the lumbar spine did not.[9,11] Both Rasch and Burke[76] and Janda[49] noted clinically that patients with weak abdominal muscles who attempted a sit-up developed spinal hyperextension. This is the effect one expects as the psoas hyperextends the lumbar spine when it and the iliacus tilt the pelvis forward without restraint by the rectus abdominis during a sit-up. This effect is sometimes called the psoas paradox.[76]

Rotation of the Thigh. Basmajian and Deluca[9] concluded that, from a functional point of view, the question of whether the iliopsoas rotates the thigh is not worth pursuing. After careful mechanical analysis of the axis of rotation in 11 specimens, Hooper[45] substantiated their conclusion with the finding that the iliopsoas does not play a significant role in rotation of the normal femur because its tendon is aligned with the axis of rotation in most cases.

However, the effect of rotation on the muscle could influence the optimal stretch position. Electrophysiological studies revealed that neither the iliacus nor the psoas was activated during medial rotation of the thigh at the hip, but both muscles often were active during lateral rotation.[9,11] Electrical stimulation of either muscle while the subject was standing or supine produced a slight lateral rotation.[22]

Based on these results, the optimal stretch position would avoid lateral rotation and would place the limb either in neutral or in medial rotation. Evjenth and Hamberg[26] recommend stretching by extension with medial rotation of the thigh. In the psoatic gait of a shortened iliopsoas, the thigh is laterally rotated.[66,67]

Abduction or Adduction of the Thigh. In one study of 13 subjects,[11] abduction of the thigh in the standing position generally recruited activity in the psoas muscle; although it, too, was monitored with fine-wire electrodes, no mention was made of activity in the iliacus muscle.[11] Close[20] reported EMG activity of the psoas during abduction, but not until other muscles had initiated abduction against gravity. However, in Greenlaw's study of 10 subjects,[39] neither abduction nor adduction activated the psoas muscle; only abduction activated the iliacus muscle. It appears that the optimum stretch position avoids abduction.

Psoas Minor. The psoas minor, when present, ordinarily should have little or no effect on movement of the thigh but should assist the psoas major in extending the normal lordotic curve of the lumbar spine while flexing the lumbosacral articulation. The latter movement would have the effect of elevating the front of the pelvis on the same side. No functional studies of this muscle have been found.

In summary, the optimal stretch position for the iliopsoas muscle is extension of the thigh, most likely without abduction and with either neutral or medial rotation.

Functions

When a person is standing or sitting, the psoas muscle may be continuously active and plays a significant role in maintaining upright posture. The iliacus shows minimal activity during standing. During walking, the iliacus is continuously active, but the psoas is active only shortly preceding and during early swing phase, when it would accelerate forward movement of the limb. Running induced vigorous iliacus activity during flexion of the thigh. Some individuals showed vigorous iliacus activity throughout a sit-up, whereas the iliacus muscles of others became active only after the first 30° of the sit-up. Testing of patients without an iliacus muscle and some sit-up data indicate that the muscle is most effective as a hip flexor after the first 30° of hip flexion.

Standing or Sitting. In electromyographic (EMG) studies during quiet standing, the iliacus showed only intermittent short bursts of marked activity at irregular intervals,[9] or no activity,[56] whereas the psoas showed continuous slight activity.[9] Nachemson[68] inserted wire electrodes directly into the lumbar psoas muscle from a posterior approach and reported that it was continuously active during standing and sitting. Activity was increased by holding 10-kg weights in each hand during sitting or standing and was decreased when the subject leaned forward. He[68] concluded that the lumbar psoas plays a significant role in maintaining upright posture.

Locomotion. During the walking cycle, the iliacus acts continuously with two peaks of activity, the greatest during the swing phase and the other in midstance. The psoas has two peaks of EMG activity that correspond with those of the iliacus and a third peak midway through the cycle (during stance phase).[10] An earlier study found that psoas muscle activity began shortly before toe-off and persisted only during the initial 40% of swing phase. This activity occurred exactly when it would be needed to accelerate forward movement of the limb.[51]

During jogging, running, or sprinting, vigorous activity appeared in the iliacus while the thigh was being flexed at the hip. This movement was forceful and imparted the major force for forward propulsion.[62] The psoas was not monitored in this study.

Sit Ups. There is general agreement that, after the first 30° of upward movement of a sit-up, the iliacus is vigorously active.[9,36,56] LaBan and coworkers[56] saw no activity in five subjects through the first 30° when the legs were straight, but did observe activity when the knees were bent. Flint[36] found mild to moderate activity in three subjects throughout that 30° angle. Apparently, some individuals depend on the rectus femoris muscle without help from the iliacus and others use both muscles when initiating a sit-up.

Scoliosis. Among the nearly 1500 subjects examined radiographically for back pain or prior to job placement, 80% of those who had 5° or more of scoliosis showed a visible psoas shadow on the convex side, but only 30% showed a visible shadow on the concave side, and none had a visible shadow only on the concave side.[13] This raises a question as to how important a role asymmetrical psoas development and activity play in scoliosis.

Extirpation. Removal of the iliopsoas muscle in two patients produced only slight loss of either isometric or isokinetic strength of hip flexion at 30°.[63] Isometric strength dropped sharply as the angle increased to 90°. Isokinetic strength decreased only slightly to moderately beyond 30°. This observation, in conjunction with the data on reduced or no electrical activity of the iliacus through the first 30° of flexion, as noted previously, suggests that the iliacus becomes significantly more effective as the prime flexor at the hip after the first 30° of hip flexion.

5. FUNCTIONAL (MYOTATIC) UNIT

Synergists to the iliopsoas for flexion of the thigh at the hip are the rectus femoris and pectineus muscles assisted by the sartorius, tensor fasciae latae, gracilis, and by the three adductors—longus, brevis, and middle part of the magnus. The antagonists to these hip flexors are primarily the gluteus maximus, the hamstring muscles, and the posterior part of the adductor magnus.

Bilaterally, the two iliopsoas muscles work as a team, synchronizing their activity for some functions and alternating it for others.

During a sit-up, additional agonists include the rectus abdominis and psoas minor muscles.

6. SYMPTOMS

Patients who have unilateral iliopsoas TrPs complain primarily of low back pain; when describing the pain, they run the hand vertically up and down the spine rather than horizontally. When bilateral iliopsoas muscles have active TrPs, the patient may perceive the pain as running across the low back, as also felt with bilateral quadratus lumborum TrPs. Pain is worse when the patient stands upright, but may remain as a slight nagging backache when the patient is recumbent. A frequent additional complaint is pain in the front of the thigh.

Patients are likely to have difficulty getting up from a deep-seated chair and are unable to do sit-ups. In severe cases, mobility may be reduced to crawling on the hands and knees.

Constipated patients with tender psoas TrPs may experience referred pain evoked by the passage of a bolus of hard feces that presses against the TrPs. A hypertrophied psoas muscle can compress the neighboring large bowel, as demonstrated by a barium study of the colon in a sportswoman.[23]

In a review of six patients with iliopsoas myofascial dysfunction, Ingber[47] also found that they experienced aggravation of their low back pain during antigravity activity and alleviation of the pain when recumbent. The most comfortable recumbent positions were side-lying in a nearly fetal position or lying supine with hips and knees flexed.

Tightness (loss of full extension range of motion) of the iliopsoas muscle initiated a chain of catastrophic effects in some ballet dancers as they tried to compensate for the loss of that muscle's function. Performing the arabesque was painful and the dancers were plagued by reduced turnout.[6]

The psoas minor syndrome[86] is caused by a tense psoas minor muscle and tendon. This syndrome was described by a surgeon, who observed it most often on the right side in 15- to 17-year-old girls with a diagnosis of suspected appendicitis. The author attributed the tension of the muscle to its failure to keep pace with the growth of the pelvis. He could palpate a "strand" of psoas minor (that he interpreted as tendon) through the abdominal wall in most patients. In almost all cases, the patients complained of pain in the lower right quadrant of the abdomen and the pain was aggravated by palpation of the taut "tendon." Consistently, the appendix was normal and tenotomy of the psoas minor relieved the symptoms. The tenotomy also relieved scoliosis of the lumbar spine (convex to the side opposite the taut psoas minor muscle) in several patients.

Disproportionate growth would be an exceptional cause of symptoms from a muscle. The previously described findings suggest that myofascial TrPs in the psoas minor may have contributed to the pain, tenderness, and muscle shortening. If so, they demonstrate that pain is referred from this muscle locally to the corresponding lower abdominal quadrant. The predominance of right-sided symptoms may have resulted from the fact that patients with similar pain and tenderness on the left side usually would not be seen by a surgeon for suspected appendicitis.

In the psoas minor syndrome, limited extension at the hip frequently impaired ambulation. Since the psoas minor normally extends only to the pelvis and not to the femur, the reason for this limitation is not immediately obvious. Several possibilities deserve consideration: *(a)* Vos[86] noted that the lateral fibers of the psoas minor tendon that join the iliac fascia can sometimes be followed as far as the lesser trochanter. In this case, the corresponding muscle fibers, which act across the hip joint, would be particularly vulnerable to stress overload. The tightness of the muscle would increase with extension of the thigh. *(b)* The shortened muscle, by producing abnormal lumbar curvature,[86] would limit pelvic motion. *(c)* The psoas minor TrPs may activate secondary TrPs in the iliopsoas, which, in turn, limit hip extension. Appropriately directed physical examination should determine which of these mechanisms is responsible.

Differential Diagnosis

TrPs in a number of muscles other than the iliopsoas refer pain in patterns that may be confused with the pain arising from iliopsoas TrPs. Low back pain can also be referred from TrPs in the quadratus lumborum, lowest section of the rectus abdominis, longissimus thoracis, rotatores, gluteus maximus, and gluteus medius muscles. Iliopsoas TrPs do not cause pain on coughing and deep breathing as do those in the quadratus lumborum muscle,[81] described in Chapter 4 of this volume. When the patient indicates that pain spreads horizontally across the low back, the pain is much more likely to be referred from TrPs bilaterally in the quadratus lumborum muscles or from the lowest portion of the rectus abdominis (Volume 1, Fig. 49.2*A*, p. 664).[83] These rectus abdominis TrPs are often associated with TrPs in the iliopsoas muscle.

Thigh and groin pain may also be due to TrPs in the tensor fascia latae, pectineus, vastus intermedius, adductores longus and brevis, or the distal parts of the adductor magnus muscle. Of these muscles, only the pectineus and tensor fasciae latae should restrict extension at the hip. Physical examination readily distinguishes the more superficial TrP tenderness of the last two muscles from the deep tenderness of the iliopsoas muscle.

Ingber[47] reported on several patients with persistent backache following laminectomy for lumbar discopathy, and one suffering discopathy who had not undergone surgery. Injecting their iliopsoas TrPs and instituting extension exercises relieved them of their symptoms.

The psoas major muscle seems peculiarly vulnerable to developing hematoma in association with anticoagulation therapy,[25,38,53,64,65,73] and sometimes following minor trauma in teenagers.[41] The hematoma causes local pain and swelling, difficulty in walking, and often seriously compromises femoral nerve function. Hematoma in the iliacus muscle induced by anticoagulation therapy can also produce femoral neuropathy.[85] The diagnosis of hematoma can be made by computed tomography[73] or by ultrasound scanning.[38,41]

A patient with pyogenic iliopsoas myositis showed no evidence of femoral nerve compression, but had local pain, local tenderness, and a limp.[55] Other abnormalities of the iliopsoas muscle visualized by computed tomography included atrophy, hypertrophy, neurofibroma, metastatic cancer, primary tumor, lymphoma,[46,73] and abscess.[42,73]

Iliopsoas bursitis is unusual, but it can cause a tender mass in the groin area with persistent diffuse pain in the lateral hip region that may extend to the knee. It is usually, but not always, seen in conjunction with underlying rheumatoid arthritis.[43]

A patient with a posteriorly displaced lesser trochanter on one side developed a painfully disabling snapping iliopsoas tendon syndrome. The tendon snapped across the iliopectineal eminence. Tenotomy gave relief.[80]

7. ACTIVATION AND PERPETUATION OF TRIGGER POINTS

Activation

The TrPs in the iliopsoas muscle are generally activated secondarily to TrPs in other muscles of the functional unit. They may be activated simultaneously with TrPs in these other muscles by sudden overload in a fall. Iliopsoas TrPs also may be activated and are perpetuated by prolonged sitting with the hips in the jackknifed position (acutely flexed), which shortens the muscle. This position is assumed often while riding in an automobile, but problems can develop whenever one sits with the buttocks pushed backward so that the torso must lean forward, placing the knees higher than the hips. Truck drivers, in particular, are vulnerable to backache because of this shortened position of the iliopsoas. They should routinely perform a hip extension exercise at every stop on the road.

Patients often report that their first awareness of pain referred from these TrPs is when they get out of bed in the morning. Sleeping in the fetal position, with the knees drawn up to the chest, can activate latent iliopsoas TrPs.

Lewit[57,59] associates TrP tenderness of the psoas with articular dysfunction in the thoracolumbar region, T_{10}-L_1. The dysfunction is identified clinically by impaired trunk rotation and side bending in this region. He associates TrP tenderness of the iliacus with dysfunction of the lumbosacral junction.[57]

Back pain caused by iliopsoas TrPs is common in pregnancy. Dobrik[21] believed that a viscerosomatic reflex was probably responsible for the close association that he observed between painful dysfunctions of the internal female genitalia and increased tension of the iliopsoas muscle. He[21] did not clarify how important he considered the reverse process: somatovisceral reflex aggravation of gynecological symptoms by iliopsoas TrPs.

Klawunde and Zeller[54] reported in 12 men and nine women that a marked relationship existed between the voluntarily recruitable electrical activity of the iliacus muscle and blocked movement of the ipsilateral sacroiliac and upper cervical joints. The iliacus muscle clinically showed increased tonus on the same side as the sacroiliac blockage, but maximum voluntary activation of the muscle was inhibited whereas the recruitable activity of the iliacus on the contralateral side was increased. Manipulation of blocked joints in the high cervical spine on the ipsilateral side reduced this difference to 25% and manipulation of the blocked sacroiliac joint reduced it further. Following treatment, the restoration of activity on the involved side nearly equaled the reduction of electrical hyperactivity on the uninvolved side.

Increased tension and inhibition of maximal contraction are typically found in muscles with myofascial TrPs.[83] It is unfortunate that the iliacus muscles of the patients in the study were not examined specifically for TrP phenomena. It is not clear whether the relation observed was due to an arthromuscular reflex that caused the effects directly or whether the joint restriction perpetuated TrPs that were secondarily inactivated by the manipulative procedure. However, it is difficult to understand why a reflexly *inhibited* muscle would show increased tension unless an additional mechanism for non-electrogenic muscular contraction, such as that produced by TrPs, was present.

Perpetuation

Overloading the psoas muscle by the repetitive vigorous concentric contraction required to perform sit-ups can perpetuate its active TrPs. The muscle is more tolerant of the eccentric contraction of slow let-backs or sit-backs (*see* Volume 1, Chapter 49, Fig. 49.11).[83]

Tightness of the rectus femoris muscle that prevents full hip extension can perpetuate TrPs in the iliopsoas muscle.

TrPs in this muscle group can be perpetuated by a lower limb-length inequality or by a small hemipelvis. The symptomatic muscles most commonly occur on the longer side, but not always.

8. PATIENT EXAMINATION (Fig. 5.3)

Patients with active TrPs that shorten the iliopsoas muscle significantly are likely to stand with the weight on the uninvolved limb and the foot of the involved limb forward with the knee bent slightly to lessen iliopsoas tension. They are also likely to stand with the torso leaning slightly toward the involved side. When asked to bend forward while standing, they lean farther to the involved side through approximately the first 20° of trunk flexion and then become centered as they continue to flex.[40]

Patients with active or latent iliopsoas TrPs tend to walk with a stooped posture, have a forward tilt of the pelvis, and exhibit hyperlordosis of the lumbar spine. Together, these factors can reduce the standing height several centimeters (an inch or more). These patients must extend the head and neck to see where they are going and may be forced to use a cane because of the stooped forward posture and low back pain. Michelle[66,67] characterizes the patient with a psoatic limp (or gait), which minimizes loading by shortening the iliopsoas muscle, as holding the thigh in flexion, abduction, and lateral rotation (the foot toes out).

The supine patient can be checked for shortening of the iliopsoas by simply testing the hip for extension range of motion with the thigh positioned over the end of the examining table, as illustrated and described in Figure 5.3. The patient grasps the thigh of the limb not being tested and pulls it toward the chest to flatten the back and stabilize the pelvis, preventing an increase in lumbar lordosis. In Figure 5.3*A*, the fully rendered right lower limb

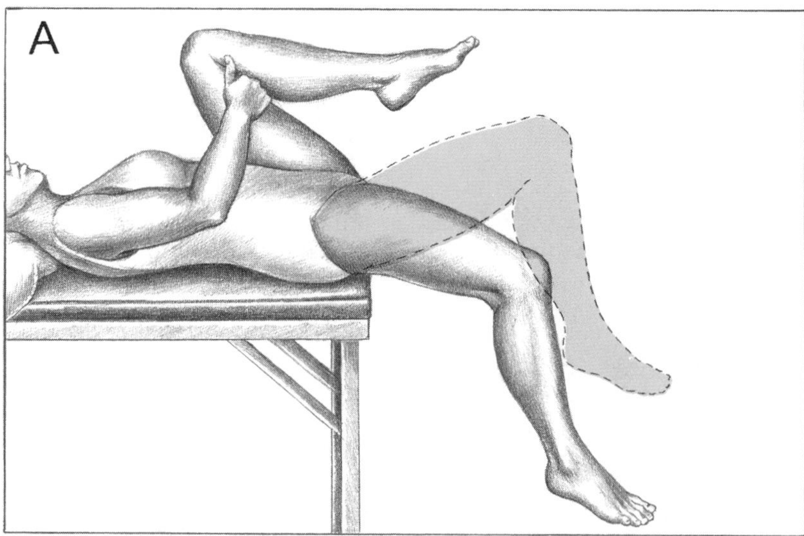

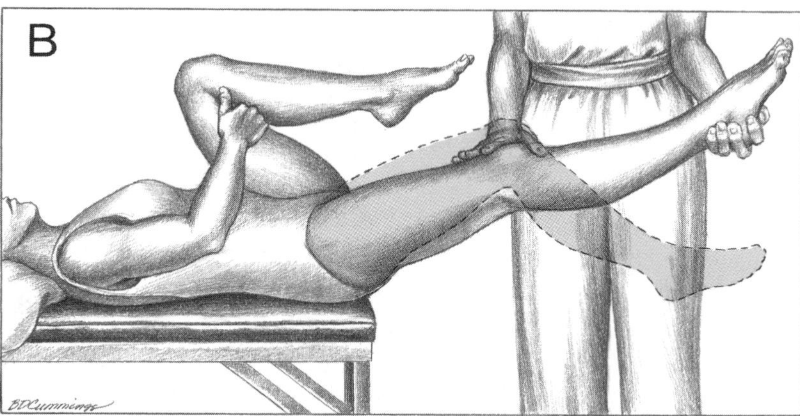

Figure 5.3. Testing the right iliopsoas muscle for tightness. *A*, the *fully rendered* right lower limb shows the normal stretch position without excessive tension. The *red limb* depicts the effect of a severely shortened iliopsoas muscle with an apparently normal-length rectus femoris. The hip remains flexed against gravity, the thigh is elevated, and the leg hangs freely, without the extension that would be seen from a tight rectus femoris muscle. *B*, the *red* right limb indicates both hip flexor and knee extensor tightness that could be due to shortening of both the iliopsoas and rectus femoris muscles, or of the rectus femoris only. The effect of a shortened rectus femoris is neutralized in the *fully rendered limb*. When the ankle is raised to straighten the knee, the hip becomes more extended, but not fully extended as in *A*. A tight rectus femoris may have contributed to the original hip flexion, but iliopsoas tightness probably causes the hip flexion remaining after the rectus femoris is relaxed. This test does not distinguish tightness of the iliopsoas from that of the tensor fascia latae muscle; such a test is described in the text. (Adapted from Kendall and McCreary.[52])

shows the normal stretch position without muscle tightness. The hip is extended and the leg hangs freely with normal knee flexion. The red limb depicts the effect of a severely shortened iliopsoas muscle (in the presence of a rectus femoris of apparently normal length). In this figure, the hip remains flexed against gravity, so the thigh is elevated. The leg hangs freely, without the excessive knee extension that would be seen if there were a tight rectus femoris muscle.

When the limb being tested remains in excessive hip flexion and excessive knee extension (*red right limb* in Fig. 5.3*B*), the position could be due to shortening of both the iliopsoas and rectus femoris muscles, or of the rectus femoris only. The effect of a shortened rectus femoris can be neutralized by putting the limb in the position shown in the *fully rendered limb* in Figure 5.3*B*. When elevating the ankle to straighten the knee allows the hip to become more extended, but not completely extended, it suggests that a tight rectus femoris contributes to some limitation of hip extension while iliopsoas tightness causes the remainder. Conversely, if there is no change in hip flexion in response to passive knee extension, there is probably no component of rectus femoris tightness.[58]

This test (Fig. 5.3*B*) does not distinguish tightness of the iliopsoas from tightness of the tensor fascia latae muscle. Passively straightening the knee with the thigh abducted and medially rotated releases tightness in the tensor fasciae latae. Iliopsoas tightness then probably causes any remaining restriction of extension at the hip.

Increasing the stretch on an iliopsoas muscle that has tightness due to TrPs is likely to cause referred pain in the sacroiliac region.

Muscle balance is necessary for good body mechanics. The iliopsoas works in harmony with the rectus abdominis; if this abdominal muscle is weak, the psoas is likely to develop problems trying to compensate. Full function of the abdominal musculature is confirmed if the patient can do a curl-up with the knees bent and without foot support.[50]

Porterfield points out that the pelvic stress added by a shortened iliopsoas muscle during hip extension while walking can cause an anterior torsion of either ilium.[74] The iliacus and psoas attachments suggest that a shortened iliacus could provoke anterior torsion of the ipsilateral ilium and a shortened psoas major could induce anterior torsion of the contralateral ilium via the contralateral SI joint.

By examining 547 unselected young military recruits for hamstring and iliopsoas tightness three times over a period of 4 years, Hellsing[44] found that 21% had restricted stretch range of motion throughout their 4-year enlistment. No significant correlation was found between this iliopsoas tightness and any back pain these recruits had before or during enlistment. The author interpreted this as showing that iliopsoas tightness does not consistently produce backache in this population, and that there are usually other important causes of backache in addition to an iliopsoas source. If the iliopsoas tightness were due to latent TrPs, the tightness would not cause backache unless the TrPs were aggravated by examination of the muscle.

9. TRIGGER POINT EXAMINATION (Fig. 5.4)

The spot tenderness of iliopsoas TrPs can be detected by palpation in three locations (Fig 5.4). In two of the three locations, the muscle fibers can be palpated directly beneath the skin without other muscle intervening. The nails of the palpating fingers and thumb must be clipped short for these examinations to avoid causing cutaneous pain.

In the supine patient, pressure can be exerted on the psoas musculotendinous junction and on iliacus muscle fibers by pressing against the lateral wall of the femoral triangle, as depicted in Figure 5.4*A* (*see* also Fig. 13.4). Pain from TrPs in this part of the muscle is referred to the low back and usually to the anteromedial aspect of the thigh and to the groin. Since the femoral nerve is on the medial side of the muscle,[33] one is less likely to apply pressure to that nerve when palpating the muscle if the thigh is abducted (Fig. 5.4*A*). If the iliacus is very tight, it may be necessary to flex the thigh slightly by supporting it with a pillow for patient comfort and to avoid excessive tension on the muscle. A local twitch response is evoked only rarely by digital examination at this site, and even less frequently at the other two sites.

At the second location, one palpates the proximal fibers of the iliacus muscle inside the iliac crest of the pelvis (Fig. 5.4*B*), through the aponeurosis of the external abdominal oblique muscle. The patient must relax the abdominal muscles, and be positioned so that the skin of the abdominal wall becomes slackened. The fingers reach inside the crest of the ilium starting in the region behind the anterior superior iliac spine and slide back and forth parallel to the iliac crest while pressing against the bone, palpating across the fibers of the iliacus muscle. Occasionally, palpation reveals taut bands and their associated spot tenderness. Pain

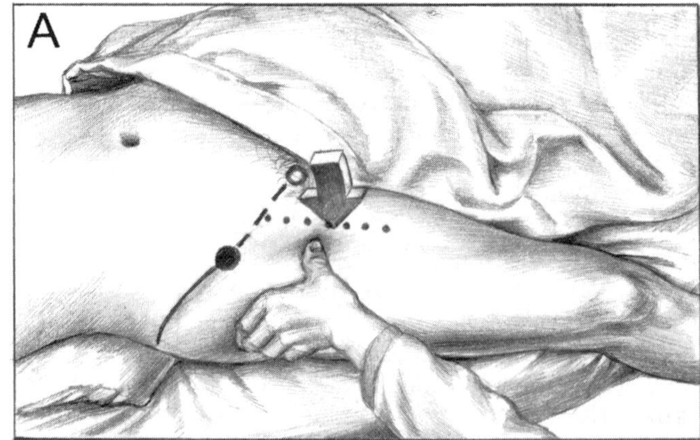

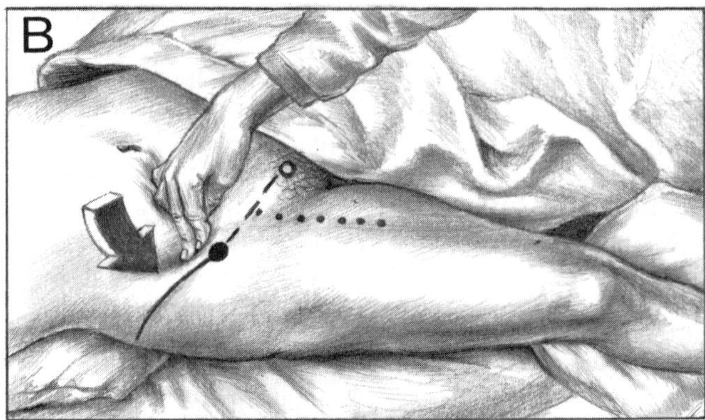

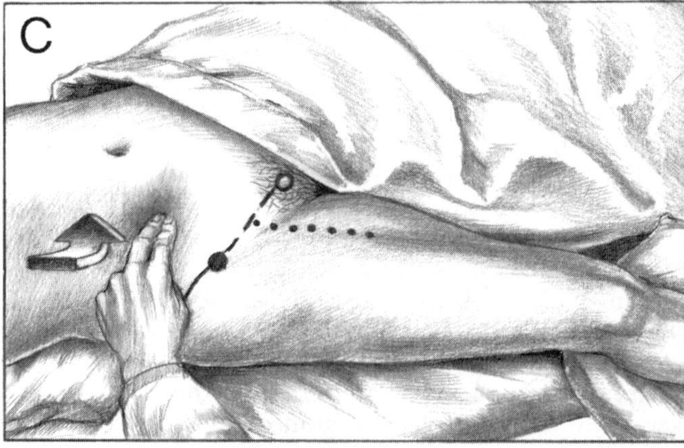

Figure 5.4. Palpation of trigger points in the right iliopsoas muscle at three locations. The *arrows* indicate the direction of pressure. The *solid circle* covers the anterior superior iliac spine; the *open circle* marks the pubic tubercle. The *solid line* marks the iliac crest; the *dashed line* locates the inguinal ligament; the *dotted line* follows the course of the femoral artery. *A*, palpation of the distal iliopsoas trigger-point region deep along the lateral wall of the femoral triangle, just above the distal attachment of the muscle to the lesser trochanter. *B*, palpation of iliacus trigger points inside the brim of the pelvis behind the anterior superior iliac spine. *C*, digital pressure on proximal psoas trigger points applied first downward beside, and then medially, beneath, the rectus abdominis muscle toward the psoas muscle. This second direction of pressure compresses the psoas fibers against the lumbar spine.

evoked from these TrPs is more likely to refer to the low back and sacroiliac region than to the thigh.

Indirect palpation of the psoas major muscle at the third location, through the abdominal wall (Fig. 5.4*C*), is remarkably effective when properly done. The patient must be comfortable and the abdominal wall relaxed. The psoas major is palpable for tenderness along the entire length of the lumbar spine. If tenderness is present, it can usually be elicited at approximately the level of the umbilicus or slightly lower. The palpating fingers are placed on the abdominal wall with the fingertips just lateral to the lateral border of the rectus abdominis muscle. Downward pressure is slowly, gradually, gently exerted to depress the fingers below the level of the rectus abdominis muscle. If the pressure is exerted directly downward with no medial component, it elicits only tenderness of other abdominal contents. At this point, therefore, the examiner exerts slowly increasing pressure medially toward the spinal column. The intervening abdominal contents transmit the pressure to the psoas muscle against the lumbar spine. It is amazing how a little pressure elicits so much pain when the psoas harbors active TrPs. One usually cannot palpate the tension of the muscle itself but, in thin patients with loose skin, one may be able to palpate its tension. Pain elicited from this part of the psoas refers chiefly to the low back.

When the clinician finds active TrPs in one iliopsoas muscle, the contralateral iliopsoas needs to be examined, since they function together. This contralateral muscle frequently also requires treatment. Usually, TrPs are more active in one iliopsoas muscle than in the other.

10. ENTRAPMENTS

The iliohypogastric, ilioinguinal, lateral femoral cutaneous, and femoral nerves all emerge from the lateral border of the psoas major muscle.[19] The obturator nerve emerges from its medial border.[17] The genitofemoral nerve passes anteriorly through the center of the belly of the muscle, emerging on its anterior surface.[1,15–17,27,30,72,78] Sometimes, the iliohypogastric nerve[16] and the ilioinguinal nerve[1,78] also pass through the belly of this muscle.

Although symptoms of entrapment of these sensory lumbosacral nerves have not been specifically related to TrPs in the psoas major, this possibility should be considered when a patient suffers enigmatic pain and disturbance of sensation in the distribution of one or more of these nerves. For example, entrapment of the genitofemoral nerve by taut TrP bands in the psoas muscle could cause pain and paresthesias in the groin, scrotum or labia, and proximal anterior thigh.[47]

Lewit[57] suggests the possibility that the lateral femoral cutaneous nerve may be entrapped by an iliopsoas muscle that is enlarged (in spasm) as it passes through the lacuna musculorum where nerve and muscle exit the pelvis together (*see* Section 2). The femoral nerve and the femoral branch of the genitofemoral nerve also pass through this foraminal space.[70] Since at this level the psoas is mostly tendon and the iliacus is still largely fleshy, it is more likely that such an entrapment would be caused by TrP shortening or reflex spasm of the iliacus than of the psoas muscle. Some enigmatic femoral nerve entrapments may arise in this way.

A number of space-occupying lesions in and around the psoas muscle also can cause symptoms of lumbosacral plexopathy. Such lesions were diagnosed by computed tomography and included intrapsoas hemorrhage in a patient receiving anticoagulant therapy, a retroperitoneal hematoma, an abscess involving the left psoas muscle, and multiple enlarged abdominal nodes due to lymphoma.[64]

11. ASSOCIATED TRIGGER POINTS

This "Hidden Prankster" can cause distorted posture that overloads back and neck muscles, perpetuating TrPs in them. The victimized muscles may include the hamstring, gluteal, thoracolumbar paraspinal, and posterior cervical muscles.

Iliopsoas TrPs are usually associated with TrPs in other muscles and rarely present as a single-muscle myofascial syndrome. The iliopsoas and the quadratus lumborum muscles are usually involved together through their stabilizing action on the lumbar spine and the occasional extensor action of the psoas muscle. Therefore, for lasting relief of an iliopsoas syndrome, TrPs in both the quadratus lumborum and iliopsoas muscles must be inactivated. Bilateral involvement of the psoas leads to bilateral involvement of the quadratus lumborum, but one side is usually more severely affected than the other. The quadratus lumborum and the posterior portion of the iliacus muscle may form a continuous sheet of fibers where both attach along the crest of the ilium.[77]

Synergistic muscles likely to exhibit myofascial TrPs in association with iliopsoas involvement include the rectus abdominis,[47] quadratus lumborum,[47] rectus femoris, tensor fasciae latae,[47] pectineus, lumbar paraspinal muscles, and the contralateral iliopsoas. When the rectus femoris is shortened because of TrPs, the iliopsoas also remains in a shortened position, making it more susceptible to TrPs. The reverse is also true; patients with patellofemoral dysfunction from a tight rectus femoris are sometimes greatly benefitted by a concomitant iliopsoas stretch program.[48]

Antagonists to the iliopsoas include the gluteus maximus and hamstring muscles. Tightness of the latter is generally of key importance to most low back pain patients. Functional shortening of the hamstrings causes an unnatural posterior tilt of the pelvis that tends to overload the psoas muscle, thus facilitating the development and perpetuation of TrPs in that muscle.

12. INTERMITTENT COLD WITH STRETCH
(Fig. 5.5)

Iliopsoas muscles should not be treated for myofascial TrPs by stretching until one identifies any coexisting lumbar spine articular dysfunction. If present, both must be treated since each can prevent recovery of the other.

It is important to apply intermittent cold with stretch to the iliopsoas bilaterally; the muscle on one side rarely develops TrPs without the other also doing so.

The hamstrings are so important in myofascial pain syndromes of the low back that it is wise to always start with bilateral release of the hamstrings (*see* Chapter 16, pages 315–338) even though the iliopsoas seems to be the muscle that is primarily involved. The remarkable increase in straight-leg raising that usually follows this hamstring release procedure removes a source of stress on the iliopsoas muscle.

The technique for using ice to apply intermittent cold is described in Chapter 2 of this volume, page 9; the technique for using vapocoolant spray is on pages 67–74 of Volume 1;[83] and techniques to augment relaxation and stretch are in Chapter 2 of this volume, on page 11.

For intermittent cold with stretch of the iliopsoas muscle (Fig. 5.5) the patient lies on the side opposite to the limb to be treated, with the low back close to the edge of the treatment table. The thigh of the limb to be treated is gently extended at the hip (Fig. 5.5*A*). After two or three initial sweeps of ice or vapocoolant spray over the muscle, the operator gradually extends the thigh and rotates it medially (Fig. 5.5*B*) while continuing to apply unidirectional parallel sweeps of cold. Each sweep successively covers the abdomen, groin, and anterior thigh on the affected side. Sweeps of coolant are then applied to the back and buttock, as shown in Figure 5.5*C*, to cover the posterior pain referral pattern.

Immediately following intermittent cold with stretch, a moist heating pad is applied to the cooled skin. When the skin has been thoroughly rewarmed, the patient actively moves the thigh slowly through full flexion and extension at the hip several times.

When re-examined following this bilateral procedure, the patient stands taller. The stooped posture induced by hip flexion has been replaced by a more erect posture. Remarkably, older individuals who have no pain complaint, but stand bent forward due to latent iliopsoas TrPs accumulated during many years, can gain several centimeters (an inch or more) of stature. They may appear to be a decade younger simply by the release of their iliopsoas TrP tension.

In the early 1950s, when ethyl chloride was the only vapocoolant spray available, the senior author observed no release of iliopsoas tension with the spray-and-stretch technique by applying the spray to the skin over the back where pain was felt.[84] Later, she suspected that the skin representation of this muscle might be over the abdomen, rather than over the low back. Spray and stretch then proved remarkably effective when she directed sweeps of the spray downward over the abdomen parallel to the midline. This emphasizes the critical importance of cooling specifically the skin area where the cutaneomuscular reflexes relate to the muscle being passively stretched, rather than cooling only where the patient complains of pain.

Postisometric relaxation[60,61] was found effective for release of iliopsoas muscle tightness associated with low lumbar discopathy[82] and is very useful for inactivating myofascial TrPs in this muscle. Deep massage and hip extension exercises may also be helpful in relieving the pain referred from iliopsoas TrPs.[47,79]

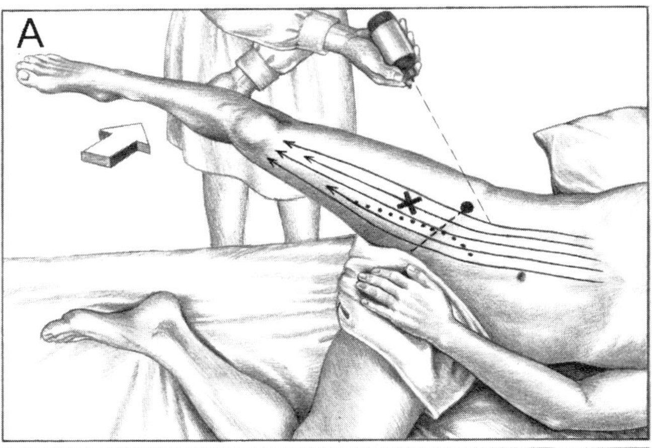

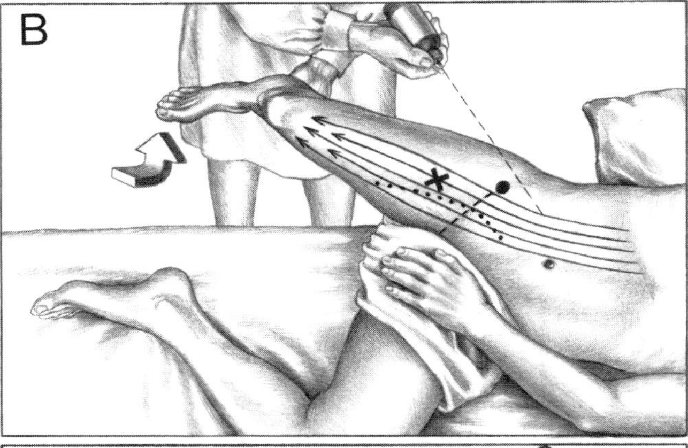

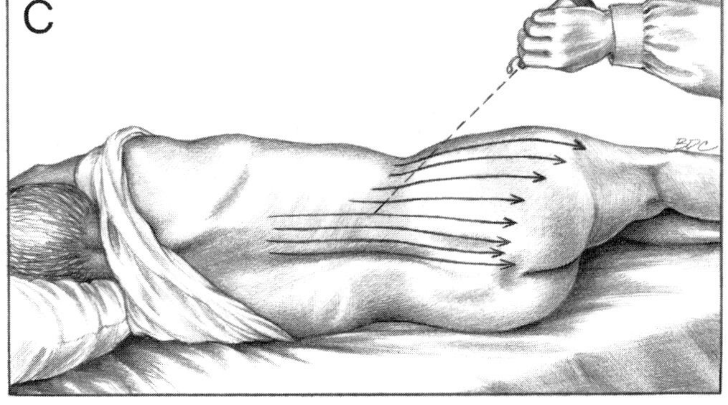

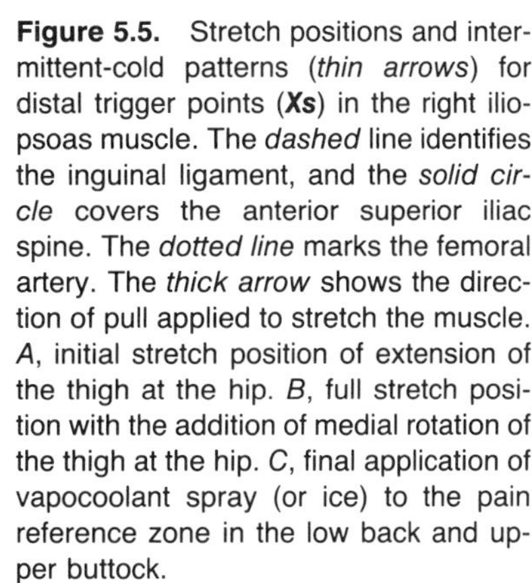

Figure 5.5. Stretch positions and intermittent-cold patterns (*thin arrows*) for distal trigger points (**Xs**) in the right iliopsoas muscle. The *dashed* line identifies the inguinal ligament, and the *solid circle* covers the anterior superior iliac spine. The *dotted line* marks the femoral artery. The *thick arrow* shows the direction of pull applied to stretch the muscle. *A*, initial stretch position of extension of the thigh at the hip. *B*, full stretch position with the addition of medial rotation of the thigh at the hip. *C*, final application of vapocoolant spray (or ice) to the pain reference zone in the low back and upper buttock.

Before leaving the clinician's office, the patient should be trained in a stretching exercise for use at home, as described in Section 14 of this chapter.

13. INJECTION AND STRETCH
(Fig. 5.6)

Only the distal end of the psoas major muscle is accessible by ordinary injection techniques. Generally, injection of this muscle should await the inactivation of associated TrPs in the quadratus lumborum, rectus abdominis, rectus femoris, hamstring, and gluteal muscles. Then, the iliopsoas TrPs can usually be inactivated by applying intermittent cold with stretch combined with Lewit's postisometric relaxation (*see* Chapter 2, pages 10–11). Occasionally, TrPs remain that require injection.

If injection of TrPs in the psoas muscle is attempted before the associated TrPs in the functionally related muscles have

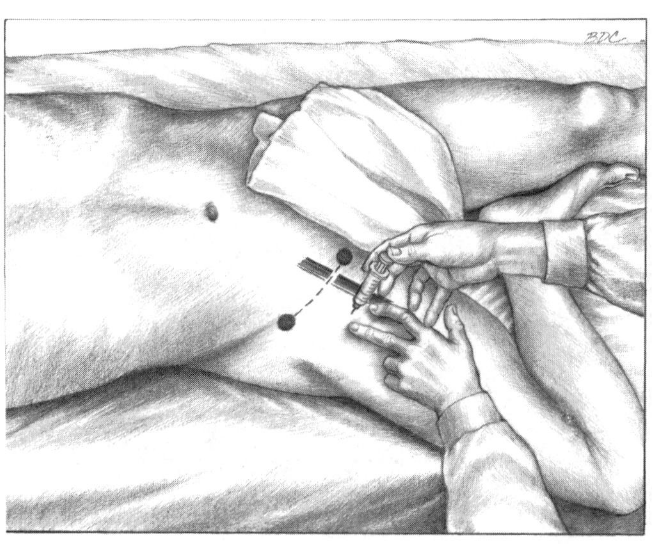

Figure 5.6. Injection of distal trigger points in the right iliopsoas muscle. The *solid circles* cover the anterior superior iliac spine and the pubic tubercle. Between them, the inguinal ligament lies beneath the *dashed line*. The femoral artery is *red*. The thigh is abducted and laterally rotated to separate the iliopsoas muscle and the femoral artery. The needle is directed toward the trigger point tenderness close to the lesser trochanter, laterally, away from the femoral artery. The pulsation of the artery is usually palpable. The femoral nerve lies close and lateral to the artery.

been eliminated, patients are prone to experience severe local soreness and increased disability for several days afterward. They complain of increased difficulty in standing and walking. The associated TrPs should be identified and inactivated before injecting the iliopsoas TrPs, because tautness of the involved iliopsoas fibers provides protective splinting for the other muscles of its functional unit. Removal of protective splinting supplied by the iliopsoas muscle, without first inactivating TrPs in the muscles that it is protecting, frequently aggravates their myofascial pain syndromes. In this situation, the increased severity of symptoms due to TrPs in the other muscles overshadows the relief obtained from the pain that had been referred from TrPs in the iliopsoas muscle. This paradoxical response to treatment also occurs in other functional units.

The distal iliacus fibers and fibers of the psoas muscle at its musculotendinous junction are accessible to injection in the femoral triangle. The position of the muscle with regard to the femoral nerve and artery must be taken into account; it has been well illustrated.[3,72] The tender areas to be injected are located by palpation just proximal to the attachment of the muscle on the lesser trochanter, as described under Section 9, Trigger Point Examination. This attachment is located on the medial aspect of the femur (Fig. 5.2).

For this injection, the thigh is extended and then abducted and laterally rotated to separate the iliopsoas muscle as far as possible from the femoral nerve and artery (Fig. 5.6). Usually, the thigh should lie flat against the examining table or else the iliopsoas muscle is likely to be undesirably slack. The pulsating femoral artery is identified by palpation medial to the TrP tenderness in the muscle fibers. However, the clinician must be aware that the femoral nerve lies between the iliopsoas muscle and the femoral artery.

While injecting these iliopsoas TrPs, one finger (the index finger of the left hand in Fig. 5.6) is held just lateral to the femoral artery, over the femoral nerve. A needle usually 50 mm (2 in) long is directed into the tender area and angled to avoid the femoral nerve and artery. Because the muscle lies so deep, only occasionally is a local twitch perceptible when the needle penetrates a TrP. The pain response of the patient (jump sign), however, is unmistakable. If the patient is asked before injection to note the location of pain elicited by the needle, he or she can report the specific pattern of referred pain evoked by the injection of that active TrP.

Performing intermittent cold with stretch after injection helps to ensure inactivation of any residual TrPs.

Application of a moist heating pad to both the abdomen and upper anterior thigh follows the intermittent cold with stretch. When the skin has been rewarmed, the patient performs *full* active range of motion in flexion and extension of the hip slowly through several cycles.

Dry needling of iliopsoas TrPs in this femoral triangle area was also reported to be effective. When the needle reached the TrP it induced a "fasciculation" (local twitch response) that could be felt by the patient and by the examiner's hand as it rested gently on the area.[47]

Inactivation of these distal iliopsoas TrPs may occasionally eliminate the more proximal psoas TrPs.

Iliacus TrPs close to the iliac crest may be injected, with special care, via a lower abdominal approach. The upper iliac fossa is palpated for taut bands and TrP tenderness, as described in Section 9, Trigger Point Examination. A spinal needle 67–87 mm (2½–3½ in) long is inserted inside the crest of the ilium and directed to the taut bands with TrP tenderness. The needle must travel close to the inner surface of the ilium to avoid penetrating abdominal contents. Occasional contact with bone ensures that the needle is still within the muscle. A pain response by the patient usually indicates that the needle encountered a TrP. Local twitch responses rarely reveal themselves here. Again, application of moist heat and active range of motion follows intermittent cold with stretch to complete the procedure.

Although no report was found that described a posterior approach for injecting psoas TrPs beside the lumbar spine, needles have been placed in that muscle from behind for other reasons. Awad[5] described and illustrated this approach to perform motor point blocks of the lumbar psoas muscle and Nachemson[68] described it for intramuscular EMG monitoring of its activity. For those accustomed to performing lumbar sympathetic blocks, this should not be especially difficult. Normally, the aorta lies anterior to the iliopsoas muscle and is shielded by the vertebral bodies from needles introduced posteriorly.

14. CORRECTIVE ACTIONS
(Figs. 5.7 and 5.8)

The initial corrective actions are to inactivate associated TrPs (*see* Section 11) and to correct any mechanical and systemic perpetuating factors (*see* Volume 1, Chapter 4).[83]

When iliopsoas TrPs are causing pain that demands emergency relief, the patient should be instructed to apply moist heat to the abdomen over the entire length of the muscle from the rib cage to the lesser trochanter. Patients need an explanation as to why this positioning of hot packs is used for a muscle that is located beside the backbone and causes pain in the back. Its musculocutaneous reflex area is the skin of the abdomen, not of the back.

If upright ambulation is prohibitively painful, a degree of mobility may be achieved temporarily by suggesting that the patient try to move around on the hands and knees. This position relieves the iliopsoas of its erect postural responsibilities.

Body Asymmetry

A lower limb-length inequality and/or a small hemipelvis should be corrected by appropriate lifts (Chapter 4, pages 77–78).

A locked sacroiliac joint is likely to aggravate TrPs in the iliacus muscle[54] and may be corrected by appropriate manipulation (Chapter 2, pages 16–17). Lewit associates iliacus TrPs with dysfunction at the lumbosacral junction,[57] while thoracolumbar restriction aggravates TrPs in the psoas muscle.[57,59]

Postural and Activity Stress

A position on the hands and knees can provide at least temporary relief of pain, often greater than can be obtained in any recumbent position. This observation is useful diagnostically and therapeutically. On awakening from sleep, it may be the only way a person who is alone and experiencing an acute attack of pain can reach the bathroom.

When sitting, the patient should maintain an open angle at the hips by avoiding the jackknifed position, at least 10° beyond a right angle. Raising the back of the seat so that the thigh slopes downward toward the front of the seat produces this desirable effect. Leaning back against a slightly reclining backrest is also helpful.

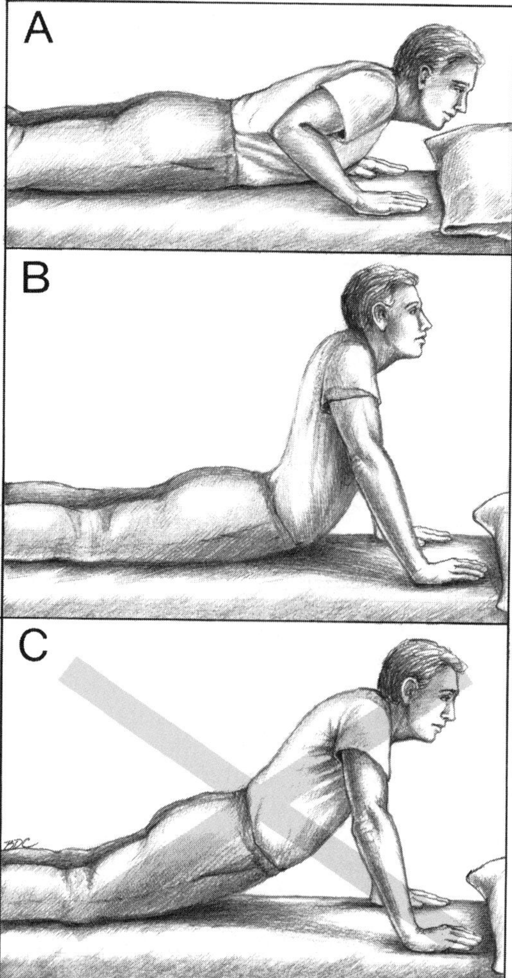

Figure 5.7. Exercise for mobilizing extension of the lumbar spine and for stretching the hip flexor muscles. This exercise is applicable only to selected patients who have no neck and shoulder-girdle problems. *A*, starting position. *B*, correct extension position with hips flat against the table. *C*, incorrect position (*red* **X**) that fails to extend the lumbar spine and tends to overload the extensor musculature.

If the jackknifed seated position is unavoidable, then standing up frequently to extend the hips and stretch the iliopsoas muscles avoids immobility in the shortened position for too long a period.

Sustained immobility in any seated position is likely to impair circulation and aggravate iliopsoas TrPs. On long automobile trips, cruise control provides an opportunity for the driver to change positions and improve the mobility of the muscles.

The habit of paradoxical breathing (*see* Volume 1, Fig. 20.13)[83] can seriously impede recovery from iliopsoas TrPs. Patients who exhibit paradoxical breathing should practice abdominal breathing until they habitually breathe in the normal pattern of coordinated chest and abdominal movements during inhalation and exhalation.

For sleeping, the patient may place a small pillow under the knees when lying on the back, or under the hips when sleeping prone. This produces some hip flexion that lessens tension on the iliopsoas muscles sufficiently to improve sleep. The patient should avoid side lying in a tight fetal position that excessively shortens the iliopsoas muscles.

A bed that sags like a hammock may place the iliopsoas in too shortened a position and aggravate pain. In this situation, moving the mattress to the floor for the night can temporarily solve the problem. A bed board offers a more permanent solution (*see* Chapter 4, page 79).

Exercise Therapy
(Figs. 5.7 and 5.8)

A hip extension exercise to stretch the iliopsoas muscle passively is illustrated in Figure 5.7. Patients are reminded to keep the thighs and pelvis solidly against the table (or floor) as they hyperextend the lumbar spine and hips. For maximum stretch of the iliopsoas, it is helpful for some patients also to medially rotate the thigh at the hip on the involved side.

Another exercise for relieving tension of the iliopsoas muscle employs the postisometric relaxation technique, which was described and illustrated for this muscle by Lewit.[57] This technique is remarkably effective and is easy for the patient to do. It is performed in the position for examination that is illustrated in Figure 5.3*A*. The lower limb on the side of the iliopsoas muscle to be stretched is allowed to hang freely with the knee bent. If the thigh needs more support, the patient moves up on the examining table. Tension is increased by pulling the other knee to the chest. This position also loads a sufficiently shortened rectus femoris muscle.

A variation of the Lewit relaxation-and-stretch method has the patient lie supine on a stair landing and gradually "walk"

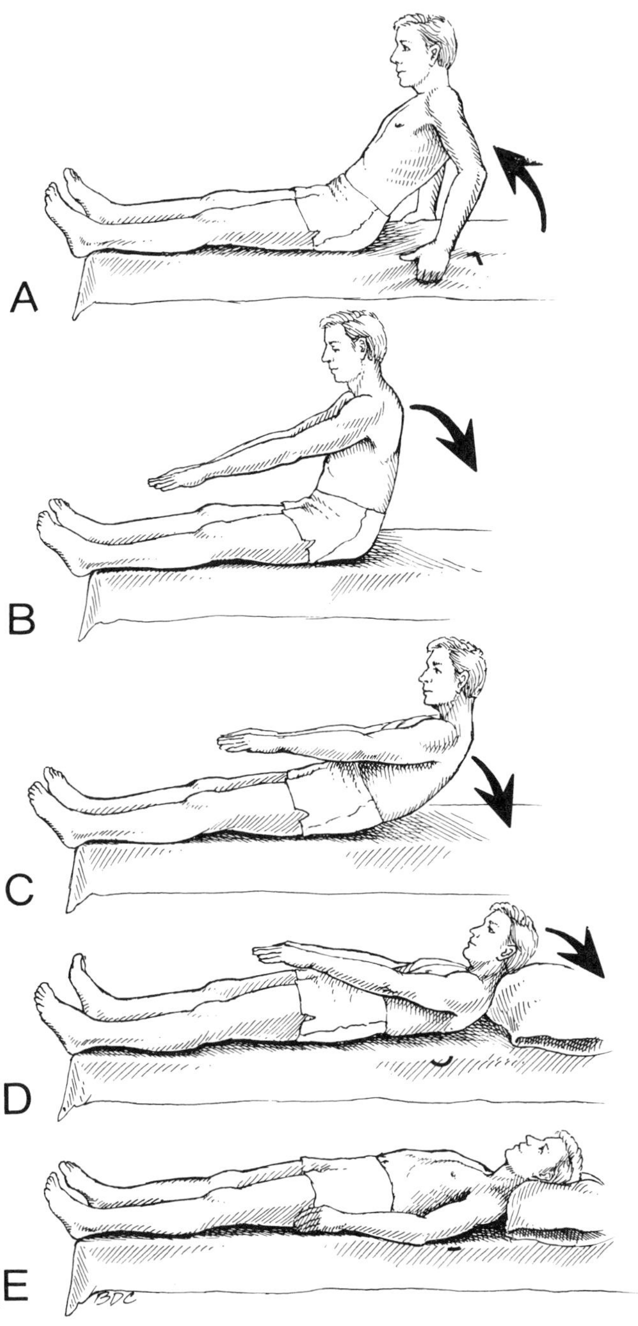

Figure 5.8. Slow Sit-back Exercise to improve strength and coordination of the abdominal and hip flexor muscles as the spine "rolls down" on the table. This exercise requires a less demanding lengthening contraction, rather than the shortening contraction of a sit-up. *A*, pushing the torso up (*arrow*) with the arms from the supine to the seated position. This avoids loading the flexor muscles of the trunk and hips. *B*, beginning of the slow sit-back, lumbar spine flexed. *C*, rolling the back down onto the table, maintaining spinal flexion so that each spinal segment reaches the table in succession. *D*, completion of slow sit-back. *E*, period of full relaxation with abdominal (diaphragmatic) breathing. Three cycles of this slow sit-back exercise should be performed daily to provide full benefit.

the foot of the involved limb downstairs while holding the knee of the uninvolved limb close to the chest (Personal communication, Mary Maloney, PT, 1990).

The In-doorway Stretch Exercise (*see* Volume 1, Fig. 42.10)[83] also provides effective stretch of the iliopsoas muscle, if the patient makes a point of swinging the hips forward, alternately. Keeping the knee of the rear leg straight emphasizes hip extension.

In the office, another effective stretch of the iliopsoas is to grasp a file cabinet with one hand for stability, then place one foot well behind and extend that thigh at the hip while bending the opposite knee placed in front. The office worker can also provide a hip flexor stretch by simply sitting on the side edge of the chair seat (without armrests), with one buttock off the edge and the knee flexed, then sliding that leg posteriorly to extend the hip.

Following a program of muscle lengthening, the iliopsoas and rectus abdominis muscles should be conditioned together in a coordinated strengthening exercise. This program should start with slow sit-backs (Fig. 5.8, and Volume 1,[83] Fig. 49.11). Then, as the muscles gain strength, the patient can reverse the process and start doing a few sit-ups safely and comfortably. This exercise program can, however, aggravate TrPs in the sternocleidomastoid and scalene muscles by overloading them in the shortened position.

It is also important to warn patients what not to do. Some patients aggravate iliopsoas TrPs in the long-sitting position while performing the In-bathtub Stretch Exercise that is illustrated in Volume 1, Figure 48.13.[83] Leaning forward, they strongly contract the iliopsoas muscles in the fully shortened position in an effort to reach their toes, which can seriously aggravate iliopsoas TrPs and induce severe pain. The patient should learn to perform this stretch by leaning forward and allowing gravity to pull the head, torso, and arms forward without vigorous muscular effort. Patients who are unable to learn to relax in this way should be discouraged from doing the In-bathtub Stretch Exercise.

References

1. Anderson JE: *Grant's Atlas of Anatomy*, Ed. 8. Williams & Wilkins, Baltimore, 1983 (Fig. 2–119).
2. *Ibid.* (Fig. 2–125).
3. *Ibid.* (Fig. 4–22).
4. *Ibid.* (Figs. 4–23, 4–24).
5. Awad EA: Phenol block for control of hip flexor and adductor spasticity. *Arch Phys Med Rehabil 53*:554–557, 1972.
6. Bachrach RM: The relationship of low back/pelvic somatic dysfunctions to dance injuries. *Orthop Rev 17*:1037–1043, 1988.
7. Bardeen CR: The musculature, Sect. 5. In *Morris's Human Anatomy*, edited by C. M. Jackson, Ed. 6. Blakiston's Son & Co., Philadelphia, 1921 (p.489).
8. Basmajian JV, Deluca CJ: *Muscles Alive*, Ed. 5. Williams & Wilkins, Baltimore, 1985 (pp. 234–235).
9. *Ibid.* (pp. 310–313).
10. *Ibid.* (p. 380).
11. Basmajian JV, Greenlaw RK: Electromyography of iliacus and psoas with inserted fine-wire electrodes. *Anat Rec 160*:310–311, 1968.
12. Bogduk N, Twomey LT: *Clinical Anatomy of the Lumbar Spine*. Churchill Livingstone, New York, 1987 (pp. 72–73).
13. Bloom RA, Gheorghiu D, Verstandig A, *et al.*: The psoas sign in normal subjects without bowel preparation: the influence of scoliosis on visualisation. *Clin Radiol 41*:204–205, 1990.
14. Carter BL, Morehead J, Wolpert SM, *et al.*: *Cross-Sectional Anatomy*. Appleton-Century-Crofts, New York, 1977 (Sects. 30–42, and 44–48).
15. Clemente CD: *Anatomy. A Regional Atlas of the Human Body*. Lea & Febiger, Philadelphia, 1975 (pp. 231, 235).
16. *Ibid.* (p. 232).
17. Clemente CD: *Gray's Anatomy of the Human Body*, American Ed. 30. Lea & Febiger, Philadelphia, 1985 (pp. 557–558).
18. *Ibid.* (p. 564, Fig. 6–70).
19. *Ibid.* (pp. 1227–1232).
20. Close JR: *Motor Function in the Lower Extremity*. Charles C Thomas, Springfield, 1964 (p. 128).
21. Dobrik I: Disorders of the iliopsoas muscle and its role in gynecological diseases. *J Man Med 4*: 130–133, 1989.
22. Duchenne GB: *Physiology of Motion*, translated by E.B. Kaplan. J. B. Lippincott, Philadelphia, 1949 (pp. 259–260).
23. Duprat G Jr., Lévesque HP, Séguin R, *et al.*: Bowel displacement due to psoas muscle hypertrophy. *J Can Assoc Radiol 34*:64–65, 1983.
24. Durianová: [Spasm of the m. psoas in the differential diagnosis of pain in the lumbosacral region.] *Fysiatr Reumatol Vestn 52*:199–203, 1974.
25. Ekelund L, Jónsson G, Rünow A: [Compartment syndrome in the iliopsoas region with compression of the femoral nerve.] *Lakartidningen 77*: 4539–4540, 1980.
26. Evjenth O, Hamberg J: *Muscle Stretching in Manual Therapy, A Clinical Manual*. Alfta Rehab Førlag, Alfta, Sweden, 1984 (p. 102).
27. Ferner H, Staubesand J: *Sobotta Atlas of Human Anatomy*, Ed. 10, Vol. 2. Urban & Schwarzenberg, Baltimore, 1983 (Fig. 91).
28. *Ibid.* (Fig. 137).
29. *Ibid.* (Fig. 152).
30. *Ibid.* (Fig. 261).
31. *Ibid.* (Fig. 351).
32. *Ibid.* (Fig. 404).
33. *Ibid.* (Fig. 410).
34. *Ibid.* (Figs. 416, 417).
35. *Ibid.* (Fig. 421).
36. Flint MM: An electromyographic comparison of the function of the iliacus and the rectus abdominis muscles. *J Am Phys Therap Assoc 45*: 248–253, 1965.
37. Fujiwara M, Basmajian JV: Electromyographic study of two-joint muscles. *Am J Phys Med 54*: 234–242, 1975.
38. Graif M, Olchovsky D, Frankl O, *et al.*: Ultrasonic demonstration of iliopsoas hematoma causing femoral neuropathy. *Isr J Med Sci 18*: 967–968, 1982.
39. Greenlaw RK: *Function of Muscles About the Hip During Normal Level Walking.* Queen's University,

Kingston, Ontario, (thesis) 1973 (*see* pp. 108–111).

40. Grice A: Personal communication, 1991.
41. Giuliani G, Poppi M, Acciarri N, *et al.*: CT scan and surgical treatment of traumatic iliacus hematoma with femoral neuropathy: case report. *J Trauma 30*:229–231, 1990.
42. Haines JD, Chop WM Jr, Towsley DK: Primary psoas abscess: an often insidious infection. *Postgrad Med 87*:287–288, 1990.
43. Helfgott SM: Unusual features of iliopsoas bursitis. *Arthritis Rheum 31*:1331–1333, 1988.
44. Hellsing A-L: Tightness of hamstring and psoas major muscles. *Ups J Med Sci 93*:267–276, 1988.
45. Hooper ACB: The role of the iliopsoas muscle in femoral rotation. *Irish J Med Sci 146*:108–112, 1977.
46. Imamura K, Ashida H, Ishikawa T. *et al.*: Human major psoas muscle and sacrospinalis muscle in relation to age: a study by computed tomography. *J Gerontol 38*:678–681, 1983.
47. Ingber RS: Iliopsoas myofascial dysfunction: a treatable cause of "failed" low back syndrome. *Arch Phys Med Rehabil 70*:382–386, 1989.
48. Ingber RS: Personal communication. 1989.
49. Janda V: *Muscle Function Testing*. Butterworths, London, 1983 (p. 29).
50. Jull GA, Janda V: Muscles and motor control in low back pain: assessment and management, Chapter 10. In *Physical Therapy of the Low Back*, edited by L. T. Twomey and J. R. Taylor, Churchill Livingstone, New York, 1987 (pp. 253–278 *see* p. 271).
51. Keagy RD, Brumlik J, Bergan JJ: Direct electromyography of psoas major muscle in man. *J Bone Joint Surg [Am]48:*1377–1382, 1966.
52. Kendall FP, McCreary EK: *Muscles, Testing and Function*, Ed. 3. Williams & Wilkins, Baltimore, 1983 (pp. 160–163).
53. Klammer A: [Fascia compartment syndrome of the iliacus-psoas compartment.] *Z Orthop 121*: 298–304, 1983.
54. Klawunde G, Zeller H-J: Elektromyographische Untersuchungen zum Hartspann des M. iliacus (Sagittale Blockierungen im lumbo-iliosakralen Bereich). *Beitr Orthop Traumatol 22*:420–430, 1975.
55. Kvernebo K, Stiris G, Haaland M: CT in idiopathic pyogenic myositis of the iliopsoas muscle: a report of 2 cases. *Eur J Radiol 3*:1–2, 1983.
56. LaBan MM, Raptou AD, Johnson EW: Electromyographic study of function of iliopsoas muscle. *Arch Phys Med Rehabil 46*:676–679, 1965.
57. Lewit K: *Manipulative Therapy in Rehabilitation of the Motor System*. Butterworths, London, 1985 (pp. 138, 276, 315).
58. *Ibid.* (p. 153, Fig. 4.42).
59. Lewit K: Muscular pattern in thoraco-lumbar lesions. *Manual Med 2*:105–107, 1986.
60. Lewit K: Postisometric relaxation in combination with other methods of muscular facilitation and inhibition. *Manual Med 2*:101–104, 1986.
61. Lewit K, Simons DG: Myofascial pain: relief by post-isometric relaxation. *Arch Phys Med Rehabil 65*:452–456, 1984.
62. Mann RA, Moran GT, Dougherty SE: Comparative electromyography of the lower extremity in jogging, running, and sprinting. *Am J Sports Med 14*:501–510, 1986.
63. Markhede G, Stener B: Function after removal of various hip and thigh muscles for extirpation of tumors. *Acta Orthop Scand 52*:373–395, 1981.
64. Massey EW: CT evaluation of lumbosacral plexus disorders. *Postgrad Med 69*:116–118, 1981.
65. Mastroianni PP, Roberts MP: Femoral neuropathy and retroperitoneal hemorrhage. *Neurosurgery 13*:44–47, 1983.
66. Michele AA: The iliopsoas muscle. *Clin Symp 12*: 67–101, 1960 (Plates I, III, VI, pp. 67, 70, 87, 89).
67. Michele AA: *Iliopsoas*. Charles C Thomas, Springfield, 1962 (pp. 195, 282, 489-491).
68. Nachemson A: Electromyographic studies on the vertebral portion of the psoas muscle. *Acta Orthop Scand 37*:177–190, 1966.
69. Netter FH: *The Ciba Collection of Medical Illustrations*, Vol.8, Musculoskeletal System. Part I: Anatomy, Physiology and Metabolic Disorders. Ciba-Geigy Corporation, Summit, 1987 (p. 86).
70. *Ibid.* (pp. 77, 89).
71. *Ibid.* (p. 87).
72. *Ibid.* (p. 89).
73. Nino-Murcia M, Wechsler RJ, Brennan RE: Computed tomography of the iliopsoas muscle. *Skel Radiol 10*:107–112, 1983.
74. Porterfield JA: The sacroiliac joint, Chapter 23. In *Orthopaedic and Sports Physical Therapy*, edited by J.A. Gould III and G.J. Davies, Vol. II. CV Mosby, St. Louis, 1985 (p. 553).
75. Rab GT, Chao EYS, Stauffer RN: Muscle force analysis of the lumbar spine. *Orthop Clin North Am 8*:193–199, 1977.
76. Rasch PJ, Burke RK: *Kinesiology and Applied Anatomy*, Ed. 6. Lea & Febiger, Philadelphia, 1978 (pp. 243–244).
77. Rohen JW, Yokochi C: *Color Atlas of Anatomy*, Ed. 2. Igaku-Shoin, New York, 1988 (p. 417).
78. *Ibid.* (p. 308).
79. Saudek CE: The hip, Chapter 17. In *Orthopaedic and Sports Physical Therapy*, edited by J.A. Gould III and G.J. Davies, Vol. II. CV Mosby, St. Louis, 1985 (pp. 365–407, *see* p. 406, Fig. 17–48).
80. Silver SF, Connell DG, Duncan CP: Case report 550. *Skel Radiol 18*:327–328, 1989.
81. Simons DG, Travell JG: Myofascial origins of low back pain. 2. Torso muscles. *Postgrad Med 73*:81–92, 1983 (*see* pp. 91, 92).
82. Stodolny J, Mazur T: Effect of post-isometric relaxation exercises on the ilio-psoas muscles in patients with lumbar discopathy. *J Manual Med 4*:52–54, 1989.
83. Travell JG, Simons DG: *Myofascial Pain and Dysfunction: The Trigger Point Manual*. Williams & Wilkins, Baltimore, 1983.
84. Travell J: Ethyl chloride spray for painful muscle spasm. *Arch Phys Med Rehabil 33*:291–298, 1952.
85. Uncini A, Tonali P, Falappa P, *et al.*: Femoral neuropathy from iliac muscle hematoma induced by oral anticoagulation therapy. *J Neurol 226*:137–141, 1981.
86. Vos PA: The psoas minor syndrome. *J Int Coll Surg 44*:30–36, 1965.

CHAPTER 6
Pelvic Floor Muscles
Bulbospongiosus, Ischiocavernosus, Transversus Perinei, Sphincter Ani, Levator Ani, Coccygeus, and Obturator Internus

"Pain in the Rear"

HIGHLIGHTS: The levator ani and coccygeus muscles afford a unique opportunity to palpate directly with minimal intervening tissue the taut band and tender attachment phenomena associated with trigger points (TrPs). **REFERRED PAIN** from TrPs in the bulbospongiosus and ischiocavernosus muscles usually projects to the perineum and adjacent urogenital structures. Sphincter ani TrPs induce pain in the posterior pelvic floor. The levator ani and coccygeus muscles refer pain and tenderness to the sacrococcygeal region. The levator ani may also refer pain to the vagina. The TrPs of the obturator internus cause pain in the anococcygeal region and in the vagina, with a spillover pattern to the thigh posteriorly. **ANATOMICAL ATTACHMENTS** of the bulbospongiosus muscle in the male are to the perineal body, below, and to the corpus spongiosus and corpus cavernosus, which they enclose, above. In the female, this muscle also attaches to the perineal body and then surrounds the vagina on its way to the corpora cavernosa clitoridis. The ischiocavernosus muscle anchors laterally to the ischial tuberosity in both men and women. Medially in the male, it blends with the crura of the penis and in the female with the crus clitoridis. The more anterior and medial pubococcygeus muscle of the levator ani forms a sling around the rectum and urogenital structures; it anchors in front to the pubis and behind to the anococcygeal and perineal bodies. The deeper iliococcygeus muscle of the levator ani forms a hammock across the pelvic floor and is anchored laterally to the tendinous arch of the levator ani muscle along the wall of the pelvis and centrally to the anococcygeal body and the last two segments of the coccyx. The coccygeus muscle usually covers the inner surface of the sacrospinous ligament. Together, these two muscles span the space between the spine of the ischium laterally and the coccyx and sacrum medially. The obturator internus covers, and is attached to, the anterolateral wall of the pelvis including the obturator foramen. It exits the pelvis through the lesser sciatic foramen to end on the greater trochanter of the femur. **INNERVATION** of these muscles is supplied by spinal nerves from L_5 to S_5. The **FUNCTION** of the anal sphincter is to serve as gate keeper of the rectum. The bulbospongiosus in the female constricts the vagina. Both the bulbospongiosus and ischiocavernosus muscles enhance tumescence of the penis in the male and of the clitoris in the female. The levator ani supports the pelvic floor and assists the anal and urethral sphincters. It helps to constrict the vagina in the female. The coccygeus flexes the coccyx inward toward the pelvis and exerts rotatory tension on the sacroiliac joint. The obturator internus laterally rotates the extended thigh and abducts the thigh when it is in 90° of flexion. **SYMPTOMS** of patients with myofascial TrPs in one or several of these pelvic muscles are remarkably similar to the symptoms of many patients categorized by other authors as having coccygodynia, levator ani syndrome, proctalgia fugax, and tension myalgia of the pelvic floor. **PATIENT EXAMINATION**, when low back or pelvic floor pain suggests the possibility of intrapelvic TrPs, should include examination of the coccyx for tenderness and mobility. The thigh should be tested for restriction of medial rotation caused by obturator internus TrP tension. **TRIGGER POINT EXAMINATION** of all of these intrapelvic muscles requires either a rectal or vaginal approach. Some muscles are more effectively examined by one of these routes, other muscles by the other. The examiner identifies each muscle by locating appropriate bony and ligamentous landmarks and carefully relates the direction of palpation to the direction of the muscle fibers. The **INTERMITTENT COLD WITH STRETCH** procedure is not applicable to these muscles, but other methods of treatment include massage, stretch, postisometric relaxation, high voltage pulsed galvanic stimulation, ultrasound, and correction of seated posture. **INJECTION** of TrPs in the perineal muscles employs surface techniques, but injection of myofascial TrPs of other muscles within the pelvis requires a bimanual approach. **CORRECTIVE ACTIONS** include consideration of mechanical and systemic perpetuating factors, seated posture, dysfunction of pelvic articulations, internal hemorrhoids, and chronic pelvic inflammatory conditions.

1. REFERRED PAIN
(Fig. 6.1)

Trigger points (TrPs) in muscles of the posterior half of the pelvic floor, including the sphincter ani, superficial transverse perinei, levator ani, and coccygeus muscles refer poorly localized pain. Patients are often uncertain whether to call it tailbone, hip, or back pain.[77] The pain centers in the region of the coccyx but often includes the anal area and the lower part of the sacrum (Fig. 6.1*A*). Both the levator ani and coccygeus muscles typically refer pain to the region of the coccyx.[88] This referred pain pattern is often called coccygodynia, although the coccyx itself is usually normal and not tender.[33,62,94,95] Since the levator ani is the muscle most commonly involved, pain in the region of the coccyx is also called the levator ani syndrome.[62]

The TrPs in the anterior half of the pelvic floor muscles, the ischiocavernosus and bulbospongiosus, are likely to refer pain to genital structures, the vagina and the base of the penis beneath the scrotum. Vaginal pain can also arise from TrPs in the levator ani and has been reproduced by pressure on the tender sites in that muscle.[94]

In addition, Goldstein found that injection of obturator internus TrPs relieved pain in the vagina.[45] Obturator internus TrPs also refer pain to the anococcygeal region and may have a spillover pattern to the upper portion of the posterior thigh (Fig. 6.1*B*).[88]

The obturator internus syndrome causes pain and a feeling of fullness in the rectum and some pain referred down the back of the ipsilateral thigh.[56] This additional thigh pain can be caused also by piriformis muscle involvement (*see* Fig. 10.1), so that muscle too should be examined for TrPs.

2. ANATOMICAL ATTACHMENTS AND CONSIDERATIONS
(Figs. 6.2 and 6.3)

As the previous descriptions of referred pain show, knowing only the patient's referred pain pattern in the pelvic region is not sufficient to identify which muscle harbors TrPs that are responsible for the pain. Therefore, a thorough knowledge of the anatomy of the muscles and their relationships is essential if one is to identify by palpation which muscle is responsible. This knowledge is valuable also for massaging TrPs in these muscles, and critically important if one wishes to inject the TrPs to inactivate them.

This section first presents the major intrapelvic muscles in the sequence of the physical examination. Then, it reviews the less commonly involved superficial perineal muscles, and, lastly, considers variable, but occasionally clinically important, intrapelvic muscles.

Sphincter Ani Muscles
(Fig. 6.2)

The sphincter ani internus and externus consist, in all, of four concentric layers or rings of muscle. The innermost ring, the sphincter ani internus, comprises autonomically innervated involuntary muscle fibers of the anal wall.[39] The remaining three layers are the deep, superficial, and subcutaneous laminae of the sphincter ani externus. The external sphincter is under vol-

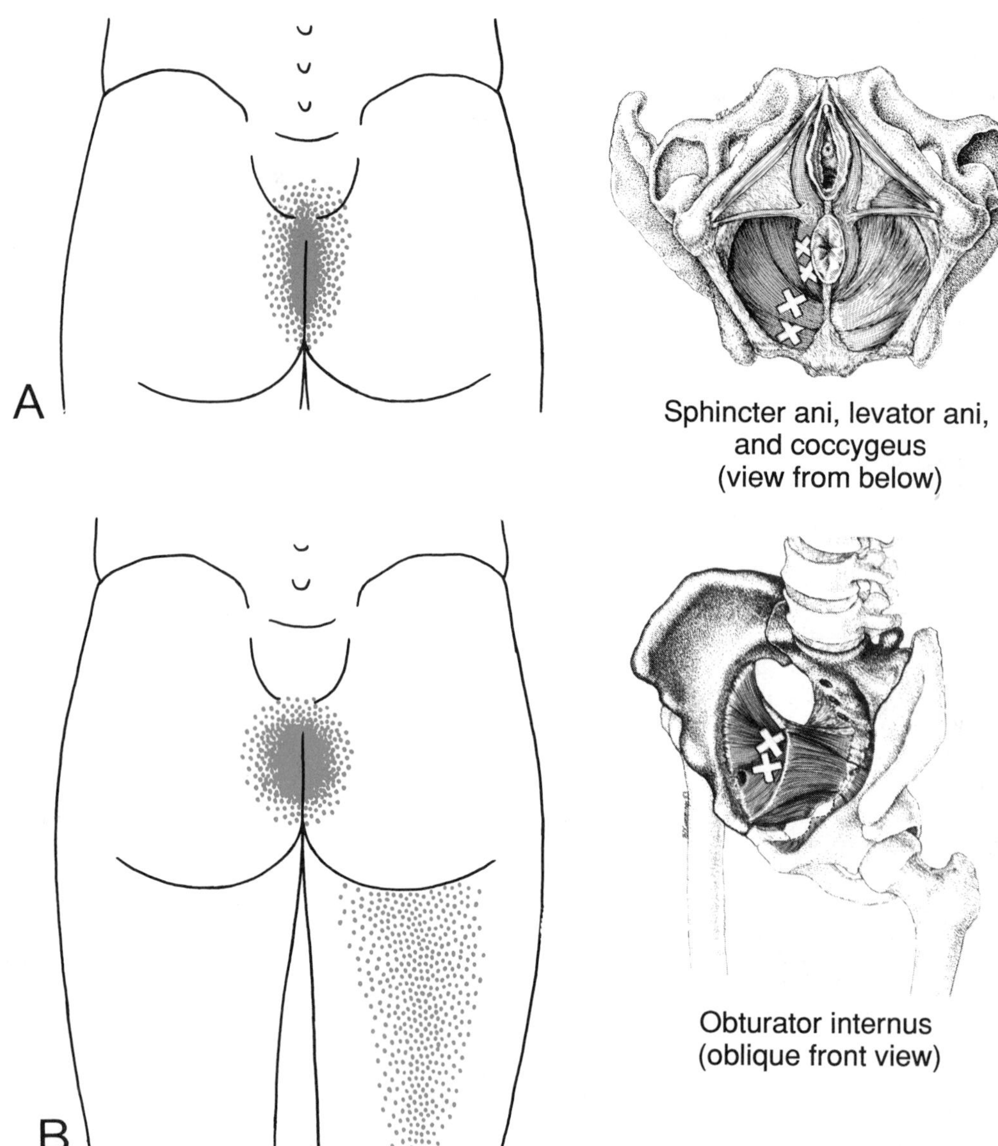

Figure 6.1. Referred pain patterns (*solid red and red stippling*) generated by trigger points (**X**s), *A*, in the right sphincter ani, levator ani, and coccygeus muscles and *B*, in the right obturator internus muscle. Pain referred from this muscle sometimes spills over to include the posterior proximal region of the thigh.

untary control. This sphincter is elliptical in shape, extending three or four times as far anteroposteriorly as it does laterally, and surrounds the last 2 cm of the anal canal. The superficial (middle) lamina of the external sphincter ani contains the bulk of the muscle. This superficial lamina is anchored posteriorly to the tendinous anococcygeal body and anteriorly to the tendinous perineal body—where it is joined by the levator ani, bulbospongiosus, and transversus perinei superficialis muscles (Fig. 6.2). The deep layer of the external sphincter ani is closely associated with the slinglike puborectalis portion of the levator ani, which is the most posterior, lateral, and deepest section of the pubococcygeal part of the levator ani (Fig. 6.2).[73]

Levator Ani Muscle
(Fig. 6.3)

The paired levator ani muscles meet in the midline to form a muscular sheet, the pelvic diaphragm, across most of the floor

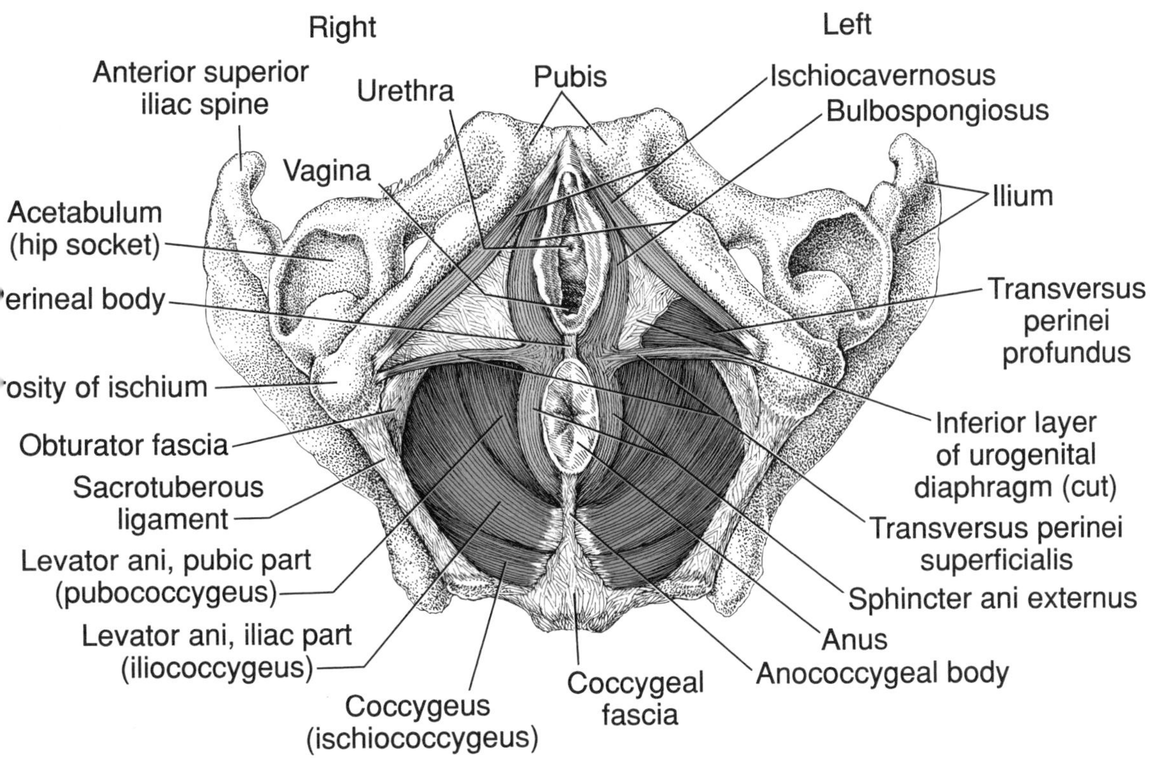

Figure 6.2. Pelvic floor muscles as seen from below in the supine female subject. The muscles of the pelvic diaphragm are *dark red* and the associated pelvic muscles are *light red*. On the subject's left side, part of the deep fascia of the urogenital diaphragm has been cut and removed to reveal the transversus perinei profundus muscle.

of the lesser pelvis. This diaphragm is perforated by the urogenital hiatus and the anal hiatus (Fig. 6.3). The levator ani is composed of two distinct muscles: the more anterior (lower in the pelvis) pubococcygeus and the more posterior (higher in the pelvis) iliococcygeus.

The pubococcygeus muscle attaches along the dorsal surface of the pubic bone from the symphysis to the obturator canal (Fig. 6.3). It forms a sling around the anus, prostate gland or vagina, and the urethra. The two halves of the pubococcygeus meet in the midline, some at the perineal body, and most at the anococcygeal body[26] (Figs. 6.2 and 6.3).

The most anterior (medial) fibers of the pubococcygeus that meet bilaterally at the perineal body in front of the anus are called the levator prostatae in the male. In the female, these anterior fibers are called the pubovaginalis muscle and serve as an important sphincter of the vagina. The more posterior fibers of the pubococcygeus (the puborectalis part) form a sling around the rectum. The closest that any of the pubococcygeus fibers come to the coccyx is usually their attachment to the anococcygeal body.[26]

Tichý[97] illustrates well how embryologically the levator ani develops as a series of telescoping rings and slings.

The posterior section of the levator ani, the iliococcygeus muscle, anchors ***above*** to the tendinous arch of the levator ani muscle and to the spine of the ischium. The tendinous arch of the levator ani anchors to the spine of the ischium posteriorly and attaches anteriorly either to the anterior margin of the obturator membrane or to the pubic bone just medial (farther anterior) to the margin of the membrane. This tendinous arch is firmly attached to the fascia covering the obturator internus muscle.[27] As seen from inside the pelvis, the levator ani covers the lower one-half to two-thirds of the obturator internus muscle and essentially all of the obturator foramen.

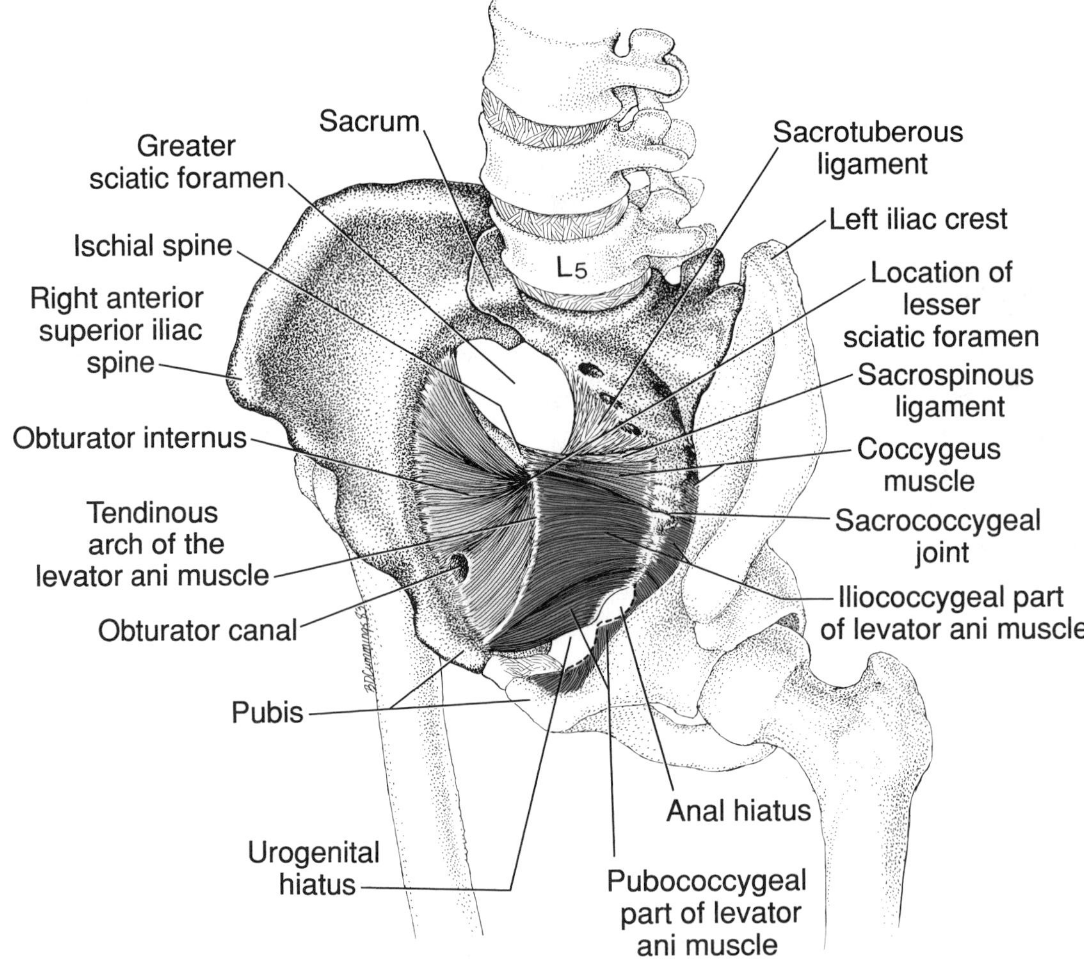

Figure 6.3. Pelvic floor muscles palpable on the right side of the pelvis by intrapelvic examination with the patient lying on the right side. The muscles are seen obliquely from above and diagonally from the left side looking down inside the pelvis. The levator ani muscle is *dark red*. The coccygeus muscle is *medium red* and the obturator internus muscle is *light red*.

Below, the iliococcygeus attaches to the anococcygeal body and to the last two segments of the coccyx.[2]

The adjacent margins of the pubococcygeus and iliococcygeus muscles may be separated or may overlap. The iliococcygeus may be replaced by fibrous tissue. Its upper border lies adjacent to the sacrospinous ligament and the overlying coccygeus muscle (Fig. 6.3).[26]

Coccygeus Muscle
(Fig. 6.3)

The coccygeus muscle, sometimes called the ischiococcygeus, lies cephalad and adjacent to the iliococcygeus muscle of the levator ani. The two muscles often form a continuous plane (Fig. 6.3). The coccygeus muscle covers (internally) the sturdy sacrospinous ligament (Fig. 6.3). ***Laterally*** the apex of this triangular muscle is anchored to the spine of the ischium and to fibers of the sacrospinous ligament. ***Medially*** it fans out to end on the margin of the coccyx and on the side of the lowest piece of the sacrum.[26]

Obturator Internus Muscle

The anatomy of the part of the obturator internus that lies outside of the pelvis and attaches to the greater trochanter of the femur is considered in Chapter 10 of this volume. Here we are concerned with the intrapelvic portion that covers the anterolateral wall of the lesser pelvis, where it surrounds and covers the greater part of the obturator foramen (Fig. 6.3). The obturator internus is fan shaped and the direction of its fibers spans an arc of roughly 135°. Its muscle fibers form an anterior and posterior mass, one in front of and the other behind the obturator canal. That canal allows nerves and vessels to penetrate the obturator membrane along the anterior margin of the obturator foramen, on the side opposite to the lesser sciatic foramen.

Inside the pelvis, the obturator internus muscle attaches to the inner pelvic brim, to the margin of the obturator foramen, and to much of the obturator membrane stretched across that bony foramen. The fibers of the muscle converge toward the lesser sciatic foramen and end in four or five tendinous bands. As the muscle exits the pelvis through the lesser sciatic foramen, it makes a right angle bend around the grooved surface between the spine and tuberosity of the ischium. This bony pulley is covered with cartilage; the passage of the tendon is also assisted by the ischiadic bursa of the obturator internus.[10] As the tendon crosses the capsule of the hip joint, it is cushioned by the subtendinous bursa of the obturator internus (*see* also Chapter 10, Section 2).[32] The exit of the obturator internus from the pelvis through the lesser sciatic foramen is marked by palpable ligaments that form two borders of that foramen: the sacrotuberous ligament posteriorly and the sacrospinous ligament above.[25] Since the fibers of the two ligaments intermingle as they cross at the upper end of the foramen,[25] the foramen is a tightly enclosed space that leaves no room for expansion of the muscle. The structures forming the lesser sciatic foramen are illustrated in Figure 10.5. That figure serves as a valuable reference throughout this chapter because it clarifies relations of intrapelvic muscles and ligaments.

Bulbospongiosus, Ischiocavernosus, and Transversus Perinei Muscles

Female Anatomy

In the female, the bulbospongiosus, ischiocavernosus, and transversus perinei superficialis muscles on each side of the body form a triangle (Fig. 6.2). The medial leg of the triangle, the bulbospongiosus (also known as the bulbocavernosus or the sphincter vaginae), surrounds the orifice of the vagina. The muscle attaches ***anteriorly*** to the corpora cavernosa clitoridis with a muscular fasciculus that also crosses over the body of the clitoris and compresses its deep dorsal vein. ***Posteriorly*** the bulbospongiosus anchors to the perineal body where it blends with the external anal sphincter and the transversus perinei superficialis (Fig 6.2).[28]

The ischiocavernosus of the female (formerly called the erector clitoridis) forms the lateral side of the triangle (Fig. 6.2). The muscle is located along the lateral boundary of the perineum next to the bony ridge of the anterior pubic ramus, extending between the symphysis pubis and the ischial tuberosity. ***Above*** and ***anteriorly*** the ischiocavernosus ends in an aponeurosis that blends with the sides and undersurface of the crus clitoridis. ***Below*** and ***posteriorly*** it is anchored to the surface of the crus clitoridis and to the ischial tuberosity.[28]

The transversus perinei superficialis muscle forms the base of the triangle. The two muscles together span the perineum laterally between the ischial tuberosities, joining the sphincter ani and bulbospongiosi in the midline at the perineal body (Fig. 6.2). The transversus perinei profundus lies deep to the superficialis; it is a broader muscle that courses between the ischial tuberosity and the vagina (Fig. 6.2).[28]

Male Anatomy

In the male, the bulbospongiosus is more complex than in the female and essentially wraps around the corpus spongiosum of the penis, which is the central erectile structure through which the urethra passes. As illustrated,[4,29,39] the two symmetrical parts of this muscle begin ***below*** at the perineal body and along the median raphe. The fibers extend outward and upward in a pennate fashion to enclose the bulk of the corpus spongiosum penis posteriorly and the corpus cavernosum penis anteriorly. ***Above***, some of the fibers end in a tendinous expansion that covers the dorsal blood vessels of the penis.[28] After 5 months of fetal gestation, this muscle wraps around the bulb of the penis.[73]

The ischiocavernosus muscle in the male is similar to that in the female, but is usually larger. On each side, the muscle attaches posteriorly to the ischial tuberosity and angles across the perineum anteriorly toward the penis. After coursing lateral to the bulbospongiosus, it ends in an aponeurosis that blends with the sides and undersurface of the crura as they become the body of the penis.[4,28,39]

The transversus perinei profundus attaches ***laterally*** to the ischial tuberosity as in the female, but in the male, the muscles interlace in the ***midline*** at a tendinous raphe deep to the bulbospongiosus muscle.[28,29,39]

Sacrococcygeus Ventralis Muscle

The sacrococcygeus ventralis (anterior) muscle is variable and was found in 102 of 110 adult bodies. It often is vestigial, consisting mainly of tendinous bands with only short muscle fibers.[37] When well developed, it extends vertically from the sides of the fourth and fifth sacral vertebrae, from the front of the first coccygeal vertebra, and from the sacrospinous ligament to the second to fourth coccygeal vertebrae and to the anterior sacrococcygeal ligament.[13,37,43,80]

The sacrococcygeus ventralis muscle may divide into medial and lateral fiber bundles. When this has happened, the lateral fibers have been identified as the sacrococcygeus ventralis (depressor caudae lateralis) muscle and the medial fibers as the infracoccygeus (depressor caudae medialis) muscle.[37] These fibers are probably phylogenetic remnants of tail-wagging muscles.

Supplemental References

Sphincter Ani Muscles

The sphincter ani is depicted from below,[4,5,29,39] in cross section,[23] in sagittal section,[1,42,81] and in coronal section.[27,83]

Levator Ani Muscle

The levator ani is shown schematically by layers in relation to other perineal muscles for both men and women.[3] It is illustrated from below[5,29,39] and from above,[2] where it is presented as having three divisions: the pubococcygeus, iliococcygeus, and the (ischio)coccygeus. The levator ani is presented in cross section,[21] in sagittal section,[1] and in frontal section.[27,38,83] Its bony attachments are depicted.[44]

Coccygeus Muscle

Midline sagittal sections provide a medial view of the coccygeus muscle from inside the pelvis.[7,43,66,68] It is shown in cross section[22] and its bony attachments are marked.[44,65]

The sacrospinous ligament, which is useful for orientation when palpating muscles deep within the pelvis, is described and illustrated.[8,25]

Obturator Internus Muscle

The usual anatomical view of this muscle is a midline sagittal section seen from inside the pelvis.[7,43,66,68] This view also includes the coccygeus muscle. It is presented in one cross section through the hip joints,[11] in a cross section through the prostate and ischial tuberosities,[82] in a series of cross sections that includes all of the muscle,[18] and in frontal sections.[27,38,83] The bony attachments of the obturator internus muscle are identified[9,44,70,72] and the ischiadic bursa of the obturator internus is illustrated.[10]

Bulbospongiosus, Ischiocavernosus, and Transversus Perinei Muscles

The bulbospongiosus, ischiocavernosus, and transversus perinei superficialis muscles are presented schematically in relation to other layers of the perineum for both men and women,[3] and bony attachments are identified.[70] The three muscles are illustrated from below without nerves or vessels for men[4,29,41] (except for the superficial transverse perinei muscle[84]) and for women.[6,30,41,86] They are shown from below with nerves and vessels for men[40,69] except for the superficial transverse perinei muscle.[85] The ischiocavernosus is shown in cross section for men and women[19] and the bulbospongiosus in cross section for a male.[20] The bulbospongiosus is illustrated in midline sagittal sections of males.[1,67]

Sacrococcygeus Ventralis Muscle

The vestigial sacrococcygeus ventralis muscle (an anterior remnant of tail-wagging muscles) may be seen looking down into the pelvis in cross section,[80] in sagittal section,[43] and in frontal section.[13,37]

3. INNERVATION

The external anal sphincter is innervated by a branch of the fourth sacral nerve and by twigs from the inferior rectal branch of the pudendal nerve. The internal sphincter is innervated by fibers of the autonomic nervous system.[31]

The obturator internus muscle is supplied by its own nerve, which carries fibers from the L_5, S_1, and S_2 segments.[32]

The levator ani muscle is innervated by fibers of the S_4 segment and sometimes of the S_3 or S_5 segments via the pudendal plexus.[26] Stimulation of the S_3 ventral root produced nearly 70% of closure pressure by the external sphincter urethrae and the remaining 30% was provided by stimulating the S_2 and S_4 spinal nerve roots.[50]

The coccygeus muscle derives its innervation from fibers of the S_4 and S_5 segments via the pudendal plexus.[26]

All of the perineal muscles (including the bulbospongiosus, the ischiocavernosus, and both the superficial and deep transverse perinei) are innervated by the second, third, and fourth sacral nerves via the perineal branch of the pudendal nerve.[28]

Fibers from the S_4 and S_5 segments usually innervate the sacrococcygeus ventralis muscle.[37]

4. FUNCTION

The only references found that concerned electromyographic (EMG) studies applied to the more superficial pelvic floor muscles and the sphincters. Understandably, no references to motor electrical stimulation experiments were located.

Sphincter Ani

Clinical experience shows and EMG studies[15] confirm that the sphincter ani is in a state of constant tonic contraction, which is increased by straining, speaking, coughing, laughing, or weight-lifting. The tonic contraction falls to a very low level during sleep and is strongly inhibited during defecation. It is strongly recruited by voluntary effort, which is accompanied by general contraction of the perineal muscles, especially the sphincter urethrae.[15,16]

Levator Ani Muscle

In general, both the pubococcygeus and iliococcygeus muscles of the levator ani support and slightly elevate the pelvic floor, resisting increased intra-abdominal pressure.[26] In the male, the more anterior (medial) pubococcygeal portion, sometimes called the levator prostatae muscle, forms a sling around the prostate and specifically applies upward pressure on it. The corresponding fibers in the female, also known as the pubovaginal muscle, constrict the vaginal orifice. The more posterior puborectalis fibers of the pubococcygeus form a sling around the anus that is structurally continuous with the sphincter ani and constricts the anus when contracted.[34] Strong contraction of this part of the levator ani can help to eject a bolus of feces. Contraction of the more anterior periurethral fibers helps empty the urethra at the end of urination and is thought to prevent incontinence during coughing or sneezing.

Histological comparison of the perianal and periurethral regions of the pubococcygeus muscle revealed that, although most fibers were type 1 (oxidative metabolism) fibers, in the periurethral region, only 4% were type 2 (glycolytic) fibers, while in the perianal region, 23% were type 2 fibers. This higher percentage of type 2 fibers in the perianal region suggests that it is used for occasional forceful contractions, as compared to more sustained contractions in the periurethral region.[34] A later study by this same group[46] reported only type 1 fibers in the external (voluntary) sphincter urethrae muscle.

In a more recent study,[53] a greater proportion of type 1 (slow-twitch) fibers was associated with improved support of the pelvic viscera, especially under conditions contributing to increased intra-abdominal pressure. A greater proportion of type 2 (fast-twitch) fibers improved the periurethral continence mechanism, providing increased urethral closure during mechanical pressure stress.

In an EMG study of 24 normal women, about half of whom had delivered babies, none was able to relax the pubococcygeal part of the levator ani muscle in the lithotomy position, whereas some were able to relax the sphincter urethrae completely.[16]

Coccygeus Muscle

Anatomically, the coccygeus muscle pulls the coccyx forward and is said to support the pelvic floor against intra-abdominal pressure.[26] It also stabilizes the sacroiliac joint[64] and has powerful leverage for rotating that joint. Therefore, abnormal tension of the coccygeus muscle could easily hold the sacroiliac joint in a displaced position.

Obturator Internus Muscle

The obturator internus is a lower-limb muscle that serves no motor function in the pelvis. As noted in Chapter 10 of this volume, the obturator internus is most strongly a lateral rotator of the thigh when the thigh is extended; the muscle becomes increasingly an abductor at the hip as the thigh is flexed.[32]

Bulbospongiosus, Ischiocavernosus, and Transversus Perinei Muscles

Contraction of the bulbospongiosus in the male serves to empty the urethra at the end of urination.[28] Erection of the penis is primarily a vascular response under autonomic control,[12,75] but the anterior and middle fibers of the bulbospongiosus and the ischiocavernous muscles contribute to erection by reflex and voluntary contraction that compresses the erectile tissue of the bulb of the penis and also its dorsal vein.[17,28,51] In the female, contraction of this voluntary muscle constricts the orifice of the vagina and contributes to erection of the clitoris by compression of its deep dorsal vein.[28]

In the male, contraction of the ischiocavernosus serves to maintain and enhance penile erection by retarding the return of blood through the crus penis. During erection, intracavernous pressure correlated strongly with the duration of voluntary EMG activity in the ischiocavernosus muscle.[54] Change of pressure on the glans reflexly activates the ischiocavernosus muscle. This substantiates the clinical impression that pressure stimulation of the glans penis during coitus contributes to the erectile process.[55]

In the female, the ischiocavernosus acts similarly to maintain erection of the clitoris by retarding return flow from the crus clitoridis.[28]

The two pairs of transverse perinei form a muscular sling that cradles the perineal body between the two ischial tuberosities. Bilateral contraction of the superficial and deep transversus perinei muscles serves to fix the perineal body in the midline between the anus and genitalia and to support the pelvic floor. In both men and women, all of these perineal muscles are generally contracted as a unit. EMG studies indicate that selective contraction of individual perineal muscles is difficult, if not impossible.[15,16]

5. FUNCTIONAL (MYOTATIC) UNIT

The pelvic floor muscles, especially the anal and urethral sphincters and the levator ani, function closely together. Contractions of the genital bulbospongiosus and ischiocavernosus muscles are scarcely, if at all, voluntarily separable from sphincter activation.

The iliococcygeus and upper pubococcygeus muscles of the levator ani are strong flexors of the coccyx. The equally powerful antagonist to this movement is the gluteus maximus; it attaches to the dorsolateral surface of the coccyx[65] with fibers that are directed laterally and form the gluteal cleft. Working together, the levator ani and gluteus maximus provide more powerful elevation (closure) of the anus than the levator ani could provide alone. When maximum voluntary effort is required to close the anal aperture, the gluteus maximus is powerfully recruited.

The obturator internus muscle functions in concert with other lateral rotators of the thigh, as described in Chapter 10 of this volume.

6. SYMPTOMS

Patients with TrPs in the sphincter ani muscle complain primarily of poorly localized aching pain in the anal region and may experience painful bowel movements.

In women, TrPs in the bulbospongiosus muscle cause dyspareunia, particularly during entry, and aching pain in the perineal region. In men, these TrPs cause pain in the retroscrotal region, discomfort when sitting erect, and sometimes a degree of impotence.

Ischiocavernosus TrPs likewise cause perineal pain but are less likely to interfere with intercourse.

Involvement of the obturator internus can cause pain and a feeling of fullness in the rectum, with occasional extension of pain down the back of the thigh.[56] This muscle may also refer pain into the vagina.[53]

The levator ani muscle is the most widely recognized source of referred pain in the perineal region. Its referred pain may be described as pain in the sacrum,[62] coccyx,[62,77,94,95] rectum,[62,71,87] pelvic floor or perirectal area,[62,71] vagina,[95] or low back.[77] Referred pain from this muscle makes sitting uncomfortable.[71,77,87] The pain may be aggravated by lying on the back,[94] and by defecation.[87]

Myofascial TrPs in the coccygeus muscle were identified as the cause of pain similar to that ascribed to TrPs in the levator ani, and referred to the coccyx, hip, or back. This pain also limited sitting.[77] TrPs in this muscle are likely to cause myofascial backache late in pregnancy and early in labor. Tenderness and "spasm" (tension) of the coccygeus muscle were usually the key factors responsible for low back pain suffered by 1350 women seen for infertility.[64]

Differential Diagnosis

The following deals with causes of coccygodynia and intrapelvic pain that are not explained by the findings obtained with the usual examination and diagnostic procedures.

The muscle outside the pelvis most likely to refer pain within the pelvis is the adductor magnus (Chapter 15, Fig. 15.2).

Numerous authors have used a variety of names to describe what would appear, on thoughtful consideration, to be largely myofascial pain syndromes of the pelvic musculature: tender coccyx,[57] coccygodynia,[33,35,77,94,95,100] coccygeal spasm,[64] levator syndrome,[47,74,76,87,92] levator ani syndrome,[71] levator spasm syndrome,[91] levator ani spasm syndrome,[62,103] tension myalgia of the pelvic floor,[89] pelvic floor syndromes,[63] pelvic pain syndrome,[90] proctalgia fugax,[36,49,79,93,96,101] and obturator internus spasm.[56]

Coccygodynia

Although the dictionary definition of coccygodynia is "pain in the coccygeal region,"[14] several authors[57,59,77] draw a sharp distinction between what they consider "true" coccygodynia resulting from traumatic injury to the coccyx and conditions elsewhere that refer pain or tenderness to the coccygeal region. One such condition is a myofascial pain syndrome.

Authors have associated pain in the region of a non-tender coccyx (dorsal surface) with abnormal tension and marked tenderness of the levator ani,[59,77,87,94] coccygeus,[64,77,94] and gluteus maximus muscles.[59] Pace[77] and Long[63] explicitly recognized that coccygeal pain is referred from myofascial TrPs in the pelvic muscles.

Levator Ani Syndromes

Several of the conditions causing pelvic pain are specifically identified with the levator ani muscle: *levator spasm syndrome*,[91] *levator ani spasm syndrome*,[62,103] *levator syndrome*,[47,87] and *pelvic floor syndromes*.[63]

For example, the levator ani spasm syndrome[62] causes pain in the sacrum, coccyx, rectum, and pelvic diaphragm. It is diagnosed by finding on rectal examination "spastic," tender muscles in the pelvic floor (puborectalis, iliococcygeus, and coccygeus). The piriformis muscle is not included in this group; it refers pain in the buttock and down the thigh.[33,62,63,91,95]

This levator ani syndrome[62] was identified in 31 patients on a Physical Medicine Service. As in other studies, most of the patients with this syndrome were women (90%). The pain was located in the sacrum (100% of patients), pelvic diaphragm (90%), anal region (68%), and in the gluteal region (only 13%). The levator ani was tender and "spastic;" these signs were bilateral in 55%. All patients experienced sharp pain in the sacral area lasting 5–10 minutes after digital examination. Of the women who attempted intercourse during the illness, 43% suffered dyspareunia. Forty percent of all patients reported disturbed bowel function (constipation or frequency) but none experienced painful bowel movements. Twenty percent complained of pain when sitting. Only 10% of the patients failed to respond to massage therapy of the levator ani muscle and 74% became symptom-free or had only very slight residual symptoms.

Patients with pelvic floor syndromes[63] experienced pain referred in various combinations to the buttock, underneath the sacrum, in the hip laterally, and the thigh posteriorly, from the piriformis, coccygeus, or levator ani muscles. The patients complained of pain when seated on hard surfaces and when sitting down on or standing up from a chair. Digital examination of an involved muscle revealed trigger areas with local soreness and a tight, fibrous, nodular feel of the involved muscle.

Proctalgia Fugax

Proctalgia fugax is defined as "painful spasm of the muscle about the anus without known cause."[14] It is characterized by paroxysms of anorectal pain in the absence of identifiable local lesions.[79] It is not a rare condition; 13–19% of apparently healthy persons surveyed have symptoms of proctalgia fugax, although most experience fewer than seven episodes per year.[79] The pain usually occurs irregularly in bouts that generally show no correlation to activity or to the condition of the patient.[79] Proctalgia can begin as early as 13 years of age.[101] A physician with this condition wrote an eloquent description of it.[93]

As we have learned more about most "idiopathic" diseases, they have turned out to represent a number of conditions lumped together under one rubric. Proctalgia fugax appears to be no exception. The levator ani syndromes, noted previously, and coccygodynia, as described by Thiele,[94,95] bear a remarkable resemblance to proctalgia fugax.

Two studies found evidence of specific causes for proctalgia fugax. One study[49] reported pressures in the rectum and sigmoid colon measured by inserting instrumented balloons while two patients were experiencing recurrent pain. The small changes in pressure observed in the rectum did not correlate with the episodes of pain, but the intermittent peaks of pressure observed in the sigmoid colon did. The greater the pressure peaks, the more likely the subject was to identify pain, which began a short time before a peak. This study strongly suggested that the pain resulted from muscular contraction of the wall of the sigmoid colon, not from pressure within the lumen.

TrPs stimulated by tension may exist in smooth muscle, interstitial connective tissue, or the lining of the bowel wall. It is also possible that increased intraluminal pressure aggravates TrPs located in the bowel mucosa when there is something within the gut that can press against them. This may be an example of intestinal TrPs that are amenable to experimental study.

In the other study, Douthwaite[36] reported 10 physicians who examined themselves during attacks of proctalgia fugax. None detected spasm of the anal sphincter. They did palpate a tense, tender band on one or the other side of the rectum, which they located in the levator ani. These findings are consistent with TrPs in the levator ani.

A few patients experience attacks of proctalgia following coitus. Peery[79] postulates that the pain derives from exaggerated or prolonged contraction of the rectal sphincter after orgasm. This pain might also derive from TrPs in the sphincter ani, bulbospongiosus, or ischiocavernosus muscles.

Oral clonidine was helpful[93] and inhaled salbutamol has also been recommended.[102]

Tension Myalgia Of The Pelvic Floor

Sinaki and associates[89] consolidated the various syndromes of the pelvic musculature (piriformis syndrome, coccygodynia, levator ani spasm syndrome, and proctalgia fugax) under one umbrella, tension myalgia of the pelvic floor. They saw the patients in the Department of Physical Medicine and Rehabilitation at the Mayo Clinic. Nearly all of the 94 patients were between 30 and 70 years of age; most were between 40 and 50 years. Women constituted 83% of the group, which is about the usual percentage of women patients with a levator ani syndrome.[91] Pain in the coccygeal area and a heavy feeling in the rectal or vaginal region were the most prominent symptoms occurring in 82% and 62%, respectively. Defecation caused pain in 33%. All patients had tenderness of the pelvic floor muscles on rectal examination. This examination elicited localized tenderness of the piriformis, coccygeus, levator ani muscles, sacrococcygeal ligaments, and of muscular attachments to the sacrum and coccyx, or some combination of these. It is likely that many of these patients had myofascial TrPs in the tender muscles, but no mention was made of the presence or absence of taut bands or referral of pain when pressure was applied to a tender spot.

Integumentary Trigger Points

Although TrPs in the scar tissue produced by a surgical incision are well known,[99] those occurring in the vaginal cuff following hysterectomy apparently are particularly troublesome.[90] These TrPs are usually associated with additional TrPs in the vaginal wall. Vaginal wall TrPs were reported as referring pain to the lower abdomen and uterine paracervical area. The pain was usually described by the patient in terms of a familiar condition, such as "ovarian pain," "menstrual cramps," or "bladder spasms." Pressure applied to these TrPs reproduced the presenting symptom.[90] Vaginal wall TrPs may be analogous to cutaneous TrPs or to colon TrPs (considered previously in this section under Proctalgia Fugax).

Non-myofascial TrPs in subcutaneous adipose tissue have been described.[57] Dittrich[35] identified TrPs in the fat pads overlying the sacrum that referred pain to the coccygeal region (coccygodynia). Pace and Henning[78] described episacral "lipomas" that were identifiable as tender, palpable nodules; they referred pain down the lateral aspect of the thigh. Slocumb[90] reported that TrPs in the tissues over the sacrum responded to injection therapy, especially if pressure on them reproduced the same pain caused by stimulation of abdominal wall and vaginal TrPs.

Articular Dysfunction

Muscle spasm and tenderness secondary to articular dysfunction at the sacroiliac joint are likely to be associated with coccygeal and low back pain. Conversely, tension of the muscles attached to the coccyx can destabilize the sacroiliac joint.[64] Ventral coccygeal tenderness is often associated with a blocked sacroiliac joint.[57] Lewit[59] found that only one-fifth of the patients who had tenderness on palpation of the ventral surface of the coccyx complained of coccygeal pain. The majority suffered primarily from low back pain.

Upslip, or innominate shear dysfunction,[48] (upward displacement of an innominate bone in relation to the sacrum) is an important source of low back and groin pain. Among 63 patients in a private orthopaedic medicine practice who were examined because of pain and found to have an innominate upslip dysfunction, the most common site of the chief pain complaint was the low back and groin (50%).[52]

The pain characteristic of dysfunctional low lumbar facet joints is discussed and illustrated in Chapter 3, page 26 and may be similar to the pain referred from intrapelvic muscles.

7. ACTIVATION AND PERPETUATION OF TRIGGER POINTS

TrPs in these pelvic floor muscles are sometimes activated by a severe fall, an automobile accident, or by surgery in the pelvic region. Often, the patients cannot identify a specific initiating event. In only one-fifth of the patients with low back pain and a tender coccyx ventrally was an injury identified as the cause of the pain.[59]

Levator ani TrPs are certainly perpetuated, and perhaps activated, by sitting in a slumped posture for prolonged periods of time. Thiele[95] demonstrated radiographically the acute angulation of the coccygeal joints caused by sitting on a hard surface in a slumped posture. Apparently the compressed gluteus maximus muscle transmits the pressure to the coccyx. Thiele attributed coccygodynia to this posture in 32% of 324 patients. Cooper[33] considered prolonged sitting in a slouched position watching television as the factor responsible for coccygodynia in 14% of 100 patients. Lilius and Valtonen[62] regarded this posture as an important cause of levator ani spasm syndrome.

In those patients with no known initiating event, possible causes for the muscle hyperirritability and TrPs are nutritional inadequacies and/or other systemic perpetuating factors (Chapter 4, Volume 1).[98]

Articular dysfunctions of the sacroiliac joints,[57] sacrococcygeal articulation, and the lumbosacral junction may be potent aggravating sources of TrPs in these pelvic floor muscles.

Chronic hemorrhoids can aggravate symptoms in the related muscles.[62] Chronic inflammatory conditions within the pelvis, such as endometritis, chronic salpingo-oophoritis, chronic prostatovesiculitis,[62] and interstitial cystitis[61] may evoke referred pain and tenderness of the pelvic floor, and have been associated with the levator ani spasm syndrome.[62] However, other coexistent pelvic disease, including ovarian cysts, pelvic adhesions, and fibroids, did not prevent a successful response to local injection of TrPs in the levator ani and coccygeus muscles and in posthysterectomy vaginal cuff scars.[90]

8. PATIENT EXAMINATION

Patients with TrPs in the pelvic floor musculature are likely to walk somewhat stiffly and sit down cautiously, often on one buttock close to the edge of the chair seat.[94,95] The patient shifts sitting position frequently and, after prolonged sitting, the act of arising from the chair often causes obvious pain and requires increased effort.[95]

If the obturator internus muscle harbors active TrPs, the stretch range of motion will show some restriction. The clinician tests this in the supine patient by looking for restricted medial rotation of the thigh with the hip straight. A considerably greater stretch of the obturator internus is obtained by flexing the thigh 90° and then adducting it. This maneuver, however, also exerts tension on the piriformis, gemelli, and obturator externus muscles.

Normally, the sacrococcygeal joint is freely movable. The coccyx normally extends through an arc of about 30°, and bends laterally to bring the tip about 1 cm from the midline. Mobility is greater in women than in men.[95] Bilateral tension of the coccygeus muscles tends to flex the sacrococcygeal joint. Unilateral coccygeus muscle tension pulls the coccyx toward one side.[95]

Lewit[57,59] emphasizes how frequently patients who complain of low back pain have marked tenderness inside the tip of the coccyx. In such cases, the coccyx is kyphotic (pulled in toward the pelvis) but is not tender to pressure on its dorsal surface and movement at the sacrococcygeal joint is not painful. Because of this kyphotic curvature and the hypertonus of the adjacent gluteus maximus muscles, it is difficult for the examiner to reach beneath the tip of the coccyx to where the ventral surface is so tender;[57] therefore, this tenderness is easily overlooked. However, when present, it is a strong indication for the need to determine the cause by doing an intrapelvic examination, as described in the next section.

It is helpful to screen for a tilted pelvis and for pelvic asymmetries, as described in Chapter 4 of this volume, and to screen for pelvic articular dysfunctions.[48]

9. TRIGGER POINT EXAMINATION

For the purpose of locating myofascial TrPs within the pelvis, the pelvic muscles can be considered in three categories: perineal muscles, pelvic floor muscles, and pelvic wall muscles. The intrapelvic muscles are examined through the rectum. Unfortunately, the conventional rectal examination does not include the identification of muscles.[24] The special features of the vaginal examination are considered subsequently. For the rectal examination, the patient may lie supine in the lithotomy position, or, if footrests are not available, semiprone in Sims's position. It is best to begin examination with the hand that supinates toward the symptomatic side. If TrPs are found on that side, it is wise to examine the opposite side of the pelvis for comparison, which is most effectively done with the other hand. It is difficult and awkward to perform an adequate rectal examination of the muscles on both sides of the pelvis with one hand.

Pelvic Floor Muscles

The pelvic floor muscles commonly afflicted with TrPs, and the ones to become well acquainted with first, are the sphincter ani, levator ani, and coccygeus muscles. Although the levator ani and coccygeus muscles cover most of the pelvic floor, the intrapelvic rectal digital examination begins with the sphincter ani.

Sphincter Ani

If the patient has TrPs in the anal sphincter, insertion of the finger can be distressing even when done very carefully. First, the clinician should examine the anal orifice for internal hemorrhoids, which can perpetuate TrPs of the anal sphincter. Lubricant is liberally applied to the examining gloved finger and the anal orifice. Ordinarily, as the examiner inserts the finger, he or she would *gently* apply pressure toward one side of the anus to help relax the sphincter. However, if one inadvertently presses on TrPs in the muscle, this aggravates the pain. In the presence of excessive sphincter tension or tenderness, instead of the clinician applying side pressure, the patient may bear down on the rectum to enhance relaxation of the sphincter ani as the clinician slowly inserts the examining finger directly into the anal orifice.

By gently flexing the tip of the finger, the examiner can feel when it has passed the sphincters. The finger first encounters the external and then the internal sphincter ani. The finger should be withdrawn to halfway along the sphincters and pressure *gently* applied to the muscle at every one-eighth of a circle (positions at 12:00, 1:30, 3:00, etc.) to find any TrP tenderness. When the finger locates tenderness in one direction, the muscle is explored to determine where the spot of maximum tenderness occurs. An associated taut band may be identified, if the TrP is not too tender and the patient can tolerate the additional pressure. If the muscle is strongly contracted, the patient can relax it by bearing down, making the contrast between the taut band and relaxed fibers more clearly evident. A taut band, when present, usually extends from one-quarter to halfway around the anus. These bands are often multiple.

When an anal sphincter harbors very active TrPs, their tenderness may preclude further rectal examination of the intrapelvic muscles. The movement and additional pressure of the finger may be intolerable. In a woman, the vaginal examination may then be substituted. Otherwise, the anal sphincter TrPs must be inactivated before the patient can be examined for intrapelvic TrPs.

Orientation Inside the Pelvis

Establishing relevant bony and ligamentous landmarks for reference helps greatly in identifying the intrapelvic muscles by palpation. For orientation purposes, it is helpful to identify the structures that border the levator ani muscle (Figs. 6.2, 6.3, and 10.5).[2]

Usually, no muscles are found in the midline on the ventral surface of the coccyx and sacrum. When the patient is examined rectally, only the rectal wall lies between the examining finger and these bones. In the midline below (distal to) the tip of the coccyx, the anococcygeal body (which usually is not distinguishable by palpation) extends to the sphincter ani and serves as the attachment for much of the pubococcygeus muscle of the levator ani. Just anterior to the rectum is an analogous structure, the perineal body, to which the bulbospongiosus, transverse perinei, and sphincter ani muscles anchor.

It is relatively easy to examine the range of motion of the coccyx. One grasps the coccyx between the finger inside the rectum and the thumb outside to flex, extend, and bend it laterally, testing for tenderness at its articulations. All of the coccygeal joints may be mobile. The most proximal joint that exhibits mobility is usually the sacrococcygeal joint.

A firm, tendinous edge crossing the pelvis at about the level of the sacrococcygeal joint (Fig. 6.3) identifies the lower border of the sacrospinous ligament. This border nearly always is sharply delineated. It lies close to the sometimes overlapping borders of the iliococcygeal muscle of the levator ani, below, and the coccygeus muscle, above. Laterally, the ligament ends at a palpable, hard, bony prominence, the spine of the ischium, to which the tendinous arch of the levator ani also anchors.[2] At least the posterior half of this tendinous arch is palpable as it swings around the pelvis to attach anteriorly to the body of the pubis. The arch may become indistinguishable near the anterior margin of the obturator membrane. This arch serves as the lateral attachment of the iliococcygeal part of the levator ani muscle; therefore, this part of the levator ani lies below it. The obturator internus muscle extends above and below the arch of the levator ani. The obturator internus muscle can be palpated directly anywhere above the arch, but below the arch, it can be palpated only through the levator ani.

Just caudal to the tip of the ischial spine, a soft spot felt through the levator ani muscle locates the opening of the lesser sciatic foramen.

Levator Ani

The most medial and anterior portion of the pubococcygeus muscle loops around the urogenital tract and serves to constrict the vagina in women (pubovaginal muscle) and to elevate the prostate in men (levator prostatae). The most posterior portion of the pubococcygeus (the puborectalis) loops around the rectum at the level of the external anal sphincter; it elevates and helps constrict the anus. Bilaterally, the iliococcygeus part of the levator ani forms a sling between the ilium and coccyx that supports the pelvic floor and pulls the coccyx inward. Contraction of the muscle can be palpated during the rectal or vaginal examination.

Palpation of the levator ani starts by feeling the ends of the muscle fibers for tenderness. The examiner then moves the finger across the midbelly of the muscle from the region of the perineal body to the middle of the sacrospinous ligament, feeling for local tenderness and taut bands indicative of TrPs. By sweeping the finger from side to side through an arc of 180° at successively higher levels, the examiner can palpate all of the fibers of the levator ani and of the coccygeus muscle as well.[95] Thiele[95] illustrated this examination technique. He commented on how frequently individual fascicles stood out like tight cords with areas of relaxed muscle between them and reported that sometimes the entire levator ani was tense and felt like a firm sheet of muscle stretched from its tendinous arch to the sacrum, coccyx, and anococcygeal body.[95] A similar examination of the piriformis muscle is illustrated in Figure 10.5 with useful anatomical landmarks. Pressure on levator ani TrPs nearly always reproduces the patient's pain complaint, usually in the region of the coccyx.

When the examiner finds tender spots that seem to be in the lateral portions of the levator ani below this muscle's tendinous arch, care must be exercised to be sure that the tenderness is not due to TrPs in the underlying obturator internus. The two muscles can be distinguished by palpating while asking the patient to squeeze the finger in the rectum (levator ani activation), relax, and then abduct the flexed thigh or laterally rotate the extended thigh on that side against resistance (obturator internus activation). The increase in muscle tension identifies the contracting muscle.

Coccygeus

The coccygeus muscle is palpable mainly at the level of the sacrococcygeal joint (Fig. 6.3).[2] Much of the muscle lies between the examining finger and the underlying sacrospinous ligament. In some persons the muscle is intertwined with the ligament, the caudal border of which is usually distinctly palpable. Against this firm ligamentous foundation, taut bands and their TrPs are usually readily identified by palpation across the muscle fibers.

Occasionally, a thick band of coccygeus muscle fibers crosses the midline; here it is readily palpable against the lowest part of the sacrum or uppermost region of the coccyx.

The gluteus maximus attachment to the outer margins of the sacrum and coccyx corresponds closely to the coccygeus muscle's attachment on the inner margins of these bones.[65]

Malbohan and associates[64] found that, among 1500 patients examined for low back pain, only a small percentage did not experience pain during internal extension pressure against the coccyx. The authors attributed this discomfort to the increased tension placed on the coccygeus muscle. However, this maneuver simultaneously stretches the iliococcygeal portion of the levator ani, which also attaches to the coccyx. Tenderness along the margin of the coccyx suggests tenderness of either levator ani musculotendinous junctions, coccygeus musculotendinous junctions (Fig. 6.3), or of a sacrococcygeus ventralis muscle[13,37] (when present).

Pelvic Wall Muscles

One pelvic wall muscle, the obturator internus, covers the anterolateral wall of the lesser pelvis. Looking into the pelvis from above, one sees that much of this muscle is covered by the levator ani (*see* Fig. 10.5). The obturator internus exits the pelvis through the lesser sciatic foramen, which is bounded on two sides by the sacrospinous and sacrotuberous ligaments. The sacrotuberous ligament attaches to the externally identifiable ischial tuberosity. The other major intrapelvic muscle, the piriformis, is found cephalad to the sacrospinous ligament and is considered in Chapter 10 of this volume. The sacrococcygeus ventralis muscle, when present, is palpable as longitudinal fibers along the margins of the lower sacrum and coccyx.

Obturator Internus

A view of the pelvis from above shows that the posterior portion of the obturator internus must be palpated through the levator ani muscle[2] (*see* Fig. 10.5). A frontal section through the anus[27] likewise illustrates this and shows the relation of these muscles to the tendinous arch. A frontal section[82] and a cross section[83] through the prostate depict how one must palpate the thick posterior part of the obturator internus through a thin layer of the levator ani muscle on either side of the prostate (or vagina).

When running the finger around the lateral wall of the pelvis above the tendinous arch of the levator ani from the ischial spine to the pubis, any observed tender spots or taut bands are in the obturator internus. The obturator internus muscle exits the pelvis through the lesser sciatic foramen. This point of exit lies below (caudal to) the tip of the ischial spine beneath the tendinous arch. Since this is an area of musculotendinous junction where most of the obturator internus muscle fibers are represented, it is a critical point to examine for tenderness to determine if TrPs are likely to be present anywhere in the muscle. Tenderness at this location is comparable to that in the region of the musculotendinous junction of the psoas major muscle just above its attachment to the lesser trochanter (*see* Chapter 5).

Piriformis

See Chapter 10 in this volume for a description of the intrapelvic examination of the piriformis muscle. Its rectal examination is illustrated in Figure 10.5.

Sacrococcygeus Ventralis

If the sacrococcygeus ventralis (when present) has TrPs, the examiner will find spot tenderness along the lower sacrum or the coccyx in a taut band running parallel to the axis of the spine. The fibers of the levator ani and coccygeus also can cause tenderness at the edge of the coccyx, but lie more nearly at right angles to the spine. Pressure on an active sacrococcygeus TrP is likely to reproduce the pain in the coccyx.

Vaginal Examination

In the female, the bulbospongiosus muscle can be satisfactorily examined for TrPs only by vaginal examination. The patient should be placed in the lithotomy position for this approach. The bulbospongiosus and levator vaginae portions of the levator ani muscle enclose the introitus. They can be located and their strength assessed by having the patient squeeze the examining finger. Myofascial TrPs weaken them. These muscles are examined for TrPs by gentle pincer palpation at about the middle of each lateral wall of the introitus. When present, the taut bands are clearly delineated, are tender, and contain TrPs that, when compressed, usually refer an ache to the vaginal and perineal regions, reproducing the patient's pain complaint.

The clinician examines the ischiocavernosus muscle by pressing directly laterally from within the distal vagina against the edge of the pubic arch. This muscle and the crus clitoridis that it covers are normally not tender. When compressed, active TrPs in this muscle refer pain to the perineal region.

Vaginal examination has the advantage that one can reach farther into the pelvis to examine the coccygeus and piriformis muscles than one can reach rectally. If the examiner places two fingers against the lateral wall of the pelvis just beyond the inside margin of the pubic arch over the obturator membrane, the upper finger overlies the anterior portion of the obturator internus while the lower finger palpates the levator ani. These muscles can be identified as described previously in the discussion of the levator ani in this section. Furthermore, one can distinguish the backward angulation of the anterior obturator internus fibers from the transverse orientation of the levator ani fibers; this is more difficult to do by rectal examination. Higher in the pelvis, the examiner palpates the bulky posterior portion of the obturator internus muscle anterior to the ischial spine.

The coccygeal region and coccygeus muscle are more difficult to palpate from the vagina than from the rectum because one must palpate through two layers of rectal mucosa and one of vaginal mucosa. An optimum localization of all the intrapelvic musculoskeletal structures requires both rectal and vaginal examinations.

Perineal Muscles

The perineal muscles—the transverse perinei, bulbospongiosus, and ischiocavernosus—are the most superficial and contribute some support to the pelvic floor. None of these muscles is likely to be identifiable unless it has taut bands, which lie parallel to the direction of the muscle fibers. In both sexes, the bilateral ischiocavernosus muscle frames the pubic arch that borders the perineum beneath the symphysis pubis.

External Examination, Male

Ideally, the patient should be placed in the lithotomy position with the feet in stirrups. If that is not practical, then he can lie supine, pulling his knees up toward the armpits. The testicles are lifted out of the way with a towel used as a sling.[4,39]

The bulb of the penis is palpable in the midline, between the anus and the base of the shaft of the penis, through the skin of the scrotum between the testicles. The bulbospongiosus muscle fibers angle around the bulb in a pennate fashion, more circumferential than longitudinal. Taut bands and TrP tenderness are most readily detectable if the bulb is at least partially tumescent so there is a firmer base against which to perform flat palpation. The ischiocavernosus muscles angle in and upward on either side of the bulb.

The transversus perinei superficialis is not usually distinguishable by palpation unless it contains taut bands. The muscle fibers extend from the ischial tuberosity on each side to the fibrous perineal body that lies between the anus and the bulb of the penis. To feel these taut bands and localize the TrP spot tenderness, it sometimes helps to provide counterpressure against the external palpating finger by one finger in the rectum.

External Examination, Female

In a woman, the lithotomy position with the feet in stirrups is likewise the most satisfactory for examining the superficial pelvic floor muscles. Usually, only the ischiocavernosus and transversus perinei superficialis muscles are identifiable by external palpation, and then only if they have taut bands and tender TrPs. The relationships of these muscles are clearly drawn[30,41] and realistically depicted.[6]

The ischiocavernosus muscle and its TrPs are more readily located by vaginal examination. The ischiocavernosus lies close to, and along most of the length of, the perineal margin of the pubic bone below the pubic symphysis. On vaginal examination, taut bands become evident when compressed by flat palpation against the margin of the pubic bone at the midvaginal level and at right angles to the direction of the muscle fibers.

As in the male, the transversus perinei superficialis on each side spans the distance between the perineal body centrally and the ischial tuberosity laterally. Palpation must be at right angles to the direction of the fibers and the muscle must be under slight tension to identify taut bands most effectively.

10. ENTRAPMENTS

No nerve entrapments by these pelvic muscles have been demonstrated. However, the situation at the lesser sciatic foramen with regard to potential entrapment of a nerve appears analogous to sciatic nerve compression at the greater sciatic foramen, as discussed in Chapter 10 of this volume. The lesser sciatic foramen has firm, unyielding boundaries: the bony ischium on one side and heavy ligaments, the sacrotuberous and the sacrospinous, on the other sides. Since these two ligaments fuse as they pass one another,[25] there is no space available for pressure relief if the foramen becomes completely filled. The pudendal nerve, the internal pudendal vessels, and the obturator internus muscle with its tendon pass through the foramen. At this point, the obturator muscle usually has become mainly tendinous, but there may be a sufficient number of muscle fibers passing through the foramen to compress the pudendal nerve and vessels if the muscle develops TrPs, shortens, and bulges. This is a possibility that deserves investigation when perineal pain or dysesthesia is unexplained.

11. ASSOCIATED TRIGGER POINTS

Myofascial TrPs in the perineal muscles (namely, the bulbospongiosus, ischiocavernosus, and transverse perinei) are likely to present as single muscle syndromes. On the other hand, pelvic floor muscles (for instance, the sphincter ani, levator ani, and coccygeus) are much more likely to exhibit multiple muscle involvement. Increased tension of the levator ani often occurs in conjunction with increased tension of the gluteus maximus muscle.[58,60]

The obturator internus and piriformis are lower-limb muscles and, as such, are prone to develop TrPs together, and in association with other lateral rotators of the hip (i.e., the gemelli, obturator externus, and quadratus femoris muscles).

12. INTERMITTENT COLD WITH STRETCH

Intermittent cold with stretch is not applicable for the management of intrapelvic TrPs. However, other therapeutic techniques have been found effective in these muscle syndromes: massage, stretch, postisometric relaxation, high voltage pulsed galvanic stimulation, ultrasound, and posture correction.

Massage

Thiele[95] presented the classic illustrated description for the examination and treatment by massage of the levator ani and coccygeus muscles via the rectum. He recommended rubbing the muscle fibers along their length, from origin to insertion, with a stripping motion (as when sharpening a straight razor), applying as much pressure as the patient could tolerate with moderate pain. The patient was instructed to "bear down" during massage to relax these muscles. The massage motion was repeated 10 to 15 times on each side of the pelvis, and this treatment was repeated daily for 5 or 6 days. Massage only once or twice a week was found to be ineffective. Of the 223 patients with coccygodynia who were treated in this way, 64% were "cured" and 27% improved.[95]

Malbohan and associates also reported successful use of massage of these two muscles in the treatment of nearly 1500 patients with low back pain attributed to coccygeal spasm.[64] Cooper[33] reported that 81% of 62 coccygodynia patients were relieved of pain by the Thiele type of massage, but careful instruction about proper sitting posture relieved an even higher percentage of 28 other patients. Grant and associates[47] found that two or three levator ani massages spaced 2–3 weeks apart, in conjunction with heat and diazepam, provided good results in 63% of patients with the levator syndrome.

Stripping massage is a powerful tool for the inactivation of these accessible myofascial TrPs. Massage is painful but it can be effective when other modalities have failed. One is able to identify the taut bands and TrPs requiring attention and literally to put one's finger on the source of the pain, treating its source until the problem is resolved.

Stretch

Two authors referred to treatment by stretching the levator ani muscle in terms of "stretching the spastic muscles,"[62] and "retropulsion of the coccyx."[64] Dorsal mobilization of the coccyx to stretch the levator ani can be included as part of the massage procedure.

Postisometric relaxation is a more sophisticated stretch technique that is considered next.

Postisometric relaxation

The principles of postisometric relaxation (or contract-relax only at mild effort) are discussed in Chapter 2, pages 10–11 of this volume. Lewit[58] describes and illustrates a valuable application for patients who have pain in the coccygeal region with a tender coccyx and who exhibit increased tension of both the levator ani and gluteus maximus muscles. The patient lies prone with the heels rotated outward, which places the gluteus maximus on partial stretch. The clinician stands beside the patient's thigh, crosses the forearms and places one palm on each buttock at the level of the anus to provide isometric resistance. The patient is instructed to press the buttocks together with very little force, to maintain this pressure for about 10 seconds, and then to "let go." During relaxation, the clinician feels the initial tension in the gluteus maximus muscles diminish. After this cycle has been repeated three to five times, external palpation of the ventral surface of the coccyx is then usually accomplished more easily and has become painless. The patient can apply this isometric contraction technique as self-treatment in a home program. The portion of the gluteus maximus that attaches to the coccyx is embryologically separate from the rest of the gluteus maximus;[97] this fact may relate to the effectiveness of postisometric therapy for this part of the muscle.

Malbohan and associates[64] outline a combined program for coccygeal pain. In addition to the postisometric relaxation described previously and massage of the levator ani and coccygeus muscles, they employ isometric relaxation of the muscles attached to the coccyx. This is performed by contraction of the muscles forming the pelvic diaphragm followed by manually assisted retropulsion (dorsal displacement) of the coccyx during relaxation. This technique passively stretches the parts of the levator ani that attach to the coccyx and anococcygeal body.

High Voltage Pulsed Galvanic Stimulation

Several reports on the levator ani syndrome describe the effectiveness of high voltage pulsed galvanic stimulation applied through an electrode inserted into the rectum. Stimulation frequency was set between 80 and 120 Hz with the maximum patient-acceptable voltage ranging between 100 and 400 V. Most authors reported a treatment time of 1 hour repeated every day or every few days for three to eight times. The details of these studies were summarized by Morris and Newton.[71] Either good or excellent therapeutic results were reported for 43–90% of patients.[92] Consistently, those patients who proved not to have the levator ani syndrome or in whom it was a secondary diagnosis responded poorly. None of these studies was controlled.

The reason why this form of electrical stimulation should inactivate myofascial TrPs is cloudy. The rhythmical contractions may increase local blood flow and help equalize sarcomere lengths. The stimulation of muscle afferent nerve fibers may help disrupt feedback loops that sustain the local TrP mechanism. These factors need to be investigated.

Ultrasound

Lilius and Valtonen[62] reported that 75% of 24 patients treated for levator ani spasm syndrome with ultrasound became symptomless or had only mild continuing symptoms. They applied 1–2.5 W/cm^2 of ultrasound to the perineum around the anus for 5–10 minutes on 15–30 successive days.

Seated Posture

Because he could demonstrate acute angulation of the coccyx radiographically when the patient was seated in the slumped posture, and because his patients responded so well to correction of this poor posture, Thiele[95] strongly emphasized the therapeutic importance of sitting posture in patients with coccygodynia. He considered it the cause of the patients' symptoms in 31% of 324 cases. Cooper[33] found that slumping posture was responsible for the pain in 14% of his 100 cases with coccygodynia. Other authors have made a point of teaching their coccygodynia patients who slump while sitting to sit up straight.[62]

13. INJECTION

Generally, only the perineal muscles and sphincter ani are accessible for injection therapy. It should be employed only if the TrP and its taut band are unmistakably palpable and precisely located. The principles of TrP injection are covered in Volume 1, pages 74–86.[98] For injection of the ischiocavernosus in either sex and of the bulbospongiosus in the male, the clinician uses flat palpation to localize the TrP. In a female patient, a taut band and TrP in the bulbospongiosus muscle are localized and held between the fingertip in the vagina and the tip of the thumb on the labium majorus and then injected through the labium using the other hand.

Massage of TrPs in the sphincter ani muscle is rarely satisfactory by itself, but these TrPs may be responsive to pulsed electrical stimulation or ultrasound, as described previously. Injection is painful but may be quickly effective.

Injection of the sphincter ani is performed bimanually. A 10-mL syringe with a 63-mm (2½-in) 21-gauge needle is loaded and gloves donned. A palpating finger localizes the taut band and its TrP in the anal sphincter. Before the needle is inserted, the skin area to be penetrated is cleansed with antiseptic and then sprayed for 6 seconds or less (just short of frosting) with vapocoolant applied for brief local anesthesia; the mucous membrane of the anal opening should be protected from the spray, since here the vapocoolant can produce burning pain. Before the skin can rewarm, the needle is inserted parallel to and at one side of the anus. When the needle approaches the sphincter ani muscle, its tip is felt by the finger in the rectum; that finger then directs the needle precisely to the TrP. Frequently there is a cluster of TrPs to be inactivated. The muscle should be thoroughly palpated for any remaining TrPs, and these should be injected before the needle is withdrawn.

Long[63] recommended injection of intrapelvic TrPs located in the levator ani or coccygeus muscles close to the coccyx when they were refractory to massage and involved a small area. He, too, used a bimanual method, palpating rectally to check the position of the needle tip. Waters[100] injected 2–10 ml of 2.0% procaine solution into tender spots in the perineum for coccygodynia.

14. CORRECTIVE ACTIONS

When patients with myofascial TrPs fail to respond to specific local treatment or when the beneficial results are only transient, the clinician should aggressively investigate the possibility of nutritional inadequacies or other systemic perpetuating factors for myofascial TrPs, which are discussed in detail in Chapter 4 of Volume 1.[98]

For the patient with TrPs in the coccygeus and levator ani muscles, the clinician should identify and, if possible, correct any articular dysfunctions of the sacroiliac joints and sacrococcygeal or lumbosacral articulations. Also in such cases, resolution of any chronic inflammatory condition within the pelvis, such as endometritis, chronic salpingo-oophoritis, chronic prostatovesiculitis, interstitial cystitis, and urinary tract infections may be critical to pain relief. A slumped seated posture must be corrected, as noted previously in Section 12.

Sphincter ani TrPs are likely to be refractory when painful internal hemorrhoids are present. Conservative approaches to relief of hemorrhoidal pain include increased liquid intake and/or a stool softener, a diet with more fiber, local application of an analgesic hemorrhoid preparation, restoration of the internal hemorrhoids to their protected position within the anal sphincter after defecation, and an enema of 30–60 gm (½–1 oz) of pediatric liquid petrolatum given the last thing before retiring at night to help lubricate passage of the stool. If conservative measures fail, banding or surgical removal of internal hemorrhoids needs to be considered.

References

1. Anderson JE: *Grant's Atlas of Anatomy*, Ed. 8. Williams & Wilkins Baltimore, 1983 (Figs. 3–10, 3–39).
2. *Ibid.* (Fig. 3–12).
3. *Ibid.* (Fig. 3–16).
4. *Ibid.* (Fig. 3–17).
5. *Ibid.* (Fig. 3–19).
6. *Ibid.* (Fig. 3–33).
7. *Ibid.* (Fig. 3–55).
8. *Ibid.* (Fig. 3–57).
9. *Ibid.* (Fig. 4–40).
10. *Ibid.* (Fig. 4–43).
11. *Ibid.* (Fig. 4–46).
12. Bard P: Control of systemic blood vessels, Chapter 10. In *Medical Physiology*, Ed. 12, Vol. 1, edited by V.B. Mountcastle. C. V. Mosby Company, St. Louis, 1968 (pp. 150–177, *See* 168–169).
13. Bardeen CR: The musculature, Sect. 5. In *Morris's Human Anatomy*, edited by C. M. Jackson, Ed. 6. Blakiston's Son & Co., Philadelphia, 1921 (p. 481, Fig. 424).
14. Basmajian JV, Burke MD, Burnett GW, *et al.* (eds.): *Stedman's Medical Dictionary*, 24th ed. Williams & Wilkins, Baltimore, 1982 (pp. 293, 1143).
15. Basmajian JV, Deluca CJ: *Muscles Alive*, Ed. 5. Williams & Wilkins, Baltimore, 1985 (pp. 399–400).
16. *Ibid.* (pp. 402–403).
17. Benoit G, Delmas V, Gillot C, *et al.*: The anatomy of erection. *Surg Radiol Anat 9*:263–272, 1987.
18. Carter BL, Morehead J, Wolpert SM, *et al.*: *Cross-Sectional Anatomy*. Appleton-Century-Crofts, New York, 1977 (Sects. 38–41, 44–46).
19. *Ibid.* (Sects. 41–42–male, Sect. 47–female).
20. *Ibid.* (Sect. 42).
21. *Ibid.* (Sects. 40–42, 46).
22. *Ibid.* (Sects. 40, 44).
23. *Ibid.* (Sects. 42, 47–48).
24. Clemente CD: *Gray's Anatomy of the Human Body,* American Ed. 30. Lea & Febiger, Philadelphia, 1985 (p. 96).
25. *Ibid.* (pp. 361–363).
26. *Ibid.* (pp. 498–500).
27. *Ibid.* (pp. 500, 501, Fig. 6–36).
28. *Ibid.* (pp. 508–511).
29. *Ibid.* (p. 509, Fig. 6–40).
30. *Ibid.* (p. 510, Fig. 6–41).
31. *Ibid.* (pp. 511–512).
32. *Ibid.* (pp. 568–570).
33. Cooper WL: Coccygodynia: an analysis of one hundred cases. *J Internat Coll Surg 33*:306–311, 1960.
34. Critchley HOD, Dixon JS, Gosling JA: Comparative study of the periurethral and perianal parts of the human levator ani muscle. *Urol Int 35*:226–232, 1980.
35. Dittrich RJ: Coccygodynia as referred pain. *J Bone Joint Surg [Am] 33*:715–718, 1951.
36. Douthwaite AH: Proctalgia fugax. *Br Med J 2*: 164–165, 1962.
37. Eisler P: *Die Muskeln des Stammes*. Gustav Fischer, Jena, 1912 (pp. 447, 449–451, Fig. 65).
38. Ferner H, Staubesand J: *Sobotta Atlas of Human Anatomy*, Ed. 10, Vol. 2. Urban & Schwarzenberg, Baltimore, 1983 (Fig. 152).
39. *Ibid.* (Fig. 292).
40. *Ibid.* (Fig. 295).
41. *Ibid.* (Figs. 320, 328, 329).
42. *Ibid.* (Fig. 325).
43. *Ibid.* (Fig. 404).
44. *Ibid.* (Fig. 420).
45. Goldstein J: Personal communication, 1990.
46. Gosling JA, Dixon JS, Critchley HOD, *et al.*: A comparative study of the human external sphincter and periurethral levator ani muscles. *Br J Urol 53*:35–41, 1981.
47. Grant SR, Salvati EP, Rubin RJ: Levator syndrome: an analysis of 316 cases. *Dis Colon Rectum 18*:161–163, 1975.
48. Greenman PE: *Principles of Manual Medicine*. Williams & Wilkins, Baltimore, 1989 (pp. 234, 236).
49. Harvey RF: Colonic motility in proctalgia fugax. *Lancet 2*:713–714, 1979.
50. Juenemann KP, Lue TF, Schmidt RA, *et al.*: Clinical significance of sacral and pudendal nerve anatomy. *J Urol 139*:74–80, 1988.
51. Karacan I, Hirshkowitz M, Salis PJ, *et al.*: Penile blood flow and musculovascular events during sleep-related erections of middle-aged men. *J Urol 138*:177–181, 1987.
52. Kidd R: Pain localization with the innominate upslip dysfunction. *Manual Med 3*:103–105, 1988.
53. Koelbl H, Strassegger H, Riss PA, *et al.*: Morphologic and functional aspects of pelvic floor muscles in patients with pelvic relaxation and genuine stress incontinence. *Obstet Gynecol 74*: 789–795, 1989.
54. Lavoisier P, Courtois F, Barres D, *et al.*: Correlation between intracavernous pressure and contraction of the ischiocavernosus muscle in man. *J Urol 136*:936–939, 1986.
55. Lavoisier P, Proulx J, Courtois F: Reflex contractions of the ischiocavernosus muscles following electrical and pressure stimulations. *J Urol 139*:396–399, 1988.
56. Leigh RE: Obturator internus spasm as a cause of pelvic and sciatic distress. *Lancet 1*:286–287, 1952.
57. Lewit K: *Manipulative Therapy in Rehabilitation of the Motor System*. Butterworths, London, 1985 (pp. 113, 174, 311).
58. *Ibid.* (pp. 223; 278, Fig. 6.97).
59. *Ibid.* (pp. 306–307).
60. Lewit K: Postisometric relaxation in combination with other methods of muscular facilitation and inhibition. *Manual Med 2*:101–104, 1986.
61. Lilius HG, Oravisto KJ, Valtonen EJ: Origin of pain in interstitial cystitis. *Scand J Urol Nephrol 7*:150–152, 1973.
62. Lilius HG, Valtonen EJ: The levator ani spasm syndrome: a clinical analysis of 31 cases. *Ann Chir Gynaecol Fenn 62*:93–97, 1973.
63. Long C, II: Myofascial pain syndromes: Part III–Some syndromes of trunk and thigh. *Henry Ford Hosp Med Bull 4*:102–106, 1956.

64. Malbohan IM, Mojíšová L, Tichý M: The role of coccygeal spasm in low back pain. *J Man Med 4*:140–141, 1989.
65. McMinn RMH, Hutchings RT: *Color Atlas of Human Anatomy*. Year Book Medical Publishers, Chicago, 1977 (p. 81).
66. *Ibid*. (p. 245).
67. *Ibid*. (p. 248).
68. *Ibid*. (p. 252A).
69. *Ibid*. (p. 256).
70. *Ibid*. (pp. 266, 273).
71. Morris L, Newton RA: Use of high voltage pulsed galvanic stimulation for patients with levator ani syndrome. *Phys Ther 67*:1522–1525, 1987.
72. Netter FH: *The Ciba Collection of Medical Illustrations*, Vol. 8, Musculoskeletal System. Part I: Anatomy, Physiology and Metabolic Disorders. Ciba-Geigy Corporation, Summit, 1987 (p. 86).
73. *Ibid*. (pp. 142–143).
74. Nicosia JF, Abcarian H: Levator syndrome: a treatment that works. *Dis Colon Rectum 28*:406–408, 1985.
75. Nocenti MR: Reproduction, Chapter 48. In *Medical Physiology*, Ed. 12, Vol. 1, edited by V.B. Mountcastle. C.V. Mosby Company, St. Louis, 1968 (pp. 992–1028, *see* 1024–1025).
76. Oliver GC, Rubin RJ, Salvati EP, *et al*.: Electrogalvanic stimulation in the treatment of levator syndrome. *Dis Colon Rectum 28*:662–663, 1985.
77. Pace JB: Commonly overlooked pain syndromes responsive to simple therapy. *Postgrad Med 58*:107–113, 1975.
78. Pace JB, Henning C: Episacroiliac lipoma. *Am Fam Phys 6*:70–73, 1972.
79. Peery WH: Proctalgia fugax: a clinical enigma. *South Med J 81*:621–623, 1988.
80. Pernkopf E: *Atlas of Topographical and Applied Human Anatomy*, Vol. 2. W.B. Saunders, Philadelphia, 1964 (Fig. 306).
81. Rohen JW, Yokochi C: *Color Atlas of Anatomy*, Ed. 2. Igaku-Shoin, New York, 1988 (p. 311).
82. *Ibid*. (p. 316).
83. *Ibid*. (p. 317).
84. *Ibid*. (p. 322).
85. *Ibid*. (p. 323).
86. *Ibid*. (p. 332).
87. Salvati EP: The levator syndrome and its variant. *Gastroenterol Clin North Am 16*:71–78, 1987.
88. Simons DG, Travell JG: Myofascial origins of low back pain. 3. Pelvic and lower extremity muscles. *Postgrad Med 73*:99–108, 1983.
89. Sinaki M, Merritt JL, Stillwell GK: Tension myalgia of the pelvic floor. *Mayo Clin Proc 52*:717–722, 1977.
90. Slocumb JC: Neurological factors in chronic pelvic pain: trigger points and the abdominal pelvic pain syndrome. *Am J Obstet Gynecol 149*: 536–543, 1984.
91. Smith WT: Levator spasm syndrome. *Minn Med 42*:1076–1079, 1959.
92. Sohn N, Weinstein MA, Robbins RD: The levator syndrome and its treatment with high-voltage electrogalvanic stimulation. *Am J Surg 144*: 580–582, 1982.
93. Swain R: Oral clonidine for proctalgia fugax. *Gut 28*:1039–1040, 1987.
94. Thiele GH: Coccygodynia and pain in the superior gluteal region. *JAMA 109*:1271–1275, 1937.
95. Thiele GH: Coccygodynia: cause and treatment. *Dis Colon Rectum 6*:422–436, 1963.
96. Thompson WG, Heaton KW: Proctalgia fugax. *J R Coll Physicians Lond 14*:247–248, 1980.
97. Tichý M: Anatomical basis for relaxation of the muscles attached to the coccyx. *Manual Med 4*: 147–148, 1989.
98. Travell JG and Simons DG: *Myofascial Pain and Dysfunction: The Trigger Point Manual*. Williams & Wilkins, Baltimore, 1983.
99. *Ibid*. (p. 19).
100. Waters EG: A consideration of the types and treatment of coccygodynia. *Am J Obstet Gyncecol 33*:531–535, 1937.
101. Weizman Z, Binsztok M: Proctalgia fugax in teenagers. *J Pediatr 114*:813–814, 1989.
102. Wright JF: Inhaled solbutamol for proctalgia fugax. *Lancet 2*:659–660, 1985.
103. Wright RR: The levator ani spasm syndrome. *Am J Proctol 6*:477, 1969.

CHAPTER 7
Gluteus Maximus Muscle

"Swimmer's Nemesis"

HIGHLIGHTS: The gluteus maximus is a large muscle composed predominantly of the "work-horse" type 1 (slow-twitch) muscle fibers. These fibers depend primarily on oxidative metabolism and are suited for continuous use, but at a small percentage of maximal strength. The weight of the gluteus maximus is several times that of the gluteus medius and gluteus minimus together. The large size and the anatomic orientation of the gluteus maximus of humans are unique and are an important anatomic basis of upright posture. The evolutionary changes in this muscle have been associated with the distinctive intelligence and manual dexterity of humans among primates. **REFERRED PAIN** from trigger points (TrPs) in the gluteus maximus projects to the buttock region, rarely to a considerable distance. The proximal **ANATOMICAL ATTACHMENTS** of this muscle are to the posterior iliac crest, lateral sacrum, and coccyx. Distally, the fibers are secured to the iliotibial band of the fascia lata and to the femur. **INNERVATION** derives from the L_5, S_1, and S_2 spinal roots via the inferior gluteal nerve. **FUNCTION** of the gluteus maximus includes powerful extension of the thigh at the hip during strenuous activities: running, jumping, climbing stairs, and arising from the seated position. During the stance phase of ambulation, the gluteus maximus restrains the tendency toward hip flexion and helps regain body position over the forward foot. This muscle helps maintain an erect posture and assists lateral rotation at the hip. **SYMPTOMS** from TrPs in this muscle commonly include restlessness and pain on prolonged sitting, increased pain when walking uphill in a bent-forward posture, and pain induced by swimming the crawl stroke. The TrPs of the gluteus maximus are distinguished from TrPs in the gluteus medius by location and are distinguished from TrPs in the deep gluteus minimus by the latter's more distant referred pain patterns. **ACTIVATION AND PERPETUATION OF TRIGGER POINTS** may result from a direct blow on the muscle, from walking uphill, from sleeping in an incorrect position, or from sudden overload during a fall or near-fall that induces a vigorous lengthening contraction. **PATIENT EXAMINATION** usually reveals an antalgic gait, impaired sitting tolerance, and restricted flexion of the thigh at the hip. **TRIGGER POINT EXAMINATION** is performed with the involved thigh of the side-lying patient flexed about 90°. The TrPs may be found in three areas and their vigorous local twitch responses are clearly visible. **INTERMITTENT COLD WITH STRETCH** is accomplished with the patient side lying by gently bringing the knee of the affected side toward the opposite axilla while parallel sweeps of the ice or vapocoolant are applied downward from the waist over the buttock to midthigh. During passive stretch, relaxation is enhanced by rhythmic slow exhalation. Application of moist heat and slow, active, full range of motion must follow. For **INJECTION AND STRETCH**, the more cephalad TrPs are identified and pinned down for injection by flat palpation; the most caudal TrPs are fixed by pincer palpation. Injection is followed by intermittent cold and muscle lengthening, moist heat, and active range of motion. **CORRECTIVE ACTIONS** include restriction of uninterrupted sitting to 15 or 20 minutes, use of a soft doughnut cushion with the hole centered under the ischial tuberosity of the painful side, and placement of a pillow between the knees when sleeping. Self-stretch exercises that are augmented with post-isometric relaxation and with coordinated exhalation are important. Lying on a tennis ball provides effective ischemic compression. Overloading the gluteus maximus by long uphill hiking and by swimming the crawl stroke should be avoided.

1. REFERRED PAIN
(Fig. 7.1)

Myofascial trigger points (TrPs) in the gluteus maximus muscle refer pain locally in the buttock region and rarely, if ever, to the considerable distance characteristic of TrPs in the deepest gluteal muscle, the gluteus minimus (Chapter 9).[74,86]

There are three common sites of TrPs in the gluteus maximus muscle. The composite pain pattern for these TrPs has been reported previously.[73,75]

Myofascial TrPs of the gluteus maximus, found adjacent to the sacrum in the region marked TrP_1 in Figure 7.1*A*, refer a crescent of pain and tenderness beside the gluteal cleft. The upper end of this pain pattern includes the sacroiliac joint. A patch of pain along and above the gluteal fold may spill over slightly onto the adjacent posterior thigh. Apropos of gluteus maximus TrP_1, Kelly[44] noted that a tender muscular lesion of the gluteus maximus in the sacroiliac region caused low backache, and Lange[47] observed that myogelosis at the origin of the gluteus maximus along the medial crest of the ilium caused lumbago.

The TrP_2 region (Fig. 7.1*B*), slightly above the ischial tuberosity, is the most common location of TrPs in the gluteus maximus muscle. Myofascial TrPs in this area usually refer pain to the entire buttock and also refer tenderness deep within the buttock, which can easily lead to the false conclusion that the deeper gluteal muscles are involved. The TrP_2 is likely to refer pain that covers the entire lower sacrum and projects laterally below the crest of the ilium. Pain from TrP_2 does not include the anal region or coccyx. Pressure on TrP_2 can produce such intense local pain when the patient sits on a hard seat that, depending on the sitting position, he or she may feel as if a nail is pressing into the bone.

Gluteus maximus TrP_3 (Fig. 7.1*C*) is located in the most medial and inferior muscle fibers. These fibers lie close to the coccyx, to which this TrP refers pain. Therefore, TrP_3 is a source of coccygodynia, which also may arise from TrPs in the coccygeus muscle (Chapter 6).

The patients with pain referred to the coccyx from gluteus maximus TrP_3 frequently insist that there is pressure on the coccyx when they are sitting, because that is where it hurts. However, ordinarily, the coccyx does *NOT* touch the chair seat; one can easily slip a finger between the coccyx and the seat, except when the individual slumps down in the chair to recline the torso. A rubber ring or "doughnut" is often prescribed to relieve this nonexistent coccygeal pressure; however, the rubber ring can aggravate the pain if it concentrates pressure on TrP_3. More effective use of this device is described in Section 14.

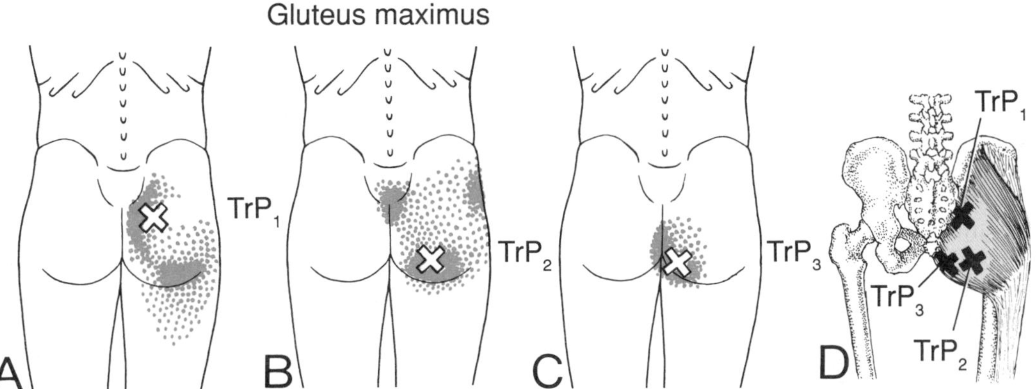

Figure 7.1. Referred pain patterns (*solid red* and *stippled areas*) of trigger points (TrPs) (**Xs**) in the gluteus maximus muscle. Trigger points are located in: *A*, the superior medial portion of the muscle (TrP_1). *B*, the lower midportion overlying the posterior surface of the ischial tuberosity (TrP_2). *C*, the most medial inferior portion (TrP_3). *D*, location of TrP_1, TrP_2 and TrP_3 in the gluteus maximus muscle.

A few authors identified tender spots in the gluteus maximus muscle as the origin of sciatica or sciaticlike pain.[32,35,44,45,47] These writers may have been describing TrPs in the posterior part of the gluteus minimus, which can refer sciaticlike pain down the back of the thigh and the calf (Chapter 9). None of these authors appears to have distinguished specifically among the three gluteal muscles, as described below in the section on Differential Diagnosis and as described in the next chapter. We have not observed a sciaticlike referred pain pattern from gluteus maximus TrPs.

Occasionally, one finds TrPs located in the gluteus maximus along its lateral border or along its attachment to the crest of the ilium. These TrPs also refer pain and tenderness chiefly over the muscle itself.

The referred *tenderness* in the regions that match the pattern of referred pain causes the patient to point out these reference zones as painful spots because they hurt when pressed or bumped. As emphasized by Kelly[43], these zones of referred tenderness should be clearly distinguished from their TrP origins and not treated as primary sites of pain.

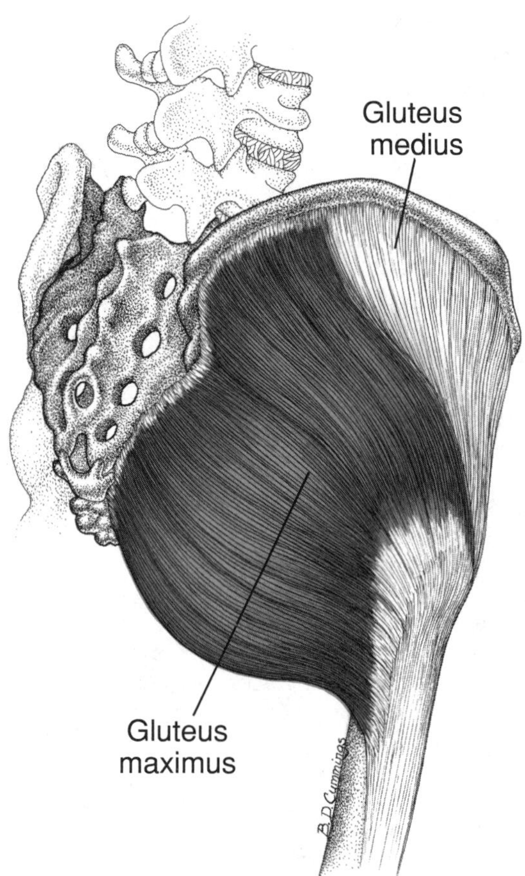

Figure 7.2. Attachments of the right gluteus maximus muscle (*red*) in the posterolateral view. The gluteus maximus muscle covers the posterior portion of the gluteus medius muscle, but not its anterior portion.

2. ANATOMICAL ATTACHMENTS AND CONSIDERATIONS
(Fig. 7.2)

From an evolutionary point of view, upright walking by true bipedal plantigrade progression has been singled out as the unique feature of human locomotion.[38] Humans alone, among mammals, can place the center of gravity of the head, arms, and torso over the hips.[6] This function has been associated with evolutionary changes in the skeleton and gluteus maximus muscle that are uniquely human. These changes include shortening and tilting of the pelvis to permit extension of the thigh at the hip to 180°, angulation of gluteus maximus fibers more horizontally,[6] and enlargement of the muscle to more than twice the size of the gluteus medius.[63] These evolutionary changes, which were well illustrated by Hunter,[37] presumably freed the hands for other activities and were considered by Bollet to be crucial to the development of the intelligence and unique manual dexterity of humans.[6]

Anatomically, the gluteus maximus forms the prominence of the buttock and is a remarkably large muscle. It is twice as heavy (844 gm) as the gluteus medius and gluteus minimus together (421 gm),[97] and it often measures more than 2.5 cm (1 in) in thickness. ***Proximally***, it attaches to the posterior border of the ilium and to the posterior iliac crest, the posterolateral surface of the sacrum, the side of the coccyx, the aponeurosis of the erector spinae muscles, the length of the sacrotuberous ligament, and to the fascia covering the gluteus medius muscle (Fig. 7.2). ***Distally***, about three-fourths of the muscle (all of its upper fibers and its superficial lower fibers) attaches to the thick tendinous aponeurotic sheet that crosses the greater trochanter and joins the iliotibial band of the fascia lata. The remaining deep lower fibers of the gluteus maximus are attached to the gluteal tuberosity of the femur between the attachments of the vastus lateralis and adductor magnus muscles;[9,78] the more horizontal course of these posterior deep fibers is clearly depicted elsewhere.[68] The most distal fibers of the gluteus maximus that arise from the coccyx originate embryologically as a separate muscle and fuse with the sacral portion before birth.[81]

The large trochanteric bursa separates the flat tendon of the gluteus maximus muscle from the greater trochanter.[21] An inconstant ischial bursa permits smooth gliding of the muscle over the ischial tuberosity. A third bursa separates the gluteus maximus tendon from that of the vastus lateralis muscle.[9,24]

Apropos of TrP_2, which is located in the lower border of the gluteus maximus close to the ischial tuberosity, it should be noted that the muscle covers the tuberosity when a person stands or walks, but slides upward when he or she is seated. The ischial tuberosity in the upright seated posture is padded by fibrous tissue, skin, and sometimes a bursa,[79] but not by muscle (this is easily confirmed by palpating the tuberosity while seated). However, as one slouches down on the seat and reclines further against the backrest, the hip extends, the muscle slides down, and the weight-bearing region shifts upward around the curve of the ischial tuberosity. At some point, the muscle and pressure meet, compressing TrP_2.

Several external coccygeal muscles with variable degrees of development may lie adjacent to the medial (posterior) fibers of the gluteus maximus. The sacrococcygeus dorsalis muscle,[4,11,16] when present, may span as many as five sacral and one or two coccygeal vertebrae, as illustrated by Toldt.[84] It often attaches proximally to the posterior inferior iliac spine.[16] How frequently it is found depends on how carefully the caudal musculature is dissected. Eisler[16] reports that, in three series of dissections, this muscle was found in one of 36, one of 16, and two of 122 bodies, respectively. In contrast, Lartschneider[48] (cited by Eisler) considered it a normal structure because it was missing in only six of 100 adult cadavers. Lartschneider[48] also found remnants of three "tail-wagging" muscles: the extensor coccygeus medialis in 58% of cases, the extensor coccygeus lateralis in 43%, and the abductor coccygeus dorsalis in 87%. These dorsal coccygeal muscles, although usually vestigial, may attain considerable bulk in some people; their TrPs cause coccygodynia.

Autopsy samples of normal adult gluteus maximus muscles from individuals under age 44 years showed that 68% of fibers were slow-twitch (type 1) and 32% were fast-twitch (type 2) muscle fibers. The muscle had essentially the same composition in two groups of persons older than 44 years: 70% of the fibers were type 1 and 30% were type 2. Although individual variability was great, the percentage of type 1 fibers (which depend largely on oxidative metabolism) always exceeded the number of type 2 (rapidly fatiguing) fibers that utilize chiefly glycolytic energy pathways.[76]

Supplemental References

Other authors illustrate the gluteus maximus muscle as seen from behind,[1,12,26,64,68,70,77] from behind with overlying nerves,[53] obliquely from behind,[85] from the side,[18,69,83] from the side with overlying nerves,[60] from below,[3,9,66] and as seen in sagittal section.[23,52] Other illustrations map its bony attachments,[27] schematically portray its bony attachments and fiber direction,[2,68] and show its attachment to the iliotibial tract distally.[54,61] It is portrayed in cross sections through the prostate,[65] the head of the femur,[67] the distal part of the hip joint,[25] at the neck of the femur,[62] at the apex of the femoral triangle,[10] and in eight equally spaced cross sections.[8] It is seen in coronal section through the femoral heads.[67]

3. INNERVATION

The gluteus maximus muscle is innervated by the inferior gluteal nerve, which arises from the dorsal portions of spinal roots L_5, S_1, and S_2. This nerve usually exits the pelvis through the restricted space of the greater sciatic foramen between the piriformis muscle and the sacrospinous ligament; it is accompanied by the inferior gluteal artery and vein. The nerve then passes between the gluteus medius and gluteus maximus muscles, and innervates the gluteus maximus through its deep surface. In 15% of 112 subjects, the inferior gluteal nerve exited the pelvis *through*, instead of below, the piriformis muscle en route to the gluteus maximus muscle. In every such case, the peroneal branch of the sciatic nerve accompanied the inferior gluteal nerve through the piriformis muscle.[82]

PART 1

4. FUNCTION

When the foot is fixed, the gluteus maximus muscle frequently functions through lengthening contractions to *control* (decelerate or restrain) movement, such as when an individual is stooping, bending, sitting down from a standing position, or descending stairs. During ambulation, this muscle functions shortly after heel-strike to restrain the tendency toward hip flexion. It also helps regain body position over the forward foot and stabilizes the pelvis. In some activities, the gluteus maximus undergoes a shortening contraction to assist extension of the trunk indirectly through its pull on the pelvis.

Actions

When tested with the pelvis fixed and the lower limb free to move, the gluteus maximus muscle is active only when moderate to heavy efforts are exerted in the movements classically ascribed to this muscle.[5,9] It can powerfully assist extension[5,9,19,34,63] and lateral rotation[5,9,19,63] of the thigh at the hip. During balanced standing and easy walking, the gluteus maximus shows minimal activity.[5,20,34,36] It is more active during running and jumping.[9,36,42]

All fibers of the muscle extend and laterally rotate the thigh.[9] Abduction of the thigh is assisted primarily by the upper fibers;[30] the lower fibers help to abduct the thigh against heavy resistance with the thigh flexed.[5]

Functions

An understanding of the specific functions of the gluteus maximus helps the clinician and the patient identify activities and stress situations that may have initiated and then perpetuated TrPs in this muscle.

Activity of the gluteus maximus that reaches only 30% of its maximum contractile force can be supported by aerobic metabolism. This level of activity does not depend on anaerobic metabolism, which depletes the muscle's energy reserves and is only 1/13th as efficient as aerobic metabolism.[50]

During quiet ambulation, limited electromyographic (EMG) activity appears chiefly in the upper and lower parts of the gluteus maximus in a biphasic pattern with one small peak near the end of swing phase and the other peak at heel strike. Motor unit activity in the middle part of the muscle is likely to be triphasic with an additional peak from terminal stance to immediately after toe-off.[5] These findings are highly variable among individuals.[50] The lower portion of the gluteus maximus appears to be the part that functions primarily to stabilize the flexed hip during the stance phase in ambulation. Greenlaw[34] reported detailed analysis of gluteus maximus activity during ambulation and other movements. During locomotion, electrical activity of the gluteus maximus consistently increases in intensity and duration with increased rate and load.

One study showed electrical activity to be maximum during stair ascension and to disappear during stair descension.[50] Gluteus maximus activity showed no remarkable difference when subjects wore high heels as compared with low heels.[41]

The gluteus maximus is not usually used in relaxed sitting, squatting, and quiet standing,[28] including swaying forward at the ankle while standing.[40] This muscle braces the fully extended knee by acting through the iliotibial tract.[9] Less than 10% of its maximum activity is observed when the subject is standing and bending forward at the hips, and while kneeling.[28,58]

The gluteus maximus shows considerably more activity when the subject lifts a load from the floor while using the safer straight-back, flexed-knee posture than it does when employing a forward-flexed, straight-knee lift (Fig. 22.16).[56]

This largest of the gluteal muscles was reported to be inactive during exercise on a stationary bicycle.[28] Another study[17] reported minimal electromyographic evidence of activity during bicycling; while this activity increased with increased workload and pedalling rate, it showed no remarkable difference with change in saddle height or with use of a posterior foot position on the pedal.[17]

The gluteus maximus becomes active, but is less active than the hamstrings, during 13 vigorous sport skills[7] and when jumping.[42] The observation that, electromyographically, the hamstrings are more active than the gluteus maximus in producing hip extension during ambulation and running may relate to the fact that the hamstrings are two-joint muscles that have nearly twice the skeletal leverage available at the hip than at the knee in the walking position.[50]

With the lower limb fixed and the pelvis free to move, as when rising from the seated position,[36] climbing stairs, or walking up a grade,[36] the gluteus maximus assists extension of the trunk through traction on the pelvis.[9] Activity in this muscle increases as the standing individual leans forward and flexes at the hip to about 45°.[63] Sudden forward-flexion movements at the hip are checked by the gluteus maximus.[57] When the thigh is fixed, this muscle forcefully tilts the pelvis posteriorly (rocks the pubis anteriorly), as during sexual intercourse.

During vigorous back extension in the prone position, the gluteus maximus becomes moderately active as an assistant to other muscles.[59]

Absence of the gluteus maximus due to disease[15] or to surgery[36] causes no limping during ordinary ambulation and little impairment of several ordinary activities. Compared with the intact side, only slight reduction in isometric and isokinetic hip extension strength (6% and 19%) occurred unless the hamstrings had also been removed.[51] This remarkable retention of strength probably reflects compensatory hypertrophy of the hamstring muscles.

5. FUNCTIONAL (MYOTATIC) UNIT

The longissimus and iliocostalis are long paraspinal muscles that work closely with the hamstrings and the gluteus maximus; functioning together as a unit, they extend the trunk. Together, they help restore upright posture from forward flexion in the standing position and help execute forced extension of the back and hip. The hamstrings (except the short head of the biceps femoris) and the posterior portions of the gluteus medius and minimus also extend the thigh at the hip. The piriformis muscle, which is parallel to the lower gluteus maximus fibers and has adjacent attachments, is a partner of the gluteus maximus in lateral rotation of the thigh.

Antagonists to the extensor function of the gluteus maximus at the hip are the hip flexors, chiefly the iliopsoas and rectus femoris muscles. The hip adductors are the chief antagonists to the lateral rotation function of the gluteus maximus and to the abduction function of its uppermost fibers. The tensor fasciae latae opposes the lateral rotation and extension effects of gluteus maximus contraction, although the two muscles share abductor function and share a common attachment to the fascia lata.

6. SYMPTOMS

Pain referred from most gluteus maximus TrPs is aggravated by walking uphill, especially in the forward-bent posture. Pain from TrPs in this muscle is intensified by vigorous contraction in the shortened position, as when swimming the crawl stroke. This cramp pain is more likely to occur in cold water. In deep water, the development of cramps together with this pain can be paralyzing and life-threatening.

Patients with an active TrP_2 near the ischial tuberosity are often uncomfortable and restless when seated. Patients with coccygodynia that is referred from TrP_3 may be observed to squirm during prolonged sitting in an attempt to avoid the local tenderness and referred pain produced by pressure on the TrPs. The connective tissue and skin over the ischial tuberosity become uncomfortably ischemic after prolonged upright sitting. As the individual slides down and forward on the seat to decrease this pressure, weight is increased on TrP_2 as described previously in Section 1. Since neither seated position gives relief, no chair seems comfortable.

Differential Diagnosis

Gluteus maximus TrPs are distinguished from TrPs in the underlying gluteus medius and gluteus minimus muscles by their topographical location in the buttock, by the distribution of the referred pain, by the depth of TrP tenderness and direction of palpable bands, and by what movement is restricted.

The topographic relationships of the three gluteal muscles are drawn in Figure 8.5. The most inferior gluteus maximus fibers are distal to the other gluteal muscles, and the most superior fibers are more horizontal than are the underlying gluteus medius fibers. The gluteus maximus rarely refers pain to the thigh, and then only for a few inches. The gluteus medius may refer pain to midthigh, and the gluteus minimus commonly refers pain that extends below the knee.

Except for the most anterior gluteus medius fibers (Fig. 7.2), TrP tenderness and taut bands palpated immediately beneath the skin in gluteal musculature belong to the gluteus maximus muscle. Other gluteal fibers must be palpated deep to at least one other layer of muscle.

Tension of the gluteus maximus restricts flexion at the hip; tension of the other two gluteal muscles restricts adduction.

As long as active gluteus maximus TrPs remain, the tenderness they refer may, on examination, obscure detection of TrP involvement in other gluteal muscles.

Swezey[80] described pseudoradiculopathy in subacute trochanteric bursitis of the subgluteus maximus bursa. The subgluteus maximus bursa lies deep to the converging fibers of the tensor fasciae latae and the gluteus maximus muscles where their fibers join to form the iliotibial tract. This bursa separates these converging fibers from the greater trochanter and from the origin of the vastus lateralis muscle. Schapira and associates[71] describe trochanteric bursitis as a common clinical problem. Inflammation of the trochanteric bursa produces intense local pain with radiation to the lateral thigh area; pain sometimes extends cephalad to the buttock and distally below the knee.[80] It is aggravated by ambulatory activities and relieved by rest.[71] Pain is also caused by pressure applied over the bursa at the junction of the lower edge of the greater trochanter and the shaft of the femur. In addition, pain is frequently elicited by medial rotation and/or abduction at the hip; but there is no loss of hip mobility. Infiltration of the sensitive area with 3 mL of 1% lidocaine[80] or 3 mL of lidocaine-methylprednisolone solution[71] caused prompt and marked reduction of the clinical manifestations of bursitis.[80]

It is possible that some persons with trochanteric tenderness that is relieved by injection of a local anesthetic have TrPs in the gluteus maximus instead of, or in addition to, bursitis. Subacute trochanteric bursitis has been commonly associated with low back pain, hip disease, and/or leg length discrepancies, which are conditions that are often associated with myofascial TrPs of the gluteal musculature. However, the location of the bursa is more lateral than the area where gluteus maximus TrPs are usually found. If present, TrPs in this superficial muscle should be detectable by their taut bands and local twitch responses.

The gluteus maximus is one of the muscles attached to the sacrum that commonly develops TrPs after sacroiliac joint displacement.[95] Recently Gitelman[31] reinforced this observation by noting that the gluteus maximus often shows hypertonicity during sacroiliac fixation. This asymmetrical tension with strong leverage on the sacrum would tend to maintain the sacral displacement until the gluteal tension was released.

The pain referred by lumbar zygapophysial (facet) joints is described and illustrated in Chapter 3 on pages 25–26.

Another disorder, fibrosis of the superficial lumbosacral fascia, was described by Dittrich.[14] The lumbar fascia serves as the aponeurotic anchor for the latissimus dorsi and gluteus maximus muscles. The cause of the fibrosis was believed to be tearing of the fascia due to excessive muscular tension. The treatment recommended was resection of the connective tissue at the exact site of tenderness; effectiveness of surgery was thought to be due to denervation of the fascial structures from which the pain arose. If this condition does in fact occur, it might be caused by the sustained tension placed on the tendinous attachments of taut muscle fibers associated with myofascial TrPs. If so, inactivation of the TrPs might be a simpler and equally effective treatment.

7. ACTIVATION AND PERPETUATION OF TRIGGER POINTS

Activation

Myofascial TrPs in the gluteus maximus muscle are often activated by acute stress overload during a fall or a near-fall. Activation of TrPs is especially likely to occur if the muscle sustains a vigorous lengthening contraction in an effort to prevent the fall. The impact of a direct blow on one buttock, as in a backward fall onto a low wooden fence, has been responsible for initiating gluteus maximus TrPs.

Prolonged uphill walking while leaning forward can overload the gluteus maximus.

Sleeping on one side with the thigh of the upper limb sharply flexed over the lower limb can overstretch the uppermost gluteus maximus muscle and activate its TrPs. These active TrPs can induce referred pain that seriously disturbs sleep. On the other hand, sleeping on the back with the legs straight places the muscle in the shortened position, which, if prolonged, also activates latent TrPs. Corrective actions are discussed at the end of this chapter.

Another common, but avoidable, cause of activation of latent gluteal TrPs is the injection of an irritant medication intramuscularly into the gluteal area.[86] As the most superficial gluteal muscle, the gluteus maximus is the most likely to be injected. Persons giving such injections should palpate the muscles for TrPs and avoid any tender spots. Diluting the material to be injected with an equal quantity of 2% procaine solution may prevent activation of a latent TrP in the event that the medication is accidentally injected into the region of the TrP.

Perpetuation

Physical activities that can perpetuate gluteus maximus TrPs include swimming with the crawl stroke, which requires hyperextension of the lumbar spine in addition to hip extension. This forceful contraction of the gluteus maximus and the lower paraspinal extensors in a strongly shortened position can activate and perpetuate their TrPs. A similar cause of gluteus maximus overload may be conditioning exercises (leg lifts) that hyperextend the low back and hip, either in the prone or standing position. Repetitious tasks, such as frequently leaning over and lifting a baby out of the playpen, have been known to perpetuate gluteus maximus TrPs.

Sitting too long in one position perpetuates TrPs in this muscle, especially when the individual is partially reclining with the knees straight, which compresses gluteus maximus TrPs and restricts circulation of blood in the muscle.

The head-forward position with thoracic kyphosis, in standing postures that increase hip flexion, is likely to overload the gluteus maximus and perpetuate TrPs in it.

A short first metatarsal bone (Morton foot structure or Dudley J. Morton foot configuration)[74] may perpetuate TrPs in the more horizontal fibers of the gluteus maximus. This anatomical variant of foot structure frequently induces medial rotation of the hip during the stance phase in walking, and this movement is counteracted to some extent by the horizontal fibers of the gluteus maximus. A corrective pad placed in the shoe under the head of the short first metatarsal bone (described in Chapter 20) frequently corrects medial rotation and reduces overload irritation of TrPs in the lower posterior fibers of the gluteus maximus.

Sitting on a wallet placed in a long hip pocket that extends under the buttock can perpetuate and aggravate TrPs in the gluteal muscles by concentrating pressure on them. The resultant low back and buttock pain is likely to be erroneously attributed to nerve pressure and has been called "back pocket sciatica."[33] However, pain referred from TrPs in the gluteus maximus muscle alone would not have a full sciatic nerve distribution.

Although a small hemipelvis does not directly perpetuate gluteus maximus TrPs, the correction of this body asymmetry to lighten the load on other muscles may aggravate and intensify the activity of gluteus maximus TrPs. The seated patient may not tolerate the firmness of an ischial ("butt") lift placed on a chair seat under the muscle with TrPs. Patients with gluteus maximus TrPs usually want pressure distributed around the ischial

PART 1

tuberosity, not concentrated on it, which happens when a TrP or an area of referred tenderness is compressed by the ischial lift.

8. PATIENT EXAMINATION

The examiner may obtain relevant information by observing the patient's seated and ambulatory posture. Patients with active TrPs in the gluteus maximus muscle are likely to walk with an antalgic gait marked by a brief single-limb support phase on the painful side with a correspondingly brief swing phase of the contralateral limb. When seated, these patients shift position frequently to relieve pressure on their gluteus maximus TrPs.

Tightness of the gluteus maximus muscle is tested in the supine patient by bringing the knee passively toward the opposite axilla and medially rotating the thigh at the hip. Normally, the thigh should rest firmly against the chest at full range of motion. Gluteus maximus TrPs can reduce this range by as much as 35°.

Palpation of the muscular attachments and bony prominences in the areas of referred pain frequently reveals tenderness, as pointed out by Kelly.[43] The tenderness along the musculotendinous junction, at the origin of the gluteus maximus muscle below the iliac crest, may well be caused by the sustained tension produced by the taut bands associated with TrPs and may be referred tenderness from TrPs.

Although the common standing test of trying to touch the fingers to the toes while bending forward with knees straight is usually interpreted as a test of hamstring tightness, tightness of the gluteus maximus due to TrPs can also be responsible for limitation of this movement. A test that distinguishes between these muscles is leaning forward with knees bent while sitting in a chair; this movement is restricted by gluteus maximus shortening, but not by hamstring muscle tension.

The strength of the gluteus maximus can be tested selectively by placing the patient prone with the knee bent to minimize hamstring action and having the patient lift the knee up from the examining table while a resisting force is applied downward on the back of the thigh at the knee.[39,46] When active TrPs are present in the gluteus maximus muscle this test characteristically reveals inconsistent (ratchety) weakness (caused by inhibition). If the patient with active TrPs in this muscle exerts sufficient effort against fixed resistance in the shortened position, additional pain is likely to appear in the muscle and in the reference zone.

9. TRIGGER POINT EXAMINATION (Figs. 7.3 and 7.4)

Taut bands in this superficial gluteal muscle are relatively easy to palpate, and local twitch responses are vigorous and often visible.

The patient lies on the side with the muscle to be examined uppermost and with that thigh flexed sufficiently to take up the slack. In some patients, a greater degree of flexion (within the comfort zone) may increase the hypersensitivity of the TrPs to palpation. Both TrP_1 and TrP_2 of the gluteus maximus muscle are best examined by flat palpation. The finger is rubbed transversely across the fibers, which lie nearly parallel to the *dashed line* in Figure 7.3. The padding placed under the hip in Figure 7.3 may be needed to relieve weight-bearing pressure on the bony prominences of the pelvis and femur, especially when the patient lies on a hard examining table. One locates TrP_1 (cephalad **X** in Fig. 7.3) lateral to the sacral attachment of the gluteus maximus. Palpation of TrP_2 is illustrated in Figure 7.3; this TrP usually is found slightly cephalad to the ischial tuberosity.

Examination for TrP_3, in the lower border of the muscle, may be done by pincer palpation (Fig. 7.4) or by flat palpation against the ischium. One of this group of TrPs is located in the most medial fibers of the gluteus maximus muscle and is adjacent to and closely associated with the vestigial coccygeal muscles described in Section 2. These gluteal fibers and the coccygeal muscle fibers both attach to the coccyx and their TrPs refer pain to the coccyx. Examination sometimes distinguishes between these muscles since the gluteus maximus fibers course distally and laterally toward the fascia lata and the posterior margin of the muscle often can be grasped between the fingers.

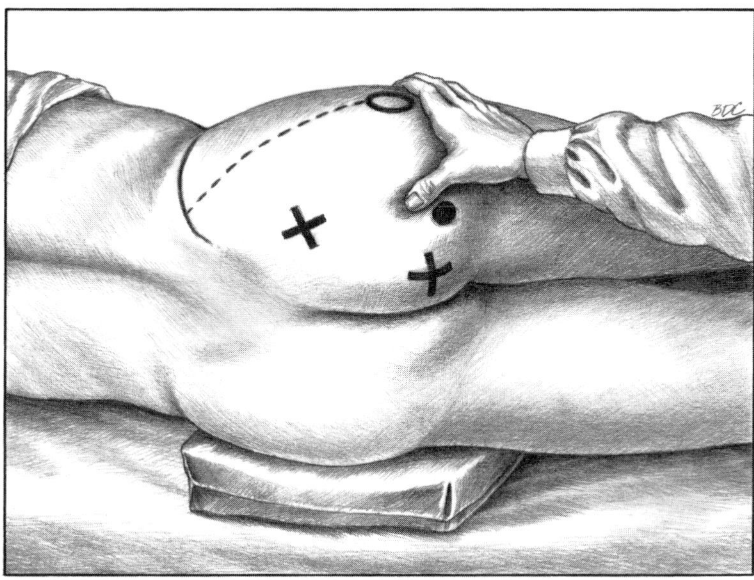

Figure 7.3. Flat palpation of a trigger point (TrP_2) in the right gluteus maximus muscle. The *open circle* marks the greater trochanter. The *solid circle* covers the ischial tuberosity. The *solid line* identifies the crest of the ilium, and the *dashed line* locates the upper border of the gluteus maximus muscle. The **X**s mark the two trigger-point areas not being palpated; TrP_1 is most cephalad, and TrP_3, most distal.

10. ENTRAPMENTS

No nerve entrapments due to myofascial TrPs in the gluteus maximus muscle have been identified. However, the middle cluneal nerves, which supply the skin over the posterior portion of the gluteus maximus muscle, penetrate that muscle near its attachments along the crest of the ilium.[22] The middle cluneal nerves, therefore, could suffer entrapment by the taut bands of gluteus maximus TrPs. The upper cluneal nerves avoid penetrating the muscle (and entrapment) by descending over the crest of the ilium; the lower cluneal nerves supply skin over the gluteus maximus muscle by swinging around its lower border.[13]

11. ASSOCIATED TRIGGER POINTS

The posterior section of the gluteus medius is the muscle most likely to develop TrPs in association with gluteus maximus TrPs. The posterior part of the gluteus minimus and the hamstring muscles on the same side are the next most likely to become involved. Occasionally, the lower ends of the long paraspinal muscles may develop secondary TrPs.

Recognition of associated TrPs in the gluteus medius and gluteus minimus muscles is important because tension caused by these TrPs is not likely to be released effectively by the stretch position used for the gluteus maximus muscle. Myofascial TrPs in the lower lumbar paraspinal muscles and in the hamstrings distort pelvic mechanics and tend to overload the gluteus maximus, thus interfering with restoration of its normal function and range of motion.

The antagonistic iliopsoas and rectus femoris muscles may also develop TrPs that require treatment to achieve release of gluteus maximus TrP tightness and to attain full upright posture.

12. INTERMITTENT COLD WITH STRETCH
(Fig. 7.5)

Details concerning use of intermittent cold with stretch for restoring full active range of motion are found in Volume 1[88] for the stretch-and-spray technique and in Chapter 2 on page 9 of this volume for the application of ice instead of vapocoolant spray.

A primary goal in the management of myofascial pain syndromes is teaching

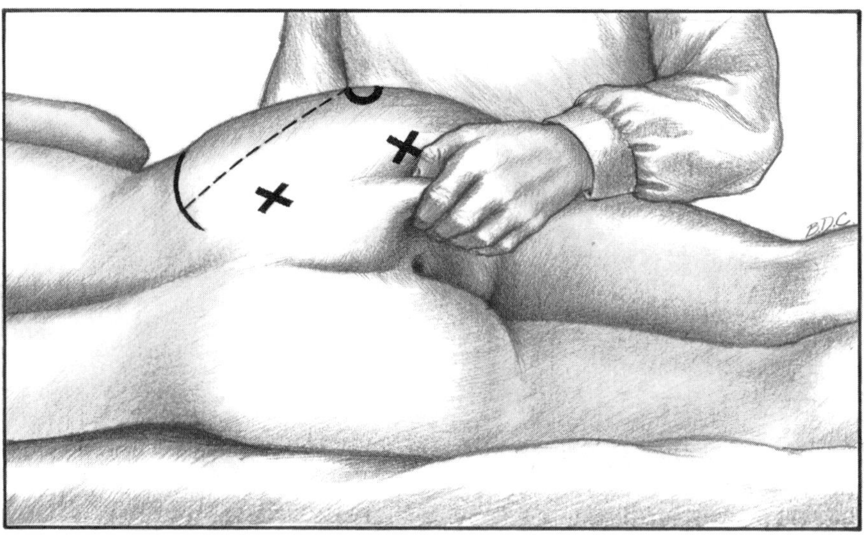

Figure 7.4. Examination by pincer palpation for trigger points in the most medial fibers of the right gluteus maximus muscle (TrP_3 region). The TrP_3 is being compressed between the thumb and fingers and characteristically refers pain to the coccyx. The ***X*s** mark the location of the more cephalad TrP_1 and the more lateral TrP_2 in the gluteus maximus muscle. The *solid line* locates the crest of the ilium; the *dashed line*, the upper margin of the gluteus maximus muscle; and the *open circle*, the greater trochanter.

the patient that the pain and disability are of *muscular* origin. The patient is asked to note and compare the range of motion before and after treatment. When release of a tight gluteus maximus is combined with release of the hamstrings (Chapter 16), the remarkable increase in range of hip flexion often permits the patient, when sitting with knees straight, to reach the toes, or to reach much closer to the toes than before. The patient can readily feel the release of muscular tension and relate it to the improvement in comfort and muscle function.

For treatment by intermittent cold with stretch, the relaxed patient lies on the side opposite to the involved gluteus maximus muscle. If the patient lies supine, a significant part of the spray pattern over the muscle and zone of referred pain (Fig. 7.5) cannot be covered by the vapocoolant. To start, the hip is flexed to the limit of comfort with the knee on the treatment table. This position also stretches tight piriformis and posterior gluteus medius or minimus fibers, but incompletely. If these muscles are involved, the intermittent cold also should cover the areas that correspond with their referred pain patterns.

The jet stream of spray or the ice is applied in slow parallel sweeps downward from the crest of the ilium and midline of the sacrum to midthigh (Fig. 7.5*A*). As the muscle tension releases, the operator gently increases flexion at the hip to take up the slack, but is careful not to cause pain and involuntary muscle contraction. The thigh should ordinarily rest firmly against the chest when full stretch of the gluteus maximus has been achieved unless the lower lumbar paraspinal muscles are also involved.

Having achieved full release of the gluteus maximus, the clinician applies moist heat over the buttock and the patient performs several cycles of active range of motion (full flexion and full extension of the hip).

Alternative Methods

Correction of ilial rotations and ilial flares[55] may be required before the hip can be taken into full flexion to release the gluteus maximus TrPs.

By having the patient grasp the thigh behind the knee and take up the slack (Fig. 7.7), he or she gains experience in passive self-stretch and can often judge better than the operator how much force to apply without causing pain. It is wise

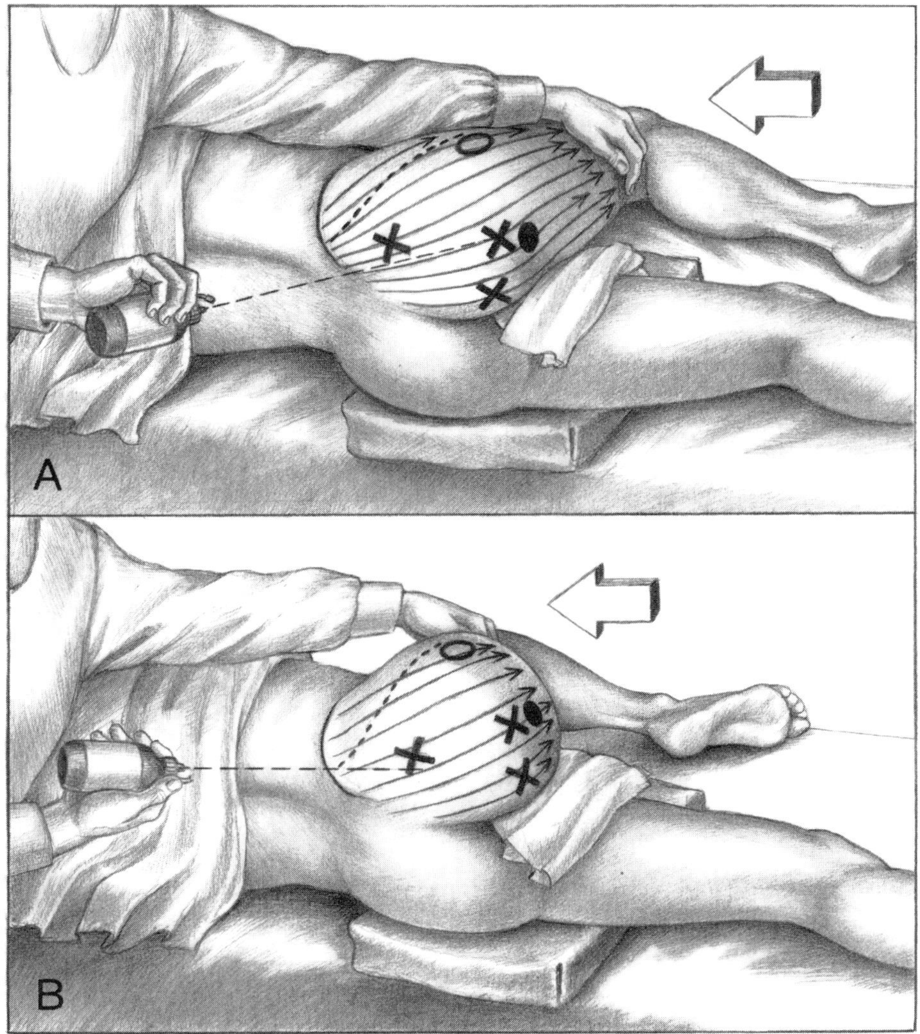

Figure 7.5. Stretch position and the spray or ice-application pattern (*thin black lines and small arrows*) for three trigger points—TrP_1, TrP_2, TrP_3—in the right gluteus maximus muscle. The ***X**s* are positioned over the three major TrP areas. The *dashed line* marks the upper border of the muscle. The *open circle* locates the greater trochanter. The *solid line* marks the crest of the ilium, and the *solid circle*, the ischial tuberosity. On a hard examining table, a pad to soften the surface is placed under the opposite greater trochanter. The *thick white arrows* show the direction of pull by the operator. *A*, initial stretch position. *B*, more advanced stretch position.

to concentrate on releasing TrP_1 and TrP_2 first; they are the ones most likely to create confusion with the myofascial pain picture caused by TrPs in other gluteal muscles.

An alternative stretch position is to have the patient seated as for a long paraspinal stretch with feet on the floor, leaning forward with the arms hanging between the knees (Volume 1[93]). This position allows for release of tension in the lower paraspinal and the gluteus maximus muscles by directing the ice or spray downward, starting at the lower thoracic region, and then covering the length of the buttock as the patient leans far forward. Relaxation can be enhanced by having the patient first inhale slowly while looking upward to encourage *very* gentle contraction and then exhale slowly during the relaxation phase as the ice or vapocoolant spray is applied.

Another method of treatment is postisometric relaxation of the gluteus maximus, as described and illustrated by Lewit.[49] The patient lies prone; isometric contraction is synchronized with inhalation and the relaxation phase is synchronized with exhalation. The clinician palpates the muscles bilaterally to ensure symmetrical and uniform contraction. Lewit notes that for this muscle with this technique, no stretch of the muscle is required; he notes also that this technique relieves tension in tender pelvic floor muscles. It is not clear whether the tension being released is due to myofascial TrPs or is the result of articular dysfunction.

13. INJECTION AND STRETCH
(Fig. 7.6)

Details of the injection-and-stretch technique are presented on pages 74–86 in Chapter 3 of Volume 1.[87]

After gluteus maximus TrPs have been identified, their injection is relatively easy except in those patients with an extremely thick padding of subcutaneous fat. For thin individuals, a 21- or 22-gauge, 37-mm (1½-in) needle is sufficient, but for some patients, a 21-gauge, 50-mm (2-in) or longer needle may be necessary to penetrate the subcutaneous fat and the full thickness of the gluteus maximus muscle.

Gluteus maximus TrP_1 (Fig. 7.6*A*) and TrP_2 (Fig. 7.6*B*) are each identified by flat palpation and then are pinned down between the fingers of one hand so that the TrP can be impaled by the injection needle on the syringe held in the other hand. One expects to observe a local twitch response of the muscle and/or a jump response of the patient when the TrP is penetrated by the needle. Frequently, multiple TrPs in an area require fanning of the needle with serial probing motions (Volume 1[89]). Deep probing for TrP_2 that extends too far laterally can reach the sciatic nerve and should be avoided. At the level of the gluteal fold, this large nerve usually lies near the midpoint between the nearest palpable borders of the ischial tuberosity and the greater trochanter.

TrP_3 is localized for injection by either pincer palpation (Fig. 7.6*C*) or flat palpation. When pincer palpation is used, the TrP is grasped firmly and the needle inserted into the tender spot where the clinician feels the firm band; the resulting twitch response can be felt between the fingers.

For all gluteus maximus TrPs, injection is followed by passive stretch usually combined with ice or vapocoolant spray application, and then by unhurried active range of motion of the muscle through both the fully lengthened (thigh to chest) and the fully shortened (thigh extended) positions, at least two or three times. Quick jerky movements should be avoided. Finally, with the patient recumbent in a relaxed, comfortable, warm situation, a moist heating pad or hot pack is applied to the buttock for 5 or 10 minutes to reduce postinjection soreness.

The patient should be warned of the likelihood of postinjection soreness for a few days, following which, full benefit of the TrP injection should be realized.

Fisk[29] reported that 10% of his patients with low back pain demonstrated at least a 10° restriction of straight leg raising on the painful side as measured by his "Passive Hamstring Stretch Test." Palpation of the gluteal musculature on the restricted side revealed trigger areas sufficiently tender to cause the patient to respond with a "jump sign." Application of therapeutic pressure on these TrPs and their injection with a local anesthetic improved the restricted hip flexion of his patients.

14. CORRECTIVE ACTIONS
(Figs. 7.7 and 7.8)

When patients present with chronic myofascial pain syndromes characterized by proliferation of TrPs over a period of time and by poor or transient response to specific local therapy, perpetuating factors should be thoroughly explored. Systemic perpetuating factors, as described in Volume 1,[92] may activate TrPs in any muscle, including the gluteus maximus. Mechanical perpetuating factors, in addition to those discussed below, are considered in Volume 1.[91]

Corrective Posture and Activities

A lower limb-length discrepancy of 5 mm (¼ in) or more that causes a functional scoliosis in a patient with active gluteus

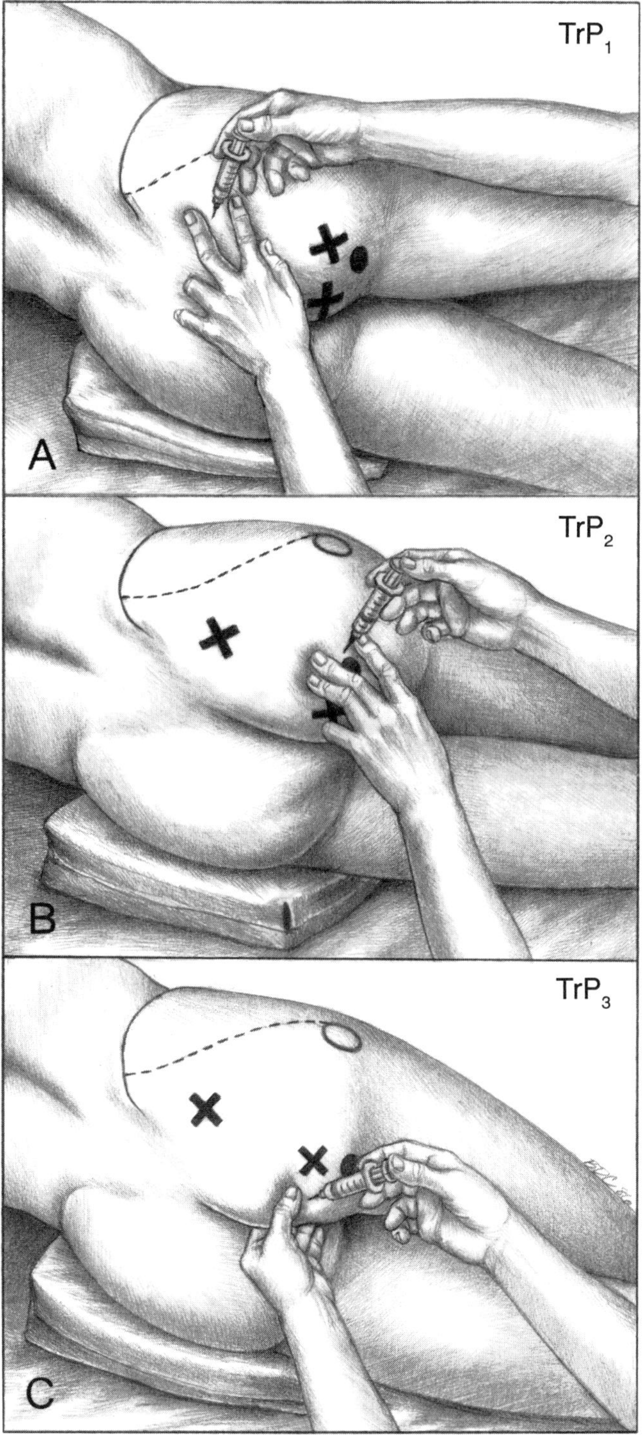

Figure 7.6. Injection of TrPs (**X**s) in the right gluteus maximus muscle. The *open circle* marks the greater trochanter. The *solid circle* covers the ischial tuberosity. The *solid line* identifies the crest of the ilium, and the *dashed line* locates the upper border of the gluteus maximus muscle. *A*, injection of TrP_1. *B*, injection of TrP_2 directly against the side of the ischial tuberosity. *C*, injection of TrP_3 using pincer palpation.

maximus TrPs should be identified and corrected, as described in Chapter 4, pages 77–78. When sacroiliac joint displacement and active TrPs of the gluteus maximus muscle are present together, both must usually be treated for lasting relief.

Patients with active gluteus maximus TrPs should be taught to limit continuous sitting to 15 or 20 minutes and then to get

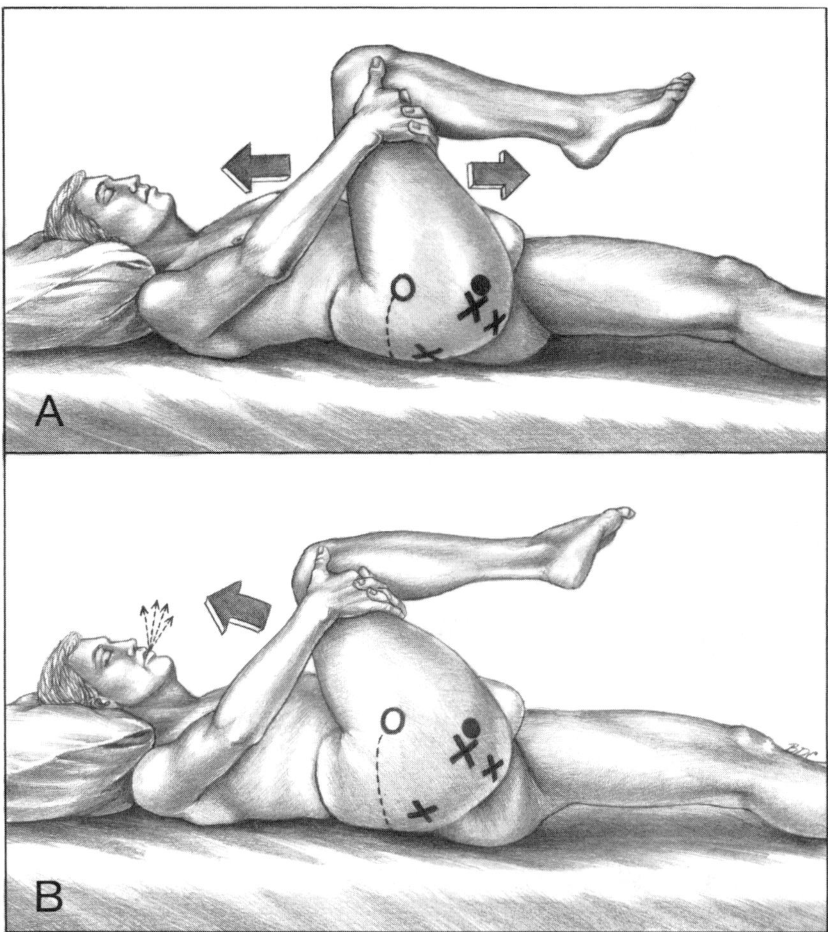

Figure 7.7. Supine passive self-stretch of the right gluteus maximus muscle (upper border outlined by *dashed line*) combined with the Lewit technique. Trigger points in this muscle are marked by ***X*s**. The *open circle* identifies the greater trochanter; the *solid circle* overlies the ischial tuberosity; and the *solid line* outlines the crest of the ilium. The *arrows* show the direction of pull or push by the patient. The Lewit technique has two phases. *A*, the individual first pulls the knee cephalad in order to flex the hip by grasping the distal thigh (not the leg). This hold avoids excessive flexion pressure on the knee joint. To complete the first phase of the Lewit technique, the subject uses the hands to resist a gentle voluntary effort by the lower limb muscles to extend the thigh at the hip. *B*, to help achieve complete muscular relaxation during the second phase, a full breath is metered out slowly (*small arrows*) through pursed lips (avoiding any exhalation effort) as the patient relaxes the hip extensors and passively moves the thigh gently into further flexion to take up the slack. This contract-relax-stretch sequence can be repeated.

up and walk around before sitting again. An interval timer placed across the room can remind the patient to get up, walk across the room, turn off the timer, reset it, and return to the chair with minimal distraction.

A soft cushion with a hole in the center (doughnut cushion) can be used to reduce sitting pressure on gluteal TrPs on one side by centering the hole under TrP_2 or TrP_3 of the affected muscle. The patient should not center the hole under the coccyx and sacrum just because that is where he or she feels the referred pain and tenderness.

When the patient sleeps on the back, a roll or small pillow under the knees prevents full shortening of the gluteus maximus muscle. When side lying, a pillow should be placed between the knees to prevent the uppermost thigh from assuming an excessively flexed and adducted position; such incorrect positioning can place the affected gluteus maximus on painful,

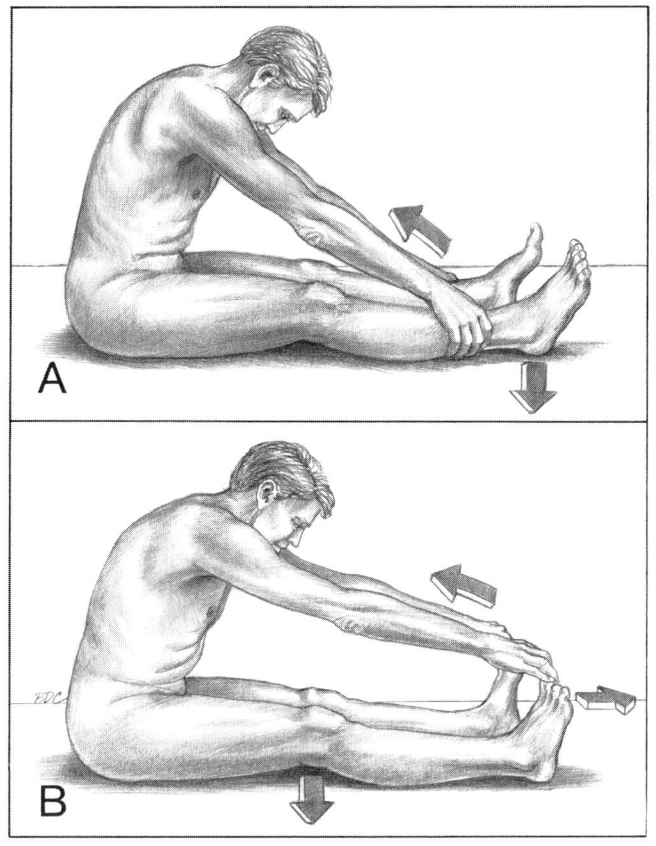

Figure 7.8. Technique for passive self-stretch of the gluteus maximus and hamstring muscles and, if desired, the gastrocnemius muscles in the seated position. Effectiveness of the stretch is enhanced by use of postisometric relaxation as follows: *A*, while reaching forward as far as possible with only slight discomfort, the patient firmly grasps the legs or ankles. He or she simultaneously pushes the heels down against the floor and gently pulls upward against the legs with the hands (*arrows*). A few seconds of this isometric gluteus maximus contraction is followed by relaxation that is enhanced by a full slow exhalation. During this prolonged period of enhanced relaxation, the individual reaches forward to pick up any slack that has developed, providing further lengthening of the muscles. With sufficient repetitions, the hands should reach the toes. *B*, final position that includes the gastrocnemius passive stretch by pulling up on the feet. Then, the isometric contraction phase must include simultaneous voluntary efforts to push down with the knees and to gently plantar flex the feet at the ankles while using the hands to resist movement of the feet.

sleep-disturbing stretch. For an illustration of proper positioning, see Figure 10.10.

Hiking up steep hills, which involves leaning forward at the hips, can overload the muscle to exhaustion and should be limited. Leaning forward to paint a wall or canvas while reaching with the paint brush can create a similar strain and should be limited or avoided. The torso should be held erect and the knees bent, if necessary.

Back-pocket sciatica[33] is avoided by moving the wallet from the back pocket to a front pocket or a shoulder bag.

The head-forward posture should be corrected to establish an erect posture that unloads the extensor muscles. See Chapter 28 for techniques to correct the head-forward posture.

Corrective Exercises

Patients with gluteus maximus TrPs are routinely taught the gluteus maximus passive self-stretch procedure, illustrated in Figure 7.7. The effectiveness of this self-stretch is improved by using postisometric relaxation,[49] which is based on the hold-relax principle[96] and is described in detail in Chapter 2. The patient should be encouraged to gain at least some improvement in range of motion at each treatment session until the thigh can be brought to the chest (with the knee near the opposite axilla) without pain.

An alternative, seated technique for passive self-stretch of the gluteus maximus, which includes stretch of the hamstring muscles, is illustrated and described in Figure 7.8. This procedure can be modified to include gastrocnemius muscle self-stretch and can be combined to advantage with the Lewit technique for enhancing relaxation of the affected muscles.

During stretching of the gluteus maximus, the antagonistic rectus abdominis and iliopsoas muscles become unusually shortened. If these muscles harbor TrPs, they may suddenly cramp. This painful reactive cramping is relieved by stretching the antagonist iliopsoas and rectus abdominis muscles in turn, as illustrated in Figure 5.5, and in Volume 1.[94]

Many patients find self-treatment by ischemic compression with a tennis ball useful for this muscle. The technique is similar to that illustrated in Figure 8.9 for the gluteus medius muscle. When a TrP has been identified, the patient lies on a tennis ball to apply ischemic compression to the TrP; the tennis ball is placed on a hard surface like the floor or on a firm large book on the mattress. The principles of ischemic compression are described in Volume 1.[90]

Patients may have been told always to bend at the knees, not at the waist,[72] in order to protect the back. That is good advice to reduce pressure on the intervertebral discs and to avoid overload of the paraspinal, quadratus lumborum, and hamstring muscles. However, lifting by bending at the knees greatly increases the load on the gluteus maximus. Therefore, if TrPs in the gluteus maximus are causing the pain and dysfunction, one should rise from stooping or rise from a chair by placing one hand on the thigh, as illustrated in Figure 22.16, to reduce the load on the gluteus maximus.

Although swimming is one of the best forms of exercise, the crawl stroke and sometimes the breast stroke are likely to aggravate TrPs in the gluteus maximus muscle. The backstroke or sidestroke should replace the other strokes.

References

1. Anderson JE: *Grant's Atlas of Anatomy*, Ed. 8. Williams & Wilkins, Baltimore, 1983 (Fig. 4–31).
2. *Ibid*. (Fig. 4–32B).
3. *Ibid*. (Fig. 3–57).
4. Bardeen CR: The musculature, Sect. 5. In: *Morris's Human Anatomy*, edited by C. M. Jackson, Ed. 6. Blakiston's Son & Co., Philadelphia, 1921.
5. Basmajian JV, Deluca CJ: *Muscles Alive*, Ed. 5. Williams & Wilkins, Baltimore, 1985 (pp. 315–316, 380–381).
6. Bollet AJ: The relationship of the gluteus maximus to intelligence. *Medical Times 112*:109–112, 1984.
7. Broer MR, Houtz SJ: *Patterns of Muscular Activity in Selected Sports Skills*. Charles C Thomas, Springfield, 1967.
8. Carter BL, Morehead J, Wolpert SM, *et al*.: *Cross-Sectional Anatomy*. Appleton-Century-Crofts, New York, 1977 (Sects. 37–43, 64).
9. Clemente CD: *Gray's Anatomy of the Human Body*, American Ed. 30. Lea & Febiger, Philadelphia, 1985 (pp. 566–567).
10. *Ibid*. (p. 108, Fig. 3–42).
11. *Ibid*. (p. 500).
12. *Ibid*. (p. 566, Fig. 6–72).
13. *Ibid*. (p. 1236).
14. Dittrich RJ: Soft tissue lesions as cause of low back pain. *Am J Surg 91*:80–85, 1956.
15. Duchenne GB: *Physiology of Motion*, translated by E.B. Kaplan. J. B. Lippincott, Philadelphia, 1949.
16. Eisler P: *Die Muskeln des Stammes*. Gustav Fischer, Jena, 1912 (pp. 451–455, Fig. 66).
17. Ericson MO, Nisell R, Arborelius UP, *et al*.: Muscular activity during ergometer cycling. *Scand J Rehab Med 17*:53–61, 1985.
18. Ferner H, Staubesand J: *Sobotta Atlas of Human Anatomy*, Ed. 10, Vol. 2. Urban & Schwarzenberg, Baltimore, 1983 (Figs. 7, 413).
19. *Ibid*. (p. 288).
20. *Ibid*. (Fig. 292).
21. *Ibid*. (Figs. 331 and 419).
22. *Ibid*. (Fig. 402).
23. *Ibid*. (Fig. 404).
24. *Ibid*. (Fig. 406).
25. *Ibid*. (Fig. 410).
26. *Ibid*. (Fig. 412).
27. *Ibid*. (Fig. 420).
28. Fischer FJ, Houtz SJ: Evaluation of the function of the gluteus maximus muscle. *Am J Phys Med 47*:182–191, 1968.
29. Fisk JW: The passive hamstring stretch test: clinical evaluation. *NZ Med J 1*:209–211, 1979.
30. Furlani J, Berzin F, Vitti M: Electromyographic study of the gluteus maximus muscle. *Electromyogr Clin Neurophysiol 14*:379–388, 1974.
31. Gitelman R: A chiropractic approach to biomechanical disorders of the lumbar spine and pelvis, Chapter 14. In *Modern Developments in the Principles and Practice of Chiropractic*, edited by S. Haldeman. Appleton-Century-Crofts, New York, 1980 (pp. 297–330, see p. 307).
32. Good MG: Diagnosis and treatment of sciatic pain. *Lancet 2*:597–598, 1942.
33. Gould N: Back-Pocket Sciatica. *N Engl J Med 290*:633, 1974.
34. Greenlaw RK: *Function of Muscles About the Hip During Normal Level Walking*. Queen's University, Kingston, Ontario, 1973 (thesis).
35. Gutstein M: Diagnosis and treatment of muscular rheumatism. *Br J Phys Med 1*:302–321, 1938.
36. Hollinshead WH: Anatomy for Surgeons, Ed. 3., Vol. 3, *The Back and Limbs*. Harper & Row, New York, 1982.
37. Hunter WS: Contributions of physical anthropology to understanding the aches and pains of aging. In *Advances in Pain Research and Therapy*, edited by J.J. Bonica and D. Albe-Fessard, Vol I, Raven Press, New York, 1976 (pp. 901–911).
38. Inman VT: Human locomotion. *Can Med Assoc J 94*:1047–1054, 1966.
39. Janda V: *Muscle Function Testing*. Butterworths, London, 1983 (p. 166).
40. Joseph J, Williams PL: Electromyography of certain hip muscles. *J Anat 91*:286–294, 1957.
41. Joseph J: The pattern of activity of some muscles in women walking on high heels. *Ann Phys Med 9*:295–299, 1968.
42. Kamon E: Electromyographic kinesiology of jumping. *Arch Phys Med Rehabil 52*:152–157, 1971.

43. Kelly M: Lumbago and abdominal pain. *Med J Austral 1*:311–317, 1942.
44. Kelly M: The nature of fibrositis. II. A study of the causation of the myalgic lesion (rheumatic, traumatic, infective). *Ann Rheum Dis 5*:69–77, 1946.
45. Kelly M: Some rules for the employment of local analgesic in the treatment of somatic pain. *Med J Austral 1*:235–239, 1947.
46. Kendall FP, McCreary EK: *Muscles, Testing and Function*, Ed. 3. Williams & Wilkins, Baltimore, 1983.
47. Lange M: *Die Muskelhärten (Myogelosen)*. J.F. Lehmanns, München, 1931 (pp. 32, 91, 106, 137, 152).
48. Lartschneider J: Die Steissbeinmuskulatur des Menschen und ihre Beziehungen zum M. levator ani und zur Beckenfascie. *Denkschr K Akad d Wiss, Wein 62*, 1895.
49. Lewit K: Postisometric relaxation in combination with other methods of muscular facilitation and inhibition. *Manual Med 2*:101–104, 1986.
50. Lyons K, Perry J, Gronley JK, Barnes L, Antonelli D: Timing and relative intensity of hip extensor and abductor muscle action during level and stair ambulation. *Phys Ther 63*:1597–1605, 1983.
51. Markhede G, Stener B: Function after removal of various hip and thigh muscles for extirpation of tumors. *Acta Orthop Scand 52*:373–395, 1981.
52. McMinn RMH, Hutchings RT: *Color Atlas of Human Anatomy*. Year Book Medical Publishers, Chicago, 1977 (p. 245).
53. *Ibid*. (p. 292).
54. *Ibid*. (p. 295).
55. Mitchell FL, Moran PS, Pruzzo NA: *Evaluation and Treatment Manual of Osteopathic Manipulative Procedures*. Mitchell, Moran & Pruzzo Associates, Manchester, MO, 1979, (pp. 361–382).
56. Németh G: On hip and lumbar biomechanics. A study of joint load and muscular activity. *Scand J Rehabil Med (Supp.1) 10*: 1–35, 1984.
57. Oddsson L, Thorstensson A: Fast voluntary trunk flexion movements in standing: motor patterns. *Acta Physiol Scand 129*:93–106, 1987.
58. Okada M: An electromyographic estimation of the relative muscular load in different human postures. *J Human Ergol 1*:75–93, 1972.
59. Pauly JE: An electromyographic analysis of certain movements and exercises: 1. some deep muscles of the back. *Anat Rec 155*:223–234, 1966.
60. Pernkopf E: *Atlas of Topographical and Applied Human Anatomy*, Vol. 2. W.B. Saunders, Philadelphia, 1964 (Fig. 312).
61. *Ibid*. (Fig. 327).
62. *Ibid*. (Fig. 329).
63. Rasch PJ, Burke RK: *Kinesiology and Applied Anatomy*, Ed. 6. Lea & Febiger, Philadelphia, 1978 (pp. 273–274).
64. Rohen JW, Yokochi C: *Color Atlas of Anatomy*, Ed. 2. Igaku-Shoin, New York, 1988 (p. 204).
65. *Ibid*. (p. 316).
66. *Ibid*. (pp. 322–323).
67. *Ibid*. (p. 328).
68. *Ibid*. (p. 418).
69. *Ibid*. (p. 419).
70. *Ibid*. (pp. 440).
71. Schapira D, Nahir M, Scharf Y: Trochanteric bursitis: a common clinical problem. *Arch Phys Med Rehabil 67*:815–817, 1986
72. Sheon RP: A joint-protection guide for nonarticular rheumatic disorders. *Postgrad Med 77*: 329–338, 1985.
73. Simons, DG: Myofascial pain syndromes, part of Chapter 11. In *Medical Rehabilitation*, edited by J.V. Basmajian and R.L. Kirby. Williams & Wilkins, Baltimore, 1984 (pp. 209–215, 313–320).
74. Simons DG, Travell JG: Myofascial origins of low back pain. Parts 1,2,3. *Postgrad Med 73*:66–108, 1983.
75. Simons DG, Travell JG: Myofascial pain syndromes, Chapter 25. In *Textbook of Pain*, edited by P.D. Wall and R. Melzack, Ed 2. Churchill Livingstone, London, 1989 (pp. 368–385).
76. Sirca A, Susec-Michieli M: Selective type II fibre muscular atrophy in patients with osteoarthritis of the hip. *J Neurol Sci 44*:149–159, 1980.
77. Spalteholz W: *Handatlas der Anatomie des Menschen*, Ed. 11, Vol. 2. S. Hirzel, Leipzig, 1922 (p. 357).
78. Stern JT: Anatomical and functional specializations of the human gluteus maximus. *Am J Phys Anthrop 36*:315–340, 1972.
79. Swartout R, Compere EL: Ischiogluteal bursitis, the pain in the arse. *JAMA 227*:551–552, 1974.
80. Swezey RL: Pseudo-radiculopathy in subacute trochanteric bursitis of the subgluteus maximus bursa. *Arch Phys Med Rehabil 57*:387–390, 1976.
81. Tichý M, Grim M: Morphogenesis of the human gluteus maximus muscle arising from two muscle primordia. *Anat Embryol 173*:275–277, 1985.
82. Tillmann B: Variations in the Pathway of the Inferior Gluteal Nerve. (Germ.) *Anat Anz 145*:293–302, 1979.
83. Toldt C: *An Atlas of Human Anatomy*, translated by M.E. Paul, Ed. 2, Vol. 1. Macmillan, New York, 1919 (p. 338).
84. *Ibid*. (p. 288).
85. *Ibid*. (p. 339).
86. Travell J: Factors affecting pain of injection. *JAMA 158*:368–371, 1955.
87. Travell JG, Simons DG: *Myofascial Pain and Dysfunction: The Trigger Point Manual*. Williams & Wilkins, Baltimore, 1983.
88. *Ibid*. (Chapter 3, pp. 63–74).
89. *Ibid*. (Chapter 3, pp. 84–85, Fig. 3.12).
90. *Ibid*. (Chapter 3, pp. 86–87).
91. *Ibid*. (Chapter 4, pp. 103–114).
92. *Ibid*. (Chapter 4, pp. 114–156).
93. *Ibid*. (Chapter 48, p. 648, Fig. 48.6A).
94. *Ibid*. (Chapter 49, p. 676, Fig. 49.6).
95. Travell J, Travell W: Therapy of low back pain by manipulation and of referred pain in the lower extremity by procaine infiltration. *Arch Phys Med 27*:537–547, 1946 (see p. 540).
96. Voss DE, Ionta MK, Myers BJ: *Proprioceptive Neuromuscular Facilitation: Patterns and Techniques*, Ed. 3. Harper & Row, Philadelphia, 1985 (pp. 304–305).
97. Weber EF: Ueber die Längenverhältnisse der Fleischfasern der Muskeln in Allgemeinen. *Berichte über die Verhandlungen der Königlich Sächsischen Gesellschaft der Wissenschaften zu Leipzig 3*: 63–86, 1851.

PART 1

CHAPTER 8
Gluteus Medius Muscle

"Lumbago Muscle"

HIGHLIGHTS: The posterior portion of the gluteus medius muscle lies deep to the gluteus maximus and its lower part covers the gluteus minimus muscle. The gluteus medius is usually at least twice the weight of the gluteus minimus and is less than half as heavy as the gluteus maximus. Its myofascial trigger points (TrPs) cause **REFERRED PAIN** that is commonly identified as low back pain or lumbago. Its three TrP regions together refer pain and tenderness primarily along the posterior crest of the ilium, to the sacrum, and to the posterior and lateral aspects of the buttock. Pain and tenderness may extend to the upper thigh. Its **ANATOMICAL ATTACHMENTS** are, proximally, along the anterior three-fourths of the iliac crest and, distally, to the greater trochanter. **INNERVATION** is supplied from spinal roots L_4, L_5, and S_1 via the superior gluteal nerve. The main **FUNCTION** of this abductor of the thigh is stabilization of the pelvis during single-limb stance. Myofascial TrPs in this muscle cause **SYMPTOMS** of pain when walking, when lying on the back or on the affected side, and when sitting slouched down in a chair. Sacroiliac joint dysfunction is an important differential diagnosis. **PATIENT EXAMINATION** should include looking for the Morton foot structure, observing the patient's gait, and testing for restricted adduction of the thigh at the hip. **TRIGGER POINT EXAMINATION** is concentrated along and below the iliac crest. The muscle's anterior and middle TrPs lie between skin and bone. The posterior TrP_1 region lies deep to the gluteus maximus muscle; TrPs in this region are not as likely to produce detectable local twitch responses as are the anterior TrPs. Gluteus medius **ASSOCIATED TRIGGER POINTS** may occur as satellites to quadratus lumborum TrPs. **INTERMITTENT COLD WITH STRETCH** of TrPs in fibers of the *anterior* gluteus medius requires extension and adduction of the thigh behind the uninvolved lower limb. *Posterior* fibers are passively lengthened by flexing and adducting the involved thigh in front of the other lower limb. Sweeps of ice or vapocoolant spray extend from the crest of the ilium over the sacrum and over the buttock to midthigh. The release of tight anterior and posterior fibers is followed by active range of motion and moist heat. Ischemic compression and deep massage provide helpful manual therapy. When the **INJECTION-AND-STRETCH** technique is used, a local twitch may be palpated, but is rarely seen when the needle encounters the TrP. **CORRECTIVE ACTIONS** include sleeping on the uninvolved side with a pillow between the knees, avoidance of prolonged immobility, use of the seated position when putting on pants, and appropriate placement of first metatarsal pads to correct for a Morton foot structure. Injection of irritating medications into TrPs should be avoided. The Abductor Self-stretch Exercise is recommended for a home program. Home use of an exercise bicycle while in the semireclining position provides a convenient and comfortable conditioning activity. Self-administered ischemic compression is easily applied to TrPs in either the anterior or posterior fibers while the patient lies on a tennis ball.

1. REFERRED PAIN
(Fig. 8.1)

Myofascial trigger points (TrPs) in the gluteus medius muscle are a commonly overlooked source of low back pain.[56] Pain projected from these TrPs is generally restricted to the immediate vicinity of the muscle. This nearby distribution is similar to the referral of pain from TrPs in the del-

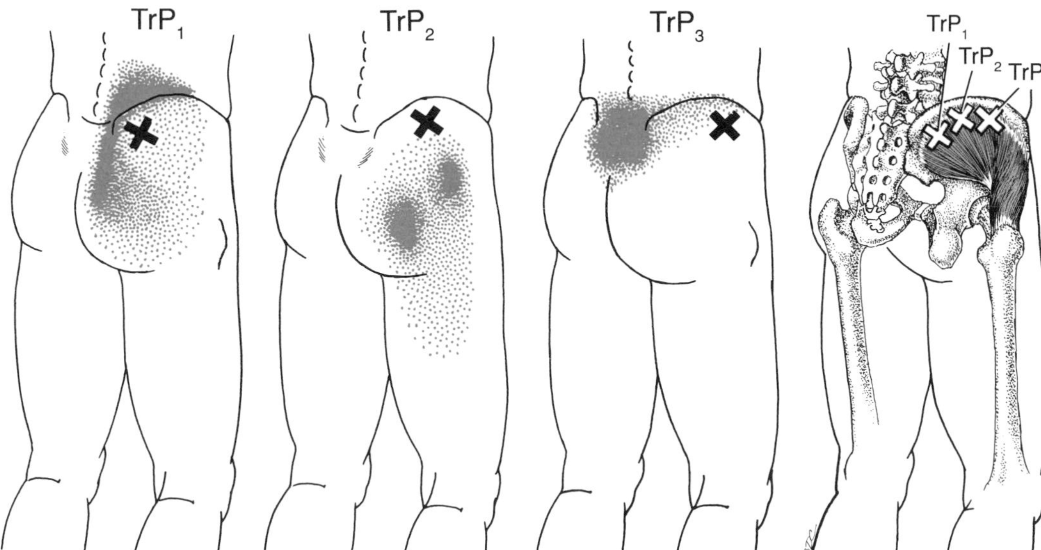

Figure 8.1. Pain patterns (*bright red*) referred from trigger points (TrPs) (***X**s*) in the right gluteus medius muscle (*darker red*). The essential pain pattern is *solid red*, and the spillover pattern is *stippled*. The most medial TrP_1 refers pain primarily to the crest of the ilium, to the region of the sacroiliac joint, and to the sacrum. The TrP_2 area is located more cephalad and laterally, and refers pain caudally to the buttock and to the upper thigh posteriorly and laterally. The most anterior TrP_3 occurs less often and refers pain bilaterally over the sacrum and into the lowest lumbar region.

toid muscle.[74] Like the deltoid, the gluteus medius also has three portions (posterior, middle, and anterior) where its TrPs are likely to be found. The region of gluteus medius TrP_1 (Fig. 8.1) is close to the iliac crest in the posterior portion of the muscle near the sacroiliac joint. TrP_1 refers pain and tenderness primarily along the posterior crest of the ilium, to the region of the sacroiliac joint, and over the sacrum on the same side; pain may also extend over much of the buttock (Fig. 8.1, TrP_1).

The region where TrP_2 is found (Fig. 8.1, TrP_2) is also just below the iliac crest, nearly centered along the length of the crest. Pain referred from TrP_2 is projected more laterally and to the midgluteal region; it may extend into the upper thigh posteriorly and laterally.

The region of rarely seen TrP_3 (Fig. 8.1, TrP_3) is likewise just below the iliac crest, but is near the anterior superior iliac spine. Pain from TrP_3 is projected primarily along the iliac crest, over the lowest lumbar region, and bilaterally over the sacrum.

In previous publications, the individual pain patterns of these three TrPs (Fig. 8.1) were consolidated into one composite pattern.[54–57,66,68] Occasionally, TrPs are found in other parts of the gluteus medius muscle.

Other authors illustrate[4,28,60] or describe[78] similar patterns of referred pain from this muscle. Two papers describe referral of pain after injection of the gluteus medius muscle with hypertonic saline.[29,63] Bates[7] illustrates referral patterns in children that are similar to the patterns observed in adults. Sola[60] describes gluteus medius referred pain as extending into the posterior thigh and calf; we believe this pattern of pain probably arises from TrPs in the underlying gluteus *minimus* muscle (Chapter 9). He[60] also notes that the gluteus medius is a frequent cause of hip pain in the later stages of pregnancy. Kelly[30] has also identified the gluteus medius as a likely source of lumbago. Others[23,31,60] reported that it may contribute to, or simulate, sciatica.

2. ANATOMICAL ATTACHMENTS AND CONSIDERATIONS
(Fig. 8.2)

The thick, fan-shaped gluteus medius lies deep to the gluteus maximus muscle and superficial to the gluteus minimus muscle

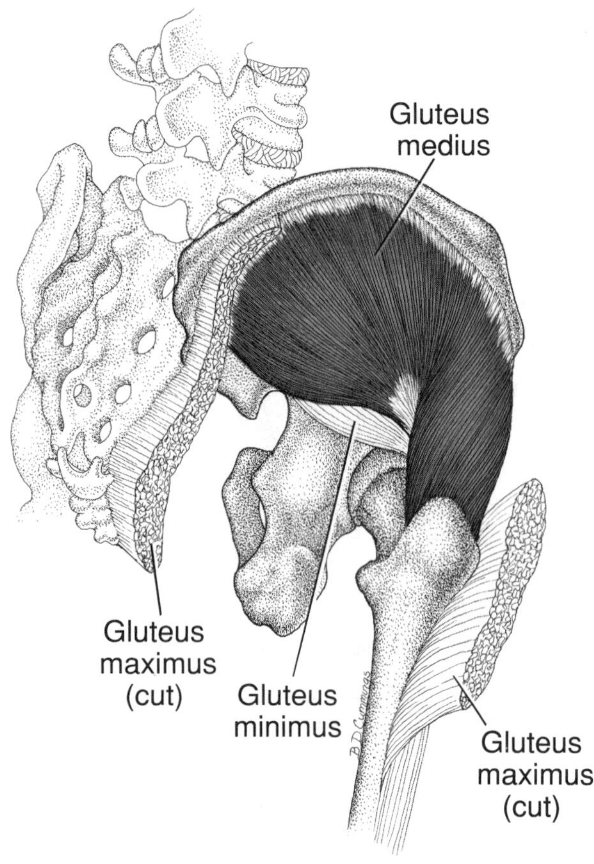

Figure 8.2. Attachments of the right gluteus medius muscle (*red*) in the posterolateral view. The gluteus maximus muscle has been cut and removed; its distal end is reflected.

on the outer surface of the pelvis. The gluteus medius is attached ***proximally*** to the external surface of the ilium along the anterior three-fourths of the iliac crest, between the anterior and posterior gluteal lines,[1,5] and to the gluteal aponeurosis that covers the anterolateral two-thirds of the muscle.[1,10] The gluteus medius attaches ***distally*** to both sides of a broad tendon anchored to the posterosuperior angle and the external surface of the greater trochanter[5] (Fig. 8.2). As they approach their femoral attachment, fiber bundles of the superficial layer cross obliquely those of the deeper posterior portion. The direction of the posterior fibers and the direction of the force that they exert are at right angles to the direction of the most anterior fibers (Fig. 8.2). Occasionally, the gluteus medius is divided into two distinct portions, or it may be fused with the piriformis muscle or with the gluteus minimus muscle.[5]

The trochanteric bursa of the gluteus medius separates the tendon of that muscle from the surface of the greater trochanter over which the tendon glides. The bursa lies between the trochanteric attachments of the gluteus minimus proximally and the gluteus medius distally, as illustrated in the Sobotta Atlas.[16,19]

Autopsy samples[58] of gluteus medius muscles in normal adults under age 44 years showed 58% slow-twitch type 1 fibers and 42% fast-twitch type 2 muscle fibers. A relative (8%) loss of type 2 fibers in the gluteus medius was observed in persons with osteoarthritis of the hip. Another adult group[58] was divided equally between individuals older and younger than 65 years of age; although individual variability was great in both groups, in every subject the number of slow-twitch type 1 fibers, which depend largely on oxidative metabolism, exceeded the number of fast-twitch type 2 fibers, which utilize glycolytic energy pathways.

Supplemental References

Other authors have illustrated the gluteus medius as seen from behind: by itself,[16,50] in relation to the gluteus maximus,[2,15,44,62,64] and in relation to the gluteus minimus.[19,44,51,65] It is also shown from in front,[18,61] in cross section,[9,17] and in coronal section.[14,41]

Its attachments to the ilium and to the femur are clearly illustrated,[20,40,49] as also is its extensive proximal aponeurotic attachment.[3,64]

3. INNERVATION

The gluteus medius muscle is innervated by the inferior branch of the superior gluteal nerve, which passes between the gluteus medius and gluteus minimus, sending branches to each muscle. The superior gluteal nerve carries fibers from the fourth and fifth lumbar and the first sacral nerves.[10,11]

4. FUNCTION

The gluteus medius is the abductor chiefly responsible for stabilizing the pelvis during single-limb weight bearing. During ambulation, the gluteus medius and other abductors prevent the pelvis from dropping excessively (tilting laterally) toward the unsupported side.

Actions

The gluteus medius muscle is generally recognized as the most powerful abductor of the thigh.[6,10,25–27,46] The anterior fibers of this muscle also assist medial rotation of the thigh. The flexion and lateral rotation functions of this muscle are either minimal or are highly dependent on positioning of the thigh.[22]

Inman[26] reported that the gluteus medius usually weighs about twice as much as the gluteus minimus, which, in turn, is nearly twice as large as the only other major abductor at the hip, the tensor fasciae latae. Weber[76] found the gluteus medius to be more than four times as heavy as the gluteus minimus.

Anatomically, the two-layer overlap arrangement of the gluteus medius (Fig. 8.2) should improve the effectiveness of the posterior fibers in producing lateral rotation and the anterior fibers in producing medial rotation, as compared with the simple fan arrangement of the gluteus minimus fibers (Fig. 9.3).

Electromyographic (EMG) studies[6,22,26,39,77] have confirmed the observations of Duchenne[12] and the conclusion of anatomists[5,10,62] that the gluteus medius is primarily an abductor of the thigh. Duchenne[12] found that stimulation of the anterior, middle, or posterior portions of the gluteus medius produced abduction at the hip. Stimulation of the anterior fibers first strongly rotated the thigh medially. Stimulation revealed that only a few posterior fibers produced weak lateral rotation.

Greenlaw monitored the anterior and posterior fibers with fine-wire electrodes and found that both groups of fibers were active during medial (internal) rotation. The posterior fibers were not active during lateral (external) rotation.[22] Duchenne's report[12] of *weak* lateral rotation by stimulation of *selected* posterior fibers is not altogether inconsistent with Greenlaw's report, because Greenlaw may not have been monitoring those fibers. Observation of a skeleton makes it clear that any gluteus medius fibers capable of producing lateral rotation of the thigh would be converted to medial rotators as the thigh moves from full extension toward flexion.

The anterior fibers showed increasing EMG activity as the degree of active flexion of the thigh increased. These anterior fibers were also active during straight leg raising or when sitting up from the supine position. Posterior fibers were inactive during flexion of the thigh and only minimally active during an effort to maximally extend the thigh.[22]

Functions

The primary function of the gluteus medius is to stabilize the pelvis during the single-limb stance phase of ambulation[6,10] and thereby to prevent the contralateral side of the pelvis from dropping. This stabilization function requires about 10% of its maximum effort.[26] The evolution of this muscle from a propulsive muscle to a stabilizing one is well described and illustrated.[37]

Using fine-wire electrodes in the anterior and in the posterior portions of the muscle during slow and fast ambulation, Greenlaw[22] found that the two portions of the muscle had similar activity patterns at both speeds. Lyons and co-workers[39] also found that activity was greatest immediately before and through the first half of stance phase on the same side. Activity then faded out until a brief burst appeared with toe-off; another brief burst anticipated heel-strike. The posterior portion of the muscle showed considerably less activity than the anterior portion during all phases of ambulation.[22]

The normal "fan" sign of the gluteus medius is observed as a more rapid ebbing of electrical activity in the posterior fibers as compared to the anterior fibers during the stance phase of free walking.[53,59] This sign was lost in patients with severe osteoarthritis of the hip[53] and reflects the distortion of normal sequencing of fiber activity due to joint dysfunction.

At times, differences in the onset, duration, and degree of EMG activity appeared among the anterior, middle, and posterior fibers of this muscle during activities of walking, crawling, stair ascending and descending, shoe tying, sitting, and single-limb standing while leaning forward. This independence of activity justifies a three-segment conceptual model of this muscle.[59]

Electrical activity of the gluteus medius was increased during ergometer cycling when the workload, pedalling rate, or saddle height was increased and when the posterior foot position on the pedal was used.[13]

As expected, carrying a load in the ipsilateral hand reduces activity of the gluteus medius muscle, and carrying the load on the opposite side increases its activity.[45] Ghori and Luckwill found that walking with a load of 20% of body weight in the contralateral hand or on the back significantly prolonged EMG activity of the gluteus medius muscle.[21]

In only one of seven subjects was the gluteus medius more than minimally active when the subject lifted a 12.8-kg box from the floor in three different ways.[43] Therefore TrPs in this muscle should not usually compromise lifting.

Loss of strength due to surgical removal of the gluteus medius and gluteus minimus muscles was reported[42] in one case when the only abductor remaining was the sartorius muscle and, in another case, when only the abducting part of the gluteus maximus remained. In both cases, nearly half of maximal abduction strength was retained, but without endurance.[42] These gluteal muscles are essential for endurance and full strength.

5. FUNCTIONAL (MYOTATIC) UNIT

The muscles that assist the abduction function of the gluteus medius are the gluteus minimus, tensor fasciae latae, and, to a lesser extent, the sartorius, piriformis,[24] and part of the gluteus maximus[42] muscle. Janda[27] also includes the iliopsoas muscle as assisting abduction.

6. SYMPTOMS

Patients with active gluteus medius TrPs are likely to complain of pain on walking, especially if they have an uncorrected Morton foot structure (Chapter 20, Sections 7 and 8).

Patients with gluteus medius TrPs have difficulty sleeping on the affected side. To avoid this pressure on the TrPs, they sleep on the back or on the other side. However, lying on the back may painfully compress posterior gluteus medius TrPs. When lying on the side opposite to the gluteus medius TrPs, a pillow should be placed between the knees to prevent excessive adduction that painfully stretches taut bands in the muscle. The best sleeping position may be half-supine, that is, turned halfway between lying on the unaffected side and on the back, with the torso supported by a pillow.

Patients with active gluteus medius TrPs are also uncomfortable when sitting in a slumped position, rolled back on the buttocks so that body weight compresses these TrPs.

Differential Diagnosis

Although the referred pain patterns from gluteus *maximus* and gluteus *medius* TrPs overlap, it is essential to distinguish between them for therapy that employs stretch. Tightness of the gluteus maximus due to TrPs restricts flexion at the hip; tightness of the gluteus medius restricts adduction. Careful attention to the location of the TrPs in the buttock, as well as to restriction of motion, helps establish their identification (*see* Section 9, Fig. 8.5). In the anterior superior portion of the buttock, only the gluteus medius muscle lies between the skin and the ilium.[44] Elsewhere in the buttock, the gluteus maximus is the superficial muscle; the gluteus medius lies deep to it.

Therapeutically, distinguishing between gluteus *medius* and gluteus *minimus* TrPs is less critical, except for the extent of the spray pattern or the depth of needle penetration required for TrP injection. Anatomically[44] and functionally, these two muscles are hard to differentiate; however, a pain reference zone extending over the full length of the thigh, and sometimes as far as the ankle, clearly identifies gluteus minimus TrPs. The TrPs of the *piriformis* muscle are not likely to cause low back pain over the sacrum, but they do refer pain over the buttock and sometimes into the thigh posteriorly.

Reynolds[48] reminds us that the pain referred from gluteus medius TrPs may be confusingly like the pain originating from **sacroiliac joint dysfunction and disease**. The diagnosis of sacroiliac joint locking and its management by manipulation has been described with detailed case reports[75] and is reviewed in Chapter 2. This dysfunction is more likely to be associated with gluteus minimus TrPs than with gluteus medius TrPs, but should be considered.[75]

Lumbar facet joints can refer pain to the buttock region that may be mistaken for gluteal TrPs. The recognition of this articular source of referred pain is reviewed in Chapter 3, pages 25–26.

Inflammation of the subgluteus medius bursa at the greater trochanter can be a cause of pain and tenderness in the region of the greater trochanter.[52] This pain must be distinguished from pain referred by gluteus medius TrPs. This tenderness must be distinguished from musculotendinous tenderness at the greater trochanteric attachment of taut bands associated with gluteus medius TrPs. This distinction can be made by examining for the TrPs.

Chronic pain following **spinal surgery for low back pain** is not uncommon. It may be due to overlooked TrPs and it can then be resolved by identifying the responsible TrPs and managing them appropriately. Another source of pain is the postmyelogram or postoperative complication, **arachnoiditis or arachnoradiculitis**. One important part of an effective management program for this condition is inactivation of TrPs in the gluteal muscles and in other muscles in the regions that are involved.[47]

Since the pain of **intermittent claudication** is related to muscular activity, the patient's history may not clearly distinguish between pain of vascular origin and pain of myofascial TrP origin. Arcangeli and associates[4] emphasized that the pain of claudication often was similar in character to that referred from TrPs. They noted that patients with stenosis or occlusion of the aorta, common iliac, or hypogastric (internal iliac) artery could have TrPs in the gluteus medius and tensor fasciae latae muscles. When TrPs were present, ischemia caused pain in their reference zones. In some of the patients, walking tolerance was related more to the severity of myalgic spots (TrPs) than to the decrease in blood flow.

Vascular occlusion is identified by decreased pulses, impaired skin circulation, and by ultrasound or contrast dye studies. On the other hand, TrPs are identified by their specific referred pain patterns and by restricted range of motion of the affected muscles; palpation of the muscles reveals spot tenderness in taut bands and may elicit a local twitch response. Referred pain that appears in predictable patterns is evoked by pressure on the tender spot, a TrP.

7. ACTIVATION AND PERPETUATION OF TRIGGER POINTS (Fig. 8.3)

Events and activities likely to initiate TrPs in the gluteus medius muscle include sudden falls, sports injuries, running, lengthy tennis matches, aerobics, long walks on a soft sandy beach, weight bearing on only one limb for an extended period of time, and injection of medications into the muscle. Such injections may activate latent TrPs.[67] Injection of irritating medications in the immediate vicinity of latent or active TrPs enhances their activity and can cause severe referred pain.[67]

Sola[60] identifies a discrepancy of at least 1 cm in leg length as a cause of unilateral low back pain and of TrPs in the gluteus medius muscle. Pelvic distortion can produce an apparent lower limb-length discrepancy (*see* Chapter 4, Section 8 for more on this important issue).

The long second (short first) metatarsal of the Morton foot structure, which is described in detail in Chapter 20, Sections 7 and 8, commonly perpetuates and can activate TrPs in the gluteus medius muscle. The abnormal weight distribution on the foot usually causes excessive pronation, as illustrated in Figure 8.3*B*. The resultant medial rotation and adduction of the thigh at the hip tend to overload the glu-

PART 1

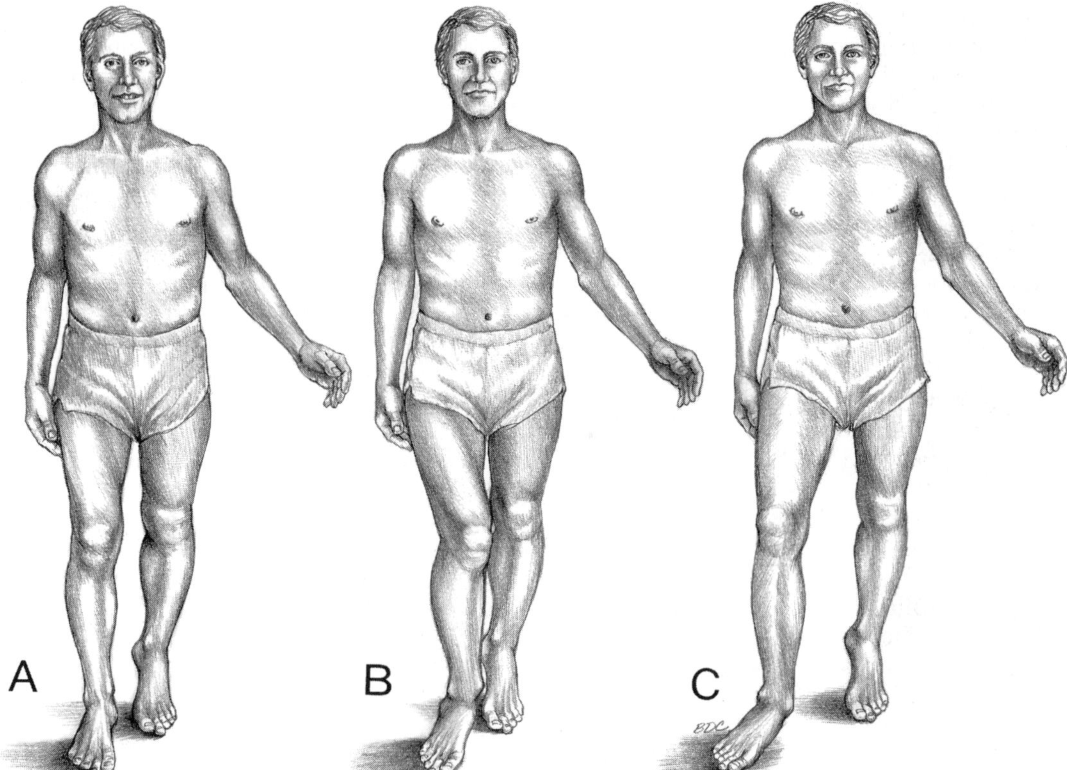

Figure 8.3. Strain of the right gluteus medius muscle during ambulation caused by the relatively long second and short first metatarsal bones of the Morton foot structure. *A*, ambulation with normal foot alignment, not out-toeing. *B*, pronation of the right foot as the ball of the foot rocks inward and weight bearing progresses from the heel to the knife-edge of the protruding head of the long second metatarsal bone at toe-off. This produces the appearance of genu valgum with adduction and medial rotation of the thigh at the hip. *C*, patient's attempt to relieve the resultant gluteal muscle strain by laterally rotating and abducting the lower limb at the hip and by further everting the foot to provide a more balanced two-point support on the first and second metatarsal heads at toe-off. This reduction of medial rotation and adduction at the hip minimizes the compensatory strain of hip abductors, chiefly the gluteus medius muscle.

teus medius and vastus medialis muscles. Rocking of the foot laterally during ambulation often overloads the peroneal muscles. Some individuals compensate by laterally rotating the thigh and further everting the foot (Fig. 8.3*C*), which imposes additional stress on the foot itself but is less stressful on the gluteus medius muscle.

Displacement of the articular surfaces of the sacroiliac joint can help perpetuate gluteus medius TrPs and, if present, should be corrected for lasting response to therapy.[75]

Established active or latent TrPs in the gluteus medius muscle are aggravated by prolonged flexion at the hip, as when sleeping in the fetal position, sitting in a low chair with feet on the floor and knees flexed, or sitting with the seat bottom inclined backward and thus flexing the thighs acutely at the hip.

Although a head-forward kyphotic posture is more likely to perpetuate gluteus maximus TrPs, it can be a significant factor in the perpetuation of gluteus medius TrPs.

Sitting on a credit-card-filled wallet placed in a deep hip pocket can concentrate pressure on gluteus medius TrPs inducing referred pain from them, producing a form of "credit-card-wallet" sciatica.[38]

8. PATIENT EXAMINATION

If the pain distribution suggests gluteus medius TrPs, the patient's gait should be

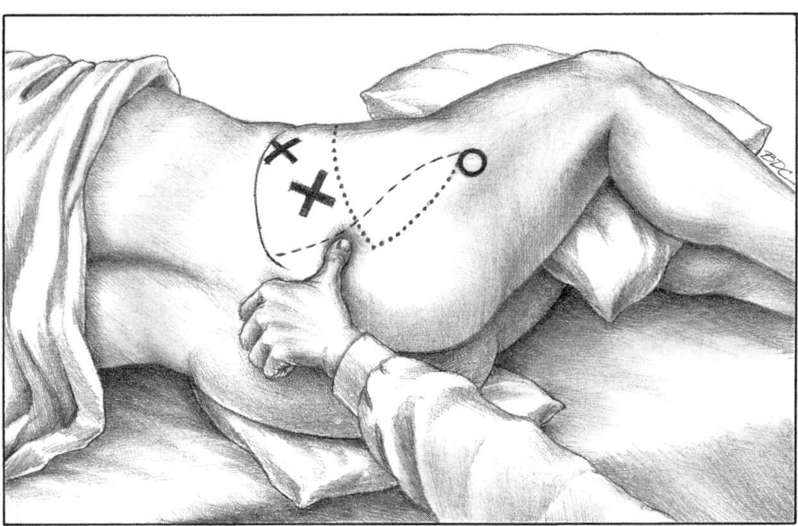

Figure 8.4. Palpation of the posterior trigger point (TrP_1) in the right gluteus medius muscle. The *open circle* locates the greater trochanter; the *solid line* marks the crest of the ilium (also the upper margin of the gluteus medius); the *dotted line* delineates the upper and posterior borders of the gluteus minimus muscle; and the *dashed line* identifies the upper (anterior) border of the gluteus maximus, which also approximates the direction of the gluteus medius fibers at this TrP. Palpation is performed with the **tip** of the examining digit moved perpendicularly to the *dashed line.*

observed for the distortions illustrated in Figure 8.3 and the feet should be examined for the long second metatarsal bone (*see* Chapter 20, Section 8). The examiner may observe that the patient stands with the weight predominantly on one leg in order to relieve tension caused by a lower limb-length inequality or to relieve discomfort caused by posterior ilial torsion of the pelvis with displacement of the sacroiliac joint on the opposite side. The patient should be examined for other evidence of lower limb-length discrepancy; *see* Volume 1[70] and Section 8 of Chapter 4 in this volume. The senior author described examination and treatment for sacroiliac joint displacement.[75]

During the examination for evidence of shortening of the gluteus medius muscle because of TrPs, the patient lies on the uninvolved side and the uppermost thigh is flexed to 90°; normally, the knee should drop onto the examining table. Failure of the knee to reach the table indicates restriction of hip adduction that may be caused by TrP tension in the gluteus medius muscle and also by increased tension in the fascia lata.

During the examination for weakness of this muscle due to TrPs, the patient lies on the uninvolved side as described previously, but with the uppermost thigh extended as illustrated by Kendall and McCreary.[32] Moderate and ratchety or "break-away" weakness is likely, as compared to the uninvolved side.

With the patient lying supine on the examining table, lateral rotation of the lower limb on the affected side may be caused by shortening due to TrPs in one or all of the following: the posterior part of the gluteus medius and gluteus minimus muscles, the piriformis, and the gemelli-obturator-quadratus femoris group of muscles. In the supine position, the lower limb on the side of a posterior ilial torsion is rotated outward, if nothing else complicates the situation.

9. TRIGGER POINT EXAMINATION (Figs. 8.4 and 8.5)

All TrPs in the gluteus medius muscle are examined while the patient lies on the side opposite to the affected muscle. Figure 8.4 illustrates the examination by flat palpation of TrP_1, which has the most posterior location of gluteus medius TrPs. A pillow placed between the knees helps prevent painful stretch of exquisitely sensitive TrPs in this muscle. The same patient position is used for examination of the more anterior TrP_2 and TrP_3, which are marked by **X**s in Figure 8.4. The latter two TrPs are covered only by skin and subcutaneous tissue. To find the taut bands of TrP_2 and TrP_3, the muscle fibers are rolled against the underlying bone by rubbing the examining finger*tip across* the fibers (perpendicular to fiber direction), using the deep tissue technique of moving the skin with the fingertip. Local twitch responses elicited in the posterior and distal parts of the gluteus medius muscle are rarely visible through the overlying gluteus maximus, but may be detected by palpation with the fingers of the other hand.

Sola[60] points out that, with extensive involvement, gluteus medius fibers along the entire gluteal ridge from the sacroiliac joint to the anterior superior iliac spine may contain painful TrPs.

Deep gluteus maximus TrPs may be difficult to distinguish from gluteus medius TrP_1, where the two muscles have similar fiber directions.[44] Taut bands in the superficial fibers of the gluteus maximus clearly feel as if they are just under the skin. Taut bands that feel deeper may be in deeper gluteus maximus fibers or in underlying muscle. If TrPs are found in the gluteus maximus, additional deeper TrPs may not be distinguishable until the overlying TrPs have been inactivated. One should apply therapy for TrPs in both muscles when in doubt as to which is involved.

All three of the common gluteus medius TrPs are located cephalad to the gluteus minimus muscle (Fig. 8.4). Thus, location of the TrP, as well as extensiveness of the pain pattern, helps distinguish gluteus medius TrPs from gluteus minimus TrPs.

In order to identify by palpation the muscle in which a TrP lies, a schematic drawing showing the limits of each muscle and where the gluteal muscles overlap is helpful (Fig. 8.5*A*). The gluteus medius is limited superiorly by the rim of the pelvis, in front by a line from slightly behind the anterior superior iliac spine to the greater trochanter, and below (posteriorly) by the piriformis line (Fig. 8.5*B*), which runs along the upper border of the piriformis muscle (Fig. 8.5*A*). The gluteus maximus covers much of the posterior portion of the gluteus medius, and the gluteus minimus lies deep to the distal two-thirds of the gluteus medius.

10. ENTRAPMENTS

No nerve entrapment by the gluteus medius muscle has been identified.

11. ASSOCIATED TRIGGER POINTS

When the posterior fibers of the gluteus medius harbor TrPs, secondary TrPs are likely to develop in the piriformis and posterior part of the gluteus minimus, which are closely related functionally, and sometimes in the gluteus maximus muscle. When the anterior fibers of the gluteus medius are involved, the tensor fasciae latae, as part of that functional unit, may also develop secondary TrPs.

The gluteus medius commonly develops satellite TrPs in response to active quadratus lumborum TrPs, because the gluteus medius lies in the pain reference zone of that muscle. This relationship can be so close that pressure on quadratus lumborum TrPs induces not only referred pain over the posterior gluteus medius muscle (referral pattern of quadratus lumborum TrPs), but also referred pain that extends over the upper thigh (gluteus medius TrP referred pain pattern) as well. Pressure on the satellite TrP in the gluteus medius induces pain only in its characteristic reference zone. Inactivation of only this satellite gluteal TrP usually provides merely temporary relief. On the other hand, inactivation of the quadratus lumborum TrPs may eliminate the gluteus medius satellite TrPs as well. In other cases, both the quadratus lumborum TrPs and their satellite TrPs in the gluteus medius must be inactivated individually for complete lasting relief.

Furthermore, Sola[60] reports the reverse situation, that gluteus medius TrPs can induce TrPs in the quadratus lumborum muscle. He notes that these gluteal TrPs may also interact with muscles in the cervical area and thus contribute to cervical pain and headache. We suggest that a mechanism for this interaction may be a postural compensation for tilted pelvic and shoulder-girdle axes that are caused by weak gluteal function. Sola[60] states

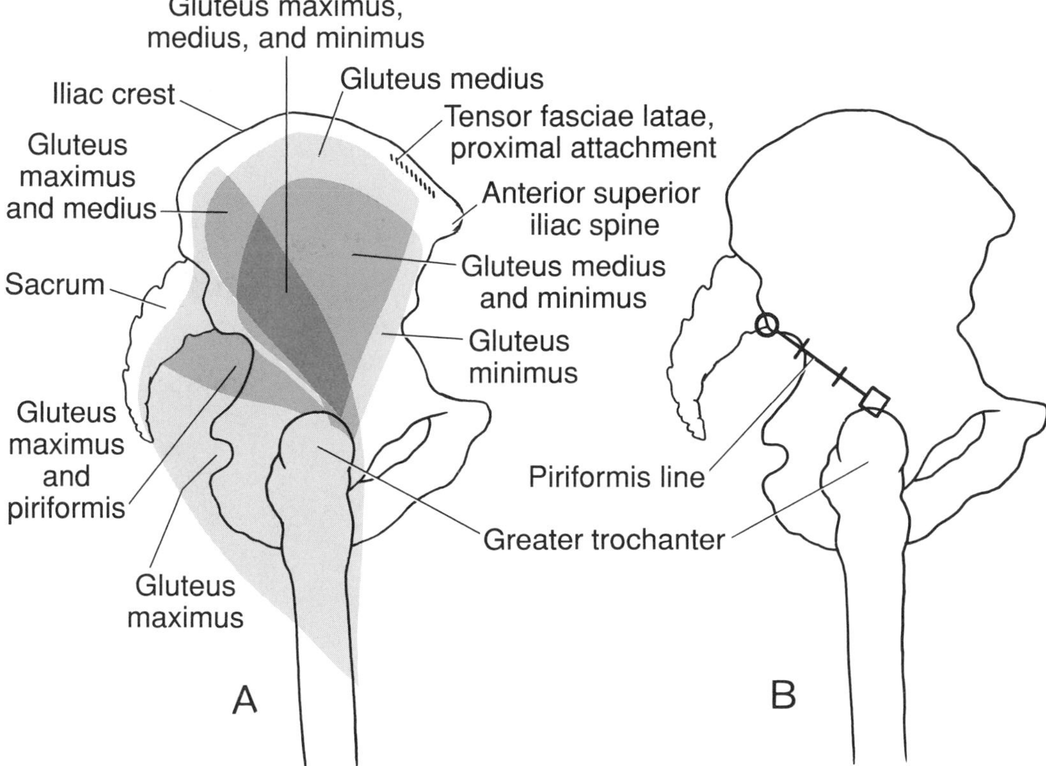

Figure 8.5. Schematic drawing that shows overlap of gluteal and piriformis muscles from a slightly posterior, nearly lateral view. *A*, *light red* identifies the areas where only a single gluteal muscle may be palpated, except for the anterior part of the gluteus minimus that is covered also by the tensor fasciae latae muscle (the iliac attachment is marked by *hatched line* and is labeled). In these single-muscle areas, there is little likelihood of encountering misleading tenderness from another gluteal muscle or from the piriformis muscle. *Medium red* on the left side of *A* illustrates where either the gluteus medius or piriformis may be palpated through the gluteus maximus in an area free of deeper gluteus minimus sensitivity; *medium red* on the right side of *A* illustrates where the gluteus medius overlies the gluteus minimus. *Dark red* shows where three muscle layers—gluteus maximus, gluteus medius, and gluteus minimus—are present. Note that the upper border of the piriformis corresponds closely with the lower borders of the gluteus medius and gluteus minimus muscles. The gluteus medius sometimes overlaps the piriformis. *B*, the piriformis line that corresponds closely to the upper border of the piriformis muscle runs from the proximal end of the greater trochanter (*open square*) to the upper end of the palpable free border of the sacrum where it joins the ilium (*open circle*). The piriformis line is divided into thirds for convenience in locating TrPs in the posterior part of the gluteus minimus and in the piriformis muscle.

that the gluteus medius seldom causes pain as a single muscle syndrome, but usually is involved with other muscles as part of a functional unit.

Posterior ilial torsion is commonly associated with shortening and TrP activity of the posterior part of the gluteus medius muscle and of the parallel piriformis. The patient is unlikely to experience prolonged relief unless TrPs in *both* the gluteus medius and piriformis muscles are inactivated *and* the ilial torsion is corrected.

12. INTERMITTENT COLD WITH STRETCH
(Fig. 8.6)

Details of intermittent cold with stretch appear in Volume 1, pages 63–74 for the stretch-and-spray technique and in Chapter 2 on page 9 of this volume for the application of ice instead of vapocoolant.

To restore full, active range of motion that is restricted because of active TrPs in the gluteus medius muscle, the sequence of intermittent cold with stretch is ap-

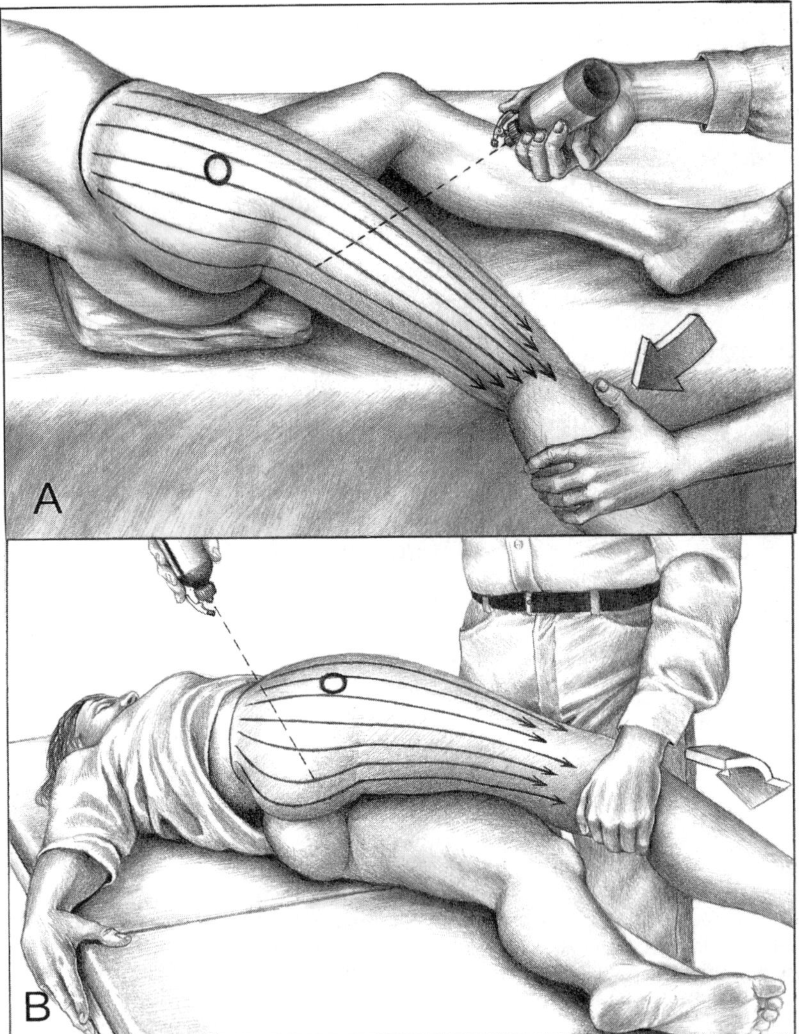

Figure 8.6. Stretch position and intermittent cold pattern (*thin arrows*) for TrPs in the right gluteus medius muscle. The *solid line* marks the crest of the ilium. The *open circle* marks the greater trochanter. The *large arrows* show the direction of passive movement required to lengthen the muscle. *A*, intermittent cold with stretch of the anterior fibers (TrP_3). To lengthen the muscle passively, the operator lifts the thigh backward toward extension so that it can be eased over the edge of the examining table and allowed to drop toward the floor gently. The force of gravity gradually enhances the stretch into adduction. *B*, intermittent cold with stretch of the posterior fibers (TrP_1 and TrP_2). While applying the vapocoolant spray or ice, the operator's hand brings the thigh forward to about 30° of flexion at the hip. As parallel sweeps of the cold release muscle tightness, the operator lowers the limb to adduct the thigh (*large curved arrow*).

plied with the patient lying comfortably on the uninvolved side. A small pillow or towel roll may be needed under the patient's waist for positioning the lumbar spine, or under the lower hip for comfort. For gluteus medius TrPs, parallel sweeps of ice or vapocoolant spray are applied in one direction distalward over the muscle and over its referred pain pattern followed by gentle passive stretch (Fig 8.6). The intermittent cold is applied to nearly the same area of skin for treatment of either anterior or posterior gluteus medius TrPs (Fig. 8.6*A* and *B*).

When releasing tension of anterior gluteus medius fibers, the operator should also apply ice or spray to the skin over the tensor fasciae latae muscle. To stretch the *anterior* section of the gluteus medius (or minimus), after several sweeps of ice or spray, the thigh should be extended and then adducted, as shown in Figure 8.6*A*. Taut bands with TrPs in the tensor fasciae latae muscle also restrict extension and adduction; lateral rotation should be added to the extension and adduction for a complete stretch of the tensor fasciae latae (*see* Chapter 12). Caution: this maneuver can overstress the sacroiliac joint if done too vigorously or held too long.

In this region, as in all regions of the body, treatment by lengthening to the full range of motion is not attempted if the patient is hypermobile in joints involved in the stretch procedure (*see* page 18 in Chapter 2 regarding hypermobility). When this problem is encountered, one can effectively treat the muscle non-invasively by using either ischemic compression or stripping massage for local stretching of the taut band (*see* page 9 in Chapter 2).

When applying intermittent cold for posterior gluteus medius TrPs, the sweeps should also cover the skin over the piriformis muscle. To lengthen the *posterior* fibers of the gluteus medius (or minimus) to full range of motion, the thigh is flexed to approximately 30° and then adducted (Fig. 8.6*B*). In this position, medial or lateral rotation has little effect on stretch of the posterior fibers.

Thigh flexion to 90° significantly alters the function of posterior fibers in the gluteus medius muscle. In this position, muscle length is changed very little by adduction, but posterior gluteus medius and minimus fibers are stretched by lateral rotation. For practical purposes, however, that movement is often blocked by other soft tissues, including the articular capsule. The most effective stretch of these fibers is achieved by adduction of the thigh at 30° of flexion.

Alternative body positioning for passive stretch is presented in Chapter 9 (Fig. 9.6). A passive stretch technique using postisometric relaxation with the patient supine is described and illustrated by Lewit[34] and described in Chapter 2 of this volume.

Following release of TrP tension, the patient actively moves the limb slowly through full adduction and abduction range of motion several times. Moist heat is applied promptly over the area of the TrP and its major pain pattern.

When releasing either anterior or posterior gluteus medius fibers by intermittent cold with stretch, it is important to prevent reactive cramping (TrP kickback) by stretching antagonists that harbor TrPs. This precaution applies to the gluteus maximus and hamstring muscles as antagonists for anterior gluteus medius TrPs and to the adductor group of muscles as antagonists for posterior gluteus medius TrPs.

Active TrPs, especially those in the more *anterior*, superficial fibers of the gluteus medius muscle, are also responsive to deep massage and to ischemic compression, which can be applied directly with the thumbs.

When gluteus medius TrPs have not been completely inactivated by intermittent cold with stretch and these other modalities, the patient may be able to increase the level of functional activity by wrapping an elastic bandage or sacroiliac (pelvic) belt firmly around the pelvis over the anterior gluteal and hip musculature. In principle, the effect of this technique may be analogous to the reflex effect of pinching the skin over the sternocleidomastoid muscle.[8,72]

13. INJECTION AND STRETCH (Fig. 8.7)

For injection, as for intermittent cold with stretch, the patient lies on the uninvolved side. The taut band is located and the spot tenderness of the posterior TrP_1 is positioned between the fingers (Fig. 8.7*A*). The probing needle is inserted directly toward the region of deep tenderness. It is sometimes possible to detect by palpation a local twitch response through the overlying thick gluteus maximus muscle.

Similarly, the more anterior TrP_2 (Fig. 8.7*B*) and TrP_3 (Fig. 8.7*C*) are injected as shown. The clinician is likely to *feel* a local twitch response when the needle penetrates one of these TrPs. Since the most visible twitch tends to occur at the distal end of the gluteus medius fibers where they lie under the gluteus maximus muscle, the response is rarely seen. The pa-

PART 1

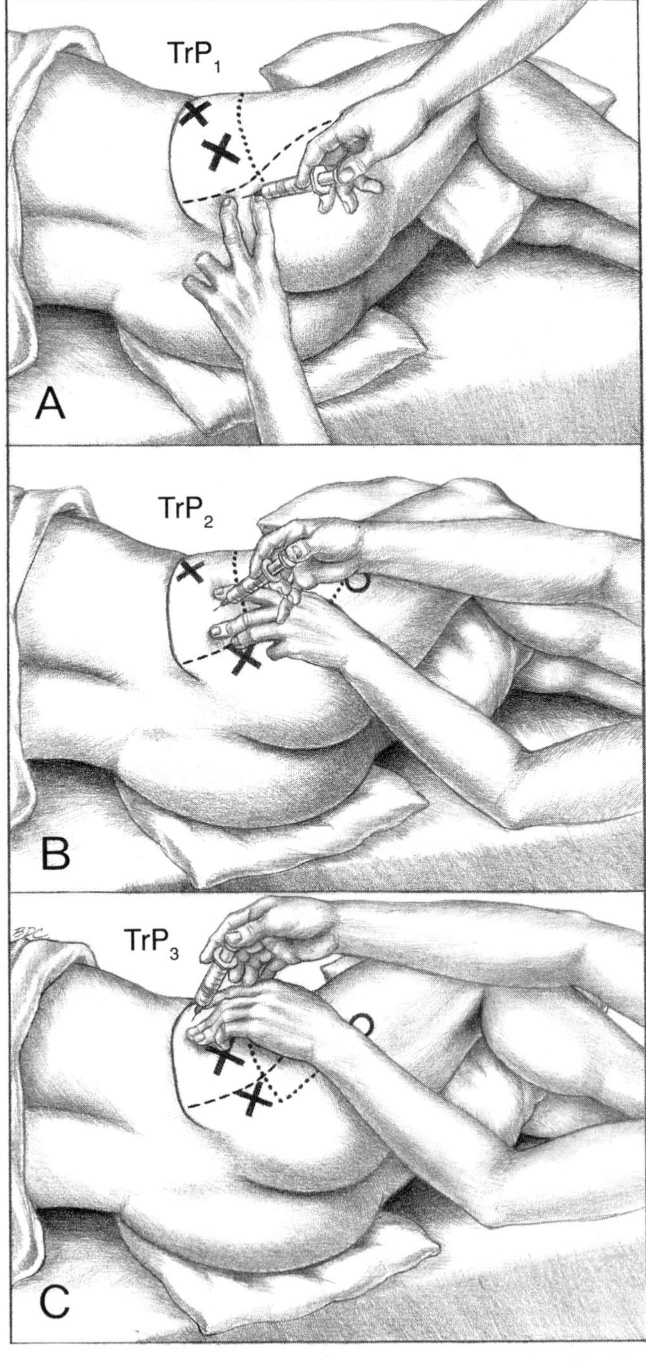

Figure 8.7. Injection of TrPs (***Xs***) in the posterior, middle, and anterior portions (TrP_1, TrP_2, TrP_3, respectively) of the right gluteus medius muscle. The *solid line* locates the crest of the ilium. The *dashed line* shows the anterior border of the gluteus maximus, and the *dotted line* delineates the upper and posterior borders of the gluteus minimus muscle. The *open circle* marks the greater trochanter. *A*, injection of TrP_1. *B*, injection of TrP_2. *C*, injection of TrP_3.

tient may or may not be aware of a twitch. Application of intermittent cold with stretch of the involved muscle follows TrP injection. The limb is then actively moved through full range of motion several times, and moist heat is applied over the injected muscle.

If these muscle-lengthening and TrP injection approaches produce only temporary results, one should examine for overlooked TrPs in functionally related muscles and also evaluate perpetuating factors (*see* Section 7 of this chapter and Volume 1[69]).

14. CORRECTIVE ACTIONS (Figs. 8.8–8.10)

Body Mechanics

For gluteus medius TrPs that were activated or perpetuated by a Morton foot structure, the shoe should be corrected temporarily by inserting a first metatarsal pad. Installation of a wedge (Chapter 20, Section 14) in the sole of the shoe provides a more permanent correction. This wedge is known as a "Flying Dutchman."

Posture and Activities (Fig. 8.8)

When a person who is prone to gluteus medius TrPs sleeps on the side, a pillow should be placed between the knees, as illustrated for the quadratus lumborum muscle in Figure 4.31.

One should avoid sitting too long in any one position. When driving a car, use of a cruise control permits more freedom of movement. At home, use of a rocking chair reduces immobility and encourages muscular relaxation. One should avoid placing a wallet full of credit cards in a deep hip pocket.[38]

Individuals prone to gluteal TrPs should not cross the legs when sitting; this position shortens the anterior gluteus medius fibers on the uppermost side and often compresses the peroneal nerve against the knee underneath. Some individuals tend to cross the lower limbs in lieu of using an appropriate ischial lift to correct a small hemipelvis; they should learn to use an ischial ("butt") lift instead, as described in Volume 1.[71]

Individuals should be warned to sit (Fig. 8.8*A*) or lean against a wall while putting on pants or socks; they should never put them on while standing up without additional support (Fig. 8.8*B*). If the person catches a foot in the pants and loses balance, sudden acute overload of the gluteal muscles is likely to activate TrPs, even though the person does not fall.

When giving intramuscular medication in the gluteal area, it is necessary to avoid TrPs that might be activated by the injected solution. The muscle is first palpated for taut bands and tender spots that are likely to be TrPs, so that those locations can be avoided.[67] The medication can be diluted with sufficient 2% pro-

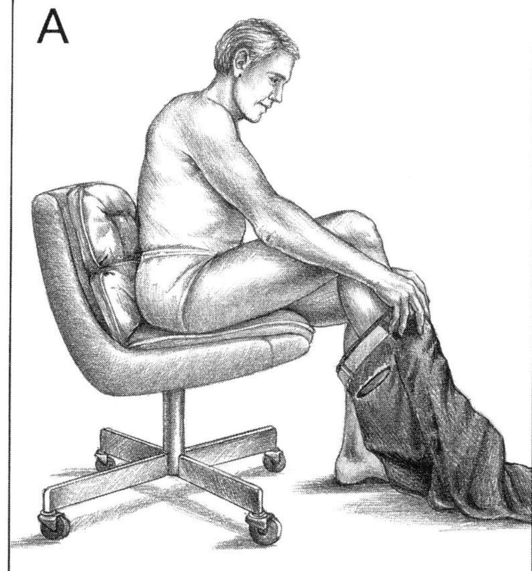

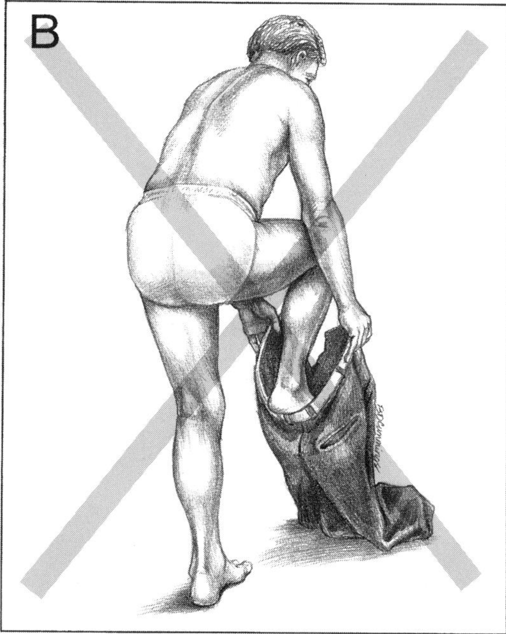

Figure 8.8. Safe and unsafe dressing positions. *A*, safe position, seated. The individual can also lean against a wall to provide body support and avoid the necessity of balancing on one lower limb. *B*, hazardous way (*red* **X**) balancing on one foot, leaning forward and sideways, and overloading the gluteal muscles on the weight-bearing side. This position also runs the risk of catching the foot in the clothing, thereby suddenly straining the muscles to maintain balance and avoid falling.

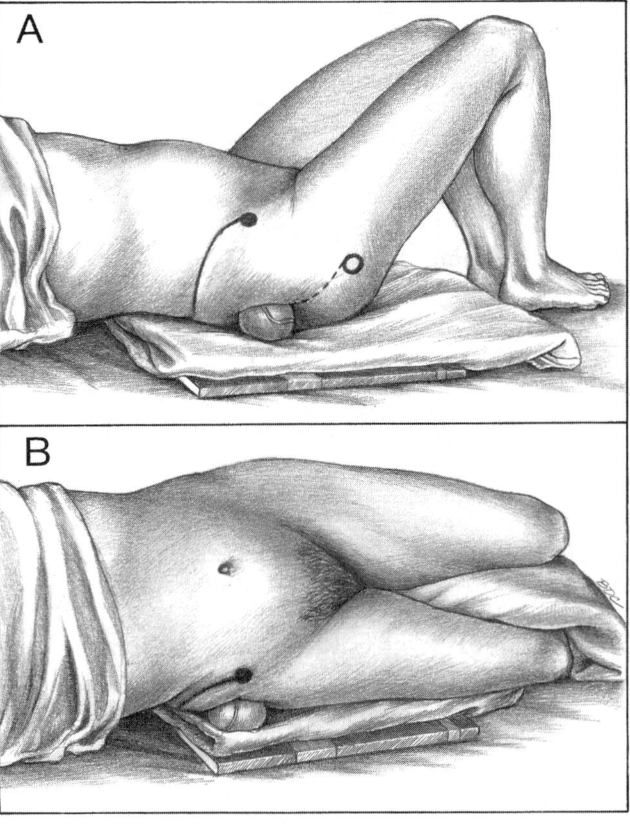

Figure 8.9. Ischemic compression applied to the gluteus medius and gluteus minimus TrPs using a tennis ball for self-administered therapy. A padded book or board is required when the patient lies on a soft compressible surface. The *solid circle* locates the anterior superior iliac spine; the *solid line*, the crest of the ilium; the *dashed line*, the anterior border of the gluteus maximus muscle; and the *open circle*, the greater trochanter. *A,* tennis ball placed under TrPs in the midportion of the gluteus medius and gluteus minimus muscles. *B*, pressure applied to TrPs in the anterior part of the gluteus medius and gluteus minimus muscles by rolling the body weight onto the ball.

caine to make the injected solution 0.5% procaine. The addition of procaine greatly reduces the chance of activating a latent TrP, should it be exposed accidentally to the medication.

Corrective Exercises
(Figs. 8.9 and 8.10)

The patient should perform postisometric relaxation[36] and synchronous respiration[35] (Chapter 2) as part of the Abductor Self-stretch Exercise for the middle and posterior fibers of the gluteus medius. This technique employs the stretch position of Figure 8.6*B* and has also been described and illustrated for this muscle by Lewit.[34] To lengthen the muscle, the side-lying patient places the involved limb in adduction in front of the other limb with the knee straight and with the thigh in approximately 30° of flexion at the hip; the patient stabilizes the pelvis by holding onto the edge of the table. Then the patient performs slow inhalation, which induces a gentle contraction of the abductors; relaxation during slow exhalation permits enhancement of the force of gravity to take up any slack that develops. Self-stretch of anterior gluteus medius fibers is performed in the position of Figure 8.6*A*.

The patient may be taught to lie on a tennis ball, as illustrated in Figure 8.9*A* to inactivate TrPs in the middle fibers, and in Figure 8.9*B* for TrPs in the anterior fibers of the gluteus medius muscle. The tennis ball technique is described in Volume 1.[73] Effectiveness of this treatment is increased when the patient rolls the ball along the taut band over the TrP, as described in Section 14, Chapter 9 of this volume.

If the abductors remain weak following inactivation of their TrPs, they can be safely strengthened first under supervision and then at home. In order to use a lengthening contraction and to avoid a shortening contraction of the gluteus medius at this stage, the patient lies on the uninvolved side and first elevates the involved lower limb (with the knee and

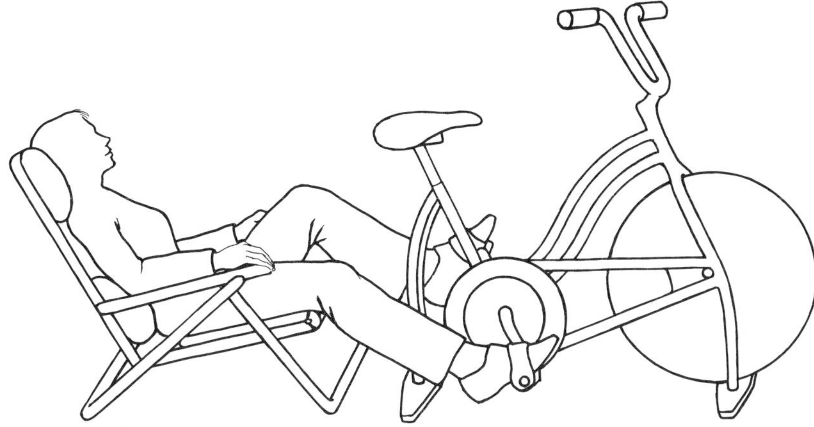

Figure 8.10. Outline drawing of bicycle exercise performed in the semireclining position using a patio recliner with the leg-rest portion folded back. The angle of the back support (amount of hip flexion) is adjusted to the comfort of the individual patient. This arrangement practically eliminates back and gluteal muscle overload while it improves venous return from the lower limbs.

hip straight) in "false" abduction (thigh laterally rotated). The elevation movement in this position activates primarily the thigh flexors. The patient then medially rotates the thigh to the *neutral* position (true abduction) and lowers the limb, using both the tensor fasciae latae and the gluteal muscles in lengthening contractions, resisting gravity. These motions are described and illustrated by Lewit.[33]

Use of an exercise bicycle at home helps to recondition muscles suffering from disuse. However, the upright seated position may aggravate gluteus medius TrPs. Positioning the bicycle to allow the patient to reach the pedals from behind it, while partially reclining with the lower limbs horizontal, can avoid overloading the gluteus medius and postural trunk muscles (Fig. 8.10). To accomplish this, a low chair or folding lounge chair is placed behind the bicycle with the chair seat at the level of the pedals. Pillows or cushions are added, as needed, to support the patient's back at a comfortable angle. Frequent moderate exercise for short periods is more effective than infrequent periods of strenuous exercise. A controlled slowly incremented program permits steady progress with minimum likelihood of overload and relapse.

References

1. Anderson JE: *Grant's Atlas of Anatomy*, Ed. 8. Williams & Wilkins, Baltimore, 1983 (Fig. 4–24).
2. *Ibid.* (Fig. 4–31).
3. *Ibid.* (Fig. 4–38).
4. Arcangeli P, Digiesi V, Ronchi O, *et al.*: Mechanisms of ischemic pain in peripheral occlusive arterial disease. In *Advances in Pain Research and Therapy*, edited by J. J. Bonica and D. Albe-Fessard, Vol. 1. Raven Press, New York, 1976 (pp. 965–973).
5. Bardeen CR: The musculature, Sect. 5. In *Morris's Human Anatomy*, edited by C. M. Jackson, Ed. 6. Blakiston's Son & Co., Philadelphia, 1921.
6. Basmajian JV, Deluca CJ: *Muscles Alive*, Ed. 5. Williams & Wilkins, Baltimore, 1985 (pp. 258, 316–317).
7. Bates T, Grunwaldt E: Myofascial pain in childhood. *J Pediatr 53*:198–209, 1958.
8. Brody SI: Sore throat of myofascial origin. *Milit Med 129*:9–19, 1964.
9. Carter BL, Morehead J, Wolpert SM, *et al.*: *Cross-Sectional Anatomy*. Appleton-Century-Crofts, New York, 1977 (Sects. 35–41, 44–46).
10. Clemente CD: *Gray's Anatomy of the Human Body*, American Ed. 30. Lea & Febiger, Philadelphia, 1985 (pp. 567–568).
11. *Ibid.* (p. 1236)
12. Duchenne GB: *Physiology of Motion*, translated by E.B. Kaplan. J. B. Lippincott, Philadelphia, 1949 (pp.249–252, 254).
13. Ericson MO, Nisell R, Arborelius UP, *et al.*: Muscular activity during ergometer cycling. *Scand J Rehabil Med 17*:53–61, 1985.
14. Ferner H, Staubesand J: *Sobotta Atlas of Human Anatomy*, Ed. 10, Vol. 2. Urban & Schwarzenberg, Baltimore, 1983 (Fig. 152).
15. *Ibid.* (Figs. 331, 403).
16. *Ibid.* (Fig. 406).
17. *Ibid.* (Fig. 410).
18. *Ibid.* (Figs. 415–417).
19. *Ibid.* (Figs. 418, 419).
20. *Ibid.* (Fig. 420).
21. Ghori GMU, Luckwill RG: Responses of the lower limb to load carrying in walking man. *Eur J Appl Physiol 54*:145–150, 1985.

22. Greenlaw RK: *Function of Muscles About the Hip During Normal Level Walking.* Queen's University, Kingston, Ontario, 1973 (thesis) (pp. 87–89, 132–134, 157, 191).
23. Gutstein-Good M: Idiopathic myalgia simulating visceral and other diseases. *Lancet 2*:326–328, 1940 (p. 328, case 6).
24. Hollinshead WH: *Functional Anatomy of the Limbs and Back*, Ed. 4. W.B. Saunders, Philadelphia, 1976 (pp. 297–298, Fig. 18–2).
25. Hollinshead WH: *Anatomy for Surgeons*, Ed. 3., Vol. 3, *The Back and Limbs*. Harper & Row, New York, 1982 (pp. 664–666).
26. Inman VT: Functional aspects of the abductor muscles of the hip. *J Bone Joint Surg 29*:607–619, 1947 (Fig. 4, p. 610).
27. Janda V: *Muscle Function Testing*. Butterworths, London, 1983 (p.172).
28. Kellgren JH: A preliminary account of referred pains arising from muscle. *Br Med J 1*:325–327, 1938 (see p. 327).
29. Kellgren JH: Observations on referred pain arising from muscle. *Clin Sci 3*:175–190, 1938 (pp. 176, 177, Fig. 1).
30. Kelly M: Lumbago and abdominal pain. *Med J Austral 1*:311–317, 1942 (p. 313).
31. Kelly M: Some rules for the employment of local analgesic in the treatment of somatic pain. *Med J Austral 1*:235–239, 1947.
32. Kendall FP, McCreary EK: *Muscles, Testing and Function*, Ed. 3. Williams & Wilkins, Baltimore, 1983 (p. 169).
33. Lewit K: *Manipulative Therapy in Rehabilitation of the Motor System*. Butterworths, London, 1985 (p. 148, Fig. 4.36, p. 285).
34. *Ibid*. (p.281, Fig. 6.101b).
35. Lewit K: Postisometric relaxation in combination with other methods of muscular facilitation and inhibition. *Manual Med 1*:101–104, 1986.
36. Lewit K, Simons DG: Myofascial pain: relief by post-isometric relaxation. *Arch Phys Med Rehabil 65*:452–456, 1984.
37. Lovejoy CO: Evolution of human walking. *Sci Am 259*:118–125, (November) 1988.
38. Lutz EG: Credit-card-wallet sciatica. *JAMA 240*: 738, 1978.
39. Lyons K, Perry J, Gronley JK, *et al*.: Timing and relative intensity of hip extensor and abductor muscle action during level and stair ambulation. *Phys Ther 63*:1597–1605, 1983.
40. McMinn RMH, Hutchings RT: *Color Atlas of Human Anatomy*. Year Book Medical Publishers, Chicago, 1977 (pp. 264, 273, 274).
41. *Ibid*. (p. 302).
42. Markhede G, Stener B: Function after removal of various hip and thigh muscles for extirpation of tumors. *Acta Orthop Scand 52*:373–395, 1981.
43. Németh G, Ekholm J, Aborelius UP: Hip load moments and muscular activity during lifting. *Scand J Rehab Med 16*: 103–111, 1984.
44. Netter FH: *The Ciba Collection of Medical Illustrations*, Vol.8, Musculoskeletal System. Part I: Anatomy, Physiology and Metabolic Disorders. Ciba-Geigy Corporation, Summit, 1987 (p.85).
45. Neumann DA, Cook TM: Effect of load and carrying position on the electromyographic activity of the gluteus medius muscle during walking. *Phys Ther 65*:305–311, 1985.
46. Rasch PJ, Burke RK: *Kinesiology and Applied Anatomy*, Ed. 6. Lea & Febiger, Philadelphia, 1978 (pp. 275–276).
47. Rask MR: Postoperative arachnoradiculitis. *J Neurol Orthop Surg 1*:157–166, 1980.
48. Reynolds MD: Myofascial trigger point syndromes in the practice of rheumatology. *Arch Phys Med Rehabil 62*:111–114, 1981.
49. Rohen JW, Yokochi C: *Color Atlas of Anatomy*, Ed. 2. Igaku-Shoin, New York, 1988 (p. 418).
50. *Ibid*. (pp. 418–419).
51. *Ibid*. (p. 441).
52. Schapira D, Nahir M, Scharf Y: Trochanteric bursitis: a common clinical problem. *Arch Phys Med Rehabil 67*:815–817, 1986.
53. Schenkel C: Das Fächersymptom des M. glutaeus medius bei Hüfttotalendoprothesen. *Z Orthop 110*: 363–367, 1972.
54. Simons, DG: Myofascial pain syndromes, Part of Chapter 11. In *Medical Rehabilitation*, edited by J.V. Basmajian and R.L. Kirby. Williams & Wilkins, Baltimore, 1984 (pp. 209–215, 313–320).
55. Simons DG: Myofascial pain syndrome due to trigger points, Chapter 45. In *Rehabilitation Medicine* edited by Joseph Goodgold. C. V. Mosby Co., St. Louis, 1988 (pp. 686–723).
56. Simons DG, Travell JG: Myofascial origins of low back pain. 3. Pelvic and lower extremity muscles. *Postgrad Med 73*:99–108, 1983.
57. Simons DG, Travell JG: Myofascial pain syndromes, Chapter 25. In *Textbook of Pain* edited by P.D. Wall and R. Melzack, Ed. 2. Churchill Livingstone, London, 1989 (pp. 368–385).
58. Širca A, Sušec-Michieli M: Selective type II fibre muscular atrophy in patients with osteoarthritis of the hip. *J Neurol Sci 44*:149–159, 1980.
59. Soderberg GL, Dostal WF: Electromyographic study of three parts of the gluteus medius muscle during functional activities. *Phys Ther 58*: 691–696, 1978.
60. Sola AE: Trigger point therapy, Chapter 47. In *Clinical Procedures in Emergency Medicine*, edited by J.R. Roberts and J.R. Hedges. W.B. Saunders, Philadelphia, 1985 (pp. 674–686, *see* p. 683).
61. Spalteholz W: *Handatlas der Anatomie des Menschen*, Ed. 11, Vol. 2. S. Hirzel, Leipzig, 1922 (p. 350, Fig. 428).
62. *Ibid*. (p. 358, Fig. 436).
63. Steinbrocker O, Isenberg SA, Silver M, *et al*.: Observations on pain produced by injection of hypertonic saline into muscles and other supportive tissues. *J Clin Invest 32*:1045–1051, 1953.
64. Toldt C: *An Atlas of Human Anatomy*, translated by M.E. Paul, Ed. 2, Vol. 1. Macmillan, New York, 1919 (p. 340).
65. *Ibid*. (p. 341).
66. Travell J: Basis for the multiple uses of local block of somatic trigger areas (procaine infiltration and ethyl chloride spray). *Miss Valley Med J 71*:13–22, 1949 (see pp. 19–20).
67. Travell J: Factors affecting pain of injection. *JAMA 158*:368–371, 1955.
68. Travell J, Rinzler SH: The myofascial genesis of pain. *Postgrad Med 11*:425–434, 1952.
69. Travell JG, Simons DG: *Myofascial Pain and Dysfunction: The Trigger Point Manual*. Williams & Wilkins, Baltimore, 1983 (pp. 103–164).
70. *Ibid*. (pp. 104–110, 651–653).

71. *Ibid.* (pp. 109–110, 651–653).
72. *Ibid.* (p. 209).
73. *Ibid.* (p. 386)
74. *Ibid.* (p. 432).
75. Travell J, Travell W: Therapy of low back pain by manipulation and of referred pain in the lower extremity by procaine infiltration. *Arch Phys Med 27*:537–547, 1946 (pp. 544–545).
76. Weber EF: Ueber die Längenverhältnisse der Fleischfasern der Muskeln in Allgemeinen. *Berichte über die Verhandlungen der Königlich Sächsischen Gesellschaft der Wissenschaften zu Leipzig 3*: 63–86, 1851.
77. Wilson GL, Capen EK, Stubbs NB: A fine-wire electrode investigation of the gluteus minimus and gluteus medius muscles. *Res Q Am Assoc Health Phys Educ 47*:824–828, 1976.
78. Winter Z: Referred pain in fibrositis. *Med Rec 157*:34–37, 1944.

PART 1

CHAPTER 9
Gluteus Minimus Muscle

"Pseudo-Sciatica"

PART 1

HIGHLIGHTS: The **REFERRED PAIN** from trigger points (TrPs) in the anterior part of the gluteus minimus muscle extends over the lower lateral buttock, down the lateral aspect of the thigh, knee, and leg to the ankle. The TrPs in the posterior fibers of this muscle have a similar but more posterior pattern that projects pain over the lower medial aspect of the buttock, and down the back of the thigh and calf. The **ANATOMICAL ATTACHMENTS** of the gluteus minimus are similar to, but less extensive in length than, those of the overlying gluteus medius. The primary **FUNCTION** of this abductor of the thigh is to help keep the pelvis level during single-limb weight bearing. The TrPs in this muscle cause **SYMPTOMS** of pain in a characteristic pattern, especially when arising from a chair or when walking. To distinguish these symptoms from similar ones caused by radiculopathy, the responsible TrPs must be positively identified. **ACTIVATION** of TrPs in the gluteus minimus can be caused by acute or chronic overload, by displacement of the sacroiliac joint, and by nerve root irritation. They may be perpetuated by these factors and also by prolonged immobility or by sitting on a wallet in the back pocket. The position for **TRIGGER POINT EXAMINATION** is side lying on the unaffected side. To locate TrPs in the anterior fibers of this muscle, the borders of the tensor fasciae latae muscle are identified distal to the anterior superior iliac spine. The gluteus minimus is palpated for spot tenderness deep to the tensor fasciae latae muscle. To locate TrPs in the posterior fibers, the line corresponding to the lower border of the gluteus minimus is identified and the region above this line explored for localized deep tenderness. The clinician should consider **ASSOCIATED TRIGGER POINTS** in the quadratus lumborum as perpetuators of satellite gluteus minimus TrPs. To apply **INTERMITTENT COLD WITH STRETCH** to this muscle, the involved (uppermost) thigh of the side-lying patient is adducted over the side or end of the examining table and the intermittent cold is applied over the muscle fibers and their referred pain zones. Added extension emphasizes lengthening of anterior fibers, and flexion to 30° emphasizes lengthening of posterior fibers. The **INJECTION-AND-STRETCH** approach first requires localization of the focal tenderness characteristic of TrPs in the tight muscle. Useful **CORRECTIVE ACTIONS** include loss of excessive body weight, keeping the body warm, changing hip position frequently, appropriate body positioning at night, correction of sacroiliac joint displacement, avoidance of strenuous unaccustomed physical activities, and avoidance of the injection of medications into the muscle. A home self-stretch program should be established for most patients with this myofascial pain syndrome.

---

1. REFERRED PAIN
(Figs. 9.1 and 9.2)

Pain referred from gluteus minimus TrPs can be intolerably persistent and excruciatingly severe. The TrP source of the pain is so deep in the gluteal musculature and much of the pain is so remote from the muscle that its true origin is easily overlooked.

Travell, in 1946, first distinguished the pain patterns of TrPs in the anterior and posterior portions of the gluteus minimus muscle. These portions refer pain down the lateral and posterior aspects of the lower limb, respectively.[56]

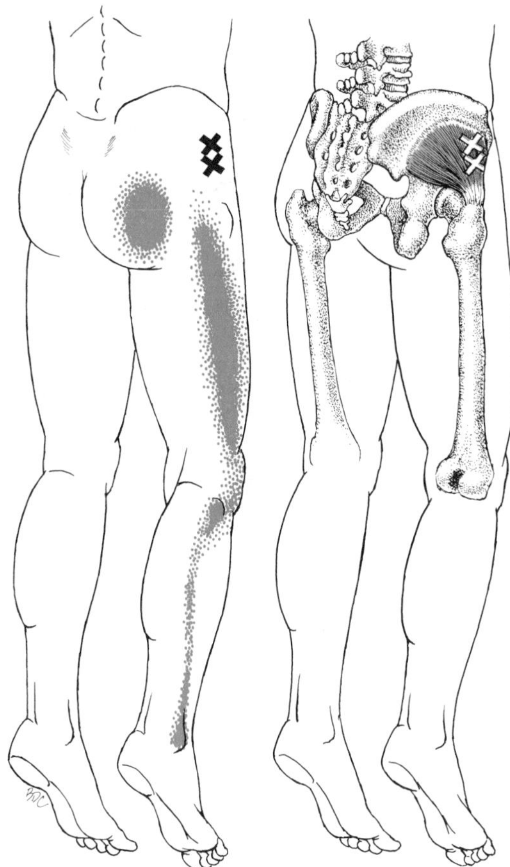

Figure 9.1. Pattern of referred pain from trigger points (TrPs) (***X**s*) in the anterior portion of the right gluteus minimus muscle (*light red*). The essential pain pattern is *solid red* and the spillover extension found when the muscle is more severely involved is *stippled*.

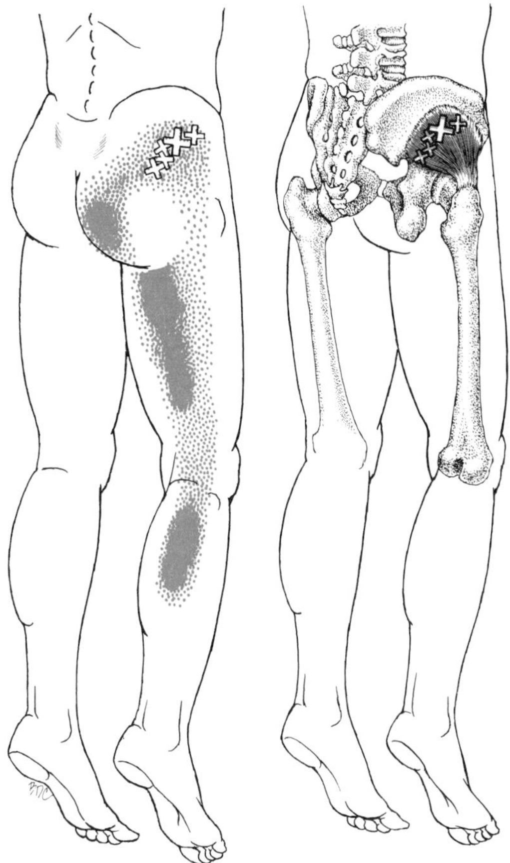

Figure 9.2. Composite pain pattern (*bright red*) referred from TrPs (***X**s*) in the posterior part of the right gluteus minimus muscle (*darker red*). The essential pain pattern is *solid red* and the spillover pattern is *stippled*. The *large* **X** marks the most common location of TrPs in the posterior part of this muscle. The most anterior *small* ***X*** lies at the junction of the anterior and posterior portions of this muscle.

These patterns, unlike those of the two more superficial gluteal muscles, may extend to the ankle, as also reported subsequently.[43–47,53,54,61]

The TrPs in the anterior portion of the gluteus minimus project both pain and tenderness (Fig. 9.1) to the lower lateral part of the buttock, the lateral aspect of the thigh and knee, and to the peroneal region of the leg as far as the ankle. Ordinarily, gluteus minimus referred pain does not extend beyond the ankle.[56] Rarely, however, it may include the dorsum of the foot.[53]

Myofascial TrPs located in the posterior part of the gluteus minimus muscle refer pain and tenderness (Fig. 9.2) in a pattern that includes most of the buttock (concentrating on its lower medial aspect), and that covers the posterior aspect of the thigh and calf. This referred pattern of pain sometimes includes the back of the knee. Referral of tenderness to the gluteal portion of this pain pattern may account for the diffuse tenderness of the gluteus maximus muscle that is observed in many patients with posterior gluteus minimus TrPs.

Good[18] described pain in the sciatic distribution as commonly arising from tender spots in gluteal muscles, without specifying which muscle. Kellgren[24] found that in 55 of 70 patients seen for "sciatica" the pain was of ligamentous or muscular origin, commonly from the gluteal musculature.

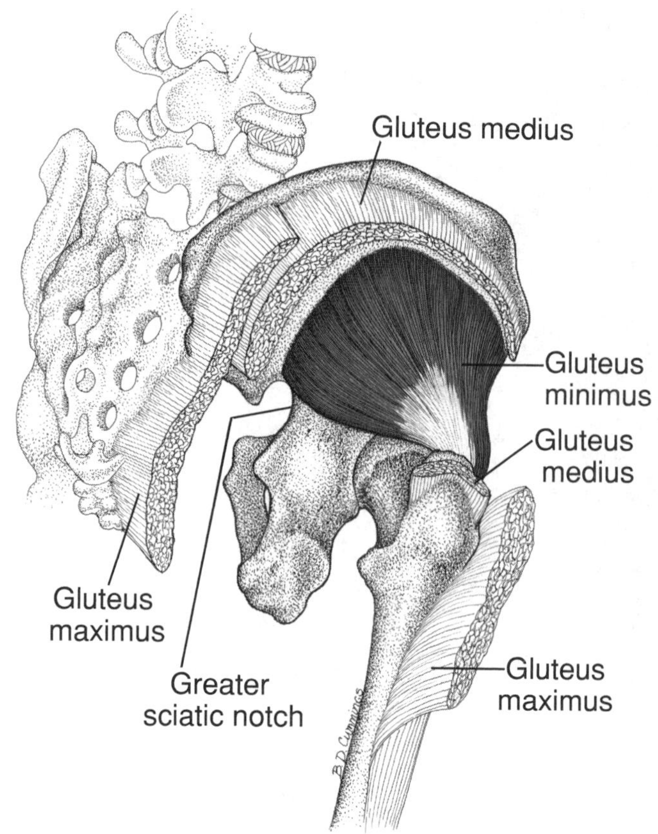

Figure 9.3. Attachments of the right gluteus minimus muscle (*red*) in the posterolateral view. To a large extent, the overlying gluteus maximus and gluteus medius muscles have been removed.

2. ANATOMICAL ATTACHMENTS AND CONSIDERATIONS

(Figs. 9.3 and 9.4)

The gluteus minimus, the deepest of the three gluteal muscles, is also the smallest in length and lightest in weight.[58] Its fan shape conforms closely to the overlying gluteus medius (Fig. 9.3). ***Proximally***, its fibers attach to the pelvis along the outer surface of the ilium between the anterior and inferior gluteal lines. This attachment closely approaches the greater sciatic foramen (Fig. 9.3) through which the piriformis muscle exits the pelvis[50] (*see* Fig. 10.2). ***Distally***, the fibers of the gluteus minimus converge onto its tendon, which attaches to the femur at the uppermost part of the anterior surface of the greater trochanter,[8,22] deep and anterior to the attachment of the piriformis muscle.[30,31,50]

The relative thickness of the gluteus minimus and its anatomical relation to the tensor fasciae latae are shown in the serial cross sections of Figure 9.4. The greater thickness of the anterior part of the gluteus minimus, as compared with its posterior part, is not generally appreciated. This difference in thickness is seen in the lowest section of Figure 9.4, the plane of which lies approximately midway between the anterior superior iliac spine and the anterior inferior iliac spine. That cross section also illustrates how one can palpate the anterior part of the gluteus minimus both behind the posterior margin of the tensor fasciae latae and between the tensor's anterior margin and the anterior border of the ilium.

The trochanteric bursa of the gluteus minimus, which lies between the anterior part of the muscle's tendon and the greater trochanter, facilitates gliding movement of the tendon over the trochanter.[8,22] This gliding movement of the tendon is necessary for the anterior fibers of the muscle to reach full stretch range of motion.

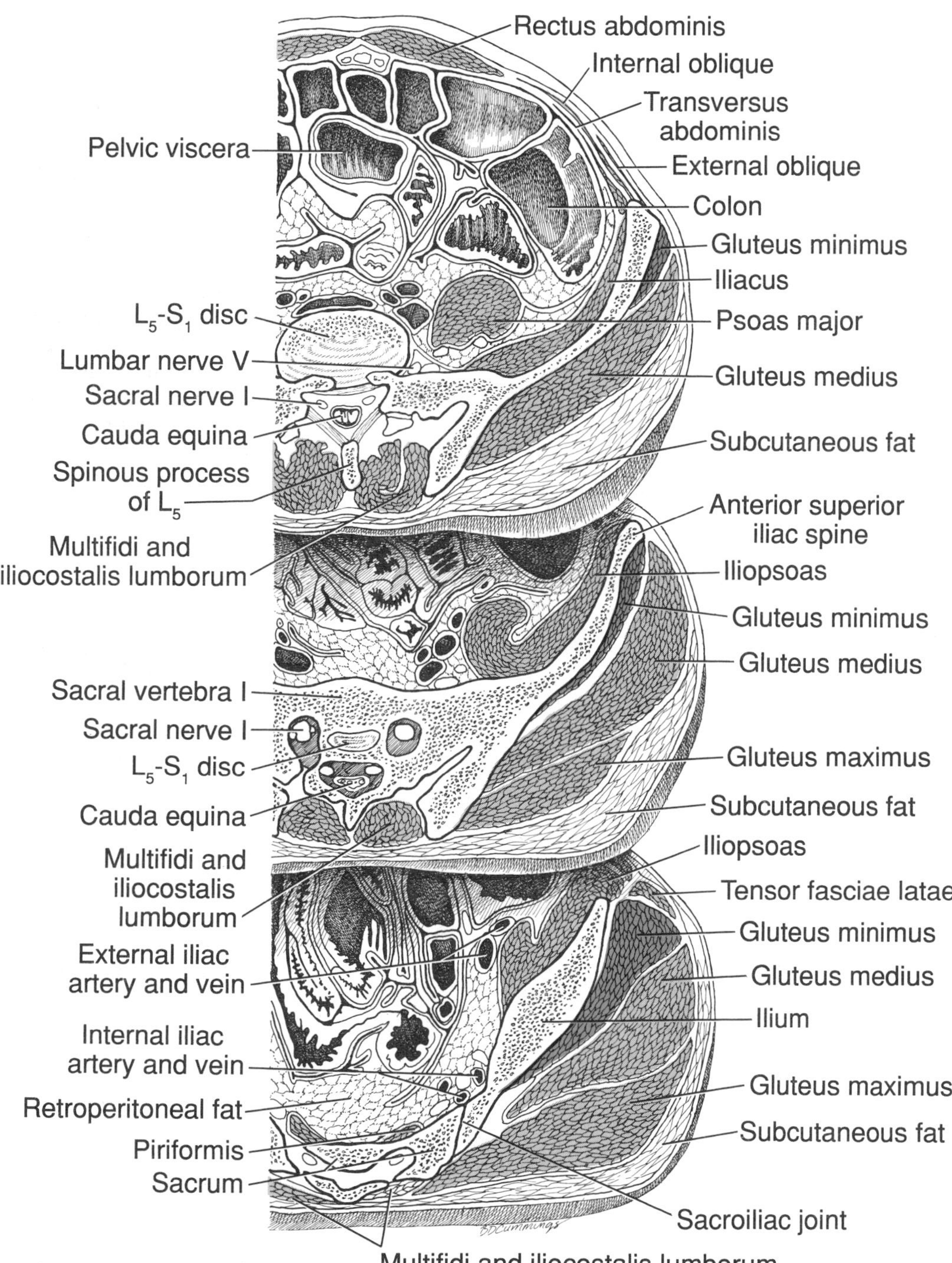

Figure 9.4. Serial cross sections through the pelvis that show the gluteus minimus muscle (*dark red*). The three sections show the relation of the anterior portion of this muscle to the ilium, to neighboring muscles (*light red*) and to the skin. The level of the middle section passes through the anterior superior iliac spine. The plane of the lowest section lies between the anterior superior iliac spine and the anterior inferior iliac spine. At the latter level, the thickest part of the anterior portion of the gluteus minimus muscle may be subcutaneous between the tensor fasciae latae and the gluteus medius muscles. This anterior portion is palpated for TrPs along the posterior margin of and deep to the tensor fasciae latae muscle.

Supplemental References

The entire gluteus minimus muscle is presented in serial cross sections.[7] Frontal sections through the hip joint show the relation of the distal portion of this muscle to the other two gluteal muscles.[12]

Just below the level of the anterior inferior iliac spine, tenderness in the anterior gluteus minimus can be palpated only by exerting deep pressure between the tensor fasciae latae muscle on one side and the rectus femoris tendon and sartorius muscle on the other. A section through, and perpendicular to, the axis of the neck of the femur[14,36] shows why.

The gluteus minimus and piriformis muscles are seen from behind,[1,15,49,50] with vascular supply,[13] and in relation to the other two gluteal muscles.[34] Seen from the side,[3] the thick anterior portion of the gluteus minimus is readily apparent. Seen from in front,[51] the potential for palpating the anterior portion deep to the anterior or posterior edge of the tensor fasciae latae muscle can be appreciated. This approach can be visualized by noting the attachment of the tensor fasciae latae on the ilium in relation to the attachments of the gluteus medius and minimus muscles.[2,30,35]

3. INNERVATION

The gluteus minimus muscle is innervated by both the superior and inferior branches of the superior gluteal nerve. The superior gluteal nerve passes between the gluteus medius and gluteus minimus muscles as it sends branches to both of these muscles. This nerve carries fibers from the L_4, L_5, and S_1 spinal nerves.[9]

4. FUNCTION

Actions

All fibers of the gluteus minimus muscle contribute to abduction of the thigh when the distal part of the lower limb is free to move. The fan-shaped arrangement of fibers in this muscle corresponds closely to the fiber arrangement in the overlying gluteus medius. Both muscles attach to the same bones at adjacent locations; therefore, the actions of corresponding anterior or posterior fibers of the gluteus minimus and gluteus medius muscles are similar.

As with the gluteus medius, the anterior fibers of the gluteus minimus are considered much more effective in producing medial rotation of the thigh than the posterior fibers are in producing lateral rotation.[5,22] This conclusion is reinforced by examination of an articulated skeleton and noting the location of the muscle's attachments.

Functions

The functions of the gluteus minimus are usually lumped with those of the gluteus medius. Authors generally agree that all of the gluteus minimus fibers assist the gluteus medius muscle in its stabilizing function of maintaining the pelvis level during ambulation.[5,8,20,37] It thus helps prevent the pelvis from dropping excessively (tilting laterally) toward the unsupported side.

Duchenne[10] identified no subject in whom the gluteus medius had atrophied and the gluteus minimus remained. He assumed that the responses to stimulation of the anterior and posterior portions of the gluteus medius applied equally to the gluteus minimus. Although Greenlaw[20] recorded electrical activity separately from the anterior and posterior portions of the gluteus medius muscle, he monitored the gluteus minimus in only one location, 3.7 cm (1½ in) above the tip of the greater trochanter, probably sampling its middle fibers. Thus, this study provides limited EMG data on the contribution by the gluteus minimus muscle to medial and lateral rotation of the thigh. In another EMG study,[60] fine-wire electrodes were placed in the gluteus minimus 5 cm (2 in) posterior to the anterior superior iliac spine, which would be among the anterior or middle fibers of the muscle. These authors reported activity with abduction and medial rotation of the thigh, as would be expected of the anterior fibers, but not with lateral rotation.

The functional relationship of the gluteus minimus to the gluteus medius is also influenced by the fact that the gluteus minimus is considerably smaller than the gluteus medius muscle. Inman[23] found that, in five cadavers, the weight ratio between the gluteus minimus and gluteus medius was nearly 1:2. Weber[58] in one specimen and Voss[57] in 12 specimens reported that the weight ratios of gluteus minimus to gluteus medius to gluteus maximus closely approximated 1:3:6. Mean fiber lengths for the gluteus minimus and gluteus medius were 4.8 cm and 6.8 cm, respectively.[58]

The evolutionary transition of the gluteus medius and gluteus minimus from propulsive to stabilizing muscles of ambulation is well described and illustrated.[29]

5. FUNCTIONAL (MYOTATIC) UNIT

Medial rotation at the hip by the anterior gluteus minimus and tensor fasciae latae muscles is assisted by the anterior fibers of the gluteus medius muscle. This action is opposed chiefly by the gluteus maximus and piriformis muscles, together with the lateral rotator group: the quadratus femoris, the two gemelli, and the two obturator muscles.

Agonists for the hip abduction function of the gluteus minimus muscle are the gluteus medius and tensor fasciae latae.[23] Abduction is countered primarily by the four major adductor muscles: the adductores magnus, longus, and brevis with the pectineus muscle and, to a lesser extent, by the gracilis muscle.

6. SYMPTOMS

Patients complain of hip pain that may cause a limp during walking. Lying on the affected side may be so painful that rolling over onto that side during the night interrupts sleep. After sitting for a while, patients with active TrPs in the anterior gluteus minimus often have difficulty rising from the chair and standing up straight[56] because the movement becomes painful.

The pain from TrPs in this muscle can be constant and excruciating. The patient may not be able to find a stretching movement or change of position that relieves the pain and can neither lie down comfortably nor walk normally.

Differential Diagnosis

The pain referred from gluteus minimus TrPs should be distinguished from that of gluteus medius and piriformis TrPs; an L_4, L_5, or S_1 radiculopathy; trochanteric bursitis; and from the pain of articular ("somatic") dysfunction. *Sciatica is a symptom, not a diagnosis; its cause should be identified.*

If the myofascial pain is referred deep into the hip joint, the source is probably TrPs in the tensor fasciae latae muscle rather than in the gluteus minimus. Low back pain in the sacral and sacroiliac regions is more likely to be due to TrPs in the gluteus medius than in the gluteus minimus muscle; the latter rarely, if ever, causes pain in this area.

Other Myofascial Syndromes

Distinguishing gluteus minimus TrPs from those in the piriformis and the overlying gluteus medius depends partly on the differences in their pain patterns and partly on where in the buttock the TrPs are located. The gluteus minimus and piriformis lie beside each other with occasional overlap, have adjacent attachments, and generate somewhat similar distributions of referred pain. The piriformis pain pattern may occasionally extend as far distally as the knee, whereas the gluteus minimus pattern usually includes the calf in addition to the thigh. A line drawn to divide the gluteus minimus from the piriformis is shown in the previous chapter, Figure 8.5*B*. This piriformis line extends from the upper border of the greater trochanter to the upper end of the palpable free border of the sacrum, where the palpating finger encounters the ilium near the caudal end of the sacroiliac (SI) joint.

Pain referred from the gluteus medius is less likely to involve the thigh; gluteus maximus TrPs restrict flexion at the hip, while piriformis TrPs restrict medial rotation. TrPs in the gluteus minimus are difficult to distinguish by palpation from those in the overlying gluteus medius throughout their large area of overlap (Fig. 8.5*A*).

Radiculopathy

The gluteus minimus is a potent myofascial source of pseudoradicular syndromes.[39] The symptoms produced by TrPs in the anterior fibers of the muscle may be mistaken for an L_5 radiculopathy,[38,53] and symptoms from the posterior fibers mimic an S_1 radiculopathy.[38] Knee pain that suggests an L_4 radiculopathy is not characteristic of gluteus minimus TrPs. Sensory or motor deficits and paresthesias in a nerve-distribution pattern, imaging of the spine, and electrodiagnostic tests distinguish neurogenic from TrP-referred pain. The latter is recognized by locating the TrPs and identifying their associated phenomena. However, a lancinating pain is more likely to be indicative of radiculopathy or sciatic nerve entrapment by the piriformis muscle.

Bursitis

The pain radiating from trochanteric bursitis travels from the buttock along the lateral aspect of the thigh to the knee[28,40] and should not be confused with myofascial referred pain. In the patient who has bursitis and is side lying with the hip partially flexed, distinct tenderness is elicited over the bursa; digital pressure on the bursa reproduces the patient's pain complaint. In the presence of trochanteric bursitis, the gliding movement of the gluteal tendons over the greater trochanter during stretching of the anterior part of the gluteus minimus or the tensor fascia latae muscle becomes exquisitely painful. One must determine by physical examination for TrPs whether the deep tenderness is referred, at least in part, from the gluteal and/or quadratus lumborum muscles.

Articular Dysfunction

Another associated disorder, blockage of movement of the SI joint, may be sustained by the persistent asymmetrical muscle tension on the pelvis caused by gluteus minimus TrPs. When this combination of SI joint dysfunction and gluteus minimus TrPs appears with restricted mobility of the lowest two intervertebral joints of the lumbar spine and tenderness of the L_4-S_1 spinous processes, this group of findings is characterized by Lewit[26] as a chain reaction. However, tenderness of the spinous processes may also be referred from TrPs in the adjacent multifidi and rotatores paraspinal muscles.

The pain referred by lumbar facet joints is described and illustrated in Chapter 3 on pages 25–26. It often overlaps the pain pattern of gluteus minimus TrPs.

Sciatica

Sciatica is a non-specific term commonly applied to the symptom of pain radiating downward from the buttock over the posterior or outer side of the lower limb.

The pain may be either myofascial or neurological in origin. Myofascial TrPs in the posterior gluteus minimus muscle can be a common source of sciatica.[47,53] This cause of sciatica is easily overlooked if the clinician does not examine the muscles.

Sciatica is usually assumed to be caused by compression of a nerve. A common neurological cause of this pain is entrapment of the sciatic and/or posterior femoral cutaneous nerves by the piriformis muscle as the nerves exit the pelvis through the greater sciatic foramen (*see* Chapter 10). Other neurogenic sciaticas include nerve root compression by spinal tumors,[41] by spinal stenosis,[25] or, rarely, by variant fascial bands,[4,48] and compression of the cauda equina by a herniated lumbar disc (radiculopathy).[6,17,25,42,53] Compression and pain may also be caused by an aneurysm.[21,59]

Negrin and Fardin[33] reported on the follow-up results of 41 patients with acute sciatica (lumbosciatalgia) and electromyographically proven monoradicular denervation. Of these, 19 underwent surgery and 22 were treated medically. Three to eight years later, among the operated patients with severe motor impairment, 33% recovered and 33% improved motor function; in the non-operated group, the initial paralysis remained largely unchanged. However, no significant difference was reported in pain relief between the operated and non-operated groups. The patients were more concerned about their pain than about their motor deficits.[33] The pain of these patients apparently was caused as much by associated TrPs, or other disorders of muscles and fasciae, as by the nerve compression.

Sheon and associates[42] suggest that "pseudosciatica" is a more appropriate diagnosis than "sciatica" when sensory and motor neurological findings are normal. In these cases, they suggest that bursitis and myofascial pain probably cause the symptoms. Kellgren[24] reported, as noted in Section 1, that, in 50 of 70 cases of sciatica, the pain was caused by ligamentous and muscular lesions. Others note that many of the patients designated as having sciatica without evidence of neurological disease probably suffer pain of myofascial origin.[38,61]

7. ACTIVATION AND PERPETUATION OF TRIGGER POINTS

Myofascial TrPs in the gluteus minimus muscle may be activated or perpetuated by sudden acute or repetitive chronic overload, SI joint dysfunction, injection of medications into the muscle, and nerve root irritation. Perpetuating factors may include prolonged immobility, tilting the pelvis by sitting on a wallet, and unstable equilibrium when standing.

Activation of Trigger Points

Gluteus minimus TrPs may be activated by an acute overload imposed by a fall; by walking too far or too fast, especially on rough ground; or by overuse in running and sports activities, such as tennis and handball. Distortion of the normal gait sufficient to induce gluteus minimus TrPs was caused in one case by a painful blister on the foot and, in another case, by walking extensively for 2 days while limping on a painful knee.

In the senior author's experience,[56] referred pain in the lower limbs following SI joint displacement results most frequently from TrPs located in the gluteus minimus muscle. The next most likely muscles to be involved with SI joint dysfunction are the erector spinae, quadratus lumborum, gluteus medius, gluteus maximus, piriformis, and, less frequently, the adductors of the thigh.[56]

The gluteus minimus is the least desirable of the gluteal muscles as a site for intramuscular injection of irritant medication; neither the gluteus maximus nor the gluteus medius muscle is as prone to develop TrPs following medication injections as is the gluteus minimus.[52] The minimus is too deep to permit easy identification of spot tenderness caused by latent TrPs. Latent TrPs in this muscle, when activated by injection of irritant medications, can refer severe "sciatica" that may last for months. The gluteus minimus muscle and the nearby sciatic nerve can be avoided by injecting the medication into the gluteus medius muscle in the upper outer quadrant of the buttock, or into the deltoid muscle.

The post-lumbar laminectomy pain syndrome[39] is frequently caused by residual myofascial TrPs that had been activated by the radiculopathy, for which a successful laminectomy had been performed. These active TrPs remain like dust on the shelf that must be wiped clean. Such residual gluteus minimus TrPs are particularly confusing when they mimic the pain for which the laminectomy was performed.

Perpetuation of Trigger Points

Prolonged immobility is a potent source of aggravation of TrPs. Since the position of the right foot is fixed on the accelerator when one drives a car, the right hip muscles are effectively immobilized unless a special effort is made to reposition the thigh and hip. Automatic cruise control permits safe intermittent repositioning of the foot, knee, and hip.

The gluteus minimus and gluteus medius muscles are relatively immobilized during prolonged standing, as when waiting in line or when standing at a cocktail party. Unless the individual frequently shifts weight from one lower limb to another, the latent TrPs may become active.

Sacroiliac joint dysfunction can both activate and perpetuate these gluteal TrPs.

Sitting on a wallet placed in a long back pocket can impinge on gluteus minimus TrPs and produce referred pain in a sciaticlike distribution.[19]

When standing, if the feet are placed close together, the base of support is reduced. For those who have suffered a loss of equilibrium, the resultant unsteadiness can increase the demands on the gluteus minimus and gluteus medius muscles, chronically overloading them.

8. PATIENT EXAMINATION

Patients with gluteus minimus TrPs exhibit some degree of antalgic gait, which may be so severe that they must either limp awkwardly or walk with a cane. When the TrPs are very hyperirritable, the seated patient is unable to cross the affected leg over the opposite knee because of painfully restricted adduction. Passive stretch of the involved muscle is

PART 1

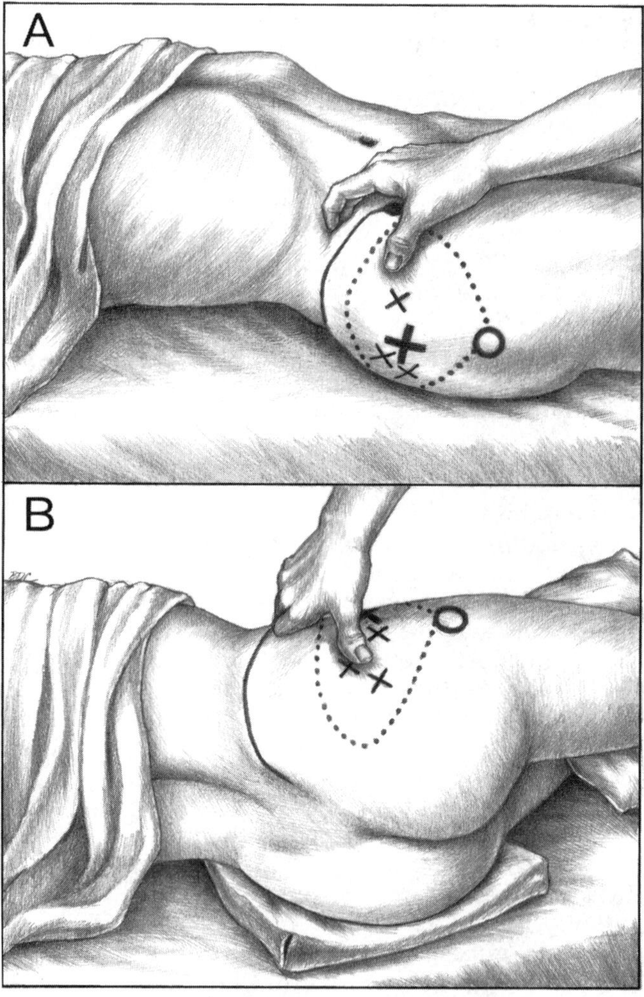

Figure 9.5. Flat palpation of TrPs in the anterior and posterior portions of the right gluteus minimus muscle. The *open circle* marks the greater trochanter. The *solid circle* identifies the anterior superior iliac spine and terminates the *solid line*, which follows the crest of the ilium. The *dotted line* outlines the gluteus minimus muscle and the ***X**s* locate its trigger points. *A*, palpation of an anterior gluteus minimus TrP deep to the posterior border of the tensor fasciae latae muscle, with the patient supine. The adjacent *small* ***X*** is an intermediate TrP between the anterior and posterior parts of the muscle. The *large* ***X*** locates the most common TrP in the posterior part of the muscle. *B*, with the patient side lying, palpation of the most frequent posterior TrP (*large* ***X*** in *A*). The two most posterior *small* ***X**s* locate less common posterior TrPs. The more anterior *small* ***X*** is the intermediate trigger point noted above in *A*. The most anterior, incomplete *large* ***X*** identifies the most common anterior trigger point. The uppermost thigh is positioned in about 30° of flexion and in as much adduction as is comfortable, using the *pillow* to support the uppermost thigh.

limited in range and is painful; active contraction is likely to elicit "ratchety" weakness. Altered sensations of pain, dysesthesia, or numbness may be elicited in the pain reference zone. Otherwise, no neurological deficits are observed due to gluteus minimus TrPs.

9. TRIGGER POINT EXAMINATION (Fig. 9.5)

Myofascial TrPs in the gluteus minimus muscle usually lie deep to both the gluteus maximus and the gluteus medius muscles or deep to the tensor fasciae latae. Therefore, taut bands in the gluteus minimus are unlikely to be palpable, but TrP spot tenderness can be clearly localized. Occasionally, if the overlying gluteal muscles are fully relaxed, one can feel the tension of taut bands deep in the buttock, and snapping palpation of active TrPs in the posterior fibers of the gluteus minimus may rarely induce a thigh jerk caused by a local twitch response. Occasionally, the referred pain pattern can be induced by sustained pressure on the tender TrP, but pain referred from this muscle usually is evoked only by a needle encountering its TrPs.

Anterior Trigger Points

For examination of anterior gluteus minimus TrPs, the patient lies supine, as illustrated in Figure 9.5*A*, with the thigh of the affected limb extended to the limit of comfort. If necessary, the knee is supported by a pillow. The anterior superior iliac spine is palpated at the anterior end of the iliac crest. The tensor fasciae latae muscle is identified by asking the patient to try to rotate the thigh medially against resistance while the clinician palpates to locate the tensed muscle that lies just under the skin.

The anterior fibers of the gluteus minimus are then explored for TrP tenderness by palpating deeply, first anterior to and then posterior to the tensor fasciae latae muscle, just distal to the level of the anterior superior iliac spine. In some patients, a thin layer of gluteus medius muscle may cover all of this anterior portion of the gluteus minimus.[35] In other patients, the gluteus medius may cover the gluteus minimus muscle deep to the posterior border, but not the anterior border, of the tensor fasciae latae muscle.[2,16,30] Thus, examining deep to the anterior border of the tensor fasciae latae muscle is usually more satisfactory when palpating for the spot tenderness of anterior gluteus minimus TrPs.

The accessibility of the anterior fibers of the gluteus minimus muscle to direct palpation depends on the location of the overlying fibers of the tensor fasciae latae, and possibly the gluteus medius muscle, in that individual (*see* Section 2). The lowest cross section in Figure 9.4 shows how spot tenderness in the gluteus minimus may be elicited by deep palpation applied along either the anterior or posterior margin of the tensor fasciae latae muscle. Which site is most useful depends on individual anatomical variations of the ilial attachments of these two muscles. The ilial attachments portrayed by McMinn and Hutchings[30] would permit direct access to the gluteus minimus only along the anterior border of the tensor fasciae latae slightly lateral and distal to the anterior superior iliac spine.

Posterior Trigger Points

To locate strongly active TrPs in the posterior portion of the gluteus minimus, the patient lies on the uninvolved side with the uppermost thigh adducted and slightly *flexed* to about 30° (Fig. 9.5*B*).

The lower posterior (medial) border of the gluteus minimus muscle is identified by locating the piriformis line that represents its common boundary with the upper border of the piriformis muscle (*see black line* in Chapter 8, Fig. 8.5*B*). The piriformis line begins 1 cm (½ in) cephalad to the upper edge of the palpable protuberance of the greater trochanter (attachment of piriformis tendon) and runs to the upper end of the palpable border of the sacrum just below the SI joint, where the piriformis muscle enters the pelvis.

The region of the most posterior TrPs in the gluteus minimus muscle can be estimated by use of the black (piriformis) line in Figure 8.5*B*. These TrPs are found superior to that line between its midpoint and the junction of its middle and lateral thirds (Fig. 9.5*B* and Fig. 8.5*B*). The most inferior (posterior) *dotted line* in Figure 9.5 is in the same location as the piriformis line of Figure 8.5*B*.

10. ENTRAPMENTS

No neurological entrapments have been identified as being due to tension induced by TrPs in this muscle.

11. ASSOCIATED TRIGGER POINTS

Active myofascial TrPs in the gluteus minimus muscle rarely present as a single-muscle syndrome. The TrPs in this muscle are most often observed in association with TrPs in the piriformis, gluteus medius, vastus lateralis, peroneus longus, quadratus lumborum, and, sometimes, the gluteus maximus muscle.

The two muscles that are most closely associated functionally with the gluteus minimus (the gluteus medius and the piriformis) are also the most likely to develop secondary TrPs. The posterior fibers of the gluteus minimus and the piriformis muscle frequently develop associated TrPs. Similarly, the anterior fibers of the gluteus minimus and the tensor fasciae latae are closely related functionally and may develop associated TrPs. The fact that the flexion and extension functions of the gluteus minimus are inconstant and variable[37] accounts for the lack of associated functional unit TrPs in the hamstring and calf muscles.

The vastus lateralis may develop TrPs that are *satellites* to those in the anterior part of the gluteus minimus muscle.

Myofascial TrPs commonly develop in the posterior portion of the gluteus

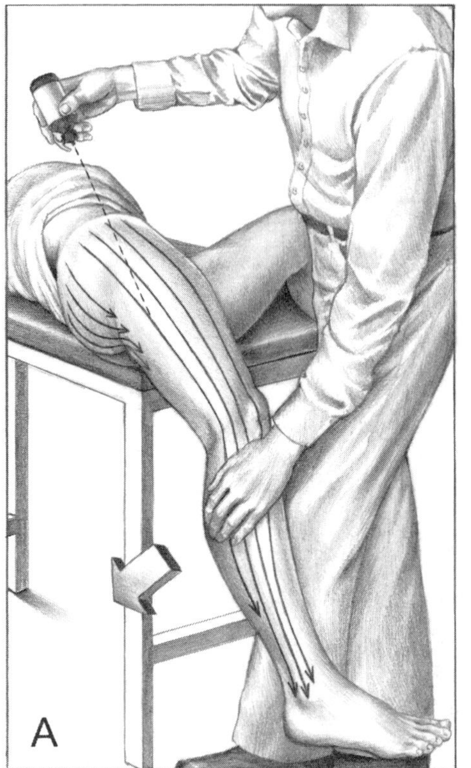

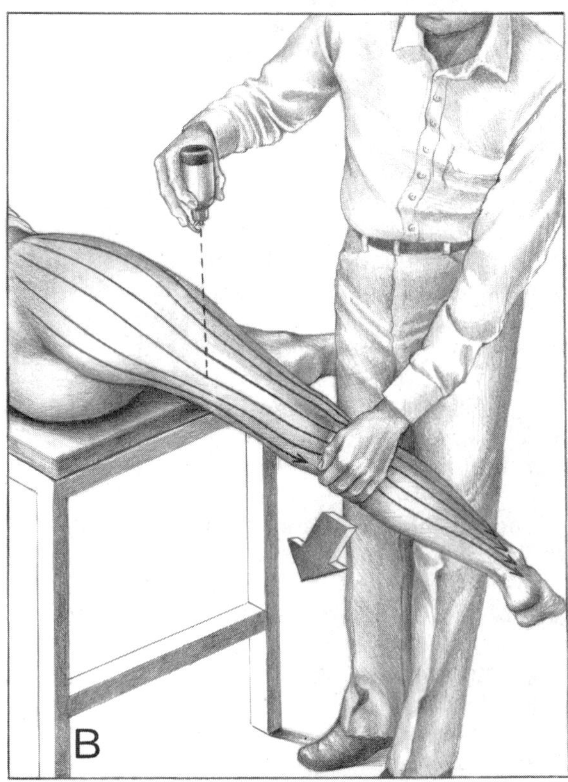

Figure 9.6. Stretch positions and intermittent cold patterns (*thin arrows*) for TrPs in the anterior and posterior portions of the gluteus minimus muscle. The jet stream of the vapocoolant spray or ice covers first the TrP region of the muscle and then its referred pain pattern. The *thick arrows* identify the direction of movement to stretch the muscle passively. In the stretch position shown, the lower limb extends beyond the end of the table. *A,* for inactivation of anterior TrPs, the thigh is gradually extended while it is adducted by the pull of gravity, fully elongating the anterior portions of the gluteus minimus and gluteus medius. *B*, to inactivate posterior TrPs, the thigh is flexed 30° at the hip, medially rotated, and then adducted by the pull of gravity as intermittent cold is applied. An alternative position is to swing the lower limb over the side of the treatment table as illustrated in Figure 8.6 for the gluteus medius; the intermittent cold pattern illustrated in this figure is also used with the alternative position.

minimus muscle, and less frequently in the anterior portion, as satellites to quadratus lumborum TrPs. This coupling can be so strong that pressure exerted on the quadratus lumborum TrPs induces not only the expected referred pain in the buttock but also unexpected pain referred down the back of the lower limb. This additional pain results from activation of satellite TrPs in the posterior part of the gluteus minimus; pressure applied to these gluteal TrPs elicits the same lower limb pain. Sometimes elimination of the quadratus lumborum TrPs inactivates the satellite gluteal TrPs. In other patients, TrPs in the two muscles must be inactivated separately.

Similarly, the peroneus longus, which lies in the pain reference zone of the anterior part of the gluteus minimus, has been seen to develop satellite TrPs from that part of this gluteal muscle.

12. INTERMITTENT COLD WITH STRETCH
(Fig. 9.6)

Details of using intermittent cold with stretch are found in Volume 1 on pages 63–74 for the stretch-and-spray technique and in Chapter 2 on page 9 of this volume for the application of ice instead of vapocoolant spray.

Intermittent cold with stretch can be applied to the gluteus minimus muscle with the patient lying on the uninvolved side and the buttocks close to the end of the treatment table (Fig. 9.6*A* and *B*). The lower limb to be treated extends over the end of the table, but is supported by the operator to avoid overloading the involved muscle. The patient may grasp the side of the table for stabilization.

For intermittent cold with stretch, one must first determine whether the TrPs are located in the anterior or the posterior fibers of the gluteus minimus.

Anterior Fibers

To release TrP tension in the anterior fibers, the thigh of the opposite (noninvolved) lower limb is flexed at the hip to stabilize the patient's pelvis (Fig. 9.6*A*). If the knee of the limb being treated is flexed about 90° (not shown in the figure), gravity tends to produce some lateral rotation of the thigh, which helps to elongate the anterior fibers of the muscle.

The edge of a plastic-wrapped block of ice or the jet stream of vapocoolant spray is applied in parallel sweeps first over the anterior half of the muscle and then over the pain reference zones—the buttock, lateral thigh, and leg—as depicted in Figure 9.6*A*. The anterior fibers are passively lengthened by first moderately extending the thigh and then adducting it by *gently* allowing the foot to ease further downward toward the floor, assisted by gravity. At first, the operator may need to support part of the weight of the limb. As TrP tension eases, the full effect of gravity is tolerated. Finally, for some patients, *gentle* pressure may be added to assist the pull of gravity. The patient can look upward during inhalation, which encourages gentle isometric contraction, and then look downward and "let go" during exhalation to augment relaxation.

Other muscles that form a functional unit with the anterior part of the gluteus minimus include the anterior fibers of the gluteus medius and the tensor fasciae latae. All three muscles have overlapping pain patterns and similar stretch positions and should be released by intermittent cold with stretch of the gluteus minimus. However, for full lengthening of the tensor fasciae latae muscle, the thigh should be rotated laterally.

Posterior Fibers

For TrPs in the posterior fibers (Fig. 9.6*B*), the patient lies on the uninvolved side with the involved limb hanging over the end of the table. The thigh of the limb to be treated is flexed to only about 30°. This positions the trochanteric attachment of the gluteus minimus so that adduction at the hip produces maximum lengthening. The pull of gravity is either lessened or augmented as described previously for the anterior part of the muscle.

Alternative positions for intermittent cold with stretch of the anterior and posterior parts of the gluteus minimus are presented in Section 12 of Chapter 8 (Fig. 8.6*A* and *B*), and have been described elsewhere.[43,45]

Parallel sweeps of vapocoolant or ice are applied over the posterior portion of the muscle and continued distalward over the posterior buttock, thigh, and calf to the ankle, covering all of the pain reference zones. As the thigh is gently lowered into adduction, relaxation is augmented, as described previously, by asking the patient to exhale slowly while parallel sweeps of intermittent cold are applied. This intermittent-cold-with-stretch sequence is repeated until full range of motion is reached or until no further gains occur.

After the procedure has been completed, the skin is rewarmed promptly with a moist heating pad. Then the patient actively moves the limb slowly through the full range of motion in abduction and adduction at least three times to help restore normal muscle function.

Other muscles in the functional unit of the posterior part of the gluteus minimus are the posterior fibers of the gluteus medius, which have an overlapping pain pattern and a similar stretch position, the piriformis, and the gluteus maximus. However, the gluteus maximus pain reference zone and intermittent cold pattern may include the sacral region; also, the gluteus maximus requires full flexion of the thigh at the hip for its complete passive stretch (*see* Fig. 7.5 in Chapter 7).

Alternative Methods

Another stretch position is portrayed by Evjenth and Hamberg.[11] They strap the

PART 1

side-lying patient to a plinth with the patient lying on the involved gluteus minimus, which renders the muscle and referred pain pattern inaccessible to spray and requires the operator to stretch the muscle by lifting the lower limb against gravity. The positions that we prefer instead for passive lengthening of the muscle are assisted by gravity, and the patient can be taught to use these positions, which are shown in Figures 9.6 and 9.8, in a home self-stretch program.

In many patients, the gluteus minimus is too deep to permit effective digital ischemic compression. If compression is tried, it usually requires the pressure of two hands applied with one thumb on top of the other. Some operators recommend use of the elbow; we consider this less desirable because the operator may not feel the nature of the tissues being compressed, resulting in less precise localization of pressure and in the application of excessive force. Application of pressure distal and medial to the gluteus minimus muscle over the sciatic nerve may cause a tingling, painful sensation and possibly neurapraxia. Production of these nerve compression symptoms should be avoided.

The tennis-ball technique described and illustrated in the previous chapter for TrPs in the gluteus medius muscle (Chapter 8, Section 14 and Fig. 8.9) enables the patient to apply ischemic compression to himself or herself (Section 14, this chapter).

13. INJECTION AND STRETCH (Fig. 9.7)

For injection, gluteus minimus TrPs must be precisely localized and their relation to the sciatic nerve identified. It is preferable to inject any gluteus maximus and gluteus medius TrPs before attempting to inject gluteus minimus TrPs. The increased TrP tension of the overlying muscles and their additional tender spots make the precise localization of gluteus minimus TrPs unnecessarily difficult.

Anterior Fibers

For injection of TrPs in the anterior fibers, the patient is propped up partly side lying (Fig. 9.7*A*) or lies supine (Fig. 9.7*B*). The method of locating the most anterior gluteus minimus TrPs has been described in Sections 2 and 9 of this chapter.

The clinician localizes a TrP in the anterior gluteus minimus muscle by deep palpation and notes carefully the precise direction of pressure that elicits maximum tenderness. When inactivating gluteal TrPs by injection, distinguishing whether the tender spot is in the gluteus medius or the gluteus minimus is not critical. Usually, multiple probing movements of the needle in a fanlike pattern in the region of maximum tenderness are required to inactivate a cluster of TrPs. It is essential that the needle penetrate far enough in the direction of spot tenderness to reach the deepest gluteus minimus fibers. A 50-mm (2-in) or 62-mm (2½-in) needle may be required.

In this muscle, needle contact with the TrP usually evokes the predictable pattern of referred pain that the patient can describe in detail, if requested ahead of time to note any pain radiation.

If the needle passes through the gluteus minimus, the needle encounters either the ilium or the capsule of the hip joint. The needle should be replaced immediately if contact with bone has bent its tip and its movement through the muscle produces a scratchy sensation. Such encounters with the periosteum are usually painful to the patient only momentarily.

Posterior Fibers

For injection of TrPs in the posterior fibers, the patient is placed fully side lying on the uninvolved side (Fig. 9.7*C*). Frequently, there are multiple TrPs in this part of the muscle. Posterior TrPs are located by palpation as noted in Section 9. The lower posterior border of the gluteus minimus is located by defining the upper limit of the piriformis muscle. Directing the needle *above*, not below, this line and in an upward direction normally eliminates the risk of accidentally penetrating the sciatic nerve as it exits the pelvis through the sciatic foramen. Injection is then performed essentially as described previously for the anterior fibers.

After completion of each probing by the needle, prompt hemostasis is applied by the palpating hand as the needle is with-

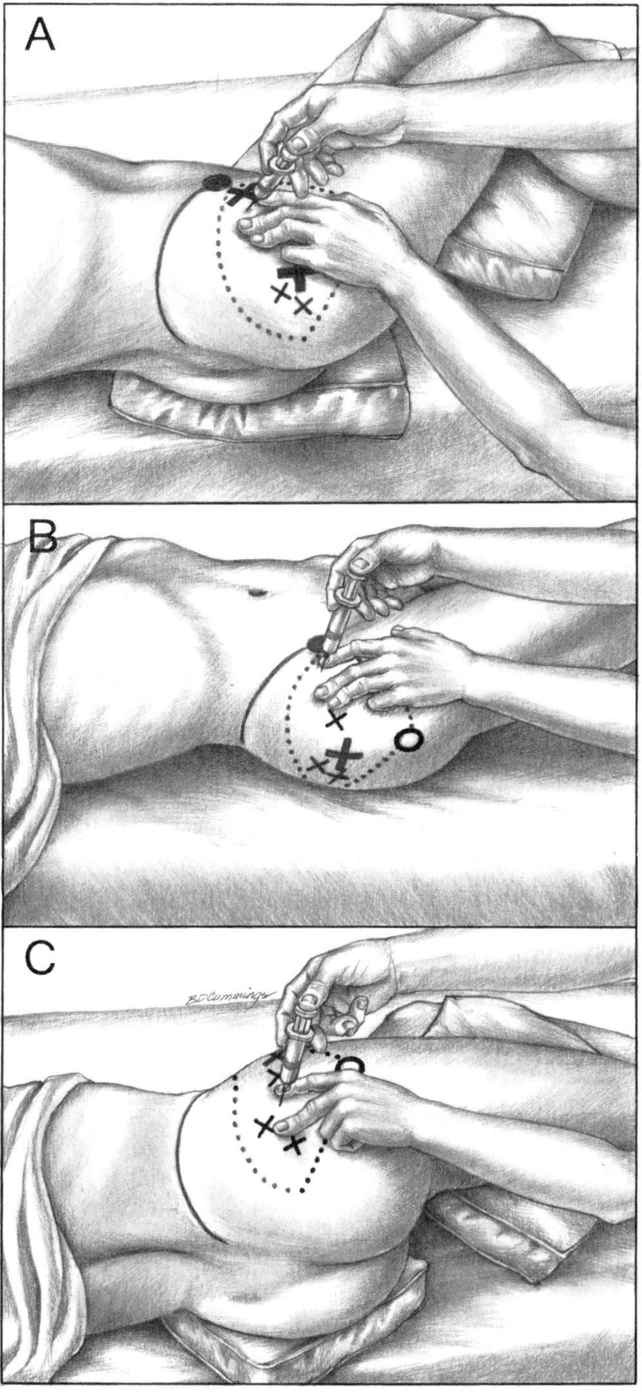

Figure 9.7. Injection of TrPs (***X**s*) in the anterior and posterior parts of the right gluteus minimus muscle. The *solid line* follows the crest of the ilium to the anterior superior iliac spine (*solid circle*). The *dotted line* marks the borders of the gluteus minimus muscle and indicates its attachment to the greater trochanter (*open circle*). *A*, probing close to the **posterior** border of the tensor fasciae latae muscle to locate anterior gluteus minimus TrPs (*anterior large **X***). *B*, probing under the **anterior** border of the tensor fasciae latae muscle to inject the trigger-point location shown in *A* by the large anterior **X**. *C*, injection of the most common posterior gluteus minimus TrPs (in the area marked by the *posterior large **X*** in *A* and *B*).

drawn. Prolonged superficial capillary oozing may indicate low tissue reserves of ascorbic acid. If possible, aspirin medication should be discontinued several days before TrP injection to reduce local bleeding.

All Fibers

After injection, the clinician should reexamine the site for residual tenderness to detect any remaining active TrPs. Injection is followed by passive stretch, then by active abduction and adduction through full range of motion at the hip. The application of a moist heating pad or hot pack also helps restore normal function of the muscle and minimize postinjection soreness.

Immediately following injection, one can conclude that the TrP was probably penetrated and inactivated if: (*a*) injection elicited a local twitch response, (*b*) deep spot tenderness at the site of injection disappears within a few minutes, (*c*) spontaneous pain and tenderness in the reference zone disappear or diminish, and (*d*) there is an appreciable increase in the range of motion.[56] Surprisingly, reproduction of the patient's referred pain pattern during injection is not conclusive; the needle may only be pressing against the outside of the TrP, thus setting off the referred pain. A similar (usually more intense) pain is experienced when the needle actually penetrates the TrP and inactivates it.

When a very active TrP in this muscle is injected, a sensation of heaviness or weakness of the limb may ensue within a minute or two. The muscle is capable of a brief contraction in response to voluntary effort, but is unable to maintain the contraction. If the patient attempts to stand on the injected limb immediately, the hip may "give way" and the patient may fall. When 0.5% procaine solution is used, this weakness should last, at most, 15 or 20 minutes.[56] Precautions should be taken by allowing the patient to rest for a suitable period of time following the injection, while moist heat is applied, and by testing the motor power of the limb before weight bearing is attempted. This weakness is similar to that which would occur if some of the local anesthetic solution reached the sciatic nerve.

14. CORRECTIVE ACTIONS
(Fig. 9.8)

The obese patient should undertake a weight-loss program, but not by excessive exercise that overloads the gluteal muscles. The wide-based waddling gait adopted by very obese patients reduces demands on the gluteus minimus and gluteus medius muscles.

The patient with gluteus minimus TrPs should keep the body warm. Latent TrPs in the gluteal muscles are readily activated not only by direct chilling of these muscles, but also by cooling of the body as a whole.

If intramuscular medicinal injections must be given in the buttock, they should not be injected as deep as the gluteus minimus muscle.

Corrective Posture and Activities

For patients with active gluteus minimus TrPs, standing is more painful than sitting. They should be encouraged to sit whenever possible, especially in situations where one usually stands, as when working in the kitchen. If standing is unavoidable, weight should be shifted regularly from one foot to the other. Relief by this alternation of weight bearing and change of position is enhanced if one foot is placed on a footrest that is elevated 5–7.5 cm (2 or 3 in). The feet should be separated to widen the base of support. Even when sitting, it is helpful to change positions every 15 or 20 minutes by standing up, moving around the room, and sitting down again. An interval timer placed across the room is a helpful reminder to change positions when a person is preoccupied with a task.

When an individual sleeps on the side with the thighs flexed, a pillow between the knees and legs helps maintain the uppermost thigh horizontal and the involved gluteus minimus muscle in a neutral position, as illustrated in the following chapter in Figure 10.10.

A hemipelvis that is small in the anteroposterior diameter can be a significant perpetuating factor for gluteus minimus and gluteus medius TrPs, causing a twisting tilt of the pelvis whenever the patient is lying supine. This should be corrected by an ischial lift, as illustrated in Figure 4.12*B*.

Displacement of the sacroiliac joint should be corrected by mobilization[32] or manipulation[55,56] techniques.

Patients with symptoms from posterior gluteus minimus TrPs should carry the wallet elsewhere than in the back pocket. The wallet can cause "back-pocket sciatica"[19] when sitting on it compresses a gluteus minimus TrP, and it can also tilt the pelvis (*see* Chapter 4).

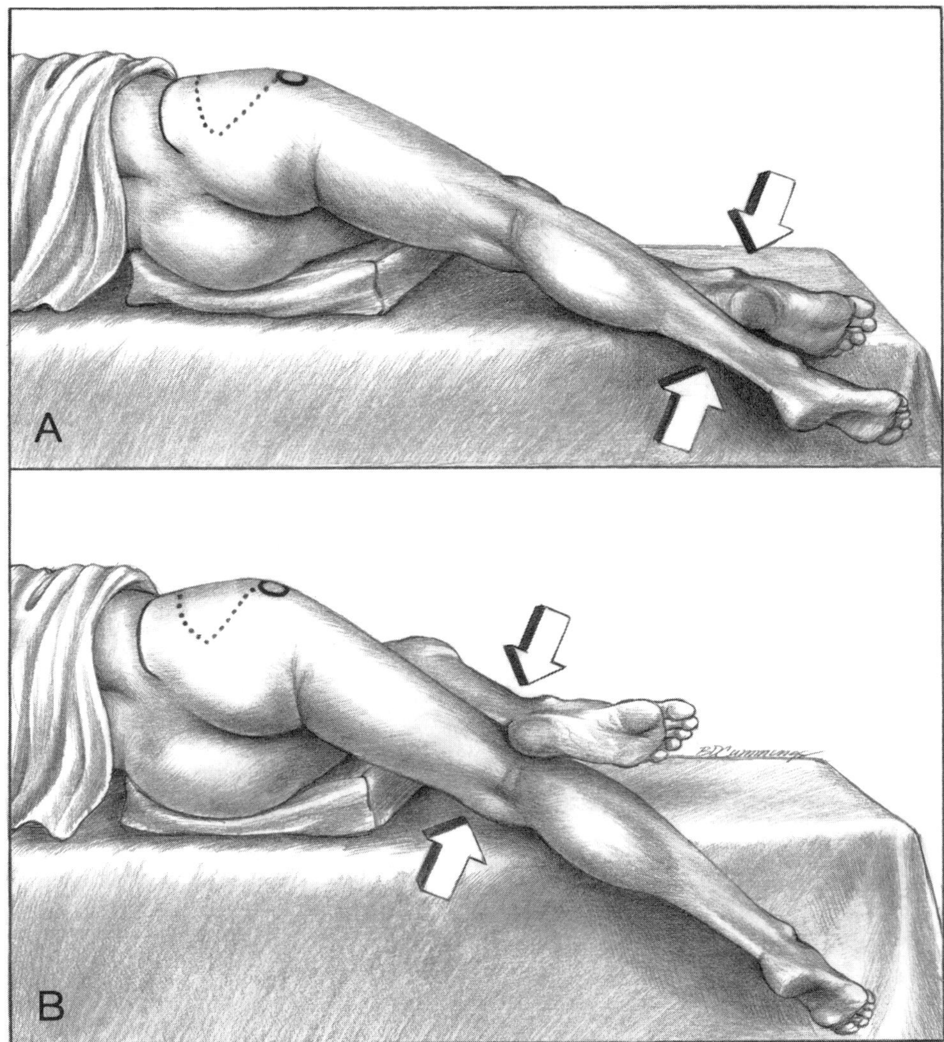

Figure 9.8. Self-stretch of the **anterior** fibers of the right gluteus minimus muscle. The *dotted line* identifies the posterior and the superior borders of the gluteus minimus muscle; these borders are closely related to the greater trochanter (*open circle*), and to the crest of the ilium (*solid line*). *A*, starting position. The individual contracts the muscle *gently* to press the right leg upward against resistance provided by the left heel. Following 5 seconds of balanced pressure (*large arrows*), or after simply holding the weight of the thigh against the pull of gravity, the person relaxes and allows the right leg to drop downward over the edge of the table. This movement into adduction takes up the slack and lengthens the anterior part of the muscle. *B*, final stretch position after several cycles of the procedure described in *A*.

Activities that impose unaccustomed stress on the muscle, such as vigorous sports and hiking, should either be avoided or be trained for by incremental conditioning.

Home Therapeutic Program

The patient frequently benefits by learning to use a tennis ball for self-application of ischemic compression to anterior and posterior gluteus minimus TrPs; this is shown in Figure 8.9 of the previous chapter. The patient can use body weight to achieve deep pressure precisely on these gluteus minimus TrPs.

The response to this ischemic compression on the posterior TrPs is enhanced if the patient slides the buttock over the tennis ball slowly to produce a stripping massage. This is done by placing the ball under the tender area closest to the greater trochanter, and sliding the body slowly in a downward direction. The tennis ball should roll slowly at a rate of about 2.5 cm (1 in) every 10 seconds toward either the iliac crest or the sacrum, following the direction of the gluteus minimus fibers. This rolling technique may be accomplished more readily by leaning against a smooth wall than by lying on the floor. Three repetitions are sufficient at one session. It is wise to follow the stripping massage promptly with moist heat. This therapy may be repeated daily until the TrP tenderness disappears, or every other day if local soreness develops.

A self-stretch that is effective for inactivating *anterior* gluteus minimus TrPs is illustrated and described in Figure 9.8. This should be coordinated with respiration so that the patient inhales during the isometric contraction phase and exhales during the relaxation phase.[27] The position illustrated in Figure 9.6*A* also can be employed with this contraction-relaxation technique. In this case, the contraction during inhalation should support the weight of the lower extremity without lifting it. During exhalation, the patient relaxes and allows gravity to lengthen the muscle.

A comparable self-stretch for the fibers of the *posterior* gluteus minimus is obtained by *flexing* the thigh approximately 30° and letting it hang over the end of a table or bed, as in Figure 9.6*B*. Resistance of gravity alone during inhalation produces the desired gentleness of contraction of the involved muscle. Then, during exhalation, gravity is a desirable and effective force to encourage gentle release of the tight fibers.

Attempts to self-stretch this muscle in the standing position are difficult and awkward. It is necessary to place the thigh alternately in adduction-flexion and adduction-extension. While weight bearing, the patient must try to relax these postural gluteal muscles and maneuver to stretch them. If one attempts this standing self-stretch, it is essential to hold onto something substantial, such as a file cabinet or dresser, for support and balance.

References

1. Anderson JE: *Grant's Atlas of Anatomy*, Ed. 8. Williams & Wilkins, Baltimore, 1983 (Figs. 4–33, 4–34).
2. *Ibid*. (Fig. 4–24).
3. *Ibid*. (Fig. 4–41).
4. Banerjee T, Hall CD: Sciatic entrapment neuropathy. *J Neurosurg 45*:216–217, 1976.
5. Basmajian JV, Deluca CJ: *Muscles Alive*, Ed. 5. Williams & Wilkins, Baltimore, 1985 (pp. 316–317, 381).
6. Bullock RG: Treatment of Sciatica (letter). *Br Med J 282*:70–71, 1981.
7. Carter BL, Morehead J, Wolpert SM, *et al*.: *Cross-Sectional Anatomy*. Appleton-Century-Crofts, New York, 1977 (Sects. 36–40, 44–46).
8. Clemente CD: *Gray's Anatomy of the Human Body*, American Ed. 30. Lea & Febiger, Philadelphia, 1985 (p. 568).
9. *Ibid*. (p. 1236).
10. Duchenne GB: *Physiology of Motion*, translated by E.B. Kaplan. J. B. Lippincott, Philadelphia, 1949 (p. 246).
11. Evjenth O, Hamberg J: Muscle Stretching in Manual Therapy, A Clinical Manual. Alfta Rehab Førlag, Alfta, Sweden, 1984 (p. 107).
12. Ferner H, Staubesand J: *Sobotta Atlas of Human Anatomy*, Ed. 10, Vol. 2. Urban & Schwarzenberg, Baltimore, 1983 (Fig. 152).
13. *Ibid*. (Fig. 405).
14. *Ibid*. (Fig. 410).
15. *Ibid*. (Fig. 418).
16. *Ibid*. (Fig. 420).
17. Gainer JV, Chadduck WM, Nugent GR: Causes of sciatica. *Postgrad Med 56*:111–117, 1974.
18. Good MG: What is "fibrositis"? *Rheumatism 5*: 117–123, 1949.
19. Gould N: Back-pocket sciatica. *N Engl J Med 290*: 633, 1974.
20. Greenlaw RK: *Function of Muscles About the Hip During Normal Level Walking*. Queen's University, Kingston, Ontario, 1973 (thesis) (pp. 89–92, 134–135).
21. Gutman H, Zelikovski A, Gadoth N, *et al*.: Sciatic pain: A diagnostic pitfall. *J Cardiovasc Surg 28*:204–205, 1987.
22. Hollinshead WH: *Anatomy for Surgeons*, Ed. 3., Vol. 3, *The Back and Limbs*. Harper & Row, New York, 1982 (pp. 664–666).
23. Inman V: Functional aspects of the abductor muscles of the hip. *J Bone Joint Surg 29*:607–619, 1947.
24. Kellgren JH: Sciatica. *Lancet 1*:561–564, 1941.
25. Lewinnek GE: Management of low back pain and sciatica. *Int Anesthesiol Clin 21*:61–78, 1983.
26. Lewit K: Chain reactions in disturbed function of the motor system. *Manual Med 3*:27–29, 1987.
27. Lewit K, Simons DG: Myofascial pain: relief by post-isometric relaxation. *Arch Phys Med Rehabil 65*:452–456, 1984.
28. Little H: Trochanteric bursitis:a common cause of pelvic girdle pain. *Can Med Assoc J 120*:456–458, 1979.
29. Lovejoy CO: Evolution of human walking. *Scientif Am 259*:118–125, 1988.
30. McMinn RMH, Hutchings RT: *Color Atlas of Human Anatomy*. Year Book Medical Publishers, Chicago, 1977 (pp. 264, 273, 274).
31. *Ibid*. (p. 293A).
32. Mitchell FL Jr, Moran PF, Pruzzo NA: *An Evaluation and Treatment Manual of Osteopathic Muscle Energy Procedures*. Mitchell, Moran and Pruzzo,

Associates, Valley Park, MO, 1979 (pp. 425–435).

33. Negrin P, Fardin P: Clinical and electromyographical course of sciatica: prognostic study of 41 cases. *Electromyogr Clin Neurophysiol 27*: 225–127, 1987.
34. Netter FH: *The Ciba Collection of Medical Illustrations*, Vol.8, Musculoskeletal System. Part I: Anatomy, Physiology and Metabolic Disorders. Ciba-Geigy Corporation, Summit, NJ, 1987 (p. 85).
35. Pernkopf E: *Atlas of Topographical and Applied Human Anatomy*, Vol. 2. W.B. Saunders, Philadelphia, 1964 (Fig. 316).
36. *Ibid.* (Fig. 329).
37. Rasch PJ, Burke RK: *Kinesiology and Applied Anatomy*, Ed. 6. Lea & Febiger, Philadelphia, 1978 (p. 276).
38. Reynolds MD: Myofascial trigger point syndromes in the practice of rheumatology. *Arch Phys Med Rehabil 62*:111–114, 1981.
39. Rubin D: An approach to the management of myofascial trigger point syndromes. *Arch Phys Med Rehabil 62*:107–110, 1981.
40. Schapira D, Nahir M, Scharf Y: Trochanteric bursitis: a common clinical problem. *Arch Phys Med Rehabil 67*:815–817, 1986
41. Scott M: Lower extremity pain simulating sciatica: tumors of the high thoracic and cervical cord as causes. *JAMA 160*:528–534, 1956.
42. Sheon RP, Moskowitz RW, Goldberg VM: *Soft Tissue Rheumatic Pain*, Ed. 2. Lea & Febiger, Philadelphia, 1987 (pp. 165, 168–169).
43. Simons, DG: Myofascial pain syndromes, part of Chapter 11. In *Medical Rehabilitation*, edited by J.V. Basmajian and R.L. Kirby. Williams & Wilkins, Baltimore, 1984 (p. 319).
44. Simons DG: Myofascial pain syndromes due to trigger points: 2. Treatment and single-muscle syndromes. *Manual Med 1*:72–77, 1985.
45. Simons DG: Myofascial pain syndrome due to trigger points, Chapter 45. In *Rehabilitation Medicine*, edited by Joseph Goodgold. C. V. Mosby Co., St. Louis, 1988 (pp. 686–723).
46. Simons DG, Travell JG: Myofascial origins of low back pain. 3. Pelvic and lower extremity muscles. *Postgrad Med 73*:99–108, 1983.
47. Simons DG, Travell JG: Myofascial pain syndromes, Chapter 25. In *Textbook of Pain*, edited by P.D. Wall and R. Melzack, Ed 2. Churchill Livingstone, London, 1989 (pp. 368–385).
48. Søgaard IB: Sciatic nerve entrapment. *J Neurosurg 58*:275–276, 1983.
49. Spalteholz W: *Handatlas der Anatomie des Menschen*, Ed. 11, Vol. 2. S. Hirzel, Leipzig, 1922 (p. 359).
50. Toldt C: *An Atlas of Human Anatomy*, translated by M.E. Paul, Ed. 2, Vol. 1. Macmillan, New York, 1919 (pp. 341, 342).
51. *Ibid.* (p. 353).
52. Travell J: Factors affecting pain of injection. *JAMA 158*:368–371, 1955.
53. Travell J: Symposium on mechanism and management of pain syndromes. *Proc Rudolf Virchow Med Soc 16*:126–136, 1957 (p. 133, Fig. 5).
54. Travell J, Rinzler SH: The myofascial genesis of pain. *Postgrad Med 11*:425–434, 1952.
55. Travell W, Travell J: Technique for reduction and ambulatory treatment of sacroiliac displacement. *Arch Phys Ther 23*:222–246, 1942.
56. Travell J, Travell W: Therapy of low back pain by manipulation and of referred pain in the lower extremity by procaine infiltration. *Arch Phys Med 27*:537–547, 1946.
57. Voss H: Tabelle der Muskelgewichte des Mannes, berechnet und zusammengestellt nach den Untersuchungen von W. Theile (1884). *Anat Anz 103*:356–360, 1956.
58. Weber EF: Ueber die Längenverhältnisse der Fleischfasern der Muskeln in Allgemeinen. *Berichte über die Verhandlungen der Königlich Sächsischen Gesellschaft der Wissenschaften zu Leipzig 3*: 63–86, 1851.
59. Werner A, Gaitzsch J: Hypogastric artery aneurysm: a very rare cause of sciatica (and a tricky diagnostic problem!) *Surg Neurol 10*:89–91, 1978.
60. Wilson GL, Capen EK, Stubbs NB: A fine-wire electromyographic investigation of the gluteus minimus and gluteus medius muscles. *Res Quart 47*:824–828, 1976.
61. Zohn DA: *Musculoskeletal Pain: Diagnosis and Physical Treatment*, Ed. 2. Little Brown and Company, Boston, 1988 (p. 212).

PART 1

CHAPTER 10
Piriformis and Other Short Lateral Rotators
Gemelli, Quadratus Femoris, Obturator Internus, and Obturator Externus Muscles

"Double Devil"

HIGHLIGHTS: The piriformis muscle is responsible for the symptoms of the piriformis syndrome and is a "double devil" because it causes as much distress by nerve entrapment as it does by projecting pain from trigger points (TrPs). **REFERRED PAIN** from a TrP in the piriformis muscle may radiate to the sacroiliac region, laterally across the buttock and over the hip region posteriorly, and to the proximal two-thirds of the posterior thigh. Pain patterns of the other five short lateral rotators of the hip have not been distinguished from those of the piriformis muscle. The intrapelvic portion of the obturator internus is considered in Chapter 6. **ANATOMICAL ATTACHMENTS** of the piriformis muscle medially are primarily to the inner surface of the sacrum. The piriformis exits the pelvis through the greater sciatic foramen. Laterally, its tendon, with those of the other short lateral rotators, attaches to the greater trochanter of the femur. Medially, the two gemelli and the quadratus femoris muscles attach to the ischium; the obturator internus attaches to the inner surface of the obturator membrane and to the rim of the obturator foramen. The obturator externus attaches medially to the outer surface of the obturator membrane and to the rim of the obturator foramen. **INNERVATION** of the piriformis muscle is directly from the first and second sacral nerves. The obturator externus is supplied by the obturator nerve from spinal nerves L_3 and L_4. The remaining short lateral rotators receive innervation through motor nerves that may arise from spinal nerves L_4 to S_3. **FUNCTION** of the piriformis in the non-weight-bearing limb is primarily lateral rotation of the thigh with the hip extended; it also acts in abduction when the hip is flexed 90°. The remaining five short deep rotator muscles are primarily lateral rotators in either position. In weight-bearing activities, the piriformis restrains vigorous or excessive medial rotation of the thigh. **SYMPTOMS** of the piriformis syndrome may be caused by referral of pain from TrPs in the muscle, by nerve entrapment and/or vascular compromise when neurovascular structures are compressed by the muscle against the rim of the greater sciatic foramen, and by sacroiliac joint dysfunction. The myofascial pain component of this syndrome includes pain in the low back, buttock, and posterior thigh that usually is increased by sitting, standing, and walking. **ACTIVATION** of TrPs in the piriformis muscle results from acute overload, as when catching oneself from a fall or when restraining vigorous and/or rapid medial rotation of the weight-bearing limb (for example, during running). Sustained overload perpetuates these TrPs, as when holding the thigh flexed in abduction for prolonged periods while driving a car. **PATIENT EXAMINATION** reveals a tendency for the seated patient to squirm and shift position frequently. The Pace Abduction Test is usually positive. In the supine position, the foot of the involved side is laterally rotated, and medial rotation of that limb is restricted in range as compared with the normal side. In the prone position, pelvic asymmetry may be noted. Standing examination may reveal an apparent lower limb-length inequality and a tilted sacral base. Bone scan scintigraphy may image a piriformis muscle with active TrPs. Additional evidence for entrapment of nerves passing through the greater sciatic foramen supports the diagnosis of a piriformis syndrome. The piriformis muscle is accessible to **TRIGGER POINT EXAMINATION** indirectly outside of the pelvis by palpation through the gluteus maximus muscle and directly inside the pelvis by rectal or vaginal examination. The remaining five short lateral rotators are all palpable through the gluteus maximus from outside the pelvis; the obturator internus can also be palpated from within the pelvis. **ENTRAPMENTS** are numerous. The nerves and blood vessels that pass through the greater sciatic foramen along with the piriformis are subject to entrapment when the muscle is sufficiently enlarged to fill the foramen. The vulnerable structures include the superior and inferior gluteal nerves and blood vessels, the sciatic nerve, the pudendal nerve and vessels, the posterior femoral cutaneous nerve, and the nerves supplying the gemelli, obturator internus, and quadratus femoris muscles. **INTERMITTENT COLD WITH STRETCH** of the piriformis muscle can best be accomplished with the patient side lying and the involved thigh uppermost, flexed to 90° at the hip. The muscle is lengthened by adducting the flexed thigh as vapocoolant spray or ice is applied distalward across the buttock over the piriformis muscle and the posterior thigh. This is followed by full active abduction and adduction of the thigh and application of moist heat. Postisometric relaxation, ischemic compression, massage, and ultrasound, alone or in combination, also may inactivate these TrPs. The **INJECTION-AND-STRETCH** procedure for piriformis TrPs is accomplished either by a completely external approach or with guidance from intrapelvic palpation. The lateral TrPs are located for injection by flat palpation through the gluteus maximus muscle. Medial TrPs near the greater sciatic foramen are so deep and close to the sciatic nerve that it is best to palpate them directly through the rectum or vagina; the needle is then directed toward the finger that is palpating the TrP. Injection is followed by passive stretch. **CORRECTIVE ACTIONS** include correcting the asymmetry produced by a lower limb-length inequality and/or a small hemipelvis, and restoring normal movement to a blocked sacroiliac joint. Postural stress is reduced by maintaining a comfortable sleep position, using a rocking chair, and by changing seated position regularly and stopping to walk at intervals when driving a car for prolonged periods. Mechanical overload of the muscles must be avoided. A self-stretch home program is established. This program may include ischemic compression of the TrPs, but with great care to avoid nerve compression.

---

1. REFERRED PAIN
(Fig. 10.1)

Piriformis trigger points (TrPs) frequently contribute significantly to complex myofascial pain syndromes of the pelvic and hip regions.

The myofascial pain syndrome of the piriformis muscle is well recognized.[43,68,69,71,94,95,109] Additional pain referred from TrPs in the adjacent members of this lateral rotator group may be difficult to distinguish from pain originating in the piriformis TrPs.

The TrPs in the piriformis muscle refer pain primarily to the sacroiliac region, to the buttock generally, and over the hip joint posteriorly; the referred pain sometimes also extends over the proximal two-thirds of the posterior thigh (Fig. 10.1). The pattern of pain referred by the more lateral TrP_1 and that referred by the more medial TrP_2 are similar.[87,88,90]

Other authors have associated the piriformis syndrome with pain in the buttock[42,80,95] and down the back of the thigh.[43,56,80,100] Pain caused by the piriformis muscle has been described as having a sciatic radiation[109] and as causing lumbago[86] or low back pain.[109] Some authors localized this pain in the region of the coccyx.[56,100] Pain was also noted in the inguinal area and at the greater trochanter.[99]

Many investigators have attributed the pain of the piriformis syndrome to compression by the muscle of the sciatic and other nerves as they pass through the greater sciatic foramen with the piriformis.[1,20,43,50,64,66,72,80,93,95,99] This nerve-entrapment pain has a different origin than the myofascial pain referred by active TrPs in the piriformis muscle; however, the two often occur together. The neurogenic pain may extend down the entire

PART 1

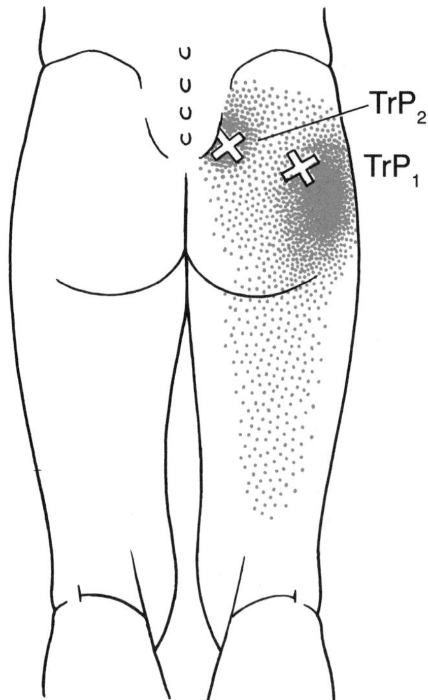

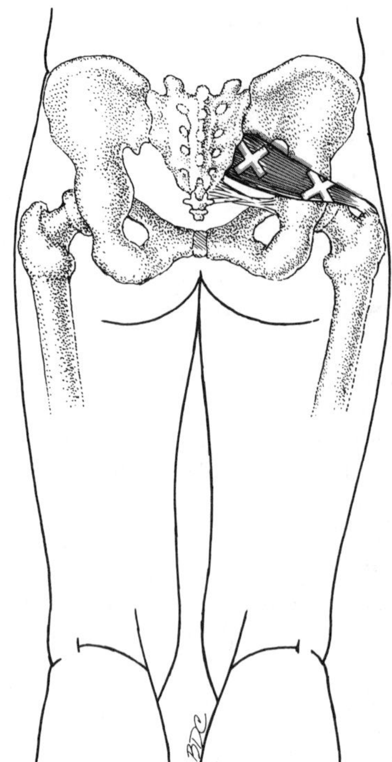

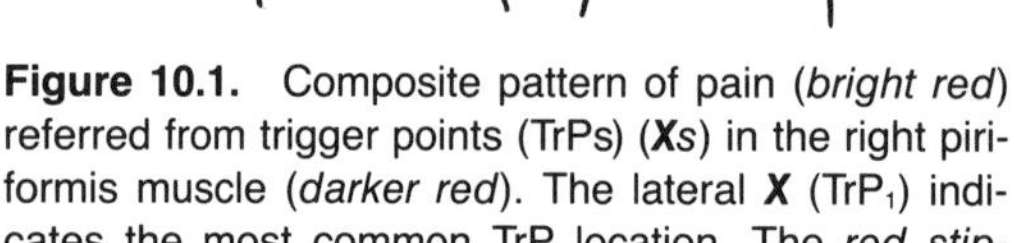

Figure 10.1. Composite pattern of pain (*bright red*) referred from trigger points (TrPs) (***X**s*) in the right piriformis muscle (*darker red*). The lateral ***X*** (TrP_1) indicates the most common TrP location. The *red stippling* locates the spillover part of the pattern that may be felt as less intense pain than that of the essential pattern (*solid red*). Spillover pain may be absent.

posterior thigh and the calf, and to the sole of the foot.

2. ANATOMICAL ATTACHMENTS AND CONSIDERATIONS

(Figs. 10.2 and 10.3)

Muscles

The piriformis is a thick and bulky muscle in most individuals; it is occasionally thin and is rarely absent.[10,108] The piriformis muscle can be small with only one or two sacral attachments. Conversely, it can be so broad that it joins with the capsule of the sacroiliac joint above and also with the anterior surface of the sacrotuberous[19,40] and/or sacrospinous[40] ligaments below.[19]

The name of the piriformis is derived from the Latin *pirum* (pear) and *forma* (shape); it was coined by Adrian Spigelius, a late 16th and early 17th century Belgian anatomist.[30] This muscle is anchored ***medially*** to the anterior (internal) surface of the sacrum usually by three fleshy digitations between the first, second, third, and fourth anterior sacral foramina (Fig. 10.2*A*). Some fibers may attach to the margin of the sciatic foramen at the capsule of the sacroiliac joint[40,41,68] and some fibers to the sacrospinous ligament.[19,40] ***Laterally***, the muscle is secured by a rounded tendon onto the greater trochanter on the medial side of its superior surface (Figs. 10.2*B* and 10.6). This tendon often blends with the common tendon of the obturator internus and gemelli muscles.[19]

Variations of the piriformis muscle include additional medial attachments to the first and fifth sacral vertebrae and to the coccyx. It may fuse with the gluteus medius or minimus above, or with the superior gemellus below. In fewer than 20% of bodies it is divided into two distinct portions through which part or all of the sciatic nerve passes (*see* Section 10).[10,66]

The piriformis muscle exits the inside of the pelvis through the greater sciatic foramen. This rigid opening is formed anteriorly and superiorly by the posterior part of the ilium, posteriorly by the sacro-

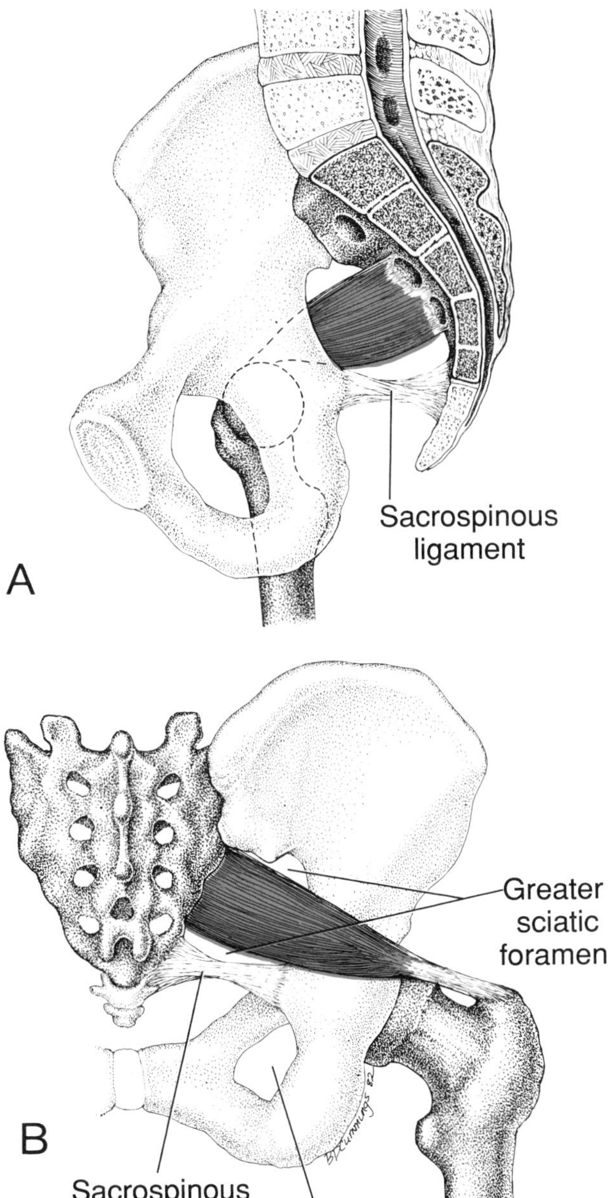

Figure 10.2. Attachments of the right piriformis muscle (*red*). *A*, seen from inside the pelvis in midsagittal view showing the attachment of the muscle on the inside of the sacrum, usually between the first four anterior sacral foramina. The fourth foramen is not shown. *B*, seen from behind (posterior view). In this figure, a relatively small muscle exits the pelvis through a relatively large sciatic foramen. Its rounded tendon attaches laterally to the superior surface of the greater trochanter. The muscle traverses the greater sciatic foramen just above the sacrospinous ligament. Most of the muscle is accessible to external palpation and nearly half of the muscle belly is accessible to palpation inside the pelvis.

tuberous ligament, and inferiorly by the sacrospinous ligament.[20] When the muscle is large and fills this space, it has the potential of compressing the numerous vessels and nerves that exit the pelvis with it.

The other short lateral rotators of the thigh at the hip, the four "GOGO" muscles (superior **g**emellus, **o**bturator internus, inferior **g**emellus, and **o**bturator externus) and the quadratus femoris, lie distal to the piriformis muscle. Like it, they are deep to the gluteus maximus muscle, but in contrast to the usual position of the piriformis, they pass anterior to the sciatic nerve (Fig. 10.3). To locate these muscles in patients, it is helpful to note that deep to the gluteus maximus, the piriformis and the upper three "GOGO" muscles form a fanlike arrangement spreading out from the upper end of the greater trochanter.

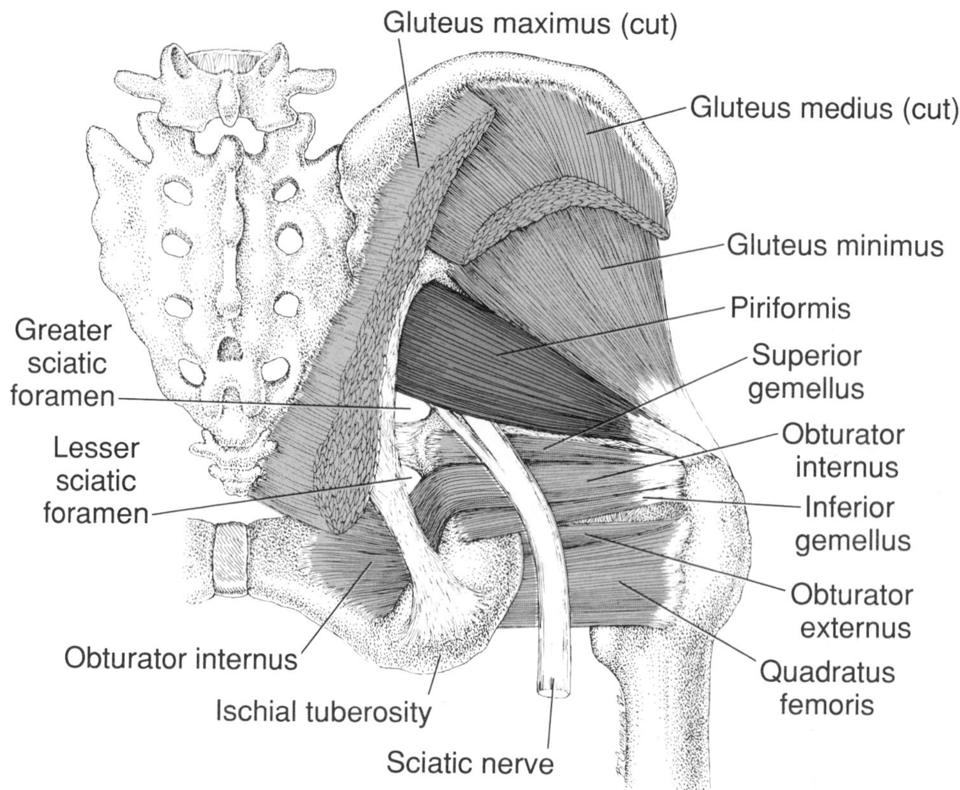

Figure 10.3. Piriformis muscle, regional anatomy: Posterior view of anatomical relations of the right piriformis muscle (*dark red*) to neighboring muscles (*light red*). The gluteus maximus and gluteus medius muscles have been cut and removed; the distal cut ends of these gluteal muscles are not shown since they would obscure the attachment of the piriformis to the femur.

The **superior and inferior gemelli muscles** attach ***medially*** to the ischium and ***laterally*** to the medial surface of the upper part of the greater trochanter, proximal to and nearly parallel with the quadratus femoris muscle (Fig. 10.3).

Between the two gemelli lies the **obturator internus**, which is partly an intrapelvic muscle and partly a hip muscle (Fig. 10.3). ***Medially***, it is attached to and covers the inner surface of the obturator membrane and attaches to the rim of the obturator foramen, except where the obturator nerve and vessels leave the pelvis through the lateral part of the membrane.

The obturator internus muscle exits the pelvis through the lesser sciatic foramen. ***Laterally***, the fiber bands of the obturator internus converge onto a tendon that is usually shared with the gemelli muscles. This tendon inserts on the anterior part of the medial surface of the greater trochanter proximal to the trochanteric fossa of the femur and attaches on the greater trochanter near but distal to the piriformis tendon.

The subtendinous bursa of the obturator internus muscle lies between its tendon and the capsule of the hip joint and may communicate with the ischiadic bursa between the obturator internus muscle and the ischium.

The **quadratus femoris** is a rectangular muscle with parallel fibers that attach ***medially*** to the anterolateral surface of the ischium, caudad to the inferior gemellus and posterior to the obturator externus. ***Laterally***, it attaches to the femur on the quadrate tubercle and along the intertrochanteric crest, which extends longitudinally about halfway between the greater and lesser trochanters (Fig. 10.3).[22,46]

The **obturator externus** muscle is considered part of the adductor group by Hollinshead;[46] however, he notes that its primary action would be lateral rotation and not adduction of the thigh. ***Laterally***, the obturator externus attaches to the femur at the trochanteric fossa deep to the quadratus femoris; it passes across the distal part of the capsule of the hip joint to anchor ***medially*** to the external surface of the obturator membrane. From the posterior view it is nearly covered by the quadratus femoris[34,36,82] (Fig. 10.3). A bursa often intervenes where the obturator externus crosses the lesser trochanter.

Nerves in the Greater Sciatic Foramen

Of critical importance to understanding piriformis entrapment syndromes is knowledge of the distribution of the neurovascular structures that exit the pelvis with the muscle through the unyielding greater sciatic foramen. The **superior gluteal nerve and blood vessels** usually pass between the superior border of the piriformis and the upper (sacroiliac) rim of the foramen. This nerve supplies the gluteus medius, gluteus minimus, and tensor fasciae latae muscles.[25] The **sciatic nerve** usually exits between the piriformis muscle and the rim of the greater sciatic foramen (Fig. 10.3). It supplies the skin and muscles of the posterior thigh and most of the leg and foot. Also exiting the pelvis along the lower border of the piriformis are the **pudendal nerve and vessels**. The pudendal nerve then crosses the spine of the ischium and reenters the pelvis through the lesser sciatic foramen, which is identified in Figure 10.3. It supplies the external anal sphincter muscle and helps supply the skin of the posterior thigh and scrotum or labia majora. This nerve also innervates the bulbocavernosus, ischiocavernosus, and sphincter urethrae membranacea muscles; the skin and corpus cavernosus of the penis in the male; and the corresponding structures of the clitoris in the female.[26] Innervation of these structures is essential to normal sexual function. The **inferior gluteal nerve**, which exclusively supplies the gluteus maximus muscle,[25] the **posterior femoral cutaneous nerve**, and the **nerves to the gemelli, obturator internus, and quadratus femoris muscles** also pass through the greater sciatic foramen with the piriformis muscle.

Collectively, these nerves are responsible for all gluteal muscle sensation and function, anterior perineal sensory and motor function, and nearly all of the sensation and motor function in the posterior thigh and calf. It is apparent that chronic compression of these nerves would cause buttock, inguinal, and posterior thigh pain, as well as pain lower in the limb.

PART 1

Supplemental References

Atlases of anatomy show the attachment of the piriformis muscle to the most proximal surface of the greater trochanter,[7,37,60] to the sacrum,[38,57] and to the ilium.[37,59] The muscle is presented in cross section[18] and as seen from above inside the pelvis.[2]

The side view from within the pelvis[3,21,35,58,103] portrays the structures palpated on internal examination. One view shows how the sacral roots of the sciatic nerve lie between the piriformis muscle and the examining finger.[4] The posterior view shows special relations for the piriformis, the "GOGO" muscles, and the quadratus femoris, and is useful when palpating tender areas in the lower lateral buttock.[5,82,102] Similar views that include the sciatic nerve serve to orient needle insertion into these muscles in relation to the greater trochanter and the sciatic nerve.[6,34,61,73,83]

Authors[73,102] have illustrated the large bursa that cushions the obturator internus as it turns sharply around the smooth bone of the lesser sciatic notch. The location of the obturator externus can be seen with the overlying quadratus femoris removed.[36]

3. INNERVATION

The piriformis muscle is usually supplied by both the first and second sacral nerves as they emerge from the anterior sacral foramina, but sometimes it is supplied by only one nerve, either S_1 or S_2.[19]

One nerve carrying fibers from L_5-S_2 or S_1-S_3 supplies the obturator internus and the superior gemellus.[46] The nerve to the quadratus femoris sends a twig to the inferior gemellus and contains fibers from L_4, L_5, and S_1.[19] Unlike all the other short lateral rotators, the obturator externus receives its innervation from a branch of the obturator nerve. This branch comes either from the obturator nerve before it divides into anterior and posterior branches or from the posterior branch. The posterior branch pierces the muscle.[23]

All of these nerves (except the innervation to the piriformis muscle itself and the nerve to the obturator externus) are vulnerable to compression as they pass through the greater sciatic foramen together with the piriformis muscle.

4. FUNCTION

In weight-bearing activities, the piriformis is often needed to *restrain* (control) vigorous and/or rapid medial rotation of the thigh, for example, during the early stance phase of walking and running. The piriformis muscle is also thought to stabilize the hip joint and to assist in holding the femoral head in the acetabulum.[19]

The six "short lateral rotators" comprise the piriformis, the superior and inferior gemelli, the obturator internus and externus, and the quadratus femoris. The piriformis is primarily a lateral rotator with the hip neutral or extended. It also abducts the thigh when the hip is flexed 90°. The remaining five short lateral rotator muscles are almost exclusively lateral rotators[77] in either flexion or extension.

Examination of an articulated skeleton makes it apparent that the degree of flexion of the thigh profoundly affects the function of the piriformis muscle. At 90° of flexion it produces horizontal abduction of the thigh.[19,46,76] However, with full flexion at the hip, it appears to rotate the thigh medially. The action of the other short lateral rotators is less influenced by flexion of the thigh at the hip. The degree of hip flexion is an important factor when considering the optimal stretch position.

No electromyographic (EMG) study of the functional kinesiology of any of these muscles was found. The actions of the piriformis, gemelli, and quadratus femoris muscles were studied by Duchenne using electrical stimulation.[29] Stimulation of the piriformis with the thigh neutral produced lateral rotation of the thigh with some extension and slight abduction. Stimulation of the superior gemellus, obturator internus, and inferior gemellus as a group caused pure lateral rotation of the thigh, as did stimulation of the quadratus femoris.

Mitchell[63] noted that the piriformis exerts an oblique force on the sacrum. The plane of the muscle closely approximates the frontal plane and lies at an angle of approximately 30° to the plane of the adjacent sacroiliac (SI) joint. As illustrated by Retzlaff and associates,[80] the lower fibers of the piriformis muscle are able to produce a strong rotary shearing force on the SI joint. This force would tend to displace the ipsilateral base of the sacrum anteriorly (forward) and the apex of the the sacrum posteriorly.[80]

5. FUNCTIONAL (MYOTATIC) UNIT

The piriformis and the other five short lateral rotator muscles, together with the gluteus maximus, are the prime lateral rotators of the thigh.[45,77] They are assisted by the long head of the biceps femoris, the sartorius, posterior fibers of the gluteus medius, sometimes by the posterior fibers of the gluteus minimus, and by the iliopsoas, the last particularly in infants.[45]

The antagonists that produce medial rotation of the thigh combine other functions and are relatively weak rotators, namely, the semitendinosus and semimembranosus, tensor fasciae latae, pectineus, and the most anterior fibers of the gluteus medius and gluteus minimus muscles.[45,77] The role of the adductors in this regard has been considered controversial;[45] however, EMG studies have shown that the adductores longus and magnus are activated during medial rotation but not during lateral rotation of the thigh at the hip.[12]

6. SYMPTOMS

Piriformis Syndrome

Retzlaff noted, "The piriformis muscle syndrome frequently is characterized by such bizarre symptoms that they may seem unrelated".[80] Pain (and paresthesias) may be reported in the low back, groin, perineum, buttock, hip, posterior thigh and leg, foot, and, during defecation, in the rectum. Symptoms are aggravated by sitting, by a prolonged combination of hip flexion, adduction, and medial rotation, or by activity. In addition, the patient may complain of swelling in the painful limb and of sexual dysfunction, dyspareunia in females, and impotence in males.

Prevalence

The patients seen on a Back Service who suffered from piriformis syndrome were greater in number than the patients with nerve root deficit caused by disc protrusion. The ratio of female to male patients with piriformis syndrome was 6:1.[71] Kipervas and co-workers[50] considered spasm of the piriformis muscle to be one of the most frequent myotonic reflexes in lumbar osteochondrosis (used by these authors to mean musculoskeletal low back pain). The gynecologist, Shordania,[86] reported that 8.3% of 450 women attending a polyclinic for lumbago had a hard, swollen, extremely tender piriformis muscle, which he considered responsible for their pain. This syndrome is not a common cause, but it is a significant and treatable cause of otherwise enigmatic pain.

Popelianskii and Bobrovnikova[75] found a piriformis syndrome in 105 (43.7%) of 240 patients with signs and symptoms of lumbosacral radiculitis. Patients with evidence of S_1 nerve root compression responded to piriformis muscle therapy much better than did patients with evidence of L_5 root compression.

Three Components

It now appears that three specific conditions may contribute to the piriformis syndrome: *(a)* myofascial pain referred from TrPs in the piriformis muscle; *(b)* nerve and vascular entrapment by the piriformis muscle at the greater sciatic foramen, and *(c)* dysfunction of the SI joint.

The original, now classic, descriptions by Pace[69] and by Pace and Nagle[71] of the piriformis syndrome as a myofascial pain syndrome due to TrPs have been reinforced or confirmed by subsequent authors.[11,43,68,75,92,94,95,109] The taut bands and shortened muscle fibers associated with TrPs represent one mechanism that would, in effect, place the muscle in sustained tension with bulging of its diameter.

Historically, many authors have recognized the potential for entrapment of the nerves and vessels passing through the greater sciatic foramen by the piriformis muscle.[1,11,40,41,43,56,64,68,75,78,93,94] Freiberg, in 1934,[40] clearly described these critical anatomical relations and, in 1937,[41] first described surgical release of the piriformis to relieve the syndrome. In 1941,[42] he was still perplexed as to what caused the muscle to be too large for the foramen. Some authors[14,85,89,94,106] have assumed that anatomical variations in the position of the sciatic nerve relative to the piriformis muscle predispose that nerve to compression by the muscle.

When actively contracting and shortening, any muscle markedly increases its girth and becomes tense. (A shortening muscle fiber must increase in diameter as its actin and myosin filaments increasingly overlap each other side by side.) Therefore, when the piriformis muscle at rest snugly fills the limited space available in the greater sciatic foramen, the accompanying nerves and vessels must be compressed whenever the muscle is shortened or contracted.

A relatively small muscle in a large greater sciatic foramen could develop pure myofascial pain without an entrapment component. Conversely, a relatively large muscle that fills the foramen and then shortens because of active TrPs would be expected to produce entrapment symptoms in addition to myofascial referred pain.

In the past, inflammation of the piriformis has been thought to be the cause of the syndrome. Freiberg,[42] however, in his summary of 12 operations on the piriformis, noted that in no instance was excised piriformis tissue reported as diseased. This substantiates Pace's contention that applying the term "piriformitis"[86] to this condition is a confusing misnomer, with which we agree.

Dysfunction of the SI joint has been considered a common and important component of the piriformis syndrome.[44,51,80,95,106] Displacement of the SI joint may interact with myofascial TrPs of the piriformis muscle to establish a self-sustaining relation. The sustained tension of the muscle caused by the TrPs could maintain displacement of the joint,[51] and the dysfunction induced by the joint displacement apparently perpetuates piriformis TrPs. In this situation, both conditions must be corrected.

Origin of Symptoms

The three components of the piriformis syndrome, myofascial TrPs, neurovascular entrapments, and articular dysfunction, are responsible for different but often overlapping symptoms.

Pain directly attributable to myofascial TrPs in the piriformis muscle includes low back pain,[64,69,71,80] buttock pain,[1,11,43,71,75] hip pain,[80] and posterior thigh pain.[43,69,71,80] This same myofascial cause is implicated when pain is increased by sitting,[43,80,94] by arising from the sitting position,[43] or while standing.[80] Pressure of a hard bolus of feces against TrPs in a patient's left piriformis muscle caused "rectal" pain during defecation when the patient was constipated.[68] Pain is typically aggravated by sitting, by prolonged hip flexion, adduction, and medial rotation, and by activity.[11] Recumbency may not provide relief from a myofascial piriformis syndrome[80] if the TrPs are more than moderately irritable.

Compression of the superior and inferior gluteal nerves and vessels could contribute to the nearly universal complaint of buttock pain.[1,43,71,78,93,94] More severe compromise of these nerves would explain gluteal muscle atrophy.[78]

Pain in the region of the SI joint may be due to dysfunction of that joint.[68,80,99,105,106]

Pressure on the sciatic nerve or on the posterior femoral cutaneous nerve in the greater sciatic foramen is a likely additional source of posterior thigh pain.[1,43,56,64,69,71,80,93,94] Sciatic nerve entrapment can be responsible for the pain and paresthesias projecting to the leg (calf) and often to the foot.[1,11,40,43,64,80,93,94] Numbness of the foot[43,64] and loss of position sense producing a broad-based, ataxic gait have also been noted.[94]

Pain on prolonged slouched sitting,[1,43,80] particularly on a hard surface,[94] may be due to pressure on piriformis TrPs or to additional pressure on the sciatic nerve at its point of entrapment, or to both.

Piriformis entrapment of the pudendal nerve may evoke perineal pain and sexual dysfunction. Female patients are likely to complain of painful intercourse (dyspareunia).[71,80,93] Simply spreading the thighs apart may be distressingly painful.[68,71] Pudendal nerve entrapment may cause impotence in men.[80] A patient of either sex may experience inguinal (groin) pain.[1,71]

Pain immediately posterior to the greater trochanter can be the result of entrapment of the nerves to the gemelli, obturator internus, and quadratus femoris muscles. The presence of local tenderness should lead one to look for TrPs in these muscles.

Differential Diagnosis

The piriformis myofascial pain syndrome is recognized by the characteristic pain pattern projected by its TrPs, by pain and weakness on resisted abduction of the thigh with the hip flexed 90°, by eliciting tenderness of the piriformis muscle using external palpation, and by palpating taut bands and tenderness via intrapelvic examination. The piriformis syndrome may be the cause of a "postlaminectomy syndrome" or of coccygodynia.[79]

Nerve entrapment is suggested by paresthesias and dysesthesias in the distribution of nerves passing through the greater sciatic foramen and by sensory disturbance extending well beyond midthigh. Malignant neoplasm, neurogenic tumors, and local infection can compress the sciatic nerve at the greater sciatic foramen. These conditions have been identified by CT scanning.[27] Sacroiliac joint displacement is likely to coexist with a piriformis myofascial syndrome,[44,51,99,106] and is recognized by the physical signs of pelvic torsion noted in Section 8 of this chapter.

Another source of pain referred to the buttock and *lateral* thigh is an episacroiliac lipoma.[70] These herniated nodules of fat are exquisitely tender to palpation and are responsive to injection of a local anesthetic. Sometimes they require surgical removal under local anesthesia for lasting relief.

Symptoms of the piriformis syndrome are easily confused with those of a herniated intervertebral disc. Absence or marked weakness of the Achilles tendon reflex,[42] and motor denervation shown by electromyography, suggest a disc lesion. Conversely, slowing of conduction velocity in the sciatic nerve through the pelvis suggests piriformis entrapment. Palpation for piriformis muscle tenderness is essential to confirm or rule out entrapment and should be performed in all cases of "sciatica." Recognition of the piriformis syndrome may avoid needless laminectomy.

Incidental radiographic reports of "narrowing of the disc space" or "degenerative changes with spur formation" are not by themselves sufficient to account for the pain characteristic of the piriformis syndrome. Degenerative changes occur in the spine with aging and do not correlate well with symptoms.[96]

Symptoms of a facet syndrome with low back pain and sciatica (*see* Chapter 3, Fig. 3.2) may be difficult to distinguish from a myofascial piriformis syndrome until the muscle is examined.[11] A facet block may relieve the back pain of a facet syndrome, but only successful inactivation of the piriformis muscle TrPs relieves the limp and the buttock and posterior thigh pain of myofascial and related entrapment origin.[71]

When the pain and pelvic wall tenderness are bilateral, spinal stenosis should be considered.[71]

Piriformis syndrome may develop secondary to sacroiliitis (sacroiliac arthritis). The diagnosis of sacroiliitis is confirmed by radiography.[68] Sacroiliitis affects one or both SI joints and may cause pain and tenderness in the low back, buttock, and lateral thigh that may also extend as far as the ankle on one or both sides. Patients with sacroiliitis are usually young people who are HLA-B27 positive and may have ankylosing spondylitis[32] (usually bilaterally symmetrical sacroiliitis[81]), psoriatic arthritis or Reiter's disease (usually asymmetrical sacroiliitis[81]), or arthritis related to inflammatory bowel disease.[74,81]

7. ACTIVATION AND PERPETUATION OF TRIGGER POINTS

Activation

Any unaccustomed overload can activate myofascial TrPs in a related muscle. One man overloaded the piriformis while spreading his knees maximally and lowering one end of a large container between his knees and onto the floor.[71] Catching oneself in a fall can overload many muscles, including the piriformis. One might hear, "My foot slipped as I ran around the swimming pool, but I caught myself and didn't fall."[71] Other movements producing overload are twisting sideways while bending and lifting a heavy weight,[68] or forceful rotation with the body weight on one leg.[71,80] The second author treated one young man who activated TrPs in this muscle by turning his body repeatedly to lift and throw pieces of firewood behind him.

The piriformis can become overloaded when it undergoes a strong lengthening contraction to *restrain* vigorous and/or rapid medial rotation of the weight-bearing limb; this occurs at times during running.

Repetitive strain can activate piriformis TrPs. One woman, a masseuse at a spa, repeatedly used her piriformis to block the movement of her body after throwing her weight to one side over the client.[71]

Placing a muscle with a latent TrP in the shortened position for a prolonged period of time is likely to activate the TrP. Flexing the thighs at the hips with the knees spread apart for obstetrical or urological procedures, or for coitus, does just this to the piriformis muscle; this position has been associated with onset of the piriformis syndrome.[68,80]

Direct trauma by striking the buttock over the piriformis muscle with a hard object may be responsible for activating piriformis TrPs.[15,68,80] The unaccustomed muscle strain of an accidental overcorrection of a lower limb-length inequality can activate latent piriformis TrPs.

Baker[9] examined 34 muscles, including the piriformis, in 100 patients who had experienced a first-time motor vehicle accident. The piriformis muscle evidenced myofascial TrPs in one-third to one-half of the patients. Among both drivers and passengers, impact on the driver's side produced the largest percentage of piriformis involvement; impact from behind produced the lowest percentage.

Piriformis TrPs are likely to be activated by the same stresses that activate TrPs in the posterior divisions of the gluteus minimus and gluteus medius muscles. TrPs in the piriformis seem unlikely to develop as satellites of TrPs in other muscles.

Perpetuation

Immobilization of an involved muscle tends to perpetuate its TrPs. Driving a car with the foot in place on the accelerator for long periods or sitting on one foot[80] are activities that can perpetuate piriformis TrPs.

Chronic infections are known to perpetuate TrPs. Specifically, chronic pelvic inflammatory disease[86] and infectious sacroiliitis[68] have been identified in the piriformis syndrome. Other conditions that may perpetuate piriformis TrPs include arthritis of the hip joint and conditions requiring total hip replacement.[71]

The Morton foot structure (mediolateral rocking foot) tends to increase medial rotation and adduction of the thigh during walking. The piriformis assists in compensating for this excessive medial rotation and thereby is overworked, leading to perpetuation of existing TrPs. Hyperpronation of the foot from other causes and also lower limb-length inequality can perpetuate piriformis TrPs.

8. PATIENT EXAMINATION

When more than an uncomplicated myofascial piriformis syndrome is suspected, a careful neurological examination of the lower limbs is valuable. Additional observations and tests are presented here, arranged by patient position during examination.

Patient Upright

The patient with entrapment of primarily the peroneal portion of the sciatic nerve may evidence only mild foot drop with weakness of dorsiflexion at the ankle. With more extensive entrapment of the sciatic nerve, the patient may limp by dragging the leg on the affected side.[71] Patients with severe piriformis syndrome may be unable to ambulate.[49,51]

While standing, the patient can be examined for SI joint mobility on each side by the technique described and illustrated by Kirkaldy-Willis.[51] The painful limb may be measurably larger in girth.

Patient Seated

When seated, patients with a piriformis syndrome tend to squirm and frequently shift position. They are likely to have difficulty crossing the involved thigh over the other knee when asked to do so. Resisted isometric contraction of the muscle is tested as described (and illustrated) by Pace[69] and by Pace and Nagel:[71] "... the examiner places his hands on the lateral aspects of the knees and asks the patient to push the hands apart. Faltering, pain, and weakness will be observed on the affected side."[71] This Pace Abduction Test has subsequently been highly regarded.[11,16,79,109]

Patient Supine

With the patient resting in the supine position, one is likely to see persistent lateral rotation of the thigh on the affected side that is evidenced by an outward rotation of the foot of at least 45°. This test was illustrated by Retzlaff and associates[80] and also described by other authors.[76,99] This position indicates shortening of the piriformis or other lateral rotators, unless due to the pelvic asymmetry of a hemipelvis that is small in the anteroposterior direction, as described in Chapter 4.

Painfulness and limitation of passive medial rotation of the affected thigh with the hip straight in the supine patient was first described by Freiberg;[41] this test was illustrated by TePoorten,[99] and is frequently mentioned,[33,71,76,99,100,109] often as Freiberg's Sign. This movement increases the tension on an already tight piriformis muscle.

Popelianskii and Bobrovnikova[75] found that pain in a sciatic distribution in response to the combination of medial rotation and adduction (Bonnet's sign) was characteristic of piriformis syndrome.

Evjenth and Hamberg[33] illustrate and describe a variation of the medial rotation test with the patient supine; the thigh of the side to be tested is flexed to 60° at the hip. Tightness of the posterior fibers of the gluteus medius and gluteus minimus muscles would limit medial rotation more in this flexed position than when the hip is straight.

Patients with the piriformis syndrome have a variable degree of restriction of straight-leg raising that is probably more dependent on compression of nerves in the greater sciatic foramen than on myofascial TrP tension of the muscle.

Examination of the supine patient at times reveals apparent shortening of the limb on the involved side[80,99] that can result from distortion of the pelvic axis caused by increased tension of the piriformis. Conversely, the piriformis syndrome may be aggravated by a lower limb-length inequality that overloads the piriformis muscle. Examination for this lower limb asymmetry is described fully in Chapter 4.

Patient Side Lying

With the patient lying on the uninvolved side, palpation of the uppermost buttock consistently reveals exquisite tenderness over and just lateral to the greater sciatic foramen[18,75,109] and often along the entire length of the piriformis. From this external approach, all of the muscle must be palpated through the gluteus maximus muscle.[11,80,99]

Popelianskii and Bobrovnikova,[75] in their study of 105 patients with piriformis syndrome, found that tenderness over the area where the sciatic nerve exits from beneath the piriformis muscle was often attributable to either or both the sciatic nerve and the piriformis muscle. They saw a number of patients without backache whose buttock pain and tenderness at this site was associated with no nerve tenderness at the crease of the buttock but who did have a tense piriformis muscle.

A test for tightness of the piriformis that is more specific than that of Freiberg, because it is influenced less by the other lateral rotators of the hip, was described and illustrated by Saudek.[84] She placed the patient side lying with the side to be tested uppermost, stabilized the pelvis with one hand, flexed the uppermost thigh to 90°, and tested for painful limitation of passive adduction of the thigh at the hip.

Patient Prone

Tightness of the piriformis may subject the sacrum to abnormal rotary stress that exacerbates pelvic dysfunction.[76] Specifically, shortening of the right piriformis muscle produces left oblique axis rotation of the sacrum. The sacral base on the right is more anterior (depressed) in relation to the adjacent posterior superior iliac spine. The sacral sulcus is deepened, as illustrated by Retzlaff and associates.[80] They found that the apex (distal tip) of the sacrum is displaced to the left of the midline and that the sulcus on the left appears more shallow.[80] This torsion of the pelvis is likely to be associated with malalignment at the symphysis pubis.

Other Tests

We agree with those who consider examination of the patient for lower limb-length inequality to be important in the piriformis syndrome.[11,43] However, clinical assessment for inequality in the supine or standing patient is subject to multiple errors. Standing radiograms to identify causes for asymmetry of the lumbar spine, including lower limb-length inequality, can be helpful when carefully taken and interpreted. Methods of measurement and interpretation are described in Chapter 4.

The myofascial piriformis syndrome is often associated with entrapment of the sciatic nerve, with signs and symptoms of L_5 and S_1 nerve root involvement. Electrodiagnostic tests for denervation and examination of the nerve roots by computed tomography (CT) scan and magnetic resonance imaging (MRI) help confirm or exclude compression at the nerve root level. They also may help detect nerve entrapment in the greater sciatic foramen.

Fishman[39] examined 24 patients with piriformis syndrome for H (Hoffman) reflex changes when the affected lower limb was moved from a neutral position to 90° of hip flexion with 30-45° of adduction and medial rotation. In this stretch position for the piriformis muscle, the sum of the H reflex and M wave latencies increased between 2.5 and 13 millisec without change in the values of the opposite lower limb in 15 of 24 (63%) of his patients. His results support the view that nerve entrapment contributes significantly to the symptoms in a high percentage of patients with the piriformis syndrome and that the electrodiagnostic response to stress positioning can be helpful in confirming the diagnosis.

A nuclear bone scan using Tc-99m methylene diphosphonate imaged the muscle in an acute piriformis myofascial syndrome.[49] The patient had

PART 1

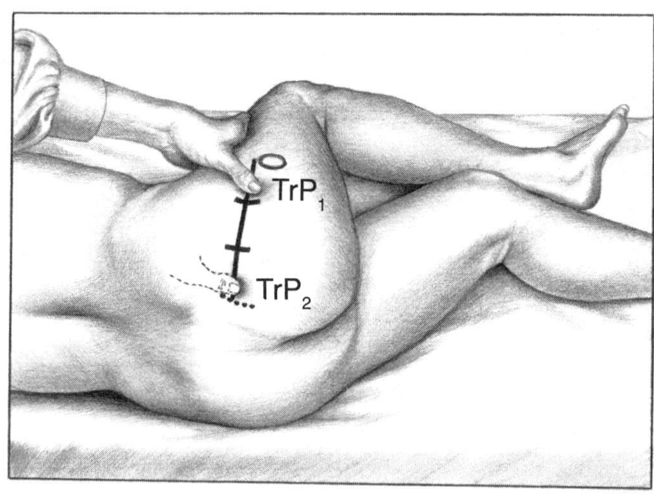

Figure 10.4. External palpation to elicit trigger-point tenderness in the right piriformis muscle through a relaxed gluteus maximus muscle. The *solid line* (piriformis line) overlies the superior border of the piriformis muscle and extends from immediately above the greater trochanter to the cephalic border of the greater sciatic foramen at the sacrum. (The technique for locating the piriformis line is illustrated in Figure 8.5*B*.) The line is divided into equal thirds. The *dotted line* marks the palpable edge along the lateral border of the sacrum, which corresponds closely to the medial margin of the greater sciatic foramen. The *fully rendered thumb* presses on the point of maximum trigger-point tenderness at TrP_1, which is usually found just lateral to the junction of the middle and lateral thirds of the line. The *outlined thumb* presses on the location of TrP_2 tenderness at the medial end of the line.

presented with a 3-day history of left buttock and thigh pain so severe that walking was impossible. The pain began immediately following a particularly strenuous tennis serve. Neurological examination was normal. When the scintigram suggested the diagnosis of piriformis muscle syndrome, "further physical evaluation revealed a TrP in the left piriformis muscle that reproduced the pain exactly. This TrP was injected . . . with immediate and permanent relief. The CT scan and myelogram were canceled."[49]

9. TRIGGER POINT EXAMINATION (Figs. 10.4 and 10.5)

Examination of this group of lateral rotator muscles for TrPs is complicated by the fact that all of them lie deep to the gluteus maximus muscle, as seen in Figure 10.3. The piriformis muscle can be examined through the gluteus maximus for most of its length. Its medial end is accessible to nearly direct palpation by rectal or vaginal examination. The femoral (lateral) ends of the gemelli and obturator internus muscles are not individually distinguishable by external palpation, but much of the intrapelvic obturator internus is directly palpable from inside the pelvis, as discussed and illustrated in Chapter 6. Tenderness in the femoral end of the quadratus femoris may be palpable through the gluteus maximus muscle. Using this approach, tenderness is less likely to be palpable in the underlying obturator externus. Obturator externus tenderness is best located by palpating between and deep to the pectineus and adductor brevis muscles in the groin, thereby exerting pressure on the muscle against the external surface of the obturator membrane.

Piriformis Muscle

The location of the piriformis muscle is determined for external examination by drawing a line (see piriformis line, Fig. 8.5*B*) from the uppermost border of the greater trochanter through the sacroiliac (cephalad) end of the greater sciatic foramen (Figs. 10.4 and 8.5*B*). When the gluteus maximus muscle is relaxed, the greater trochanter may be located by circular deep palpation with the flat of the hand over the hip laterally, revealing the underlying bony prominence. The crescent-shaped medial boundary of the sciatic foramen along the lateral border of the sacrum (*dotted line*, Fig. 10.4) is palpable inferior to the posterior inferior iliac spine through the relaxed gluteus maximus muscle.

The structure palpated along this border is the long posterior sacroiliac ligament. Its fibers extend from the ilium to the sacrum close to the SI joint and descend to become continuous with the sacrotuberous ligament.[20] The palpable border of this ligament along the sacrum corresponds closely to the medial border of the greater sciatic foramen.

The outline of a tense piriformis muscle is sometimes palpable along the piriformis line, and the muscle may show marked tenderness throughout its length.[80,99] Figure 10.3 illustrates how closely the lower borders of the gluteus medius and gluteus minimus muscles approximate the upper border of the piriformis, permitting palpation of the piriformis without interference from them. If one palpates too far cephalad, the gluteus medius and gluteus minimus, not the piriformis, are being palpated deep to the gluteus maximus.

The lateral TrP_1 region of the piriformis is usually located just lateral to the junction of the middle and lateral thirds of the piriformis line (Fig. 10.4). This lateral TrP is accessible only by external palpation. The medial TrP_2 region is markedly tender when pressure is applied medially over the region of the greater sciatic foramen, illustrated by the outlined thumb in Figure 10.4, and as noted also by others.[56,71,109] These medial TrPs are exquisitely tender when examined from within the pelvis.

Kipervas and associates[50] establish the location for palpating the piriformis muscle through the skin somewhat differently. They select the junction of the middle and lower thirds of a line drawn between the anterior superior iliac spine and the ischiococcygeus muscle.

If any doubt exists as to the cause of tenderness over the greater sciatic foramen, the medial end of the piriformis should be palpated within the pelvis by the rectal or vaginal route.[11,50,52,69,71,85,100] This examination is performed more readily if the examiner has a long finger (Fig. 10.5). The technique is also illustrated by Thiele.[100] The patient is placed side lying with the affected side uppermost and with that knee and hip flexed. The transversely oriented sacrospinous ligament[21] is felt as a firm band stretching between the sacrum and the ischial spine and is normally covered by fibers of the coccygeus muscle[109] that also can harbor TrPs. The piriformis muscle lies just cephalad to this ligament and, if involved, is tender and feels tense.[50,62,71,95,100] The patient is likely to exclaim that, for the first time, someone has found "my pain."[71]

One can often examine the muscle bimanually, with one hand pressing externally on the buttock while the other hand palpates internally. The greater sciatic foramen presents an unmistakable soft spot through which palpation pressure from one finger outside the pelvis can be transmitted to another finger inside the pelvis. To confirm identification of the piriformis muscle, the examiner palpates for contractile tension in the muscle while having the patient attempt to abduct the thigh by trying to lift the uppermost knee.

The sacral nerve roots lie between the examiner's finger and the piriformis muscle (Fig. 10.5). If the nerve roots are irritated by entrapment at the greater sciatic foramen, they, too, may be tender and are likely to project pain in a sciatic distribution.

Kipervas and co-workers[50] reported EMG findings in 23 patients with a piriformis muscle injury syndrome associated with lumbar osteochondrosis. The number of patients who had symptoms of radiculopathy in addition to myofascial changes in the piriformis muscle was not stated. Eight (35%) showed spontaneous resting activity in the involved piriformis muscle, indicating a tendency first to develop muscle spasm.

Eleven patients (48%) had a low discharge rate on voluntary contraction (25–30 Hz), compared with a normal value of 50–70 Hz in the contralateral uninvolved piriformis and the overlying ipsilateral gluteus maximus.[50] The mean motor unit duration for the involved piriformis muscles was significantly increased to 7 millisec (normal side 6.3 millisec) ($p < 0.01$). These changes are characteristic of neuropathy.

On the other hand, 15 (65%) of involved muscles produced low amplitude motor unit action potentials of only 80 μV (normal 450 μV). The amplitude range of interference pattern EMG was decreased to 107–190 μV (normal side 166–276 μV). These changes are more likely to be seen in myopathic diseases, unless the potentials were

PART 1

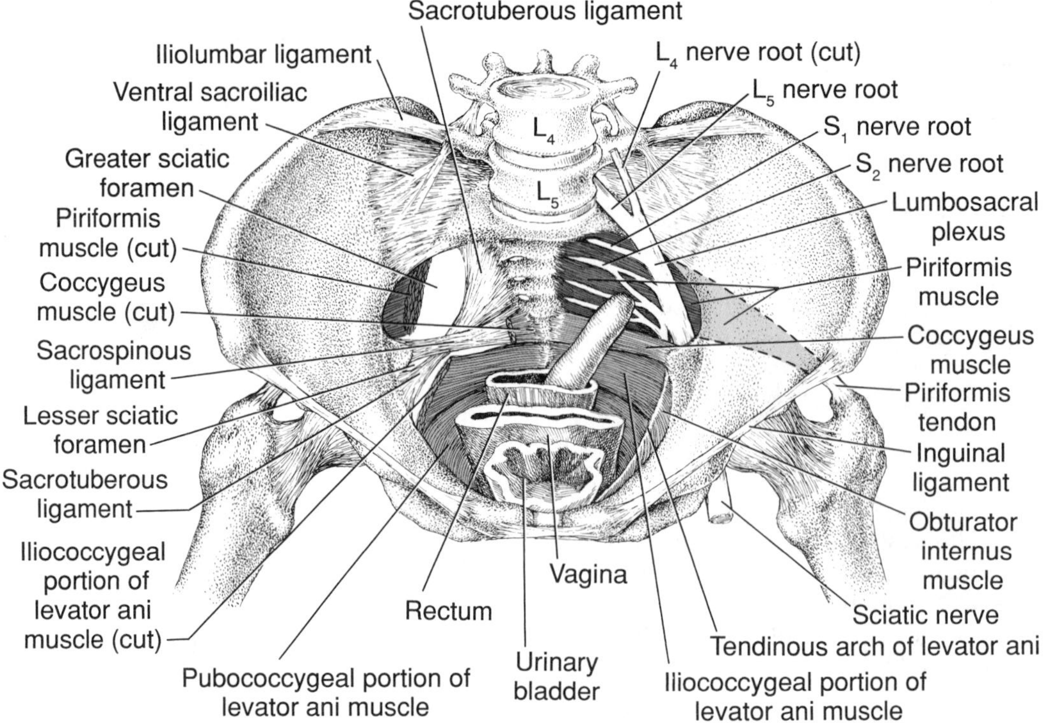

Figure 10.5. Internal palpation of the left piriformis muscle (*dark red* within the pelvis and *light red* outside the pelvis) via the rectum, viewed from in front and above. The levator ani is *medium red*; the coccygeus and obturator internus muscles are *light red*. The sacrospinous ligament (covered by the coccygeus muscle) is the last major transverse landmark identified by the palpating finger before it reaches the piriformis muscle. The sacrospinous ligament attaches cephalad mainly to the coccyx, which is usually easily palpated and mobile. The posterior wall of the rectum and the S_3 and S_4 nerve roots lie between the palpating finger and the piriformis muscle.

produced by recently reinnervated motor units. The gluteus maximus did not show any of these changes.[50]

The thickness of the involved piriformis muscle in a patient scheduled for operation was estimated to be 11 mm by measuring the depth of penetration of the needle through which voluntary motor unit activity was observed. This estimate was proven accurate at operation.[50]

Gemelli and Obturator Internus

Figure 10.3 shows that, in the anatomical position, all of the piriformis muscle lies above the level of its attachment to the uppermost part of the greater trochanter. Deep tenderness (deep to the gluteus maximus) inferior to the piriformis—at the level of and medial to the upper one-third of the greater trochanter—is most likely tenderness of one of the gemelli or of the obturator internus muscle. If TrPs in the obturator internus are responsible for this tenderness, it can be palpated directly by rectal or vaginal examination, as described in Chapter 6.

Figure 10.3 reminds one that the sciatic nerve is also compressed as pressure is applied medial to a point midway between the greater trochanter and the ischial tuberosity. The nerve usually emerges between the piriformis and superior gemellus muscles and continues its course superficial to the superior gemellus, obturator internus, inferior gemellus, obturator externus, and quadratus femoris muscles.

Quadratus Femoris and Obturator Externus

Figure 10.3 shows that deep tenderness medial to the lower two-thirds of the greater trochanter probably arises in the quadratus femoris or, possibly, in the even deeper obturator externus muscle. The sciatic nerve may also be tender.

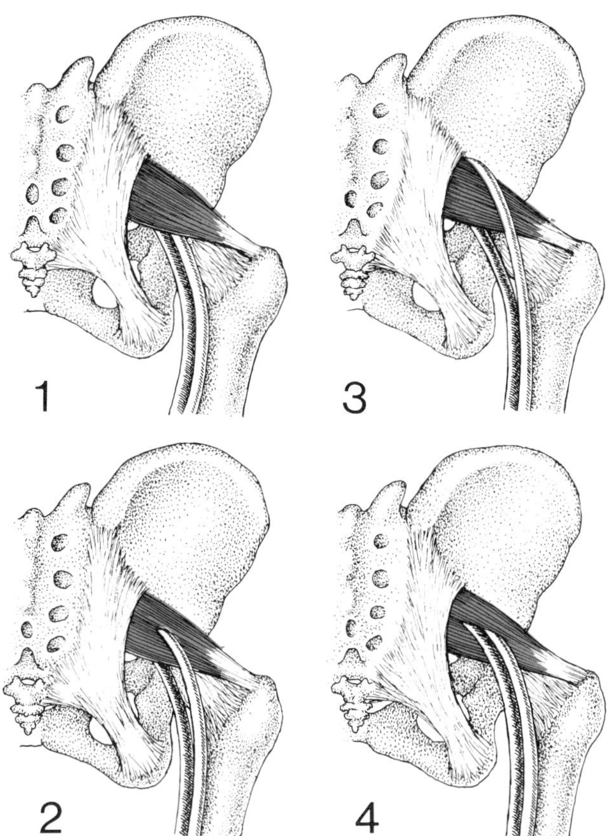

Figure 10.6. Four routes by which portions of the sciatic nerve may exit the pelvis: *(1)* the usual route, in which all fibers of the nerve pass anterior to the piriformis between the muscle (*red*) and the rim of the greater sciatic foramen, seen in about 85% of cadavers; *(2)* the peroneal portion of the nerve passes through the piriformis muscle and the tibial portion travels anterior to the muscle, as seen in more than 10% of cadavers; *(3)* the peroneal portion of the sciatic nerve loops above and then posterior to the muscle and the tibial portion passes anterior to it; both portions lie between the muscle and the upper or lower rim of the greater sciatic foramen, as seen in 2–3% of cadavers; *(4)* an undivided sciatic nerve penetrates the piriformis muscle in less than 1% of cadavers. (After Beaton and Anson,[14] with permission.)

Tenderness due to TrPs in the obturator externus muscle may be detected also in the groin. One must first palpate the superficial pectineus and adductor brevis to confirm that they do not harbor tender TrPs that would obscure a deeper source of tenderness. Deep pressure is then applied between the pectineus and adductor brevis against the outer surface of the obturator membrane, which is covered by the obturator externus muscle.

10. ENTRAPMENTS
(Fig. 10.6)

Conduction of compound action potentials by the sciatic nerve is remarkably sensitive to gentle but prolonged pressure.[28] In rabbits, these compound action potentials of the intact sciatic nerves decreased to 50% of initial value after the application of only a 10-g (⅙-oz) weight directly to the nerve for 45 minutes. The response decreased also to 50% after a sustained application of 20 g (⅓ oz) for a shorter time, 10–15 minutes. The larger (faster conducting) fibers were selectively susceptible to pressure. In these relatively brief experiments, loss of circulation was not responsible for the nerve conduction loss; stagnation of blood flow without nerve compression did not measurably affect neural conduction for up to 2 hours.[28] These experimental observations are confirmed clinically for both motor and sensory nerves when one tries to get up after sitting immobile for too long on a hard toilet seat.

The value of nerve conduction studies that examine the segment that passes through the **greater sciatic foramen** was demonstrated by Nainzadeh and Lane.[67] Although routine EMG studies of root levels L_3 through S_1 were normal, somatosensory-evoked potential studies of root levels S_2 through S_4 by stimulation of the pudendal nerve showed increased P40(P1) latencies of 47 millisec. This led to the diagnosis of piriformis muscle syndrome. Tenolysis of the piriformis muscle relieved the patient's symptoms and the

Table 10.1.
How Often the Peroneal and Tibial Portions of the Sciatic Nerve Go Around or Through the Piriformis Muscle (Percent of Limbs)

Authors	Both* Below Muscle (%)	Peroneal** through Tibial below (%)	Peroneal*** above, Tibial below (%)	Both**** through (%)	Both above (%)	Peroneal above, Tibial through (%)	Number of limbs
Anderson[8]	87.3	12.2	0.5	0	0	0	640
Beaton and Anson[14]	90	7.1	2.1	0.8	0	0	240
Beaton and Anson[13]	89.3	9.8	0.7	0.2	0	0	2250
Lee and Tsai[52]	70.2	19.6	1.5	1.8	3	1.2	168
Pećina[72]	78.5	20.7	0.8	0	0	0	130

* Illustrated in Panel 1 of Fig. 10.6.
** Illustrated in Panel 2 of Fig. 10.6.
*** Illustrated in Panel 3 of Fig. 10.6.
****Illustrated in Panel 4 of Fig. 10.6.

P40(P1) response returned to a normal latency of 40 millisec. Synek[97,98] established the diagnosis of piriformis syndrome by evidence of chronic denervation of the muscles in the nerve distribution below the sciatic notch, with slowing and decreased amplitude of somatosensory evoked potentials from those nerves in the portion passing through the greater sciatic foramen. The authors of these papers apparently had not explored the possibility (and likelihood) of myofascial TrPs causing these piriformis syndromes.

Two kinds of entrapments may occur as part of the piriformis syndrome: vascular[41] or nerve[41,43,66,72] entrapment between the piriformis muscle and the rim of the greater sciatic foramen and, possibly, nerve entrapment within the muscle.[85,89,106]

The first kind of entrapment has been well documented at surgery for the sciatic nerve[1,94] and for the superior gluteal nerve[78] (see Section 6). Freiberg[41] noted that a rich vascular plexus from the inferior gluteal vessels lies between the sciatic nerve and the piriformis muscle. Compression within the greater sciatic foramen could cause distal venous engorgement of the sheath of the trunk of the sciatic nerve, which he observed at operation. Both the blood vessels and nerves were subject to compression by the piriformis muscle as they passed through the greater sciatic foramen. Those affected structures are described in Section 2, and the symptoms attributable to the resulting compression are covered in Section 6. The vulnerable structures include the superior gluteal, inferior gluteal, and pudendal nerves and vessels; the sciatic and posterior femoral cutaneous nerves; and the nerves supplying both gemelli, the obturator internus, and the quadratus femoris muscles.

Figure 10.6 depicts the second kind of entrapment that would depend on variations in how the sciatic nerve passes beside or through the piriformis muscle. Table 10.1 summarizes reports documenting these variations. Generally, the peroneal division of the sciatic nerve has been reported to penetrate the muscle in 10–20% of limbs, probably about 11%.

Table 10.2 summarizes nine papers that report 40 piriformis operations with 35 confirmed as piriformis syndrome by relief of symptoms. Two patients were described as having engorgement of the veins distal to the foramen;[1] two reports described thinning of the sciatic nerve at the foramen with distal swelling;[1,94] and two surgeons noted tightness that prevented probing into the greater sciatic foramen.[1,78] None of the papers noted passage of any part of the sciatic nerve through the substance of the piriformis muscle. Of the 40 case reports describing

Table 10.2.
Reports of Operative Treatment of Piriformis Syndromes and Relation of Sciatic Nerve to the Piriformis Muscle as it Exits Pelvis

Source	Number of muscles	Nerve position
1934 Freiberg and Vinke[40]	1	Below
	1	NR
1937 Freiberg[41]	12	NR
1976 Mizuguchi[64]	14	NR
1976 Kipervas *et al.*[50]	1	Below
1980 Adams[1]	4	Below
1980 Rask[78]	1	AR
1981 Solheim *et al.*[93]	2	AR
1983 Stein and Warfield[94]	1	AR
1988 Cameron and Noftal[17]	3	NR

NR - No remarks about the sciatic nerve in report.
AR - Appearance of nerve reported, but anatomical configuration not stated.

surgical sectioning of the piriformis muscle, normal anterior passage of the nerve deep to and inferior to the muscle was explicitly described in five patients;[1,40,50] anterior passage was implied in one;[1] fifteen operations were described as freeing the sciatic nerve with no comment on a variant pathway.[50,64,93] For the remaining 19 operations, no mention was made of the nerves. It is considered unlikely that a surgeon would section the piriformis muscle before locating *all* of the sciatic nerve. It also seems unlikely that a variant configuration of the nerve would have been observed and not reported. Many of the papers on this subject by surgeons make special note of how frequently part or all of the sciatic nerve passes through the belly of the piriformis muscle in anatomical studies, but apparently none of these variations was a factor in the patients who obtained relief by sectioning the piriformis muscle.

These surgical reports suggest that anatomical variations in the position of the nerve may, contrary to the usual opinion, possibly reduce the risk of compression. Accepting an incidence of 11% variation in nerve configuration, for the cases reported in Table 10.2 one would have expected to see about four (4.4) variant sciatic nerve configurations among the 40 surgical cases. The fact that none was reported raises a question as to whether the variant configurations through the muscle may be protective of the nerve rather than a source of entrapment. Taut bands of muscle are probably more resilient than the unyielding bony and ligamentous foramen boundaries.

A similar variation in the pathway of the inferior gluteal nerve has also been observed. The inferior gluteal nerve penetrated the piriformis muscle on its way to the gluteus maximus muscle in 8.9% of 224 limbs.[101]

The posterior branch of the obturator nerve normally reaches the thigh by piercing the **obturator externus muscle.**[23,24] This branch supplies the obturator externus as it penetrates the muscle, and, as the nerve terminates, it supplies the adductor magnus and part of the adductor brevis muscle.[24] Entrapment of this nerve might be caused by taut TrP bands in the obturator externus muscle, but no case is known in which this entrapment was identified clinically.

11. ASSOCIATED TRIGGER POINTS

The piriformis rarely presents as a single-muscle pain syndrome. TrPs in this muscle are most likely to be associated with TrPs in adjacent synergists. The posterior part of the gluteus minimus is nearly parallel to and attaches close to the attachments of the piriformis muscle. Adjacent, on the lower edge of the piriformis, lie three of the lateral rotator group: the two gemelli and the obturator internus. Pace and Nagle[71] noted the concurrent involvement of these latter muscles and also warned that the levator ani and coccygeus muscles are commonly involved with the piriformis muscle. The piriformis fibers that are attached to the lower sacrum sometimes intermingle with the coccygeus fibers when the latter fibers cover the sacrospinous ligament.

When multiple gluteal muscles are involved, piriformis spot tenderness may not be apparent until TrPs in the overlying gluteus maximus and in the posterior

PART 1

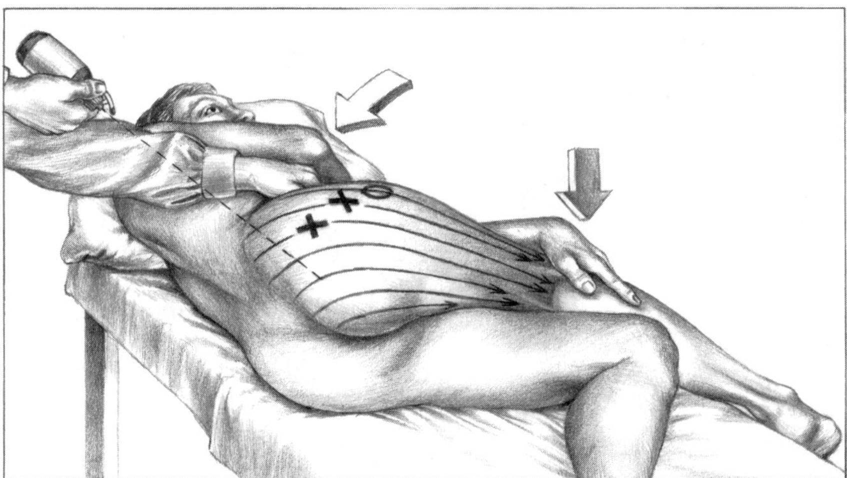

Figure 10.7. Stretch position and intermittent cold pattern (*parallel lines with thin arrows*) for TrPs in the right piriformis muscle. The *thick arrows* show the directions of force exerted by the operator and by the patient. The *open circle* marks the greater trochanter. The ***X*s** mark the regions where TrPs are located. The uppermost thigh is flexed nearly 90° at the hip. The patient anchors the greater trochanter by holding the distal thigh down against the table, assisted by gravity, while the operator progressively adducts the thigh at the hip by pulling backward on the crest of the ilium.

fibers of the adjacent gluteus medius and gluteus minimus muscles have been inactivated. However, a rectal or vaginal examination should reveal tenderness at the medial end of the piriformis muscle.

12. INTERMITTENT COLD WITH STRETCH

(Figs. 10.7 and 10.8)

Stretching of the piriformis muscle augmented by vapocoolant spray or ice application has been found by the authors and by others[11] to be effective in the management of the piriformis syndrome. Because of ozone layer concerns, the use of Fluori-Methane as the vapocoolant spray has been questioned and alternatives recommended.[91] Details of the original stretch-and-spray technique are found on pages 63–74 in Volume 1 of this manual; a method of substituting ice for vapocoolant spray appears on page 9 in Chapter 2 of this volume.

Since the piriformis muscle is primarily a lateral rotator of the thigh together with the other five short lateral rotators, all can be stretched by medial rotation of the thigh with the hip straight, as illustrated by Evjenth and Hamberg.[33] However, because the piriformis tendon attaches to the femur at the level of the axis of rotation of the hip joint, it changes from a lateral rotator to an abductor of the thigh when the hip is flexed to 90°. The best leverage on and the most effective stretch of the piriformis are obtained when the muscle is lengthened by adducting the thigh with the hip flexed to 90° (Fig. 10.7).

Figure 10.7 illustrates the single-operator, patient-assisted passive stretch technique for intermittent cold with stretch of the piriformis muscle. The patient lies on the uninvolved side with the uppermost thigh flexed to a right angle. The clinician pulls back on the pelvis while the subject assists by pushing down on the distal thigh of the side being treated. The operator applies several parallel sweeps of ice or vapocoolant spray from the TrP distalward over the muscle and over the pain pattern as shown in Figure 10.7. It is not necessary to extend sweeps of intermittent cold below the knee to cover an area of pain caused by nerve entrapment, but only as far as the muscle's referred pain pattern extends down the thigh.

The intermittent cold-with-stretch procedure can be effectively combined with postisometric relaxation, as described below and in Chapter 2 on page 11. Vapocoolant spray has been recommended by other authors for facilitating the release of tension in this muscle.[95,99] Steiner and associates[95] recommended ethyl chloride spray to those who prefer its more rapid cooling effect and Fluori-Methane to those who prefer the safety of its non-flammability (and non-anesthetic effect) for inactivation of piriformis TrPs. We expect Fluori-Methane to be replaced by a comparable, but environmentally safe product.

Intermittent cold with stretch is repeated until full muscle length is achieved or until no further gains are apparent. The skin is rewarmed with a moist heating pad and the thigh actively moved through full adduction-abduction while it is flexed 90°, and through full medial and lateral rotation when the hip is straight.

Prompt reactivation of piriformis TrPs following a good response to intermittent cold with stretch (or injection) may be due to associated displacement of the SI joint. This displacement must be corrected by mobilization of the joint (Chapter 2). Several patients, immediately following restoration of normal function of both the SI joint and the piriformis muscle, developed *acute* subcostal pain along the lower margin of the rib cage in the vicinity of the diaphragm. Each of these patients exhibited paradoxical breathing[90,104] and responded to myofascial release procedures that lifted the lower rib cage up and outward, exerting traction on the lateral abdominal wall muscles and the diaphragm.

Stretch Techniques

Effective stretch or massage for treatment of any muscle with myofascial TrPs depends strongly on the completeness of the patient's relaxation achieved before and during elongation of the muscle. Reciprocal inhibition and contract-relax are effective relaxation techniques. Postisometric relaxation combines both relaxation and muscle elongation.

Massage may be considered a form of localized stretch in the region of the TrP. It is most effective for inactivation of TrPs if the muscle is passively lengthened to the point of taking up all of the slack but remains fully relaxed.

Retzlaff and associates[80] recommended several stretch techniques including reciprocal inhibition, which, for the piriformis, is most effectively done by contracting the antagonistic medial rotator muscles without allowing any medial rotation movement of the thigh, and then after relaxation, passively taking up the slack in the piriformis by increasing medial rotation. Reciprocal inhibition can be alternated with postisometric relaxation, and the intermittent cold applied during the relaxation and take-up-slack phase.

The technique of postisometric relaxation reported by Lewit and Simons[55] is similar in principle to that described as contract-relax by Voss *et al.*[107] and is described in detail in Chapter 2. Postisometric relaxation is facilitated in the piriformis muscle by coordinating the gentle voluntary contraction phase (against the resistance of gravity) with inhalation while looking up, and coordinating the relaxation phase with exhalation while looking down.[54] This facilitation technique may be used alone or with the application of intermittent cold during the relaxation phase.

Some clinicians may prefer alternative stretch positions that have been recommended by other authors. The stretch technique for the piriformis described and illustrated by Lewit[53] affects all short lateral rotators. For this method, the patient is placed prone with the hip extended and the knee flexed. As the foot swings outward, the leg provides gravity-assisted medial rotation of the thigh. This approach stretches all of the short lateral rotators including the piriformis. In this technique, the knee is vulnerable to injury if pressure is applied to the foot or ankle to assist stretch. Another technique illustrated by Evjenth and Hamberg[33] applies adduction to the thigh with the patient supine and with both the hip and knee flexed. This position has the advantage of placing the hip in flexion and provides a convenient method of self-stretch. However, it loses some of the assistance by gravity and makes the referred pain pattern inaccessible to the application of vapocoolant or ice.

Following ischemic compression of the piriformis muscle using the elbow method (see below), TePoorten[99] placed the patient supine and flexed the affected leg on the thigh and the thigh on the abdomen; he then straightened the lower limb while adducting the thigh. After repeating

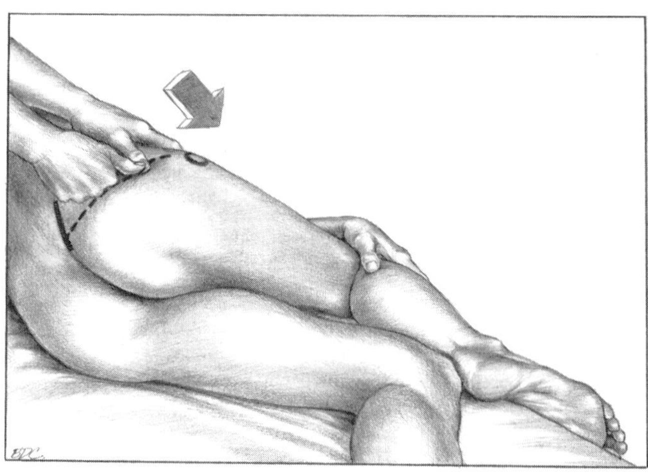

Figure 10.8. Ischemic compression by bimanual thumb pressure to inactivate a TrP in the lateral part of the right piriformis muscle, the upper marginal fibers of which lie deep to the *dotted line*. The uppermost thigh is flexed. The thumb is placed slightly lateral to the junction of the lateral and middle thirds of the distance from the greater trochanter (*open circle*) to the border of the sacrum (*solid line*). Firm application of pressure toward the femur is usually required to project force (*thick arrow*) through the overlying gluteal muscles, which must remain fully relaxed for this technique to be effective. Meanwhile, increasing slack in the piriformis muscle is taken up by adducting the thigh to the limit of the patient's comfort and by asking the patient to hold the knee to prevent it from moving while the operator maintains backward traction on the pelvis. The clinician should avoid pressure that produces tingling in the lower limb due to nerve compression.

this two or three times, he found that it often corrected pelvic and lower limb-length imbalance and relieved the piriformis syndrome.

Julsrud[48] presented a case report of a female athlete with piriformis syndrome who, with daily stretching exercises of the piriformis muscle, resumed running without pain.

Ischemic Compression (Fig. 10.8)

Ischemic compression may be applied externally, as described in Volume 1,[104] with the addition that, for the piriformis, pressure is applied bimanually with the thumbs (Fig. 10.8) over each area of TrP tenderness in the muscle. These areas are located beginning at the lateral end of the muscle, to avoid applying pressure on the sciatic nerve. Other authors[31,80,99] have described and illustrated[80] the application of external pressure on piriformis TrPs by the bent elbow. This technique is attractive because it provides strong leverage, but it may be hazardous because it reduces the operator's sensation of underlying structures and increases the risk of injuring the sciatic nerve. If this elbow technique is used, it should be used with caution in this region.

Direct digital pressure has been applied rectally on rigid tender piriformis muscles near the medial attachment of the muscle and complete pain relief reported.[44] Effectiveness of these compression techniques is improved if the muscle is placed on moderate stretch during treatment.

Massage

In 1937, Thiele[100] described internal massage of the piriformis muscle. With full-length insertion of the finger in the rectum, the fibers of the piriformis are felt immediately beyond (superior to) the sacrospinous ligament. Lateral motion of the finger proceeds lengthwise on that portion of the belly of the muscle lying within the pelvis. The massage is begun lightly to avoid irritating extremely tender tense muscles. In subsequent treatments, the massage pressure is increased. If increased pain is experienced, the clinician returns to lighter massage; pressure is increased as tenderness subsequently decreases. Müller[65] strongly recommended this method of treatment for the piriformis syndrome.

Other Methods of Treatment

Hallin[43] reported that six to ten ultrasound treatments over the tender piriformis muscle at $1\frac{3}{4}$–2 W/cm^2 for 5–6 minutes daily usually relieved the piriformis syndrome pain in 2 weeks. Some physical therapists have found a special transvaginal ultrasound applicator effective. Barton *et al.*[11] recommended ultrasound therapy prior to stretching the piriformis muscle.

Shortwave diathermy was reported to be helpful in conjunction with a full course of physical therapy.[47] Clinical experience (Personal communication, Mary Maloney, P.T.) has shown that pulsed diathermy (Magnatherm Model 1,000. International Medical Electronics, Ltd., 2805 Main, Kansas City, MO 64108) applied in sequential 10-minute periods of relatively high, low, high intensity is a valuable substitute in deeply placed muscles for a heating pad following intermittent cold with stretch. This is most useful in severe acute myofascial TrP syndromes when all intensities must be reduced. As recovery progresses and the patient's tolerance increases, or in chronic myofascial pain syndromes, it becomes preferable to use the pulsed diathermy with a moving head technique at a sustained higher level with appropriate precautions (Personal communication, Mary Maloney, P.T.).

For diathermy to be effective, one would expect that it must increase circulation proportionately more than it increases metabolism in the region of the TrP. Studies are needed to determine the specific effects of diathermy on TrPs.

Reconditioning exercises for the piriformis should follow stretch therapy. One such exercise is described in Section 14 of this chapter.

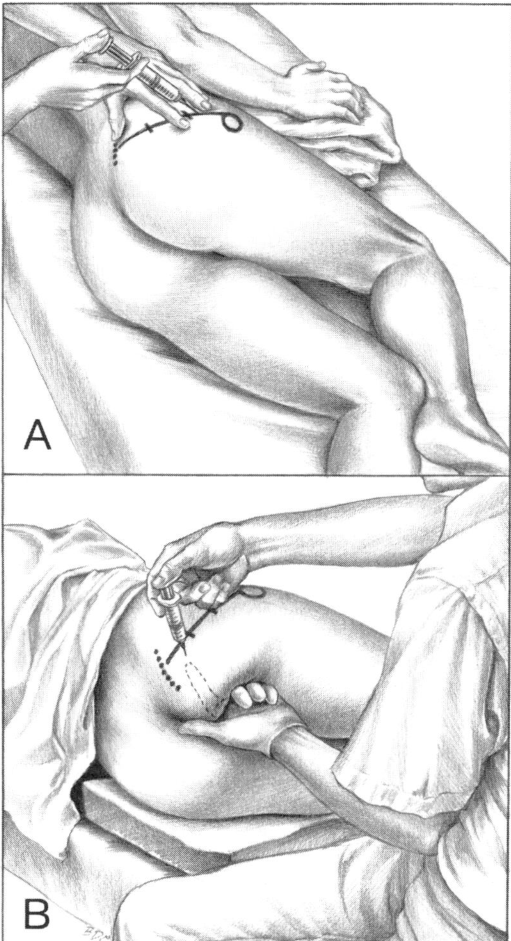

Figure 10.9. Injection of TrPs in the right piriformis muscle. The *open circle* locates the greater trochanter; the *dotted line*, the palpable margin along the edge of the sacrum; and the *solid line*, marked in thirds, overlies the upper (cephalad) margin of the piriformis muscle. *A*, injection of TrP_1 using the usual, completely external, approach. *B*, injection of TrP_2 using a bimanual technique. The left hand locates the trigger-point tenderness via intrapelvic palpation, and the right hand directs the needle toward that fingertip.

13. INJECTION AND STRETCH (Fig. 10.9)

Piriformis Muscle

Details of the examination technique for locating piriformis TrPs are found in Section 9 of this chapter. Details of the injection technique are presented in Section 13 of Chapter 3 in Volume 1.[104]

The lateral TrPs located in the TrP_1 area should be injected before injecting those in the medial TrP_2 area. The lateral TrPs are readily reached externally through the skin and are not in the vicinity of a major nerve trunk. The inactivation of the lateral TrP_1 may also eliminate TrP_2 activity.

Lateral Trigger Point (TrP_1)

To inject the more lateral TrP_1 (Fig. 10.9*A*), the patient lies on the uninvolved side with the uppermost thigh flexed to approximately 90°. The superior border of the piriformis muscle is located by marking a line (see Figure 8.5) that runs from just above the greater trochanter to the point where the palpable border of the sacrum encounters the ilium at the inferior border of the sacroiliac joint. This piriformis line, shown in Figure 10.9, is divided into thirds and the piriformis muscle is palpated just inferior to it for tender spots, as described in Section 9, Trigger Point Examination. The TrP_1 area is lateral and just inferior to the junction of the lateral and middle thirds of the piriformis line. When an active TrP is located, application of digital pressure usually reproduces the myofascial portion of the patient's pain distribution. The spot tenderness of the most sensitive TrP is localized between the fingers of the palpating hand.

Usually a 22-gauge, 50-mm (2-in) needle is used on a 10-mL syringe for the lateral TrP location. In a thin person, a 22-gauge, 1½-inch needle may be sufficient to reach through the skin, gluteus maximus, and piriformis muscle to the joint capsule. This depth of penetration is necessary to ensure penetrating all of the TrPs in this portion of the piriformis muscle. In obese patients, a longer 63- to 75-mm (2½- to 3-in) needle may be required. A solution of 0.5% procaine is prepared by diluting 2% procaine with isotonic saline for injection.

When the TrP tenderness has been localized, the needle is inserted through the skin directly toward the point of maximum tenderness. In pain-sensitive patients, dribbling a small amount of procaine solution during progression of the needle minimizes pain when the TrP is encountered. When a TrP is impaled, the region several millimeters to either side of and above and below the TrP is then explored by peppering with the needle in probing steps, searching for additional TrPs in that vicinity. Needle encounter with a TrP is recognized by the pain response of the patient, and particularly if the encounter reproduces the patient's referred pain. Penetration of the TrP is confirmed when the needle evokes sharp pain and a local twitch response of the muscle.

Before withdrawing the needle completely, the skin at its entry point is slid to one side and the area is palpated for deep tenderness to ensure that no residual TrPs remain.

Following injection, intermittent cold with stretch is applied, as described previously, to eliminate any TrPs that may have been missed. This is followed by active range of motion, with the patient slowly fully shortening and then fully lengthening the muscle by moving the thigh through medial and lateral rotation with the hip straight. This is repeated two or three times to reestablish full range of motion and normalize muscle function. A moist heating pad is then applied to rewarm the skin.

Others[95,99] have also recommended treating the piriformis syndrome by injecting TrPs or tender spots in this lateral musculotendinous portion of the muscle.

Medial Trigger Point (TrP_2)

The authors recommend that injection of TrPs in the medial TrP_2 region be accomplished bimanually. One finger palpates the inner surface of the medial third of the piriformis muscle using the rectal or vaginal route; the other hand inserts the needle externally, directing the needle toward the intrapelvic palpating fingertip, and injects the local anesthetic solution. With sufficient finger-reach, it is possible to palpate both the pelvic inner surface of the piriformis muscle and the pelvic sciatic nerve against the sacrum, as well as the area of the greater sciatic foramen.

Namey and An[68] emphasized that when a long-acting local anesthetic is injected, the physician should warn the patient of possible numbness and weakness in the distribution of the sciatic nerve following injection. The patient should not leave unassisted nor attempt to drive a car until any such local anesthesia has disappeared. When using 0.5% procaine, nerve block rarely lasts longer than 20 minutes.

Others[16,69,71,95] have recommended injection of the piriformis near the lateral border of the sacrum. Pace[69] described passing a long spinal needle just below the edge of the ilium and encountering the piriformis muscle as it exits through the greater sciatic foramen. He guided the direction of the needle by a finger that was palpating the TrP through the vagina or rectum and aimed the needle at the finger until he could feel the needle distend the tissues over the TrP. We localize the TrP in the same way.

Pace[69] then injected 1% lidocaine and waited 5 minutes to establish that the sciatic nerve had not been infiltrated and that the patient was not experiencing a pins-and-needles sensation down the leg. Then, he injected 6 mL of a mixture containing 4 mL of 1% lidocaine and 2 mL (20 mg) of triamcinolone acetonide.[71] We inject only 0.5% procaine and, therefore, need no 5-minute waiting period.

As described previously, Pace recommended a long spinal needle.[69] We also find that, for this approach, a 75- or 90-mm (3- or 3½-in) spinal needle is required in most patients. It was the clinical impression of Pace and Nagle[71] that the addition of corticosteroid provided more complete and more lasting relief. We prefer to inject only 0.5% procaine, since accidental infiltration of the nerve with this solution causes only transient paresthesia and weakness. With either technique, the needle must be replaced immediately if it encounters bone that curls the tip of the needle to produce a hook. A hook on the needle produces a scratchy sensation of roughness when the needle is withdrawn even slightly.

Gynecologists may prefer to use a paravaginal approach.[16,71,109] Wyant[109] notes that the muscle is easier to reach for examination in the female using the vaginal rather than the rectal route. He described a method of introducing the needle through the perineum medial to the ischial tuberosity and advancing it paravaginally under tactile control into the piriformis TrP. It is also possible to reach the piriformis from the lateral fornix of the vagina, by an approach similar to that for paracervical block. Wyant[109] recommended injection of 8 mL of 0.5% lidocaine mixed with 80 mg of triamcinolone.

Among the 84 patients with piriformis syndrome who received injections of 10-mL of 0.5% solution of procaine,[75] 55% of them had prompt amelioration of angiospastic signs and symptoms. The lower extremity oscillogram improved and the chilly feeling in the leg disappeared. In many, weak Achilles reflexes were restored and the extent and intensity of hypalgesia were improved.

Surgical Release

Having first[41] reported surgical release of the muscle, Freiberg later[42] expressed frustration with a lack of rationale for this procedure. Since histological examination of surgical specimens showed no abnormality, he assumed that the muscle was not primarily responsible. He was, however, apparently unaware of myofascial TrPs. Surgical release is still performed for piriformis syndrome.[64,93] If symptoms are caused by myofascial TrPs, then surgery is unnecessary as shown by recent reports of successful medical treatment of the piriformis syndrome.[15,43,68,69,71,94,95,109] Pace stated unequivocally, "surgical resection is not indicated;"[69] Barton *et al.* consider it the last resort.[11]

Other Short Lateral Rotators

No literature was found that described the identification and injection of TrPs in the remaining five short lateral rotators. When TrPs occur there, the location is established as described in Section 9. For practical purposes, localization to a specific muscle is not necessary and one need only distinguish two groups of muscles: the two gemelli and the lateral part of the obturator internus compose one group; the quadratus femoris and the underlying obturator externus compose the other.

When TrP tenderness is identified in one of these muscle groups and injection is deemed necessary, the physician must consider the path of the sciatic nerve as it crosses over these muscles, usually midway between the ischial tuberosity and the greater trochanter (Fig. 10.3). Tenderness of taut bands caused by piriformis TrPs extends almost horizontally across the lower buttock. Tenderness of the sciatic nerve extends vertically along the path of the nerve.

The lateral (peroneal) portion of the sciatic nerve can be located precisely in order to avoid it during injection by observing motor responses to stimulation of the anterior tibial nerve in the region of the injection site. Either a magnetic ring or an EMG needle can be used for stimulation. The former is not invasive and is less painful. A Teflon-coated hypodermic needle of the type used for motor point blocks can be used both for localized stimulation and then injection at another location. Sensory response is unreliable. Stimulation of a TrP elicits pain in its referral pattern, which, in these muscles, may mimic neurogenic pain.

The technique for injection of these muscles is essentially the same as that described for the TrP_1 area in the lateral part

PART 1

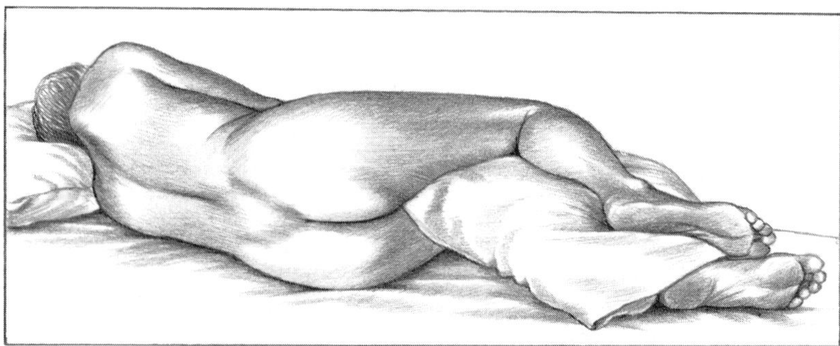

Figure 10.10. Correct lower-limb position to improve sleep when lying on the unaffected side. A pillow is placed between the knees and ankles in order to avoid adduction of the uppermost thigh at the hip, which would place painful stretch on a tense piriformis, as well as on other short lateral rotator, and/or tense gluteal muscles.

of the piriformis, except that one selects a more distal location of needle entry.

14. CORRECTIVE ACTIONS
(Figs. 10.10 and 10.11)

Body Asymmetry

Whenever a lower limb-length inequality or a small hemipelvis produces a compensatory functional scoliosis, the inequality should be corrected. A heel (shoe) lift, as noted by Hallin,[43] corrects the former and an ischial (butt) lift, as described on pages 77–78 in Chapter 4, corrects the latter. See Chapter 4 for a review of the relation between lower limb-length inequalities and pelvic distortions.

Postural and Activity Stress
(Fig. 10.10)

When sleeping on the side, the patient should place a pillow between the knees with the support extending to the ankles to avoid prolonged adduction at the hip with the thigh flexed, which may painfully stretch the taut piriformis muscle and seriously disturb sleep. The recommended position is illustrated in Figure 10.10.

The patient who has myofascial syndromes of these lateral rotator muscles should avoid prolonged immobilization of the involved lower limb when driving a car for a long distance; this can be accomplished by stopping and walking briefly every 20–30 minutes. Sitting on one foot can aggravate TrPs in the hip muscles on that side and should be avoided by those prone to piriformis TrPs.

When sitting at home or at work, the patient should be instructed to change position often. The use of a rocking chair helps to prevent immobility of the muscles, including the piriformis, for prolonged periods of time.

Mechanical Stress

The patient with an involved piriformis muscle should be warned against either making a strong lateral rotatory effort or the braking (restraining) of strong medial rotatory momentum when bearing weight on the involved limb. Such strong rotations often occur when a person plays vigorous tennis, soccer, or volleyball, or engages in competitive running; these rotations are likely to reactivate piriformis TrPs.

In 1947, the senior author and her father[106] reported the importance in some patients of reducing sacroiliac displacement in addition to inactivating the piriformis TrPs to achieve lasting relief. More recently, Hinks[44] emphasized that when sacroiliac subluxation occurs together with the piriformis syndrome, both the subluxation *and* the muscle tension must be restored to normal.

The presence of a Morton foot structure (mediolateral rocking foot) should be identified and corrected as described in Sections 8 and 14 of Chapter 20, to avoid imposing repetitive compensatory strain on the lateral rotator muscles of the hip.

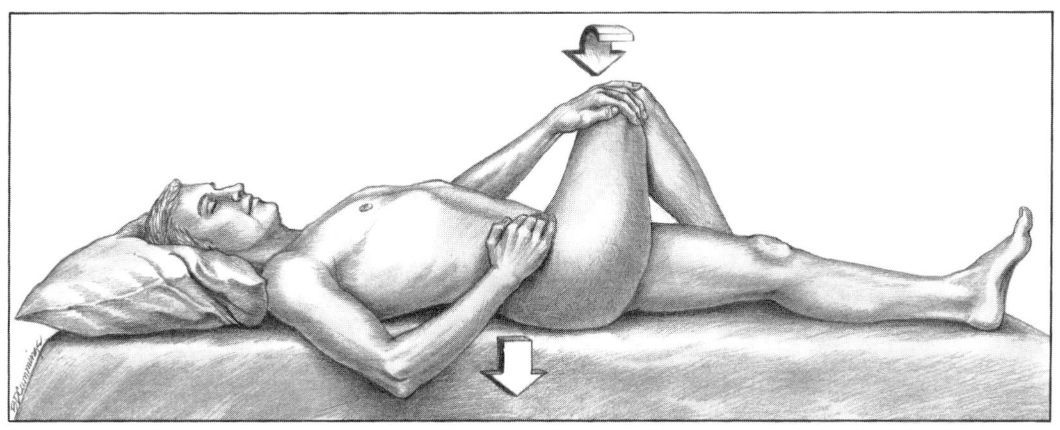

Figure 10.11. Self-stretch of the right piriformis muscle. The right thigh is flexed nearly 90° at the hip with the right foot on the treatment table. To adduct the thigh at the hip, pressure is exerted downward with both hands (*large arrows*), one on the thigh and the other on the pelvis, pulling against each other. To perform postisometric relaxation, the individual then attempts to abduct the thigh by pressing it *gently* against the resisting left hand for a few seconds (isometric contraction of abductors), then relaxes and gently moves the thigh into adduction, which gradually lengthens the piriformis muscle.

Attention should also be given to other causes of a hyperpronated foot.

Self-therapy
(Fig. 10.11)

We have found, as have others,[11] that a home program of prolonged piriformis stretching can be essential for complete and lasting relief. To perform the piriformis muscle passive self-stretch, the supine patient (Fig. 10.11) crosses the leg of the involved side over the opposite thigh, and rests the opposite hand on the knee of the uppermost affected limb. This hand is used, when needed, to assist gravity in adducting the involved thigh, which is flexed about 90°. The patient stabilizes the hip on the involved side by pressing down on the iliac crest with the ipsilateral hand. Release of muscle tension is augmented by the patient "thinking" of gently lifting the weight of the adducted leg (but not moving it) during slow inhalation; then, during slow exhalation, having the muscle "let go" and allowing the piriformis to elongate, as described by Lewit.[54,55]

Saudek[84] illustrates a side-lying version of piriformis self-stretch similar to the supine technique described above. She also illustrates self-stretch of this muscle in the seated position.

A tennis ball may be used for self-application of ischemic compression to the piriformis muscle while side lying in a manner similar to that described in Section 14 of Chapter 8 for the gluteus medius muscle and as shown in Figure 8.9. This treatment can be helpful for lateral piriformis TrPs and for the other five short lateral rotators. The tennis ball must be placed far enough laterally (anteriorly) to avoid the sciatic nerve where pressure causes numbness and tingling below the knee.

Steiner and associates[95] describe and illustrate a valuable "loosening" exercise in which the standing patient performs a rhythmic full rotation of the hips, letting the trunk and arms loosely follow. They recommend performing this exercise three to six times (every few hours) throughout the day.

Stretching of the piriformis should be followed by reconditioning exercises, starting with the subject lying on the unaffected ("normal") side with the uppermost (affected) thigh flexed to 90°. It is particularly beneficial if an assistant can first passively abduct the patient's thigh and then allow the patient to lower the thigh slowly to the treatment table, activating the piriformis in a lengthening contraction. Using this same position, progression can be made to shortening contractions by active abduction of the flexed thigh against the resistance of gravity.

References

1. Adams JA: The piriformis syndrome—report of four cases and review of the literature. *S Afr J Surg 18*:13–18, 1980.
2. Anderson JE: *Grant's Atlas of Anatomy*, Ed. 8. Williams & Wilkins, Baltimore, 1983 (Fig. 3–12).
3. *Ibid*. (Fig. 3–55).
4. *Ibid*. (Fig. 3–73).
5. *Ibid*. (Fig. 4–32*A*).
6. *Ibid*. (Fig. 4–36).
7. *Ibid*. (Fig. 4–40).
8. *Ibid*. (Fig. 4–127*A*).
9. Baker BA: The muscle trigger: evidence of overload injury. *J Neurol Orthop Med Surg 7*:35–44, 1986.
10. Bardeen CR: The musculature, Sect. 5. In *Morris's Human Anatomy*, edited by C. M. Jackson, Ed. 6. Blakiston's Son & Co., Philadelphia, 1921 (p. 493).
11. Barton PM, Grainger RW, Nicholson RL, *et al.*: Toward a rational management of piriformis syndrome. *Arch Phys Med Rehabil 69*:784, 1988.
12. Basmajian JV, Deluca CJ: *Muscles Alive*, Ed. 5. Williams & Wilkins, Baltimore, 1985 (p. 319).
13. Beaton LE, Anson BJ: The relation of the sciatic nerve and its subdivisions to the piriformis muscle. *Anat Rec 70* (Suppl.):1–5, 1937.
14. Beaton LE, Anson BJ: The sciatic nerve and the piriformis muscle: their interrelationship a possible cause of coccygodynia. *J Bone Joint Surg [Br] 20*:686–688, 1938.
15. Brown JA, Braun MA, Namey TC: Pyriformis syndrome in a 10-year-old boy as a complication of operation with the patient in the sitting position. *Neurosurgery 23*:117–119, 1988.
16. Cailliet R: *Low Back Pain Syndrome*. Ed. 3. F.A. Davis, Philadelphia, 1981 (pp. 192–194).
17. Cameron HU, Noftal F: The piriformis syndrome. *Can J Surg 31*:210, 1988.
18. Carter BL, Morehead J, Wolpert SM, *et al.*: *Cross-Sectional Anatomy*. Appleton-Century-Crofts, New York, 1977 (Sects. 38, 39, 44, 45).
19. Clemente CD: *Gray's Anatomy of the Human Body*, American Ed. 30. Lea & Febiger, Philadelphia, 1985 (pp. 568–571).
20. *Ibid*. (Figs. 5–29 and 5–30, pp. 361–363).
21. *Ibid*. (Fig. 6–74, p. 569).
22. *Ibid*. (p. 570).
23. *Ibid*. (p. 571, Fig. 6–75).
24. *Ibid*. (pp. 1230–1231).
25. *Ibid*. (p. 1236).
26. *Ibid*. (p. 1244).
27. Cohen BA, Lanzieri CF, Mendelson DS, *et al.*: CT evaluation of the greater sciatic foramen in patients with sciatica. *AJNR 7*:337–342, 1986.
28. De Luca CJ, Bloom LJ, Gilmore LD: Compression induced damage on in-situ severed and intact nerves. *Orthopedics 10*:777–784, 1987.
29. Duchenne GB: *Physiology of Motion*, translated by E.B. Kaplan. J.B. Lippincott, Philadelphia, 1949 (255, 256).
30. Dye SF, van Dam BE, Westin GW: Eponyms and etymons in orthopaedics. *Contemp Orthop 6*:92–96, 1983.
31. Edwards FO: Piriformis Syndrome. *Academy of Osteopathy Yearbook*, 1962 (pp. 39–41).
32. Ehrlich GE: Early diagnosis of ankylosing spondylitis: role of history and presence of HLA-B27 Antigen. *Internal Medicine for the Specialist 3*(3):112–116, 1982.
33. Evjenth O, Hamberg J: *Muscle Stretching in Manual Therapy, A Clinical Manual*, Vol. 1, The Extremities. Alfta Rehab Førlag, Alfta, Sweden, 1984 (pp. 97, 122, 172).
34. Ferner H, Staubesand J: *Sobotta Atlas of Human Anatomy*, Ed. 10, Vol. 2. Urban & Schwarzenberg, Baltimore, 1983 (Figs. 331, 403, 406).
35. *Ibid*. (Fig. 404).
36. *Ibid*. (Fig. 419).
37. *Ibid*. (Fig. 420).
38. *Ibid*. (Fig. 421).
39. Fishman LM: Electrophysiological evidence of piriformis syndrome—II. *Arch Phys Med Rehabil 69*:800, 1988.
40. Freiberg AH, Vinke TH: Sciatica and the sacroiliac joint. *J Bone Joint Surg 16[Am]*:126–36, 1934.
41. Freiberg AH: Sciatic pain and its relief by operations on muscle and fascia. *Arch Surg 34*:337–350, 1937.
42. Freiberg AH: The fascial elements in associated low-back and sciatic pain. *J Bone Joint Surg [Am]23*:478–480, 1941.
43. Hallin RP: Sciatic pain and the piriformis muscle. *Postgrad Med 74*:69–72, 1983.
44. Hinks AH: Letters: Further aid for piriformis muscle syndrome. *J Am Osteopath Assoc 74*:93, 1974.
45. Hollinshead WH: *Functional Anatomy of the Limbs and Back*, Ed. 4. W.B. Saunders, Philadelphia, 1976 (pp. 299–301).
46. Hollinshead WH: *Anatomy for Surgeons*, Vol. 3, *The Back and Limbs*, Ed. 3. Harper & Row, New York, 1982 (pp. 666–668, 702)
47. Jan M-H, Lin Y-F: Clinical experience of applying shortwave diathermy over the piriformis for sciatic patients. *Taiwan I Asueh Hui Tsa Chih 82*:1065–1070, 1983.
48. Julsrud ME: Piriformis syndrome. *J Am Podiatr Med Assoc 79*:128–131, 1989.
49. Karl RD, Jr., Yedinak MA, Hartshorne MF, Cawthon MA, Bauman JM, Howard WH, Bunker SR: Scintigraphic appearance of the piriformis muscle syndrome. *Clin Nucl Med 10*: 361–363, 1985.
50. Kipervas IP, Ivanov LA, Urikh EA, Pakhomov SK: [Clinico-electromyographic characteristics of piriformis muscle syndrome] (Russian) *Zh Nevropatol Psikhiatr 76*:1289–1292, 1976.
51. Kirkaldy-Willis WH, Hill RJ: A more precise diagnosis for low-back pain. *Spine 4*:102–109, 1979.
52. Lee C-S, Tsai T-L: The relation of the sciatic nerve to the piriformis muscle. *J Formosan Med Assoc 73*:75–80, 1974.
53. Lewit K: *Manipulative Therapy in Rehabilitation of the Motor System*. Butterworths, London, 1985, (pp. 278, 279).

54. Lewit K: Postisometric relaxation in combination with other methods of muscular facilitation and inhibition. *Manual Med 1*:101–104, 1986.
55. Lewit K, Simons DG: Myofascial pain: relief by post-isometric relaxation. *Arch Phys Med Rehabil 65*:452–456, 1984.
56. Long C: Myofascial pain syndromes: Part III—some syndromes of trunk and thigh. *Henry Ford Hospital Bulletin 3*:102–106, 1955 (p. 104).
57. McMinn RMH, Hutchings RT: *Color Atlas of Human Anatomy*. Year Book Medical Publishers, Chicago, 1977 (p. 81).
58. *Ibid*. (p. 245).
59. *Ibid*. (p. 264).
60. *Ibid*. (pp. 273, 274).
61. *Ibid*. (p. 293).
62. Mirman MJ: Sciatic pain: two more tips. *Postgrad Med 74*:50, 1983.
63. Mitchell FL: Structural pelvic function. *Academy of Applied Osteopathy Yearbook 2*:178–199, 1965.
64. Mizuguchi T: Division of the pyriformis muscle for the treatment of sciatica. *Arch Surg 111*: 719–722, 1976.
65. Müller A: Piriformitis? *Die Medizinische Welt 24*: 1037, 1937.
66. Myint K: Nerve compression due to an abnormal muscle. *Med J Malaysia 36*:227–229, 1981.
67. Nainzadeh N, Lane ME: Somatosensory evoked potentials following pudendal nerve stimulation as indicators of low sacral root involvement in a postlaminectomy patient. *Arch Phys Med Rehabil 68*:170–172, 1987.
68. Namey TC, An HS: Emergency diagnosis and management of sciatica: differentiating the non-diskogenic causes. *Emergency Med Reports 6*:101–109, 1985.
69. Pace JB: Commonly overlooked pain syndromes responsive to simple therapy. *Postgrad Med 58*:107–113, 1975.
70. Pace JB, Henning C: Episacroiliac lipoma. *Am Fam Physician 6*:70–73, 1972.
71. Pace JB, Nagle D: Piriform syndrome. *West J Med 124*:435–439, 1976.
72. Pećina M: Contribution to the etiological explanation of the piriformis syndrome. *Acta Anat 105*:181–187, 1979.
73. Pernkopf E: *Atlas of Topographical and Applied Human Anatomy*, Vol. 2. W.B. Saunders, Philadelphia, 1964 (Fig. 314).
74. Pope MH, Frymoyer JW, Anderson G (eds): *Occupational Low Back Pain*. Praegar, New York, 1984.
75. Popelianskii Ia. Iu., Bobrovnikova TI: [The syndrome of the piriformis muscle and lumbar discogenic radiculitis.] (Russian) *Zh Nevropatol Psikhiatr 68*:656–662, 1968.
76. Porterfield JA: The sacroiliac joint, Chapter 23. In *Orthopaedic and Sports Physical Therapy*, edited by J.A. Gould and G.J. Davis. The C.V. Mosby Co., St. Louis, 1985 (pp. 550–580, see 553, 565–566).
77. Rasch PJ, Burke RK: *Kinesiology and Applied Anatomy*, Ed. 6. Lea & Febiger, Philadelphia, 1978 (p. 278).
78. Rask MR: Superior gluteal nerve entrapment syndrome. *Muscle Nerve 3*:304–307, 1980.
79. Reichel G, Gaerisch F Jr: Ein Beitrag zur Differentialdiagnose von Lumbago und Kokzygodynie. *Zent bl Neurochir 49*:178–184, 1988.
80. Retzlaff EW, Berry AH, Haight AS, Parente PA, Lichty HA, *et al*. The piriformis muscle syndrome. *J Am Osteopath Assoc 73*:799–807, 1974.
81. Rodnan GP: *Primer on the Rheumatic Diseases*. Arthritis Foundation, 1983 (pp. 87, 179, 181).
82. Rohen JW, Yokochi C: *Color Atlas of Anatomy*, Ed. 2. Igaku-Shoin, New York, 1988 (pp. 418, 419).
83. *Ibid*. (p. 441).
84. Saudek CE: The hip, Chapter 17. In *Orthopaedic and Sports Physical Therapy*, edited by J.A. Gould III and G.J. Davies, Vol. 2. CV Mosby, St. Louis, 1985 (pp. 365–407, see Figs. 17–31, 17–42, 17–43).
85. Sheon RP, Moskowitz RW, Goldberg VM: *Soft Tissue Rheumatic Pain*, Ed. 2. Lea & Febiger, Philadelphia, 1987 (pp. 168–169).
86. Shordania JF: Die chronischer Entzündung des Musculus piriformis—die piriformitis—als eine der Ursachen von Kreuzschmerzen bei Frauen. *Die Medizinische Welt 10*:999–1001, 1936.
87. Simons, DG: Myofascial pain syndromes, part of Chapter 11. In *Medical Rehabilitation*, edited by J.V. Basmajian and R.L. Kirby. Williams & Wilkins, Baltimore, 1984 (pp. 209–215, 313–320).
88. Simons DG: Myofascial pain syndrome due to trigger points, Chapter 45. In *Rehabilitation Medicine*, edited by Joseph Goodgold. C.V. Mosby Co., St. Louis, 1988 (pp. 686–723, see 709, 711).
89. Simons DG, Travell JG: Myofascial origins of low back pain. 3. Pelvic and lower extremity muscles. *Postgrad Med 73*:99–108, 1983.
90. Simons DG, Travell JG: Myofascial pain syndromes, Chapter 25. In *Textbook of Pain*, edited by P.D. Wall and R. Melzack, Ed 2. Churchill Livingstone, London, 1989 (pp. 364, 365, 377).
91. Simons DG, Travell JG, Simons LS: Protecting the ozone layer. *Arch Phys Med Rehabil 71*:64, 1990.
92. Sinaki M, Merritt JL, Stillwell GK: Tension myalgia of the pelvic floor. *Mayo Clin Proc 52*:717–722, 1977.
93. Solheim LF, Siewers P, Paus B: The piriformis muscle syndrome. *Acta Orthop Scand 52*:73–75, 1981.
94. Stein JM, Warfield CA: Two entrapment neuropathies. *Hosp Pract*:100A–100P, January 1983.
95. Steiner C, Staubs C, Ganon M, *et al*.: Piriformis syndrome: pathogenesis, diagnosis and treatment. *J Am Osteopath Assoc 87*:318–323, 1987 (p. 322, Fig. 3).
96. Stimson BB: The low back problem. *Psychosom Med 9*:210–212, 1947.
97. Synek VM: Short latency somatosensory evoked potentials in patients with painful dysaesthesias in peripheral nerve lesions. *Pain 29*:49–58, 1987.
98. Synek VM: The piriformis syndrome: review and case presentation. *Clin Exper Neurol 23*:31–37, 1987.

99. TePoorten BA: The piriformis muscle. *J Am Osteopath Assoc 69*:150–160, 1969.
100. Thiele GH: Coccygodynia and pain in the superior gluteal region. *JAMA 109*:1271–1275, 1937.
101. Tillmann VB: Variation in the pathway of the inferior gluteal nerve. *Anat Anz 145*:293–302, 1979.
102. Toldt C: *An Atlas of Human Anatomy*, translated by M.E. Paul, Ed. 2, Vol. 1. Macmillan, New York, 1919 (p. 341).
103. *Ibid*. (pp. 346, 347).
104. Travell JG, Simons DG: *Myofascial Pain and Dysfunction: The Trigger Point Manual*. Williams & Wilkins, Baltimore, 1983 (pp. 74–86, 86–87, 364–365).
105. Travell W, Travell J: Technique for reduction and ambulatory treatment of sacroiliac displacement. *Arch Phys Ther 23*:222–232, 1942.
106. Travell J, Travell W: Therapy of low back pain by manipulation and of referred pain in the lower extremity by procaine infiltration. *Arch Phys Ther 27*:537–547, 1946.
107. Voss DE, Ionta MK, Myers BJ: *Proprioceptive Neuromuscular Facilitation*, Ed.3. Harper & Row, Philadelphia, 1985 (pp. 304–305).
108. Wood J: On some varieties in human myology. *Proc R Soc Lond 13*:299–303, 1894.
109. Wyant GM: Chronic pain syndromes and their treatment. III. The piriformis syndrome. *Can Anaesth Soc J 26*:305–308, 1979.

PART 1

PART 2

CHAPTER 11
Hip, Thigh, and Knee Pain-and-Muscle Guide

INTRODUCTION TO PART 2

This second part of THE TRIGGER POINT MANUAL includes all of the thigh muscles not included in Part 1 of Volume 2: the quadriceps femoris, the hamstrings, all adductors including the pectineus, the tensor fasciae latae, sartorius, and popliteus muscles. Differential diagnosis of an individual muscle's referred pain pattern is considered under Section 6, Symptoms, in each muscle chapter.

PAIN GUIDE TO INVOLVED MUSCLES

This guide lists the muscles that may be responsible for referred pain in each of the areas shown in Figure 11.1. These areas, which identify where patients may complain of pain, are listed alphabetically below. The muscles most likely to refer pain to a designated area are listed under the name of that area. One uses this chart by locating the name of the area that hurts and then by looking under that heading for the muscles that are likely to cause the pain. Then, reference should be made to the pain patterns of individual muscles; the figure and page numbers of each pattern follow in parentheses.

In a general way, the muscle listings follow the order of frequency in which they are likely to cause pain in that area. This order is only an approximation; the selection process by which patients reach an examiner greatly influences which of their muscles are most likely to be symptomatic. **Bold face** type indicates that the muscle refers an essential pain pattern to that pain area. Normal type indicates that the muscle may refer a spillover pattern to that pain area. TrP means trigger point.

PAIN GUIDE

ANTERIOR KNEE PAIN

Rectus femoris (14.1, p. 250)
Vastus medialis (14.2*A* and 14.2*B*, p. 251)
Adductors longus and brevis (15.1, p. 291)

ANTERIOR THIGH PAIN

Adductors longus and brevis (15.1, p. 291)
Iliopsoas (5.1, p. 90)
Adductor magnus (15.2*A*, p. 292)
Vastus intermedius (14.3, p. 252)
Pectineus (13.1, p. 237)
Sartorius (12.6, p. 227)
Quadratus lumborum (4.1*A*, p. 30)
Rectus femoris (14.1, p. 250)

ANTEROMEDIAL KNEE PAIN

Vastus medialis (14.2, p. 251)
Gracilis (15.3, p. 293)
Rectus femoris (14.1, p. 250)
Sartorius, lower TrP (12.6, p. 227)
Adductors longus and brevis (15.1, p. 291)

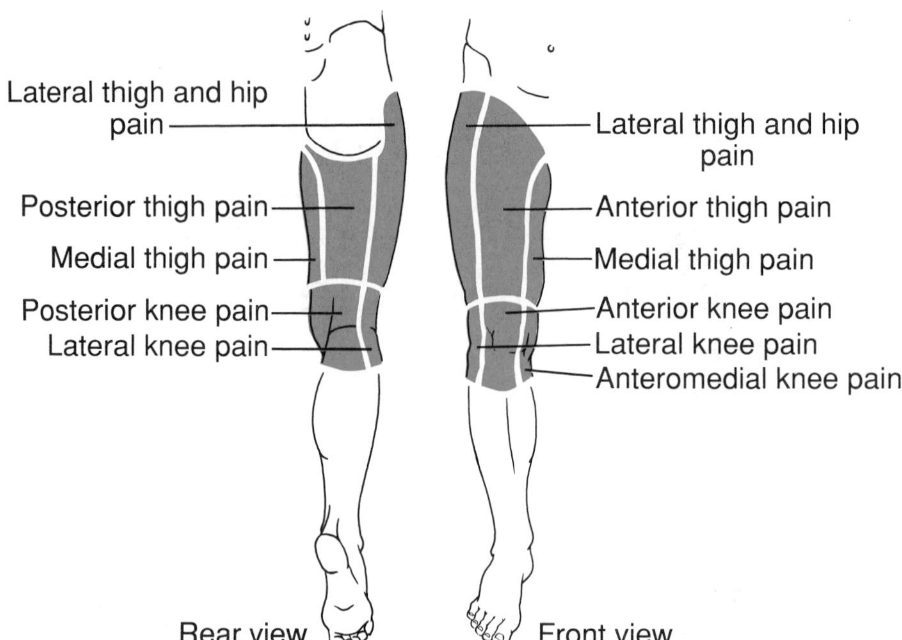

Figure 11.1. Designated areas (*red*) in the hip, thigh, and knee regions where patients may describe myofascial pain. The pain may be referred to each designated area from the muscles listed in the PAIN GUIDE on the previous page and on this page.

LATERAL KNEE PAIN

Vastus lateralis (14.4 TrP_{1-4}, p. 253)

LATERAL THIGH AND HIP PAIN

Gluteus minimus (9.2, p. 169)
Vastus lateralis (14.4 TrP_{2-5}, p. 253)
Piriformis (10.1, p. 188)
Quadratus lumborum (4.1*A*, p. 30)
Tensor fasciae latae (12.1, p. 218)
Vastus intermedius (14.3, p. 252)
Gluteus maximus (7.1*B*, TrP_2, p. 133)
Vastus lateralis (14.4 TrP_1, p. 253)
Rectus femoris (14.1, p. 250)

MEDIAL THIGH PAIN

Pectineus (13.1, p. 237)
Vastus medialis (14.2*B*, p. 251)
Gracilis (15.3, p. 293)
Adductor magnus (15.2*A*, TrP_1, p. 292)
Sartorius (12.6, p. 227)

POSTERIOR KNEE PAIN

Gastrocnemius (21.1 TrP_3, TrP_4, p. 399)
Biceps femoris (16.1, p. 317)
Popliteus (17.1, p. 340)
Semitendinosus and semimembranosus (16.1, p. 317)
Gastrocnemius (21.1 TrP_1, p. 399)
Soleus (22.1 TrP_2, p. 429)
Plantaris (22.3, p. 430)

POSTERIOR THIGH PAIN

Gluteus Minimus (9.1, p. 169)
Semitendinosus and semimembranosus (16.1*A*, p. 317)
Biceps femoris (16.1, p. 317)
Piriformis (10.1, p. 188)
Obturator internus (6.1*B*, p. 112)

CHAPTER 12
Tensor Fasciae Latae Muscle and Sartorius Muscle

"Pseudotrochanteric Bursitis" and *"Surreptitious Accomplice"*

HIGHLIGHTS—TENSOR FASCIAE LATAE: **REFERRED PAIN** and tenderness from trigger points (TrPs) in the tensor fasciae latae muscle concentrate in the anterolateral thigh over the greater trochanter and extend down the thigh toward the knee. Proximal **ANATOMICAL ATTACHMENTS** of the tensor fasciae latae are to the anterior iliac crest and anterior superior iliac spine. Distally, the anteromedial tendinous fibers of the tensor fasciae latae terminate in the lateral patellar retinaculum and in the deep fascia of the leg superficial to the patellar ligament. The posterolateral half of the muscle's tendon attaches below the knee onto the lateral tubercle of the tibia via the iliotibial tract, from which some fibers branch to the lateral femoral condyle and the linea aspera of the lower femur. **FUNCTION** of the tensor fasciae latae in normal gait is to assist hip flexion during swing and to assist in stabilization of the pelvis during stance. It acts to assist flexion, abduction, and medial rotation of the thigh (in that order of importance), and to help stabilize the knee. All fibers of the muscle may assist flexion and abduction of the thigh. The most anteromedial fibers are always involved in flexion and abduction of the thigh. The most posterolateral fibers always assist medial rotation of the thigh and stabilization of the knee. **SYMPTOMS** include pain deep in the hip and down the thigh as far as the knee. The pain prevents walking rapidly or lying comfortably on the side of the TrPs. Pain referred from this muscle mimics pain from TrPs in the anterior gluteus minimus, gluteus medius, and vastus lateralis muscles, and also is often mistakenly attributed to trochanteric bursitis. **PATIENT EXAMINATION** reveals restriction of extension at the hip and limited adduction (Ober sign). **TRIGGER POINT EXAMINATION** is conducted by flat palpation with the patient supine. Frequently, a local twitch response is evident. **ASSOCIATED TRIGGER POINTS** seen with tensor fasciae latae TrPs most often are in the anterior gluteus minimus muscle, sometimes in the rectus femoris, iliopsoas, or sartorius muscles. **INTERMITTENT COLD WITH STRETCH** for inactivating TrPs in the tensor fasciae latae is most effectively done with the side-lying patient positioned so that, as the vapocoolant or ice is applied distalward over the muscle and anterolateral thigh, the thigh is first extended. Gravity is then allowed to pull the thigh into adduction and lateral rotation. Application of a moist heating pad and slow active range of motion complete the procedure. **INJECTION** of the relatively superficial TrPs in this muscle involves no special caveats or unusual precautions. **CORRECTIVE ACTIONS** include avoiding prolonged hip flexion and, as home therapy, the patient is taught a hip extension exercise for stretching the tensor fasciae latae and other hip flexor muscles.

HIGHLIGHTS—SARTORIUS: **REFERRED PAIN** from trigger points (TrPs) in the sartorius muscle is often described as sharp or tingling, not the deep ache that usually characterizes myofascial TrP pain. The disturbing sensation appears in the general vicinity of the TrP. Proximal **ANATOMICAL ATTACHMENTS** of the sartorius muscle are to the anterior superior iliac spine, and distal attachments are to the medial surface of the upper tibia. The muscle curves diagonally across the front of the thigh. **FUNCTION** of the sartorius includes assisting hip flexion and knee flexion during walking. It assists flexion, abduction, and lateral rotation of the thigh, in that order of importance. **TRIGGER POINT EXAMINA-**

TION is performed by flat palpation of the muscle with the patient supine. Meralgia paresthetica is usually caused by **ENTRAPMENT** of the lateral femoral cutaneous nerve as it exits the pelvis at the inguinal ligament. For this muscle, **INTERMITTENT COLD WITH STRETCH** is usually less satisfactory than massage techniques or **INJECTION**, which is usually uncomplicated for the TrPs in this superficial muscle. **CORRECTIVE ACTIONS** primarily consist of avoidance of strain of the sartorius (e.g., avoid sitting in the lotus position) and avoidance of prolonged hip flexion during the day or at night.

---

1. REFERRED PAIN—TENSOR FASCIAE LATAE

(Fig. 12.1)

The term "pseudotrochanteric bursitis" applies to the pain and tenderness referred from trigger points (TrPs) in the tensor fasciae latae muscle. Patients with these TrPs often describe pain in the hip joint region and down the anterolateral aspect of the thigh (Fig. 12.1), occasionally extending as far as the knee. The pain is more severe during movement of the hip. These patients are likely to be misdiagnosed as having trochanteric bursitis.

Other authors have identified myalgic spots (TrPs) localized in the tensor fasciae latae muscle.[41,42,45] When compressed, these TrPs referred pain to the thigh,[45,57,104] along the outside of the thigh, knee, and calf,[55] and into the hip and anterolateral aspect of the thigh.[95–97] Arcangeli *et al.*[9] illustrated pain referred from TrPs in the tensor fasciae latae muscle that projected to the anterolateral portion of the thigh. Kellgren[56] induced pain referred over the lateral surface of the buttock, thigh, knee, and upper half of the anterolateral leg by injecting hypertonic saline into the tensor fasciae latae muscle.

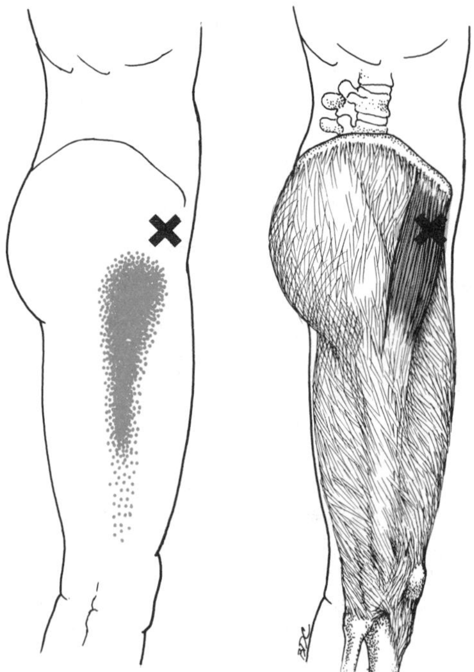

Figure 12.1. Pattern of pain (*bright red*) referred from a trigger point (***X***) in the right tensor fasciae latae muscle (*red*), fascia removed.

2. ANATOMICAL ATTACHMENTS AND CONSIDERATIONS—TENSOR FASCIAE LATAE

(Fig. 12.2)

The tensor fasciae latae muscle attaches ***proximally*** to the anterior part of the outer lip of the crest of the ilium, to the outer aspect of the anterior superior iliac spine (Fig. 12.2), and to the deep surface of the fascia lata.[23] At its upper anterior attachment, it lies between the gluteus medius and the sartorius. ***Distally***, the anteromedial part and the posterolateral part of the muscle form different attachments, which are reflected in equally distinctive functions.[85] (In other mammals, including other primates, the iliotibial tract and the fascia lata are separate structures with different functions.[85])

The tendinous fibers of the **anteromedial half** of the tensor fasciae latae muscle extend down the thigh and curve anteriorly at the level of the patella to interweave with the lateral patellar retinaculum and the deep fascia of the leg superficial to the patellar ligament. Contrary to earlier, less detailed studies, tendinous fibers of this anteromedial half of the muscle do not attach directly to the patella; most are secured at or above the knee.[85]

The tendinous fibers of the **posterolateral half** of the tensor fasciae latae muscle join the fibers of the longitudinal middle layer of the fascia lata (iliotibial

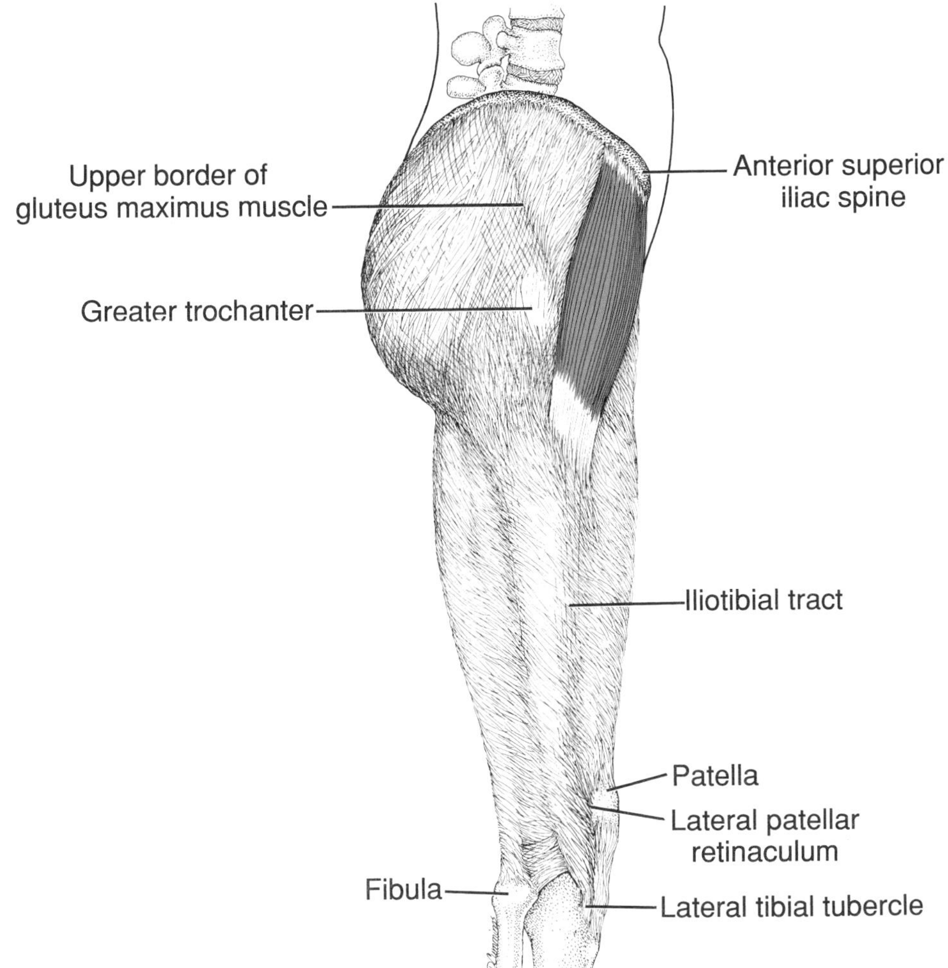

Figure 12.2. Side view of attachments of the right tensor fasciae latae muscle (*red, fascia cut*). Above, the muscle attaches along and below the crest of the ilium just posterior to the anterior superior iliac spine. Below, the anteromedial tendinous fibers attach to the fascia at the knee, and the posterolateral tendinous fibers anchor to the iliotibial tract, which continues down to the lateral tubercle of the tibia.

tract). This fibrous band attaches distally to the lateral tubercle of the tibia, but some fibers from its deep surface branch off and attach to the lateral femoral condyle and linea aspera of the femur. Traction on this band (the middle layer of the fascia lata) produced tension in the iliotibial tract that was visible all the way down to the lateral tubercle of the tibia. However, some of the force was taken up by the fascial attachments to the femur.[85]

Tendinous fibers of the superior portion of the gluteus maximus muscle also join the iliotibial tract via the superficial layer of oblique interweaving fibers.[85]

The tensor fasciae latae is a relatively small postural muscle. It is about half the weight of the gluteus minimus and one-fourth the weight of the gluteus medius.[48]

Variations in this muscle include an accessory slip to the inguinal ligament. Sometimes its fibers fuse with those of the gluteus maximus to form a muscular mass comparable to the deltoid muscle of the shoulder.[11] The tensor fasciae latae has been reported to be congenitally absent as a family trait.[70]

Supplemental References

The tensor fasciae latae is shown from in front,[3,6,76] in dissection,[89] from in front with vessels and

PART 2

nerves,[92] and in relation to the gluteus minimus.[80] It is seen from behind in dissection[90] and in relation to the gluteus minimus,[81] and from the lateral side in its entirety.[34] The muscle appears in a full series of cross sections,[20] in three cross sections of the thigh,[79] and at one level.[36] Photographs reveal its surface contours through the skin.[2,35,65] Its bony attachment is marked on the anterior iliac crest.[37,78]

3. INNERVATION—TENSOR FASCIAE LATAE

A branch of the superior gluteal nerve to the gluteus minimus muscle innervates the tensor fasciae latae muscle. The nerve derives its fibers from the fourth and fifth lumbar and the first sacral spinal nerves.[23]

4. FUNCTION—TENSOR FASCIAE LATAE

As is the case for most other lower limb muscles, the tensor fasciae latae functions during the stance phase of gait primarily to *control* movement (often at a proximal segment) rather than to produce it. This muscle assists the gluteus medius and gluteus minimus in stabilizing the pelvis (countering the tendency to fall away from the support limb).[86] The most posterolateral fibers also are involved in stabilizing the knee.[85]

Actions

In general, the tensor fasciae latae assists flexion, abduction, and medial rotation of the thigh at the hip.[14,87]

More specifically, electromyographic (EMG) findings indicate that all fibers, at times, may assist flexion and abduction of the thigh. Only the anteromedial fibers, however, are *always* involved in flexion and abduction of the thigh. Only the most posterolateral fibers are always active in medial rotation; they are also involved in locking the knee in full extension with the hip maintained in medial rotation.[85]

This muscle is a flexor of the thigh at the hip regardless of what the knee is doing.[14,38] The posterolateral fibers were active electromyographically during flexion of the thigh only when it was also rotated medially. These posterolateral fibers were active during abduction of the thigh except when it was combined with lateral rotation of the hip. The posterolateral fibers were always involved in medial rotation, but the anteromedial fibers were active during medial rotation only when the hip was also flexed, or abducted 45°. As expected, the muscle did not contribute to lateral rotation.[85] Understandably, the findings of previous authors, who made no distinction between these two groups of fibers, were frequently controversial.

Stimulation of the tensor fasciae latae muscle produced strong medial rotation and some flexion of the thigh,[29,53] but weak[53] or no[29] abduction. However, Merchant,[71] using a mechanical model, concluded that the tensor fasciae latae contributed nearly one-third of the abductor force at the hip with the pelvis and femur in neutral position, and that this force was markedly increased by lateral rotation and markedly decreased by medial rotation of the femur.

Functions

Paré and associates[85] have shown that the anteromedial half and the posterolateral half of the tensor fasciae latae muscle are active at different times for different reasons. During walking, the most anteromedial fibers were activated in the swing limb (during midswing); the most posterolateral fibers were activated in the stance limb. The posterolateral fibers are also active at heel-strike during jogging, running, or sprinting,[68,85] stepping up on a platform, and climbing a ladder. The more vigorous the activity, the more vigorous were these responses. The fact that the anteromedial portion of the muscle attaches at and above the knee and that the posterolateral portion also attaches below the knee fits with the cited EMG evidence that the anteromedial portion of the muscle acts primarily as a flexor of the thigh while the posterolateral portion acts more as a stabilizer of the knee.

In an EMG study of selected sports skills,[17] both the right and left tensor fasciae latae muscles were vigorously active during volleyball and basketball jumping activities. Both muscles were slightly to moderately active during right-handed throwing activities, during a tennis serve, and when batting a baseball.

Lifting a heavy load from the floor caused minimal EMG activity in the tensor fasciae latae muscle, but a step forward while holding the load evoked nearly 50% of the maximum voluntary level of activity,[74] consistent with the results observed by Paré and associates.[85] During bicycling,[47] this muscle was active electromyographically during the period when the hip flexors became active as the pedal progressed upward from horizontal through the top of its stroke.

Absence[53] or paralysis[72] of the tensor fasciae latae produced no changes in gait or in function at the knees or hips. However, stress testing was not reported.

5. FUNCTIONAL (MYOTATIC) UNIT—TENSOR FASCIAE LATAE

For flexion of the thigh, the tensor fasciae latae muscle works with the following agonists: the rectus femoris, iliopsoas, pectineus, anterior gluteus medius and minimus, and sartorius muscles. Its chief antagonists for this function are the gluteus maximus and hamstring muscles.

For abduction of the thigh, the agonists are the gluteus medius and gluteus minimus. This function is opposed by the adductor group of hip muscles and the gracilis.[87]

6. SYMPTOMS—TENSOR FASCIAE LATAE

Patients with active TrPs in the tensor fasciae latae muscle are aware primarily of the referred pain, usually in the hip joint, and of pain and soreness (referred tenderness) in the region of the greater trochanter. Some complain of pain extending down the thigh as far as the knee. They have poor tolerance for prolonged sitting with the hip flexed 90° or more (jackknifed position). Pain prevents them from walking rapidly.

These patients are usually unable to lie comfortably on the side of the TrPs because doing so puts body-weight pressure on the area of referred tenderness over the greater trochanter and directly on the TrPs. They are sometimes unable to lie on the opposite side without a pillow between the knees because of the tight iliotibial band. Until these patients discover the value of this pillow, they often must sleep on the back.

Differential Diagnosis

Pain referred from TrPs in the tensor fasciae latae can easily be mistaken for pain arising from TrPs in the anterior gluteus minimus, gluteus medius, or vastus lateralis muscles. Certain TrPs in the quadratus lumborum muscle also refer pain and tenderness to the greater trochanter.

An L_4 neuropathy caused by lumbar spine derangement, or the peripheral nerve entrapment of meralgia paresthetica, may produce pain distribution confusingly similar to the pattern of pain referred from tensor fasciae latae TrPs. Section 10A, which follows in this chapter, discusses meralgia paresthetica in detail. When patients have symptoms of meralgia paresthetica, they may, in addition, have active TrPs in the tensor fasciae latae muscle that are also contributing to their symptoms.

Patients with tensor fasciae latae TrPs are readily misdiagnosed as having trochanteric bursitis. These patients with TrPs do have pain and tenderness over the bursa, but these symptoms are referred from the TrPs and are not caused by disease of the bursa.

The iliotibial tract friction syndrome causes diffuse pain and tenderness of the lateral femoral condyle where the iliotibial tract rubs back and forth; this condition is common in bowlegged runners with pronated feet and is seen in those who wear shoes with worn lateral soles.[16]

Sacroiliitis (sacroiliac arthritis) refers pain and tenderness to the low back, buttock, and, like tensor fasciae latae TrPs, to the lateral thigh. However, the pain of sacroiliitis may extend beyond the knee to the ankle.[73]

7. ACTIVATION AND PERPETUATION OF TRIGGER POINTS—TENSOR FASCIAE LATAE

Activation of tensor fasciae latae TrPs may be due to sudden trauma, as when landing on the feet from a high jump, or to chronic overload. This chronic overload may be caused by jogging uphill and downhill without appropriate support for a foot with a Morton foot structure or other factor causing an excessively pronated foot.

Regular walking or running on surfaces that are sloped to one side can lead to tensor fasciae latae problems because these slants increase genu varus in one leg and genu valgus in the other. They also increase pronation on one side and limit it on the other.

Poor conditioning and inadequate warm-up stretching exercises can lead to injuries that activate or perpetuate TrPs in runners.

As in other muscles, TrPs in the tensor fasciae latae are aggravated by immobilization in the shortened position for long periods. This happens during prolonged sitting with the hip at an acute angle or while sleeping in a tightly flexed fetal position.

In a study of 100 patients with myofascial pain as the result of a first serious automobile collision, Baker[10] reported the activation of very few tensor fasciae latae TrPs regardless of the direction of impact.

8. PATIENT EXAMINATION—TENSOR FASCIAE LATAE

Patients with tensor fasciae latae TrPs tend to keep the hip slightly flexed when standing and have difficulty leaning backwards and hyperextending the hip (a movement that is restricted also by TrPs in the iliopsoas and anterior sections of the gluteus medius and gluteus minimus muscles). Ambulation with the hips flexed is not painful. Pain on walking that is caused by tensor fasciae latae TrPs disappears if the upper limbs carry the body weight (as when using crutches).

The patient may be examined for muscle tightness in the supine position with one hip held in flexion by the patient and the other limb extended over the end of the treatment table, as illustrated in Figure 5.3 of the Iliopsoas chapter. In this position, the affected thigh can be tested for restriction of adduction by pressing the thigh of the extended limb medially.[51,62] When the tensor fasciae latae muscle is tight, adduction is limited to a range of less than 15°, and the longitudinal groove on the lateral aspect of the thigh beside the fascia lata deepens. The abduction function of this muscle is tested with the patient lying on the side opposite to the one being tested; the patient is asked to raise the foot of the uppermost limb while the clinician palpates both the gluteus medius and tensor fasciae latae muscles with one hand and tests for strength by opposing the movement with the other.[61] Loading the muscle during either test is likely to cause pain in the region of that hip joint if the muscle has active TrPs.

In a common syndrome of muscle imbalance,[63] tight tensor fasciae latae and quadratus lumborum muscles overpower an inhibited or weak gluteus medius muscle. The patient stands with a forward tilt of the pelvis and accentuated lumbar lordosis. Release of TrP tension of the tight muscles must precede efforts to strengthen the gluteus medius.

A tight tensor fasciae latae and/or a tight gluteus maximus muscle can contribute to iliotibial band tightness. A tight iliotibial band causes the Ober sign;[43,83,94] with the patient lying on the side opposite to the tight band, the knee of the uppermost limb does not reach the table. Tightness of the tensor fasciae latae muscle can also produce the *appearance* of a shorter limb on the involved side when the patient is examined in the supine or prone position, in a manner similar to that illustrated for the quadratus lumborum muscle (*see* Fig. 4.9). See Chapter 4, Section 8, for details on how to determine lower limb-length inequality.

The region of the greater trochanter may be tender to palpation because of referred tenderness from TrPs and is not always a sign of trochanteric bursitis.

The authors know of no study that specifically reports the prevalence of latent TrPs in children. However, in one study,[66] 115 school children aged 8–20 years were examined for muscle tightness including tightness of the tensor fasciae latae muscle. The children were examined three times over a period of 4 years. The results showed a correlation among increasing height, increasing weight and low physical fitness, and the development of shortened muscles; it was stronger in boys than in girls.[66] The cause of the muscle tightness was not evaluated.

9. TRIGGER POINT EXAMINATION—TENSOR FASCIAE LATAE
(Fig. 12.3)

The TrPs in this superficial muscle are disclosed in the supine patient by flat palpation, as illustrated in Figure 12.3. The muscle can be located by palpating its tension while the patient rotates the thigh

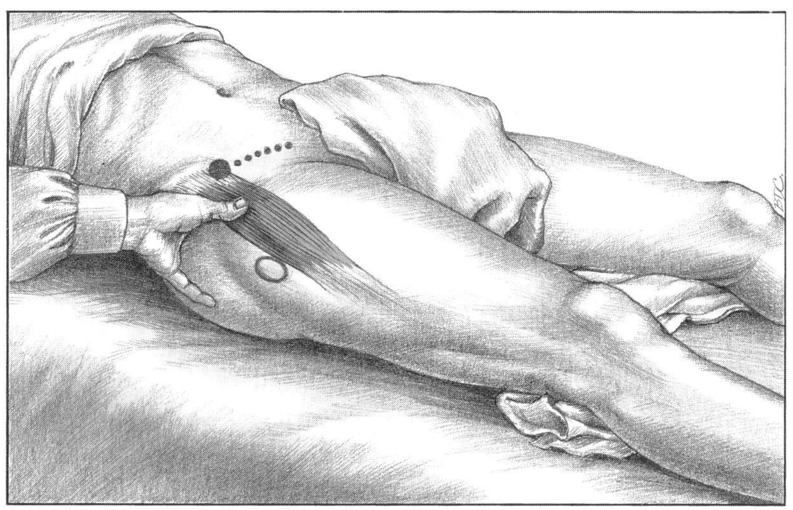

Figure 12.3. Palpation of trigger points in the right tensor fasciae latae muscle (*red*). The *solid circle* locates the anterior superior iliac spine and the *open circle* marks the greater trochanter. The *dotted line* identifies the inguinal ligament. The thumb presses at the usual location of trigger points in this muscle.

medially against resistance. When the patient is fully relaxed and the muscle is placed under slight (stretch) tension, palpation at right angles to the direction of the muscle fibers reveals taut bands and the spot of maximum tenderness (TrP) in each band. Pressure on active tensor fasciae latae TrPs sustained for up to 10 seconds augments the pain referred from them. Snapping palpation of active TrPs in this muscle usually elicits a visible local twitch response.

10. ENTRAPMENTS—TENSOR FASCIAE LATAE

No neurological entrapments are known to be associated with TrPs in this muscle.

11. ASSOCIATED TRIGGER POINTS—TENSOR FASCIAE LATAE

The TrPs in the tensor fasciae latae muscle may occur as a single-muscle syndrome or, more commonly, may develop secondary to TrPs in the anterior gluteus minimus and, sometimes, in the rectus femoris, iliopsoas, or sartorius muscles. Tensor fasciae latae TrPs cannot be eliminated if active TrPs remain in the anterior gluteus minimus muscle, which prevent its full stretch.

This muscle's TrPs do not seem to cause associated TrPs in any of the prime movers of the hip.

12. INTERMITTENT COLD WITH STRETCH—TENSOR FASCIAE LATAE (Fig. 12.4)

The use of ice for applying intermittent cold with stretch is explained on page 9 of this volume and the use of vapocoolant with stretch is detailed on pages 67–74 of Volume 1.[101] Techniques that augment relaxation and stretch are reviewed on page 11 of this volume. Full stretch is avoided in hypermobile patients. Alternative treatment methods are reviewed on pages 9–11 of this volume.

For application of intermittent cold with stretch to the tensor fasciae latae, the patient lies on the unaffected side (Fig. 12.4). Ice or vapocoolant spray is applied in slow parallel sweeps distalward from the crest of the ilium over the anterior thigh to just above the knee. Successive sweeps progress laterally to cover the muscle. Meanwhile, the thigh of the uppermost limb is extended and afterward guided by the operator as the limb is allowed to be pulled into adduction and lateral rotation by gravity. It is important to start with extension. The muscle is tightened when adduction is attempted initially in hip flexion and can snap painfully across the greater trochanter. In addition to guiding and controlling the involved limb, the clinician's hand should be placed so that it stabilizes the patella.

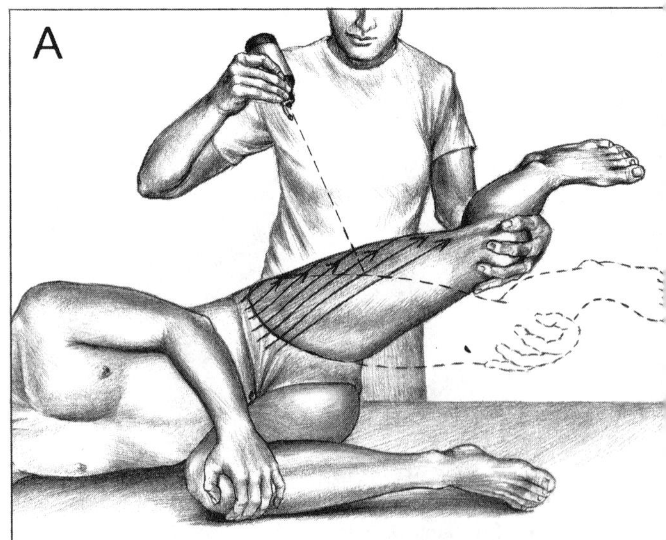

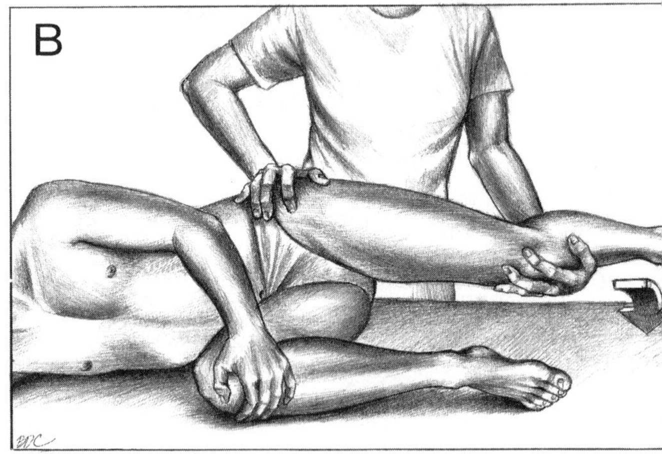

Figure 12.4. Stretch positions and ice or vapocoolant spray pattern (*thin arrows*) for trigger points in the left tensor fasciae latae muscle. To prevent the muscle from painfully impinging on the greater trochanter as the muscle is lengthened, the operator first extends the abducted thigh and then adducts it, intermittently cooling the skin over the muscle and pain reference zone. Throughout, the patient assists in stabilizing the lumbar spine and pelvis by holding the knee of the untreated limb down on the examining table. *A*, The operator applies ice or vapocoolant (*thin arrows*) downward over the muscle and also over the thigh anterolaterally while gently bringing the partly abducted thigh (*fully rendered limb*) into extension, and then starts to lower the limb gently into adduction (*outlined limb*), avoiding medial rotation of the thigh. *B*, To obtain full stretch on this muscle, the operator must stabilize the pelvis with one hand to minimize movement of the lumbar spine and pelvis while the thigh is moving into adduction. The operator's other hand supports the weight of the limb and firmly grasps the patella to stabilize it against the pull of the fascia lata. Concurrent use of augmented postisometric relaxation provides release of muscle tension since the operator has no free hand with which to apply vapocoolant. Intermittent cold can be employed at this stage if the operator releases the pelvis to apply the cold and then reestablishes pelvic positioning prior to further release of the muscle. As the muscle releases, the operator then takes up slack in the direction of lateral rotation of the thigh by allowing the lower leg to drop downward (*thick arrow*).

A two-operator technique is most effective. One clinician stabilizes the pelvis; the other applies the ice or vapocoolant with one hand while stabilizing the patella and moving the involved limb into extension and then adduction and lateral rotation with the other. A single operator can stabilize the pelvis with one arm and body weight, while using the other hand to stabilize the patella and to guide the involved lower limb into extension and adduction. In this case, the ice or vapocoolant must be applied before, not during, the stretch. The Lewit technique performed by the patient enhances relaxation of the muscle.

An alternative to stabilizing the patella manually is to use non-irritating tape for the stabilization.

Following intermittent cold with stretch, a moist, wet-proof heating pad is applied over the muscle and its pain reference zone until the skin is rewarmed. The patient then slowly mobilizes the muscle by several cycles of full active range of motion.

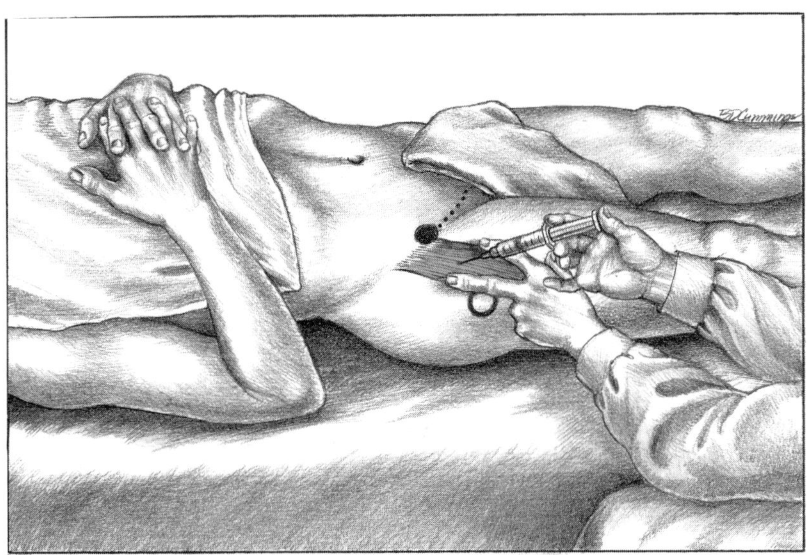

Figure 12.5. Injection of a trigger point in the right tensor fasciae latae muscle (*red*). This trigger point is quite superficial so that the needle is at a small acute angle to the skin surface. The *solid circle* locates the anterior superior iliac spine. The *dotted line* identifies the inguinal ligament. The *open circle* marks the greater trochanter.

13. INJECTION AND STRETCH—TENSOR FASCIAE LATAE
(Fig. 12.5)

A full description of the procedure for injection and stretch of any muscle appears in Volume 1, pages 74–86.[101]

Myofascial TrPs in the tensor fasciae latae muscle are injected with the patient lying supine (Fig. 12.5). The muscle is identified by asking the patient to turn the kneecap inward (medially rotate the thigh) while the region of the muscle is palpated. (If the muscle is already sufficiently tense due to its TrPs, this procedure may not be needed.) To localize the taut bands, it may be necessary to slacken the muscle slightly by placing a pillow under the knee, thus flexing the hip slightly. When the TrP tenderness has been precisely located, pressure is applied with the fingers of one hand to pin down the taut band as the needle is inserted into its TrPs with the other hand (Fig. 12.5). A few milliliters of 0.5% procaine in isotonic saline are injected into the cluster of TrPs using a 37mm (1½-in) needle; each TrP is identified by a local twitch response of the muscle, or by a pain response (jump sign) of the patient.

If the tensor fasciae latae muscle has been accurately identified, no major nerves or vessels lie in the path of the needle, which is angled nearly horizontally to penetrate this subcutaneous muscle.

Following this procedure, a few sweeps of ice or vapocoolant are applied in the manner illustrated in Figure 12.4. Then, the patient should actively move the thigh slowly through the full flexion-extension range of hip motion. Finally, moist heat is applied over the injection site to minimize postinjection soreness. Postinjection soreness can be quite annoying to patients for a few days following injection, and may be lessened by supplemental vitamin C prior to injection and by acetaminophen afterward, as needed.

The clinician should carefully examine the anterior gluteus minimus for associated TrPs and should also inactivate them at this time, if a satisfactory result is to be expected.

14. CORRECTIVE ACTIONS—TENSOR FASCIAE LATAE

In the patient with a chronic myofascial pain syndrome, it is important to identify any mechanical factors that are perpetuating the tensor fasciae latae TrPs. Systemic perpetuating factors (*see* Volume 1, Chapter 4)[101] should also be addressed.

Corrective Posture and Activities

For both this muscle and the sartorius, sitting in the cross-legged lotus position for a period of time should be avoided. It is also important to avoid prolonged flexion of the thigh at the hip caused by such positions as sitting in a jackknifed position in a chair, sleeping on the back with a large pillow under the knees, or sleeping in the fetal position with the hips and knees strongly flexed. During sleep, the hip should be kept extended beyond 90° of flexion, and preferably close to full extension.

Chairs in which the patient sits for any length of time should provide an open angle at the hips. Either the backrest should be tilted backward and the patient should lean back against it most of the time, or the front of the seat should be sloped downward. A pad of folded newspaper can be placed across the rear of the seat to achieve this desired slope.

On long trips in an automobile, cruise control permits change of position of the lower limbs; thus, the driver can avoid holding the hip flexor muscles immobilized in a shortened position for long periods.

To reduce irritability of tensor fasciae latae TrPs, it is important to avoid walking or jogging up hills, which requires leaning forward and flexing the hips. It is also important for a runner to avoid shoes that are excessively worn and to avoid running on surfaces that slope from side to side. A benefit for the runner's muscles is to run on a level track, to run on one side of the road in one direction and on the same side of the road for the return trip, or to run only on the crown of a traffic-free road.

Home Therapeutic Program

A self-stretch exercise for the tensor fasciae latae is performed by lying on the side opposite the muscle to be stretched, extending and laterally rotating the uppermost hip, and relaxing to obtain gravity-assisted adduction. Some people stretch this muscle in the standing position, using body weight shift for stretch. Patients with tensor fasciae latae TrPs should also perform hip extension exercises similar to those recommended in Chapter 5 to release the iliopsoas muscle, and in Chapter 14 for release of the rectus femoris muscle.

SARTORIUS

1A. REFERRED PAIN—SARTORIUS (Fig. 12.6)

The specific TrPs illustrated (Fig. 12.6) and their referred pain patterns up and down the muscle are examples of what can occur anywhere in the sartorius. The TrPs in this muscle produce a surprising burst of *superficial* sharp or tingling pain, not the usual deep aching pain referred from myofascial TrPs.

2A. ANATOMICAL ATTACHMENTS AND CONSIDERATIONS—SARTORIUS (Fig. 12.7)

The thin, narrow, ribbonlike sartorius is the longest muscle in the body.[24] It attaches ***proximally*** to the anterior superior iliac spine (Fig. 12.7). The muscle descends obliquely across the front of the thigh from lateral to medial, forming a roof over the femoral artery, vein, and nerve in Hunter's canal. In the lower part of the thigh, it descends nearly vertically, passing over the medial condyle of the femur. ***Distally***, the sartorius ends in a tendon that curves obliquely anteriorly to attach to the medial surface of the body of the tibia just anterior to the attachments of the gracilis and semitendinosus tendons.[24] Thus, it is the most anterior of the "pes anserinus" muscles.

The sartorius is one of four muscles in the body with inscriptions that effectively shorten the average fiber length. (The other three muscles are the rectus abdominis, gracilis,[27] and semitendinosus.[25]) The microscopic inscriptions of the sartorius are not aligned and do not form clearly defined bands across the

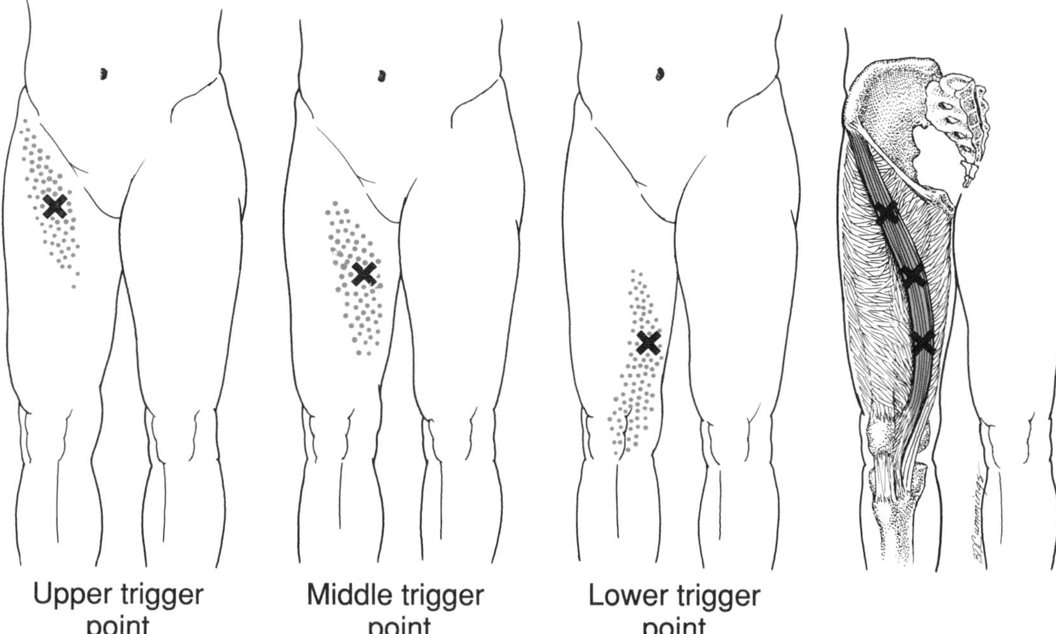

Figure 12.6. Referred pain patterns (*dark red*) of three trigger points (**Xs**) at different levels in the right sartorius muscle (*light red*), anteromedial view. The trigger points in this long thin muscle are superficial, just under the skin.

muscle, as do the inscriptions of the rectus abdominis and semitendinosus.[22,25] Therefore, sartorius myoneural junctions are also exceptional in their distribution throughout the length of the muscle.[8,21,27] Weber[103] found that, macroscopically, the apparent average length of sartorius muscle fibers was 43.5 cm (17 in). The next longest were the gracilis muscle fibers which averaged 25.5 cm (10 in) in length.

Anatomical variations of the sartorius include additional attachments to the inguinal ligament, iliopectineal line of the pubis proximally,[24] and to the ligament of the patella, tendon of the semitendinosus muscle,[24] or to the medial condyle of the femur[33] distally. This muscle may be divided longitudinally into two parallel bellies; it may be crossed by a tendinous inscription, or more rarely may have an intermediate length of tendon that divides it into upper and lower bellies similar to the division of the digastric muscle.[13]

Supplemental References

The entire sartorius muscle is shown in front view without nerves or vessels,[6,12,76,89] in relation to the vessels and nerves in the femoral triangle,[1,92] with its innervation,[75] and in relation to the lateral femoral cutaneous nerve.[1] The distal part of the muscle is also viewed from behind.[77,90] Its distal end is shown from the medial view attaching to the tibia[91] and in relation to the anserine bursa,[82] and as the muscle appears in the lateral view.[34] The muscle and its relation to surrounding structures are revealed in serial cross sections,[19] in cross sections at three levels,[79] and at one level.[5,36] Its bony attachments are marked.[4,37,78] The surface contours produced by this muscle are demonstrated photographically.[2,35,65]

3A. INNERVATION—SARTORIUS

The sartorius muscle usually is innervated by two branches that separate from the femoral nerve near the origin of the anterior cutaneous branches. This muscle is supplied by fibers of the second and third lumbar nerves.[24]

4A. FUNCTION—SARTORIUS

During the swing phase of gait, the sartorius assists the iliacus and the tensor fasciae latae in hip flexion and assists the short head of the biceps femoris in knee flexion. It may assist the vastus medialis, gracilis, and semitendinosus in support-

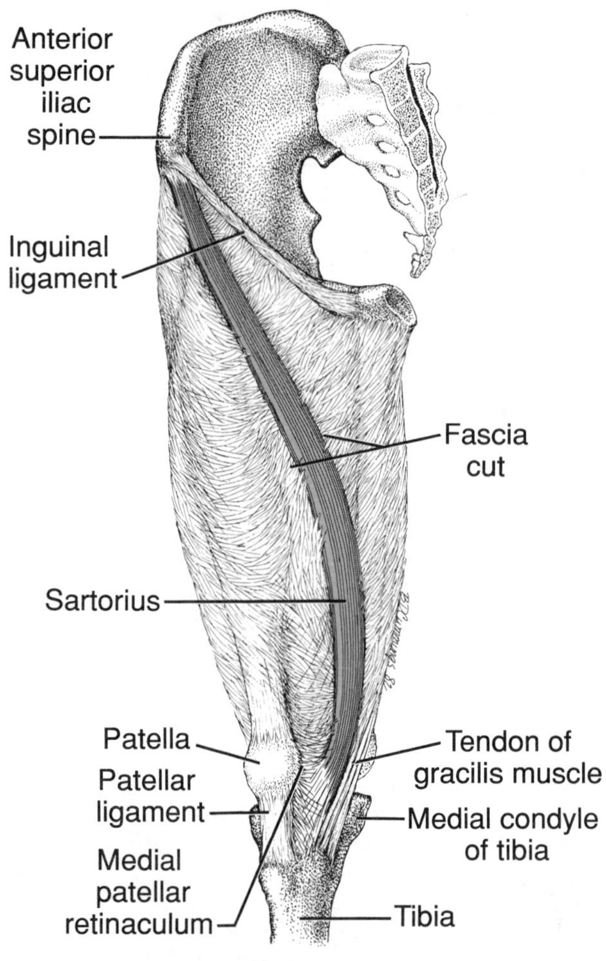

Figure 12.7. Attachments of the right sartorius muscle (*red*), viewed from in front and somewhat from the medial side. It attaches *proximally* to the anterior superior spine of the ilium and *distally* to the medial aspect of the upper tibia. The muscle lies deep to the layer of fascia shown on both sides of it, and as seen in Figure 12.8 with the fascia intact.

PART 2

ing the knee medially against the lateral thrust (valgus thrust) that occurs during single limb balance.[86]

The sartorius earned its name as the muscle that assists the hip movements necessary to assume the position of a cross-legged tailor (*sartor*, a tailor). This muscle, like the tensor fasciae latae, is a flexor and abductor of the thigh, but the sartorius rotates the thigh ***laterally*** instead of medially.[87] Electromyographically, the sartorius is activated during efforts to flex the thigh[38,50,99] and to abduct it.[50,99] This muscle is essentially not activated during medial rotation of the thigh.[50,99] During a lateral rotation effort, the sartorius is only slightly and occasionally activated,[99] except in the usual sitting position, when there is slight to moderate activity.[50] Activation of this muscle by knee flexion or extension is highly variable.[7,50] It is more likely to assist knee flexion when the hip is also flexed.[50]

In an EMG study of selected sports skills,[17] both the right and left sartorius muscles were vigorously active during volleyball and basketball jumping activities. The left sartorius was consistently more active than the right in all right-handed ball-throwing and batting activities, as well as during a tennis serve. A detailed EMG study[52] of a standing two-legged jump revealed the sartorius to be vigorously active through both the take-off phase and the landing phase of the jump.

Sartorius activity during level walking peaks in the middle of swing phase (assisting hip flexion).[50] The sartorius is active as a hip flexor during bicycling.[47]

5A. FUNCTIONAL (MYOTATIC) UNIT—SARTORIUS

The sartorius muscle assists the rectus femoris, iliopsoas, pectineus, and tensor fasciae latae muscles in flexing the thigh at the hip. This function is opposed by the gluteus maximus and hamstring muscles.

For abduction of the thigh, the sartorius assists the gluteus medius, gluteus minimus, piriformis, and tensor fasciae latae. This action is opposed by the three hip adductor muscles and the gracilis.

The lateral rotation effect of the sartorius counters the opposing medial rotation function of the tensor fasciae latae. Otherwise, they act as agonists.

6A. SYMPTOMS—SARTORIUS

The pain referred from lower sartorius TrPs may be felt up and down the thigh and in the knee region medially, but *not deep* in the knee.

In addition to referred pain, patients with upper sartorius TrPs may have symptoms of entrapment of the lateral femoral cutaneous nerve (*see* Section 10A). In that case, their symptoms of meralgia paresthetica include dysesthesia or numbness of the anterolateral aspect of the thigh (*see* Fig. 12.8).

Differential Diagnosis

Pain referred over the anteromedial portion of the knee from TrPs in the lower part of the sartorius is confusingly similar to the pain referred from TrPs in the vastus medialis muscle. However, the pain referred from the sartorius is more diffuse and superficial than the pain deep in the knee joint usually referred from the vastus medialis.

Lange[60] warned that the pain caused by myogelosis [TrPs] in the lower sartorius muscle is easily mistaken for pain originating in the knee, and he described a case report.

We find that patients rarely present with a complaint of pain caused solely by the sartorius muscle. Lange[60] made this same observation. A sartorius TrP can be discovered serendipitously during injection of a vastus medialis TrP deep to the sartorius muscle. When the needle encounters this superficial sartorius TrP, the patient reports a sharp or tingling pain felt diffusely over the adjacent thigh.

The pain from sartorius TrPs referred to the knee may also be mistaken for disease of that joint.[88]

7A. ACTIVATION AND PERPETUATION OF TRIGGER POINTS—SARTORIUS

Sartorius TrPs do not usually occur as a single-muscle syndrome, but rather occur in conjunction with TrP involvement of related muscles. Sartorius TrPs are usually activated as secondary TrPs by those in other muscles of its functional unit. Occasionally, these TrPs may be initiated by an acute overload strain in a twisting fall.

The TrPs in this muscle are perpetuated by a rocking (excessively pronating) foot, characteristic of the Morton foot structure that is described in Chapter 20.

8A. PATIENT EXAMINATION—SARTORIUS

Sartorius TrPs are usually discovered after TrPs in functionally related muscles have been inactivated. They often are the residue left behind after treatment of more obvious TrPs. The TrPs in this long slack muscle do not limit movement or cause mechanical dysfunction; range of motion is not restricted. Weakness and pain on loading the sartorius muscle can be tested with the patient in the seated position, knee bent 90°, by performing lateral rotation of the thigh at the hip against resistance, as illustrated by Saudek.[93]

In a patient with sartorius TrPs, the attachment area of the sartorius on the tibia is tender because of sustained tension and tenderness referred to that region.

9A. TRIGGER POINT EXAMINATION—SARTORIUS

The TrPs of the sartorius muscle are very superficial and easily missed. One must use flat palpation across the fiber direction, exploring along the length of the muscle, as described and illustrated by Lange.[59] The taut band is usually detected first and then the exquisite spot tenderness at the TrP. Local twitch responses

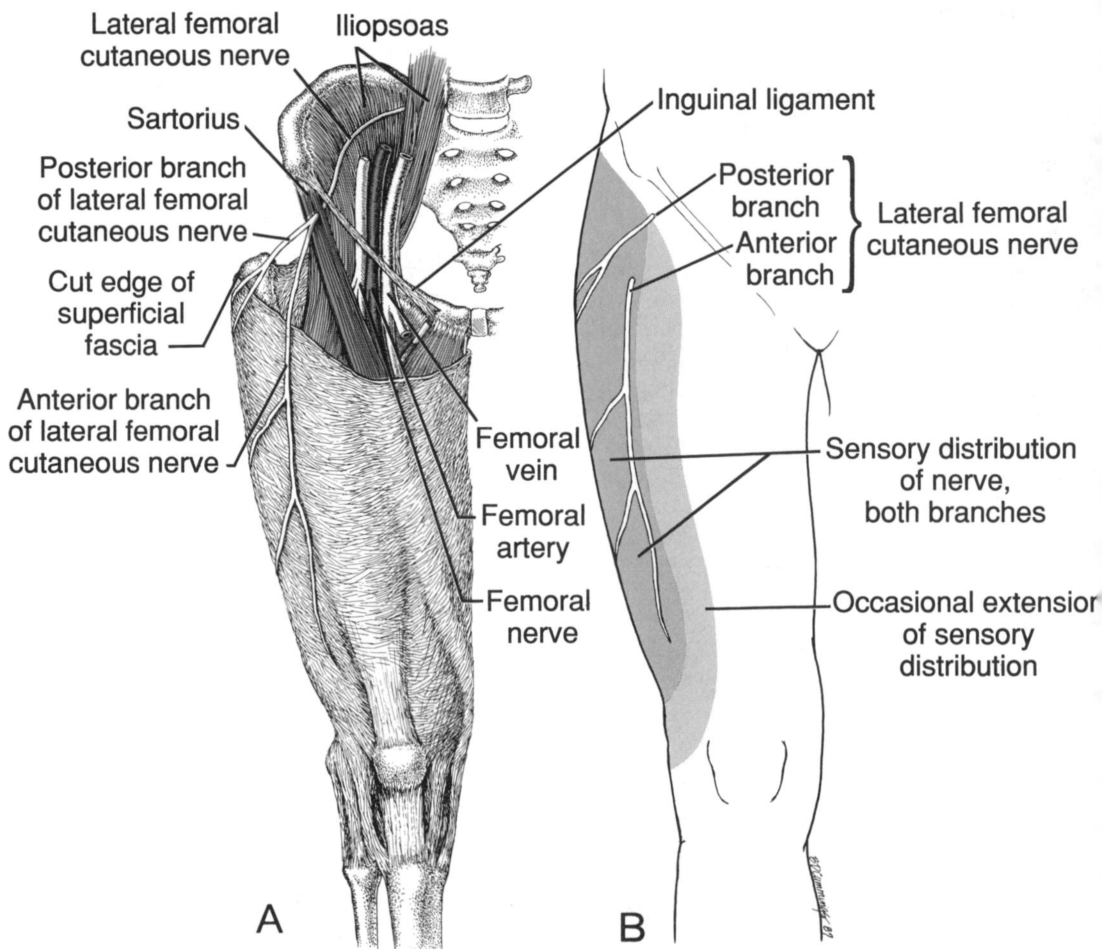

Figure 12.8. Potential entrapment of the lateral femoral cutaneous nerve when it passes through the sartorius muscle. *A*, anatomical relations of this unusual course of the lateral femoral cutaneous nerve. *B*, usual sensory distribution of this nerve, *dark gray*; occasional extension of its distribution, *light gray*.

elicited by snapping palpation at the TrP are often visible in this muscle.

10A. ENTRAPMENTS—SARTORIUS (Fig. 12.8)

The authors have observed several patients who were relieved of the symptoms of meralgia paresthetica by the injection of a tender spot in the musculature distal to the anterior superior iliac spine. The location of these tender spots was consistent with TrPs in the proximal portion of the sartorius muscle. Similarly, Teng[100] was able to relieve patients with this disorder by injecting the iliacus or quadriceps femoris muscles distal to the medial portion of the inguinal ligament. No relief was obtained when he injected abdominal wall muscles above the ligament, or muscles distal to its lateral portion. He attributed this relief to reduction of tension in the muscles, which reduced fascial tension on the inguinal ligament.

Since the cause of meralgia paresthetica is frequently not known, this topic is critically examined here in order to better understand how muscles might contribute to the symptoms of the disorder.

Meralgia Paresthetica (Fig. 12.8)

Meralgia (painful thigh) describes a pain syndrome without suggesting a cause. Historically, the etiology of this dysfunction has been enigmatic. A 1977 review[31] culled 80 purported causes from previous literature. The weight of evidence now indicates that meralgia paresthetica is usually caused by entrapment of, or trauma to, the lateral femoral cutaneous nerve as it exits the pelvis. The symptoms are burning pain and paresthesias in the distribution of this nerve, which extends down the anterolateral thigh, sometimes to the knee (Fig. 12.8).[58]

Incidence

This entrapment neuropathy is more common than is generally appreciated. The reported incidence is highly variable, however, depending on the investigator. One neurosurgeon[100] identified five patients with this disorder in the 7 years preceding 1963. Then he developed the condition himself, and became a student of the syndrome. In the subsequent 8 years, he diagnosed 297 patients as having meralgia paresthetica. If the examiner is not specifically looking for meralgia paresthetica, it is easily mistaken for radiculopathy.

Anatomy

The lateral femoral cutaneous nerve arises from the dorsal portion of the second and third lumbar spinal nerves and appears within the pelvic cavity as it emerges from the lateral border of the psoas major muscle (Fig. 12.8*A*). It proceeds obliquely across the iliacus muscle toward the anterior superior iliac spine. It exits the pelvis either above, through, or under the inguinal ligament, usually within 5 cm (2 in) of the anterior superior iliac spine. Thus, the nerve usually passes through the lacuna musculorum with the iliopsoas muscle. Keegan and Holyoke[54] noted in their study of 50 cadavers that the nerve usually passed through a tunnel in the inguinal ligament. Teng[100] described this passage as an "inguinal foramen." The nerve often makes a right-angle turn as it exits the pelvis. It then usually passes superficial to the sartorius muscle and then divides at once into anterior and posterior branches. These branches continue deep to the fascia lata for 5–10 cm (2–4 in) down the thigh before both anterior and posterior branches pierce this fascial layer to become subcutaneous.[26,54,100]

The nerve can become entrapped in several locations: beside the spinal column, where branches from the lumbar nerves join to form the femoral cutaneous nerve within the belly of the psoas major; within the abdominal cavity by pressure on the nerve against the pelvis; or where the nerve exits the pelvis. The last is usually the site of trouble.

Stookey[98] did a series of dissections of the lateral femoral cutaneous nerve and was impressed by the marked angulation of the nerve as it emerged from the pelvis. He observed that the angulation and tension of the nerve were increased by extension of the thigh[98] and decreased by thigh flexion. He also noted that the nerve usually exited superficial to the sartorius muscle, but sometimes passed through it (Fig. 12.8*A*). When the nerve passes through or deep to the sartorius muscle where it lies against the ilium, it would be vulnerable to compression by that muscle.[67] (It also sometimes crosses the crest of the ilium superior and lateral to the anterior superior iliac spine, where it would be especially vulnerable to tight clothing and impact trauma.)

Edelson and Nathan[31] examined 110 lateral femoral cutaneous nerves in 90 adult and 20 fetal cadavers for enlargement of the nerve at its pelvic exit. In 51% of adult cases and none of the fetal cases, a significant enlargement or pseudoganglion was present in the area of the nerve where it passed under the inguinal ligament to turn sharply downward onto the thigh.

In a more recent autopsy study[49] of 12 nerves from patients who had had no known disease of the peripheral nerves, five of the 12 showed unequivocal pathological changes at or just below the inguinal ligament. Changes included local demyelination and Wallerian degeneration, and microscopic increase in connective tissue components. The presence of polarized internodal swellings suggested that mechanical factors were responsible. Endoneurial vascular changes also were observed that might contribute to nerve damage.[49]

These data strongly suggest that subclinical meralgia paresthetica is far more common than has been realized and that many clinical cases probably are overlooked.

Teng[100] reported a series of 84 operations on patients with meralgia paresthetica. In 26 (31%) of the patients, the foramen through which the nerve penetrated the inguinal ligament was constricted and would not permit the passage of a probe. In 37 (44%), the nerve appeared to be compressed by the posterior fibers of the inguinal ligament and/or a tense fascia lata. Twelve (14%) revealed scarring that appeared to constrict the nerve. (In five (6%) of the patients, the lateral femoral cutaneous nerve arose either wholly or in part from the femoral nerve, and the entrapment occurred in the region of the cribriform fascia.) In none of these patients was the nerve found to pass through the sartorius muscle.

A much higher proportion of nerves was found to pass through the inguinal ligament in surgical reports than in cadaver studies. This suggests that the nerve's penetration of the inguinal ligament predisposes it to the development of meralgia paresthetica severe enough to require surgery.

Lewit[64] attributes some cases of meralgia paresthetica to entrapment of the nerve by spasm of the iliopsoas muscle in the lacuna musculorum, through which they both pass. Elimination of the iliopsoas muscle spasm by manipulation of the thoracolumbar junction, lumbosacral junction, hip, or coccyx relieved the symptoms of meralgia paresthetica in these cases.[64]

As illustrated in Figure 12.8*A*, the lateral femoral cutaneous nerve might be entrapped by the sartorius muscle as the nerve penetrates the muscle after passing deep to the inguinal ligament. This apparently is a relatively infrequent anatomical variation and has not been reported in surgical procedures for relief of meralgia paresthetica. However, Keegan and Holyoke[54] noted that the sartorius has a medial aponeurotic expansion from its tendinous attachment to the anterior superior iliac spine; this aponeurosis attaches to the inferior border of the inguinal ligament and could depress this ligament when the muscle contracts. It is conceivable that TrP tension in the sartorius could exert pressure on the nerve in this way.

Clinical Findings

The pain and/or paresthesia over the anterolateral thigh reported by patients with meralgia paresthetica is usually increased by standing or walking,[40,54,69,98] and by positions of hip extension.[31,100] In one case, it was reported after running and then bicycling when the symptomatic lower limb was 1 cm (½ in) longer than the other.[15] Running may have required additional extension at the hip on the side of the longer limb. The symptoms are generally relieved by sitting down or otherwise flexing the thigh.[40,98]

Meralgia paresthetica has been associated with an obese, pendulous, lax abdominal wall;[28,31,40] with tight, constricting garments or belts;[31,32] with shortening of the contralateral lower limb;[15,58] and, in one case, with compression from a wallet carried in a front pants pocket.[84]

On examination, patients with meralgia paresthetica have **sensory changes** in the distribution of the lateral femoral cutaneous nerve (Fig. 12.8*B*).[15,30,40,69,100] Local tenderness, sometimes with paresthesias and pain projected in the nerve distribution, may be elicited by pressure over the region where the nerve traverses the inguinal ligament.[15,40,100]

Electrodiagnostic evidence of nerve entrapment may be obtained by demonstrating a slowed sensory conduction velocity of the nerve in the region of the inguinal ligament.[18] The lateral femoral cutaneous nerve contains no motor fibers.

Treatment

Most patients with meralgia paresthetica respond to conservative therapy. Teng[100] injected every one of his 297 patients with lidocaine to block the lateral femoral cutaneous nerve at the inguinal ligament, and many experienced prolonged relief. Effective conservative therapy includes significant weight loss[46] (sometimes with as little as 5 or 10 lb),[39] avoidance of excessive extension at the hip, avoidance of constricting garments around the hips,[46] correction of a lower limb-length inequality,[15,58] injection of the nerve with lidocaine and prednisone at the spinal[44] or inguinal[102] level, and inactivation of sartorius TrPs. A steroid could alleviate symptoms by reducing the local tissue reactions to trauma. If conservative measures fail, surgery may be required.[40,100]

11A. ASSOCIATED TRIGGER POINTS—SARTORIUS

Sartorius TrPs are likely to be observed in conjunction with TrP tension in other muscles of the functional unit. The uppermost TrPs in the sartorius may develop in association with rectus femoris TrPs. Midmuscle and lower sartorius TrPs can appear in association with vastus medialis TrPs.

Sartorius TrPs also may be associated with TrPs in its antagonists, the thigh adductors.

12A. INTERMITTENT COLD WITH STRETCH—SARTORIUS

The sartorius is a uniquely long, slack muscle with multiple inscriptions. This serial arrangement of fibers makes its TrPs relatively difficult to inactivate by intermittent cold with stretch. However, if one attempts this technique, the patient lies supine with the buttocks at the end of the table and holds the thigh of the untreated leg against the chest to stabilize the pelvis and lumbar spine. As ice or vapocoolant is applied from above downward over the sartorius muscle, the clinician moves the thigh to be treated into adduction, extension, and medial rotation. The intermittent cold-with-stretch procedure is followed by moist heat and then full active range of motion.

Local injection, ischemic compression, deep friction massage, or stripping massage may be required. These techniques may be the treatment of choice, since TrPs in this muscle do not usually limit range of motion; instead, the taut bands need to be treated as a local problem.

13A. INJECTION AND STRETCH—SARTORIUS

To inject TrPs in the superficial sartorius muscle it is necessary to angle the needle tangentially, nearly parallel to the surface of the skin.

Occasionally during injection of a TrP in the vastus medialis or rectus femoris muscle, the needle penetrates an overlying sartorius TrP that had escaped notice, unexpectedly causing a twitch of the muscle and a characteristic pins-and-needles or tingling sensation projected up and down over the sartorius muscle. This referred pain is not sudden but rather a spreading pain.

14A. CORRECTIVE ACTIONS—SARTORIUS

Systemic perpetuating factors, as described in Volume 1, Chapter 4,[101] should be identified and resolved.

Corrective Body Mechanics

Since a lower limb-length inequality can perpetuate sartorius TrP activity by causing increased adduction of the longer limb at the hip during walking[58] or additional extension during running, the inequality should be corrected (*see* Chapter 4). This asymmetry tends to stretch the deep fascia and nerve at the entrapment point.[58]

Corrective Posture and Activities

The lotus position (similar to the tailor's position for which the muscle is named) places the sartorius in a shortened position and is to be avoided. Sitting in this position can generate referred pain when sartorius TrPs are active.

Sleeping in the jackknifed position with the knees and hips flexed places the muscle in a sustained shortened position and can aggravate its TrPs.

When patients with sartorius TrPs lie on either side, they find it more comfortable to place a pillow or other padding between the knees. It hurts to rest one knee against the other because of referred tenderness to the knee region. Other patients sleep on the back for relief, which may not be the best solution.

Home Therapeutic Program

Some patients may find it convenient to apply self-ischemic compression or deep friction massage to the sartorius TrPs. These techniques, which apply local stretch of the taut band, are probably more effective than an overall stretch of the muscle.

The patient may be instructed how to use gravity and postisometric relaxation (Chapter 2, page 11) to release taut bands in this muscle.

To recruit gravity for lengthening the sartorius muscle, the patient lies on the unaffected side with the buttocks at the end of the bed or examining table and pulls the thigh of the asymptomatic lower limb to the chest while allowing the uppermost involved limb to hang down over the end of the bed. Positioning of the body should be such that gravity pulls the thigh into extension and adduction. The contract-relax phases of postisometric relaxation are then synchronized with slow deep respiration.

References

1. Anderson JE: *Grant's Atlas of Anatomy*, Ed. 8. Williams & Wilkins, Baltimore, 1983 (Figs. 4–17, 4–20).
2. *Ibid.* (Fig. 4–21B).
3. *Ibid.* (Fig. 4–22).
4. *Ibid.* (Figs. 4–23, 4–65).
5. *Ibid.* (Fig. 4–26).
6. *Ibid.* (Fig. 4–28).
7. Andriacchi TP, Andersson GBJ, Örtengren R, *et al.*: A study of factors influencing muscle activity about the knee joint. *J Orthop Res 1*:266–275, 1984.

PART 2

8. Aquilonius S-M, Askmark H, Gillberg P-G, *et al.*: Topographical localization of motor endplates in cryosections of whole human muscles. *Muscle Nerve 7*:287–293, 1984.
9. Arcangeli P, Digiesi V, Ronchi O, Dorigo B, Bartoli V: Mechanisms of ischemic pain in peripheral occlusive arterial disease. In *Advances in Pain Research and Therapy*, edited by J.J. Bonica and D. Albe-Fessard, Vol. I. Raven Press, New York, 1976 (pp. 965–973, *see* Fig. 2).
10. Baker BA: The muscle trigger: evidence of overload injury. *J Neurol Orthop Med Surg 7*:35–44, 1986.
11. Bardeen CR: The musculature, Sect. 5. In *Morris's Human Anatomy*, edited by C.M. Jackson, Ed. 6. Blakiston's Son & Co., Philadelphia, 1921 (p. 491).
12. *Ibid.* (p. 500, Fig. 442).
13. *Ibid.* (p. 502).
14. Basmajian JV, Deluca CJ: *Muscles Alive*, Ed. 5. Williams & Wilkins, Baltimore, 1985 (p. 318).
15. Beazell JR: Entrapment neuropathy of the lateral femoral cutaneous nerve: cause of lateral knee pain. *J Orthop Sports Phys Therap 10:*85–86, 1988.
16. Brody DM: Running injuries: prevention and management. *Clin Symp 39*:2–36, 1987 (*see* pp. 19, 22, 23).
17. Broer MR, Houtz SJ: *Patterns of Muscular Activity in Selected Sports Skills*. Charles C Thomas, Springfield, 1967.
18. Butler ET, Johnson EW, Kaye ZA: Normal conduction velocity in the lateral femoral cutaneous nerve. *Arch Phys Med Rehabil 55*:31–32, 1974.
19. Carter BL, Morehead J, Wolpert SM, *et al.*: *Cross-Sectional Anatomy*. Appleton-Century-Crofts, New York, 1977 (Sects. 37–48).
20. *Ibid.* (Sects. 38–48, 64–72).
21. Christensen E: Topography of terminal motor innervation in striated muscles from stillborn infants. *Am J Phys Med 38*:65–78, 1959.
22. Clemente CD: *Gray's Anatomy of the Human Body*, American Ed. 30. Lea & Febiger, Philadelphia, 1985 (pp. 491, 492, Fig. 6–31).
23. *Ibid.* (pp. 559, 568).
24. *Ibid.* (pp. 561–562).
25. *Ibid.* (p. 572).
26. *Ibid.* (pp. 1229–1231).
27. Coërs C, Woolf AL: *The Innervation of Muscle.* Blackwell Scientific Publications, Oxford, 1959 (pp. 18–20).
28. Deal CL, Canoso JJ: Meralgia paresthetica and large abdomens [letter]. *Ann Intern Med 96*:787–788, 1982.
29. Duchenne GB: *Physiology of Motion*, translated by E.B. Kaplan. J. B. Lippincott, Philadelphia, 1949 (p. 259).
30. Ecker AD: Diagnosis of meralgia paresthetica. *JAMA 253*:976, 1985.
31. Edelson JG, Nathan H: Meralgia paresthetica: an anatomical interpretation. *Clin Orthop 122*:255–262, 1977.
32. Eibel P: Sigmund Freud and meralgia paraesthetica. *Orthop Rev 13*:118–119, 1984.
33. El-Badawi MG: An anomalous bifurcation of the sartorius muscle. *Anat Anz 163*:79–82, 1987.
34. Ferner H, Staubesand J: *Sobotta Atlas of Human Anatomy*, Ed. 10, Vol. 2. Urban & Schwarzenberg, Baltimore, 1983 (Figs. 7, 413).
35. *Ibid.* (Fig. 380).
36. *Ibid.* (Fig. 410).
37. *Ibid.* (Figs. 420, 421).
38. Ferraz de Carvalho CA, Garcia OS, Vitti M, *et al.*: Electromyographic study of the m. tensor fascia latae and m. sartorius. *Electromyogr Clin Neurophysiol 12*:387–400, 1972.
39. Gerwin R: Personal communication, 1990.
40. Ghent WR: Meralgia paraesthetica. *Can Med Assoc J 81*:631–633, 1959.
41. Good MG: Diagnosis and treatment of sciatic pain. *Lancet 2*:597–598, 1942.
42. Good MG: What is "fibrositis?" *Rheumatism 5*:117–123, 1949.
43. Gose JC, Schweizer P: Iliotibial band tightness. *J Orthop Sports Phys Therap 10*:399–407, 1989.
44. Guo-Xiang J, Wei-Dong X: Meralgia paraesthetica of spinal origin: brief report. *J Bone Joint Surg [Br] 70*:843–844, 1988.
45. Gutstein M: Diagnosis and treatment of muscular rheumatism. *Br J Phys Med 1*:302–321, 1938 (Case IV).
46. Hope T: Pinpointing entrapment neuropathies in the elderly. *Geriatrics 35:*79–89, 1980.
47. Houtz SJ, Fischer FJ: An analysis of muscle action and joint excursion during exercise on a stationary bicycle. *J Bone Joint Surg [Am] 41:* 123–131, 1959.
48. Inman VT: Functional aspects of the abductor muscles of the hip. *J Bone Joint Surg 29*:607–619, 1947.
49. Jefferson D, Eames RA: Subclinical entrapment of the lateral femoral cutaneous nerve: an autopsy study. *Muscle Nerve 2*:145–154, 1979.
50. Johnson CE, Basmajian JV, Dasher W: Electromyography of sartorius muscle. *Anat Rec 173*:127–130, 1972.
51. Jull GA, Janda V: Muscles and motor control in low back pain: assessment and management, Chapter 10. In *Physical Therapy of the Low Back*, edited by L.T. Twomey, J.R. Taylor. Churchill Livingstone, New York, 1987 (pp. 253–278, *see* pp. 266–267, Fig. 10.4).
52. Kamon E: Electromyographic kinesiology of jumping. *Arch Phys Med Rehabil 52*:152–157, 1971.
53. Kaplan EB: The iliotibial tract. Clinical and morphological significance. *J Bone Joint Surg [Am] 40*:817–832, 1958.
54. Keegan JJ, Holyoke EA: Meralgia paresthetica: an anatomical and surgical study. *J Neurosurg 19*:341–345, 1962.
55. Kellgren JH: A preliminary account of referred pains arising from muscle. *Br Med J 1*:325–327, 1938 (Case VII).
56. Kellgren JH: Observations on referred pain arising from muscle. *Clin Sci 3*:175–190, 1938 (Fig. 8).
57. Kelly M: The relief of facial pain by procaine (novocaine) injections. *J Am Geriatr Soc 11*:586–596, 1963 (Table 1).
58. Kopell HP, Thompson WAL: *Peripheral Entrapment Neuropathies*. Robert E. Krieger, New York, 1976 (pp. 84–88).

59. Lange M: *Die Muskelhärten (Myogelosen).* J.F. Lehmanns, München, 1931 (p. 49, Fig. 13).
60. *Ibid.* (pp. 144–145, Fig. 45, Case 27).
61. Lewit K: *Manipulative Therapy in Rehabilitation of the Motor System.* Butterworths, London, 1985 (pp. 148–149, Fig. 4.36).
62. *Ibid.* (p. 153, Fig. 4.42).
63. *Ibid.* (pp. 170–171, Fig. 4.67).
64. *Ibid.* (p. 315).
65. Lockhart RD: *Living Anatomy*, Ed. 7. Faber & Faber, London, 1974 (pp. 58, 59).
66. Máckova J, Janda V, Máček, *et al.*: Impaired muscle function in children and adolescents. *J Man Med 4*:157–160, 1989.
67. Macnicol MF, Thompson WJ: Idiopathic meralgia paresthetica. *Clin Orthop 254*:270–274, 1990.
68. Mann RA, Moran GT, Dougherty SE: Comparative electromyography of the lower extremity in jogging, running, and sprinting. *Am J Sportsmed 14*:501–510, 1986.
69. Massey EW: Meralgia paraesthetica. *JAMA 237*: 1125–1126, 1977.
70. Meberg A, Skogen P: Three different manifestations of congenital muscular aplasia in a family. *Acta Paediatr Scand 76*:375–377, 1987.
71. Merchant AC: Hip abductor muscle force: an experimental study of the influence of hip position with special reference to rotation. *J Bone Joint Surg [Am] 47*:462–476, 1965.
72. Müller-Vahl H: Isolated complete paralysis of the tensor fasciae latae muscle. *Eur Neurol 24*: 289–291, 1985.
73. Namey TC: Emergency diagnosis and management of sciatica: differentiating the non-diskogenic causes. *Emerg Med 6*:101–109, 1985.
74. Németh G, Ekholm J, Arborelius UP: Hip load moments and muscular activity during lifting. *Scand J Rehabil Med 16*:103–111, 1984.
75. Netter FH: *The Ciba Collection of Medical Illustrations*, Vol. 8, Musculoskeletal System. Part I: Anatomy, Physiology and Metabolic Disorders. Ciba-Geigy Corporation, Summit, 1987 (p. 80).
76. *Ibid.* (p. 83).
77. *Ibid.* (p. 85).
78. *Ibid.* (p. 86).
79. *Ibid.* (p. 87).
80. *Ibid.* (p. 90).
81. *Ibid.* (p. 91).
82. *Ibid.* (p. 94).
83. Ober FR: The role of the iliotibial band and fascia latae as a factor of back disabilities and sciatica. *J Bone Joint Surg [Am] 18*:65–110, 1936.
84. Orton D: Meralgia paresthetica from a wallet [letter]. *JAMA 252*:3368, 1984.
85. Paré EB, Stern JT Jr, Schwartz JM: Functional differentiation within the tensor fasciae latae. *J Bone Joint Surg [Am] 63*:1457–1471, 1981.
86. Perry J: The mechanics of walking. *Phys Ther 47*:778–801, 1967.
87. Rasch PJ, Burke RK: *Kinesiology and Applied Anatomy*, Ed. 6. Lea & Febiger, Philadelphia, 1978 (p. 282).
88. Reynolds MD: Myofascial trigger point syndromes in the practice of rheumatology. *Arch Phys Med Rehabil 62*:111–114, 1981.
89. Rohen JW, Yokochi C: *Color Atlas of Anatomy*, Ed. 2. Igaku-Shoin, New York, 1988 (p. 416).
90. *Ibid.* (p. 419).
91. *Ibid.* (p. 422).
92. *Ibid.* (p. 438).
93. Saudek CE: The hip, Chapter 17. In *Orthopaedic and Sports Physical Therapy*, edited by J.A. Gould III and G.J. Davies, Vol. II. CV Mosby, St. Louis, 1985 (pp. 365–407, *see* p. 385).
94. *Ibid.* (pp. 389–390).
95. Sola AE: Treatment of myofascial pain syndromes. In *Recent Advances in the Management of Pain*, edited by Costantino Benedetti, C. Richard Chapman, Guido Moricca. Raven Press, New York, 1984, Series title: *Advances in Pain Research and Therapy*, Vol. 7 (pp. 467–485, *see* p. 480–481, Fig. 12).
96. Sola AE: Trigger point therapy, Chapter 47. In *Clinical Procedures in Emergency Medicine*, edited by J.R. Roberts and J.R. Hedges. W.B. Saunders, Philadelphia, 1985 (pp. 674–686, *see* pp. 681–683, Fig. 47–9).
97. Sola AE, Williams RL: Myofascial pain syndromes. *Neurology 6*:91–95, 1956.
98. Stookey B: Meralgia paraesthetica. *JAMA 90*: 1705–1707, 1928.
99. Stubbs NB, Capen EK, Wilson GL: An electromyographic investigation of the sartorius and tensor fascia latae muscles. *Res Q Am Assoc Health Phys Educ 46*:358–363, 1975.
100. Teng P: Meralgia paresthetica. *Bull Los Angeles Neurol Soc 37*:75–83, 1972.
101. Travell JG, Simons DG: *Myofascial Pain and Dysfunction: The Trigger Point Manual.* Williams & Wilkins, Baltimore, 1983.
102. Warfield CA: Meralgia paresthetica: causes and cures. *Hosp Pract 21*:40A,40C,40I, 1986.
103. Weber EF: Ueber die Längenverhältnisse der Fleischfasern der Muskeln im Allgemeinen. *Berichte über die Verhandlungen der Königlich Sächsischen Gesellschaft der Wissenschaften Zu Leipzig 3*:65, 1851.
104. Winter Z: Referred pain in fibrositis. *Med Rec 157*:34–37, 1944.

CHAPTER 13
Pectineus Muscle

"The Fourth Adductor"

HIGHLIGHTS: **REFERRED PAIN** projects over the pectineus muscle just below the inguinal ligament, extends deep into the groin and perhaps the hip joint, and may travel a short distance down the anteromedial aspect of the thigh. The proximal **ANATOMICAL ATTACHMENT** of this muscle is to the pubic bone. Distally, it anchors to the back of the femur below the attachment of the iliopsoas muscle. **FUNCTION** of the pectineus muscle involves a combination of adduction and flexion of the thigh at the hip. The pectineus qualifies as the fourth adductor. The main **SYMPTOM** is persistent pain, which often becomes apparent after trigger points (TrPs) in the other three adductor and/or iliopsoas muscles have been inactivated. **ACTIVATION OF TRIGGER POINTS** may result from tripping or falling on a staircase, may follow fracture of the femoral neck or a total hip replacement, or may occur in a situation that causes strong resistance to adduction of the thigh, such as sexual activity or gymnastic exercises. **PERPETUATION OF TRIGGER POINTS** may be caused by sustained or repeated hip adduction-flexion, or by systemic factors. **PATIENT EXAMINATION** reveals little restriction of range of motion. **TRIGGER POINT EXAMINATION** elicits exquisite tenderness where this muscle lies directly under the skin. Snapping palpation across the muscle fibers may produce a vigorous local twitch response and evoke referred pain. **ASSOCIATED TRIGGER POINTS** are often found in the iliopsoas muscle and/or the other adductor muscles, especially the adductor longus and brevis. The **INTERMITTENT COLD-WITH-STRETCH** procedure entails application of the spray or ice over the muscle from its proximal to its distal end and beyond it a short distance, while the thigh is passively abducted and extended at the hip. This is followed by a moist hot pack and full active range of motion. **INJECTION AND STRETCH** may be required to inactivate TrPs fully in this muscle. The thigh of the supine patient is abducted and laterally rotated and the overlying femoral artery is located by its pulsation. The TrPs in this muscle are injected in a medial direction to avoid the femoral artery, which is continuously palpated during injection. **CORRECTIVE ACTIONS** include compensation for a lower limb-length inequality and/or a small hemipelvis; avoidance of prolonged shortening of the muscle, especially while sitting; and avoidance of vigorous activities that suddenly stretch the muscle beyond its tolerance.

---

1. REFERRED PAIN
(Fig. 13.1)

Myofascial trigger points (TrPs) in the pectineus muscle produce a deep-seated aching pain in the groin immediately distal to the inguinal ligament; the pain may also cover the upper part of the anteromedial aspect of the thigh (Fig. 13.1).[5] The pain is often described by patients as "in the groin and in the hip joint," but they may have a poor understanding of where the hip joint is located. The deep groin pain may also extend medially to the region where the adductor magnus attaches to the pelvis.

2. ANATOMICAL ATTACHMENTS AND CONSIDERATIONS
(Fig. 13.2)

The pectineus muscle attaches ***proximally*** to the pecten (crest) of the superior ramus of the pubic bone lateral to the pu-

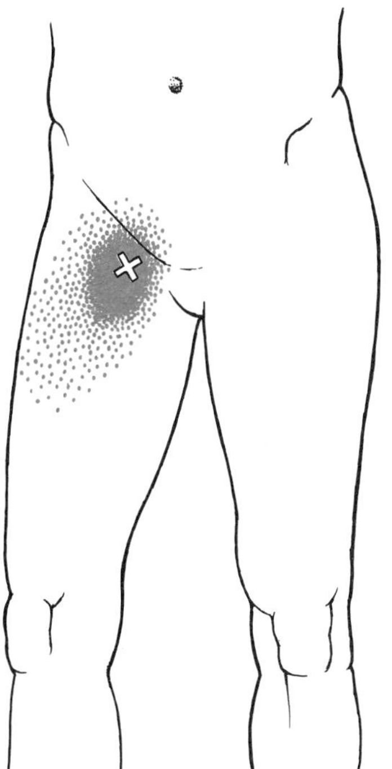

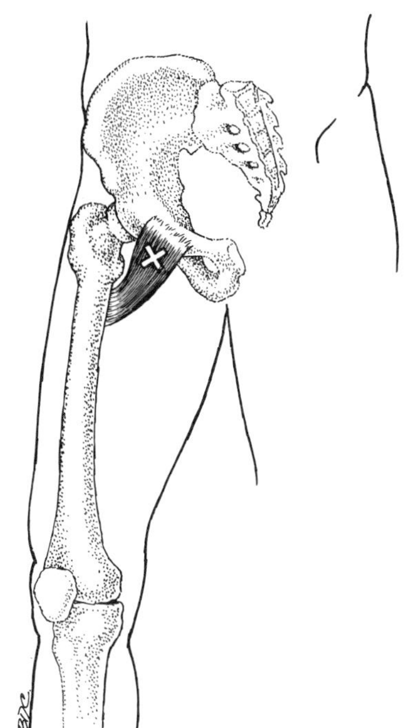

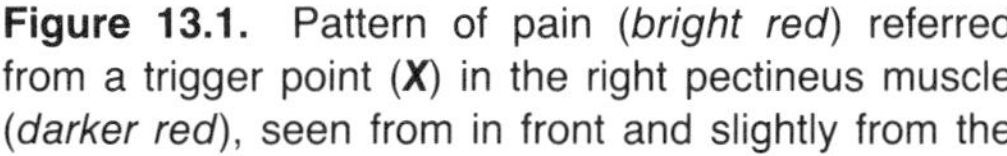

Figure 13.1. Pattern of pain (*bright red*) referred from a trigger point (**X**) in the right pectineus muscle (*darker red*), seen from in front and slightly from the medial side. The *essential* referred pain pattern is solid red, and the occasional spillover pattern is *stippled*.

bic tubercle. This attachment is caudal and deep to the inguinal ligament, which attaches medially to the pubic tubercle (Figs. 13.2 and 13.4).[6,10]

The pectineus muscle comprises most of the medial part of the floor of the femoral (Scarpa's) triangle. This triangle is bounded by the inguinal ligament above, by the sartorius muscle laterally, and by the adductor longus muscle medially. Medial to the pectineus, the floor of the triangle is completed by the adductor brevis muscle, and lateral to it, by the iliopsoas muscle.[19]

The pectineus muscle attaches ***distally*** to the pectineal line on the medial posterior aspect of the femur.[9] The pectineal line extends distally from the lesser trochanter (attachment of the iliopsoas muscle) to the linea aspera[33] (attachment of the vastus medialis, adductor longus, and adductor magnus muscles). The pectineus overlies the uppermost fibers of the adductor brevis muscle as they descend to attach to the back of the femur (*see* Fig. 13.4).[8,34] Except for its usual innervation by the femoral nerve and its more diagonally directed fibers, the pectineus is similar anatomically to the adductor brevis.

The pectineus muscle exhibits a number of variations. It may be more or less completely divided into superficial and deep, or into medial and lateral parts.[6] In the latter situation, the lateral portion is supplied by either a branch of the femoral nerve or the accessory obturator nerve, if present, and the medial portion is supplied by the obturator nerve.[10]

The obturator externus muscle lies deep to the pectineus muscle and covers the obturator foramen of the pelvis.[15,17]

Supplemental References

Other authors have illustrated the pectineus muscle, showing its relationship to surrounding muscles from the front view,[2,14,24,31,34] to major blood vessels in the femoral triangle,[1,13,26] and its attachment to the pecten of the pubic bone.[3,17,25] They show its relation to other muscles in cross section approximately at the middle of the pectineus[27] or in a series of cross sections throughout the length of the muscle.[8] Its attachment to the femur is best seen from behind.[4,16]

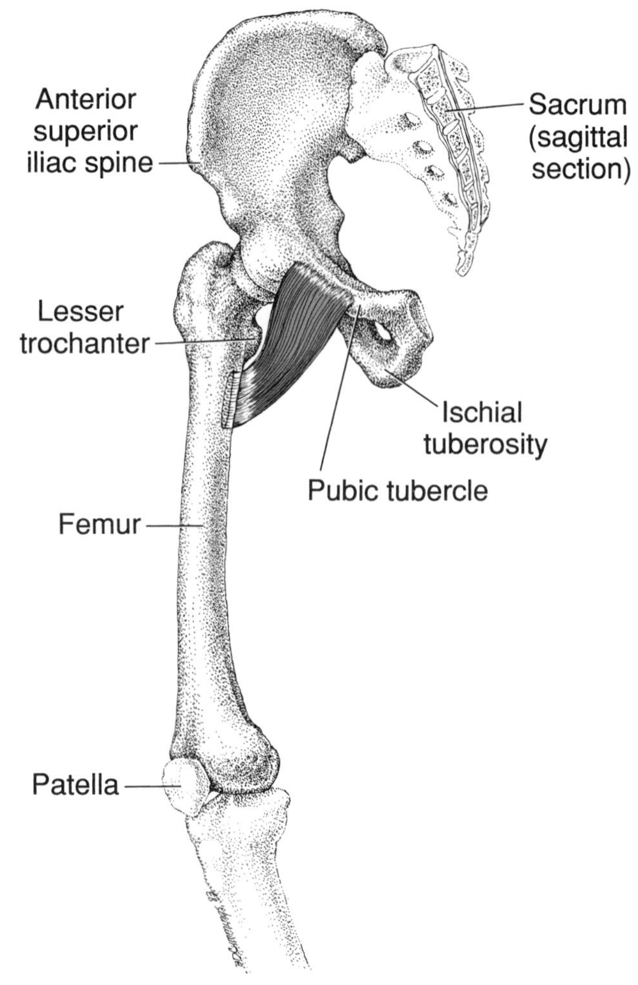

Figure 13.2. Attachments of the right pectineus muscle (*red*), seen from in front and slightly from the medial side. The muscle attaches proximally and medially to the superior ramus of the pubis, and distally it fastens to the posterior surface of the femur medial to its midline.

3. INNERVATION

The pectineus muscle is usually supplied by the femoral nerve via branches of the second to fourth lumbar spinal nerves.[10] The branch of the femoral nerve to the pectineus arises immediately below the inguinal ligament, passes beneath the femoral sheath and penetrates the anterior surface of the muscle.[11] The muscle may also receive a branch from the obturator nerve. When an accessory obturator nerve is present (about 29% of specimens), the muscle is innervated via the accessory obturator from the third and fourth lumbar nerves. Instead of passing through the obturator foramen, this accessory nerve crosses *over* and anterior to the superior ramus of the pubis to which the pectineus attaches.[11]

The pectineus muscle is the one best suited for the combined movements of adduction and flexion at the hip. It is the most proximal adductor muscle.

There is general agreement that the pectineus is both an adductor and flexor of the thigh at the hip.[10,12,20,22,28,32] It adducts more strongly as the thigh is flexed.[32] Based on his electrical stimulation experiments, Duchenne[12] concluded that the pectineus is such a strong adductor-flexor that it and the iliopsoas muscle, functioning together, can cross one thigh over the other when an individual is in the seated position.

The muscle's short lever arm and its small angle of pull of about 60° suggest

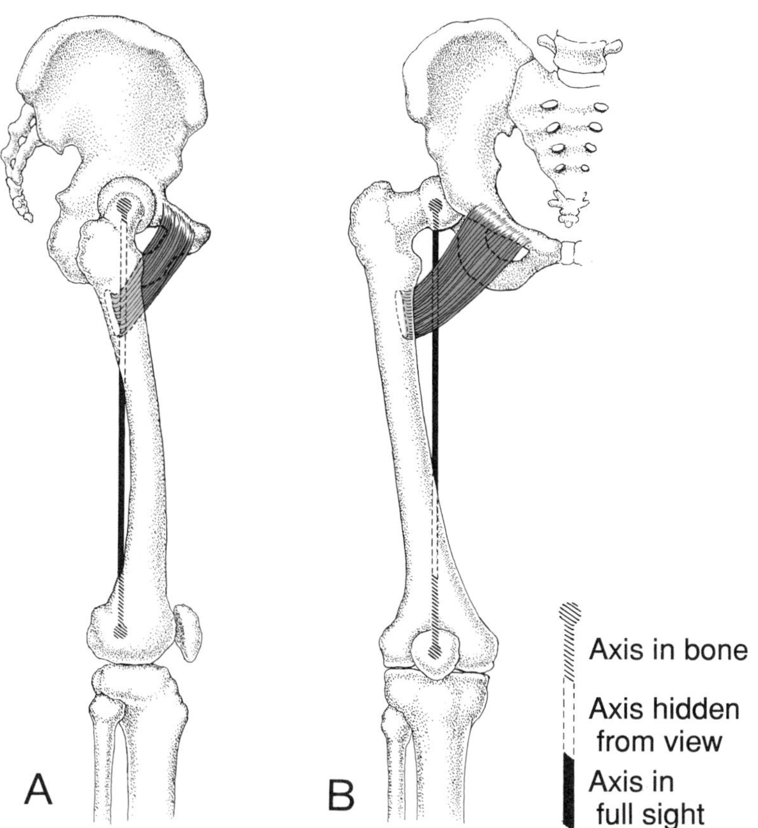

Figure 13.3. Relation of the right pectineus muscle (*red*) to the axis of rotation (*vertical bar*) of the femur in the neutral position. Within view, the muscle is *dark red*; behind bone, it is *light red*. *A*, side view, *B*, front view. Here the muscle passes close to and in front of the axis of rotation; however, it may pass either in front of or behind the axis. Whether this muscle medially or laterally rotates the thigh in this position is highly dependent on minor variations in anatomy. Adapted from Kendall and McCreary.[22]

PART 2

that its purpose is power rather than speed. Leverage improves as the thigh moves forward and inward,[28] which correlates with the increased electromyographic (EMG) activity observed in the muscle at 90° of thigh flexion.[32]

There has been general indecision[6] or disagreement[32] as to whether the muscle rotates the thigh medially[10] or laterally.[12,20,31] For passive stretching of the pectineus muscle, it is unlikely that rotation of the thigh either way produces much difference in its length in most people.

When one examines its anatomy, the controversy is not surprising. The muscle fibers run from a medial attachment on the pubis to a more lateral distal attachment *behind* the femur. At first glance it looks as if the muscle would laterally rotate the thigh. Figure 13.3, adapted from Kendall and McCreary,[22] relates these attachments to the mechanical axis of rotation of the thigh. The front view (Fig. 13.3*B*) shows how far lateral to this axis the pectineus attaches on the femur. Both front and side views show that, at least sometimes, the muscle crosses in front of the axis line. Thus, with its proximal attachment on the pubis being more anterior than its distal attachment on the femur, when the muscle passes **anterior** to the axis of rotation, it pulls the thigh toward the body, medially rotating it at the hip joint. The one reported EMG study[32] showed, in two subjects, no gross differences in the intensity of electrical activity during adduction, flexion, or medial rotation. However, essentially no electrical activity appeared in response to lateral rotation.

The second author analyzed hip rotation in 90° of hip flexion on one skeleton and used string to simulate the muscle line of pull. Remarkably little change of (simulated) muscle length occurred with either medial or lateral rotation of the femur.

However, a small change in bony configuration could easily change this result one way or the other. Poor leverage may account for the relatively large EMG response to active medial rotation.[32] An EMG study of a large number of subjects with a diversity of body builds is needed to clarify the factors that determine the rotational action of this muscle.

5. FUNCTIONAL (MYOTATIC) UNIT

Muscles that function with the pectineus in its thigh adduction-flexion action are four adductors—the adductors longus, brevis, and magnus, and the gracilis—and one flexor of the thigh, the iliopsoas muscle. The remaining hip flexors, namely, the tensor fasciae latae, sartorius and rectus femoris muscles, tend to be or clearly are abductors, not adductors.

Muscles that are the chief antagonists to adduction of the thigh by the pectineus are the gluteus medius, gluteus minimus, and tensor fasciae latae. The gluteus maximus and hamstring muscles oppose flexion.[18,21,29]

6. SYMPTOMS

Patients with pectineus TrPs complain of the referred pain, but rarely present with pain from this muscle only. Usually, additional functionally related muscles are involved. After TrPs in the three other adductors or the iliopsoas have been inactivated, the pectineus is uncovered as the cause of persistent deep-seated groin pain, especially during weight-bearing activities that cause abduction of the thigh. Therefore, the pectineus should be checked for TrP tenderness after inactivating either adductor or iliopsoas TrPs.

Patients with pectineus TrPs may also be aware of limited abduction at the hip, especially when seated in the lotus position (*see* Section 15, Case Report). Among the four muscles that act as adductors, however, TrPs in the pectineus restrict the range of abduction the least.

Differential Diagnosis

Patients with obturator nerve entrapment may present with a pain complaint suggestive of pain referred from pectineus TrPs.[7] The entrapment causes more pronounced sensory changes than the TrPs do. Also, examination of the muscle will reveal taut bands and TrP tenderness only with the myofascial syndrome.

The pain of pectineus TrPs may also be suggestive of hip joint disease, which is diagnosed by radiography.

Pubic stress symphysitis, seen in distance runners[30] and persons who compete in contact sports like ice hockey, causes pain in the region of the symphysis pubis. The pain is aggravated by sports activity. A TrP in the pectineus can aggravate the symphysitis and add confusingly similar symptoms. Pectineus TrPs can be identified by manual examination. The diagnosis is reinforced by relief of pain following inactivation of TrPs.

Tenderness at the symphysis pubis is also common when the patient has an upslip of the innominate bone.

7. ACTIVATION AND PERPETUATION OF TRIGGER POINTS

Activation

Pectineus muscle TrPs are likely to result from tripping or falling, or from any other event that causes unexpectedly strong resistance to combined adduction-flexion of the thigh at the hip. One patient[5] activated his pectineus TrPs while rapidly lifting and moving a heavy computer. Some patients have forgotten the initial incident until specifically queried about the possibility of one. Unaccustomed sexual activity that involves vigorous adductor activity can be responsible for activating pectineus TrPs. A sudden, vigorous adduction-flexion movement while performing gymnastic exercises may overload the muscle, especially when it is already fatigued. Another activity that can stress the muscle is horseback riding, when the rider uses the thighs, rather than the legs and feet, to grasp the horse.

TrPs in this muscle also develop in association with disease of the hip joint, such as advanced osteoarthritis, or with fracture of the neck of the femur, and after surgery on the hip.

Perpetuation

Repetition of a mechanical stress similar to that which previously activated the pectineus TrPs can perpetuate them. In addition, a lower limb-length inequality may impose chronic overload on this muscle. These TrPs are perpetuated also by a sustained posture that places the muscle in a shortened position, such as sitting cross-legged or with the hips in a jackknifed position; an individual with a small hemipelvis often sits cross-legged.

8. PATIENT EXAMINATION

Pectineus TrPs primarily cause pain with little weakness or restriction of motion. Some patients exhibit an antalgic gait.[5] Testing the abduction-extension range of motion usually produces only mild to moderate pain at very nearly the full range,[5] often with no further increase in pain when the thigh is medially or laterally rotated in this stretch position. (This finding applies, of course, only after concurrent iliopsoas and other adductor muscle TrPs have been inactivated.)

When the patient with an active pectineus TrP stands on the opposite leg and then attempts to swing the involved thigh into extreme adduction with flexion at the hip, groin pain occurs at the end of the movement.

9. TRIGGER POINT EXAMINATION
(Figs. 13.4 and 13.5)

The pectineus muscle can be located by first palpating the upper border of the symphysis pubis. Two or three centimeters (approximately an inch) lateral to the symphysis is the pubic tubercle (*see* Fig. 13.2), to which the medial end of the inguinal ligament attaches (Fig. 13.4). When the thigh is placed in moderate abduction without flexion, the adductor longus muscle (Fig. 13.4) should be palpable, if not visible. The adductor longus and brevis muscles lie parallel to, and are immediately medial and deeper than, the pectineus. The pectineus muscle attaches to the crest (pecten) of the superior ramus of the pubic bone just inferior to the medial portion of the inguinal ligament. By palpating lateral to the pubic tubercle, the anterior edge of the superior ramus of the pubic bone is readily felt. If there is any doubt as to the location of the pubic tubercle, one can identify the proximal attachment of the adductor longus, which is close and medial to the tubercle.

The lateral distal part of the pectineus muscle lies deep to the femoral neurovascular bundle (Fig. 13.4). The artery courses down the middle of the femoral triangle. Its pulsation is readily palpable in most patients.

The TrPs in the pectineus muscle are located just distal to the superior ramus of the pubis (*see* Fig. 13.1). These TrPs lie immediately under the palpating finger in this subcutaneous muscle. To feel the stringlike taut band in this muscle, the finger palpates in the same proximal location described above, rubbing across the fibers of the pectineus muscle parallel to the border of the superior ramus of the pubic bone. Pressure may be applied to a TrP in the pectineus in the manner shown in Figure 13.5 to elicit its spot tenderness. Flat palpation of this TrP may induce a clear referral of pain. Snapping palpation of the TrP may elicit a visible or palpable twitch of the muscle.

10. ENTRAPMENTS

No nerve entrapments are known to be caused by TrPs in the pectineus muscle.

11. ASSOCIATED TRIGGER POINTS

The TrPs in the pectineus muscle are frequently discovered in association with TrPs in the iliopsoas, the three adductors, and the gracilis muscle. When these neighboring TrPs have been inactivated, a search for the cause of the residual tenderness and deep groin pain reveals the pectineus TrPs. For this reason, it is important after eliminating any TrPs in the iliopsoas and adductor muscles, always to check for residual pain-producing active TrPs in the pectineus.

12. INTERMITTENT COLD WITH STRETCH
(Fig. 13.6)

Since the lower, more diagonal fibers of the pectineus muscle give it a major adductor function, it is essential that all the other muscles functioning as adductors be freed of TrP tightness in order to effectively release the pectineus muscle.

The use of ice for applying intermittent cold with stretch is explained on page 9 of this volume and the use of vapocoolant

PART 2

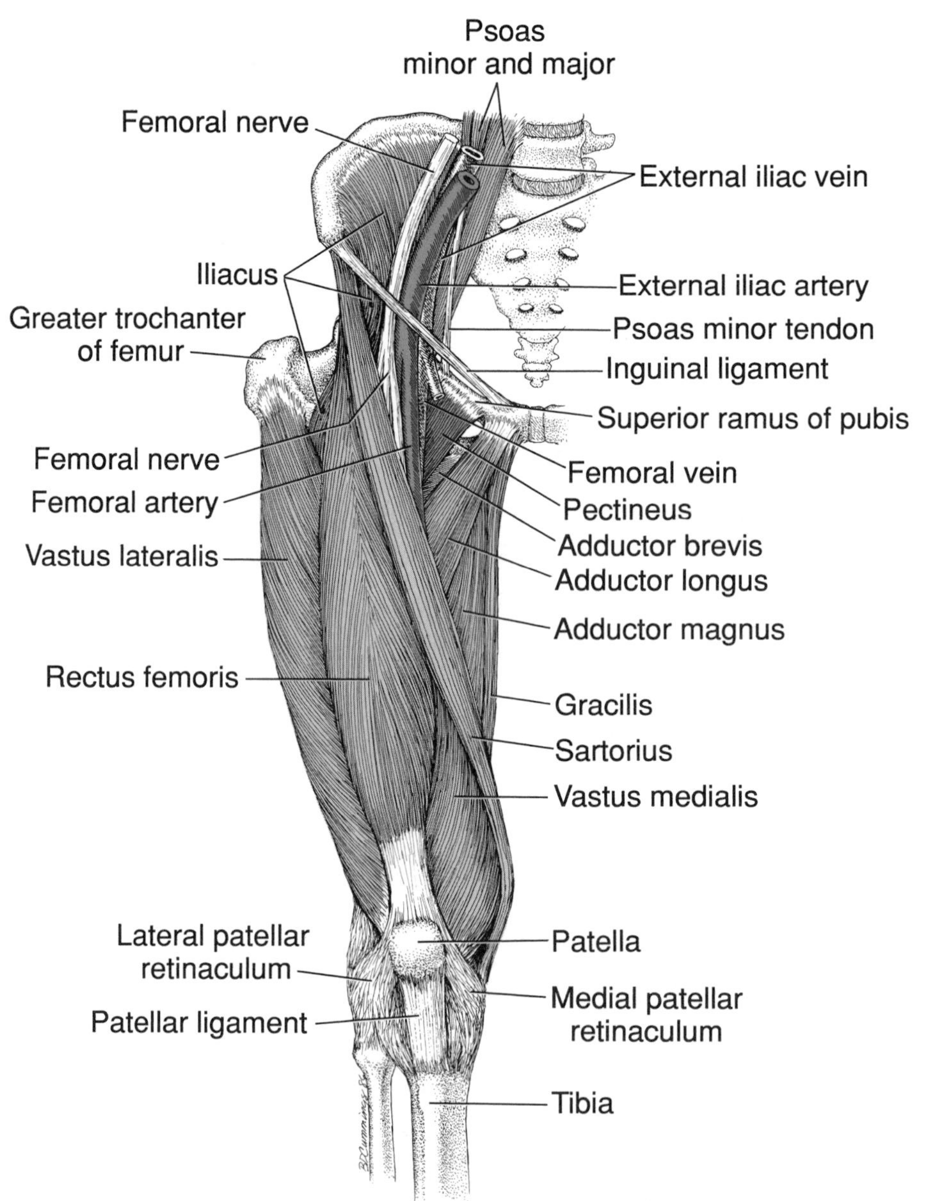

Figure 13.4. Anatomical relations of the right pectineus muscle (*medium red*) to neighboring thigh muscles (*light red*) and to the femoral (Scarpa's) triangle. This triangle is bounded by the inguinal ligament superiorly, by the sartorius muscle laterally, and the adductor longus medially. The femoral artery is *dark red*; the femoral vein has *black hatching*; and the femoral nerve is *white*.

with stretch is detailed on pages 67–74 of Volume 1.[35] Techniques that augment relaxation and stretch are reviewed on page 11 of this volume. Full stretch is avoided across hypermobile joints. Alternate treatment techniques are summarized on page 000 of this volume.

To release this entire functional unit, one starts by applying intermittent cold with stretch to the adductor magnus muscle in the manner illustrated as the first step of the procedure for the hamstring muscles, abducting the thigh of the supine patient (*see* Fig. 16.11*A*).

Next, intermittent cold with stretch is applied to the adductor longus and brevis (*see* Fig. 15.14). During the application of vapocoolant or ice, the operator gently ab-

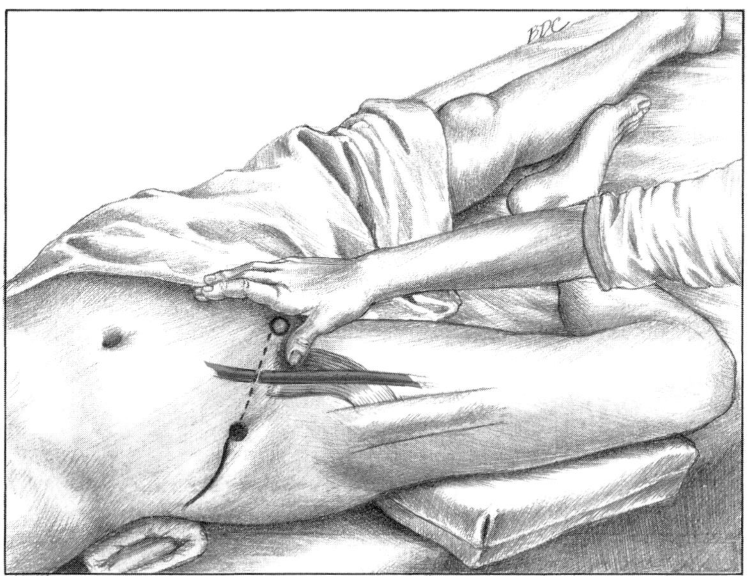

Figure 13.5. Palpation of trigger points in the right pectineus muscle (*light red*). *Dark red* marks the path of the palpable (pulsating) femoral artery, which is part of the neurovascular bundle. The *dashed line* identifies the inguinal ligament. The *open circle* marks the pubic tubercle and the *solid circle*, the anterior superior iliac spine. The *solid black line* locates the crest of the ilium. The pectineus muscle forms the upper medial floor of the femoral triangle. The *pillow* under the thigh elevates the knee slightly to relieve excessive tension on the pectineus muscle. The *rolled towel* provides lumbar support for the patient's comfort. The blanket helps to prevent chilling of the patient.

ducts the thigh at the hip, with the foot on the affected side placed against the middle of the opposite thigh of the supine patient. This position also adds some stretch to the pectineus, but is an incomplete stretch without adding hip extension.

For the final stretch, the patient's hip is placed close to the edge of the treatment table and the leg of the limb being treated is allowed to hang over the edge. For protection of the lumbar region (particularly if there is hypermobility), the pelvis should be stabilized; either the pelvis can be strapped down or the patient can hold the opposite thigh close to the abdomen (not pictured). As sweeps of ice or vapocoolant are applied as shown in Figure 13.6, the clinician, using the assistance of gravity, *gently* abducts and extends the thigh until resistance (a barrier) is reached. To include postisometric relaxation in each treatment cycle, the patient slowly inhales and *gently* tries to flex and adduct the thigh while the clinician resists the movement, maintaining the position. Then, as the patient relaxes and slowly exhales, the clinician allows gravity to help take up the slack that develops. Since this position also stretches the iliopsoas muscle, before finishing the procedure, downsweeps of vapocoolant or ice are also applied beside the midline of the abdomen as illustrated in Figure 5.5.

When the limit of this motion is reached, medial and then lateral rotation at the hip may be performed. If either movement is found to increase tension on the pectineus muscle and cause discomfort, more sweeps of vapocoolant or ice are applied during this additional rotary stretch.

Immediately following intermittent cold with stretch, the clinician applies a moist heating pad to the areas of cooled skin. When the skin has rewarmed, the patient actively moves the thigh *slowly* and *smoothly* through full flexion-adduction and then extension-abduction several times to reestablish normal active range of motion.

Instead of, or in addition to, intermittent cold with stretch, the clinician can apply ischemic compression and deep massage (*see* Chapter 2 for details). Full

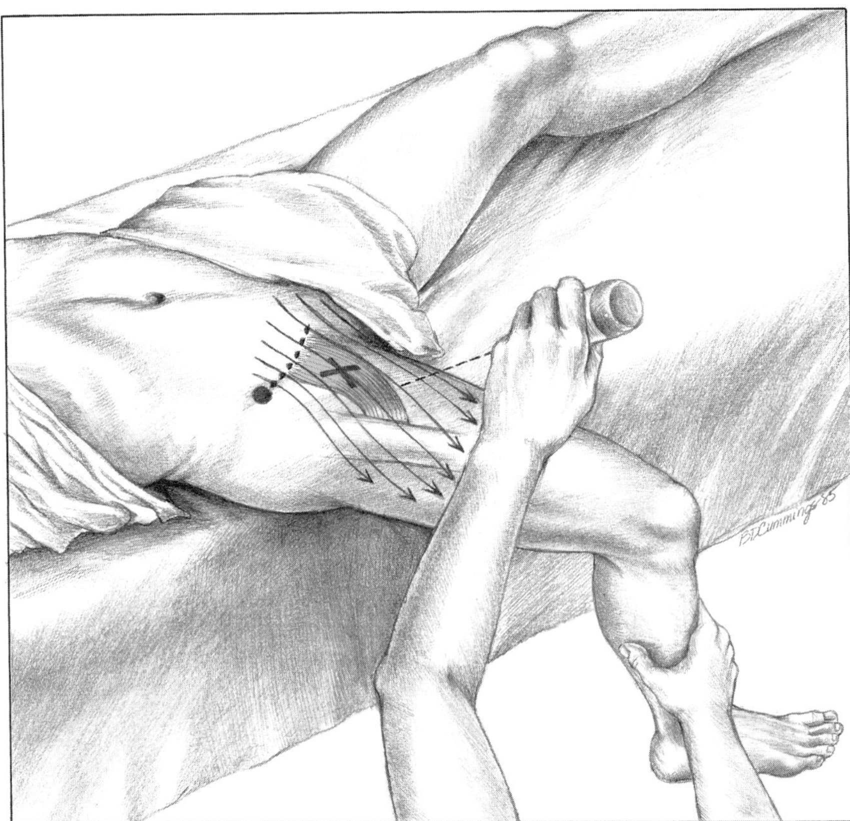

Figure 13.6. Stretch position and the ice-stroking or vapocoolant-spray pattern (*thin arrows*) for a trigger point (***X***) in the right pectineus muscle. The *dotted line* marks the inguinal ligament and the *solid circle*, the anterior superior iliac spine. To stretch the pectineus, the thigh is gradually moved outward and downward (in abduction and extension). Moving the thigh by grasping the knee instead of the leg would avoid any possible trauma to the knee. At the limit of the range, one may add pressure at the distal thigh to test first medial and then lateral passive rotation at the hip, to learn whether either movement increases the tension on the pectineus muscle.

lengthening of the muscle should follow this deep massage.

13. INJECTION AND STRETCH
(Fig. 13.7)

Before the authors learned to release the adductor magnus muscle first, spray and stretch of the pectineus was usually not effective, and it was necessary to inject the TrPs in this muscle to obtain complete relief of pain.

To inject these TrPs, the thigh of the supine patient is placed in lateral rotation, abduction, and slight flexion (Fig. 13.7). This position shifts the femoral artery toward the lateral margin of the muscle, since the vessel is fixed distally at the adductor hiatus. Injecting this muscle with the thigh in the anatomical position increases the risk of puncturing the artery. The abducted position also helps to increase the tension of the muscle fibers and to make the taut bands more readily palpable.

The TrP is palpated as described in Section 9, Trigger Point Examination. Two fingers straddle the TrP to localize it for accurate penetration by the probing needle. The femoral artery is avoided by palpating its pulsations and directing the needle away from it. In thin patients, the artery is readily palpated laterally in the femoral (Scarpa's) triangle (Fig. 13.4).

The basic technique for injection of the TrPs with 0.5% procaine solution is described and illustrated in Volume 1, Chapter 3, Section 13.[35] A 37–mm (1½-in) 21–gauge needle is directed medially pre-

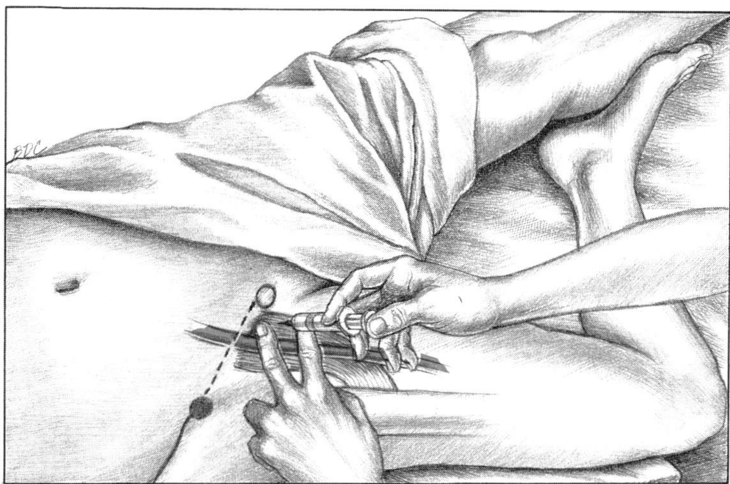

Figure 13.7. Injection of a trigger point in the right pectineus muscle (*light red*). The thigh of the supine patient is placed in abduction, lateral rotation, and slight flexion. The *solid circle* locates the anterior superior iliac spine; the *dashed line*, the inguinal ligament; and the *open circle*, the pubic tubercle. The femoral artery (*dark red*) is avoided by palpating its pulsations and directing the needle medially away from it.

cisely into the TrP and pressure applied for hemostasis as the needle is withdrawn. The effectiveness of this approach is illustrated in a case report of Baker[5] and in the case report in Section 15 of this chapter.

Injection of a TrP is followed at once by application of intermittent cold with stretch, then a moist hot pack, and finally by several cycles of active range of motion, alternating thigh extension-abduction and thigh flexion-adduction.

14. CORRECTIVE ACTIONS

In general, activities or positions that overload the thigh adductors or that immobilize the muscle in a shortened position should be avoided or modified.

Patients with persistent myofascial pain syndromes who respond poorly to specific local TrP therapy should be screened carefully for both mechanical and systemic perpetuating factors (Volume 1, Chapter 4).[35]

Corrective Body Mechanics

Any discrepancy in lower limb length or any asymmetry in hemipelvis size should be corrected. Correction of these body asymmetries is made by supplying a suitable shoe lift or ischial (butt) lift (*see* Chapter 4), assuming that malalignments, such as ilial rotations, have been previously corrected. The apparent asymmetry that is almost always caused by an ilial rotation should be corrected by mobilization and restoration of normal pelvic symmetry, not by a limb-length correction.

Corrective Posture and Activities

The patient also should avoid sitting with the knees crossed or the hips flexed acutely (in a jackknifed position) because these positions maintain the pectineus muscle in a shortened state. When sitting erect in a chair, one's knees should *not* be higher than the hips.

Some patients, especially women, may perform vigorous adduction of the thighs during sexual intercourse, which can overload the adductor muscles including the pectineus. Alternative positions should be explored or adductor-conditioning exercises gradually instituted after pain-producing TrPs have been inactivated.

When sleeping, if the patient lies on the side opposite to the involved pectineus muscle, a pillow should be placed between the knees (*see* Fig. 4.31) to prevent postural aggravation of the pectineus TrPs.

Home Therapeutic Program

The patient should be instructed in a self-stretch exercise for the pectineus muscle. This can be performed using the position shown in Figure 13.6. The patient can enhance muscle lengthening by using postisometric relaxation as described in Section 12. Looking upward while inhaling facilitates contraction of the muscle; looking downward while exhaling enhances relaxation of the muscle. Gravity takes up the slack that develops. Instructions should also be given in corrective posture and activities as described previously.

15. CASE REPORT
(Seen by David G. Simons, M.D.)

S.S., a 24-year-old male physical therapist, reported that, while fatigued, he had performed repeated martial art kicks a year earlier. This vigorous kicking movement produced marked adduction of the thigh across the front of the body with partial flexion at the hip. Suddenly, during one of these movements, he felt a twinge of pain deep in the right groin, anterior to the hip joint. As he continued the exercise, pain intensified. The ensuing intense, aching soreness caused him to avoid any ballistic kicking or sports activity that required strong adduction of the thigh. The acute phase lasted several weeks. Ordinary ambulation was painless. Conservative therapy with ice, hot packs, and ultrasound had no effect. The problem was aggravated by repeated assumption of the position of combined hip flexion, abduction, and lateral rotation (lotus position), in an attempt to work through the pain.

The patient previously was treated by two physicians and five physical therapists without any improvement. X-rays were unremarkable, revealing only minimal sclerosis around the acetabulum of the hip joint.

When first seen, the patient described the pain as annoying and worrisome, but not disabling. It restricted his recreational gymnastic activities. He had no rest pain and no pain with ordinary activities. However, when he assumed the lotus position, abduction of the thigh at the hip was restricted on the right side, and there was aching pain in the groin that increased as abduction was increased. A more abrupt pain in the same region occurred in the standing position when the right thigh was crossed over in front of the left, producing full adduction combined with some flexion.

Examination for a lower limb-length inequality and for a small hemipelvis showed no body asymmetry. Examination of muscles in the hip region revealed palpable tenseness of the entire pectineus muscle, a taut band within the muscle, and exquisite tenderness at one spot along the band. Snapping palpation at the tender spot elicited no obvious local twitch response and no distinguishable radiation of pain.

Procaine injection of TrPs in the pectineus muscle, followed at once by application of vapocoolant spray and stretch to the other adductors and the pectineus muscle, reduced the TrP sensitivity to finger pressure approximately 50%. After 2 weeks of self-administered postisometric relaxation[23] for ***gentle*** adductor stretch in the lotus position, the patient achieved a comfortable full range of motion in this position. Adduction of the flexed thigh during standing was then painless, and the patient was able to perform both concentric and isometric adduction strengthening exercises without discomfort.

Comment:

This case is unusual in that it is a single-muscle pectineus syndrome. Initial therapy by TrP injection and stretch was chosen rather than intermittent cold with stretch alone, because it was clearly a single-muscle myofascial syndrome that had been refractory to previous conservative therapy.

The non-progressive nature of the symptoms and the immediate and lasting response to therapy made further investigation for systemic perpetuating factors unnecessary.

References

1. Anderson JE: *Grant's Atlas of Anatomy*, Ed. 8. Williams & Wilkins, Baltimore, 1983 (Fig. 4–20).
2. *Ibid*. (Fig. 4–22).
3. *Ibid*. (Fig. 4–39).
4. *Ibid*. (Fig. 4–40).
5. Baker BA: Myofascial pain syndromes: ten single muscle cases. *J Neurol Orthop Med Surg 10*: 129–131, 1989.
6. Bardeen CR: The musculature, Sect. 5. In *Morris's Human Anatomy*, edited by C.M. Jackson, Ed. 6. Blakiston's Son & Co., Philadelphia, 1921 (p. 504).
7. Bowman AJ Jr, Carpenter AA, Iovino J, *et al*.: Intrapelvic complications of hip surgery: a case report of obturator nerve entrapment. *Orthopedics* 2:504–506, 1979.
8. Carter BL, Morehead J, Wolpert SM, *et al*.: *Cross-Sectional Anatomy*. Appleton-Century-Crofts, New York, 1977 (Sects. 39–43, 45–48).
9. Clemente CD: *Gray's Anatomy of the Human Body*, American Ed. 30. Lea & Febiger, Philadelphia, 1985 (pp. 278–279).
10. *Ibid*. (pp. 563–564).
11. *Ibid*. (pp. 1230–1232).
12. Duchenne GB: *Physiology of Motion*, translated by E.B. Kaplan. Lippincott, Philadelphia, 1949 (pp. 266, 267).

13. Ferner H, Staubesand J: *Sobotta Atlas of Human Anatomy*, Ed. 10, Vol. 2. Urban & Schwarzenberg, Baltimore, 1983 (Fig. 407).
14. *Ibid*. (Figs. 415, 416).
15. *Ibid*. (Fig. 417).
16. *Ibid*. (Fig. 420).
17. *Ibid*. (Fig. 421).
18. Hollinshead WH: *Functional Anatomy of the Limbs and Back*, Ed. 4. W.B. Saunders, Philadelphia, 1976 (pp. 271, 300–302, 304).
19. Hollingshead WH: *Anatomy for Surgeons*, Ed. 3., Vol. 3, *The Back and Limbs*. Harper & Row, New York, 1982 (pp. 685, 696–698).
20. Janda V: *Muscle Function Testing*. Butterworths, London, 1983 (pp. 161, 169, 176).
21. *Ibid*. (pp. 161, 164, 169, 171).
22. Kendall FP, McCreary EK: *Muscles, Testing and Function*, Ed. 3. Williams & Wilkins, Baltimore, 1983 (p. 178).
23. Lewit K, Simons DG: Myofascial pain: relief by post-isometric relaxation. *Arch Phys Med Rehabil 65*:452–456, 1984.
24. McMinn RMH, Hutchings RT: *Color Atlas of Human Anatomy*. Year Book Medical Publishers, Chicago, 1977 (p. 244).
25. *Ibid*. (p. 270).
26. *Ibid*. (p. 298).
27. Pernkopf E: *Atlas of Topographical and Applied Human Anatomy*, Vol. 2. W.B. Saunders, Philadelphia, 1964 (Fig. 329).
28. Rasch PJ, Burke RK: *Kinesiology and Applied Anatomy*, Ed. 6. Lea & Febiger, Philadelphia, 1978 (p. 272).
29. *Ibid*. (p. 282).
30. Rold JF, Rold BA: Pubic stress symphysitis in a female distance runner. *Phys Sportsmed 14*:61–65, 1986.
31. Spalteholz W: *Handatlas der Anatomie des Menschen*, Ed. 11, Vol. 2. S. Hirzel, Leipzig, 1922 (p. 349, 350).
32. Takebe K, Vitti M, Basmajian JV: Electromyography of pectineus muscle. *Anat Rec 180*:281–283, 1974.
33. Toldt C: *An Atlas of Human Anatomy*, translated by M.E. Paul, Ed. 2, Vol. 1. Macmillan, New York, 1919 (p. 132, Fig. 320).
34. *Ibid*. (p. 352).
35. Travell JG, Simons DG: *Myofascial Pain and Dysfunction: The Trigger Point Manual*. Williams & Wilkins, Baltimore, 1983.

CHAPTER 14
Quadriceps Femoris Group
Rectus Femoris, Vastus Medialis, Vastus Intermedius, and Vastus Lateralis

"Four-Faced Trouble Maker"

HIGHLIGHTS: **REFERRED PAIN** patterns of myofascial trigger points (TrPs) in the quadriceps femoris muscle group can appear on the medial, anterior, or lateral aspects of the thigh and in the knee. The common TrP in the rectus femoris occurs at the upper end of the muscle and refers to the lower anterior thigh and anterior knee regions. The TrPs in the vastus medialis refer pain to the knee anteromedially and upward along the anteromedial aspect of the thigh. The vastus intermedius pain pattern hits the middle portion of the anterior thigh, and the vastus lateralis has at least five TrP sites that can cause misery along the lateral thigh from the pelvis and greater trochanter to the lateral side of the knee. **ANATOMICAL ATTACHMENTS** of the rectus femoris are such that it crosses both the hip and the knee joints, unlike the three vasti of the quadriceps femoris, which cross only the knee joint. Proximally, the rectus femoris is anchored to the pelvis in the region of the anterior inferior iliac spine. The vastus intermedius that lies deep to it attaches to a large area of the anterolateral surface of the femur. Both the vastus medialis and vastus lateralis attach on their respective sides to the posterior aspect of the femur along the length of its shaft. Tendons of all four heads of the quadriceps femoris unite to form a strong tendon, which attaches distally to the base of the patella. The patella is anchored to the tibial tuberosity by the patellar ligament. Quadriceps **FUNCTION** frequently involves the exertion of force on the thigh (reverse action), and it often involves lengthening contractions to *control* knee flexion. Function is easily inhibited by disturbance of knee mechanics including effusion into the joint. The role of the oblique (distal, diagonal) fibers of the vastus medialis is to counter the lateral pull of the vastus lateralis on the patella, a critically important function. When the foot is free, the quadriceps femoris acts primarily to extend the leg at the knee (all four heads) and to assist flexion of the thigh at the hip (rectus femoris only). The rectus femoris forms a **FUNCTIONAL UNIT** for flexion at the hip primarily with the iliopsoas and pectineus muscles, which are opposed by the gluteus maximus and hamstring muscles. All heads of the quadriceps femoris contribute to knee extension and are opposed primarily by the hamstring muscles. **SYMPTOMS** of quadriceps femoris TrPs are chiefly pain and weakness. Since the quadriceps femoris is the only strong extensor at the knee, any TrP in that muscle group compromises knee extension. A buckling knee can be caused by TrPs in the vastus medialis and reportedly from the vastus lateralis. TrPs in either of these muscles can distort patellar balance. The TrPs in the rectus femoris, vastus medialis, and vastus lateralis are likely to disturb sleep. Vastus lateralis TrPs can cause lateral thigh pain and/or locking of the patella with the knee in the extended position. Differential diagnosis of knee pain should consider other causes of patellofemoral dysfunction, including tendinitis of the quadriceps or patellar tendons, as well as knee joint dysfunction and pathology. **ACTIVATION OF TRIGGER POINTS** in the quadriceps femoris often occurs during a fall, misstep, or trauma to the muscle, and due to injection of irritant medication into the muscle. Quadriceps femoris TrPs often are perpetuated by tightness of the hamstrings, which hinders full extension at the knee and thus imposes an excessive load on the quadriceps femoris group of muscles. Deep knee bends readily overload this muscle. **PATIENT EXAMINATION** starts with evaluation of gait for asymmetries, deviations, and malalignment of lower limb segments. Strength and range of motion are tested separately for the rectus femoris and for the three vasti. Loss of patellar mobility reveals information about the relative tightness of individual heads of the muscle. **TRIGGER POINT EXAMINATION** of the rectus femoris by flat palpation locates TrPs near its proximal attachment. The TrP that commonly causes buckling of the knee is found in the medial border of the vastus medialis near the transition to oblique fibers. The vastus intermedius harbors multiple deep TrPs that are often difficult to localize by palpation. The TrP in the distal vastus lateralis that causes a locked patella is superficial, but can be located only if the patella is moved distally to uncover the TrP for flat palpation. The clusters of deep TrPs in the middle two-fourths of the vastus lateralis are usually multiple and require deep palpation for their discovery, but they are difficult to localize. **INTERMITTENT COLD WITH STRETCH** for the rectus femoris requires simultaneous hip extension and knee flexion during and after application of ice or vapocoolant over all of the muscle and all of its referred pain pattern. Lengthening the remaining three heads of the quadriceps femoris requires only knee flexion. The patient should be in somewhat different positions for lengthening each of the heads, with cold application patterns tailored to cover each muscle and its referred pain pattern. The patella is depressed distally while fully flexing the knee when releasing the most distal TrP in the vastus lateralis. The adductor longus and brevis are generally treated by intermittent cold with passive stretch prior to stretch of the vastus medialis. The cooled skin is promptly rewarmed with a moist heating pad, and the patient performs slowly executed *full* active range of motion through several cycles. With a few exceptions, **INJECTION** of quadriceps femoris TrPs presents no special difficulties. Caution must be exercised with vastus medialis TrP_2 along the medial margin of the muscle close to the femoral artery, vein, and nerve. The vastus intermedius and vastus lateralis TrPs located deep at the midthigh level appear deceptively non-tender to flat palpation and are hard to localize for injection, but pose no particular hazard. In order to locate TrPs and inject the distal vastus lateralis TrP_1 that is responsible for the locked patella, the patella must be moved distally. **CORRECTIVE ACTIONS** include avoiding overload of the quadriceps femoris by lifting an object from ground level in a safe manner that does not strain either the thigh or back muscles, and by avoiding deep knee bends. Patients with a buckling knee TrP in the vastus medialis muscle should have an appropriate shoe insert added if their second metatarsal is longer than the first metatarsal or if they have a hyperpronated foot. Prolonged immobility should be avoided. A home self-stretch exercise program helps ensure continued relief. Lying with the vastus lateralis TrPs on a tennis ball augments their inactivation by self-massage. Strengthening exercises should begin with unweighted slow lengthening contractions; weighted shortening contractions should start only after the related muscle TrPs have been inactivated.

PART 2

---

1. REFERRED PAIN
(Figs. 14.1–14.5)

The trigger points (TrPs) in all four heads of the quadriceps femoris muscle refer pain to the thigh and knee region. Only the rectus femoris and vastus medialis TrPs produce anterior knee pain. Those in the vastus lateralis cause posterolateral knee pain. The referred pain from the rectus femoris TrPs is more likely to be felt deep in the knee joint than is the knee pain referred from the vastus medialis or the vastus lateralis.

Rectus Femoris (*two-jointed puzzler*)
(Fig. 14.1)

The TrPs in the rectus femoris muscle, like those in the long head of the triceps brachii of the upper limb, are extremely common and frequently overlooked. Neither of these two-joint muscles usually undergoes full stretch in daily activities. Seldom is either examined to determine if it restricts range of motion. The rectus femoris is a two-joint puzzler because the usual location of its TrP is at hip level, high on the thigh just below the anterior inferior iliac spine, but the pain is felt at the knee in and around the pa-

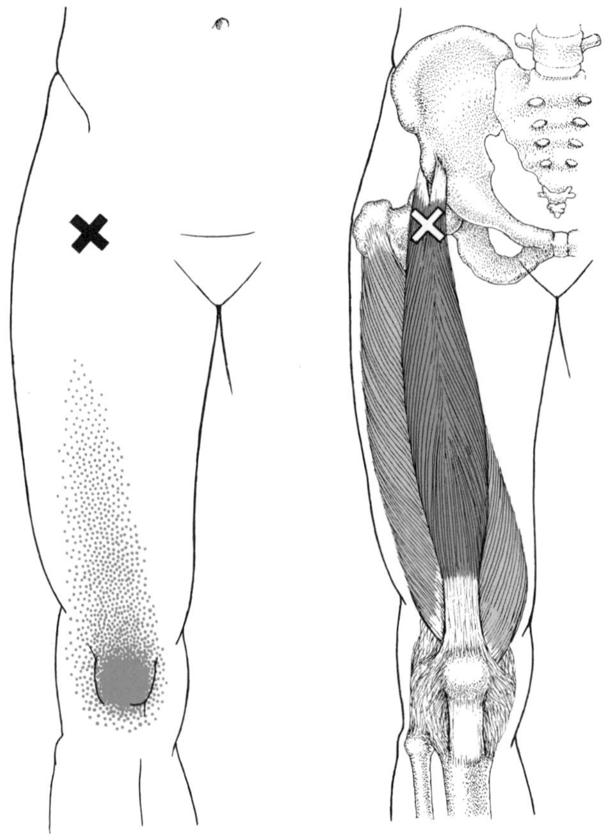

Figure 14.1. Pain pattern (*bright red*) referred from the usual trigger point (***X***) in the right rectus femoris muscle (*dark red*). Other parts of the quadriceps femoris are *light red*. *Solid bright red* denotes the essential pattern of pain experienced by nearly everyone with this trigger point. *Red stippling* indicates the occasional extension of its essential referred pain pattern.

tella (Fig. 14.1), and sometimes deep in the knee joint. Patients with these TrPs often have severe deep aching pain at night over the lower thigh above the knee anteriorly. They are unable to find a position or movement that provides relief until they learn how to stretch this muscle fully. Occasionally, a rectus femoris TrP occurs in the lower end of the muscle just above the knee near the patella and is likely to refer pain deep into the knee joint.

Vastus Medialis (*buckling knee muscle*) (Fig. 14.2)

The vastus medialis TrP_1, which is the more common of the two TrP locations in this muscle, refers pain to the front of the knee (Fig. 14.2*A*), as previously illustrated.[101,102,113] The more proximal TrP_2 refers aching pain in a linear distribution over the anteromedial aspect of the knee and lower thigh (Fig. 14.2*B*).

The TrPs in this muscle are easily overlooked because the taut muscle fibers only minimally restrict the range of motion of the knee and because the TrP may not produce pain, but only dysfunction. The vastus medialis is often a "quitter." After several weeks or months, the initial pain phase of its TrPs changes to an inhibition phase. The pain is replaced by unexpected episodes of quadriceps weakness that produce buckling of the knee. This sudden weakness may cause the individual to fall, inflicting injury.

In children, the vastus medialis was the second most frequently seen location for TrPs (11%) among 85 cases of myofascial pain.[19] The most common pain pattern referred from this muscle in children was comparable to that of TrP_1 in adults.

Vastus Intermedius (*frustrator*) (Fig. 14.3)

The vastus intermedius muscle is a "frustrator" because it develops many TrPs that cannot be palpated directly; they are hidden beneath the rectus femoris muscle. The pain pattern from these TrPs ex-

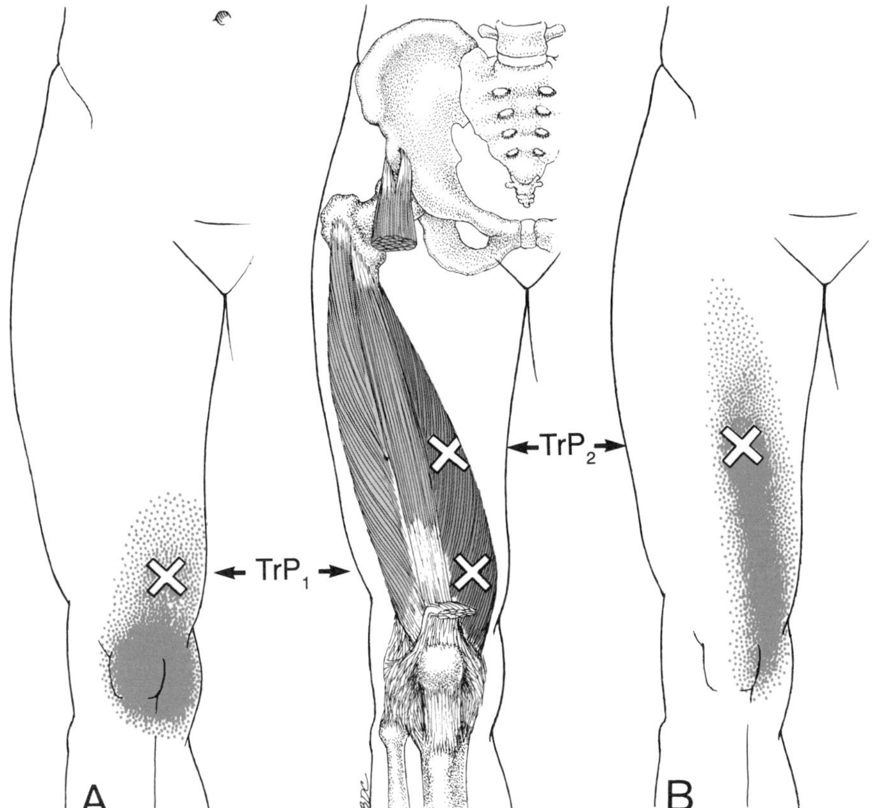

Figure 14.2. Pain patterns (*dark red*) referred from trigger points (***Xs***) in the right vastus medialis muscle (*medium red*). The remaining parts of the quadriceps femoris, which are retained for orientation, are *light red*; the rectus femoris (also *light red*) has been cut and removed. *Solid dark red* depicts the essential pattern of pain experienced by nearly everyone with these trigger points. *Red stippling* indicates the occasional extension of the essential referred pain pattern. *A*, distal TrP_1. *B*, proximal TrP_2.

tends over the front of the thigh nearly to the knee, but is most intense at midthigh (Fig. 14.3). TrPs at multiple locations in the vastus intermedius may refer pain and tenderness that extend over the upper thigh anterolaterally. The TrPs in this muscle are usually multiple, rarely solitary.

Kellgren reported that 0.1 mL of 6% hypertonic saline solution injected into the vastus intermedius muscle caused pain in the knee.[60]

Vastus Lateralis (*stuck patella muscle*) (Fig. 14.4)

The vastus lateralis characteristically develops multiple TrPs along the lateral aspect of the thigh. This muscle has the largest bulk of the four heads of the quadriceps femoris. Its five TrP locations (Fig. 14.4) can refer pain throughout the full length of the thigh laterally and to the outer side of the knee. Occasionally, the lateral thigh pain extends as high as the pelvic crest. When its TrPs are in the more superficial layers of the muscle, they are more likely to have a local pattern, whereas TrPs located deep in the muscle usually produce pain that explodes up and down the thigh. When vastus lateralis TrPs refer pain and tenderness to the proximal thigh region, the patient may be unable to lie on that side, disturbing sleep at night. Good[48] also found that myalgic spots (probably TrPs) in the lateral edge of the vastus lateralis referred pain to the knee.

A distinctive feature of TrP_1 in the vastus lateralis is a "stuck patella," in addition to pain around the lateral border of the patella that sometimes extends upward over the lateral region of the thigh

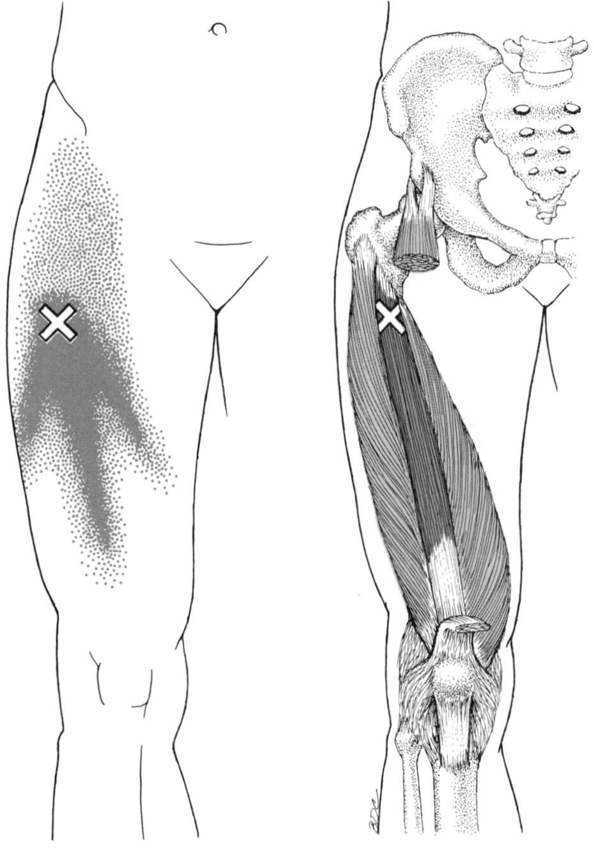

Figure 14.3. Pain pattern (*dark red*) referred from the common trigger point location (***X***) in the right vastus intermedius muscle (*medium red*). Other parts of the quadriceps femoris are *light red*. The rectus femoris has been cut and removed. *Dark solid red* denotes the essential pattern of pain felt by nearly everyone with this trigger point. *Red stippling* indicates occasional extension of the essential referred pain pattern. Additional trigger points may occur more distally in the muscle.

(Fig. 14.4). This pattern has been described in a case report by Nielsen,[87] and has been illustrated.[103,113] Pain from this TrP_1 may extend into and through the knee, and sometimes toward the back of the knee, as illustrated for children.[19] The more posteriorly located TrP_2 also causes pain lateral to the patella, but refers pain more extensively up the lateral aspect of the thigh and sometimes down the lateral aspect of the leg farther distally than the pattern of TrP_1. The TrP_3 location posterolaterally at midthigh level refers pain that travels the entire length of the posterolateral region of the thigh and includes the lateral half of the popliteal space. It is the one quadriceps TrP area that produces posterior knee pain.

A more anteriorly placed "hornets' nest" of TrPs at midthigh level in the TrP_4 region is not uncommon and is likely to cause severe pain over the entire length of the lateral thigh, slightly anterior to the pain of TrP_3, and extending upward almost to the pelvic crest. Distally, the pain referred from the TrP_4 region of the vastus lateralis swings anteriorly around the lateral border of the patella rather than posteriorly to the popliteal space. TrP_5, in the proximal end of the vastus lateralis muscle, refers pain and tenderness only to its immediate vicinity (Fig. 14.4). A composite pattern of TrP_4 and TrP_5 has been presented as the anterior vastus lateralis referred pain pattern.[101,102]

Vastus lateralis TrPs apparently are common in children. They were the TrPs most frequently found (35%) in a study of 85 children with myofascial pain syndromes.[19]

Ligamentous Trigger Point (Fig. 14.5)

The fibular (lateral) collateral ligament may harbor a ligamentous TrP that refers pain proximally to the lateral side of the knee (Fig. 14.5). This location of the pain may suggest that it arises from distal TrPs in the vastus lateralis muscle.

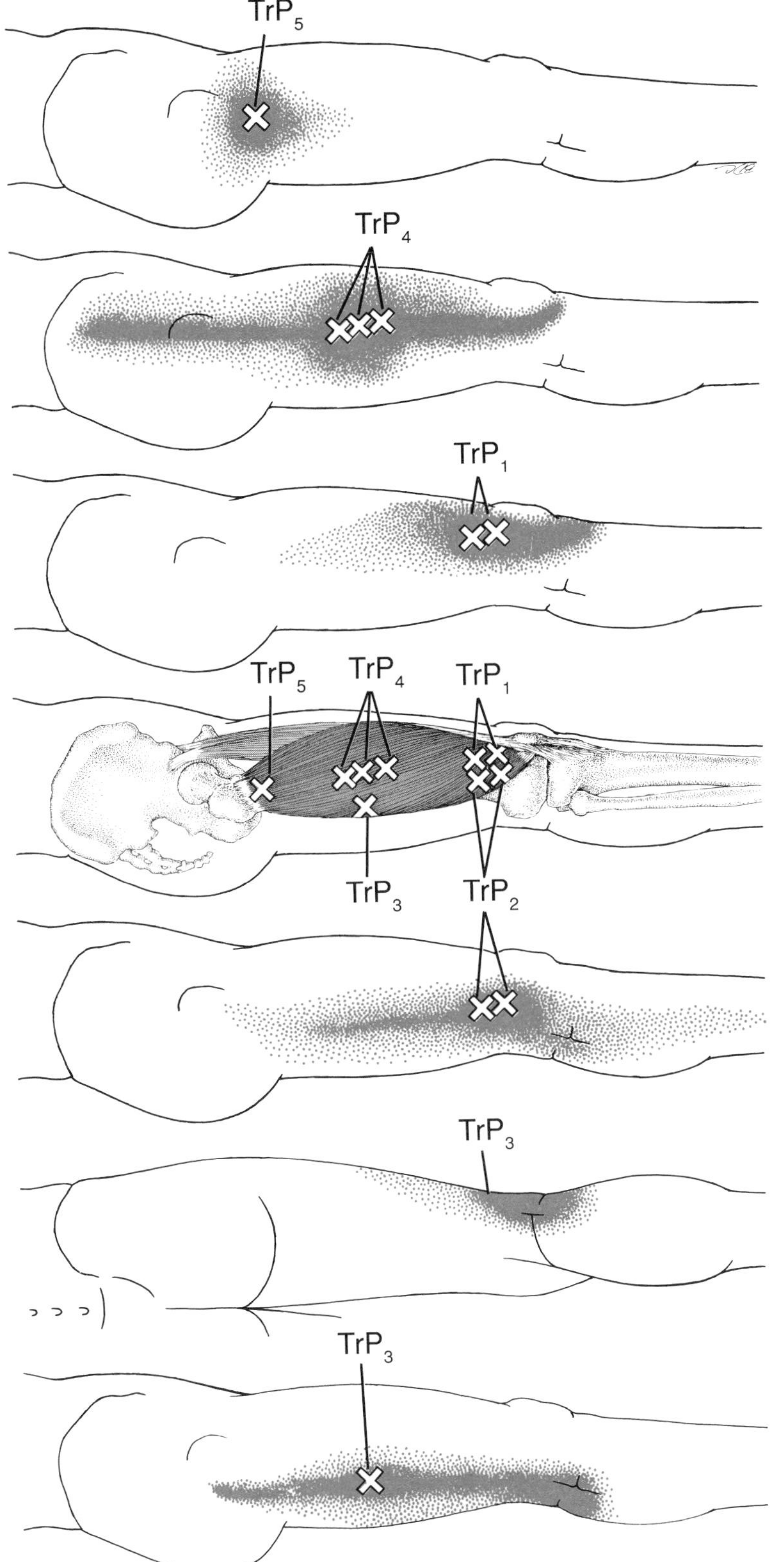

Figure 14.4. Pain patterns (*bright red*) referred from trigger points (***X**s*) in the right vastus lateralis muscle (*dark red*). The rectus femoris is *light red*. *Solid bright red* denotes the basic pain experienced by nearly everyone with these trigger points. *Red stippling* indicates the occasional extension (spillover) of the essential referred pain pattern. TrP_1 restricts patellar mobility. TrP_4 is close to the fascia lata and produces a "bolt of lightning" pain that prevents sleeping on the affected side.

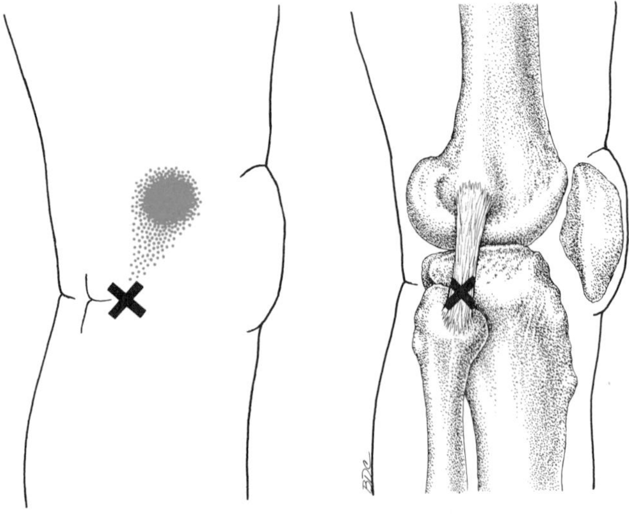

Figure 14.5. Pain pattern (*solid red* and *red stippling*) referred from a ligamentous trigger point (***X***) in the fibular collateral ligament of the right knee (lateral view).

2. ANATOMICAL ATTACHMENTS AND CONSIDERATIONS
(Figs. 14.6–14.9)

All four muscles of the quadriceps femoris group attach by a common tendon to the patella which, in turn, is attached to the tibial tuberosity by the patellar ligament (Fig. 14.6). The patella is a sesamoid bone in the tendon of the quadriceps femoris.[29] The three vasti muscles cross only the knee joint, since they attach ***proximally*** to the femur and ***distally*** through the patella and patellar ligament to the tibia. The rectus femoris, however, crosses both the knee and the hip joints; it alone of the quadriceps group attaches ***proximally*** to the pelvis. It joins the vasti to attach ***distally*** to the patella and, through the patellar ligament, to the tibial tuberosity.[10,29]

The quadriceps femoris is the largest (heaviest) muscle in the body. It may weigh 50% more (1271 gm) than the next heaviest muscle, the gluteus maximus (814 gm).[118]

Rectus Femoris
(Fig. 14.6)

The two-joint rectus femoris muscle lies between the vastus medialis and vastus lateralis, and covers the vastus intermedius (Figs. 14.6 and 14.7).

Proximally, the rectus femoris is anchored to the pelvis by two tendons, one attached to the anterior inferior iliac spine and the other to a groove above the posterior brim of the acetabulum.[3,29] ***Distally***, the muscle attaches to the proximal border of the patella and, through the patellar ligament, to the tuberosity of the tibia (Fig. 14.6). The rectus femoris extends the length of the thigh in front. Proximally, it is covered by the sartorius muscle at and just below the attachment to the anterior inferior iliac spine; more distally, the sartorius crosses diagonally to lie along the medial border of the rectus femoris,[27] covering the adductor canal that contains the femoral nerve and blood vessels.

The superficial fibers of the rectus femoris form a bipennate inverted "V" pattern,[96,97] while the deep fibers course directly down to the deep aponeurosis.[29] Together, the directions of the vastus medialis and vastus lateralis lower fibers form a diagonal pattern opposite to that of the upper fibers of the rectus femoris (Fig. 14.6).[96]

Anatomical variations of the quadriceps femoris are rare. The rectus femoris rarely may anchor to the pelvis by only one tendon. That tendon may attach either to the anterior inferior iliac spine or to the rim of the acetabulum.[11]

Vastus Medialis
(Fig. 14.7)

The vastus medialis attaches ***proximally*** along the entire length of the posteromedial aspect of the shaft of the femur,[3] to the lower half of the intertrochanteric line, the medial lip of the

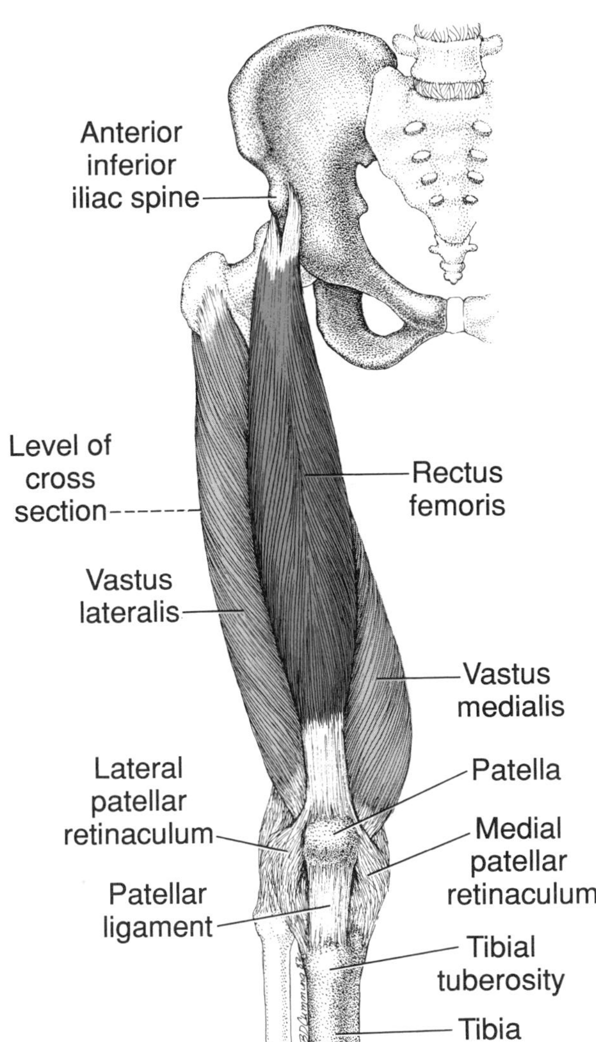

Figure 14.6. Attachments (front view) of the right rectus femoris muscle (*dark red*) in relation to the vastus lateralis and vastus medialis muscles (*light red*). Figure 14.8 shows the cross section of the thigh at the level indicated here.

linea aspera, the upper part of the medial supracondylar line, the tendons of the adductor longus and adductor magnus, and to the medial intermuscular septum.[29] Anteriorly, the vastus medialis attaches to the aponeurosis of the quadriceps femoris tendon together with the vastus intermedius muscle, and its fibers wrap around the femur angling downward from its posterior attachments (Fig. 14.7). Thus, when the muscle is freed anteriorly and pulled aside, one sees a considerable area of bare bone between it and the vastus intermedius. This contrasts with the extensive lateral attachment of the vastus intermedius to the anterior femur that underlies much of the vastus lateralis.[3,42]

The vastus medialis attaches ***distally*** not only to the medial border of the patella and through the patellar ligament to the tibial tuberosity, but also, by a slip of muscle to the medial patellar retinaculum. The distal fibers of the vastus medialis are markedly angulated as they attach in the region of the patella (Fig. 14.7) and can be clearly separated from the rest of the vastus medialis by fiber direction and by a fascial plane. These distal angulated fibers often attach proximally not to the femur, but chiefly to the adductor magnus, partly to the adductor longus, and to the medial intermuscular septum. The latter obliquely oriented fibers have been designated the **vastus medialis oblique**.[23,70]

PART 2

Vastus Intermedius (Fig. 14.8)

The vastus intermedius is at least as large as the rectus femoris and lies deep to it and also partly deep to the vastus lateralis (Figs. 14.7 and 14.8).

It attaches ***proximally*** to the anterior and lateral surfaces of the upper two-thirds of the shaft of the femur; it attaches ***distally*** to the patella and, through the patellar ligament, to the tibial tuberosity.[29] As noted previously, the vastus intermedius is clearly separated on its medial side from the vastus medialis, but laterally the vastus intermedius fibers merge with those of the vastus lateralis, as seen in cross section (Fig. 14.8).

Vastus Lateralis (Fig. 14.9)

The vastus lateralis, the largest component of the quadriceps femoris, is a much bigger, heavier muscle than is generally appreciated. Seen from in front (Fig. 14.7), it is not impressive; however, when seen from the lateral side (Fig. 14.9), its large extent becomes apparent. Its large size is also apparent in a cross section of the thigh (Fig. 14.8); at a higher level it surrounds nearly half the circumference of the femur.

Proximally, it is anchored to the lateral side of the posterior aspect of the upper three-fourths of the femur[3] by an aponeurosis that covers the inner part of the muscle.[29] The aponeurosis deep to the muscle attaches ***distally*** to the lateral border of the patella and via the patellar ligament crosses the knee. A few fibers of the muscle attach to the lateral patellar retinaculum.

PART 2

Bursae

Four bursae are associated with the quadriceps muscle and the patella at the knee.[28] The large subcutaneous *prepatellar* bursa, (shown elsewhere in cross section[27] and in sagittal section[28]) separates the patella from its overlying skin. The *suprapatellar* bursa (also shown in cross section[27]) is actually an extension of the synovial cavity of the knee joint; it lies between the femur and the portion of the quadriceps femoris tendon just above the patella. It extends deep to the aponeuroses of the vasti muscles, especially that of the vastus medialis, and is retracted during extension of the knee by the small **articularis genu muscle** that lies deep to the distal end of the vastus intermedius muscle.[7] The smaller *deep infrapatellar* bursa lies between the patellar ligament and the upper part of the tibia. The fourth bursa is the small *subcutaneous infrapatellar* bursa.[11,28]

Supplemental References

All four heads of the quadriceps femoris muscle are illustrated from in front without associated nerves or vessels,[6,84] and with nerves.[83] A similar picture that omits the vastus intermedius is accompanied by another that portrays accurately the relation of the quadriceps femoris to the sartorius muscle.[96] All heads are presented from the anteromedial view without associated nerves or vessels,[39] and with the vastus intermedius omitted.[97]

The vastus medialis is shown from the front view with the limb rotated laterally, and in relation to the saphenous nerve and femoral vessels in the adductor canal.[4]

The vastus lateralis is portrayed from behind[76] and from the lateral side.[41,44] The vastus medialis[43,77] and the rectus femoris[77] are seen from the medial side.

All four heads of the quadriceps femoris appear in a cross section high in the thigh at the level of the distal attachment of the gluteus maximus[5] and in a series of cross sections every 2 cm throughout the length of the quadriceps femoris.[27] The relationships of the four heads are revealed in a series of three cross sections.[40,86]

The skeletal attachments of both ends of the quadriceps femoris muscle are marked on the bones.[3,42,75,85]

The articularis genu muscle is seen with its attachments.[7]

The surface appearance of all heads except the vastus intermedius is revealed photographically as the quadriceps femoris is held in strong contraction.[38,72]

The relations of the suprapatellar bursa, subcutaneous prepatellar bursa, and the deep infrapatellar bursa to the patella and associated tendons of the quadriceps femoris are shown in sagittal section.[29] The suprapatellar bursa is seen from the lateral view[29] and also appears in cross section at a level through the quadriceps femoris tendon proximal to the patella.[40]

3. INNERVATION

All four heads of the quadriceps femoris and the articularis genu muscle are supplied by branches of the femoral nerve composed of fibers from the second, third, and fourth lumbar spinal nerves.[29]

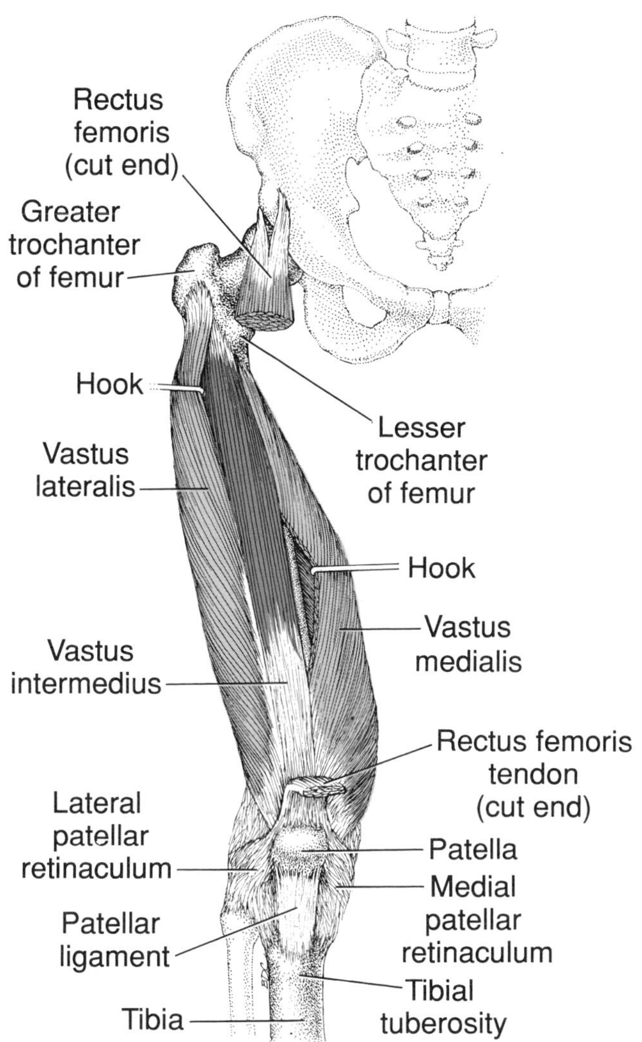

Figure 14.7. Attachments (front view) of the right vastus medialis (*light red*), vastus intermedius (*dark red*), and vastus lateralis (*light red*) muscles of the quadriceps femoris group. The bulk of the overlying rectus femoris muscle has been cut and removed. Part of the anterior attachment of the vastus medialis to the aponeurosis of the quadriceps tendon along the medial edge of the vastus intermedius has been cut and pulled aside by the lower hook. This reveals the deeper fibers of the vastus medialis as they disappear to attach behind the femur and it exposes the bare bone deep to the fibers anteriorly. The upper hook pulls the vastus lateralis aside to show the underlying portion of the vastus intermedius.

PART 2

The femoral nerve passes deep to the sartorius muscle and then travels in the adductor canal along the medial edge of the vastus medialis, which is supplied directly by branches from this nerve. The branches to the remaining three heads of the quadriceps femoris muscle pass between the rectus femoris and the vastus intermedius to their destinations (as illustrated).[83] A filament from one of the femoral nerve's branches to the vastus intermedius penetrates that muscle to supply the articularis genu muscle and the knee joint.[30]

4. FUNCTION

When the leg and foot are free to move, the four heads of the quadriceps femoris muscle act together as the prime extensors of the leg at the knee. The rectus femoris also either flexes the thigh at the hip or flexes the pelvis on the thigh, depending on which segment is fixed.[12,29] The three vasti respond simultaneously to vigorous effort. Participation of the rectus femoris also depends on demands at the hip joint. The four heads trade off among themselves in variable ways during slow increase of knee extension to maximum effort. Balanced tension on the patella between the vastus medialis and vastus lateralis maintains normal positioning and tracking of the patella.

For upright activities with the foot fixed on a supporting surface, the quadriceps muscle group exerts its pull proximally rather than distally. These muscles

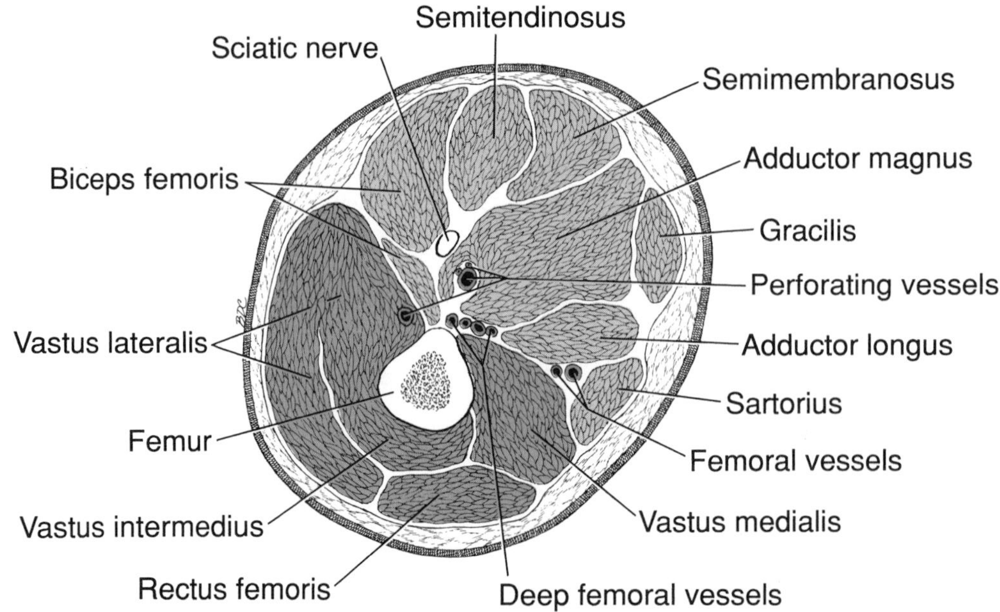

Figure 14.8. Cross sectional anatomy of the right thigh at the level indicated in Figure 14.6 and also in Figure 14.13, looking down from above. The blood vessels are *dark red* and the quadriceps muscles are *medium red*. All other muscles including the adductor group and hamstrings are *light red*. *See also* a cross section at a higher level, Figure 16.5.

frequently undergo lengthening contractions to control or decelerate movement caused by body weight.

The quadriceps femoris functions to control movements of bending backward, squatting, sitting down from the standing position, and descending stairs, but is not active in quiet standing. During walking, it is active immediately after heel-strike to control knee flexion and at toe-off to stabilize the knee in extension. It is not active during the period that the knee is extending during stance. Stance phase quadriceps activity is either prolonged or increased (or both) under certain circumstances, such as when there is significant loss of function in the plantar flexors, when heavy loads are carried on the back, when walking speed is increased, and when one wears high heels. The quadriceps femoris is *not* active in extension of the leg during the early swing phase, but it is active in the last part of swing, in preparation for weight bearing. The quadriceps femoris also serves an important function (shortening) during rising from sitting and in ascending stairs, and it functions in many sports activities. A strong peak of activity appears in the middle of the downstroke during ergometer cycling.

There is no consistent major difference in the proportion of fiber types among the four heads of the quadriceps femoris. The numbers of slow-twitch (type 1) and fast-twitch (type 2) fibers are consistently nearly equal.

Actions

In stimulation studies, as would be expected from the attachments, the rectus femoris pulled the patella in a purely proximal direction, the vastus medialis pulled it proximally and medially, and the vastus lateralis pulled it proximally and laterally.[34] Only the isolated contraction of the vastus lateralis could cause luxation of the patella (always laterally).[34] The balanced tension on the patella provided by the diagonal vectors of the vastus medialis and the vastus lateralis is important to normal tracking of the patella (and normal quadriceps function).[92]

The rectus femoris can assist in abduction of the thigh in supine subjects, but showed little activity during rotation of the leg at the knee.[8,15,92]

Electromyographically, the four heads can trade off among themselves in variable ways during a slow increase toward a maximal effort to extend the knee.[16,32] When rising from the sitting to the

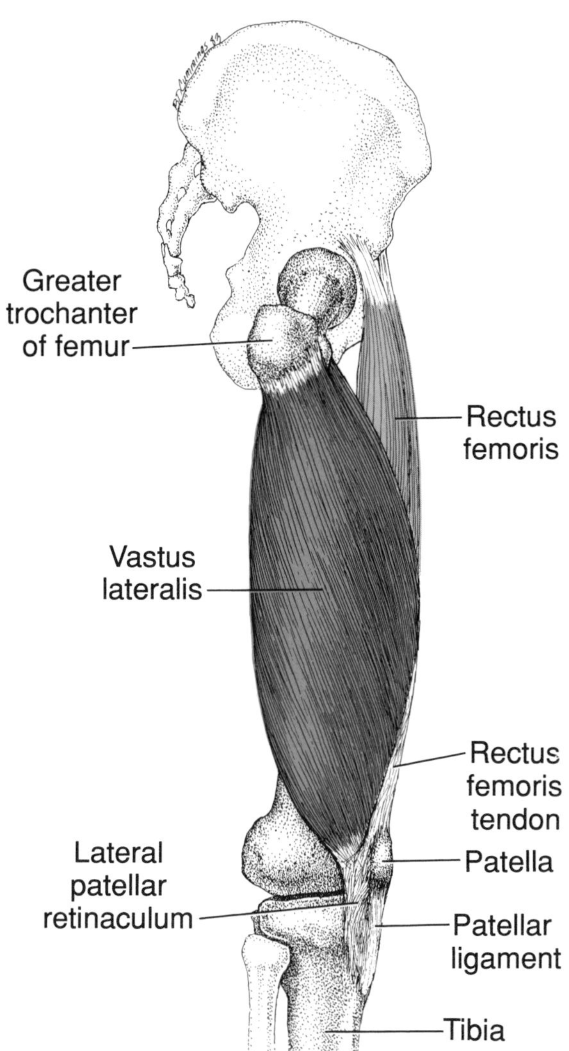

Figure 14.9. Attachments (lateral view) of the right vastus lateralis muscle (*dark red*) in relation to the rectus femoris muscle (*light red*).

PART 2

standing position and vice versa, there is no fixed sequence of relative recruitment among the four heads of the quadriceps femoris muscle.[16]

Maximum effort to extend the knee isometrically at eight positions between 0° and 90° produced similar EMG activity among the four heads of the quadriceps femoris at each position. The vastus medialis oblique produced twice the action potential count of any other part of the quadriceps at all angles.[71]

Orthopaedic texts have commonly attributed the last 15° of extension at the knee to the action of the distal diagonal fibers of the vastus medialis (**vastus medialis oblique**) described previously under Anatomical Attachments. Several studies have presented convincing evidence that this is *not* the case;[70,71,81] investigators concluded that the primary function of these diagonal fibers is to stabilize the patella and prevent its lateral dislocation.[23,59,94]

Functions

Standing and Positioning

During balanced standing, the quadriceps femoris is almost completely inactive, whether a load is placed in front of the thighs or strapped to the back.[14]

Duarte *et al.*[33] confirmed and extended an earlier study by Basmajian and associates,[18] which established when the various heads of the quadriceps femoris muscle were active in common postures and during movements. Using fine-wire electrodes, they[33] found that electromyographically the three vasti acted simultaneously, and that the most active were the vastus medialis and vastus intermedius. Late activation of the rectus femoris occurred during hip flexion, bending backwards, squatting, and sitting down. The vasti took the brunt of the load when arising from a squat position. Rectus femoris EMG activity was more prominent in high speed movement, whereas the vasti were active in opposing fixed resistance.

The quadriceps femoris works in close coordination with the rectus abdominis when fast voluntary trunk movements are performed during standing.[89]

Walking

In normal walking, activity of the quadriceps femoris group is biphasic.[17,110] Electrical activity reaches a peak after heel-strike, but before foot flat, to control the knee flexion that occurs in early stance.[55] The second peak of activity appears at toe-off to stabilize the knee in extension. Surprisingly, the quadriceps was found to be silent during the early phase of knee extension during the swing phase. Thus, extension of the leg at the knee probably occurs as the result of passive swing.[17]

Yang and Winter[121] found, in 11 healthy subjects, that the second peak of electrical activity was most prominent at higher walking speeds and much more marked in the rectus femoris than in the vastus lateralis. Another study[79] reported a sudden increase in the rate of electrical activity with increasing walking speed at speeds between 0.9 and 1.2 m/sec (3 and 4 ft/sec). EMG activity of the vastus lateralis was increasingly prolonged in the stance phase with increasingly heavy loads, up to 50% of body weight, carried on the back.[46]

During stair climbing, rectus femoris EMG activity appeared at the beginning of stance phase until the second period of double support, when the contralateral foot is placed on the step above. During descent of stairs, the rectus femoris was usually active through most of the stance phase, but most vigorously at the beginning and end of stance.[110]

Among 19 subjects, 12 of whom were trained athletes, some remarkable intersubject variability was observed in the timing of EMG activity among the rectus femoris, medial hamstrings, tibialis anterior, and gastrocnemius muscles during level walking and during ascending and descending stairs. The contraction pattern of the rectus femoris was clearly the most constant among these muscles.[110]

Six young women showed a marked increase in quadriceps femoris EMG activity during stance phase when walking in high heels, as compared to flat heels.[57]

In gait studies on five normal adults before and after tibial nerve block, Sutherland and associates found that, after the nerve block, quadriceps activity during stance was prolonged to compensate for loss of the normal contribution of the ankle plantar flexors to knee stability.[107]

Lifting

When an individual lifts a load with the trunk erect and the knees bent, a significant part of the load usually carried by the paraspinal muscles is borne by the quadriceps femoris group of muscles. With knees straight and hips flexed, the quadriceps group is inactive,[47,82] but as the knees are flexed to assume the crouched position, the rectus femoris in one study,[47] and also the vastus medialis and vastus lateralis in another,[90] showed increased electrical activity with increased knee flexion. When a load was then lifted from this crouched position, the electrical activity of the rectus femoris was more than doubled when the load was held out in front, away from the body, as compared to the activity when the load was held close to the body.

Sports and Jumping

During *right*-handed throwing and hitting in sports, the greatest electrical activity among the rectus femoris, vastus medialis, and vastus lateralis muscles consistently appeared in the *left* rectus femoris. The vigorous jumping effort of a one-foot jump volleyball spike and of a basketball layup strongly activated all of these three heads bilaterally.[25] Vigorous activity of the rectus femoris was observed during the take-off and landing phases in a detailed study of jumping.[58]

The quadriceps femoris provides an important braking action (serving as a checkrein on knee flexion) on landing after jumping. It provides a similar shock-absorbing effect during running. Such vigorous lengthening contractions can cause postexercise muscular soreness (*see* Appendix).

Ergometer Cycling

During cycling, the vastus medialis and vastus lateralis were active throughout the downstroke of the bicycle pedal, reaching a peak of nearly 50% of maximum voluntary EMG activity shortly before the middle of the downstroke. The rectus femoris reached a lower peak of 12% of maximum voluntary EMG activity shortly after the beginning of the downstroke and started to increase activity gradually halfway through the upstroke.[37] The reduced activity of the rectus femoris during downstroke reflects the fact that this hip flexor and knee extensor is inhibited from contributing to knee extension when the thigh is being extended at the hip. During standardized ergometer cycling, the knee extensors performed 39% of the positive mechanical work, and the hip flexors only 4%.[36]

Vecchiet and associates[116] injected hypertonic saline solution to test the vastus lateralis for sensitivity to the production of referred pain following 30 minutes of cycling at 70% of maximum capacity. Injection of 10% saline solution into the muscle was significantly more painful immediately after and 60 minutes following the exercise than it was prior to the exercise.

Interactions

The effect of contraction of the two-joint rectus femoris is never limited to only one joint. The action of this muscle in motion at the knee alone is closely coordinated with that of the vasti muscles; in biarticular motions it has complex relationships. As would be expected, a movement that simultaneously shortens the muscle at both joints, such as kicking a football, strongly activates it. Conversely, a movement that elongates the muscle simultaneously across both joints inhibits its contraction. Moreover, elongating the muscle at one joint inhibits its activity for shortening at the other. The rectus femoris is inactive when hip flexion is accompanied by knee flexion, even though it is active in hip flexion alone. Similarly, the muscle is electrically inactive when hip extension accompanies knee extension, whereas it is active in knee extension alone.[12]

The vastus lateralis component of the quadriceps femoris was monitored in a study of postural adjustments to a fast trunk flexion movement during standing.[89] When the subject activated the tibialis anterior to help provide forward momentum, the resultant knee flexion was controlled by a lengthening contraction of the vastus lateralis.

When the foot excessively pronates (due to a Morton foot structure, a hypermobile midfoot, ankle equinus, muscular imbalance, or some other cause), the leg and thigh deviate inward, the Q angle increases, and the vastus medialis muscle can become overloaded. The muscle may serve a role in controlling the knee angulation, protecting the medial ligaments of the knee in the process.

Fiber Types and Performance

No consistent major difference in the proportion of fiber types was observed among the four heads of the quadriceps femoris.

The vastus lateralis has been the most popular of the four heads for biopsy. Individual studies found considerable variation in fiber type distribution both within and between subjects. In one study of elite female track athletes, the proportion of slow-twitch (type 1) fibers in the vastus lateralis varied from 25 to 90%.[50] In most studies, the percent of slow-twitch fibers in the vastus lateralis has been near 50%.[35,45,49–51,54,68,69,88] One study[68] reported the distribution of fiber types throughout the entire vastus lateralis muscle in six previously healthy men who suffered sudden accidental death. Each sample represented the distribution in 1 sq mm of tissue. The proportion of type 1 fibers increased primarily as the samples were taken from greater depth (for example, 40–60% depth in one muscle). It was not unusual for individual values within one muscle to range from 33 to 65% type 1 fibers. This study warns us that studies that did not control for depth of the samples must be interpreted with caution.

With increasing age, quadriceps femoris strength decreased in both males and females between the ages of 20 and 70 years. This could be accounted for partly by a loss of motor units through loss of innervation.[106] A study of just the vastus lateralis[99] in 45 healthy, sedentary men and women 65–89 years of age also presented evidence of partial denervation, decrease in percentage of and atrophy of type 2 fibers, streaming of Z lines with rod formation, dilatation of sarcoplasmic reticulum, and increase in intracellular lipid droplets. The Z line changes are similar to those described in the repair stage following postexercise stiffness (*see* Appendix), and the increase in intracellular lipid droplets suggests impaired aerobic energy metabolism.

Painless infusion of as little as 10 mL of sterile isotonic saline into normal knee joints caused some reduction of maximum strength of the quadriceps. Larger quantities strongly inhibited the quadriceps, reducing its contraction by more than 50%.[122] Aspiration of chronic knee effusion did not immediately reduce inhibition of the quadriceps.[56] Inhibition of quadriceps strength is related more closely to effusion in the knee joint than to the painfulness of contraction.[56,122] Selective weakness and wasting of the quadriceps femoris develop following meniscal and ligamentous injuries of the knee.[122] Fourteen meniscectomy patients at 34 days postoperatively still experienced severe inhibition of contraction of the quadriceps muscle, but had little or no pain. Inhibition was greater when the knee was extended than when it was flexed.[100] Quadriceps function can be inhibited by non-painful sensory input, such as pressure from the knee joint.[13] In a therapy program, this inhibition of concentric contraction may be largely overcome by first facilitating eccentric contractions.[2]

Surgical excision of one, two, or three heads of the quadriceps femoris reduced isometric strength 22%, 33%, and 55%, respectively, and reduced isokinetic strength somewhat more. Usually only slight impairment of function was observed with less than 50% loss of strength.[74] Another study[81] reported the effects of excision of all of the vastus lateralis and 75% of the vastus intermedius; extensor torque was reduced 60% on the operated side. Although this patient had a normal vastus medialis, he still had an extensor lag.

A study of low-level static contraction of the quadriceps femoris required holding one leg in extension at 5% of maximum voluntary contraction for 1 hour. Results demonstrated that the muscle was able to maintain homeostasis with respect to energy turnover, but not with respect to intra/extracellular potassium concentration.[105] Sustained contraction, even at this low level, disturbs muscle function.

Assuming that during compression blood flow in the muscle stops when intramuscular pressure exceeds systolic pressure, onset of ischemia would occur during brief static contractions at 50% of maximum voluntary contraction for the rectus femoris.[98] This clearly becomes an increasingly limiting factor to sustained contraction at about this level of effort.

5. FUNCTIONAL (MYOTATIC) UNIT

Together, the four heads of the quadriceps femoris group compose the prime extensor of the knee. The three vasti normally work closely together. EMG activity of the rectus femoris may vary from that of the other three heads because of its additional action as a hip flexor. The primary antagonists to extension at the knee are the three hamstring muscles, which are assisted by the gastrocnemius, popliteus, gracilis, and sartorius muscles.[92]

For hip flexion, the rectus femoris acts with the iliopsoas, pectineus, tensor fasciae latae, and adductors—depending on the degree of hip flexion. The primary antagonists to hip flexion are the gluteus maximus, three hamstring muscles, and the adductor magnus.[92]

6. SYMPTOMS

Referred pain is commonly the presenting symptom with two main exceptions, the buckling knee syndrome of the vastus medialis and the locked patella syndrome of the vastus lateralis. A third exception, the buckling hip syndrome, may occasionally be seen when TrPs are present both at their usual location in the rectus femoris (just below the anterior inferior iliac spine) and high in the vastus intermedius. Hip buckling occurs when the weight-bearing patient extends the knee and the hip simultaneously.

Patients who complain of weakness of knee extension often have rectus femoris, vastus medialis, and/or vastus intermedius TrPs, active or latent. The vastus intermedius is likely to cause more trouble going up stairs, and the rectus femoris, going down stairs.

Rectus Femoris

When patients are awakened at night by pain in front of the knee cap and just above it on the anterior thigh, TrPs in the rectus femoris muscle should be suspected. This is especially true if, on awakening in a side-lying position, the knee is extended and the hip is flexed, an unusual position that fully shortens the rectus femoris. Patients rarely discover for themselves the combined position of hip extension and knee flexion that is required to stretch the rectus femoris fully in order to obtain relief.

Patients who have knee pain and a sense of weakness when going down stairs should be checked for rectus femoris TrPs.

Vastus Medialis

Distal TrPs in the vastus medialis initially produce a toothache-like pain deep in the knee joint, which often interrupts the patient's sleep. It may be misinterpreted as being due to inflammation of the knee joint.[95] The myofascial pain usually fades in a few weeks or months and is replaced by episodic inhibition of quadriceps femoris function that causes unexpected buckling (weakness) of the knee during walking.[9,111] Buckling usually occurs during walking on rough ground when sudden medial rotation of the knee places an unexpected load on the vastus medialis as the muscle lengthens during knee flexion. This buckling response may cause the individual to fall.

Baker[9] cites the case of an incapacitated 12-year-old athlete with the buckling knee syndrome who was completely relieved by inactivation of the vastus medialis TrP.

With surface electrodes over the vastus medialis of a patient with active TrPs in the muscle and disabling knee pain, the senior author observed reduced EMG activity when the seated patient lifted the foot and unsuccessfully attempted full knee extension. Following inactivation of the TrPs in the vastus medialis by local procaine injection, the muscle at once showed a marked increase in the surface EMG activity when the patient again exerted a maximum effort to extend the knee. The full range of knee extension returned; the weakness had disappeared.

Vastus Intermedius

Patients with TrPs in the vastus intermedius have difficulty fully straightening the knee, especially after it has been immobile for some time during sitting. They cannot step up onto the next stair step and then straighten the knee, or walk without a limp after arising from a chair. Their pain occurs during knee movement, rarely at rest. Driving a car is usually not a problem, since no vigorous extension at the knee is required.

The buckling knee syndrome also can result from the combination of vastus intermedius TrPs and TrPs in the two heads of the gastrocnemius muscle near their femoral attachments.

Vastus Lateralis

When the patient complains that it hurts to walk, and the pain distribution is along the lateral aspect of the thigh including the knee, TrPs in the vastus lateralis muscle may be responsible. Patients with TrPs in the vastus lateralis also complain that it hurts to lie on the involved side and that the pain disturbs their sleep.

Myofascial TrPs in the distal end of the vastus lateralis (and sometimes in the vastus intermedius also) can immobilize the patella. Partial loss of normal patellar movement causes difficulty in straightening or bending the knee after getting up from a chair. A completely locked patella immobilizes the knee joint, usually in slight flexion. The patient cannot walk, can hardly crawl, and is uncomfortable in a wheelchair if the chair has no elevating leg rests and the knee must be bent close to 90°.

Troedsson[115] found each of 35 patients with trick knees to have a tender indurated area along the lower medial border of the vastus lateralis muscle in the symptomatic limb. Twenty-four of the 25 patients who were treated with physical therapy directed to the vastus lateralis were relieved of the knee instability. (Our experience has been that the lower medial border of the vastus *medialis* is a more probable location of TrPs responsible for a buckling knee.)

Differential Diagnosis

Unexplained thigh and knee pain in children, even in infants, is more frequently due to quadriceps femoris TrPs than is generally realized.[19,20] These youngsters with thigh and knee pain should be examined for TrPs.

Knee pain in patients with disease of the hip joint, or who have had a surgical procedure on the hip joint, is often assumed to originate in the hip; however, it can also arise from quadriceps femoris TrPs. (Posterior knee pain may also be due to TrPs in the hamstring muscles.)

The lateral thigh pain characteristic of proximal vastus lateralis TrPs is commonly misdiagnosed as trochanteric bursitis because of referred pain and referred tenderness in the area of the greater trochanter. A similar pain pattern may also be caused by TrPs in the anterior part of the gluteus minimus muscle or by TrPs in the tensor fasciae latae muscle. Similarly, anterior knee and thigh pain characteristic of TrPs in the rectus femoris may actually be referred from adductor longus and/or brevis TrPs, and medial thigh pain suggestive of vastus medialis TrPs may arise from TrPs in the gracilis muscle.

Phantom limb pain may be induced by residual quadriceps femoris TrPs remaining in the stump of an above-knee amputee. Also, when a flap of quadriceps muscle that contains TrPs is used to cover the end of the bone, the patient may have difficulty ambulating on it until its TrPs are inactivated.

A so-called trick knee (one that suddenly buckles and gives way without warning) may be caused by anterior subluxation of the lateral tibial plateau, which usually requires surgical correction.[73] Probably, a more common source of this symptom is the presence of TrPs in the vastus medialis.

Knee Pain

Pain in the region of the knee can arise from articular dysfunction including ligamentous strain and tears, from a torn meniscus, from tendinitis, bursitis, myofascial problems, or compromise of nerves. Radin[91] lists 16 non-myofascial causes of anterior knee pain. When considering knee pain from the point of view of the quadriceps femoris, the patella is of special importance.

Chondromalacia patellae usually follows dislocation of the patella with chondral or osteochondral fracture, or direct trauma to the patella. It is a common cause of knee pain in runners.[64] Findings in chondromalacia that help distinguish it from myofascial knee pain include: subpatellar tenderness, which is elicited by displacing the patella medially or laterally and palpating the underside of its edges; tenderness to compression of the patella against the femur; effusion within the knee joint; quadriceps femoris muscle atrophy; and crepitus or grating during active extension of the knee.[31]

Patellofemoral dysfunction is defined as anterior knee pain coming from the patellofemoral articulation without any gross abnormality of the articular cartilage of the patella. The pain is attributed to abnormal tracking of, or pressure on, the patella.[108] Abnormal size or placement of the patella may be the cause of knee dysfunction and pain.[119]

Normal functioning of the patellofemoral joint depends largely on the dynamic balance between the medial and lateral forces exerted by the vastus medialis and vastus lateralis muscles. Lateral subluxation is more common than medial displacement of the patella, since the line of pull of the quadriceps musculature is lateral to the alignment of the patellar ligament that connects the patella to the tibial tubercle. This deviation is commonly measured as the Q angle, the angle between a line passing through the center of the patella to the anterior superior iliac spine and a line through the center of the patella to the tibial tubercle. The angle should not exceed 14° in males and 17° in females.[108] Valgus deformity of the knee and underdevelopment of the distal vastus medialis are commonly associated with lateral patellar subluxation.[64,91] Increased tension and shortening of the vastus lateralis caused by TrPs aggravate this condition.

Medial subluxation of the patella is rare, but when it is diagnosed, it may be a complication of a lateral retinacular release operation that severs the vastus lateralis tendon. Over half of the patients with this subluxation problem are reported to have had immediate relief of the knee pain for which the procedure was done. However, the subsequent medial patellar subluxation from release of the vastus lateralis tendon often becomes disabling.[53]

Pain in the medial side of the knee and proximal calf may be caused by saphenous nerve entrapment.[120]

Lateral knee pain may be caused by entrapment of the lateral femoral cutaneous nerve.[21] Lateral knee pain may also result from an iliotibial tract friction syndrome,[24] as described in Chapter 12.

Quadriceps tendinitis is characterized by pain at the upper pole of the patella, more common laterally than medially.[64] There is a relatively high probability that this symptom is actually caused by vastus lateralis TrPs.

Tendinitis of the patellar ligament, "jumper's knee," is particularly common in basketball players, high jumpers, and hurdlers.[22,64] The pain and the tenderness at the attachment of the patellar ligament to the lower pole of the patella are not likely to be myofascial in origin, unless a major portion of the quadriceps muscle group harbors TrPs.

Taylor[109] reported two cases of deep infrapatellar bursitis, one caused by *Staphylococcus aureus* infection, and the other caused by deposition of uric acid crystals of gout.

Brucini and co-workers[26] examined the EMG activity of the vastus medialis in 18 patients with osteoarthritis of the knee and in eight healthy con-

PART 2

trols. The controls showed no EMG activity at rest, supine, or as a rule during quiet standing on only one leg or on both legs. In 14 of the 18 patients, low-level involuntary EMG activity appeared at rest in the supine position with the knee straight, but was eliminated in every case by some form of active or passive lower limb movement. Also, the vastus medialis muscle showed electrical activity in proportion to the amount of weight placed on the painful knee. Before treatment, a voluntary contraction of the quadriceps femoris group of muscles, which was sustained for a few seconds, resulted in EMG activity that persisted for 2–30 seconds after the patient tried to relax. Following injection of tender areas [that had TrP characteristics] in the periarticular muscles, EMG activity ceased immediately on termination of voluntary contraction.

7. ACTIVATION AND PERPETUATION OF TRIGGER POINTS

Many patients with diabetes are taught to inject insulin into the lateral aspect or midline of the thigh, and several patients have developed TrPs in the rectus femoris or vastus lateralis muscle where they injected themselves. Injection of insulin or other drugs[112] in the region of a latent TrP can activate it. Quadriceps myofibrosis can result from repeated intramuscular injections.[1]

The quadriceps group is susceptible to activation of TrPs by an acute overload from a sudden vigorous eccentric (lengthening) contraction. Such a vigorous contraction can result from a misstep into a hole, stepping off the curb, or from stumbling. Direct trauma by impact against the femur can activate TrPs in any head of the quadriceps, but least likely in the vastus intermedius.

Acute or chronic overload can occur in an exercise program that includes deep knee bends. This exercise perpetuates quadriceps femoris TrPs, especially those in the vastus intermedius. Another exercise that is likely to perpetuate TrPs in the quadriceps is an attempt to strengthen the muscle harboring active TrPs by extending the knee in a concentric contraction with a weight placed near the ankle. A slow eccentric contraction is tolerated much better.

Quadriceps femoris TrPs are commonly perpetuated by sustained overload that is the result of tightness caused by TrPs in the antagonistic hamstring muscles. The quadriceps cannot recover until the hamstring tightness is released. The patient, however, complains of pain referred from the quadriceps femoris TrPs, not from the hamstring TrPs, which are the perpetuating factor. Quadriceps femoris TrPs are also perpetuated by overload resulting from active TrPs in the soleus muscle. Soleus TrPs restrict ankle dorsiflexion, and this can overload the quadriceps especially when lifting "correctly" with the knees bent and torso erect.

Placing any muscle in a fixed position for long periods tends to aggravate its TrPs. Immobilization is often an integral part of therapy for orthopaedic problems of the lower limb. Patients should be checked for TrPs before and after immobilization, especially if they are experiencing unexpected pain afterward.

Some people habitually sit for long periods with one foot tucked under the buttock (often subconsciously to correct a small hemipelvis). This habit can be the critical perpetuating factor that prevents recovery from the pain of quadriceps TrPs.

Rectus Femoris

Myofascial TrPs are activated in the rectus femoris muscle, as in other muscles of the quadriceps femoris group, by a fall or accident that produces a suddenly overloaded lengthening contraction, such as a high velocity skiing accident.

Sitting for a long time with a heavy weight on the lap (e.g., holding a heavy child on the lap during a long car trip) can activate TrPs in this muscle. TrPs in the rectus femoris tend to persist because the muscle does not ordinarily undergo full stretch in the course of daily activities. Full stretch requires, simultaneously, complete flexion at the knee and nearly complete extension at the hip.

The rectus femoris may develop an active TrP during recovery from hip fracture and hip surgery.

Lange[63] associated degenerative joint disease of the hip with myogelosis [TrPs] in the rectus femoris and vastus lateralis muscles. We see rectus femoris TrPs develop as the result of overload caused by abnormal hip joint mechanics, and then vastus lateralis TrPs develop because that muscle attempts to compensate for the compromised rectus femoris.

Vastus Medialis

Excessive pronation of the foot from various causes (a hypermobile midfoot, ankle equinus, muscular imbalance) can perpetuate TrPs in the vastus medialis. This member of the quadriceps femoris group often develops TrPs also because of the Morton foot structure (relatively long second, short first metatarsal). This structure, if uncorrected, results in excessive mediolateral "rocking" of the foot. See Chapter 20, Peroneal Muscles, for the diagnosis and management of this condition. With chronicity, these vastus medialis TrPs are likely to cause a buckling knee. The question often arises as to why the patient has vastus medialis TrPs in only one limb when both feet have relatively short first and long second metatarsals. Further examination often reveals that the limb on the side of the involved knee is shorter, and it is the shorter limb that sustains greater impact and push-off forces during ambulation.

Lange[62] associated the development of myogelosis in the vastus medialis with flat feet, which is accompanied by pronation of the foot.

In addition, this muscle is likely to develop TrPs as the result of strenuous athletic activity, such as jogging, skiing, football, basketball, and soccer. Vastus medialis TrPs are also activated by falls and direct trauma to the knee joint and/or the muscle (such as dashboard trauma from a motor vehicle accident when a seat belt is not worn.) Activation of TrPs in it is a common sports injury and the TrPs are generally quite responsive to specific TrP treatment, provided that perpetuating factors are corrected.

Vastus medialis TrPs may be perpetuated by prolonged kneeling on a hard surface, e.g., kneeling on the ground while gardening or beside the bathtub while bathing a baby.

Vastus Intermedius

This muscle is rarely the first quadriceps muscle to develop TrPs; it develops them secondarily as a result of overload from protecting TrPs in the other quadriceps femoris muscles, which are members of the same functional unit.

Vastus Lateralis

Vastus lateralis TrPs are activated by sudden overload of the muscle, particularly during lengthening contractions, e.g., in skiing accidents. In addition, because of the muscle's size and exposed location, TrPs may be activated in the vastus lateralis by direct trauma, e.g., as the result of a fall sideways against the edge of a step or a piece of furniture, during lurching movements in sports, or from a bullet wound in the thigh.

Vastus lateralis TrPs are perpetuated when the muscle is immobilized in a shortened position for a long period, as when sitting with the knee fully extended.

8. PATIENT EXAMINATION
(Figs. 14.10–14.12)

The patient's gait is analyzed first. A patient with a "stuck patella" from a vastus lateralis TrP will walk stiff-legged without bending one knee normally, and so tends to drag that foot. The inability both to extend fully and flex the knee freely results in a limp. The patient cannot rise from a chair while keeping the back straight, and must pitch the torso forward to lighten the load on the thigh muscles. The limp can be improved and hip buckling can be avoided if the patient walks on tiptoe on the disabled side, avoiding the need to extend the knee fully; however, this compensation leads to other problems.

While walking, if the patient toes out and complains of medial thigh pain or perhaps of a buckling knee, vastus medialis TrPs associated with a Morton foot structure should be suspected (*see* Fig. 8.3 for an illustration of this stance). Patients with vastus medialis TrPs evidence minimal restriction of knee flexion.

TrPs in the vastus intermedius muscle may be responsible, if, while walking, the patient has difficulty bending the knee to lift the foot off the ground and instead hikes the hip (pelvis) on that side to clear the foot from the floor, and if he or she has trouble climbing stairs.

PART 2

While palpating the quadriceps femoris for taut bands and TrPs, one may encounter a fibrotic mass produced by an earlier tear of the muscle. Surgical extirpation of the fibrotic tissue resulted in good return of quadriceps femoris function in all of three such cases.[93]

Examination of the Patella

For the examination of the patella, the knee should be straight and the quadriceps femoris must be completely relaxed. Quadriceps tension can restrict passive movement of the patella. Before examining for patellar mobility, the clinician should observe and palpate the patella for subluxation at rest, which nearly always occurs in the lateral direction.[78] It is important to test patellar mobility (Fig. 14.10) whenever quadriceps femoris TrPs are suspected. TrP tension in the vastus medialis restricts normal lateral mobility of the patella (Fig. 14.10*E*) but does not cause a locked patella.

With a "stuck patella" caused by a TrP in the distal vastus lateralis, the patella loses all passive movement, including its normal downward range of motion (Fig. 14.10*C*) of at least 1 cm (about ½ in) that occurs during knee flexion. A patient with a "stuck patella" is unable to extend the knee fully and may be unable to flex it more than about 5°. Attempts to move the patella passively may produce grating sounds, which may indicate abnormal pressure against the femur or damaged chondral surfaces. Less severe vastus lateralis tension from TrPs restricts only medial mobility of the patella (Fig. 14.10*D*).

Increased tension due to vastus intermedius TrPs restricts rotation of the patella in either direction (Fig. 14.10*F* and *G*). In addition, tension from the vastus lateralis restricts normal medial rotation (with reference to the upper pole) of the patella (Fig. 14.10*F*). Tension from the vastus medialis restricts corresponding lateral rotation of the patella in the frontal plane around the center of the patella (Fig. 14.10*G*).

Rectus Femoris

To test the stretch range of motion of the rectus femoris, the operator must *simultaneously* extend the hip and flex the knee. As illustrated in Figure 14.11, motion at one joint increases at the expense of the other joint when the muscle is tight. At the full range of motion, the heel should touch the buttock with the hip near full extension. Restriction of this normal range by latent TrPs in the rectus femoris occurs commonly. A tight iliopsoas muscle restricts extension at the hip, but does not affect flexion at the knee.

It is informative to test the knee jerk response, which can be inhibited by TrPs in the rectus femoris muscle. In this case, the tendon reflex returns after inactivation of these TrPs.

Three Vasti

In the mobility test for the three vasti muscles (Fig. 14.12), the operator examines the supine patient for range of knee flexion with the thigh flexed at the hip. TrPs in the **vastus intermedius** significantly restrict flexion at the knee. The heel does not reach the buttock by several fingerbreadths. However, TrPs in the **vastus lateralis** cause this restriction only if the patella is displaced or locked. TrPs in the **vastus medialis** cause, at most, only minor restriction of knee flexion. Large calf muscles or fat calves *rarely* restrict full knee flexion.

While conducting the test for range of motion, one should also test for weakness by comparing the involved and uninvolved sides. Myofascial TrPs induce an inconsistent, ratchety weakness without atrophy (except perhaps for a small amount that may be caused by disuse).[87] Marked quadriceps femoris atrophy is usually associated with disease of the knee joint.[122] The size of the quadriceps femoris muscle in children is measurable directly by ultrasound imaging.[52]

9. TRIGGER POINT EXAMINATION (Figs. 14.13–14.17)

As seen in Figure 14.13, the front of the thigh is covered mainly by the quadriceps femoris muscles, except its proximal medial region that is occupied by the hip adductors. These two groups of muscles are separated superficially by the sartorius muscle, which has been cut and reflected in this figure. The

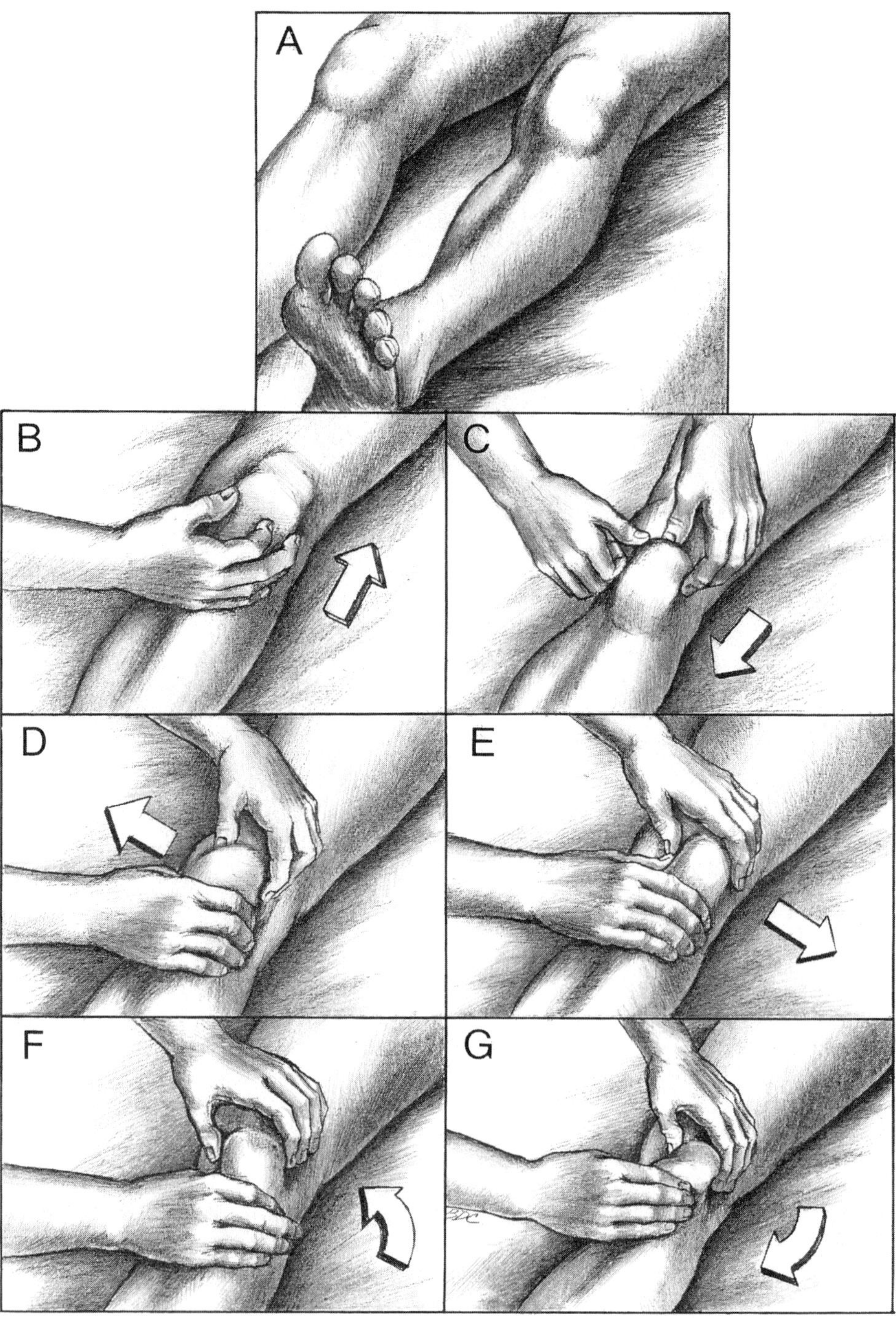

Figure 14.10. Examination of left patellar mobility, normal subject. *A*, resting position of the patella. *B*, upward displacement. *C*, downward displacement. *D*, medial displacement. *E*, lateral displacement. *F*, medial rotation (with reference to the upper pole of the patella). *G*, lateral rotation.

groove between the sartorius and the adductor longus, the adductor canal, is generally readily identifiable by deep palpation. It delineates the medial border of the quadriceps femoris throughout most of its length. The vastus lateralis covers nearly all of the lateral thigh, as seen in Figure 14.9.

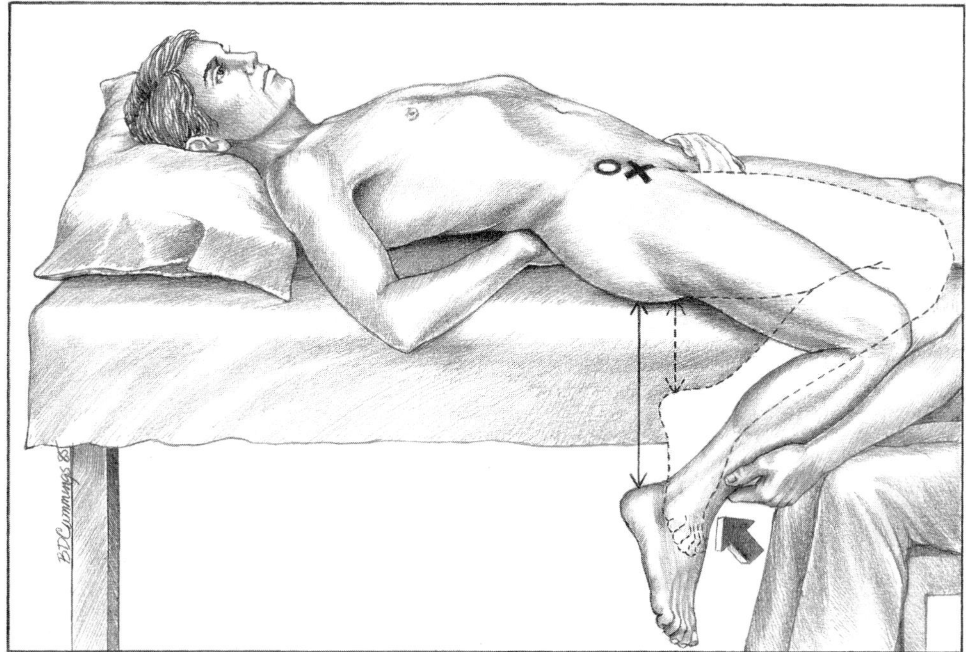

Figure 14.11. Effects of a tight right rectus femoris muscle. The *open circle* identifies the anterior superior iliac spine. The ***X*** locates the usual location of trigger points in this muscle, which crosses both the hip and knee joints. The hand of the operator presses the leg upward in the direction of the *thick arrow* to determine available flexion at the knee throughout an increasing range of hip extension. In this illustration, the tight right rectus femoris produces a pull on the pelvis that arches the back when the examiner attempts to flex the patient's knee (*fully rendered limb*). The *outlined limb* portrays an equally taut rectus femoris muscle but with increased knee flexion (*thin arrow, dotted line*) as compared to that in the fully rendered limb. This increased knee flexion is achieved at the expense of extension at the hip. For a clinical test of the stretch range of this muscle, the opposite thigh should be maintained in flexion to stabilize the pelvis and lumbar spine (*see* Fig. 14.18).

Rectus Femoris
(Fig. 14.14)

In most individuals, a cleft is palpable between the vastus medialis and the medial border of the rectus femoris (and the underlying vastus intermedius). The lateral border of the rectus femoris is usually palpable along the length of the anterolateral thigh, but there is no palpable distinction between the vastus intermedius and the vastus lateralis.

The TrPs of the rectus femoris are commonly located high (proximally) in the muscle close to the anterior inferior iliac spine and are found by flat palpation (Fig. 14.14). Lange[61] illustrated this examination using the fingertips.

The rectus femoris can be distinguished from the sartorius muscle by having the patient perform isometric knee extension (without hip flexion). Of these two muscles, only the rectus femoris extends the leg at the knee. The sartorius arises from the anterior superior iliac spine, above the attachment of the rectus femoris (Fig. 14.13) and covers its uppermost end. Local twitch responses can often be elicited from these proximal rectus femoris TrPs as well as from sartorius TrPs.

Rarely, one encounters a TrP in the distal part of the rectus femoris muscle about 10 cm (4 in) above the upper border of the patella. The TrP lies at the lateral border of the rectus femoris and is relatively superficial. It is not found in isolation, but only in conjunction with deeper TrPs clearly located in the vastus lateralis.

Vastus Medialis
(Fig. 14.15)

For examination of the vastus medialis, the patient should lie supine with the thigh on the symptomatic side placed in

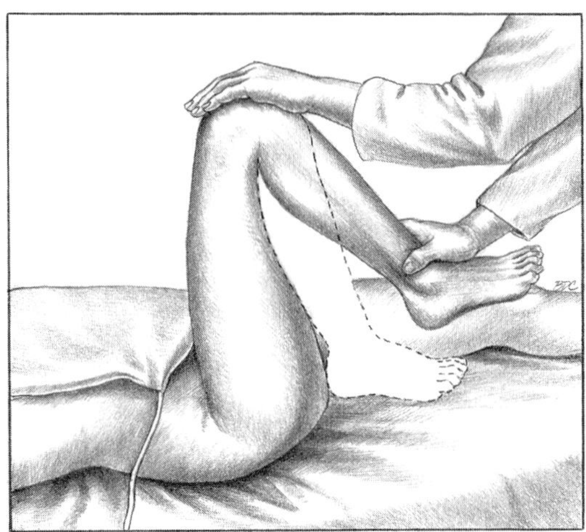

Figure 14.12. Heel-to-buttock test for flexibility of the vastus medialis, vastus intermedius, and vastus lateralis muscles of the right quadriceps femoris group. The patient should place the hand between the heel and buttock to become aware of the degree of restriction. The *fully rendered* position depicts a moderately restricted range of knee flexion, which often is due to trigger points in the vastus intermedius. Lesser degrees of limitation are more likely to be caused by trigger points in the other two vasti. The operator's test pressure is applied gently against the leg just above the ankle. The *outlined leg* showing full knee flexion (heel against buttock) confirms full normal length for all three vasti. Flexion of the thigh at the hip avoids stretching of the rectus femoris muscle. A dry heating pad is placed on the abdomen to maintain body warmth.

moderate abduction and the knee supported at about 90° of flexion (Fig. 14.15). A pad or pillow under the knee improves the patient's comfort. Flat palpation is used and most of the TrPs are usually found close to the medial border of the muscle (Fig. 14.2). The distal TrP_1 (Fig. 14.15*B*) is the most troublesome and the one most likely to cause a buckling knee. A cluster of TrPs also may be located along the medial border of the muscle about where the transition to oblique fibers would be expected. The adductor muscles are commonly involved when these distal TrPs in the vastus medialis muscle are active.

If the patient with vastus medialis TrPs has a buckling knee syndrome, a roll of skin over the TrP should be grasped and held firmly while the patient takes a few steps; during this compression test, the knee feels more secure to the patient and does not tend to buckle.

The more proximal TrP_2 (area being palpated in Fig. 14.15*A*) is likely to evoke only referred pain and not buckling. It is found at about midthigh near the medial border of the vastus medialis next to the adductor muscles (*see* Fig. 14.13). Occasionally, the taut band can be palpated close to the linea aspera where the adductor magnus also attaches. The clinician presses straight toward the femur to locate TrP spot tenderness and to evoke its pattern of referred pain. This proximal TrP_2 is rarely present in the absence of vastus medialis TrP_1. Local twitch responses are often apparent.

Vastus Intermedius (Fig. 14.16)

The reason for the "frustrator" nickname of the vastus intermedius is the inability to palpate directly the multiple TrPs that can develop along its length deep to the rectus femoris. Rarely is it possible to feel the taut bands of TrPs in this deep muscle mass. The entire muscle feels tense. When it is possible to palpate its TrPs, they are found by first locating the upper lateral border of the rectus femoris and following it a short distance distally until the fingers feel a space that permits palpation very deep, close to the femur. Only here (Fig. 14.16) is digital pressure likely to elicit the referred pain pattern of strongly active vastus intermedius TrPs. The TrPs of the vastus intermedius are found distal to the usual location of those in the rectus femoris (compare Fig. 14.1 with Fig. 14.3).

Usually, digital pressure on the muscle does not reproduce the TrP referred pain pattern, whereas needle penetration of the TrP does reproduce it. Therefore, the role of these TrPs is easily underestimated. Because of the overlying fascia and muscle, what appear to be TrPs of only slight or moderate tenderness on palpation often prove explosively painful when penetrated by a needle.

When both the rectus femoris and vastus intermedius contain TrPs, inactivating those in the rectus femoris makes it

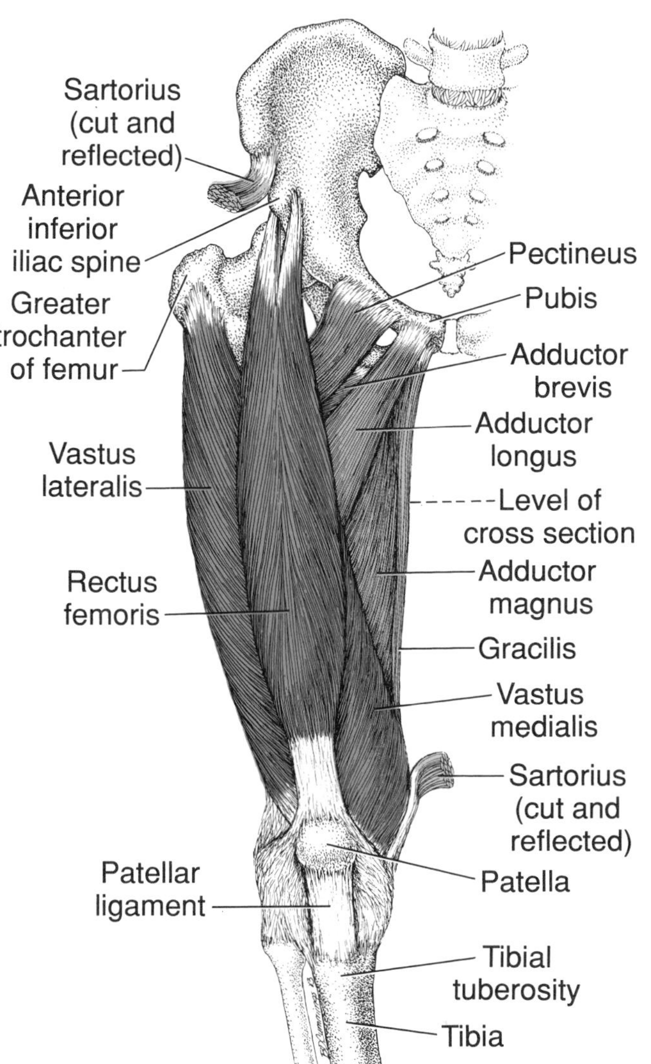

Figure 14.13. Regional anatomy (front view) of the right quadriceps femoris muscle (*dark red*); the vastus intermedius is not visible. The overlying sartorius muscle (*light red*) has been cut and reflected to more clearly reveal the relationship of the quadriceps to the adductor group, and to the pectineus and gracilis muscles (also *light red*).

easier to locate those in the vastus intermedius. The vastus intermedius is more likely than the rectus femoris to harbor TrPs located in the distal part of the muscle.

Vastus Lateralis
(Fig. 14.17)

The vastus lateralis sometimes develops a myofascial syndrome alone without involvement of other parts of the quadriceps femoris. This lateral thigh muscle, like the vastus intermedius, usually has multiple TrPs and many of them lie deep in the muscle. The taut bands of these TrPs can be located only with difficulty, if at all, and only by flat palpation directly against the underlying bone (Fig. 14.17). As one can see in this figure, and in that showing the referred pain patterns of the vastus lateralis (Fig. 14.4), TrPs may occur throughout most of the length of this muscle. This extensive distribution presents both diagnostic and therapeutic difficulties. Deep in the anterolateral part of the midthigh, where the muscle is thickest and its fibers fuse with those of the vastus intermedius (Fig. 14.8), the TrP spot tenderness cannot be clearly localized by palpation from the surface; rather, one detects a more diffuse tenderness. It is a challenging area because specific TrP spot tenderness is so hard to localize for injection.

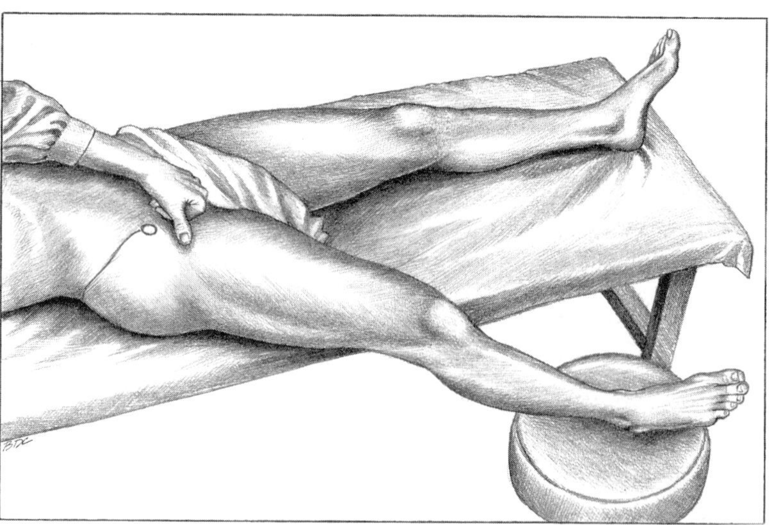

Figure 14.14. Palpation for tenderness of trigger points in the right rectus femoris muscle using thumb pressure. The *open circle* marks the readily palpable anterior **superior** iliac spine, which is just above the attachment of the rectus femoris onto the anterior **inferior** iliac spine of the pelvis. The *solid line* locates the crest of the ilium. Note how high proximally in the muscle this trigger point area is located.

The most distal TrP responsible for a locked patella often is found only by having the patient lie relaxed with the knee extended while the operator depresses the patella inferiorly and medialward to palpate the vastus lateralis in line with and close to the lateral border of the patella, in an area that the patella had covered before it was depressed. This TrP often feels like an exquisitely tender hard knot, and has been described and illustrated in a case report.[87]

10. ENTRAPMENTS

None of the quadricep femoris group is known to cause nerve entrapments associated with TrP tension of those muscles.

11. ASSOCIATED TRIGGER POINTS

Limitation of knee flexion due to TrPs in any one vastus muscle encourages the development of TrPs in the other two vasti and in the rectus femoris. Shortening of the hamstrings due to TrPs, especially in the biceps femoris, overloads the antagonistic quadriceps femoris; when the hamstrings have TrPs, usually at least part of the quadriceps group does too.

Rectus Femoris

Muscles likely to develop TrPs in association with TrPs in the rectus femoris include the three vasti and the iliopsoas muscle. The intermedius is the vastus muscle most likely to be involved also; the vastus medialis is the least likely. Proximal TrPs in the sartorius muscle may also appear. The relatively rare TrP at the distal part of the rectus femoris is found in association with deeper underlying TrPs in the vastus lateralis.

Vastus Medialis

The vastus medialis is the member of the quadriceps femoris group that is most likely to develop TrPs in the absence of TrPs in the other three heads. Such TrPs are often associated with a Morton foot structure. Also frequently associated with that foot structure are TrPs in the peroneus longus and gluteus medius muscles.

The distal vastus medialis TrP (TrP_1 in Fig. 14.2) is often associated with TrPs in the hip adductor muscles. This is the only part of the quadriceps femoris muscle group that frequently develops TrPs secondary to adductor TrPs.

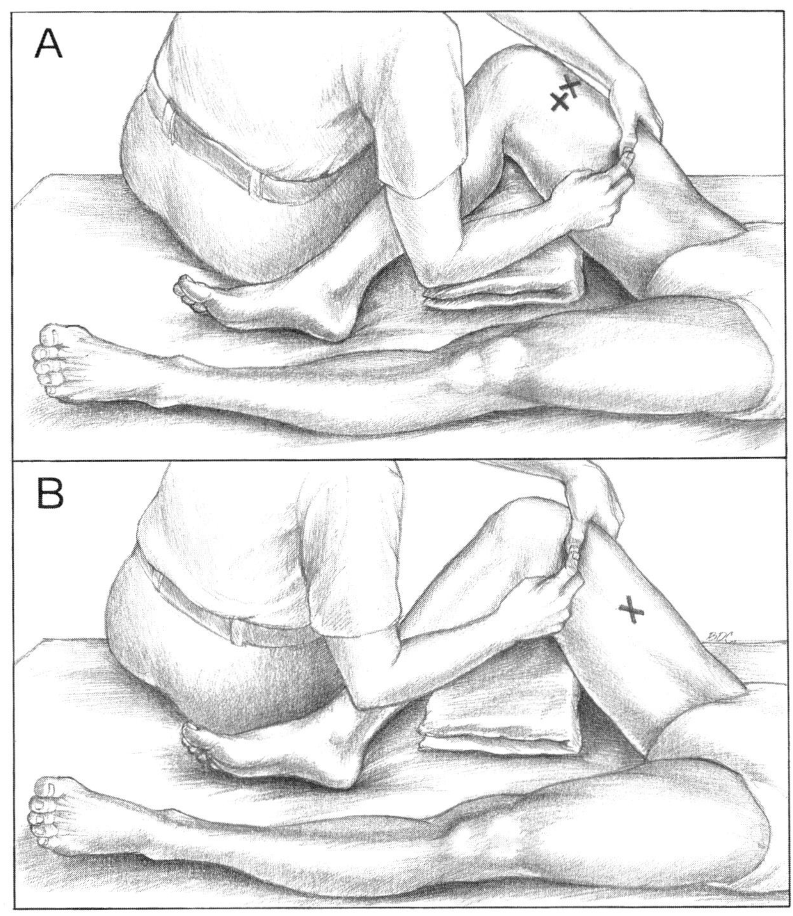

Figure 14.15. Palpation of common locations of trigger points (***X**s*) in the right vastus medialis muscle. *A*, palpation of the proximal trigger point (TrP_2) location. *B*, examination of the distal TrP_1 region.

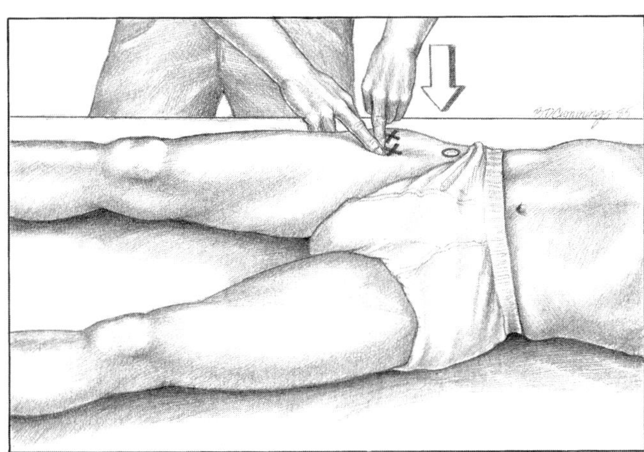

Figure 14.16. Examination of a trigger point high in the right vastus intermedius, deep to the rectus femoris muscle. The (***X**s*) show common sites of proximal trigger points in the vastus intermedius muscle. The *open circle* locates the anterior inferior iliac spine. The *arrow* indicates the downward (posterior) direction of strong pressure exerted by the operator.

TrPs in the vastus medialis can also be aggravated by active TrPs in the proximal end of the rectus femoris or in the tensor fasciae latae muscle. These other TrPs must be inactivated before the vastus medialis TrPs can be permanently eliminated.

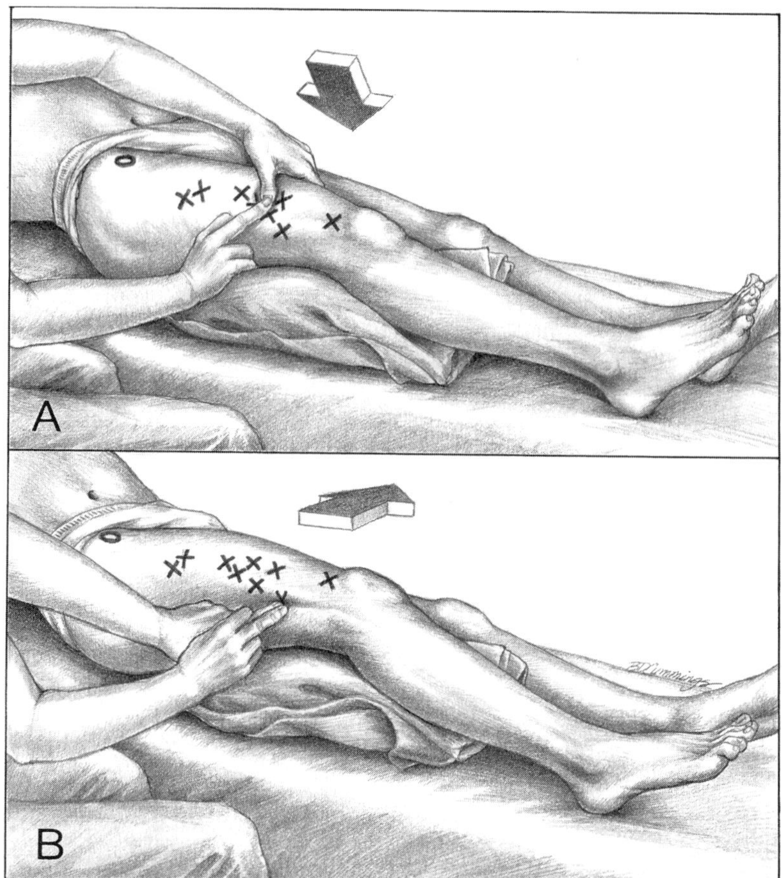

Figure 14.17. Examination by flat palpation for trigger points in the right vastus lateralis muscle. The leg is slightly flexed at the knee, a position provided here by the blanket. The ***Xs*** indicate locations of the many trigger points in this muscle. The *arrows* show the directions of pressure being applied. The *open circle* marks the anterior superior iliac spine. *A*, anterior portion of the vastus lateralis; *B*, posterior portion of the muscle.

Vastus Intermedius

The rectus femoris and vastus lateralis muscles of the quadriceps group are the agonists most likely also to be involved when the vastus intermedius develops TrPs.

Vastus Lateralis

TrPs in the anterior part of the gluteus minimus tend to activate satellite TrPs in the vastus lateralis muscle, which lies within the former muscle's pain reference zone.

12. INTERMITTENT COLD WITH STRETCH

(Figs. 14.18–14.22)

When treating the quadriceps femoris muscle, the tibiofemoral, patellofemoral, and superior tibiofibular articulations should be evaluated and released from any restriction by gentle mobilization, if possible. Normal mobility of the patella is important.

Whenever intermittent cold with stretch is applied to one of the vasti, one must be sure that TrPs in the other two vasti are not blocking the range of knee motion.

The use of ice for applying intermittent cold with passive stretch is explained on page 9 of this volume and the use of vapocoolant spray with stretch is detailed on pages 67–74 of Volume 1.[114] Techniques that augment relaxation and stretch are reviewed on page 11 of this volume and other techniques are also noted elsewhere.[104] Avoid stretching of hypermobile joints to their *full* range of motion. Alternative treatment methods are reviewed on pages 9–11 of this volume.

When treating the quadriceps femoris muscle group for TrPs, it is important to apply intermittent cold and stretch to the hamstring muscles also. Whenever any part of the quadriceps femoris harbors active TrPs, the hamstrings usually have at least latent TrPs that restrict movement. Application of intermittent cold with stretch of the quadriceps femoris causes unaccustomed sudden shortening of the hamstring muscles that can activate their latent TrPs, producing severe cramping pain. Should such a reactive cramp, or "kickback," of the hamstrings (or any other antagonistic muscle in a comparable situation) occur, the antagonist should be lengthened immediately by application of intermittent cold with stretch. This reaction can be avoided by first releasing hamstring tightness at least partially before proceeding to full release of the quadriceps femoris.

It is valuable for patients to experience the improvement that is achieved by having them note the increased range of knee motion after, as compared with before, treatment.

Muscles may respond poorly to intermittent cold with stretch if the patient becomes chilled. A dry heating pad on the abdomen, as shown in Figures 14.22 and 14.26, effectively replaces heat lost to the intermittent cold and reflexly increases blood flow to the limbs. One can feel how far distally the warmth of this reflex heating has progressed, monitoring it until the feet are warm. This feeling of comfortable warmth helps the patient relax more fully. The replacement of body heat is especially important in a cool or drafty treatment room.

Rectus Femoris
(Figs. 14.18 and 14.19)

Prior to treating the rectus femoris for myofascial TrPs, it is important to identify and correct any coexisting lumbar spine or hip articular dysfunction.

To stretch the two-joint rectus femoris muscle passively, the hip must be extended while the knee is flexed. This may be done with the patient lying on the opposite side (Fig. 14.18*A*) or lying supine with the thigh hanging over the edge of the treatment table (Fig. 14.18*B*). The uninvolved thigh should be flexed to stabilize the pelvis and lumbar spine, particularly if any lumbar hypermobility is present. Before treatment, the patient reaches down and feels the distance between the heel and buttock to measure how far apart they are. Parallel unidirectional slow sweeps of cold are applied from the iliac crest downward over the front and sides of the thigh and knee to cover all of the muscle and its referred pain pattern. With the patient in the side-lying position, the operator pulls the ankle toward the buttock to take up slack while applying parallel sweeps of cold, as described previously. The patient may assist by also pulling on the ankle, thus learning how to perform the stretch as part of a home-exercise program (Fig. 14.29). When the procedure is finished, the patient tests how close the heel now approaches the buttock and, in this way, becomes aware of the progress made.

A moist heating pad or hot pack rewarms the cooled skin (Fig. 14.19).

Following these procedures, the patient slowly exercises the rectus femoris actively through its fully lengthened and shortened ranges of motion, from hip extension combined with knee flexion to hip flexion with knee extension.

The location for application of the moist heating pad (Fig. 14.19) should be based *not* on where it *hurts* but on where the *active TrPs* are located. Although the pain is rarely felt at the upper end of the rectus femoris, its common TrP site, that is where the moist heat must be applied. The greater the extent of coverage of the entire muscle by the moist heat, the better is the result.

Generally, TrPs in the rectus femoris muscle respond well to intermittent cold with stretch when this myofascial TrP therapy is properly administered and when any perpetuating factors are managed.

Vastus Medialis
(Fig. 14.20)

Of the four heads of the quadriceps femoris, the vastus medialis most dependably

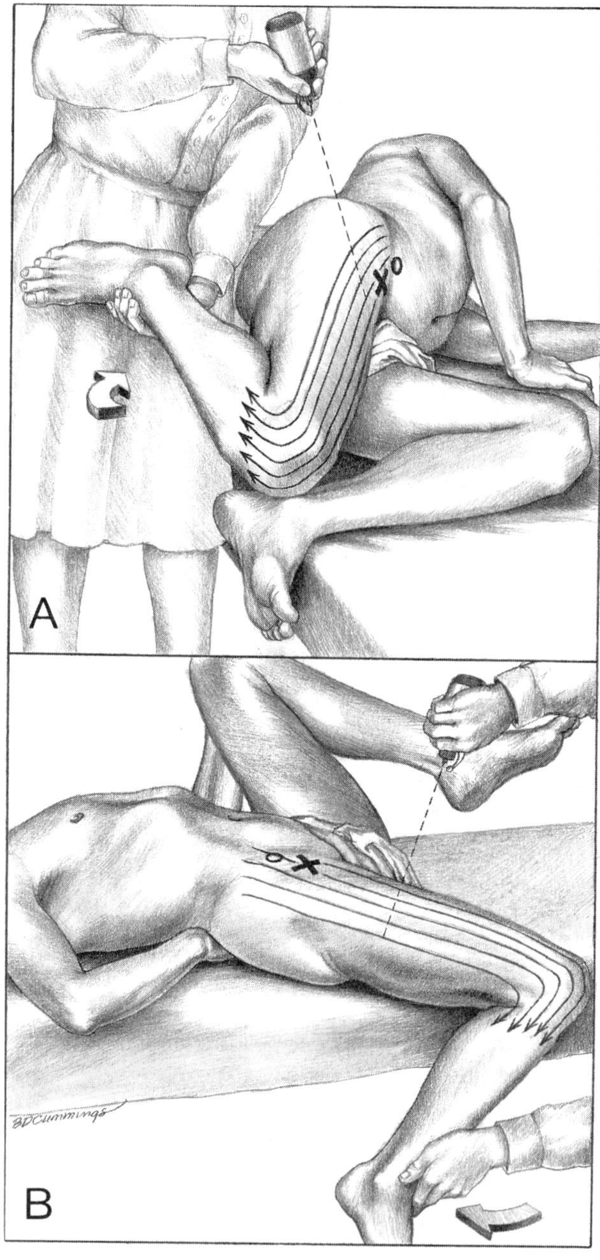

Figure 14.18. Passive stretch positions and partial intermittent cold pattern (*thin arrows*) for the right rectus femoris muscle. The parallel sweeps of ice or other coolant also extend over the front of the thigh more medially than shown here in order to cover all of the muscle and its entire referred pain pattern. The black ***X*** shows the usual location of this muscle's trigger points. The *open circle* marks the anterior **superior** iliac spine, which is above the attachment of this muscle on the anterior **inferior** iliac spine of the pelvis. *A*, side-lying position. The operator passively lengthens the rectus femoris by simultaneously extending the thigh at the hip and flexing the leg at the knee (*thick arrow*). *B*, supine position. The operator is again flexing the leg at the knee (*thick arrow*) to lengthen the muscle while the hip is extended. This two-joint stretch contrasts with the one-joint stretch of the three vasti (*see* Fig. 14.21). The patient's left hand holds the uninvolved thigh in flexion to stabilize the pelvis and prevent excessive extension of the spine.

responds to intermittent cold with stretch that incorporates postisometric relaxation. However, complete TrP inactivation may not be obtained by this procedure in stubborn chronic myofascial syndromes of this muscle or when restriction in the range of knee flexion is a minimal component. The latter is not uncommon. When complete relief is not achieved, it becomes necessary to use other modalities, such as ischemic compression, stripping massage, ultrasound, or TrP injection, to inactivate any remaining TrPs. Because of the attachment of the vastus medialis to fascia of the adductor longus and adductor magnus, release of tension in those muscles is often necessary to achieve full release of the vastus medialis.

To apply intermittent cold with stretch to the vastus medialis, the patient lies supine with the thigh abducted and the knee flexed on the affected side, as illus-

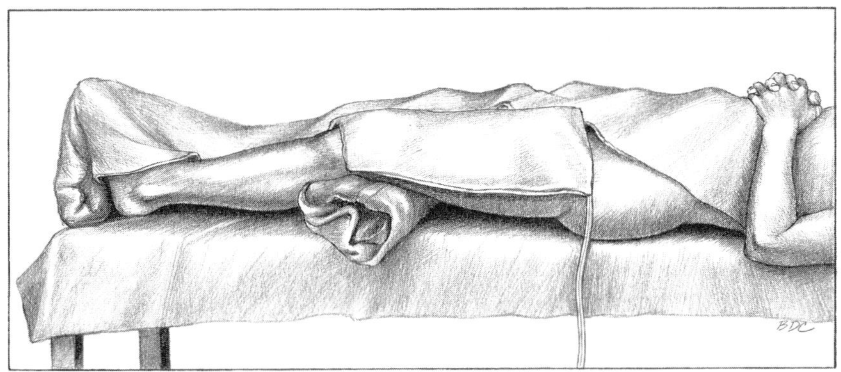

Figure 14.19. Application of a moist wet-proof heating pad to the left quadriceps femoris muscle following intermittent cold with stretch or trigger-point injection. A rolled towel is placed under the knees to lengthen the three vasti heads of the muscle slightly while applying the moist heat. Feet are supported in a neutral position. The blanket over the exposed skin not in the treatment area helps to preserve body warmth.

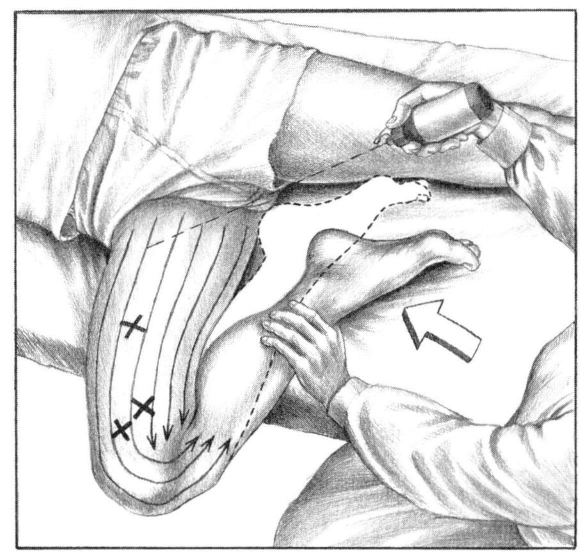

Figure 14.20. Stretch position and intermittent cold pattern (*thin arrows*) for trigger points (***X**s*) in the right vastus medialis muscle. This position simultaneously stretches the adductors, which therefore must also be covered by sweeps of ice or vapocoolant. Slack is taken up in the direction shown by the *thick arrow*. Following inactivation of the vastus medialis trigger points, the heel reaches the buttock (*outlined leg and foot*).

trated in Figure 14.20. Parallel sweeps of ice or vapocoolant spray are directed over the muscle and distally over the referred pain pattern, and then the knee is increasingly flexed as intermittent cooling is continued briefly. The application of cold should cover the adductors, since they also are stretched in this position. When the adductor longus and/or magnus also harbor active TrPs, the ice or vapocoolant should be directed so as to include all of the composite adductor pain pattern as well (*see* Figs. 15.1 and 15.2). It may be necessary to inactivate adductor TrPs in order to release the vastus medialis muscle fully.

The patient should palpate the distance between heel and buttock before and after the procedure to monitor progress. Full range of motion should bring the heel up against the buttock.

The procedure is followed by the application of a moist heating pad over the muscle with the patient placed in a com-

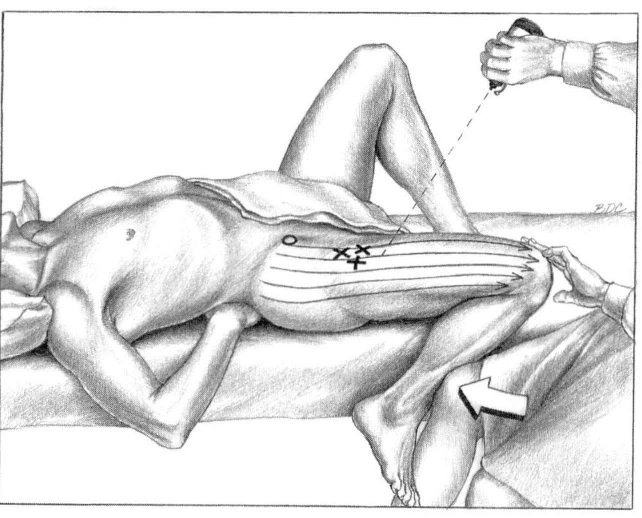

Figure 14.21. Stretch position and intermittent cold pattern (*thin arrows*) for trigger points (***X**s*) in the right vastus intermedius muscle in the supine patient. The *thick arrow* shows the direction of pressure to lengthen the vastus intermedius passively by flexing the knee. Positioning at the hip joint does not influence the stretch on this muscle, which crosses only the knee joint. This contrasts with the rectus femoris muscle (*see* Fig. 14.18*B*).

fortable position, supine with a small pillow under the knee (Fig. 14.19). After several minutes of moist heat application, the recumbent patient reestablishes full functional range of motion by slowly alternating between the treatment position of a fully lengthened vastus medialis to a fully shortened muscle.

Vastus Intermedius
(Fig. 14.21)

The TrPs in the vastus intermedius are difficult to inactivate by intermittent cold with stretch because there may be so many of them and because they tend to become fibrotic, similar to those in the subscapularis muscle in the condition "frozen shoulder" (*see* Chapter 26, Volume 1[114]). For both of these muscles, it may be necessary to resort to injection of the TrPs to inactivate them, after administration of an antifibrotic agent, such as the potassium salt of *p*-aminobenzoic acid, sold under the name Potaba. These TrPs are not readily accessible to manual pressure therapy.

To apply intermittent cold with passive stretch to the vastus intermedius muscle, the patient lies supine on the treatment table, as illustrated in Figure 14.21. Movement at the hip does not affect stretch of this muscle, but an initial stretch procedure including some knee flexion together with hip extension ensures release of the rectus femoris so that its tense fibers do not block full stretch of the vasti. (During this initial rectus femoris release, the opposite thigh is flexed to stabilize the pelvis and lumbar spine.) During application of intermittent cold, the muscle is placed on just enough gentle stretch to take up the slack. The ice or vapocoolant spray is applied in parallel sweeps as illustrated, and then slack is taken up by further flexing the knee (Fig. 14.21).

Intermittent cold with stretch can be combined effectively with the Lewit technique of postisometric relaxation.[66,67] To combine them, the relaxed patient gently extends the knee isometrically against operator resistance for at least 3 seconds and then relaxes. The operator applies intermittent cold and again passively lengthens the muscle to take up the slack that developed following isometric contraction. The addition of the Lewit technique, which is a form of contract-relax at maximal available muscle length,[117] facilitates release of tension and inactivation of TrPs in any head of the quadriceps femoris. A study of the effectiveness of this technique on the quadriceps femoris in eight normal asymptomatic men showed that knee flexion increased 4 ± 1% and that the increase persisted for 90 minutes.[80]

The intermittent cold-with-stretch procedure is followed by application of a moist heating pad over the vastus intermedius and then by several cycles of slow active movement through its fully lengthened range and fully shortened range.

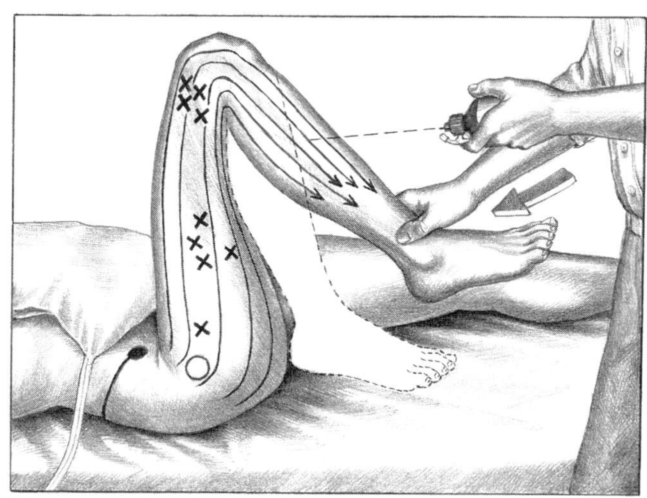

Figure 14.22. Stretch position and intermittent cold pattern for the right vastus lateralis. The ***Xs*** mark common locations of trigger points in this member of the quadriceps femoris muscle group. The *open circle* identifies the greater trochanter; the *solid circle*, the anterior superior iliac spine; and the *heavy solid line*, the crest of the ilium. The *fully rendered* right lower limb is shown in the position reached after partial release of muscle tension. The *outlined* leg and foot have reached the position of full vastus lateralis length with the heel against the buttock. The *large arrow* shows the direction of gentle pressure applied to take up slack. The vastus intermedius and the vastus medialis are also being stretched during this procedure, and the intermittent cold application should also include those muscles if they harbor TrPs. The dry heating pad on the abdomen provides reflex circulation to the limbs that compensates for heat lost to the cold application and considerable exposure of bare skin.

Vastus Lateralis
(Fig. 14.22)

To apply intermittent cold with passive stretch to the vastus lateralis, the patient lies supine with the hip flexed to approximately 90°, as illustrated in Figure 14.22. The figure shows a dry heating pad placed on the abdomen for reflex heating in a cold room. Slack is taken up in the vastus lateralis as the intermittent cold is applied in parallel sweeps distally over the muscle and over its referred pain pattern (Fig. 14.22). Then, after a pause for the patient to breathe deeply, gentle pressure is applied on the leg to increase the passive stretch while a second set of parallel sweeps of ice or vapocoolant is completed. When the distal suprapatellar TrP is of concern, one must manually depress the patella, as illustrated in Figure 14.10*C* and as described in a case report,[87] to obtain complete stretch of the vastus lateralis.

13. INJECTION AND STRETCH
(Figs. 14.23–14.27)

A full description of the procedure for injection and stretch of any muscle appears in Volume 1, pages 74–86.[114]

The solution preferred for injection of TrPs is 0.5% procaine in isotonic saline. This may be prepared in the syringe by diluting one part of 2% procaine solution with three parts of isotonic saline. The precise localization of the TrPs is described in detail for each of the four heads of the quadriceps femoris in the preceding Section 9, Examination of Trigger Points.

Injection of TrPs in any of the four heads, as described later in the subsequent paragraphs, is followed promptly by brief intermittent cold with stretch and then the application of a moist heating pad. Finally, full active movement of the muscle is performed slowly and completely through several cycles, from the fully shortened range to the fully lengthened range.

Rectus Femoris
(Fig. 14.23)

For injection of the TrPs in the rectus femoris muscle, the patient lies supine, the thigh is extended slightly, and the knee is bent slightly to eliminate excessive slack in the muscle (Fig. 14.23). The taut band is palpated and the TrP spot tenderness localized for precise infiltration. All TrPs present in this muscle should be treated. If

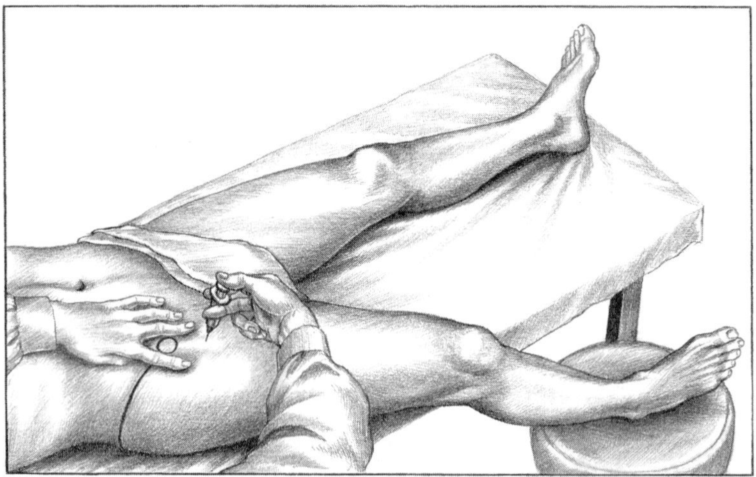

Figure 14.23. Injection of the usual trigger point high in the right rectus femoris muscle. The *open circle* locates the anterior superior iliac spine. The *solid line* marks the iliac crest. The location of this trigger point is more proximal than that of the proximal trigger points in the vastus intermedius (*see* Fig. 14.25). Usually, the patient would be covered with a blanket to prevent chilling of the body.

the involved muscle has been confirmed to be the rectus femoris and not the sartorius, there should be little likelihood of penetrating the femoral artery or nerve with the needle.

Vastus Medialis
(Fig. 14.24)

For injection of vastus medialis TrPs, the patient is positioned with the thigh flexed and abducted and the knee flexed to 90°, as illustrated in Figure 14.24, to make all its TrP areas accessible. The more distal TrP_1 region includes multiple TrPs that may cause either knee pain or buckling of the knee. They are explored with the needle as illustrated in Figure 14.24*A*.

Injection of the more proximal TrP_2 area is shown in Figure 14.24*B*. If TrPs requiring injection are found toward the medial border of the proximal TrP_2 area, one must remember that the femoral artery courses along that border. Then the needle should be angled laterally, away from the sartorius muscle and the artery.

If, after injection, the vastus medialis TrPs are still tender, the physician should examine the upper end of the rectus femoris, the tensor fasciae latae, and the adductor longus and magnus muscles for associated TrPs that may perpetuate the vastus medialis TrPs.

Vastus Intermedius
(Fig. 14.25)

Inactivating the TrPs in this muscle requires much persistence and can be frustrating because their true severity is easily underestimated. Figure 14.25 shows the position of the patient for injecting some TrPs in the vastus intermedius muscle. Localizing these TrPs for injection is difficult because they are so deep, within 3 mm (⅛ in) of the bone. If the needle is inserted far into the muscle, it contacts bone. When one encounters these TrPs with the needle deep in the vastus intermedius, they usually cause an explosion of referred pain. Before withdrawing the needle through the skin, it is important to slide the skin aside and to palpate deeply, checking that all TrP tenderness has been eliminated by the probing injection.

As shown in cross section in Figure 14.8, anatomically there is no clear delineation between the deep lateral fibers of the vastus intermedius and the deep medial fibers of the vastus lateralis. They commonly are involved together. Many of the difficulties experienced when injecting TrPs in one muscle apply to the other. When one finds TrPs that need injection in either of these heads of the quadriceps femoris, it is prudent to explore for TrPs in the other head. Some patients have

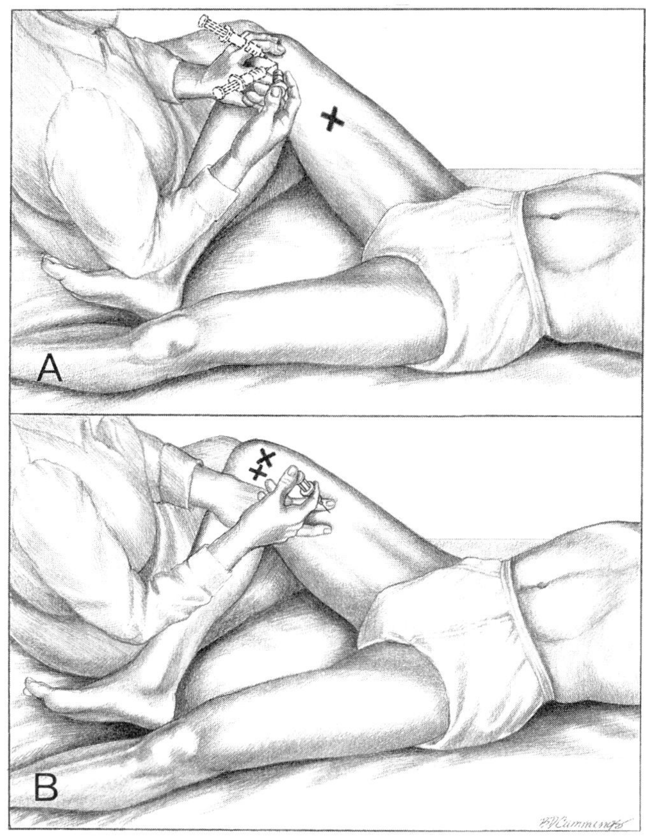

Figure 14.24. Injection of vastus medialis trigger points. *A*, *broken-line syringes* portray various probing angles for injection of the distal (TrP_1) group of trigger points shown as **X**s in *B*. These distal trigger points often cause buckling of the knee. *B*, injection of the proximal trigger point area along the medial border of the muscle, located at the **X** in *A*.

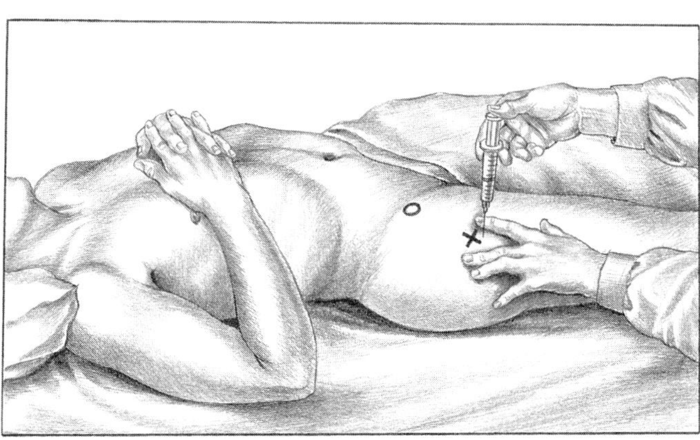

Figure 14.25. Injection of a trigger point (**X**) in the right vastus intermedius muscle. The *open circle* locates the anterior superior iliac spine. This trigger point area is located more distally and deeper than that in the rectus femoris muscle shown in Figure 14.23. The needle is directed straight downward (posteriorly) toward the underlying femur, nearly perpendicular to the skin surface.

limited tolerance for the autonomic disruption caused by the explosive impact of injecting these TrPs. This is one region for which analgesic premedication of apprehensive patients may be indicated.

Vastus Lateralis
(Figs. 14.26 and 14.27)

Effective injection of vastus lateralis TrPs usually requires the identification and inactivation of multiple TrPs (Fig. 14.26). One must identify the spots of TrP tenderness by deep palpation against the femur to localize them for injection. In average sized individuals, one may need a 63-mm (2½-in) needle to reach the deepest TrP_3, TrP_4, and TrP_5 locations (Fig. 14.4). It is often necessary to push the biceps femoris aside to reach vastus lateralis TrP_3 (Fig. 14.4), which is located posteriorly

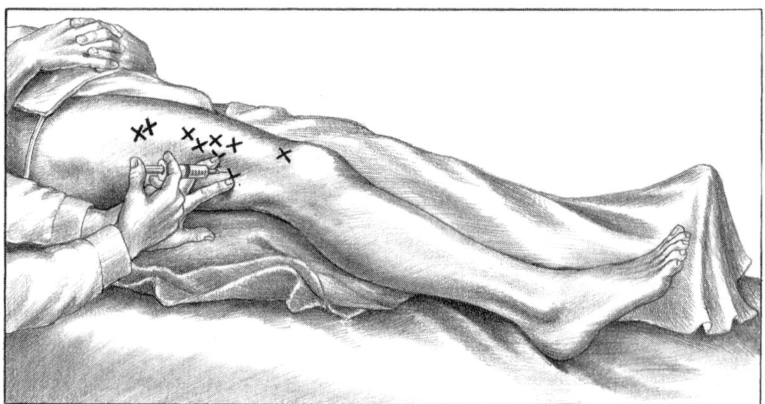

Figure 14.26. Injection of trigger points (**X**s) in the right vastus lateralis muscle. This muscle usually exhibits multiple trigger points that are difficult to localize by palpation. The needle is directed toward a trigger point in the posterior cluster of trigger points while the taut band, if palpable, is pinned down by the fingers of the opposite hand. A blanket covers the untreated lower limb to help keep the patient warm. A dry heating pad is applied to the abdomen as a convenient way to replace heat lost from the exposed lower limb.

Figure 14.27. Injection of the most distal trigger point (TrP_1) in the right vastus lateralis muscle. The *dashed line* around the patella emphasizes the fact that the patella is being pushed downward to uncover the trigger point. Tension due to a trigger point in this lowest part of the muscle consistently locks the patella upward and thus painfully blocks both flexion and extension of the knee. The middle finger of the palpating hand presses the patella downward and pins down the palpable band in the muscle, while the other hand proceeds with the injection.

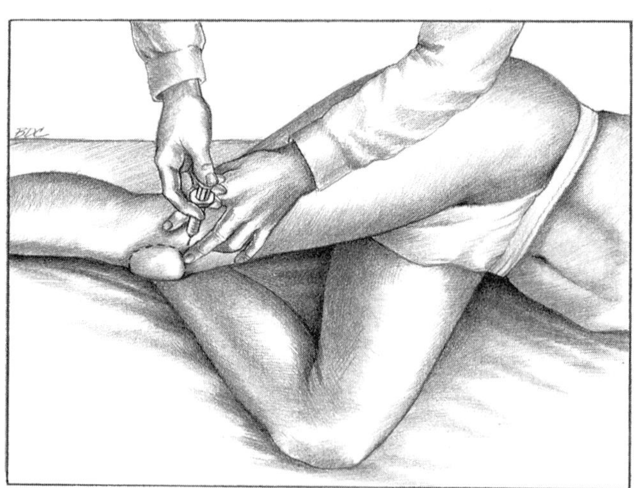

against the back of the femur. The needle must be slanted anteriorly to stay in the vastus lateralis and not enter the adjacent hamstring muscle. When penetrated, these TrPs are likely to refer pain to the back of the knee. This is a region where the needle may have to substitute for the palpating finger to find the TrPs.

Locating all of the vastus lateralis TrPs and injecting them specifically can be tedious, but becomes necessary when other methods of therapy fail to inactivate them fully.

Cryptic TrP_1 is found only by pressing the patella downward as far as it will go while palpating for a taut band and TrP tenderness just above the lateral border of the patella. A short needle, 25 mm (1 in) long, may be sufficient for injection. TrP_1 is injected as illustrated and described in Figure 14.27. It is necessary to push the patella distally to make the TrP accessible during injection. When this TrP has been responsible for limited movement at the knee, full knee function and patient mobility return immediately when it is inactivated, an unforgettably dramatic experience for the patient and the clinician.

14. CORRECTIVE ACTIONS (Figs. 14.28–14.31)

The buckling knee caused by vastus medialis (or possibly vastus lateralis)

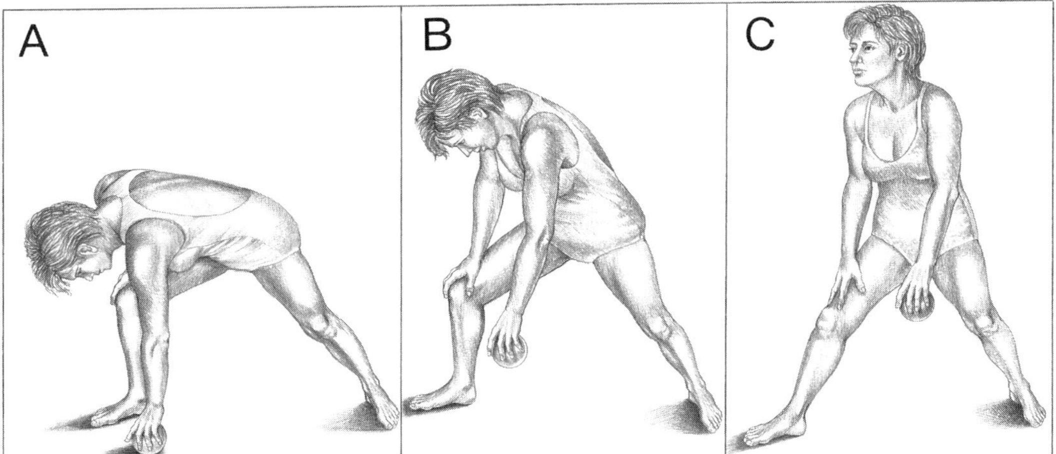

Figure 14.28. Lifting an item safely from the floor while sparing the quadriceps femoris muscles bilaterally. *A*, reaching to the floor with one hand while the other hand supports body weight on the knee. *B*, pushing up with the hand braced against the knee. *C*, torso upright, with knees straight and the quadriceps group unloaded throughout the activity. The rear limb is then moved forward under the body. Support by the arm also takes some of the load off the long paraspinal muscles of the back.

TrPs is a special threat to the elderly. Elimination of the responsible TrP is another valuable "fall-proofing" technique, especially for those who are prone to falling.

Corrective Posture and Activities
(Fig. 14.28)

Two guiding principles require attention: to avoid shortening and/or prolonged immobilization of the quadriceps femoris group of muscles.

Avoid Overload

Patients with active TrPs in any part of the quadriceps femoris muscle group must learn to lift heavy objects and pick things up from the floor in a safe manner that spares the quadriceps femoris (as well as the paraspinal muscles) from overload. This alternate to the technique usually taught is described and illustrated in Figure 14.28. This alternate method also avoids marked dorsiflexion, which becomes difficult or impossible when active TrPs in the soleus muscle limit stretch of that muscle.

Deep knee bends and *complete* squats should be *prohibited* for patients. These maneuvers can cause serious overload of the quadriceps femoris during the initial effort to rise unassisted. In the squatting position, the quadriceps femoris has a poor mechanical advantage. (This position is also a hazard for the knee ligaments.) A partial squat, or a partial knee-bend, is relatively safe if the thigh does not drop lower than the horizontal position (parallel to the floor).

Until the quadriceps muscle group has recovered from its myofascial pain syndrome, it is important for the patient to avoid overloading these muscles when arising from a chair seat. To accomplish this, the patient can use the upper limbs to assist by pushing against an armrest of the chair with one hand and against the distal thigh with the other hand; if no armrests are available, the hands push against both thighs distally.

Avoid Prolonged Immobilization

During sitting, one should avoid a jack-knifed position at the hips (acute angle of hip flexion) with the knees extended. Many automobile seats produce a jack-knifed position with the knees somewhat extended. This can be improved by using a SACRO-EASE (McCarty's SACRO-EASE, 3329 Industrial Avenue, Coeur d'Alene, Idaho 83814) or other back support and placing a lift beneath the rear of the seat portion of the back support. Automatic cruise control can be helpful by permitting more flexibility in positioning of the right foot on the accelerator pedal during long auto trips. Any long trip should be broken by a rest and stretch stop at least every hour.

Habitually sitting with one foot under the other buttock immobilizes the quadriceps femoris for long periods. This can seriously aggravate its TrPs and should be avoided.

Patients with quadriceps femoris TrPs should avoid sitting upright for a prolonged period with the legs straight out in front resting on an ottoman; this position places all parts of the quadriceps group in a markedly shortened position, aggravating any existing TrPs.

To avoid sitting with the lower limbs in a fixed position, it is wise to have the patient use a rocking chair for movement, particularly at the hips and knees. Rocking mobilizes all of the quadriceps femoris muscle group.

To avoid maintaining the quadriceps in a shortened position at night, it is important to avoid marked hip flexion for the rectus femoris and also to avoid full knee extension, especially for the vasti. When patients with vastus medialis TrPs sleep on the opposite (unaffected) side at night, a pillow placed between the knees can reduce pressure on the area of referred tenderness over the knee, as well as on the muscle itself. Patients with vastus lateralis TrPs should not sleep on the side of the affected muscle, because the resulting pressure can be enough to irritate the TrPs, but not enough to inactivate them.

When patients have TrPs in the vastus medialis, it is important to teach them not to kneel on the floor or ground during such activities as tending a baby, scrubbing or painting the floor, gardening, etc. Overload due to prolonged kneeling is a potent perpetuator of vastus medialis TrPs. These patients should sit on a low bench, or on a low substantial box, instead of kneeling.

Corrections for Structural Stress

Correction should be made for a hyperpronating foot. Patients with vastus medialis TrPs and the Morton foot structure should have the appropriate corrections made in all their shoes (*see* Chapter 20, Peroneal Muscles). The postural strain that causes pain and dysfunction of the vastus medialis is described in Chapter 8, Gluteus Medius, and illustrated in Figure 8.3*B*. A good arch support should be used if hyperpronation is caused by a hypermobile midfoot. If muscular imbalances are present, they must be corrected. A leg length inequality should be corrected to equalize foot impact.

Exercise Therapy
(Figs. 14.29–14.31)

Nearly every patient with quadriceps femoris TrPs will benefit from a home self-stretch program. Passive stretching is effective whether performed while side lying (Fig. 14.29) or while standing (Fig. 14.30). Both figures show a passive stretch suitable for the rectus femoris with the patient simultaneously pulling the leg back and upward to extend the thigh while flexing the knee. The recumbent stretch of Figure 14.29 is invaluable to patients who are awakened at night by pain arising from rectus femoris TrPs. They simply reach down, pull the leg back and upward toward the buttock, gently stretching the muscle; then they can usually sleep again in comfort.

In the standing position (Fig. 14.30), the patient is taught first to hold the ankle with the hand on the same side to achieve the passive stretch and then to repeat the stretch, holding the same ankle with the opposite hand. This exercise emphasizes stretch first of the vastus medialis, and then of the vastus lateralis. This Standing Self-stretch Exercise is most effective if done in a pool of warm water that supports most of the body weight.

A self-stretch for the rectus femoris can be performed at the workplace or elsewhere away from home as the patient sits on the side edge of a chair with the affected lower limb hanging over the edge of the chair. The patient bends the affected knee and moves the thigh posteriorly along the side of the chair while supporting the torso against the back of the chair.

One study reported that nearly all of the competitive male swimmers studied stretched the quadriceps femoris muscles, but only 5 of 16 basketball players appreciated the need to do so.[65] It is important

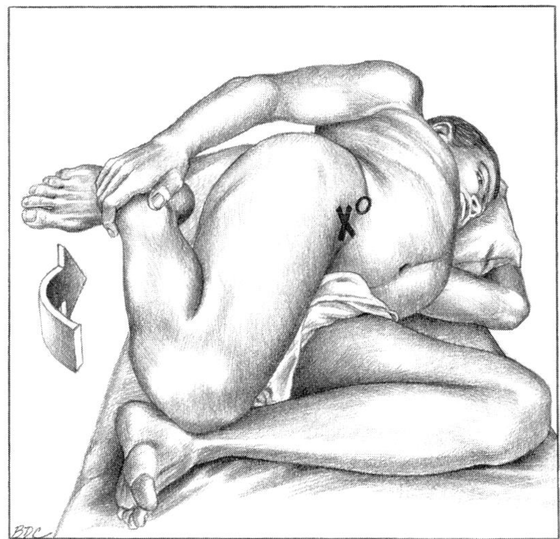

Figure 14.29. Side-lying self-stretch for a trigger point (***X***) in the right rectus femoris muscle. The *open circle* marks the anterior superior iliac spine. The patient slowly brings the heel against the buttock to flex the knee fully while maintaining and then increasing extension of the thigh at the hip by also pulling the knee and thigh posteriorly; the hand holds the ankle, not the foot. The *arrow* indicates the direction of pull. This patient has pulled the pelvis down in front, exaggerating lumbar lordosis. Such a pelvic tilt can be prevented by starting with the other thigh flexed and held against the chest. The trigger-point tension of the rectus femoris muscle responds well to incorporation of the Lewit technique of postisometric relaxation with this stretch.

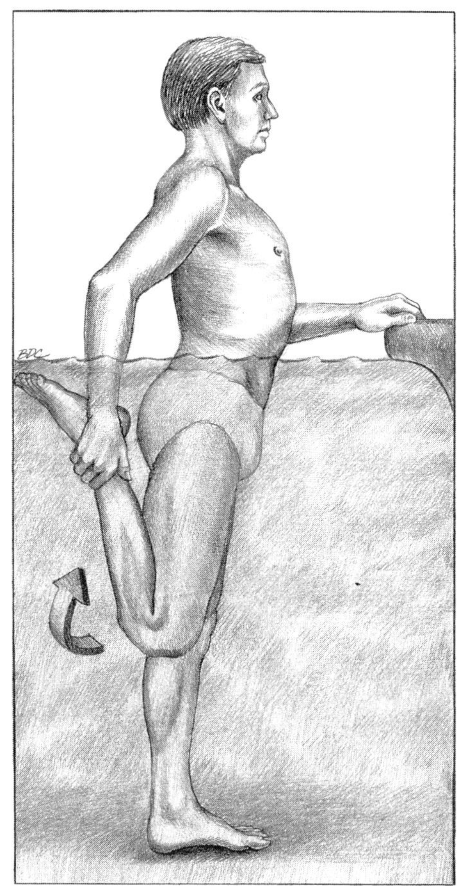

Figure 14.30. Standing Self-stretch Exercise of the right rectus femoris to fully lengthen the muscle. The *arrow* shows the direction of pull. This exercise is best done while standing at least waist deep in the warm water of a swimming pool or tank and holding onto the edge of the pool's wall for balance.

for everyone to maintain range of motion of these muscles with increasing age.

Another exercise of benefit to patients who had a locked knee caused by a vastus lateralis TrP is self-mobilization of the patella. With the knee straight, the patient consciously relaxes the quadriceps femoris and simply manually moves the patella in all directions, as illustrated for examination in Figure 14.10.

Quadriceps femoris strengthening exercises that entail knee extension with weight added at the ankle are contraindicated in patients with active TrPs in this group of muscles. The TrPs should be inactivated before the strengthening exercises are started. The first strengthening exercises should employ slow **lengthening** (eccentric) contractions, *not* shortening (concentric) contractions. Therefore, the seated patient's leg should be elevated passively, and then the patient should slowly control the return of the foot to the resting flexed position. This principle is analogous to the use of the slow sit-back rather than a sit-up for strengthening the abdominal muscles without overloading them and perpetuating their TrPs (Chapter 49, Volume 1).[114]

For patients with TrPs in the lower part of the vastus medialis, initially an elastic knee support can improve function and reduce pain. Either an elastic knee sleeve with an opening for the patella or a figure-of-eight elastic bandage can serve as a reminder that the knee needs protection. The added support gives the patient an increased sense of security until the TrPs are fully inactivated and normal function of the muscle is restored. It also serves as a form of neutral warmth to maintain

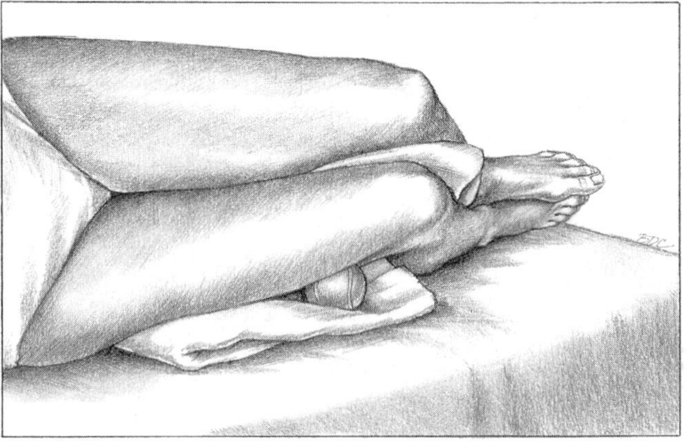

Figure 14.31. Tennis ball technique for ischemic compression to inactivate most superficial (and sometimes deep) trigger points in the right vastus lateralis muscle.

body heat and prevent chilling of the muscle.

Patients with active TrPs in the vastus lateralis muscle can use a tennis ball for self-administration of ischemic compression (Fig. 14.31). The patient controls the amount of body weight resting on the ball and rolls the ball along the muscle until it reaches a tender TrP. Ischemic compression is administered as described in Chapter 2, page 9 of this volume. The tennis ball technique is often an effective way for the patient to eliminate many of the more superficial TrPs encountered in this muscle.

References

1. Alvarez EV, Munters M, Lavine LS, *et al.*: Quadriceps myofibrosis, a complication of intramuscular injections. *J Bone Joint Surg [Am] 62*:58–60, 1980.
2. Anderson A: Personal communication, 1990.
3. Anderson JE: *Grant's Atlas of Anatomy*, Ed. 8. Williams & Wilkins, Baltimore, 1983 (Figs. 4–23, 4–24).
4. *Ibid.* (Fig. 4–25).
5. *Ibid.* (Fig. 4–26).
6. *Ibid.* (Fig. 4–28).
7. *Ibid.* (Fig. 4–66).
8. Arsenault AB, Chapman AE: An electromyographic investigation of the individual recruitment of the quadriceps muscles during isometric contraction of the knee extensors in different patterns of movement. *Physiother Can 26*:253–261, 1974.
9. Baker BA: Myofascial pain syndromes: Ten single muscle cases. *J Neurol Orthop Med Surg 10*:129–131, 1989.
10. Bardeen CR: The musculature, Sect. 5. In *Morris's Human Anatomy,* edited by C.M. Jackson, Ed. 6. Blakiston's Son & Co., Philadelphia, 1921 (p. 500).
11. *Ibid.* (p. 503).
12. Basmajian JV, Deluca CJ: *Muscles Alive*, Ed. 5. Williams & Wilkins, Baltimore, 1985 (pp. 235–239).
13. *Ibid.* (p. 243).
14. *Ibid.* (p. 258).
15. *Ibid.* (p. 322).
16. *Ibid.* (pp. 325–328, 330).
17. *Ibid.* (p. 371, Fig. 16.1, pp. 372–373, 381).
18. Basmajian JV, Harden TP, Regenos EM: Integrated actions of the four heads of quadriceps femoris: an electromyographic study. *Anat Rec 172*:15–19, 1972.
19. Bates T, Grunwaldt E: Myofascial pain in childhood. *J Pediatr 53*:198–209, 1958.
20. Baxter MP, Dulberg C: "Growing Pains" in childhood—a proposal for treatment. *J Pediatr Orthop 8*:402–406, 1988.
21. Beazell JR: Entrapment neuropathy of the lateral femoral cutaneous nerve: cause of lateral knee pain. *J Orthop Sports Phys Ther 10*:85–86, 1988.
22. Blazina ME, Kerlan RK, Jobe FW: Jumper's knee. *Orthop Clin North Am 4*:665–678, 1973.
23. Bose K, Kanagasuntheram R, Osman MBH: Vastus medialis oblique: an anatomic and physiologic study. *Orthopedics 3*:880–883, 1980.
24. Brody DM: Running injuries: prevention and management. *Clin Symp 39*:2–36, 1987.
25. Broer MR, Houtz SJ: *Patterns of Muscular Activity in Selected Sports Skills*. Charles C Thomas, Springfield, 1967.
26. Brucini M, Duranti R, Galletti R, *et al.*: Pain thresholds and electromyographic features of periarticular muscles in patients with osteoarthritis of the knee. *Pain 10*:57–66, 1981.
27. Carter BL, Morehead J, Wolpert SM, *et al.*: *Cross-Sectional Anatomy*. Appleton-Century-Crofts, New York, 1977 (Sects. 39–43, 45–48, 64–69).
28. Clemente CD: *Gray's Anatomy of the Human Body*, American Ed. 30. Lea & Febiger, Philadelphia, 1985 (pp. 404–406, Figs. 5–70, 5–71).
29. *Ibid.* (pp. 562–563).
30. *Ibid.* (p. 1233).
31. Cox JS: Chondromalacia of the patella: a review and update—Part 1. *Contemp Orthop 6*:17–30, 1983.

32. Deutsch H, Lin DC: Quadriceps kinesiology (EMG) with varying hip joint flexion and resistance. *Arch Phys Med Rehabil 59*:231–236, 1978.
33. Duarte Cintra AI, Furlani J: Electromyographic study of quadriceps femoris in man. *Electromyogr Clin Neurophysiol 21*:539–554, 1981.
34. Duchenne GB: *Physiology of Motion*, translated by E.B. Kaplan. J.B. Lippincott, Philadelphia, 1949 (pp. 275–279).
35. Edgerton VR, Smith JL, Simpson DR: Muscle fibre type populations of human leg muscles. *Histochem J 7*:259–266, 1975.
36. Ericson M: On the biomechanics of cycling. A study of joint and muscle load during exercise on the bicycle ergometer. *Scand J Rehabil Med* (Suppl) *16*:1–43, 1986.
37. Ericson MO, Nisell R, Arborelius UP, *et al.*: Muscular activity during ergometer cycling. *Scand J Rehabil Med 17*:53–61, 1985.
38. Ferner H, Staubesand J: *Sobotta Atlas of Human Anatomy*, Ed. 10, Vol. 2. Urban & Schwarzenberg, Baltimore, 1983 (Fig. 380).
39. *Ibid.* (Figs. 407–409).
40. *Ibid.* (Figs. 410–411b).
41. *Ibid.* (Fig. 413).
42. *Ibid.* (Figs. 420, 421).
43. *Ibid.* (Fig. 464).
44. *Ibid.* (Fig. 465).
45. Garrett WE Jr, Califf JC, Bassett FH III: Histochemical correlates of hamstring injuries. *Am J Sports Med 12*:98–103, 1984.
46. Ghori GMU, Luckwill RG: Responses of the lower limb to load carrying in walking man. *Eur J Appl Physiol 54*:145–150, 1985.
47. Ghosh SN, Nag PK: Muscular strains in different modes of load handling. *Clin Biomech 1*:64–70, 1986.
48. Good MG: What is "fibrositis"? *Rheumatism 5*: 117–123, 1949.
49. Green HJ, Daub B, Houston ME, *et al.*: Human vastus lateralis and gastrocnemius muscles: a comparative histochemical and biochemical analysis. *J Neurol Sci 52*:201–210, 1981.
50. Gregor RJ, Edgerton VR, Rozenek R *et al.*: Skeletal muscle properties and performance in elite female track athletes. *Eur J Appl Physiol 47*:355–364, 1981.
51. Häggmark T, Eriksson E, Jansson E: Muscle fiber type changes in human skeletal muscle after injuries and immobilization. *Orthopedics 9*: 181–185, 1986.
52. Heckmatt JZ, Pier N, Dubowitz V: Measurement of quadriceps muscle thickness and subcutaneous tissue thickness in normal children by real-time ultrasound imaging. *J Clin Ultrasound 16*:171–176, 1988.
53. Hughston JC, Deese M: Medial subluxation of the patella as a complication of lateral retinacular disease. *Am J Sports Med 16*:383–388, 1988.
54. Inbar O, Kaiser P, Tesch P: Relationships between leg muscle fiber type distribution and leg exercise performance. *Int J Sports Med 2*: 154–159, 1981.
55. Inman VT, Ralston HJ, Todd F: *Human Walking*. Williams & Wilkins, Baltimore, 1981 (p. 124).
56. Jones DW, Jones DA, Newham DJ: Chronic knee effusion and aspiration: the effect on quadriceps inhibition. *Br J Rheumatol 26*:370–374, 1987.
57. Joseph J: The pattern of activity of some muscles in women walking on high heels. *Ann Phys Med 9*:295–299, 1968.
58. Kamon E: Electromyographic kinesiology of jumping. *Arch Phys Med Rehabil 52*:152–157, 1971.
59. Kaufer H: Mechanical function of the patella. *J Bone Joint Surg [Am] 53*:1551–1560, 1971.
60. Kellgren JH: Observations on referred pain arising from muscle. *Clin Sci 3*:175–190, 1938.
61. Lange M: *Die Muskelhärten (Myogelosen).* J.F. Lehmanns, München, 1931 (p. 49, Fig. 13).
62. *Ibid.* (pp. 137–138, Fig. 43).
63. *Ibid.* (pp. 156–157, Fig. 52).
64. Leach RE: Running injuries of the knee. *Orthopedics 5*:1358–1377, 1982.
65. Levine M, Lombardo J, McNeeley J, *et al.*: An analysis of individual stretching programs of intercollegiate athletes. *Phys Sportsmed 15*: 130–136, 1987.
66. Lewit K: Postisometric relaxation in combination with other methods of muscular facilitation and inhibition. *Manual Med 2*:101–104, 1986.
67. Lewit K, Simons DG: Myofascial pain: relief by post-isometric relaxation. *Arch Phys Med Rehabil 65*:452–456, 1984.
68. Lexell J, Henriksson-Larsén K, Sjöström M: Distribution of different fibre types in human skeletal muscles: 2. A study of cross-sections of whole m. vastus lateralis. *Acta Physiol Scand 117*:115–122, 1983.
69. Lexell J, Henriksson-Larsén K, Winblad B, *et al.*: Distribution of different fiber types in human skeletal muscles: effects of aging studied in whole muscle cross sections. *Muscle Nerve 6*:588–595, 1983.
70. Lieb FJ, Perry J: Quadriceps function: an anatomical and mechanical study using amputated limbs. *J Bone Joint Surg [Am] 50*:1535–1548, 1968.
71. Lieb FJ, Perry J: Quadriceps function. *J Bone Joint Surg [Am] 53*:749–758, 1971.
72. Lockhart RD: *Living Anatomy*, Ed. 7. Faber & Faber, London, 1974 (p. 114).
73. Losee RE, Johnson TR, Southwick WO: Anterior subluxation of the lateral tibial plateau. *J Bone Joint Surg [Am] 60*:1015–1030, 1978.
74. Markhede G, Stener B: Function after removal of various hip and thigh muscles for extirpation of tumors. *Acta Orthop Scand 52*:373–395, 1981.
75. McMinn RMH, Hutchings RT: *Color Atlas of Human Anatomy*. Year Book Medical Publishers, Chicago, 1977 (pp. 264, 273–275, 277–278, 281–282).
76. *Ibid.* (p. 294).
77. *Ibid.* (p. 299).
78. Miller GM: Resident Review #24: subluxation of the patella. *Orthop Rev 9*:65–76, 1980.
79. Milner M, Basmajian JV, Quanbury AO: Multifactorial analysis of walking by electromyography and computer. *Am J Phys Med 50*:235–258, 1971.
80. Möller M, Ekstrand J, Öberg B, *et al.*: Duration of stretching effect on range of motion in lower

extremities. *Arch Phys Med Rehabil 66*:171–173, 1985.

81. Murray MP, Jacobs PA, Mollinger LA, *et al.*: Functional performance after excision of the vastus lateralis and vastus intermedius. *J Bone Joint Surg [Am] 65*:856–859, 1983.
82. Németh G, Ekholm J, Arborelius UP: Hip load moments and muscular activity during lifting. *Scand J Rehabil Med 16*:103–111, 1984.
83. Netter FH: *The Ciba Collection of Medical Illustrations*, Vol.8, Musculoskeletal System. Part I: Anatomy, Physiology and Metabolic Disorders. Ciba-Geigy Corporation, Summit, 1987 (p. 80).
84. *Ibid.* (p. 83).
85. *Ibid.* (p. 85).
86. *Ibid.* (p. 87).
87. Nielsen AJ: Spray and stretch for myofascial pain. *Phys Ther 58*:567–569, 1978.
88. Nygaard E: Skeletal muscle fibre characteristics in young women. *Acta Physiol Scand 112*: 299–304, 1981.
89. Oddsson L, Thorstensson A: Fast voluntary trunk flexion movements in standing: motor patterns. *Acta Physiol Scand 129*:93–106, 1987.
90. Okada M: An electromyographic estimation of the relative muscular load in different human postures. *J Human Ergol 1*:75–93, 1972.
91. Radin EL: Chondromalacia of the patella. *Bull Rheum Dis 34*:1–6, 1984.
92. Rasch PJ, Burke RK: *Kinesiology and Applied Anatomy*, Ed. 6. Lea & Febiger, Philadelphia, 1978 (pp. 272, 282, 292–293, 309, Table 162).
93. Rask MR, Lattig GJ: Traumatic fibrosis of the rectus femoris muscle. *JAMA 221*:268–269, 1972.
94. Reynolds L, Levin TA, Medeiros JM, *et al.*: EMG activity of the vastus medialis oblique and the vastus lateralis in their role in patellar alignment. *Am J Phys Med 62*:61–70, 1983.
95. Reynolds MD: Myofascial trigger point syndromes in the practice of rheumatology. *Arch Phys Med Rehabil 62*:111–114, 1981.
96. Rohen JW, Yokochi C: *Color Atlas of Anatomy*, Ed. 2. Igaku-Shoin, New York, 1988 (p. 416).
97. *Ibid.* (p. 417).
98. Sadamoto T, Bonde-Petersen F, Suzuki Y: Skeletal muscle tension, flow, pressure, and EMG during sustained isometric contractions in humans. *Eur J Appl Physiol 51*:395–408, 1983.
99. Scelsi R, Marchetti C, Poggi P: Histochemical and ultrastructural aspects of m. vastus lateralis in sedentary old people (age 65–89 years). *Acta Neuropathol 51*:99–105, 1980.
100. Shakespeare DT, Stokes M, Sherman KP, *et al.*: Reflex inhibition of the quadriceps after meniscectomy: lack of association with pain. *Clin Physiol 5*:137–144, 1985.
101. Simons DG: Myofascial pain syndrome due to trigger points, Chapter 45. In *Rehabilitation Medicine*, edited by Joseph Goodgold. C.V. Mosby Co., St. Louis, 1988 (pp. 686–723, see p. 710, Fig. 45–8E to 8H).
102. Simons DG, Travell JG: Myofascial pain syndromes, Chapter 25. In *Textbook of Pain*, edited by P.D. Wall and R. Melzack, Ed 2. Churchill Livingstone, London, 1989 (pp. 368–385, see p. 377, Fig. 25.8F–H).
103. *Ibid.* (p. 378, Fig. 25.9B).
104. Simons DG, Travell JG, Simons LS: Protecting the ozone layer. *Arch Phys Med Rehabil 71*:64, 1990.
105. Sjøgaard G: Muscle energy metabolism and electrolyte shifts during low-level prolonged static contraction in man. *Acta Physiol Scand 134*:181–187, 1988.
106. Stålberg E, Borges O, Ericsson M, *et al.*: The quadriceps femoris muscle in 20–70-year-old subjects: relationship between knee extension torque, electrophysiological parameters, and muscle fiber characteristics. *Muscle Nerve 12*: 382–389, 1989.
107. Sutherland DH, Cooper L, Daniel D: The role of the ankle plantar flexors in normal walking. *J Bone Joint Surg [Am] 62*:354–363, 1980.
108. Swenson EJ Jr, Hough DO, McKeag DB: Patellofemoral dysfunction. *Postgrad Med 82*:125–141, 1987.
109. Taylor PW: Inflammation of the deep infrapatellar bursa of the knee. *Arthritis Rheum 32*: 1312–1314, 1989.
110. Townsend MA, Lainhart SP, Shiavi R, *et al.*: Variability and biomechanics of synergy patterns of some lower-limb muscles during ascending and descending stairs and level walking. *Med Biol Eng Comput 16*:681–688, 1978.
111. Travell J: Pain mechanisms in connective tissue. In *Connective Tissues, Transactions of the Second Conference, 1951*, edited by C. Ragan. Josiah Macy, Jr. Foundation, New York, 1952 (pp. 86–125, see p. 116).
112. Travell J: Factors affecting pain of injection. *JAMA 158*:368–371, 1955.
113. Travell J, Rinzler SH: The myofascial genesis of pain. *Postgrad Med 11*:425–434, 1952.
114. Travell JG, Simons DG: *Myofascial Pain and Dysfunction: The Trigger Point Manual*. Williams & Wilkins, Baltimore, 1983.
115. Troedsson BS: The buckling knee syndrome. *Minn Med 55*:722–724, 1972.
116. Vecchiet L, Marini I, Colozzi A, *et al.*: Effects of aerobic exercise on muscular pain sensitivity. *Clin Ther 6*:354–363, 1984.
117. Voss DE, Ionta MK, Myers BJ: *Proprioceptive Neuromuscular Facilitation*, Ed. 3. Harper and Row, Philadelphia, 1985.
118. Weber EF: Ueber die Längenverhältnisse der Fleischfasern der Muskeln in Allgemeinen. *Berichte über die Verhandlungen der Königlich Sächsischen Gesellschaft der Wissenschaften zu Leipzig 3*:63–86, 1851.
119. Worrell RV: The diagnosis of disorders of the patellofemoral joint. *Orthop Rev 10*:73–76, 1981.
120. Worth RM, Kettelkamp DB, Defalque RJ, *et al.*: Saphenous nerve entrapment: a cause of medial knee pain. *Am J Sports Med 12*:80–81, 1984.
121. Yang JF, Winter DA: Surface EMG profiles during different walking cadences in humans. *Electroencephalogr Clin Neurophysiol 60*:485–491, 1985.
122. Young A, Stokes M, Iles JF: Effects of joint pathology on muscle. *Clin Orthop 219*:21–27, 1987.

CHAPTER 15
Adductor Muscles of the Hip
Adductor Longus, Adductor Brevis, Adductor Magnus, and Gracilis

"Obvious Problem-makers"

HIGHLIGHTS: **REFERRED PAIN** from myofascial trigger points (TrPs) in the adductor longus and adductor brevis muscles of the thigh travels upward deep in the groin and downward to the knee and shin. The TrPs at midthigh level in the adductor magnus (TrP_1 region) refer pain to the anteromedial aspect of the thigh from the groin to just above the knee. This muscle's proximal TrPs (TrP_2 region) refer severe pain deep within the pelvis. Gracilis TrPs can refer superficial pain along the length of the medial thigh. Proximal **ANATOMICAL ATTACHMENTS** of the adductor longus, adductor brevis, and two-thirds of the adductor magnus are to the lower borders of the pelvis, extending along the pubic ramus and the ischial ramus to the ischial tuberosity. Distally, these muscles attach in a vertical line along the back of the femur from the lesser trochanter to a point a short distance above the knee. The three adductor muscles overlap each other with the adductor longus in front and the adductor magnus behind. The remaining third of the adductor magnus (the ischiocondylar part) attaches proximally in the region of the ischial tuberosity and distally to the adductor tubercle on the medial condyle of the femur. The gracilis muscle overlies the adductor magnus and is attached to the pelvis medial to the ischiocondylar part of the adductor magnus. The gracilis anchors below the knee to the tibia as part of the pes anserinus. **INNERVATION** of these muscles is via the obturator nerve, except for the ischiocondylar part of the adductor magnus, which is innervated by the sciatic nerve. During the stance phase of gait, the adductors **FUNCTION** to restrain abduction of the stance limb, controlling lateral shift and adding stability. The gracilis assists other muscles in controlling the valgus angulation of the knee. During early swing phase, adductors bring the limb toward the midline (primarily by the adductor magnus); late in the swing phase, the adductors and gracilis help maintain flexion for forward reach. The primary action of all the muscles in this chapter is adduction of the thigh. The adductor longus, adductor brevis, and the anterior two parts of the adductor magnus also assist medial rotation and flexion of the thigh. The posterior (ischiocondylar or "hamstring") part of the adductor magnus is, on the other hand, an extensor of the thigh and has an equivocal effect on its rotation. The gracilis also assists flexion of the knee when the knee is extended, and medial rotation of the leg when the knee is flexed. The chief **SYMPTOM** of the patient with adductor TrPs is pain and tenderness in their referred patterns. Pectineus and vastus medialis TrPs have referral zones that partly overlap those of the adductors. In addition, in making the diagnosis, the clinician needs to consider pain caused by avulsion of the pelvic or tibial attachments of adductor muscles, stress fracture of the inferior ischial or pubic ramus of the pelvis, pubic stress symphysitis, osteoarthritis of the hip joint, nerve entrapment, and psychological stress. **PATIENT EXAMINATION** focuses on evaluating restriction of thigh abduction and on palpation of the muscles. **TRIGGER POINT EXAMINATION** of the subcutaneous adductor longus and gracilis muscles is generally satisfactory using flat palpation. However, both the adductor brevis and the bulky adductor magnus are nearly completely covered by other muscles, making localization of TrPs in them difficult and dependent on deep palpation. **EN-**

PART 2

TRAPMENT of the femoral artery and vein and the saphenous nerve can occur as they exit the adductor canal at the adductor hiatus. **INTERMITTENT COLD WITH STRETCH** of the adductor muscles generally starts with the patient supine and with the thigh flexed and moved passively toward abduction. Intermittent cold is applied in parallel sweeps over the anterior and medial thigh from midthigh upward over the groin and inguinal area, and downward from midthigh over the knee and shin to the ankle. Gentle pressure is applied to take up any slack in hip abduction. Application of a moist heating pad and full active range of motion complete the procedure. **INJECTION AND STRETCH** of the adductor longus and gracilis muscles is like that for TrPs in other superficial muscles. In addition, however, for the adductor longus as well as for the adductor brevis, the adjacent femoral artery must be considered. The adductor magnus presents serious problems in locating its TrPs and then reaching them for injection; it is a bulky muscle that, for the most part, lies underneath other muscles. **CORRECTIVE ACTIONS** for these hip adductors primarily include avoiding immobility that places them in a shortened position for long periods, correcting systemic perpetuating factors, and providing an adequate home stretch program.

---

1. REFERRED PAIN
(Figs. 15.1–15.3)

The referred pain patterns and limited function due to trigger points (TrPs) in these adductor muscles are what one might expect, with the exception of the posterior portion of the adductor magnus, hence their characterization as "obvious problem-makers." TrP involvement of the adductor longus is perhaps the most common cause of groin pain.[97,98]

PART 2

Adductor Longus and Adductor Brevis

The authors draw no distinction between the patterns of pain and tenderness referred from TrPs in the adductor longus and the adductor brevis (Fig. 15.1). These TrPs project pain both proximally and distally. The proximal pattern is consistently present; pain is experienced deep in, and proximal to, the groin and in the anteromedial portion of the upper thigh. Referral of pain from these TrPs distally focuses on the upper medial part of the knee with a spillover pattern that extends downward over the tibia (Fig. 15.1). This pain pattern has been described and illustrated previously.[93,94,97,98,100] The TrPs located in the more proximal part of the muscles usually refer pain upward to the groin and those located in the more distal part of the muscles tend to refer pain downward to the knee and the tibia.[97]

Kelly[52,53] characterized the tender spot in the adductor longus near its proximal attachment as referring pain to the knee and causing stiffness. Long[61] characterized the adductor longus syndrome caused by TrPs as producing pain in the medial thigh near the groin, in the vicinity of the medial portion of the inguinal ligament, and superficially along the medial or anterior thigh to the knee. It often was accompanied by a gelling phenomenon [taut bands].

Kellgren[51] illustrated the pain referred from the adductor longus muscle when it was injected with 0.1 mL of 6% saline solution. The pattern corresponded closely to that of Figure 15.1 except that he did not report pain extending below the knee.

In children,[17] the essential referred pain from adductor longus TrPs was illustrated distal to the inguinal ligament; its spillover pattern covered the anteromedial thigh, medial knee, and upper two-thirds of the medial aspect of the leg. Fine[46] reported inguinal pain in a 10-year-old boy caused by TrPs in the adductors of the thigh.

Adductor Magnus

The relatively common myofascial TrP location in the midportion of the adductor magnus muscle, the TrP_1 region, refers pain upward into the groin below the inguinal ligament and also downward over the anteromedial aspect of the thigh nearly to the knee (Fig. 15.2*A*). This groin pain is described as deep, almost as if it might be in the pelvis, but the patient is unable to identify pain in any specific

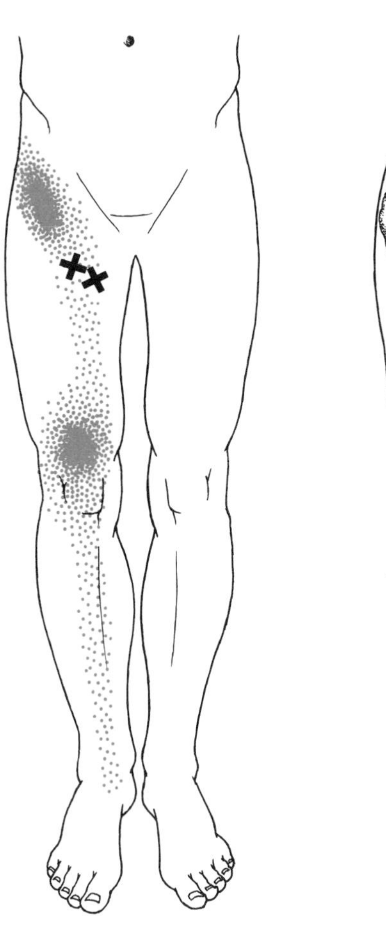

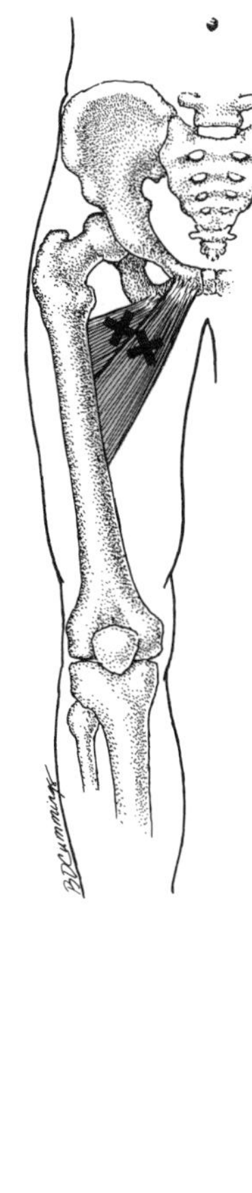

Figure 15.1. Anterior view of the right adductor longus and adductor brevis muscles and the composite pain pattern, (*dark red*) referred from TrPs (**X**s) in these two muscles (*light red*). The essential pain pattern is *solid red*; *red stippling* indicates occasional extension to a spillover pain pattern.

PART 2

pelvic structure. Many patients have a mistaken idea of where the groin is. When the patient uses that descriptive term, he or she should be asked to point to the exact location of the pain. "Groin" generally applies to the inguinal region, but may indicate the anterior crease at the junction of the thigh with the trunk.[96]

Pain referred from TrPs in the more proximal TrP_2 region of the adductor magnus is usually described as a generalized internal pelvic pain, but may be identified as including the pubic bone, vagina, rectum, or (less often) the bladder (Fig. 15.2*B*). The pain may be described as shooting up inside the pelvis and exploding like a firecracker.

Gracilis

The TrPs in the gracilis muscle produce a local, hot, stinging (not prickling), superficial pain that travels up and down along the inside of the thigh (Fig. 15.3).

2. ANATOMICAL ATTACHMENTS AND CONSIDERATIONS
(Figs. 15.4–15.8)

The adductor muscles lie in the medial thigh between the quadriceps femoris group of muscles toward the front and the hamstring muscles behind. The most anterior of the three major adductors is the adductor longus; the adductor brevis is intermediate and the adductor magnus is the most posterior.

A fourth adductor, the pectineus muscle (Chapter 13), lies partly anterior and superior to the adductor brevis. The gracilis is the only one of this muscle group that crosses two joints—the hip and the knee.

Adductor Longus and Adductor Brevis
(Figs. 15.4 and 15.5)

The **adductor longus** is the most superficial and the most prominent of the three

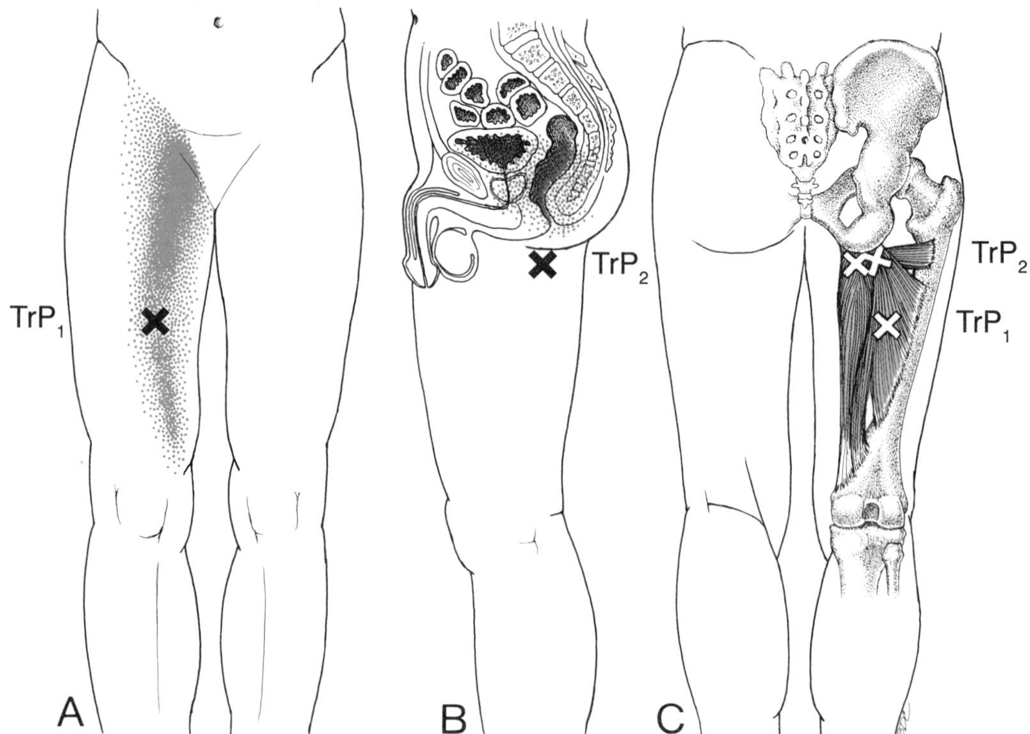

Figure 15.2. Pain pattern (*dark red*) referred from trigger points (***X**s*) in the right adductor magnus muscle (*light red*). The essential pain pattern is *solid red*; *red stippling* locates occasional extension of the referred pain in a spillover pattern. *A*, anterior view of the referred pain pattern from the midthigh TrP_1 region; *B*, midsagittal view showing the intrapelvic pain pattern referred from the TrP_2 region. These trigger points are found in the most proximal portion of the ischiocondylar part of the adductor magnus medial to or deep to the gluteus maximus muscle. *C*, posterior view, anatomy of the muscle and location of its common trigger points.

major adductor muscles in the anteromedial aspect of the thigh. It attaches ***proximally*** by a narrow flat tendon to a relatively small spot on the outer surface of the pelvis between the symphysis pubis and the obturator foramen (Fig. 15.4).[27,67] Its fibers angle downward, laterally, and posteriorly to anchor ***distally*** to the linea aspera on the middle third of the femur. The linea aspera extends down the back of the femur and also receives the vastus medialis on the medial side, and laterally, the adductor magnus, which wraps around behind the adductor longus and adductor brevis (Figs. 15.5 and 15.7). The fibers of the adductor longus often blend with those of the vastus medialis distally at their femoral attachment. The adductor longus may unite above with the pectineus, in which case they completely cover the adductor brevis from in front.

Viewed from the front, the **adductor brevis** is partly covered by the pectineus proximally and by the adductor longus distally (Fig. 15.5). It is sandwiched between these two adductor muscles anteriorly and the adductor magnus posteriorly. The attachment of the adductor brevis ***proximally*** to the inferior ramus of the pubis is surrounded by the gracilis medially, the obturator externus laterally, and, to some extent, by the adductor magnus behind.[2] The adductor brevis attaches ***distally*** to the linea aspera just lateral to and behind the adductor longus, and the adductor magnus attaches lateral to and behind the adductor brevis.[43] The vastus medialis attaches medial to all of these adductor muscles, thus covering the lower part of the adductor longus and adductor magnus from in front.[27,73]

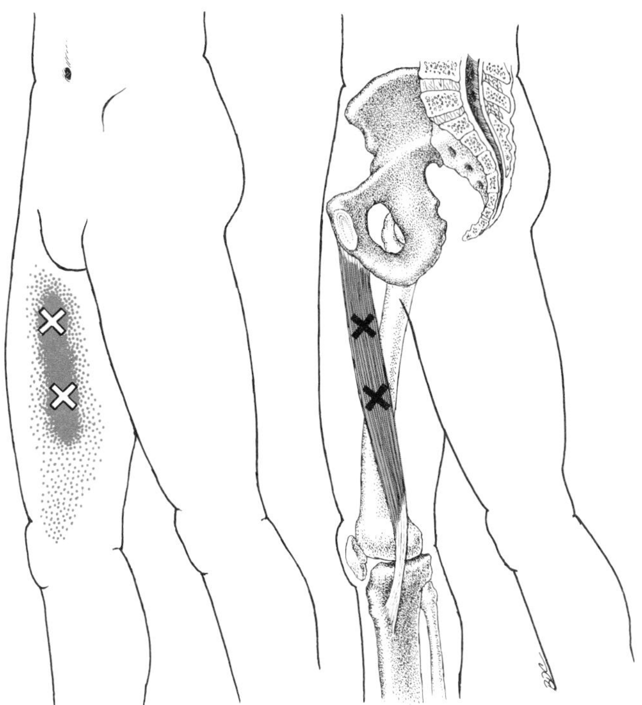

Figure 15.3. Medial view of the composite pain pattern (*dark red*) referred from trigger points (**X**s) in the right gracilis muscle (*light red*). *Solid red* denotes the essential pain pattern and *red stippling* indicates the occasional spillover pain pattern.

Adductor Magnus
(Figs. 15.6 and 15.7)

The adductor magnus is a large and, for the most part, a deeply placed muscle that is best understood as the tripartite structure described by Bardeen:[13] the most anterior and uppermost adductor minimus, the middle part, and the posteriorly placed (largely ischiocondylar) third part. This arrangement is comparable to that of the other three hip adductors (pectineus, adductor brevis, and adductor longus). The uppermost of the three parts of the adductor magnus, often known as the adductor minimus, attaches to the pelvis anterior to the attachment of the middle part, and its fibers are the most horizontal. The middle part may overlap the adductor minimus posteriorly. If so, these intermediate fibers run more diagonally. Proximally, the bulk of the third (most posterior or ischiocondylar) part attaches to the ischial tuberosity. Some of its fibers are oriented diagonally, but most are nearly vertical.

The uppermost part of the adductor magnus (adductor minimus) is the most anterior of the three parts. Its fibers lie nearly horizontal; they angle down only slightly from their ***medial*** (anterior) attachment on the inferior pubic ramus to their ***lateral*** (posterior) femoral attachment starting just below the lesser trochanter and extending down along the upper part of the linea aspera (Figs. 15.4–15.6). This anterior upper part of the adductor magnus usually constitutes a separate muscle belly.

The middle part of the adductor magnus muscle is fan shaped (Figs. 15.5 and 15.6) and may overlap the adductor minimus. Its apex attaches ***proximally*** along the ischial ramus between the ischial tuberosity and the inferior pubic ramus. From this apex, it fans out to attach ***distally*** along the linea aspera down to the tendinous (adductor) hiatus, through which the femoral vessels pass. An upward extension of this hiatus often clearly separates the middle and posterior parts of the adductor magnus (Figs. 15.5 and 15.7).[7]

Most of the fibers of the massive ischiocondylar part of the adductor magnus travel vertically (Figs. 15.6 and 15.7). The fibers attach ***proximally*** in the region of the ischial tuberosity and,

PART 2

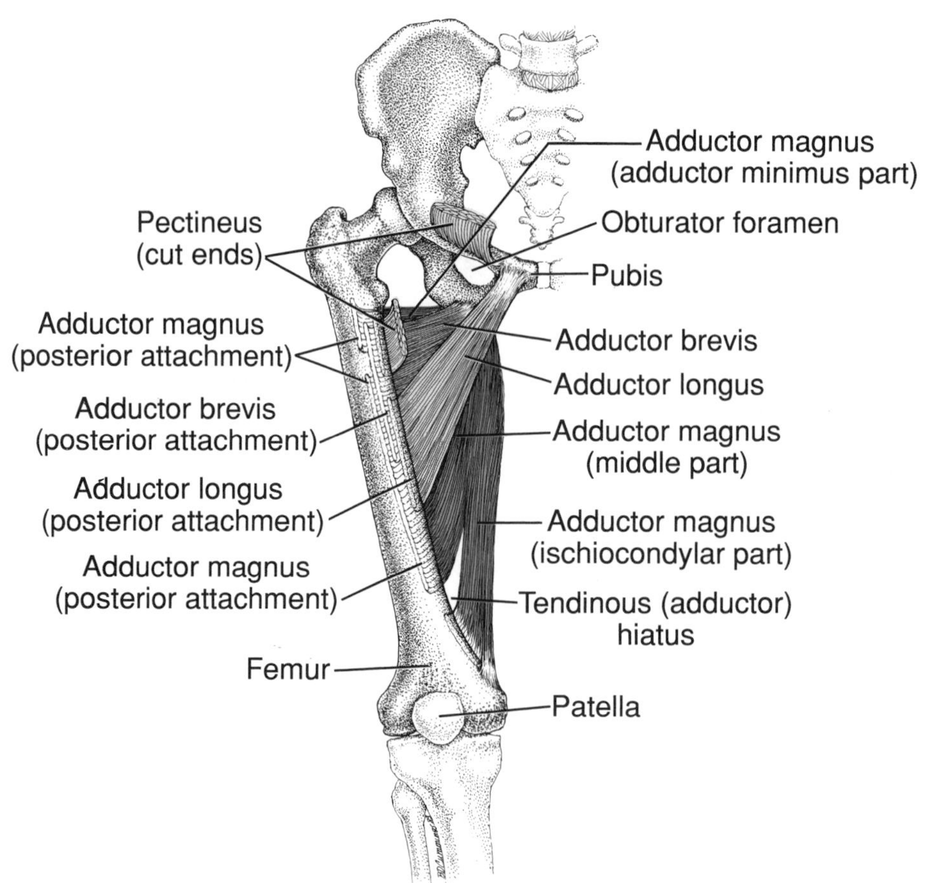

Figure 15.4. Attachments of the right adductor muscle group, front view. The pectineus muscle is cut and largely removed (*light red*). The most superficial adductor muscle, the adductor longus, is also *light red*. The adductor brevis (*medium red*) extends distally only to the middle section of the femoral attachment of the adductor longus and deep to it. The adductor magnus (*dark red*) is the deepest (most posterior) and the largest of the adductor muscles. Attachments of these muscles to the posterior aspect of the femur are rendered schematically.

to some extent, forward along the ischial ramus, largely posterior to the other two parts of the muscle. As seen in the front, back, and medial views (Figs. 15.5–15.7), the fibers along the upper medial border of this ischiocondylar part curl around the middle part. This permits concentrated attachment of most of the adductor magnus fibers in the region of the ischial tuberosity. ***Distally***, most of the large third part anchors by a thick tendon to the adductor tubercle on the medial condyle of the femur. A few fibers attach to a fibrous expansion that completes the space between the adductor tubercle and the tendinous (adductor) hiatus (Fig. 15.6).[27] This part of the adductor magnus is similar to a "hamstring" muscle except that it does not cross the knee joint; it is supplied by the sciatic nerve.

Bardeen[13] describes the adductor magnus as forming a groove in which the medial hamstring muscles (semimembranosus and semitendinosus) lie. Sometimes this is clearly evident.[8] The floor of the groove is formed mainly by the middle part, and the medial wall of the groove by the ischiocondylar part, of the adductor magnus. This configuration of the third part of the adductor magnus is poorly represented in the cross sections generally available, but is clearly seen in the cross section by Bardeen.[13] Thus, the bulk of the adductor magnus lies deep and medial to the semitendinosus and semimembranosus muscles. The anatomy

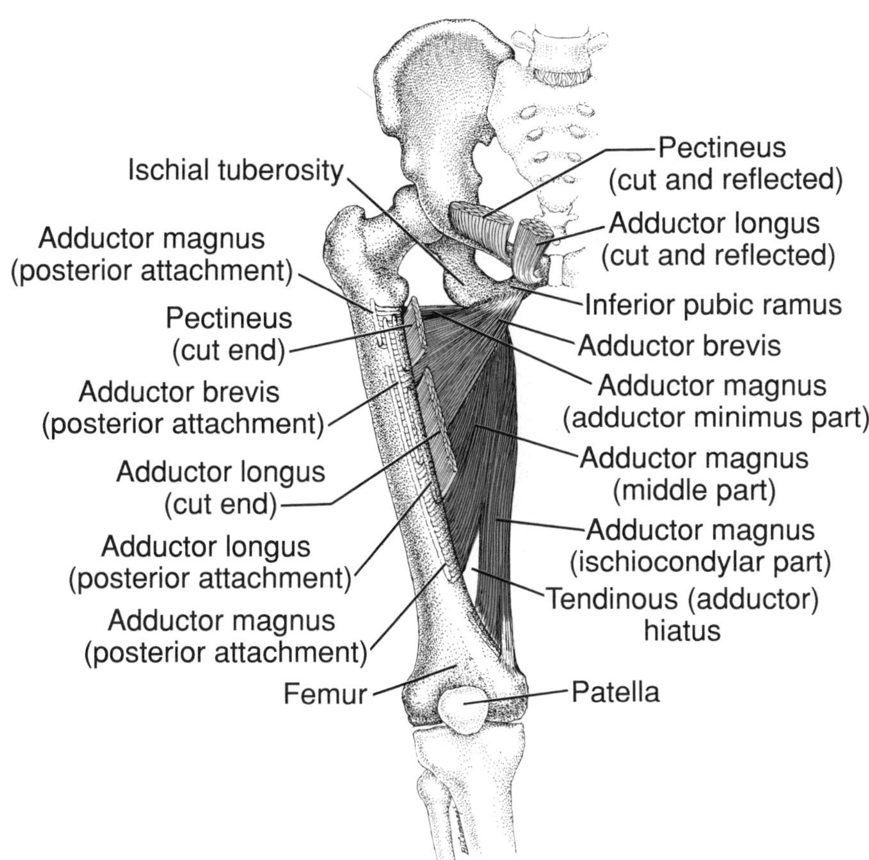

Figure 15.5. Attachments of the right deep adductor muscles, front view. The overlying pectineus and adductor longus have been cut and the ends reflected (*light red*). The adductor brevis (*medium red*) lies anterior to the larger adductor magnus (*dark red*). Attachments of the adductor muscles to the posterior aspect of the femur, not in view, are rendered schematically.

of the adductor canal and of the adductor hiatus is described in Section 10, Entrapments.

The adductor magnus is comparable in cross sectional area to the vastus lateralis in the upper and midthigh;[76] the vastus lateralis is the largest of the quadriceps femoris group of muscles. The adductor magnus is the third heaviest muscle in the body (505 gm), more than two-thirds the weight of the gluteus maximus and slightly less than the combined weight of all three hamstring muscles (638 gm).[102] Thus, this "hamstring-like" adductor is heavier than any single hamstring muscle.[102]

Gracilis
(Fig. 15.8)

The superficial gracilis muscle extends the length of the medial aspect of the thigh; it crosses two joints, the hip and the knee (Fig 15.8, medial view). Most of the muscle is seen from the front in relation to other thigh muscles in Figure 14.13 of the previous chapter, and it is seen in cross section at approximately midthigh level in Figure 14.8 of that same chapter (quadriceps). This thin, flat muscle attaches ***proximally*** to the lower rim of the outside of the pelvis at the junction of the body of the pubis and the inferior pubic ramus. The gracilis anchors ***distally*** to the medial surface of the tibia distal to the tibial condyle. Here, its tendon joins the sartorius and semitendinosus tendons to form the pes anserinus (*see* Fig. 15.8 in this chapter and Fig. 12.7 in Chapter 12). The anserine bursa lies between these tendons and the tibia.[27]

The gracilis has been identified as the second longest muscle in the body (without considering gross inscriptions) and the sartorius as the long-

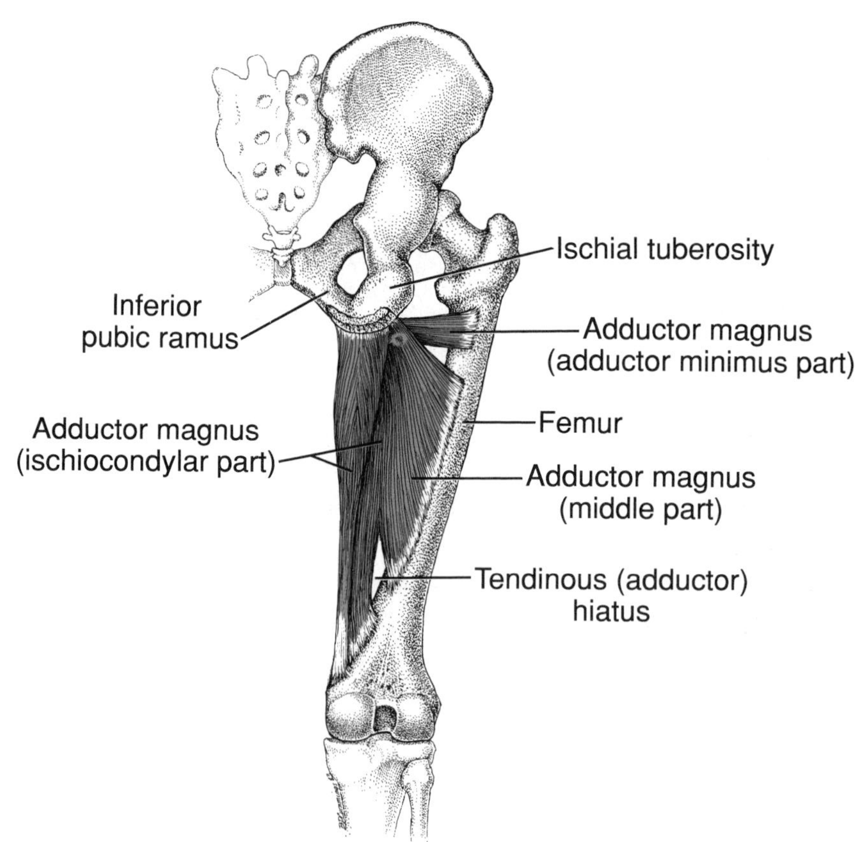

Figure 15.6. Attachments (posterior view) of the right adductor magnus muscle (*red*) showing the distinctions among its three parts.

est.[102] One report describes the gracilis as being innervated by scattered endplates, which supports the microdissection evidence that it comprises parallel bundles of short fibers linked together sequentially.[29] Another author[26] describes and illustrates two clearly distinguishable bands of endplates as if the muscle had developed from two myoblasts that subsequently fused at midmuscle. (The bellies of the rectus abdominis and semitendinosus muscles are also segmented in this manner, which limits the length of their fibers.)

Supplemental References

Adductors Longus, Brevis, and Magnus

All three adductor muscles are presented in front view with associated vessels and nerves that pass through the adductor canal[3,77] and in cross section.[1,39,76] The locations of their bony attachments are marked proximally and distally,[2,43,75] in detail just proximally at the pelvis,[67] in detail distally,[68] and all attachments are shown schematically.[5]

The adductor longus is illustrated alone from in front without neurovascular structures,[73] and with the adductor brevis.[88] The adductor longus is seen from in front with vessels and nerves in relation to the sartorius muscle[37] and from an anteromedial view in relation to the neurovascular contents of the adductor canal.[38] The adductor longus[21] and the adductor brevis[20] are shown throughout their length in serial cross sections. Photographs of the surface contours identify the adductor mass[60] and the adductor longus.[34]

As noted previously, the adductor magnus is often illustrated together with the adductor longus and adductor brevis. A photograph[89] of the adductor magnus includes its most proximal part, the adductor minimus, from in front without neurovascular structures. The three muscles are also seen from in front with neurovascular structures.[74]

Posterior views of the adductor magnus without neurovascular structures illustrate how little of the muscle is immediately subcutaneous in the upper half of the thigh[36] and throughout the length of the thigh.[42,90] One posterior view shows the entire muscle with overlying structures removed, revealing the marked division between its middle and posterior parts, between which the

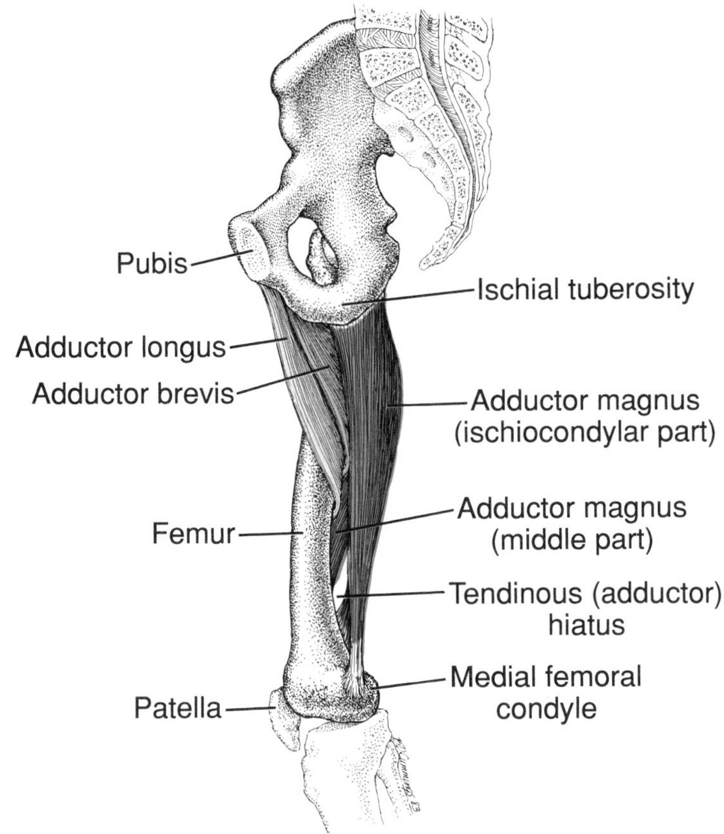

Figure 15.7. Attachments (medial view) of the right adductor longus (*light red*), adductor brevis (*medium red*), and adductor magnus (*dark red*) muscles. This unusual view shows the basis for the functional difference between the ischiocondylar part of the adductor magnus and the remaining adductor muscles, namely, its more posterior attachment to the pelvis and femur so that it can extend the thigh.

femoral artery and vein emerge.[7] The attachment of its tendon posteriorly on the medial femoral condyle appears in detail.[70]

A posterior view of the length of the thigh portrays the relationship of both the middle and the distal ends of the posterior portion of the adductor magnus muscle to the sciatic nerve and to the vessels traversing the tendinous (adductor) hiatus.[78] One posterior view shows the relationship of the adductor magnus to the overlying muscles, their relationship to the sciatic nerve, and the groove in the adductor magnus that receives the hamstring muscles.[8] The sciatic nerve is shown passing between the adductor magnus muscle in front and the hamstring muscles behind.[8,78] Serial cross sections portray the bulk of the adductor magnus[24] and also its uppermost adductor minimus part.[23] All parts of the adductor magnus are shown in sagittal section.[35,66] The schematic of the muscle in anterior and posterior views gives some indication of the overlap between its uppermost, nearly horizontal fibers and its medial fibers that are longitudinal.[49]

Gracilis

The gracilis is seen from in front without neurovascular structures in drawings[4,73] and in photographs,[88,89] and in drawings with neurovascular structures.[3,37] The muscle is presented from the medial side in full length without neurovascular structures[6,41] and in detail at its attachment below the knee.[44,79] Its rear view is portrayed without neurovascular structures.[42] Its bony attachments are marked[9,10,43,45,75] in detail at the pelvis[67] and at the knee.[69,80] The gracilis muscle is shown in a cross section,[1] in three serial cross sections,[39,76] and in a full series of cross sections.[22] Its sagittal section is presented as a drawing[35] and as a photograph.[66]

3. INNERVATION

The adductor longus, the adductor brevis, and the first (adductor minimus) and second (middle) parts of the adductor magnus

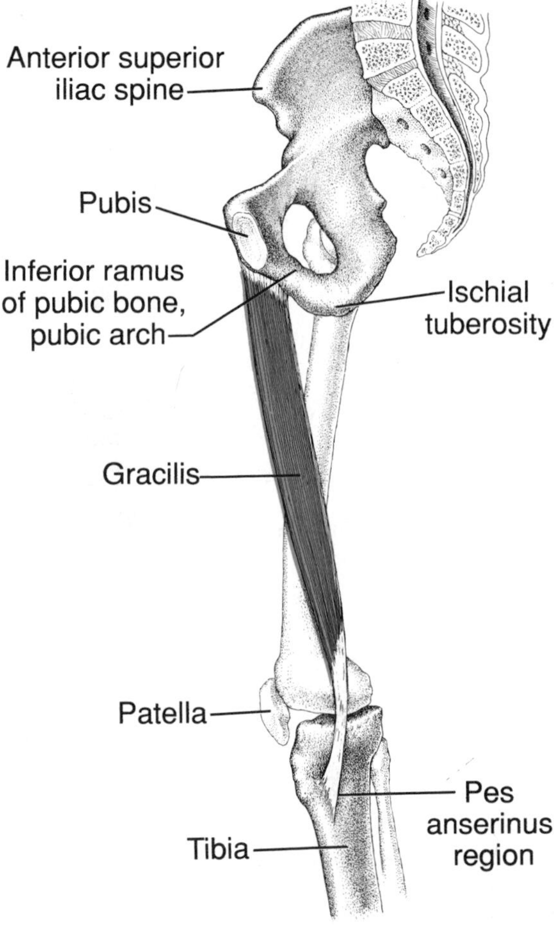

Figure 15.8. Attachments (medial view) of the right gracilis muscle (*red*).

are supplied by the anterior division of the obturator nerve (as illustrated[72]). This nerve contains fibers from the second, third, and fourth lumbar spinal nerves.[16,27] The adductor minimus part of the adductor magnus may also receive fibers from a branch of the nerve to the quadratus femoris muscle, which lies cephalad and parallel to the adductor minimus.[13] The ischiocondylar ("hamstring") part of the adductor magnus receives innervation via the sciatic nerve[27] from the fourth and fifth lumbar and first sacral spinal nerves.[40]

The anterior division of the obturator nerve also supplies the gracilis muscle, but from only the second and third lumbar nerves.[27]

4. FUNCTION

The adductor longus becomes active around the time of toe-off, and the adductor magnus around the time of heel-strike during walking, jogging, running, and sprinting. The adductor magnus becomes active during ascent of stairs, but is inactive during descent. It is also active when "stemming" during skiing and while gripping the sides of the horse with the knees when riding.

The adductors probably play several roles in walking. During the early swing phase (pick up), the adductor magnus brings the limb toward the midline; during late swing, the adductors and the gracilis help increase and maintain hip flexion for the forward reach of the limb.[84] During the earliest part of the stance phase, the gracilis may be functioning to assist the other pes anserinus muscles and the vastus medialis in controlling the valgus angulation of the knee as body weight is shifted onto that foot.[84] During early stance, the ischiocondylar part of the adductor magnus is in a position to assist the hamstrings and gluteus maximus in restraining the tendency toward hip flexion that is produced by body weight. Later in stance, as weight is shifting toward and across the midline to the other foot, the adductor longus and adductor magnus restrain abduction, controlling the weight shift and adding stability.[84]

Actions

There is general agreement that the primary action of the gracilis muscle and all three major adductors is adduction of the thigh at the hip.[14,27,30,31,85]

The adductor longus, adductor brevis, and the anterior (upper) portion of the adductor magnus assist flexion and medial rotation of the thigh.[30] The posterior (ischiocondylar, "hamstring") portion of the adductor magnus acts as an extensor of the thigh,[27,85] and was not recruited electromyographically during flexion effort.[14] Its effect on rotation is equivocal.[14]

These muscles are active in association with knee flexion or extension in children and, to a lesser degree, in adults.[14] This may serve a stabilizing function.

Among the four adductor muscles covered in this chapter, only the fibers of the gracilis cross both the hip and knee joints. The gracilis muscle is primarily an adductor of the thigh.[15,27,50,85] It assists thigh flexion to some extent.[31] It assists flexion of the knee only if the knee is extended and assists medial rotation of the tibia when the knee is flexed.[15,27,50]

Functions

During ambulation, electromyographic (EMG) recordings with fine-wire electrodes in the adductor longus consistently showed that it was active just before, during, and for a short time after toe-off (end of stance phase). The adductor magnus was active just before, during, and for a short time after heel-strike (end of swing and beginning of stance phase).[28,47,62] Which part of the adductor magnus was not explicitly stated, but it was probably the ischiocondylar part. Basmajian and Deluca[14] noted that the anterior part of the adductor magnus was active nearly continuously throughout the gait cycle, whereas the ischiocondylar part showed biphasic activity characteristic of the hamstring muscles.

With increasing speed of ambulation, the intensity and duration of the peak of EMG activity in the adductor magnus at heel-strike increased,[47] and activity appeared earlier in the cycle.[62] Leaning forward while walking markedly increased its EMG activity.[47] During stair ascension, the adductor magnus showed a strong burst of activity around the beginning of stance phase and no activity during descent.[62]

During the more strenuous activities of jogging, running, and sprinting, the adductor longus did not change its basic (walking) pattern of activity but extended its duration somewhat.[63]

Since the rationale for these ambulation activity patterns is not clear, Basmajian and Deluca[14] concluded that adductor activity is facilitated through reflexes of the gait pattern and that these muscles do not function as prime movers of the hip.

The adductor magnus is utilized for medial rotation of the thigh in such activities as "stemming" when skiing and in gripping the sides of a horse with the knees when riding.[85]

Broer and Houtz[19] found that during right-handed sports activities the EMG activity of the right gracilis muscle, recorded from surface electrodes, was always at least equal to, and usually greater than, that of the contralateral left muscle. The greatest gracilis EMG activity was seen during jumping for a one-foot volleyball spike or for a basketball layup. The activities causing the next greatest EMG response of the gracilis were the tennis serve and batting a ball. These gracilis recordings by surface electrodes may have included considerable adductor magnus EMG activity.

A patient, who had had the entire adductor longus excised, fully compensated by hypertrophy of the remaining adductor muscles and showed no loss of strength or apparent impairment of ambulation on level surfaces, on stairs, and when jumping.[64] Extirpation of the adductors longus, brevis, and magnus resulted in a 70% loss of adduction strength, but only slight or moderate impairment of walking, stair climbing, or jumping.[64]

5. FUNCTIONAL (MYOTATIC) UNIT

For thigh adduction, the major adductor muscles work with the pectineus and gracilis muscles; adduction is countered by the gluteus medius, gluteus minimus, and the tensor fasciae latae muscles. For medial rotation, the adductor group works with the anterior part of the gluteus minimus muscle and is antagonistic to the lateral rotation function of the gluteus maximus, the posterior part of the gluteus minimus, and the iliopsoas.[85]

The middle part of the adductor magnus and the short head of the biceps femoris have the same fiber direction and a contiguous attachment on the linea aspera along the back of the femur. Together they give the appearance of one muscle except for the dividing line of their common attachment to the femur.[42] Thus, when these two muscles contract at the same time, they *together* function similarly to one hamstring owing to the proximal attachment of the adductor magnus to the ischial tuberosity, and the distal attachment of the short head of the biceps femoris to the head of the fibula with an expansion to the lateral condyle of the tibia. They have the advantage of attachment to the femur so that each end of this composite "two-joint" structure can exert force independent of the other. This hip-extensor, knee-flexor function is synergistic with that of the biceps femoris (long head), semitendinosus, and semimembranosus muscles.

For hip adduction, the gracilis acts with the three primary adductors of the thigh and the pectineus. For flexion at the knee, the gracilis assists the three hamstring muscles when the knee is straight. For medial rotation of the leg at the knee, it assists the semimembranosus, semitendinosus, and popliteus muscles.[85]

6. SYMPTOMS

Adductor Longus and Adductor Brevis

Patients with TrPs in these two adductor muscles are frequently aware of the pain in the groin and medial thigh only during vigorous activity or muscular overload, rather than at rest. The pain is increased by weight bearing and by sudden twists of the hip.[61] The patients often do not realize how severely abduction of the thigh is restricted but, occasionally, they note restricted lateral rotation of the thigh.

Adductor Magnus

Patients with active TrPs in the proximal end of the adductor magnus, TrP_2, may complain of intrapelvic pain that may be specifically localized to the vagina or rectum, or may be diffuse and described only as somewhere "deep inside." In some patients, symptoms occur only during sexual intercourse. When TrP_1 is active, the patient complains primarily of anteromedial thigh and groin pain.

Patients with active adductor magnus TrPs frequently have difficulty positioning the lower limb comfortably at night. They usually prefer to lie on the opposite side with the thigh horizontal and slightly flexed at the hip, as when a pillow is placed between the knees and legs.

Gracilis

Usually, gracilis TrPs are encountered serendipitously during injection of TrPs in neighboring adductor or hamstring muscles, and the characteristic referred pain response of the gracilis is unexpectedly elicited. When patients with active TrPs in the gracilis muscle present themselves, the chief complaint is usually a superficial, hot, stinging pain in the medial thigh. The pain is rarely described as prickling. It may be constant at rest, and no change of position reduces the pain. Walking tends to relieve it.

Differential Diagnosis

Myofascial TrPs are common sources of groin and medial thigh pain. When adductor longus TrPs develop bilaterally, as may occur with strenuous horseback riding, the symmetrical distribution of referred pain can simulate a midlumbar spinal lesion.[98] In addition to TrPs in the adductor musculature, TrPs in the pectineus muscle (*see* Fig. 13.1) or in the vastus medialis (*see* Fig. 14.2) are also possible sources of the pain.

Even when a myofascial source of the pain has been located, a number of other conditions may be present at the same time, which also need attention. If no TrPs are found in the muscles, these other conditions become prime suspects. Three such conditions are overload of or trauma to musculoskeletal structures, articular dysfunction, and nerve entrapment.

In patients with stubborn chronic pain, one must expect that multiple etiologies are responsible. Ekberg and associates[32] employed a multidisciplinary approach to manage long-standing unexplained groin pain in 21 male athletes. The diagnostic medical team evaluated the athletes for inguinal hernia, neuralgia, adductor tenoperiostitis, symphysitis, and prostatitis. The evaluation included X-ray films of the pelvis and radioisotope studies of the pubic symphysis. Only two patients had just one condition, symphysitis. Ten patients had two conditions, six patients had three conditions, and three patients had four conditions. The authors did not explore the additional possibility of myofascial TrP pain.

The referred pain pattern of the gracilis muscle is somewhat like that of the sartorius, which is felt more anteriorly on the thigh. Gracilis referred pain is described as a diffuse achiness centered in the region of the muscle; the pain from sartorius TrPs is more likely to strike in heavy streaks or jolts. The patient usually obtains no relief from gracilis pain by change of position or stretching movements, as is also the case for sartorius muscle TrPs.

Mechanical Overload

Three conditions associated with chronic overload of the adductor muscles are pubic stress symphysitis (osteitis pubis), pubic stress fracture (avulsion stress fracture of the pubic bone), and adductor insertion avulsion syndrome.

Pubic Stress Symphysitis. Rold and Rold[91] emphasized that pubic stress symphysitis (osteitis pubis[18]) of athletes must be distinguished from adductor tendon avulsion at the pelvis, from fractures of the pubic or ischial rami, and from local septic conditions. Pubic stress symphysitis usually has an insidious onset with acute exacerbation during stressful sports activity. Examination reveals focal tenderness of the pubic symphysis bilaterally and pain on abduction and extension of the thighs.[91] Symphysitis sometimes is accompanied by adductor TrPs. In this situation, abduction and extension are more restricted on the side of the TrPs. The most anterior adductors, the pectineus and the adductor longus, are the most likely to be involved. This is understandable because these two adductor muscles have the most effective leverage for putting asymmetrical stress on the pubic symphysis. Radiographic evidence of sclerosis and irregularity of the pubic bones at the symphysis, and scintigraphic evidence of increased radionuclide uptake at the symphysis are confirmatory findings.[91] Brody[18] describes (and Netter illustrates[18]) shearing action on the symphysis as the cause of symphysitis. The tendency for the pelvis to seesaw up and down is aggravated by tension of the adductor muscles.[18]

Pubic Stress Fracture. Of 70 military trainees diagnosed to have pubic stress fractures during their first 12 weeks of training, 43 had fractures of one inferior pubic ramus, 11 of both inferior pubic rami, and two had ipsilateral fractures of both the inferior and superior pubic rami.[81] Many of these trainees were of short stature and they experienced pain only during marches. Marching required them to take "giant steps all day."

Stress fractures of the inferior pubic ramus, usually at the junction with the ischial ramus, occur in 1–2% of runners. In a study of 12 such runners,[83] the patients experienced groin pain aggravated by running. Diagnosis was eventually confirmed by radiography, but could be established immediately by bone scan (radionuclide scintigraphy). The lesion was thought to be a fatigue fracture in response to the tensile forces exerted by the adductor muscles on the pubic ramus.[82] Laxity of the symphysis pubis and increased muscle tension due to TrPs could be contributing factors, but apparently were not investigated.

A stress fracture of the avulsion type at the attachment of the adductor magnus to the pubic ramus in an active swimmer was confirmed by radionuclide imaging.[54]

Adductor Insertion Avulsion Syndrome. The adductor insertion avulsion syndrome ("thigh splints") developed in seven short, female, basic trainees who were required to march to the stride of taller males. Radionuclide scans revealed linear lesions in the upper or mid femur that suggested periosteal elevation. This location corresponded to the insertion of the adductor muscles.[25] In a scintigraphic study of 70 trainees with symptoms of pubic stress fracture,[81] 14 also showed a linear periosteal reaction in the region of insertion of the adductor longus and adductor brevis muscles on the femur. In the two subjects in whom roentgenograms of the femurs were obtained, both showed periosteal elevation along the medial aspect of the femur where the adductors longus and brevis attach.[81] The pain and tenderness were localized to the region of muscular attachment, aching in character, increased by activity, and relieved by rest.[81]

One would expect that the degree of overload placed on the muscle by the stress that caused these fractures and avulsions would be likely to activate TrPs in the adductor muscles of susceptible individuals. The skeletal lesions could then be further aggravated by increased muscle tension due to the TrPs.

Articular Dysfunction

Lewit[59] associates TrP involvement of the adductor muscle group with articular dysfunction of the hip joint; referred pain from the TrPs can be contributing to the patient's total pain problem. On the other hand, others[61,86] warn that the referred pain from adductor longus TrPs may be mistaken for the pain of osteoarthritis of the hip. It is easy to fall into the trap of attributing all the pain to osteoarthritis and of not checking for hip adductor TrPs. Inactivating the adductor TrPs provides satisfactory pain relief to some patients with osteoarthritis of the hip joint.[97] We find, as did Long,[61] that the pain of osteoarthritis is usually deeper in the groin, and is more likely to be referred laterally than medially.

The concept that part of the disability associated with osteoarthritis of the hip is of muscular origin was substantiated by a study[58] in which patients with osteoarthritis of the hip were given stretching exercises for the adductor musculature. The mean increase of 8.3° in range of hip abduction and the increase in the cross sectional area of type 1 and type 2 fibers in the adductors were significant ($p < 0.05$).

PART 2

Nerve Entrapment

The obturator and genitofemoral nerves may cause pain or tingling in the groin or in the medial thigh when they become entrapped.

About half of the patients who have an obturator hernia (usually elderly women) develop symptoms of entrapment of the obturator nerve: pain and/or tingling and paresthesias down the medial surface of the thigh to the knee (Howship-Romberg sign).[48,55,57,65,95] Extension of the thigh increases the pain,[55] and the adductor tendon jerk is diminished or absent. (This reflex is elicited with a reflex hammer by tapping a finger placed across the musculotendinous junction of the adductor magnus about 5 cm (2 in) above the medial epicondyle.[48])

Entrapment of the genitofemoral nerve is often caused by excessively tight clothing over the inguinal ligament. Patients with entrapment of this nerve experience pain and/or numbness in an elliptical area on the anterior aspect of the thigh immediately below the middle of the inguinal ligament. This area also shows decreased perception of pinprick and touch. Appendectomy, psoas muscle infection, and local trauma are predisposing factors.[87]

7. ACTIVATION AND PERPETUATION OF TRIGGER POINTS

Myofascial TrPs in the adductor muscles, including the gracilis, are likely to be activated by sudden overload, as when someone slips on ice and resists spreading the legs apart while trying to recover balance. A TrP in the adductor muscles was reported to have been activated in a 10-year-old boy while playing basketball.[46] Adductor TrPs may also be activated by osteoarthritis of the hip, or become apparent after hip surgery.

Myofascial TrPs were activated in the adductor longus muscle by strenuous horseback riding,[98] but were rarely activated by a motor vehicle accident.[11]

Adductor magnus TrPs are often activated by skiing or by taking an unaccustomed long bicycle trip. A latent TrP_1 in the adductor magnus can be reactivated by a simple misstep while getting into the front seat of a car.

Adductor TrPs may be perpetuated by running up hill or down hill, as is true also for TrPs in the pectineus muscle. However, patients with adductor TrPs are more likely to identify the onset of symptoms with a specific event than are patients with pectineus TrPs. Adductor TrPs may also be perpetuated by sitting in a fixed position while driving on a long auto trip, or while sitting for long periods in a chair with the hips acutely flexed and one thigh or leg crossed over the other knee.

8. PATIENT EXAMINATION (Figs. 15.9 and 15.10)

Active TrPs in the adductor longus and adductor brevis restrict abduction of the thigh[93] to a greater degree than do TrPs in the pectineus muscle. TrPs in the adductor magnus can also restrict flexion of the hip, especially in the abducted position. These restrictions are readily tested by having the supine patient place the foot of the affected limb against the oppo-

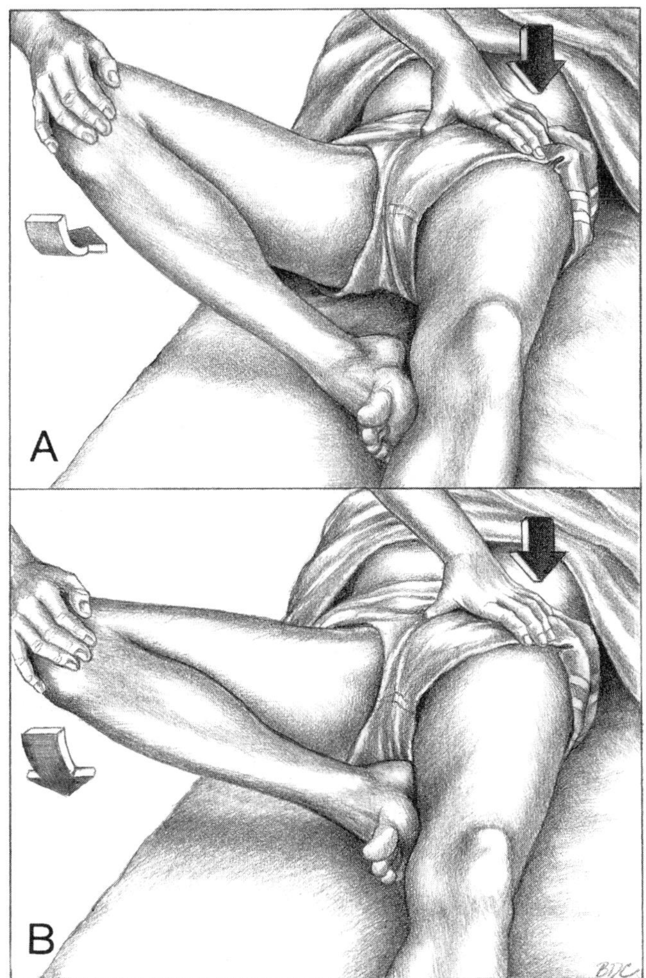

Figure 15.9. Testing stretch range of the right adductor group of muscles. The operator's left hand stabilizes the pelvis. *Arrows* indicate directions of pressure. *A*, position of restricted movement. Foot is at side of knee. *B*, essentially full range of motion. The thigh has been flexed additionally by moving the foot farther up the thigh to include testing of the ischiocondylar part of the adductor magnus, and the thigh is fully abducted to its normal range, establishing full length of all adductors.

PART 2

site knee while the operator gently abducts and then flexes the affected thigh by moving the knee outward and upward (Fig. 15.9*A*). At the same time, the clinician stabilizes the pelvis by pressure on its opposite side. With this technique, the thigh is abducted, flexed, and somewhat laterally rotated, which simultaneously tests all three of the major adductors for shortening.

Figure 15.9*A* illustrates restricted range of hip abduction and Figure 15.9*B* shows essentially full range. Moving the heel of the limb being tested farther proximally against the other thigh will cause pain and be limited by the presence of TrPs in the vasti (especially the vastus medialis, which is prone to involvement with the adductors). The purpose of that movement in this test is to increase flexion of the thigh at the hip. The movement produces this effect only in those individuals who have a relatively long leg length compared to thigh length.

An alternate procedure first tests the stretch range of the posterior (ischiocondylar) part of the adductor magnus by flexing the partially abducted thigh of the supine patient (Fig. 15.10*A*). The clinician then tests the stretch range of all three adductor muscles by further abduction of the flexed thigh (Fig. 15.10*B*). Gradual additional lowering of the abducted thigh toward the floor reveals tightness of the adductors longus and brevis.

Patients with adductor TrPs exhibit no abnormality of ordinary movement unless the TrP pain is so severe that it causes an antalgic gait with a reduced duration of stance on the affected side.

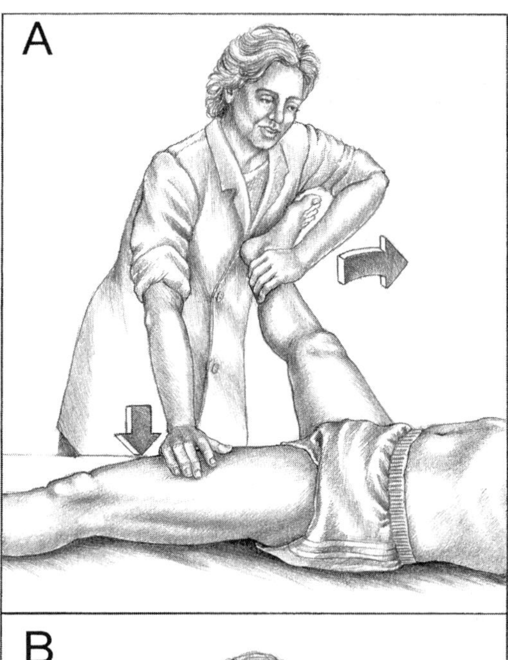

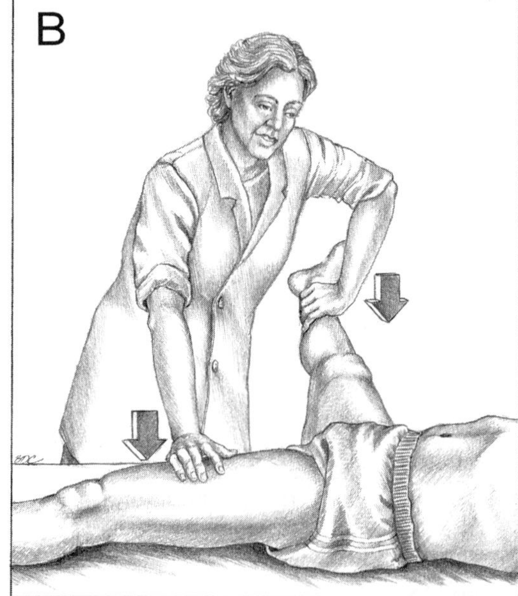

Figure 15.10. Testing the right adductor group of muscles for restricted stretch range. The left thigh is stabilized by the operator. *A*, swinging the partly abducted thigh in an arc toward the patient's head tests primarily for restriction of the adductor magnus and gracilis muscles. *B*, slowly moving the patient's abducted thigh down toward the floor, without jerking, checks for restriction chiefly of the pectineus, adductor longus, and adductor brevis muscles.

Tenderness of the tendinous attachment of the adductor magnus is elicited by pressure on the posteromedial aspect of the medial femoral condyle, which is identified in Figure 15.7. Tenderness is usually present there when the adductor magnus muscle is afflicted with active or latent myofascial TrPs.

Restriction of abduction caused by gracilis TrPs also is disclosed by the tests described previously. The increased tension of taut bands due to TrPs in the gracilis muscle is likely to cause tenderness at its tibial attachment (Fig. 15.8).[59] Similar tenderness may be caused by anserine bursitis.

9. TRIGGER POINT EXAMINATION
(Figs. 15.11 and 15.12)

Adductor Longus and Adductor Brevis
(Fig. 15.11)

The common locations of TrPs in the adductor longus and adductor brevis muscles are shown in Figure 15.1.

To examine for these TrPs, the patient is placed in a supine position with the thigh and knee partially flexed and the thigh abducted to place the adductor longus on moderate stretch (Fig. 15.11). The one-third of the adductor longus that is closest to the pelvis is best examined by pincer palpation (Fig. 15.12*A*). The distal two-thirds usually is best examined for TrPs by flat palpation against the underlying femur (Fig. 15.11).

Since the adductor brevis underlies the longus, it is reached only by deep flat palpation, and its TrPs are located primarily by the patient's pain responses (jump sign). The adductor longus rarely produces noteworthy local twitch responses to palpation, and the adductor brevis is practically inaccessible to snapping palpation, as seen in Figures 15.4 and 15.5.

Adductor Magnus
(Fig. 15.12)

Figure 15.2 shows the common locations of TrPs in the adductor magnus muscle. Posteriorly, in the proximal third of the thigh, the adductor magnus is covered by the gluteus maximus, biceps femoris, semitendinosus, and semimembranosus muscles.[36] Only in the proximal portion of the posteromedial aspect of the thigh is a triangle of the muscle accessible to sub-

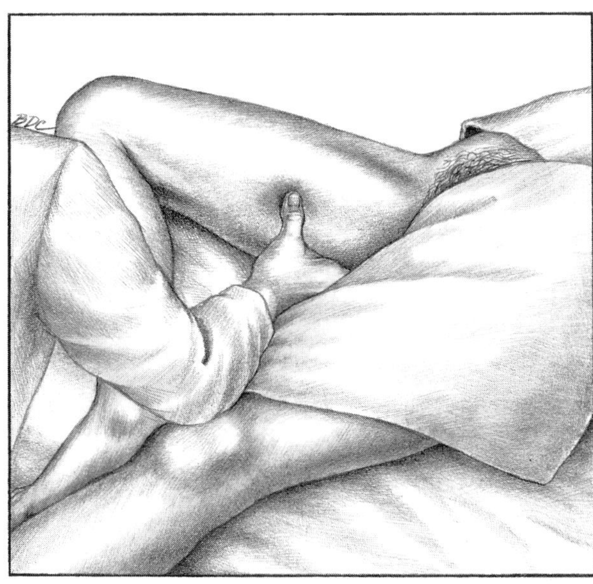

Figure 15.11. Examination by flat palpation for trigger points in the distal portion of the right adductor longus muscle. The knee is supported by a pillow to encourage voluntary relaxation while the muscle is placed on a comfortable, moderate stretch for palpation. (*See* Fig. 15.12*A* for examination of proximal trigger points in this muscle).

cutaneous palpation (Figs. 15.12*B* and 16.8). This narrow triangle is bordered by the ischial tuberosity and pubis proximally, the semimembranosus and semitendinosus muscles behind, and the gracilis muscle anteriorly.[36] This "window of palpation" may extend the length of the upper one-third of the thigh and may be several centimeters (an inch or more) across at its widest, just below the pelvis. The gracilis muscle covers the ischiocondylar (most vertical) part of the adductor magnus over most of its length.

Therefore, myofascial TrPs in the most medial portion of the ischiocondylar part of the adductor magnus in the TrP_2 region are usually best located by pincer palpation that reaches around and deep to the gracilis muscle. TrPs in the diagonal fibers (middle portion) of the adductor magnus muscle in the TrP_1 region (Fig. 15.2*C*) and TrPs in the TrP_2 region (Fig. 15.12*B*) in some patients can be reached only by flat palpation posterior to the gracilis muscle. Each TrP region produces its distinctive referred pain pattern (Fig. 15.2). Tenderness may be caused by TrPs in the adductor magnus or by TrPs in the overlying musculature, especially the gracilis muscle. Because so much of the adductor magnus lies deep to other sizeable muscles, it is often difficult to detect and locate its TrPs accurately; they are readily overlooked.

Gracilis

Myofascial TrPs in the gracilis muscle (Fig. 15.3) may be located by pincer palpation in patients who are thin or have relatively loose skin, but examination often requires flat palpation. The muscle may be indistinguishable in patients well padded with fat. Lange[56] illustrates the location of myogelosis (palpable, tender taut bands) [TrPs] in the upper third of the gracilis muscle.

10. ENTRAPMENTS

Tension due to myofascial TrPs in the adductor longus, adductor brevis, and gracilis muscles is not known to cause nerve entrapment.

A taut adductor magnus can compress the femoral vessels at their exit through the adductor (tendinous) hiatus. Sometimes, the middle and posterior parts of the adductor magnus are fused, which greatly reduces the size of the hiatus. One patient was seen who had no palpable dorsalis pedis pulse, but the pulse returned at once after inactivation of TrP_1 in the adductor magnus muscle. This may have been due to an unusual anatomical structure that facilitated compression of the femoral artery combined with a TrP taut band of adductor magnus fibers at the adductor hiatus.

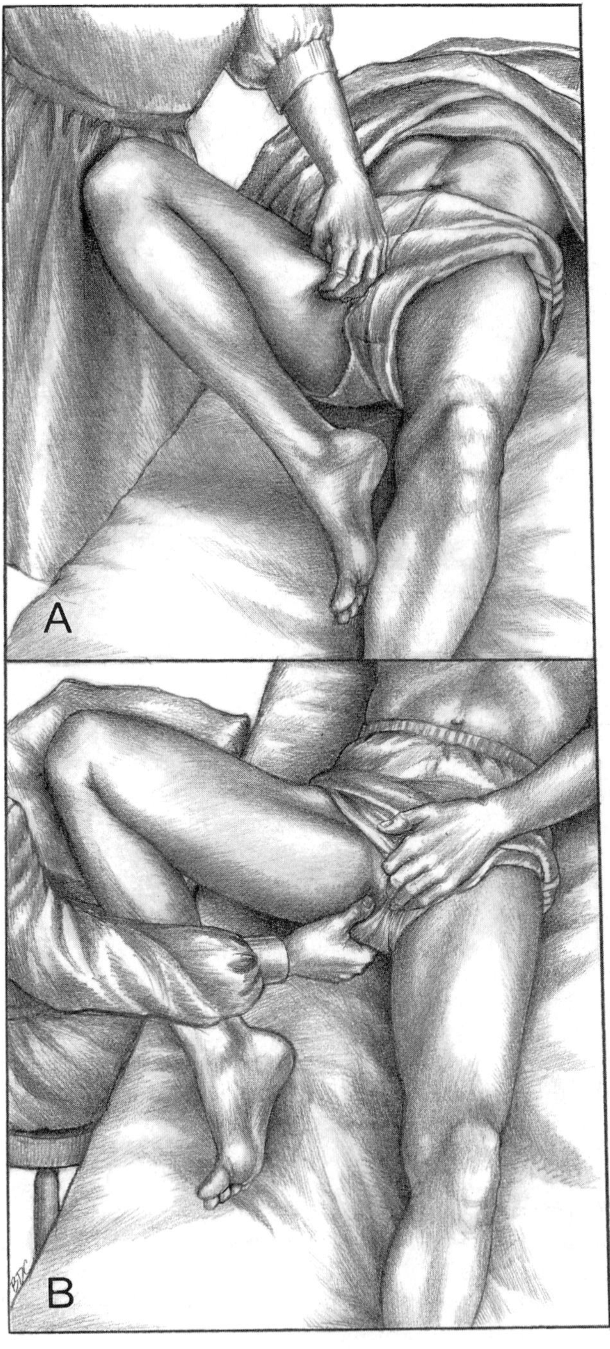

Figure 15.12. Examination for proximal trigger points in the right adductor muscles. *A*, adductor longus (and adductor brevis) by pincer palpation. The knee is supported against the operator to ensure voluntary relaxation while these muscles are placed on moderate stretch for examination. *B*, proximal end of the adductor magnus (TrP_2), examined by flat palpation against the underlying ischium posterior to the adductor longus, adductor brevis, and gracilis muscles.

Three cases of thrombosis of the superficial femoral artery at the outlet of Hunter's canal were reported in association with athletic activities.[12] The arterial injury and thrombosis were attributed in two cases to a scissorslike compression by the vastus medialis and adductor magnus tendons at this location and, in another case, to compression by a constricting tendinous band extending across the femoral artery from the adductor magnus to the vastus medialis tendon at the level of Hunter's canal outlet. These observations suggest that, in some adductor canal configurations, taut-band tension on the tendons forming the margins of the canal might cause at least venous compression at this site.

The adductor hiatus marks the distal (outlet) end of the adductor (Hunter's) canal that begins proximally at the apex of the femoral triangle. Hunter's canal is covered by a fascial layer deep to the sartorius muscle and is bounded anteriorly and laterally by the vastus medialis muscle and posteriorly by the adductor longus and adductor magnus. In addition to the femoral artery and vein, the canal contains the saphenous nerve.

11. ASSOCIATED TRIGGER POINTS

Myofascial TrPs in the adductor longus and adductor brevis may be associated with TrPs in the adductor magnus and occasionally with TrPs in the pectineus muscle. The pectineus should always be checked if the adductor muscles harbor TrPs.

Involvement of the adductor longus and adductor magnus may be associated with TrPs in the most medial fibers of the vastus medialis. Anatomically, they are literally tied together. The fascial coverings of these muscles form a thick bridge between them above the knee, which helps establish a medial pull on the patella that counters the lateral pull of the vastus lateralis.

Surprisingly, TrPs in the gracilis are rarely associated with TrPs in the primary adductors, but may be associated with TrPs in the lower end of the sartorius muscle.

12. INTERMITTENT COLD WITH STRETCH
(Figs. 15.13 and 15.14)

Usually, it is best to apply intermittent cold with stretch first to the adductor magnus and then proceed to the adductor longus and adductor brevis muscles.

The use of ice for applying intermittent cold with stretch is explained on page 9 of this volume and the use of vapocoolant spray with stretch is detailed on pages 67–74 of Volume 1.[101] Techniques that augment relaxation and stretch, as well as alternative methods of treatment, are reviewed in Chapter 2.

Adductor Magnus
(Fig. 15.13)

To inactivate TrPs in the adductor magnus, the application of intermittent cold with passive stretch is initiated with the patient in the position illustrated in Figure 15.13. The patient should be made aware of the amount of restriction of thigh range of motion before treatment, for later comparison. After initial parallel sweeps of ice or a vapocoolant jet stream, the thigh is gently abducted and flexed. The operator supports the weight of the thigh against the force of gravity while the patient inhales deeply. During slow exhalation and complete relaxation of the patient, slow parallel sweeps of ice or vapocoolant are applied upward over the medial and posteromedial aspects of the thigh including the groin. As the muscle relaxes, gentle pressure is applied to take up any slack that permits additional abduction and flexion of the thigh. This procedure may be repeated rhythmically two or three times while the patient breathes slowly and deeply. When repetition no longer increases the range of motion, a moist heating pad is applied over the adductor muscles. When the skin has rewarmed, the patient slowly performs two or three cycles of full active range of motion through hip abduction and adduction. The patient should then note the difference in range of motion as compared with the range prior to treatment.

Adductor Longus and Adductor Brevis
(Fig. 15.14)

For application of intermittent cold with passive stretch to the adductor longus and adductor brevis, the supine patient positions the heel of the limb to be treated against the opposite limb above the knee. During ice application or vapocooling, the foot is gradually moved as far up the thigh as the patient finds comfortably tolerable (Fig. 15.14). As described previously for the adductor magnus, the application of intermittent cold is synchronized with patient exhalation and relaxation. Parallel sweeps of the cold are applied with an upsweep over the thigh and groin and with a downsweep over the knee and shin to cover the pain reference

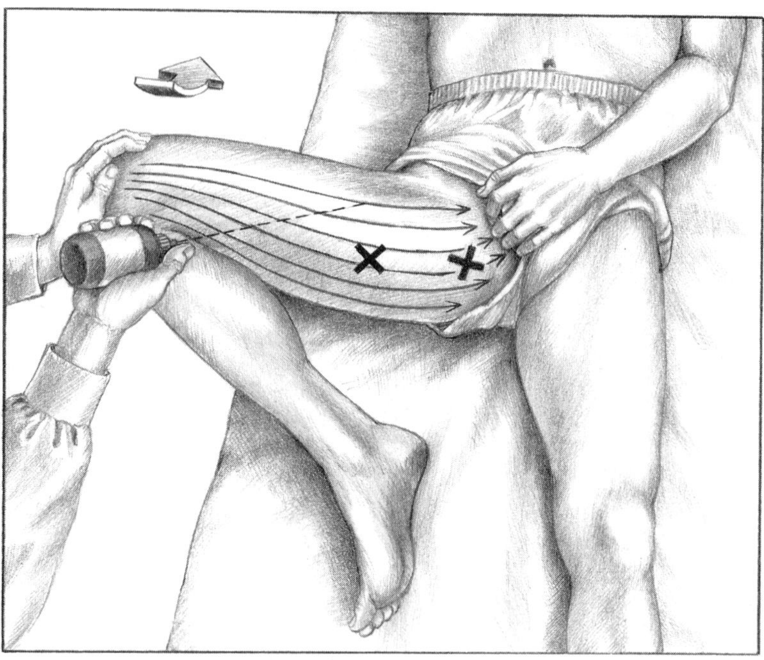

Figure 15.13. Stretch position and intermittent cold pattern (*thin arrows*) for trigger points in the right adductor magnus muscle with the patient lying supine. The **X***s* mark frequent locations of these trigger points. The intermittent cold pattern extends upward from the patella, covering the entire muscle in parallel sweeps. The *thick arrow* shows the direction of pressure downward toward the floor and cephalad, to increase the abduction-flexion passive stretch on this muscle.

zones.[93,94,97] As the muscle tension releases, the thigh drops down in abduction toward the table. Between applications of intermittent cold and gentle passive stretch, the foot of the treated side is moved upward toward the buttock as in Figures 15.9*B* and 15.16*B*. Since this technique also stretches the vasti (medialis, intermedius, and lateralis) of the quadriceps femoris, it is essential that the ice or spray application includes the anterior as well as the lateral aspect of the thigh. The stretch techniques illustrated in both Figures 15.13 and 15.14 are assisted by gravity.[98] Using this technique, the commonly associated trigger points in the vastus medialis derived from those in the adductor longus are inactivated at the same time.

An effective release of tight adductor muscles, which markedly increases the abduction range of motion, may induce a reactive cramp (kickback) by activation of latent TrPs in the gluteus medius muscle. When this muscle is thus suddenly shortened to less than its accustomed range, the patient may exclaim, "Oh, I have a pain in my back." The newly activated TrPs in the gluteus medius muscle responsible for this reactive cramping should be released immediately by intermittent cold and stretch of the cramped muscle (*see* Chapter 8).

The cold-with-stretch procedure is followed at once by application of a moist heating pad over the treated muscles and then full active range of motion through hip abduction-adduction and knee extension-flexion. Finally, the patient learns how to perform a home stretch program (*see* Section 14).

Using a contract-relax stretching technique for six muscle groups, Möller and associates[71] found that the adductor stretch was one of the most effective (17 ± 3% increase in range).

Additional stretch techniques for the adductor muscles are described and illustrated by Evjenth and Hamberg.[33]

Ultrasound is a valuable therapeutic modality for the adductor magnus because so much of the muscle is too deep to be reasonably accessible by manual treatment methods.

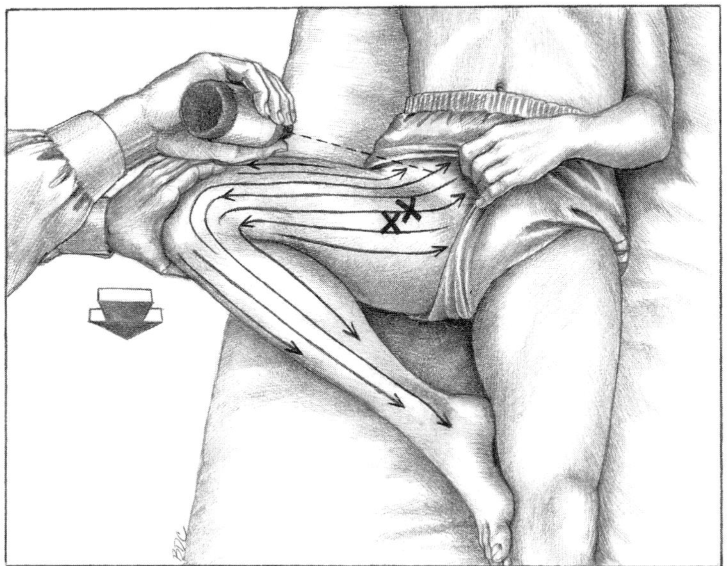

Figure 15.14. Stretch position and intermittent cold pattern (*thin arrows*) for trigger points (**X**s) in the right adductor longus and adductor brevis muscles. A vapocoolant spray or an application using ice first covers the muscle and its proximal referred pain pattern with upward parallel sweeps, and then is applied downward over the distal pain reference zone, including the knee, shin, and ankle. As the adductor muscle tension releases, the thigh and knee drop down toward the table (*thick arrow*). Sweeps of intermittent cold also cover the thigh anteriorly and laterally to release any tension of the vasti of the quadriceps femoris. The right foot is successively moved up the thigh for additional stretch, as in Figure 15.9B.

Gracilis

The stretch techniques described for the adductor group do not stretch the gracilis muscle, since bending the knee releases stretch on the gracilis.[92] A similar technique but with the knee straight, presented as the first step for intermittent cold with stretch of the hamstring muscles (*see* Figs. 16.11*A* and Fig. 15.10), releases not only the hamstring muscles but also the gracilis and the ischiocondylar part of the adductor magnus.

13. INJECTION AND STRETCH
(Figs. 15.15 and 15.16)

Adductor Longus and Adductor Brevis
(Fig. 15.15)

In cases of the adductor longus syndrome, when intermittent cold with passive stretch and other non-invasive methods fail to release the muscle, procaine infiltration is recommended.[97]

The femoral artery lies deep to the sartorius muscle lateral to the long and short adductor muscles. For this reason, one should first locate by palpation the pulsation of the femoral artery and the anterolateral border of the adductor longus and then direct the needle posteromedially from there. In this way, one injects away from, not toward, the femoral artery (Fig. 15.15*A*). Injection of the adductor longus and adductor brevis is safest and most satisfactory if one can grasp the muscle to be injected in a pincer grip. To do this, the muscle is slackened by placing the thigh in partial adduction (Fig. 15.15*B*).

If the muscle cannot be grasped, then the patient should assume the position of Figure 15.15*A* and the muscle should be placed under moderate tension for flat palpation. Figure 15.15*A* illustrates injection of TrPs in the right adductor longus muscle using a flat palpation technique. One expects to identify taut bands in this muscle, and the needle often elicits a local twitch response that is either seen as dimpling of the skin or is felt by the operator.

One does not expect to identify taut bands or local twitch responses in the underlying adductor brevis. To inject TrPs in the adductor brevis muscle in the man-

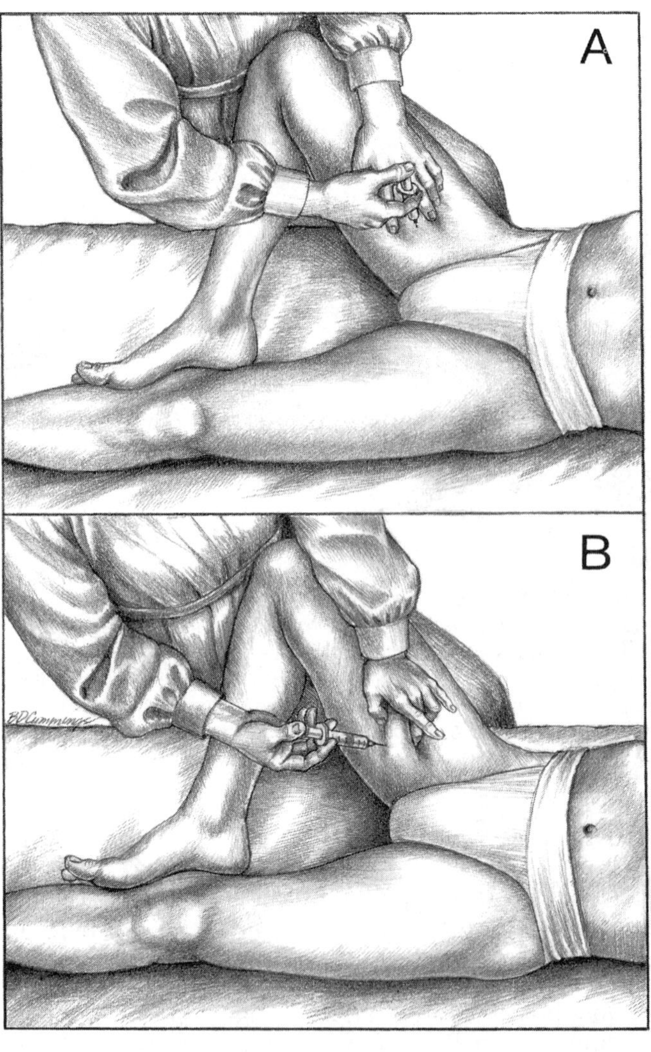

Figure 15.15. Injection of trigger points in the slackened right adductor longus and adductor brevis muscles. *A*, adductor longus using the flat palpation technique. *B*, adductor brevis using pincer palpation.

ner shown (Fig. 15.15*B*), it is possible to grasp both the adductor longus and adductor brevis in a pincer grip so that the needle is directed deep toward a finger that compresses the taut band and TrPs to be injected. In this way, there is little possibility of accidentally needling or penetrating the femoral artery since it would not be included in the pincer grasp. Using 0.5% solution of procaine in isotonic saline, 1–2 mL are injected directly into the TrP. The adjacent muscle fibers are then explored with the needle to ensure that all TrPs have been found, while hemostasis is maintained by finger pressure with the other hand.

When the injection has been completed, the muscle should be lengthened, as described previously. A moist heating pad or hot pack is then applied to the site for a few minutes to minimize postinjection soreness and to facilitate the patient's achieving full active range of motion.

Long[61] warned that injection of adductor longus TrPs must be made deeply and carefully beginning with the more tendinous upper portions of the muscle near its origin. He recommended widely infiltrating the belly of the muscle below its origin. He also observed that the adductor longus syndrome is one of the more gratifying myofascial pain syndromes to treat, when it is an isolated single-muscle syndrome.

Elimination of a disabling adductor TrP in a 10-year-old boy was reported in response to injection of 4 mL of 0.25%

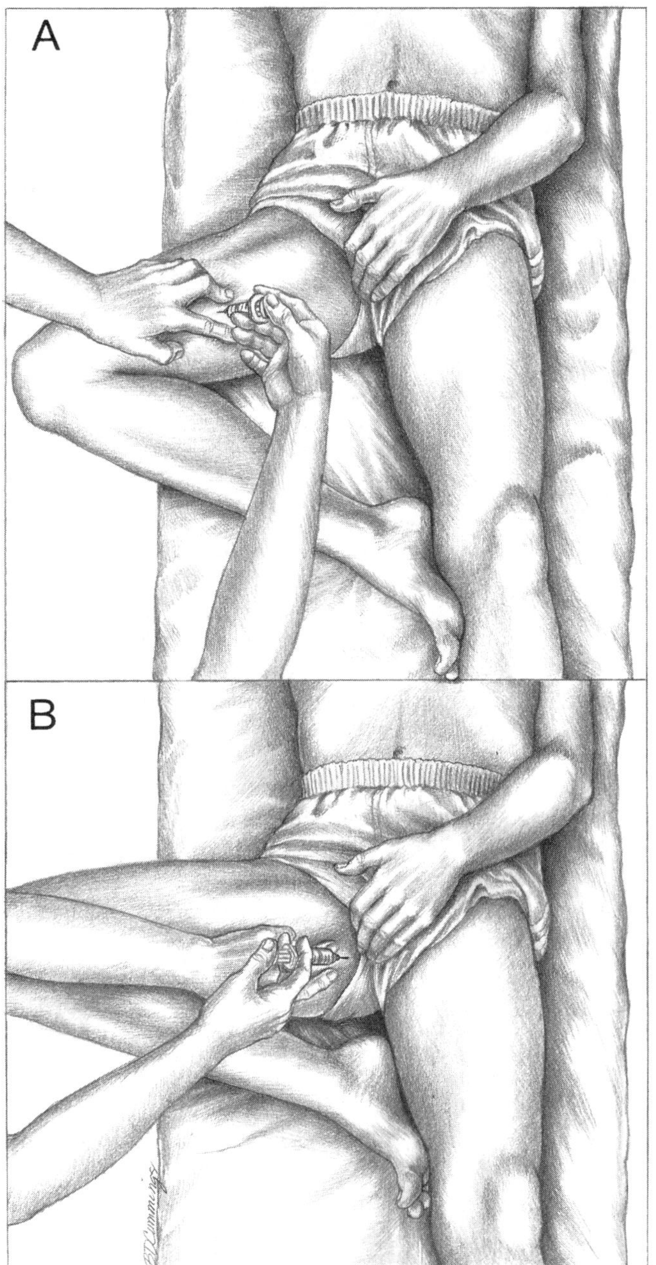

Figure 15.16. Injection of trigger points in the right adductor magnus muscle. *A*, midportion of the muscle, TrP_1 region. *B*, proximal end of the muscle in the TrP_2 region near the attachment of the adductor minimus fibers to the inferior pubic ramus. Deep to this site are the ischiocondylar fibers that form the major bulk of the muscle and attach in the region of the ischial tuberosity.

bupivicaine using a small-gauge needle.[46] We prefer procaine because of the reported myotoxic effects of bupivicaine (Chapter 3[101]).

Injection of the adductor longus TrPs in one patient produced immediate disappearance of a sharp referred pain response, but a dull aching pain remained with appearance of hyperesthesia in the reference zone over the tibia. This hyperesthesia of the reference zone subsided in 4 hours and, by that time, all sensation in the reference zone had become normal.[99]

Adductor Magnus
(Fig. 15.16)

Injection of TrPs in either the midportion TrP_1 or proximal TrP_2 region is unlikely to encounter the femoral vessels because the adductor longus muscle lies between the vessels and the anterior surface of the adductor magnus. However, when injecting from the medial aspect of the thigh (Fig. 15.16*A*), one should be aware that the sciatic nerve passes against the adductor magnus, between it and the hamstring muscles. The nerve passes deep to the ischiocondylar and middle parts of the adductor magnus. It is recommended that cross-sectional anatomy[76] be reviewed before injecting the deeper portions of this muscle.

Because of the large size of the adductor magnus muscle, and because of the access to it from the side, sometimes a needle 75-mm (3-in) long may be required to reach the deeper TrPs. Generally, the TrP spot tenderness in this muscle can be located only by deep palpation. Because of the thickness of the muscle, one is ordinarily unable to identify its taut bands or to perceive local twitch responses.

Injection of TrPs in the proximal TrP_2 region of the adductor magnus must take into account the gracilis muscle. When one has established that the TrP tenderness is beside or deep to the gracilis, one can then inject at the site of tenderness precisely in the direction in which application of pressure elicited pain. Occasionally, it is more convenient to pass the needle through the gracilis muscle to reach the adductor magnus.

When the TrP injection is finished, the muscle is lengthened, a moist heating pad is applied, and then the full active range of motion is performed, as described previously.

Gracilis

For injection of TrPs in the gracilis muscle, the patient is first positioned as in Figure 15.16*A*. If more tension is needed on the muscle, the knee is extended. When TrPs are localized by palpation of this subcutaneous muscle, they may be injected using either the pincer or flat palpation technique, depending on the looseness of the subcutaneous tissue. Taut bands are distinguishable unless the subcutaneous adipose tissue is too thick. A 37-mm (1½-in) needle should be long enough.

14. CORRECTIVE ACTIONS

Structural body asymmetry does not appear to be a major factor in the activation and perpetuation of TrPs in the adductor muscles. However, one must seriously consider the common systemic perpetuating factors of the myofascial pain syndromes, such as vitamin inadequacy, borderline anemia, chronic infections, and thyroid marginal hypofunction (Chapter 4, Volume 1).[101]

Corrective Posture and Activities

For all the hip adductors, it is important to avoid leaving the muscle in a shortened position for a long period of time. This shortened position is avoided when the patient is sleeping on one side by placing a pillow between the knees and legs. The uppermost thigh should be kept in a nearly horizontal position and not allowed to drop forward and down toward the bed, which would cause shortening of its adductor muscles. Excessive hip flexion is also avoided.

When sitting, an individual should avoid crossing one leg or thigh over the other knee. This position may be assumed to compensate for a small hemipelvis, a skeletal asymmetry that is corrected by an appropriate ischial (butt) lift (*see* Chapter 4 of this volume and Chapter 4 of Volume 1[101]). One should also avoid sitting in a chair that places the hips in a jackknifed position. Sitting immobile during a long auto trip should be minimized by frequent stops to get out and walk around, or by the driver's use of cruise control to permit active movement of the lower limbs.

Home Therapeutic Program

A simple home technique to reduce TrP activity in these adductor muscles is the regular application of moist heat over the TrPs in the groin area and just distal to it.

The clinician should instruct the patient in a home stretch program to maintain full adductor length. The simplest stretch is the one suggested by Brody[18] in which the standing patient holds onto a table or wall for stability, spreads the legs apart to nearly full range, and then swings the hips away from the side to be stretched.

With TrP involvement of any of the adductor muscles, the patient should be encouraged to do the swimming pool adductor stretch. The patient stands chest deep in warm water with the hands on the hips and the legs spread as far apart as is comfortable. With the torso erect, the patient bends one knee and slowly shifts the body weight toward that side, thus increasing passive stretch of the adductors on the side of the straight knee.

This standing adductor stretch can also be done while the patient holds onto a door jamb or a filing cabinet with one hand and places the other hand on the hip. If the adductors are involved bilaterally, the same stretch is repeated, shifting body weight toward the other side as that knee is bent. This stretch is useful for all adductor muscles.

A passive stretch technique recommended by Saudek[92] employs gravity, which enhances the effectiveness of the postisometric relaxation technique. The supine patient lies down with the buttocks up against a wall and rests the legs and feet up on the wall with the knees straight and legs spread apart; the force of gravity encourages abduction of the thighs.

References

1. Anderson JE: *Grant's Atlas of Anatomy*, Ed. 8. Williams & Wilkins, Baltimore, 1983 (Fig. 4–5, 4–26).
2. *Ibid*. (Figs. 4–23, 4–24).
3. *Ibid*. (Fig. 4–25).
4. *Ibid*. (Fig. 4–28).
5. *Ibid*. (Fig. 4–29).
6. *Ibid*. (Fig. 4–30).
7. *Ibid*. (Fig. 4–32A).
8. *Ibid*. (Fig. 4–34).
9. *Ibid*. (Fig. 4–39).
10. *Ibid*. (Fig. 4–64).
11. Baker BA: The muscle trigger: evidence of overload injury. *J Neurol Orthop Med Surg 7*:35–44, 1986.
12. Balaji MR, DeWeese JA: Adductor canal outlet syndrome. *JAMA 245*:167–170, 1981.
13. Bardeen CR: The musculature, Sect. 5. In *Morris's Human Anatomy*, edited by C.M. Jackson, Ed. 6. Blakiston's Son & Co., Philadelphia, 1921 (pp. 494, 506, Fig. 441).
14. Basmajian JV, Deluca CJ: *Muscles Alive*, Ed. 5. Williams & Wilkins, Baltimore, 1985 (pp. 319–320, 380).
15. *Ibid*. (p. 323).
16. Basmajian JV, Slonecker CE: *Grant's Method of Anatomy*, 11th Ed. Williams & Wilkins, Baltimore, 1989 (p. 282).
17. Bates T, Grunwaldt E: Myofascial pain in childhood. *J Pediatr 53*:198–209, 1958.
18. Brody DM: Running injuries. *Clinical Symposia. CIBA (No. 4) 32*:2–36, 1980 (*see* pp. 17, 28 and 29).
19. Broer MR, Houtz SJ: *Patterns of Muscular Activity in Selected Sports Skills*. Charles C Thomas, Springfield, 1967.
20. Carter BL, Morehead J, Wolpert SM, *et al.*: *Cross-Sectional Anatomy*. Appleton-Century-Crofts, New York, 1977 (Sects. 41–43, 47, 48, 64).
21. *Ibid*. (Sects. 41–43, 47, 48, 64, 65).
22. *Ibid*. (Sects. 41–43, 47, 48, 64, 66, 67–72).
23. *Ibid*. (Sects. 42, 43, 47, 48).
24. *Ibid*. (Sects. 43, 48,64, 66, 67).
25. Charkes ND, Siddhivarn N, Schneck CD: Bone scanning in the adductor insertion avulsion syndrome ("thigh splints"). *J Nucl Med 28*: 1835–1838, 1987.
26. Christensen E: Topography of terminal motor innervation in striated muscles from stillborn infants. *Am J Phys Med 38*:65–78, 1959.
27. Clemente CD: *Gray's Anatomy of the Human Body*, American Ed. 30. Lea & Febiger, Philadelphia, 1985 (pp. 563–565, Fig. 6–71).
28. Close JR: *Motor Function in the Lower Extremity*. Charles C Thomas, Springfield, 1964 (p. 79, Fig. 16).
29. Coërs C, Woolf AL: *The Innervation of Muscle*. Blackwell Scientific Publications, Oxford, 1959 (pp. 1, 18–20).
30. Duchenne GB: *Physiology of Motion*, translated by E.B. Kaplan. J. B. Lippincott, Philadelphia, 1949 (pp. 266–268).
31. *Ibid*. (pp. 286, 290).
32. Ekberg O, Persson NH, Abrahamsson PA, *et al.*: Longstanding groin pain in athletes. A multidisciplinary approach. *Sports Med 6*:56–61, 1988.
33. Evjenth O, Hamberg J: *Muscle Stretching in Manual Therapy, A Clinical Manual*. Alfta Rehab Førlag, Alfta, Sweden, 1984 (pp. 105, 109–119).
34. Ferner H, Staubesand J: *Sobotta Atlas of Human Anatomy*, Ed. 10, Vol. 2. Urban & Schwarzenberg, Baltimore, 1983 (Figs. 380, 381).
35. *Ibid*. (Fig. 404).
36. *Ibid*. (Fig. 406).
37. *Ibid*. (Fig. 407).
38. *Ibid*. (Figs. 408, 409).
39. *Ibid*. (Figs. 410, 411a, 411b).
40. *Ibid*. (p. 290).
41. *Ibid*. (Fig. 417).
42. *Ibid*. (Fig. 418).
43. *Ibid*. (Figs. 420, 421).
44. *Ibid*. (Fig. 464).
45. *Ibid*. (Fig. 468).
46. Fine PG: Myofascial trigger point pain in children. *J Pediatr 111*:547–548, 1987.
47. Green DL, Morris JM: Role of adductor longus and adductor magnus in postural movements and in ambulation. *Am J Phys Med 49*:223–240, 1970.
48. Hannington-Kiff JG: Absent thigh adductor reflex in obturator hernia. *Lancet 1*:180, 1980.
49. Hollinshead WH: *Anatomy for Surgeons*, Ed. 3., Vol. 3, *The Back and Limbs*. Harper & Row, New York, 1982 (pp. 700–701).

50. Jonsson B, Steen B: Function of the gracilis muscle. An electromyographic study. *Acta Morphol Neerl Scand 6*:325–341, 1966.
51. Kellgren JH: Observations on referred pain arising from muscle. *Clin Sci 3*:175–190, 1938 (*see* p. 186).
52. Kelly M: Some rules for the employment of local analgesia in the treatment of somatic pain. *Med J Austral 1*:235–239, 1947.
53. Kelly M: The relief of facial pain by procaine (Novocain) injections. *J Am Geriatr Soc 11*:586–596, 1963.
54. Kim SM, Park CH, Gartland JJ: Stress fracture of the pubic ramus in a swimmer. *Clin Nucl Med 12*:118–119, 1987.
55. Kozlowski JM, Beal JM: Obturator hernia: an elusive diagnosis. *Arch Surg 112*:1001–1002, 1977.
56. Lange M: *Die Muskelhärten (Myogelosen)*. J.F. Lehmanns, München, 1931 (p. 157, Fig. 52).
57. Larrieu AJ, DeMarco SJ III: Obturator hernia: report of a case and brief review of its status. *Am Surg 42*:273–277, 1976.
58. Leivseth G, Torstensson J, Reikeras O: Effect of passive muscle stretching in osteoarthritis of the hip. *Clin Sci 76*:113–117, 1989.
59. Lewit K: *Manipulative Therapy in Rehabilitation of the Motor System*. Butterworths, London, 1985 (pp. 138, 282).
60. Lockhart RD: *Living Anatomy*, Ed. 7. Faber & Faber, London, 1974 (Figs. 114–117).
61. Long C II: Myofascial pain syndromes, part III—some syndromes of the trunk and thigh. *Henry Ford Hosp Med Bull 4*:102–106, 1956.
62. Lyons K, Perry J, Gronley JK, *et al.*: Timing and relative intensity of hip extensor and abductor muscle action during level and stair ambulation. *Phys Ther 63*:1597–1605, 1983.
63. Mann RA, Moran GT, Dougherty SE: Comparative electromyography of the lower extremity in jogging, running, and sprinting. *Am J Sports Med 14*:501–510, 1986.
64. Markhede G, Stener B: Function after removal of various hip and thigh muscles for extirpation of tumors. *Acta Orthop Scand 52*:373–395, 1981.
65. Martin NC, Welch TP: Obturator hernia. *Br J Surg 61*:547–548, 1974.
66. McMinn RMH, Hutchings RT: *Color Atlas of Human Anatomy*. Year Book Medical Publishers, Chicago, 1977 (p. 245).
67. *Ibid.* (pp. 264, 270).
68. *Ibid.* (pp. 275, 277).
69. *Ibid.* (pp. 281, 282).
70. *Ibid.* (pp. 306, 307).
71. Möller M, Ekstrand J, Öberg B, *et al.*: Duration of stretching effect on range of motion in lower extremities. *Arch Phys Med Rehabil 66*:171–173, 1985.
72. Netter FH: *The Ciba Collection of Medical Illustrations*, Vol. 8, Musculoskeletal System. Part I: Anatomy, Physiology and Metabolic Disorders. Ciba-Geigy Corporation, Summit, 1987 (p. 81).
73. *Ibid.* (p. 83).
74. *Ibid.* (p. 84).
75. *Ibid.* (p. 86).
76. *Ibid.* (p. 87).
77. *Ibid.* (p. 90).
78. *Ibid.* (p. 91).
79. *Ibid.* (p. 94).
80. *Ibid.* (p. 107).
81. Ozburn MS, Nichols JW: Pubic ramus and adductor insertion stress fractures in female basic trainees. *Milit Med 146*:332–333, 1981.
82. Pavlov H: What is your diagnosis? *Contemp Orthop 10*:75–78, 1985.
83. Pavlov H, Nelson TL, Warren RF, *et al.*: Stress fractures of the pubic ramus. *J Bone Joint Surg [Am] 64*:1020–1025, 1982.
84. Perry J: The mechanics of walking. *Phys Ther 47*:778–801, 1967.
85. Rasch PJ, Burke RK: *Kinesiology and Applied Anatomy*, Ed. 6. Lea & Febiger, Philadelphia, 1978 (pp. 276–278, 282, 309).
86. Reynolds MD: Myofascial trigger point syndromes in the practice of rheumatology. *Arch Phys Med Rehabil 62*:111–114, 1981.
87. Rischbieth RH: Genito-femoral neuropathy. *Clin Exp Neurol 22*:145–147, 1986.
88. Rohen JW, Yokochi C: *Color Atlas of Anatomy*, Ed. 2. Igaku-Shoin, New York, 1988 (p. 416).
89. *Ibid.* (p. 417).
90. *Ibid.* (p. 420).
91. Rold JF, Rold BA: Pubic stress symphysitis in a female distance runner. *Phys Sportsmed 14*:61–65, 1986.
92. Saudek CE: The hip, Chapter 17. In *Orthopaedic and Sports Physical Therapy*, edited by J.A. Gould III and G.J. Davies, Vol. II. C.V. Mosby, St. Louis, 1985 (pp. 365–407, *see* pp. 389, 404).
93. Simons DG: Myofascial pain syndrome due to trigger points, Chapter 45. In *Rehabilitation Medicine*, edited by Joseph Goodgold. C.V. Mosby Co., St. Louis, 1988 (pp. 686–723) (*see* pp. 709–711, Fig. 45–8D).
94. Simons DG, Travell JG: Myofascial pain syndromes, Chapter 25. In *Textbook of Pain*, edited by P.D. Wall and R. Melzack, Ed 2. Churchill Livingstone, London, 1989 (pp. 368–385) (*see* p. 377).
95. Somell A, Ljungdahl I, Spangen L: Thigh neuralgia as a symptom of obturator hernia. *Acta Chir Scand 142*:457–459, 1976.
96. *Stedman's Medical Dictionary*, Ed. 24. Williams & Wilkins, Baltimore, 1982 (p. 608).
97. Travell J: The adductor longus syndrome: A cause of groin pain; Its treatment by local block of trigger areas (procaine infiltration and ethyl chloride spray). *Bull NY Acad Med 26*:284–285, 1950.
98. Travell J: Symposium on mechanism and management of pain syndromes. *Proc Rudolf Virchow Med Soc 16*:126–136, 1957.
99. Travell J, Bigelow NH: Role of somatic trigger areas in the patterns of hysteria. *Psychosom Med 9*:353–363, 1947.
100. Travell J, Rinzler SH: The myofascial genesis of pain. *Postgrad Med 11*:425–434, 1952.
101. Travell JG, Simons DG: *Myofascial Pain and Dysfunction: The Trigger Point Manual*. Williams & Wilkins, Baltimore, 1983.
102. Weber EF: Ueber die Längenverhältnisse der Fleischfasern der Muskeln in Allgemeinen. *Berichte über die Verhandlungen der Königlich Sächsischen Gesellschaft der Wissenschaften zu Leipzig 3*:63–86, 1851.

CHAPTER 16
Hamstring Muscles
Biceps Femoris, Semitendinosus, and Semimembranosus

"Chair-seat Victims"

HIGHLIGHTS: **REFERRED PAIN** from the myofascial trigger points (TrPs) in the semitendinosus and semimembranosus muscles concentrates in the lower buttock and adjacent thigh. From there, pain may extend down the posteromedial aspect of the thigh and knee to the upper half of the calf medially. Pain referred from TrPs in the lower half of the biceps femoris (long or short head) focuses on the back of the knee and may extend up the posterolateral area of the thigh as far as the crease of the buttock. The proximal **ANATOMICAL ATTACHMENTS** of the three true hamstring muscles (semitendinosus, semimembranosus, and long head of the biceps femoris) are to the ischial tuberosity. Distally, the medial hamstrings—the semitendinosus and semimembranosus—attach to the medial side of the tibia just below the knee. Both heads of the lateral hamstring muscle, the biceps femoris, attach below the knee to the lateral and posterior aspects of the fibula. The short head is not a true hamstring muscle; proximally, it attaches not to the pelvis but to the posterior middle third of the femur along the linea aspera. **INNERVATION** of the hamstrings is from the tibial portion of the sciatic nerve, except the short head of the biceps femoris, which is supplied by the peroneal portion of the sciatic nerve. A major **FUNCTION** of the true hamstring muscles is to restrain the tendency toward hip flexion that is produced by body weight during the stance phase of walking. They are essential for running, jumping, dancing, and bending forward. They act primarily as hip extensors and knee flexors. The short head of the biceps femoris acts only at the knee and is mainly a flexor. When the knee is flexed, the semitendinosus and semimembranosus muscles also assist medial rotation of the leg at the knee, whereas both heads of the biceps femoris help rotate it laterally. **SYMPTOMS** due to TrPs in the hamstring muscles include pain that is increased by sitting and walking and that often disturbs sleep. Part or all of the pain patterns referred by hamstring TrPs can be caused by TrPs in eight other muscles. Hamstring myofascial pain must also be distinguished from forms of sciatica, osteoarthritis of the knee, hamstring syndrome attributed to muscle tears, and insertion syndromes of the semitendinosus and semimembranosus muscles. **ACTIVATION AND PERPETUATION OF TRIGGER POINTS** in the hamstring muscles can result from acute or repetitive overload or from the chronic trauma of underthigh pressure by the high front edge of a chair seat. Prolonged bed rest with the knees flexed can aggravate hamstring TrPs. **PATIENT EXAMINATION** should include evaluation for hamstring tightness using the Straight-leg Raising Test. Hamstring tension is not the cause of pain elicited by passive dorsiflexion of the foot at the limit of straight leg raising. **TRIGGER POINT EXAMINATION** of the medial hamstring muscles is performed through the posteromedial aspect of the thigh with the patient supine. The biceps femoris is examined with the patient lying on the side opposite to the muscle being examined. Pincer palpation can often be used for the medial hamstrings, but flat palpation is usually required for the biceps femoris. For **INTERMITTENT COLD WITH STRETCH** of the hamstring muscles, one starts by releasing the posterior part of the adductor magnus muscle, applying parallel sweeps of coolant in an upward pattern as the thigh of the supine patient is abducted with the knee extended. Maintaining hip flexion from this position of abduction, intermittent cold is applied in a proximal to distal pattern over the length of the tight hamstring muscles. First, the medial and then the lateral hamstrings are released as the flexed limb is adducted through an arc from lateral to medial. The procedure is completed with application of a moist heating pad and full active range of motion. Postisometric relaxation is valuable in combination with intermittent cold with stretch, or as a separate treatment method, and as a subsequent home exercise. **INJECTION** of hamstring TrPs is best done using pincer palpation for tactile control of needle position in the muscle. It is important to know the course of the sciatic nerve and femoral artery with respect to the TrPs to be injected and the direction of needle insertion. **CORRECTIVE ACTIONS** for patients prone to hamstring TrPs include avoiding working these muscles in a shortened position without opportunity for full stretch, avoiding placing them in a fixed shortened position for prolonged periods of time, and making sure that there is adequate clearance under the front of the chair seat to prevent under-thigh compression. If the fingers can slip easily between the thigh and the front edge of the seat, clearance is adequate. The patient learns the Long-seated Reach Exercise as part of his or her home program.

---

1. REFERRED PAIN
(Fig. 16.1)

The essential referred pain pattern of trigger points (TrPs) in both the *semitendinosus* and *semimembranosus* muscles (Fig. 16.1*A*) projects upward to the gluteal fold. Spillover referred pain travels downward to the medial region of the posterior thigh and back of the knee, and sometimes to the calf medially. The upward pattern reminds one of the direction in which pain is referred by distal TrPs in the biceps brachii muscle (*see* Volume 1, Fig. 30.1).[98]

The essential pain pattern referred from TrPs in either or both heads of the *biceps femoris* (Fig. 16.1*B*) projects distalward to the back of the knee. Spillover referred pain extends downward a short distance below the knee into the calf and may also extend upward in the posterior thigh as high as the crease of the buttock. When pain is referred to the medial side of the back of the knee by semitendinosus or semimembranosus TrPs, its quality is sharper than the deep aching pain referred from the biceps femoris, which is felt more laterally in the knee. This biceps femoris pattern of referred pain and tenderness has been reported.[92,93,97]

Gutstein[45] identified pain in the knee as coming from myalgic spots in the semitendinosus and semimembranosus muscles; he commonly found the myalgic spots in the lower half of these muscles.[46] Kelly[52,53] identified tender fibrositic lesions in the upper third of the hamstring muscles as referring pain in a "sciatic" distribution. Lewit[58] attributed pain in the region of the fibular head in some patients to tension in the biceps femoris muscle.

Hamstring myofascial pain syndromes have been reported in children, in whom the pattern of pain referred by the biceps femoris was nearly the same as that found in adults. That muscle was the fourth most common site of TrPs among 85 children whose primary problem was pain caused by TrPs.[17] Aftimos[1] reported the case of a 5-year-old boy who had disabling pain in his knee caused by a TrP point in the inferior part of the biceps femoris muscle.

2. ANATOMICAL ATTACHMENTS AND CONSIDERATIONS
(Figs. 16.2–16.5)

By anatomical definition,[13] a hamstring muscle must attach to the ischial tuberosity, attach to the leg below the knee, *and* be supplied by the tibial division of the sciatic nerve. All of the muscles of this chapter except the short head of the biceps femoris meet these criteria for true hamstrings, which are two-joint muscles that cross both the hip and the knee.

The belly of the semitendinosus has unusually long muscle fibers (20 cm) compared to the relatively short fibers (8.0 cm) of the semimembranosus, that has over three times the cross-sectional area of the semitendinosus. The long head of the biceps femoris is intermediate in fiber length and cross-sectional area.[99]

PART 2

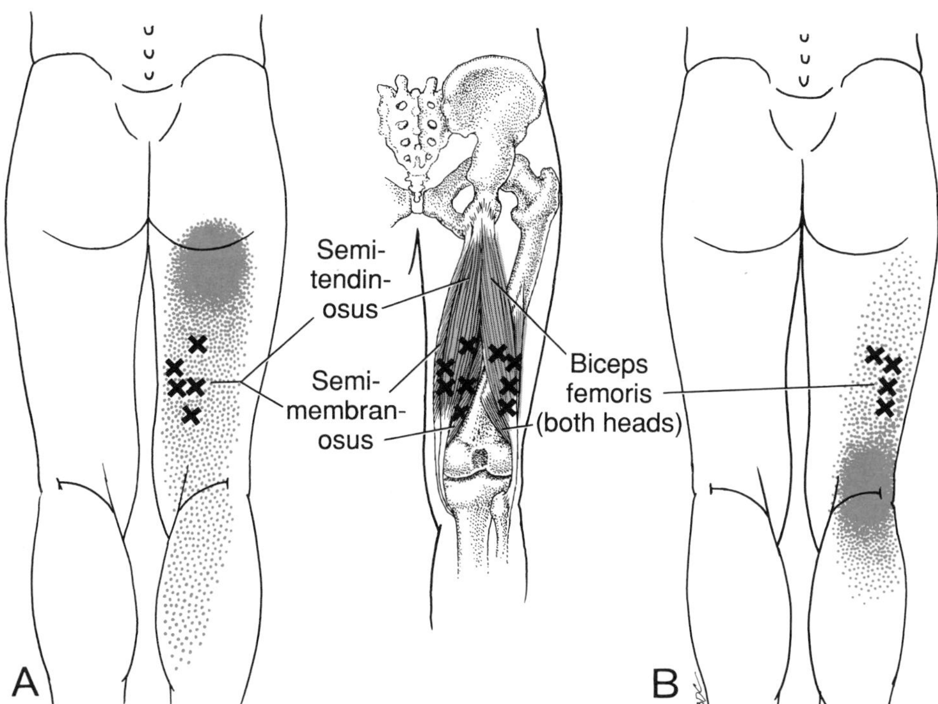

Figure 16.1. Composite pain patterns (*dark red*) referred from trigger points (***X****s*) in the right hamstring muscles. *Solid red* denotes the essential pain distribution referred from these trigger points. *Red stippling* locates the occasional extension of the pattern in some patients. *A*, semitendinosus and semimembranosus muscles. *B*, long and short heads of the biceps femoris muscle.

The short head of the biceps femoris is functionally distinct from the long head, since it crosses only the knee joint.

Semitendinosus and Semimembranosus
(Figs. 16.2–16.4)

The semitendinosus and semimembranosus muscles compose the medial hamstrings. The bulk of the fibers of the semitendinosus lies in the proximal half of the thigh and the bulk of the semimembranosus lies in the distal half. The semitendinosus overlies the deeper semimembranosus (Fig. 16.2).[89]

The semitendinosus muscle (Fig. 16.2) attaches ***proximally*** onto the posterior aspect of the ischial tuberosity by a common tendon with the long head of the biceps femoris (superficial to the semimembranosus attachment).[69] The belly of the semitendinosus muscle becomes tendinous below midthigh and also is normally divided by a tendinous inscription at about midbelly level (Fig. 16.2).[23] ***Distally***, its tendon curves around the posteromedial aspect of the medial condyle of the tibia and anchors to the tibia (*see* Fig. 16.4). The semitendinosus tendon attachment is the most distal of three tendons, the common attachment of which forms the pes anserinus.[69,82] This attachment is considerably farther from the axis of rotation of the knee joint than is that of the other hamstring muscles, giving the semitendinosus strong leverage to flex the knee after the knee is partially bent. This leverage becomes apparent when one bends the knee to a right angle, contracts the hamstrings, and palpates the relative prominence of the semitendinosus tendon.

The division of the semitendinosus muscle into two tandem segments by the tendinous inscription across the middle of the muscle (Fig. 16.2) is apparently related to its phylogenetic origin. In man, two distinct endplate bands are found in the semitendinosus muscle, one above and one below the inscription.[22] The semitendinosus muscle of the rat is di-

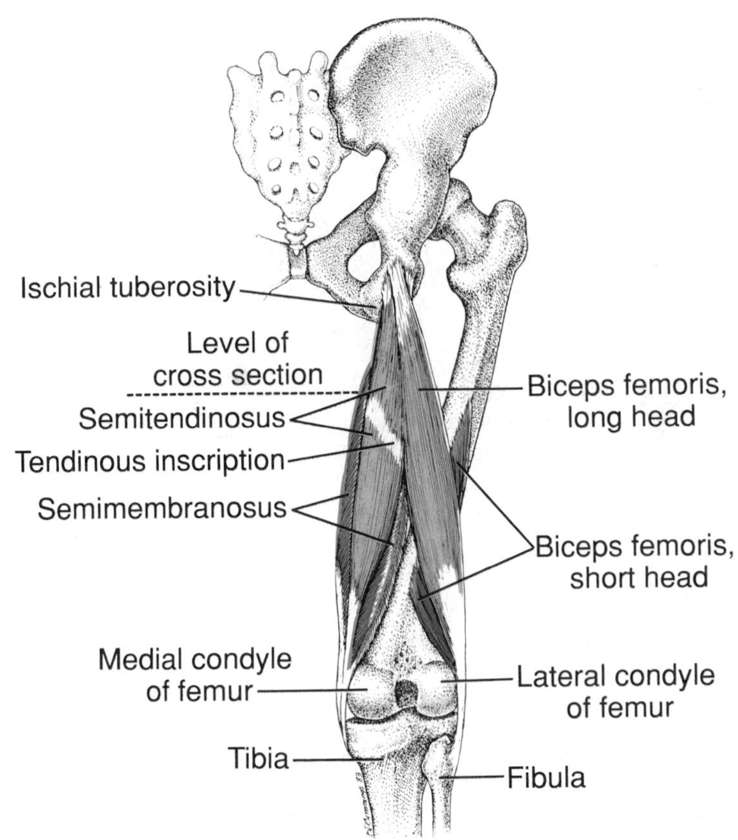

Figure 16.2. Attachments of the right superficial hamstring muscles, posterior view. The semitendinosus and long head of the biceps femoris are *light red*. The underlying semimembranosus and short head of the biceps femoris are *dark red*.

vided into three tandem segments, each innervated by separate peripheral nerves with a set of myoneural junctions at midfiber for each segment.[67] However, the spinal nerve roots supplying the muscle have fibers evenly distributed throughout all three segments. (The rat's biceps femoris muscle has two such tandem segments).[67]

The relatively broad semimembranosus muscle (Fig. 16.3) attaches ***proximally*** on the posterior aspect of the ischial tuberosity lateral and deep to the common tendon of the semitendinosus and biceps femoris muscles. This arrangement places the semimembranosus muscle anterior (deep) to the semitendinosus muscle. The short, oblique semimembranosus muscle fibers form a short, thick muscle belly mostly in the distal half of the thigh (Fig. 16.3).[12,89] ***Distally***, the medial aponeurosis of the semimembranosus becomes tendinous and attaches onto the posteromedial surface of the medial condyle of the tibia just below the joint capsule, close to the axis of rotation of the knee joint[69,82] (Fig. 16.4).

Biceps Femoris

The biceps femoris, the lateral hamstring muscle, has a long head and a short head. The long head crosses both the hip and knee joints, but the short head crosses only the knee joint.

The long head of the biceps femoris attaches ***proximally*** to the posterior aspect of the ischial tuberosity in a common tendon with the semitendinosus muscle (Fig. 16.2). In the distal thigh, the long head is joined by the short head and together they form a tendon that ***distally*** establishes a tripartite anchor to the lateral aspect of the head of the fibula.[23] It is also attached

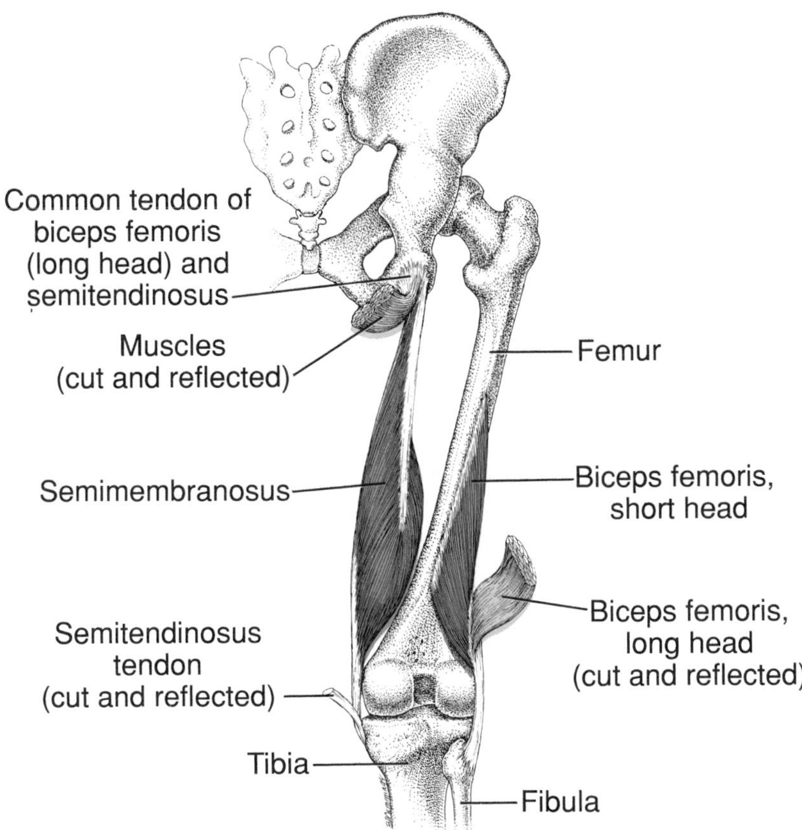

Figure 16.3. Attachments of the deep layer of right hamstring muscles, posterior view. The semimembranosus and short head of the biceps femoris are *dark red*. The cut ends of the superficial layer of hamstring muscles are *light red*.

by a small tendinous slip to the lateral aspect of the tibia.

The short head of the biceps femoris (Fig. 16.3) attaches ***proximally*** to the lateral lip of the linea aspera along nearly the same portion of the femur to which the middle part of the adductor magnus attaches. Together, these last two muscles compose a functional hamstring unit, the middle of which is anchored to the femur. ***Distally***, the short head joins the long head in a common tendon that attaches to the posterolateral aspect of the head of the fibula.

Variations

Numerous variations and anomalies are reported among the hamstring muscles.[43] The semitendinosus may be fused with neighboring muscles, and it may have two tendinous inscriptions.[12]

The extent of the belly of the semimembranosus varies considerably. It may be fused with the semitendinosus or with the adductor magnus. It may be absent, reduced, or doubled in size.[23]

The long head of the biceps femoris may be attached proximally by additional fasciculi to the sacrum, coccyx, and sacrotuberous ligament, mimicking the sacrococcygeal origin of the muscle in lower vertebrates. This attachment would give an additional reason for addressing hamstring tightness in sacral dysfunction. The long head of the biceps femoris may have a tendinous inscription similar to that of the semitendinosus muscle.[12]

The short head of the biceps femoris may be absent or doubled. Additional heads may be attached proximally to the ischial tuberosity or distally to the medial supracondylar ridge of the femur.[23]

Bursae

At the ischial tuberosity, the superior bursa of the biceps femoris frequently is present, separating the common tendon of the long head of the biceps

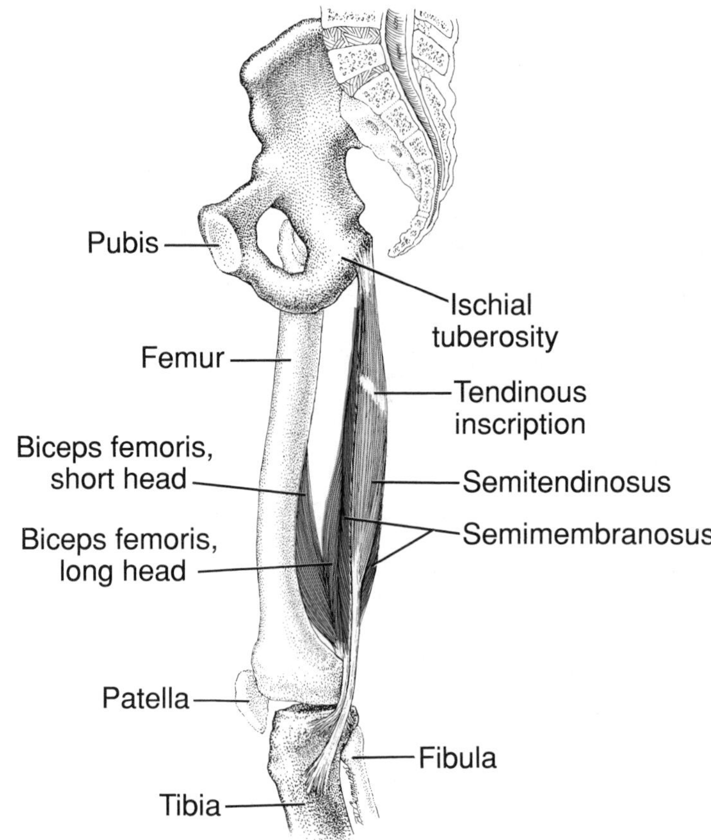

Figure 16.4. Attachments of the right hamstring muscles, medial view. The superficial semitendinosus is *light red* and the deeper semimembranosus is *dark red*. The two heads of the biceps femoris are *intermediate red*.

and the semitendinosus muscles from the deeper tendon of the semimembranosus.[12]

At the knee, the bursa of the semimembranosus muscle is a large double bursa that is consistently present. One part separates the semimembranosus muscle from the medial head of the gastrocnemius muscle; the other separates the semimembranosus tendon from the knee joint.[8,38] This deep bursa often communicates with the joint cavity.[12] The anserine bursa separates the three tendons of the pes anserinus from the underlying tibial collateral ligament of the knee joint.[23,34]

Sciatic Nerve

(Fig. 16.5)

Knowledge of the location of the sciatic nerve is important when injecting TrPs in the hamstring muscles. Throughout the thigh, the nerve lies deep to a hamstring muscle; in the upper thigh, it lies deep to the gluteus maximus muscle and the lateral side of the long head of the biceps femoris muscle, resting on the adductor magnus, as seen in cross section (Fig 16.5).[4,80] As it descends through the upper half of the thigh, the nerve crosses deep to the long head of the biceps femoris from its lateral side to its medial side (*see* Fig. 14.8). At midthigh, the nerve lies deep to the biceps femoris, between it and the semimembranosus muscle, still resting on the adductor magnus. In the distal thigh, the tibial and peroneal branches of the sciatic nerve lie deep in the space between the semimembranosus muscle and the tendon of the long head of the biceps femoris, lateral to the popliteal vessels,[31,80] well illustrated by Netter.[33]

Supplemental References

Both the superficial and the deep layers of these hamstring muscles appear from behind without nerves or vessels in drawings[35] and in photographs.[89] The muscles appear as seen from behind with vessels and nerves[78] in a manner that emphasizes their relations to the sciatic nerve.[7,30,32,76,81] The tendinous inscription of the semitendinosus shows clearly.[6,32] A

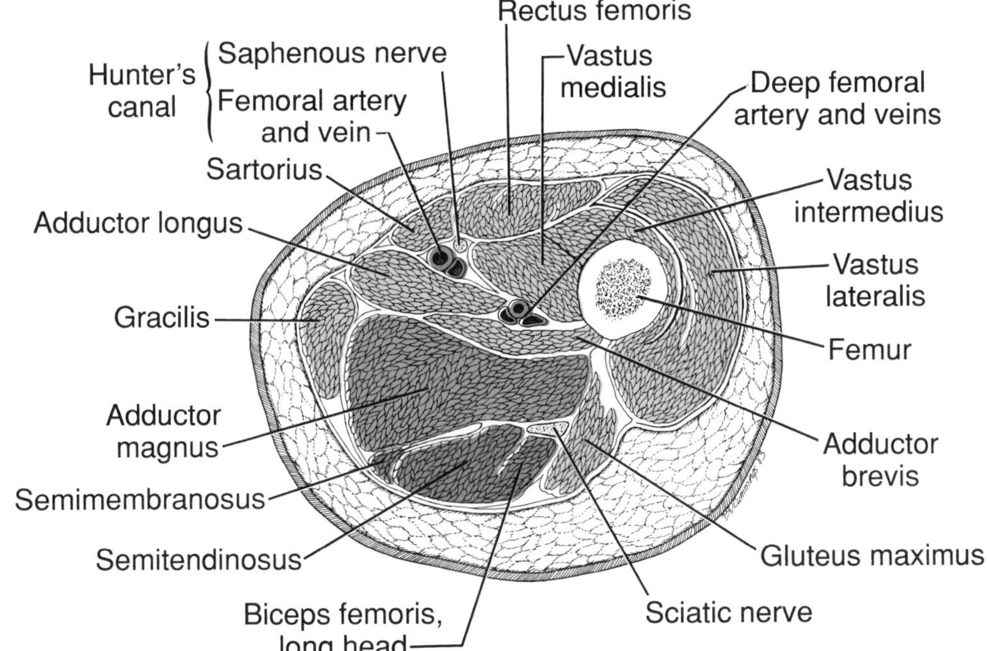

Figure 16.5. Cross section of the thigh at the junction of its upper and middle thirds. *See* Figure 16.2 for level of section. Hamstring muscles, arteries, and veins are *dark red*. At this level, the adductor magnus (*intermediate red*) is considerably larger than the hamstring group. Other muscles of the thigh are *light red*. In this section, the semitendinosus and biceps femoris appear to be fused. Redrawn with permission.[4]

photograph presents the upper half of the thigh from behind with the gluteus maximus muscle removed.[70]

Drawings portray the hamstrings in lateral view.[33,77] A medial view of the knee clearly reveals the relation of the semitendinosus tendon to the other tendons of the pes anserinus.[37] The hamstrings appear in the medial view with the gracilis muscle in place.[5]

Cross sections depict the relation among these muscles in multiple serial sections throughout their length,[21] in three cross sections of the upper, middle, and lower thigh,[31,80] or as one cross section through the upper thigh.[4]

Markings on bones identify the bony attachments for both ends of all hamstring muscles,[3,36,69,79] and in detail for the knee attachments.[9]

Photographs identify surface contours of the muscles in well-muscled subjects.[29,61,71]

A rear view illustrates the semimembranosus bursa;[10,38] the anserine bursa appears in anteromedial view and in cross section.[34]

3. INNERVATION

With two exceptions, the hamstring muscles are supplied by branches from the tibial portion of the sciatic nerve containing fibers of the fifth lumbar and first two sacral nerves. The long head of the biceps femoris receives fibers from only the first three sacral nerves and not from the fifth lumbar nerve. The short head of the biceps femoris is supplied by branches of the peroneal portion of the sciatic nerve instead of the tibial portion; it, too, receives fibers from the fifth lumbar and first two sacral nerves.[23]

4. FUNCTION

The *true* hamstrings (semitendinosus, semimembranosus, long head of the biceps femoris) extend the thigh at the hip. In ambulation, these hip extensors function indirectly to keep the trunk erect during stance (directly restraining the tendency toward hip flexion that is produced by body weight) and to decelerate the forward-moving limb at terminal swing. During standing and forward bending, they control flexion at the hip. All hamstrings flex the leg at the knee. However, the individual hamstrings do not act consistently in flexing the knee during walking. Usually, the short head of the biceps femoris is active in knee flexion for toe clearance.

Actions

The three true hamstring muscles act primarily as hip extensors and knee flexors when the thigh and leg are free to move. The medial hamstrings (semitendinosus and semimembranosus) assist medial rotation at the hip according to most (but not all[13,23]) authors. Basmajian and Deluca[15] note that these muscles are only slightly recruited by effort to rotate the thigh medially when the hip is straight. The lateral true hamstring (long head of the biceps femoris) assists lateral rotation at the hip with the hip extended.[15,86] The short head of the biceps femoris is primarily a flexor at the knee. When the knee is flexed, the semitendinosus and semimembranosus muscles also medially rotate the leg at the knee, and both heads of the biceps femoris laterally rotate it.[13,15,23,86]

In agreement with these remarks, direct electrical stimulation of the semitendinosus has been demonstrated to cause simultaneous extension and medial rotation of the thigh, and flexion of the leg at the knee.[25] When the knee was flexed and the leg placed in lateral rotation, stimulation produced medial rotation of the leg. Direct electrical stimulation of the long head of the biceps femoris also extended the thigh but laterally rotated it as the thigh became extended; this stimulation also flexed the leg at the knee. As the knee flexed, the leg increasingly rotated outward.[25] Furlani and associates[39] demonstrated electromyographically that both heads of the biceps femoris became active during flexion of the leg at the knee, but only the long head contributed to extension of the thigh at the hip.

Thirteen subjects showed no activity in the semitendinosus or semimembranosus muscles when attempting to rotate the leg medially while seated with the knee flexed to 90°.[73]

Functions

The true hamstring muscles show vigorous electromyographic (EMG) activity (controlling flexion at the hip) when the trunk is flexed while standing, and also when individuals are walking, running, jumping, or bicycling.

When the general term *hamstrings* is used in the following section, the authors being quoted did not specify which hamstring muscles they monitored electromyographically.

Posture and Postural Activities

All three of the true hamstring muscles are electromyographically quiescent during quiet standing,[15,84] even when standing on one foot.[15] Motor unit activity was observed during forward bending but not during backward bending: in the hamstrings,[50] in the biceps femoris,[40,84] and in the semitendinosus muscle.[84] Okada[84] found that any form of leaning forward activated the biceps femoris and semitendinosus muscles. Also, raising the arms activated the hamstrings.[50]

In three normal subjects, sudden voluntary trunk flexion was controlled by vigorous hamstring and other extensor activity. In these normal subjects, the hamstrings responded first, the gluteus maximus next, and the erector spinae last to produce this braking action.[83]

Walking

In walking subjects, the true hamstrings reached their peak of activity just before or at heel-strike.[16] The short head of the biceps femoris was active only through the period of toe-off.[24]

Activation of the true hamstrings toward the end of swing phase decelerates the limb.[62] The fact that the short head of the biceps femoris becomes active only at toe-off, when the knee starts flexing for swing phase, suggests that when other hamstrings become active at this time they assist knee flexion for toe clearance.

Fine-wire electrodes in the semimembranosus[62] and fine-wire[72] and surface[74,102] electrodes in the long head of the biceps femoris muscles revealed that activity started at midswing and lasted through the period of heel strike with no second peak.[62] Three of seven subjects showed activity during toe-off at slow and fast gaits.[74] Some subjects evidenced continuous or intermittent activity from toe-off through the next fifth of the gait cycle.[72] The amplitude of EMG activity increased with increased rate of walking,[74,102] and variability increased at uncomfortably slow walking speeds.[72]

The pattern of activation is consistent for any one individual at various walking speeds. The variability among subjects reported previously indicates that some people use the true hamstrings for walking in a somewhat different manner than others do.

Carrying a load of 15% or 20% of body weight in one hand (for example, a heavy suitcase) significantly increased the duration of semimembranosus and semitendinosus EMG activity on the same side. Loads carried centrally on the back had no effect on the activity of these muscles.[42]

When descending stairs, all three true hamstrings showed most, if not all, of their activity in association with toe-off at the beginning of swing phase.[62,95] However, when ascending stairs, these muscles revealed their individuality. The semimembranosus responded with peak EMG activity during the 20% of the cycle preceding heel-strike, and the long head of the biceps femoris responded with only a weak burst just preceding heel-strike but with major peaks at the beginning and end of stance phase.[62]

Running, Jumping, and Sports Activities

During jogging, running, and sprinting, EMG activity from surface electrodes appeared from both the medial and lateral hamstrings just prior to maximum hip flexion and shortly after the onset of knee extension during swing, suggesting that this muscle group, through an eccentric contraction, is helping restrain the hip joint in terminal flexion and then helps modulate the rapid extension at the knee, as well as contributing to extension at the hip joint.[66]

During a two-leg jump straight upward from a semicrouched position, surface electrodes over the hamstrings showed several bursts of EMG activity prior to take-off and also at take-off (when activity was the greatest), and finally at and after landing.[51]

Surface electrodes over the medial and lateral hamstrings during 11 right-handed sports activities consistently showed moderate to marked activity, greater on the right side than on the left, except during a left-footed one-foot jump volleyball spike with the right hand.[20]

Ergometer Cycling

Ericson[26] calculated that, together, all of the hip extensors produce 27% of the total positive mechanical work during ergometer cycling.

An average of surface electrode activity through 25 cycles of pedaling in 11 subjects[27] showed that the biceps femoris EMG activity peaked at the beginning of the backward motion of the pedal, whereas the combination of semitendinosus and semimembranosus EMG activity peaked near the end of this period. Activity of the biceps femoris increased with increased pedaling rate and with increased seat height.[27]

Additional Considerations

Németh and associates[75] used surface electrodes to record biceps femoris and semitendinosus-semimembranosus EMG activity in 15 subjects when they lifted a 12.8-kg (28-lb) box from the floor. As a group, these hamstring muscles were considerably more active during a straight-knee lift than during a flexed-knee lift.

The fiber composition of the proximal and distal portions of all three true hamstrings and of the short head of the biceps femoris in 10 autopsy subjects ranged in average composition from 50.5% to 60.4% of type 2 (fast-twitch) fibers. The only significant difference between the two ends of each muscle was the higher percentage of type 2 fibers in the distal, as compared with the proximal, portions of the semitendinosus muscle, which are separated by a tendinous raphe.[41]

In a study of muscle tightness and hypermobility in students 8–20 years of age,[64] children who were active in sports had a lower prevalence of shortened hamstring muscles and a higher prevalence of hypermobility. When an individual developed one of these conditions, it was likely to persist.

The propensity of hamstring muscles to develop tightness and hyperactivity is associated with a corresponding tendency for the gluteus maximus to become lax and inhibited.[56] This muscle imbalance contributes to musculoskeletal pain syndromes, as discussed and illustrated by Lewit.[56]

Duchenne[25] observed that patients who have lost the use of all their hamstring muscles have a tendency to fall forward when walking, and that they instinctively move the center of gravity posteriorly to maintain extension of the trunk [hips] and, thus, avoid falling. These individuals cannot walk rapidly or on uneven ground, cannot run, hop, dance, jump, or incline the trunk forward without falling.[86] Markhede and Stener[68] reported that function was not impaired, or was impaired only slightly, when only one muscle, the semitendinosus or the biceps femoris, had been surgically removed unilaterally; they reported that function was moderately impaired when all the hamstrings were removed unilaterally. This total loss of the true hamstring muscles was associated with a 25% reduction in the isometric and isotonic strength of hip extension. Additional loss of the adductor magnus muscle reduced isokinetic strength of hip extension to 50% of that on the uninvolved side.[68]

5. FUNCTIONAL (MYOTATIC) UNIT

The hip extensors in the functional unit of the true hamstrings include the gluteus maximus, which is the major extensor of the thigh against resistance, and the posterior parts of the adductor magnus. They are assisted by the posterior portions of the gluteus medius and gluteus minimus.

Flexion at the knee, accomplished by the true hamstrings and the short head of the biceps femoris, is assisted by the sartorius, gracilis, gastrocnemius, and plantaris muscles. Medial rotation of the leg at the knee is performed primarily by the semitendinosus and semimembranosus members of the hamstring muscles and by the popliteus, assisted by the sartorius and gracilis muscles. Lateral rotation of the leg at the knee is performed by the biceps femoris, unassisted.[86]

The corresponding *antagonists* to extension at the hip are primarily the iliopsoas, tensor fasciae latae, rectus femoris, sartorius, and pectineus muscles. The chief antagonist to knee flexion is the quadriceps femoris muscle group.[86]

6. SYMPTOMS

Characteristic Symptoms

The patient with TrPs in the hamstring muscles usually experiences pain on walking; he or she may even limp, because loading this group of muscles is so painful and the muscle inhibition compromises hip stability. When sitting, patients with these TrPs are likely to experience pain posteriorly in the buttock, upper thigh, and back of the knee that is reproduced by pressure on the TrPs. These patients commonly experience pain when getting up from a chair, especially after they have been sitting with knees crossed. They tend to push themselves up out of the chair with their arms (which may overload muscles in the upper limbs and shoulder girdle and thus perpetuate TrPs present in those regions). Myofascial TrPs in the biceps femoris muscle often wake patients at night, and the patients describe disturbed or nonrestful sleep.

The patient may complain only of symptoms of quadriceps femoris TrPs when the trouble actually originates in the hamstrings. The hamstring shortening that is caused by TrPs in them is likely to overload and decompensate the quadriceps muscles. This overload can activate TrPs in the quadriceps. These TrPs produce a different pattern of referred pain (*see* Chapter 14). The quadriceps femoris symptoms will not resolve until their cause, tension of the hamstrings, has been eliminated. This relation is comparable to that of the middle trapezius and rhomboids in the posterior shoulder girdle with the pectoralis major muscle on the front of the chest.

Differential Diagnosis

Myofascial Considerations

Trigger points in several other muscles refer pain and tenderness in patterns that overlap those of hamstring TrPs. Other TrP pain patterns include those of: the obturator internus and piriformis muscles; TrP_2 in the gluteus medius muscle; the posterior gluteus minimus (except that its pattern usually skips the back of the knee); TrP_3 in the vastus lateralis; the popliteus and plantaris muscles; and TrP_3 and TrP_4 in the gastrocnemius muscle.

Patients with TrPs in the hamstring muscles are often diagnosed as having "sciatica" (or pseudosciatica[55]) because pain extends down the posterior thigh within the distribution of the sciatic nerve.

Among patients with low back pain, tightness of the hamstring muscles in one or both lower limbs is common,[2] tempting one to infer a causal relationship. However, a prospective study of nearly 600 military recruits showed a high prevalence of hamstring tightness (more than ⅓ of limbs examined), but no significant correlation with low back pain.[48] Myofascial TrPs commonly responsible for hamstring shortening do not refer pain to the low back region.

Among children, the hamstrings were reported to be the fourth most common muscle group to harbor myofascial TrPs,[17] but the pain frequently had been diagnosed (or dismissed) as "growing pains."[18]

The postlaminectomy pain syndrome may be caused by active TrPs remaining after successful surgery for nerve root entrapment, and it often receives a major contribution from TrPs in the hamstring muscles.[90,96]

Myofascial TrPs in the hamstring muscles refer pain and tenderness that may be mistaken for osteoarthritis of the knee unless both the muscles and the knee joint are carefully examined.[88]

As noted by Sherman,[91] TrPs in hamstring muscles that are used to cover the end of an above-knee amputation stump can be responsible for distressing phantom limb pain, especially in the phantom knee. Like Sherman, we also found that this source of the pain was eliminated by inactivating the responsible TrPs.

Other Considerations

Articular dysfunction, particularly lack of mobility of the L_4-L_5 and L_5-S_1 vertebral joints and of the sacroiliac joint, is associated with hamstring spasm and restriction of the Straight-leg Raising Test.[59] A posteriorly rotated ilium shortens the hamstrings and an anteriorly rotated ilium increases the tension on them. Surgical fusion of the L_5-S_1 articulations aggravates hamstring tightness and makes it a more critical factor.[65]

Brody[19] ascribes symptoms of posterior thigh pain and local tenderness on bending or prolonged sitting to *strain* or *partial tear of the hamstring muscles*. The tears are attributed to inadequate stretching of these muscles before and after running. Only in the severe, acute cases of such tears in sprinters is operative intervention recommended. Conservative treatment is advised in the more common cases of recreational or long-distance runners. Activation of latent hamstring TrPs could have caused these symptoms in many of the patients who were diagnosed as having a muscle strain, but apparently the subjects were not examined for TrPs.

Puranen and Orava[85] described a *hamstring syndrome* with pain in the lower gluteal area that radiated down the posterior thigh to the popliteal space. Pain was experienced in the sitting position often causing the patient to change position frequently or stand up for relief. Activities including gymnastic exercises, sprinting, hurdling, sudden spurts by endurance runners, and kicking a soccer ball with maximum force exacerbated the pain. Tender bandlike structures were palpable in the hamstring muscles at the lateral proximal insertion area that, at operation, were adherent to and irritating the sciatic nerve. Surgical release of the band relieved the symptoms in most cases.[85] The fibrotic bands of the hamstring syndrome should be distinguished from taut bands of TrPs by the fact that they are connective tissue, not muscle tissue, and should not produce local twitch responses on snapping palpation.

Weiser[100] identified 98 women and two men as having *semimembranosus insertion syndrome* because of their complaint of pain at the medial aspect of the knee with tenderness over the attachment of the semimembranosus muscle. Pain increased during exercise, walking down stairs, marked knee bending, and lying on the side. In some patients, pain radiated up the posterior thigh and/or down the calf. Of these 100 patients, 58 were relieved by one or two injections of 2% lidocaine with 10 mg of triamcinolone into the region of the insertion of the semimembranosus tendon at the depth of the periosteum. Nine patients experienced only partial relief, 18 had no relief, and 15 were lost to follow-up. Apparently none was examined for TrPs in the semimembranosus muscle, which is a probable differential diagnosis that could account for a number of the treatment failures.

Halperin and Axer[47] reported on 172 patients treated for *semimembranous tenosynovitis*, the description of which resembles the semimembranosus insertion syndrome described previously. Ninety-eight patients had "semimembranous tenosynovitis" only and, of these, over 60% obtained complete relief with conservative treatment. Those with additional diagnoses of degenerative joint disease of the knee and pes anserinus tendinitis (at the attachment of the semitendinosus muscle) did not respond as well. As initial treatment, patients received analgesics and anti-inflammatory drugs: aspirin, indomethacin, phenylbutazone, and proprionic acid derivatives. If necessary, ultrasound and friction massage were added. If that failed, finally 1% lidocaine with either 40 or 80 mg of methylprednisolone acetate was injected locally, up to three times. The possible contribution of TrPs in these muscles was apparently not considered; this might have been helpful for cases not responding well to initial therapy.

Snapping syndrome of the semitendinosus tendon over a prominent area of the medial tibial condyle was relieved in a patient by releasing the tibial attachment of the tendon and suturing it to the semimembranosus tendon.[63] The syndrome was apparently caused by rupture of the fanned-out fibers that form part of the terminal portion of the tendon and normally hold it in place when the knee is extended.

Snapping bottom[87] is rare but disablingly painful. It is caused by luxation of the tendon of the biceps femoris muscle over the ischial tuberosity at its attachment. The one patient reported was relieved of symptoms by tenotomy.

Bursitis of the biceps femoris superior bursa, the bursa of the semimembranosus muscle, or of the anserine bursa can easily be diagnosed erroneously when local pain and tenderness referred from TrPs in the hamstring muscles are present at the site of the bursa; the two conditions may coexist.

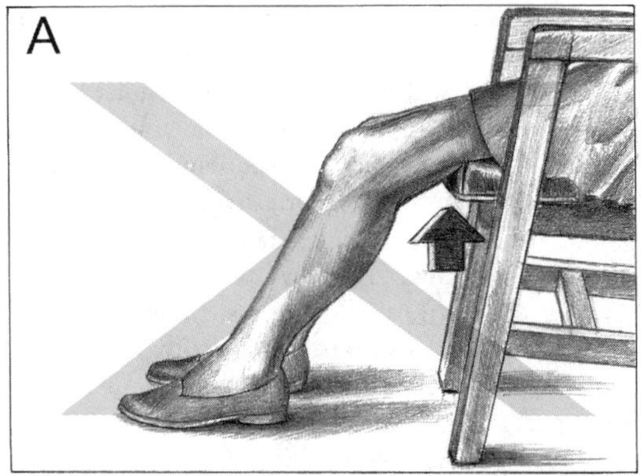

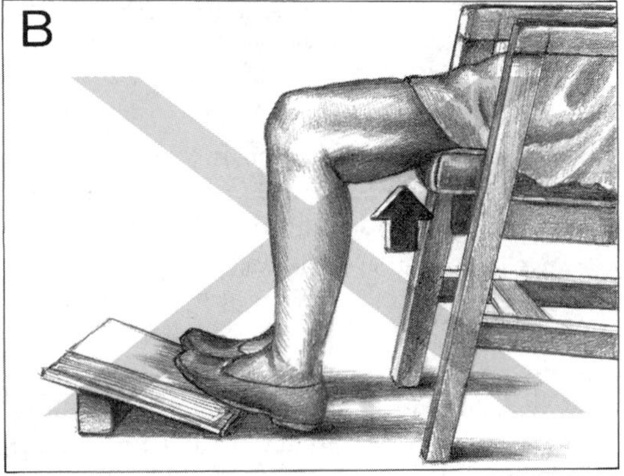

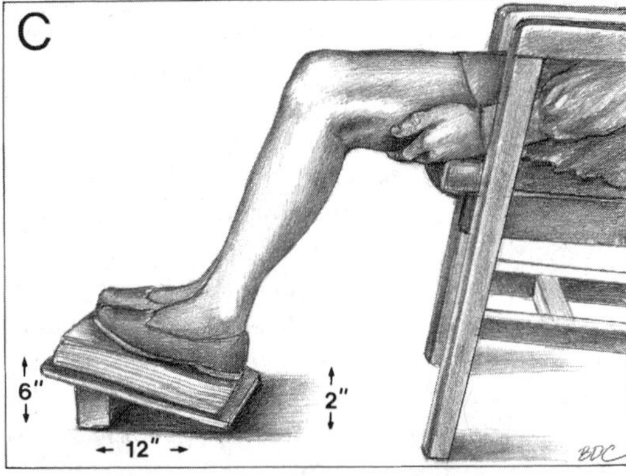

Figure 16.6. Hamstring muscle compression and shortening of soleus muscle due to incorrect seated posture. Red ***X*** emphasizes this hazardous posture. *A*, severe underthigh compression of hamstrings at *arrow* due to the high chair seat and extension of the knee. This posture also places the soleus muscles in the shortened position due to plantar flexion at the ankle. *B*, excessive plantar flexion at the ankle is eliminated, but underthigh compression is not fully corrected because of wrong positioning of heels at the footstool. *C*, full correction of both problems by a sloped footstool. Elevating the knee provides clearance for the hand to slip easily between the thigh and the front edge of the chair seat (an indication that compression is no longer a problem) and restores the foot to a neutral position at the ankle.

7. ACTIVATION AND PERPETUATION OF TRIGGER POINTS
(Fig. 16.6)

Underthigh compression by an ill-fitting chair (Fig. 16.6*A*) can both activate and perpetuate TrPs in the hamstring muscles. Short-statured patients with hamstring TrPs who sit in the customary chairs, or patients of average stature who sit in long-legged chairs with too high a seat, experience aggravation of pain because of pressure on hamstring TrPs. In addition, they may experience the tingling and numbness of neurapraxia. One solution to this problem of underthigh compression by the chair seat is to use a footstool (Fig. 16.6*C*) that supports the heels and lifts the thighs (it also should angle the feet upward to prevent prolonged shortening of the calf muscles).

Patio furniture can be particularly hazardous to the hamstrings. Manufacturers commonly attach a canvas or plastic seat to a horizontal bar across the front of the seat. The seat bottom sags and the cross bar presses firmly against the posterior thigh, causing local ischemia. This is most troublesome to individuals with relatively short legs when their heels do not rest firmly on the floor. Even the contoured plastic chairs so common in waiting rooms and meeting rooms cause this problem if the front edge of the chair seat is too high for the individual's leg length.

Children are often placed in highchairs without a footrest, or on chair seats that were raised by adding books. The lack of foot support leads to underthigh compression, which is a common cause of restlessness and irritability; these are relieved by providing adequate foot support to take pressure off the posterior thigh above the knee. Many times, the children are too young to identify or communicate the source of their distress. Many school chairs present this same problem because chairs of one size are used for children of widely different heights.

Patients with a small hemipelvis, when sitting, intuitively compensate for the small hemipelvis by leaning forward and placing the weight on the thighs instead of the buttocks, or by crossing the lower limbs to help level the pelvis. In this way, the small hemipelvis can be an important initiating or perpetuating factor for hamstring TrPs. The body structure of short upper arms in relation to torso height can also cause an individual to shift the body weight forward onto the thighs (*see* Fig. 4.13*E*).

In the past, clinicians frequently prescribed bed rest for several days to several weeks as treatment for acute low back strain. A semi-Fowler position with the hips and knees moderately flexed was common; the patient was often advised to put a pillow under the knees. When this position is maintained for days, the hamstring muscles tend to develop TrPs because they are never stretched. Fortunately, prolonged bed rest is no longer considered desirable for acute musculoskeletal low back pain.

Activation of latent TrPs in the hamstrings (reactive cramp) can result from their unaccustomed shortening during inactivation of rectus femoris TrPs by fully lengthening that muscle.

Of the 100 subjects examined by Baker[11] following their first motor vehicle accident, about one in four developed TrPs in the semimembranosus muscle regardless of the direction of impact; right and left muscles were affected about equally.

8. PATIENT EXAMINATION
(Fig. 16.7)

The clinician looks to see whether the posterior thighs are being compressed by the front of a chair seat. Are the patient's feet dangling because his or her legs are not long enough for the feet to rest fully on the floor? Are the thighs tightly compressed against the front edge of the seat bottom while the patient is sitting and giving the medical history? If the patient fidgets during this time, he or she may harbor active TrPs in the hamstring muscles, especially if pain is present in the posterior knee, thigh, or lower buttock. Patients often mistakenly refer to the buttock as the "low back."

If the patient crosses the legs when sitting or limps on walking, this further suggests hamstring TrPs. Or, the seated patient may lean forward to lighten the weight on the ischial tuberosities or to gain support for the arms; when this posture occurs, the examiner should check the patient for a small hemipelvis and also for short upper arms (*see* Chapter 4, pages 43 and 44).

Hamstring tightness is the most frequent reason why an individual cannot touch the toes when forward bending with knees extended.[57] The tightness does not restrict flexion at the hip when the knee is bent.

The TrPs in the hamstrings markedly limit motion during the Straight-leg Raising Test (Fig. 16.7*A*).[93] The pain that these TrPs cause at the limit of hip flexion may be felt in the lower buttock, the back of the thigh, or behind the knee (Fig. 16.1). The hamstrings are judged to be tight if, in this test, the thigh cannot be raised (with the knee straight) to an angle of at least 80° above the horizontal,[57] including 10° of posterior pelvic tilt.[54]

Lasègue's sign is elicited (Fig. 16.7*B*) by flexing the hip of the supine patient to the comfort tolerance with the knee straight and then dorsiflexing the foot. The test is positive if the patient experiences pain in the posterior thigh or low back. This is usually interpreted as indicating lumbar root or sciatic nerve irritation. A pain response in the calf and back of the knee, however, is also a sign of shortening of the gastrocnemius muscle (for example, due to TrPs). This dorsiflexion of the foot does not increase tension on the hamstring muscles,[55] so Lasègue's sign is absent in cases of TrPs in those muscles.

Of historical interest are the facts that Lasègue never wrote about the sign that bears his name, and that those who first connected a sign with his name did not mention dorsiflexion of the foot,[14] but only described the Straight-leg Raising Test.[94]

A crossed reflex effect from one lower limb to the other can be demonstrated when hamstring tension bilaterally restricts straight-leg raising. Release of hamstring tightness on one side by intermittent cold with stretch results immediately in a remarkable increase in the range of straight-leg raising on the opposite, untreated side. Similar crossed effects have been demonstrated experimentally.

Eight patients with *unilateral* disc protrusion confirmed by myelography showed marked *bilat-*

PART 2

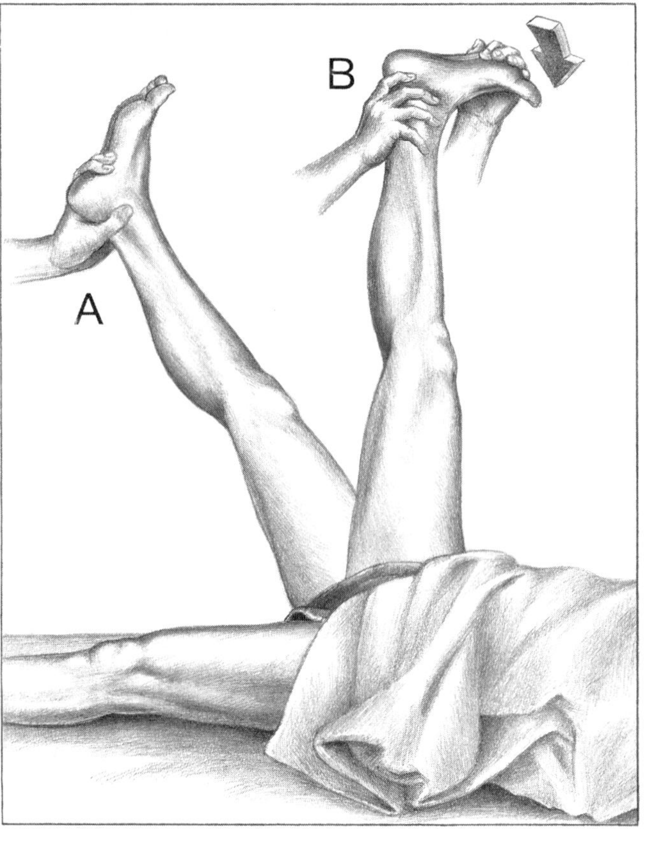

Figure 16.7. Straight-leg Raising Test for hamstring tightness before and after intermittent cold with stretch. *A*, limited range of hip flexion with knee straight, before inactivation of hamstring trigger points (positive Straight-leg Raising Test). *B*, test of ankle dorsiflexion and full range of motion following application of intermittent cold with stretch. Gastrocnemius muscle TrP tension and nerve root irritation both render the addition of dorsiflexion at the ankle painful (positive Lasègue's sign).

eral suppression of biceps femoris nociceptive flexion reflexes. The reflexes were elicited by sural nerve stimulation while pain was induced by straight-leg raising on the painful side. Straight-leg raising on the uninvolved side caused no depression of the reflex.[101]

In some muscles, active TrPs cause sufficient pain when the muscle is fully shortened that they slightly restrict the shortened range of motion as well as markedly restrict the stretch range of motion. Active TrPs in the hamstring muscles may slightly restrict the combination of active extension at the hip and flexion at the knee, giving the erroneous impression that a tight rectus femoris muscle is responsible. In this situation, inactivation of the hamstring TrPs restores range of motion.

Persons with tight hamstrings may have a posterior pelvic tilt, a flattening of the lumbar curve, and a head-forward posture, which, in turn, causes problems in the upper body musculature. Therefore, the importance of a thorough examination, even when all muscular symptoms are limited to the upper half of the body, cannot be overemphasized.[98]

We find that patients with medial hamstring TrPs and pain referred to the gluteal fold also experience *referred tenderness* at these pain referral sites. Similarly, patients with biceps femoris TrPs that refer pain to the knee also exhibit referred tenderness in the back of the knee, particularly where the tendon attaches to the fibular head (Figs. 16.2 and 16.3).

9. TRIGGER POINT EXAMINATION (Figs. 16.8–16.10)

When examining the hamstrings for injection, it helps to remember that they are nearly encased on their medial and anterior sides by the adductor magnus (Fig. 16.8). Posteriorly, the proximal attachment of the hamstring muscles is covered by the gluteus maximus (*dashed outline* in Fig. 16.8).[78] The upper lateral portion of the thigh is occupied by the gluteus maximus, adductor magnus, and vastus lateralis.

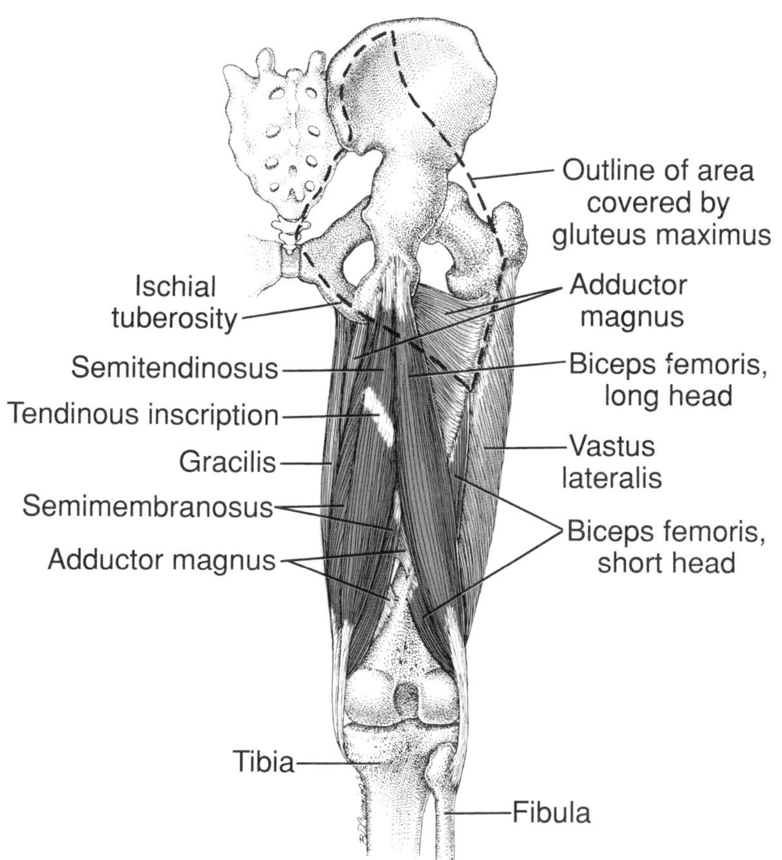

Figure 16.8. Regional anatomy of the right hamstring muscles, posterior view. The hamstrings are *dark red* and the adjacent deeper muscles are *light red*. The *broken line* encloses area covered by the gluteus maximus muscle.

The semitendinosus muscle is easily identified by locating its prominent tendon behind the knee medially when the knee is bent against resistance and then by following the tendon upward into the thigh. The semimembranosus muscle lies deep to the semitendinosus, and is muscular in the distal thigh. Its muscle fibers can be palpated on each side of the semitendinosus tendon. The semimembranosus forms the medial border of the hamstrings and is adjacent to the gracilis muscle in the lower half of the thigh (Fig. 16.8).[80]

Usually, either pincer or flat palpation can be used for examination of the medial hamstring muscles. However, it often is difficult to grasp the biceps femoris in pincer palpation, particularly in heavily-muscled and obese individuals. Then, flat palpation must be used.

To locate TrPs in the semitendinosus or semimembranosus muscles (Fig. 16.1), the muscles are approached from the medial aspect of the thigh (Fig. 16.9). The patient lies supine with the involved thigh in the abducted position, the knee bent to adjust tension on the muscles, and the lower limb supported, as shown in Figure 16.9. If the adductors are shortened, a pillow may be placed underneath the knee, as shown, or the patient can roll slightly toward that side with a pillow supporting the opposite hip. Tight adductors should be released before attempting to release tight hamstrings.

For pincer palpation, the distal medial hamstring mass is grasped 8–12 cm (3–4½ in) above the posterior knee fold (Fig. 16.9*A*) and the muscle mass is pulled away from the femur with the finger tips to ensure that all of the semitendinosus and semimembranosus musculature is included for palpation. One can then roll the muscle fibers between the thumb and

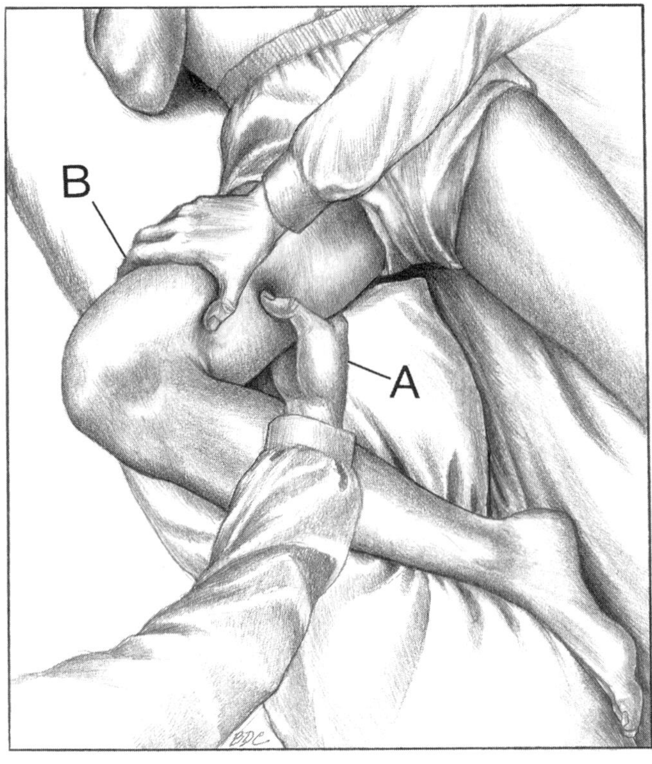

Figure 16.9. Examination for trigger points in the right semimembranosus and semitendinosus muscles, along the distal half of the femur where these trigger points are commonly found. Spot tenderness at trigger points in the underlying adductor magnus may also be elicited. Two methods of palpation are used: *A*, pincer palpation; *B*, flat palpation with the thumb pressing both of these hamstring muscles against the femur.

fingers to examine for taut bands and tender spots. Taut bands are clearly distinguishable, and snapping palpation can elicit local twitch responses in the more superficial semitendinosus muscle. Flat palpation is accomplished by direct pressure on the muscle against the underlying femur (Fig. 16.9*B*).

The pressure of flat palpation may also compress TrPs in the distal end of the underlying adductor magnus, which would require that inactivation of these TrPs by intermittent cold with stretch include abduction for restoration of the adductor magnus to full length (see Section 12 of this chapter).

When examining the biceps femoris muscle for TrPs, it is best to approach it from the posterior aspect of the thigh. The patient lies on the opposite side with the knee bent slightly, as in Figure 16.10. This figure illustrates use of the thumb for flat palpation of TrPs in the biceps femoris on the lateral aspect of the thigh, pressing against the underlying femur. The biceps femoris is difficult to grasp separately by pincer palpation because the investing fascia of the lateral border is firmly joined with that of the vastus lateralis muscle. The short head of the biceps femoris lies deep to the long head in the distal half of the thigh (Fig. 16.4), but the two heads can be distinguished by palpation because the long head becomes tense when the patient tries to extend the hip, while the short head does not change tension.

Lange[55] illustrates tender and palpably tense (myogelotic) areas [TrPs] in the medial and lateral hamstrings in the upper half of the thigh and at midthigh.

10. ENTRAPMENTS

No entrapments of nerves or blood vessels due to TrPs in the hamstring muscles have been confirmed.

However, in the *hamstring syndrome*[85] described in Section 6 on page 325, several cases were observed in which the sciatic nerve was constricted where it passed between two fibrotic bands of the hamstring muscles near the lateral proximal attachment to the ischial tuberosity. Symptoms were relieved by surgically releasing the fibrotic bands.

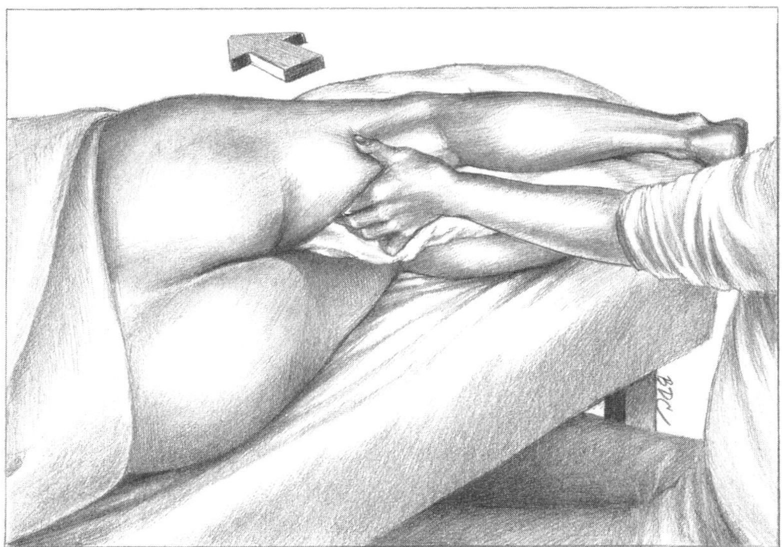

Figure 16.10. Examination for trigger points in the right biceps femoris muscle by flat palpation against the femur. The *large arrow* shows the anterior direction of thumb pressure. The knee is bent only slightly so that there is sufficient tension on the muscle for examination. Trigger points are found in the biceps femoris on the lateral side of the posterior thigh at about the same level as the semitendinosus and semimembranosus trigger points on the medial side.

11. ASSOCIATED TRIGGER POINTS

In association with TrPs in the hamstring muscles, secondary TrPs are likely to develop in the posterior (ischiocondylar) part of the adductor magnus muscle, which also extends the thigh, and which lies along the medial border of, and anterior to, the medial hamstring muscles. Probably because of its close anatomical relation to the long head of the biceps femoris, the vastus lateralis muscle is also prone to become involved. The gastrocnemius muscle, but not the soleus, tends to develop secondary TrPs in association with hamstring TrPs.

Antagonists to the hamstrings may also develop secondary TrPs, especially the iliopsoas muscle and the quadriceps.

Tight hamstrings produce a posterior tilt of the pelvis that flattens the lumbar spine and thus can induce an undesirable head-forward posture; this postural dysfunction imposes compensatory overload on a number of muscles; those likely to become involved are the quadratus lumborum, thoracic paraspinals, and rectus abdominis, in addition to shoulder-girdle and neck muscles. Hamstring tension is so often a key to low back pain of myofascial origin that even though the iliopsoas or quadratus lumborum muscles seem to be primarily involved, it is wise to start treatment by releasing the hamstrings.

12. INTERMITTENT COLD WITH STRETCH

(Fig. 16.11)

The application of intermittent cold with stretch to the hamstring muscles usually produces one of the most dramatic responses observed with this therapeutic modality. Before the clinician applies this procedure to the hamstring group, and while the patient is in the long sitting position, the patient should test how far the fingers will reach forward along the shins. Later, he or she can compare this distance with the range of motion following treatment; the patient will then realize how much release of muscular shortening was achieved.

The use of ice for applying intermittent cold with stretch is explained on page 9 of this volume and the use of vapocoolant with stretch is detailed on pages 67–74 of Volume 1.[98] Avoid stretching hypermobile joints to their full range. Techniques that augment relaxation and stretch are reviewed on page 11 and alternative treat-

PART 2

ment methods are reviewed on pages 9–11 of this volume.

Since tight lower long paraspinal muscles and tight gluteal muscles, especially the gluteus maximus, can restrict hip flexion, sometimes it is necessary to treat these muscles by intermittent cold with stretch before applying it to the hamstrings.

It is possible to start the intermittent cold with stretch of the hamstring muscles by simply flexing the thigh at the hip with the knee straight and applying the intermittent cold distally from the buttock, over the hamstrings and behind the knee. However, this is rarely effective as the first step in treatment, because any tightness of the posterior part of the adductor magnus will block full hamstring lengthening, especially of the medial hamstrings.

Therefore, the *first step* for release of the hamstrings is to lengthen the adductor magnus passively. The patient lies supine with sufficient space at the side of the treatment table to *abduct fully* the affected thigh. The operator grasps the ankle to abduct the thigh at the hip while applying ice or vapocoolant spray in parallel distal-to-proximal sweeps that cover this adductor muscle (Fig. 16.11*A*).[92,93] The thigh is held nearly parallel to the floor and the knee is kept straight. Cycles of intermittent cold application coordinated with passive abduction are repeated until no further (or full) abduction range is obtained.

The *second step* starts with the thigh abducted. The foot is gradually elevated by adducting the limb, while maintaining flexion at the hip. Now, the direction of cooling reverses: proximal-to-distal sweeps of ice or vapocoolant spray are applied over the thigh posteriorly to provide full coverage of the semimembranosus and semitendinosus muscles and their referred pain patterns (Fig. 16.11*B*). As the thigh is gradually adducted, the parallel lines of cold are applied to successively more lateral aspects, covering the biceps femoris, accessible gluteal musculature, and the vastus lateralis (Fig. 16.11*C, D*, and *E*). It is essential that the intermittent cold be applied to the skin overlying the muscle fibers that are being elongated. When asked, the patient frequently can point to an area of skin where more cooling is needed. Application of ice or vapocoolant to such an area usually results in some immediate release of muscle tightness and significantly increased range of motion.

As the *last step*, when the limb reaches a vertical position (neither abducted nor adducted) (Fig. 16.11*D*), the foot is gently dorsiflexed at the ankle (Fig. 16.7*B*) and the area to which cold is being applied is extended to cover the calf muscles. Passive hip adduction is then continued until the thigh is fully adducted in full flexion (Fig. 16.11*E*), while the parallel sweeps of ice or vapocoolant fully cover the biceps femoris, the accessible gluteal musculature, and most of the semitendinosus and semimembranosus muscles.

A moist heating pad is applied for several minutes to rewarm the skin as the patient relaxes and the opposite limb is treated. The hamstring muscles should always be released bilaterally. After rewarming, the patient performs several cycles of active range of motion by slowly moving each thigh alternately from the extended to the fully flexed position, with the knee straight, to help restore normal muscle function.

Now, when the patient in the long sitting position tests the ability to reach the feet with the fingers, the increase in range is impressive and offers an opportunity for invaluable patient education to improve compliance.

If hamstring length is restricted in both lower limbs, releasing the tightness of the hamstring muscles of one limb using intermittent cold with stretch increases the length of the *untreated* hamstrings. This response demonstrates a crossed reflex effect and the close myotatic relation between the hamstring muscles bilaterally. However, since the hamstrings of both limbs are involved, the TrPs of both need to be inactivated. The improvement in muscle length on the untreated side is likely to be short lived, and the hamstring muscles on both sides may soon tighten again if both sides are not treated directly.

Aftimos[1] recently reported successful use of vapocoolant spray (ethyl chloride) and stretch to inactivate TrPs in the biceps femoris muscle of a 5-year-old boy.

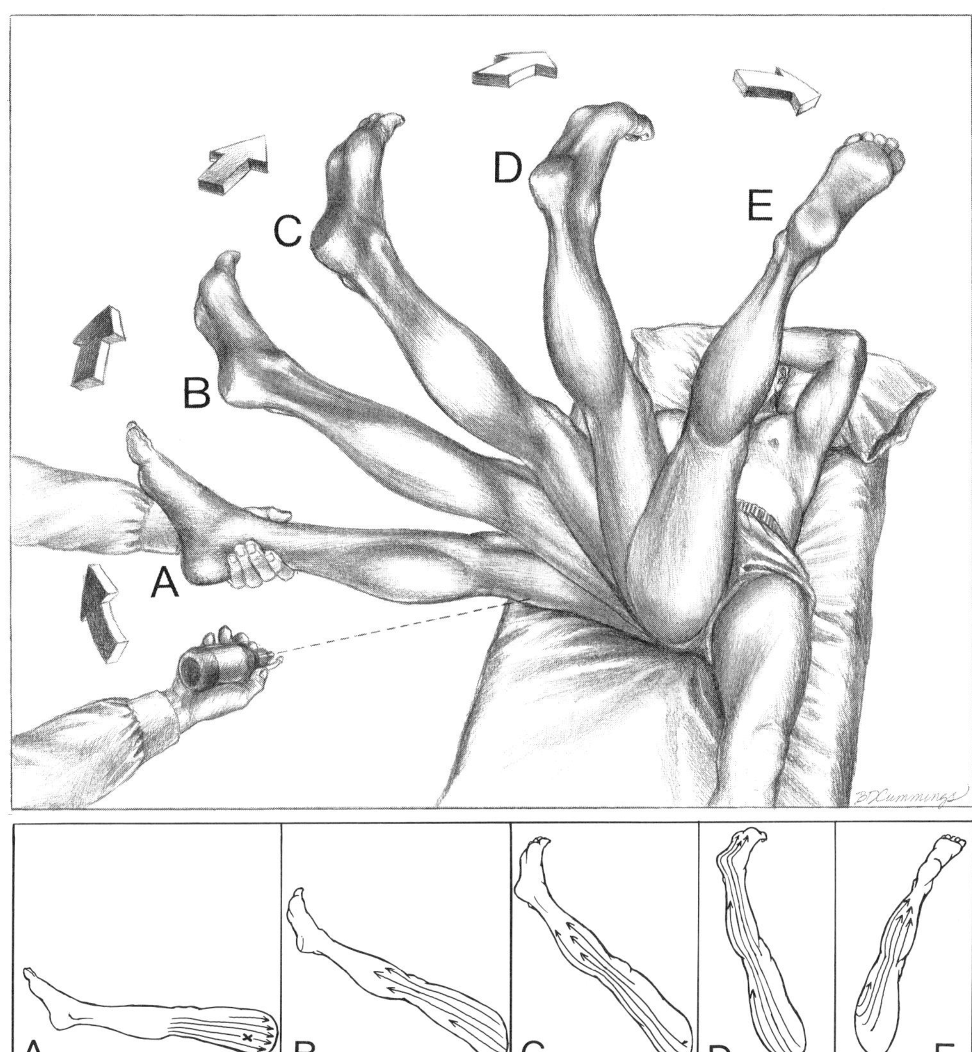

Figure 16.11. Stretch positions and intermittent cold patterns (*thin arrows*) for the right hamstring muscles. The *thick arrows* indicate the direction of pressure applied by the operator. The patient is encouraged to keep the opposite knee flat on the table. First, the thigh is abducted at the hip to release adductor magnus tightness, and then is adducted toward the midline of the body while hip flexion is maintained. Successive parallel sweeps of the ice or vapocoolant must move in sequence around the thigh posteriorly from the medial to the lateral side in order to cover the muscles then being stretched. The knee is fully extended throughout the procedure. *A*, initial abduction of the thigh at the hip; parallel sweeps of spray or ice traverse the skin over the adductor muscles from distal to proximal. *B*, start of arcuate crossing movement from abduction to adduction, while the proximal-to-distal application covers *all* hamstring muscles. Hip flexion is maintained. *C*, the thigh is moved toward pure flexion. *D*, during full hip flexion, the foot is dorsiflexed at the ankle while the gastrocnemius muscle of the calf and its referred pain zone are included in the proximal-to-distal application of cold. *E*, full flexion and adduction at the hip requires an intermittent cold pattern that includes the vastus lateralis as well as the adjacent biceps femoris and accessible gluteal muscles. This procedure is either preceded by, or followed by, intermittent cold with stretch of the paraspinal thoracolumbar and sacral muscles and all the gluteal muscles. Between cycles, a pause is usually needed to allow rewarming of the skin.

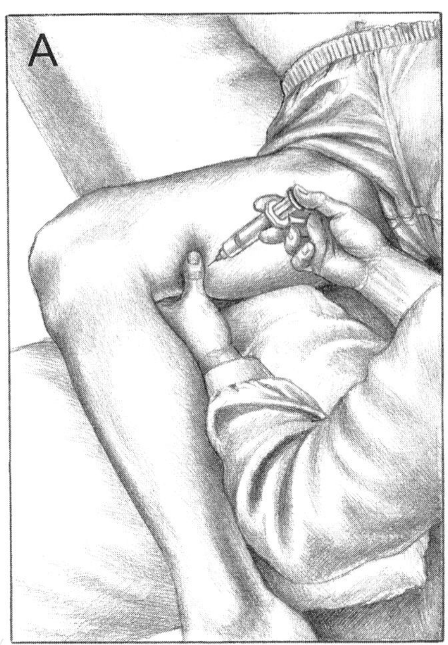

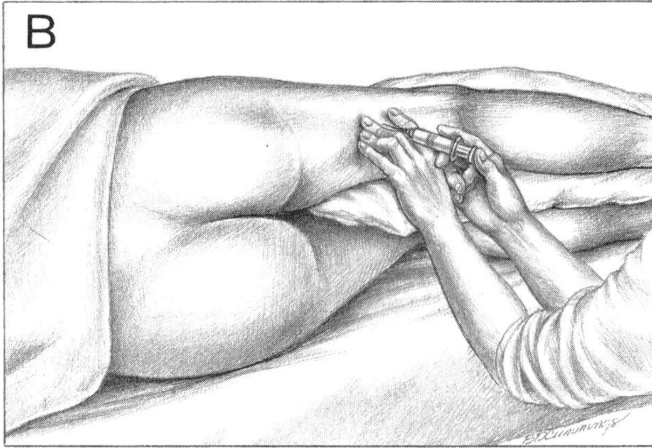

Figure 16.12. Injection of trigger points at their usual location in the right hamstring muscles (operator seated). *A*, semitendinosus and semimembranosus. *B*, biceps femoris, long head.

Other Methods

Postisometric relaxation (as described for the biceps femoris[58]) in combination with eye movement and respiration[60] is remarkably effective for releasing tight hamstrings. The basic technique is described on pages 10–11 of this volume. This procedure is especially valuable as a self-stretch procedure that can be incorporated in the Long-seated Exercise illustrated in Figure 16.13.

Evjenth and Hamberg[28] describe and illustrate a more forceful approach to stretching the hamstrings, which emphasizes the importance of releasing their tension, but may be more traumatic than the stretch techniques described here.

13. INJECTION AND STRETCH (Fig. 16.12)

When injecting hamstring TrPs, it is wise to limit treatment to only one side of the body on one visit. The patient may experience sufficient postinjection soreness to make weight bearing on the treated limb temporarily painful. Two sore lower limbs could unnecessarily restrict mobility.

Before injecting the hamstring muscles, one should review the course of the sciatic nerve. It passes down the posterior thigh underneath the long head of the biceps femoris muscle, which crosses over it about midthigh.[81] Proximally, the nerve reaches the lateral border of the long head while still deep to the gluteus maximus. Distally, at the popliteal space, the nerve's tibial portion emerges from under the medial border of the long head of the biceps femoris about where the semimembranosus muscle and the long head part company.[7,76] The femoral blood vessels join the sciatic nerve at about this same level by emerging posteriorly through the adductor canal from beneath the middle portion of the adductor magnus. The tibial neurovascular bundle then lies deep to the semitendinosus muscle fibers and passes down the limb near the midline behind the knee. The peroneal branch of the sciatic nerve follows beside or deep to the medial border of the short head of the biceps femoris to the knee.

Semimembranosus and semitendinosus TrPs can be injected with the patient lying supine, the knee bent, and the thigh partially abducted (Fig. 16.12*A*). The positioning is most convenient for injection if the patient's leg rests on the lap of the seated operator. For TrPs in the distal part of the thigh, one grasps at least the medial hamstrings (sometimes it is more effective to grasp all of the hamstrings) in a pincer grasp and pulls the medial hamstrings away from the femur. One can then roll the muscle between the tips of the fingers and thumb, examining for taut bands and spot tenderness. When the location of maximum tenderness along the taut bands has been found, this part of the band is fixed between the fingers and thumb so that the needle can be inserted precisely into the cluster of TrPs. The needle is directed laterally through the muscle mass, not toward the femur. The needle is inserted only where it remains palpable between the digits. This avoids the popliteal artery and tibial nerve, which lie close to the bone, but not within the pincer grasp. (This is remarkably similar to the technique used for grasping the long head of the triceps brachii muscle, page 473 in Volume 1.[98])

This medial approach requires a 22-gauge needle about 75 mm (3 in) long, or shorter in small individuals. A 10-mL syringe is filled with 0.5% procaine solution, gloves are donned, and the skin area to be injected is cleaned with antiseptic. Injection is performed as described on pages 74–86 in Volume 1,[98] after ruling out a possible allergy to procaine.

It is more difficult, but sometimes possible, to palpate taut bands and TrPs in the laterally located long head of the biceps femoris muscle using this pincer technique. For injection of this muscle, the patient lies on the side opposite to the involved muscle. If, as usually is the case, flat palpation must be used to locate the TrPs (Fig. 16.12*B*), the needle is inserted close to the midline of the thigh and is directed laterally, away from the tibial nerve and other major neurovascular structures. This approach also avoids the peroneal branch of the sciatic nerve, unless the most distal portion of the muscle is being injected.

Figure 16.1 serves as a reminder that frequently there are multiple TrPs in these muscles. Finding these TrPs requires considerable exploration with the needle to ensure that the operator has injected all of them. A local twitch response confirms that a TrP has been impaled. A referred pain response usually indicates needle penetration of a TrP, but may mean only that the needle pressed against the TrP without penetrating and disrupting it. Before leaving one area, the needle is withdrawn to a subcutaneous position, then moved to the side and the region palpated for residual TrP tenderness. If present, the residual TrPs are carefully localized by palpation and injected.

Because one must usually inject multiple TrPs in these muscles, it is especially important that, as the needle is withdrawn from the muscle to the skin, pressure by the palpating hand is maintained on the injection site to ensure adequate hemostasis immediately following injection. Local bleeding as a result of the needling increases postinjection soreness.

Postinjection soreness may last for several days. The prompt application of a moist heating pad over the injected area for several minutes helps reduce it. The procedure is completed by having the patient slowly move the thigh and leg through the full range of flexion and extension several times to help reestablish normal muscle function.

The patient should be trained in a home self-stretch program for these muscles.

The strong neurological interaction between the two lower limbs (crossed reflexes) was demonstrated when phantom pain in a missing lower limb was relieved by injecting areas in the other normal limb with local anesthetic solution.[44]

14. CORRECTIVE ACTIONS (Fig. 16.13)

Repetitive overuse from the crawl stroke when swimming should be avoided by individuals with hamstring muscles that are prone to develop TrPs. Also to be avoided is working the hamstrings in a shortened position without stretch, as when bicycling with too low a seat so that the knees never straighten fully.

Corrective Posture and Activities

Underthigh compression can be avoided by selecting chairs that match the leg length of the sitter, or by propping the feet up on an angled footrest placed a short distance in front of the chair (Fig. 16.6*C*). A thick handbag or other object

PART 2

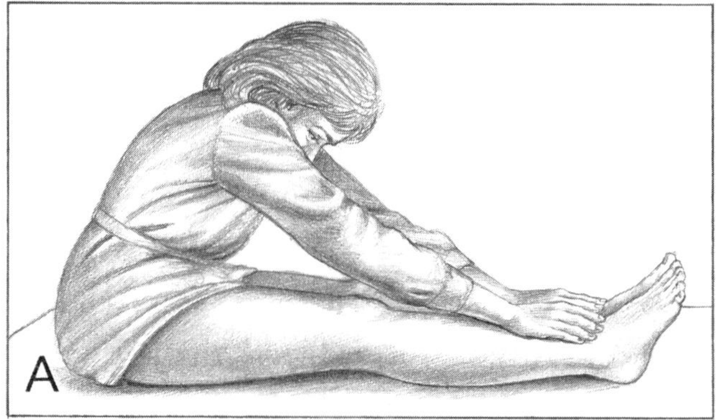

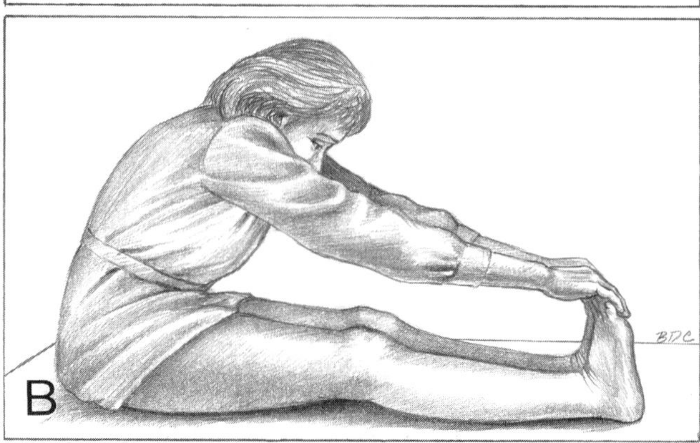

Figure 16.13. The Long-seated Reach Exercise for hamstring self-stretch. *A*, initial stretch by slowly and gently sliding the fingers down the shins, keeping the knees straight. *B*, final stretch. Postisometric relaxation coordinated with deep breathing can enhance relaxation in the hamstrings. By grasping and dorsiflexing the feet, the gastrocnemius muscles are also passively stretched. The patient should learn to do this exercise without contracting the abdominal muscles, while exhaling slowly and allowing gravity to pull the torso forward. (Contraction of the abdominal muscles in this shortened position may activate latent trigger points, if present.)

can serve as a footrest. Cloth cones filled with sand, which provide a footrest with a range of heights, can be placed under the table in front of dining room chairs.

When selecting a chair for the home, one should ensure that the front edge of its seat is rounded and well padded. The seat bottoms of patio chairs should be made of firm plastic or wood, not of canvas or webbing that sags and places the weight of the thigh on a sharp-edged bar at the front of the seat. The importance of this was emphasized by a group of apparently normal individuals who developed thrombophlebitis as the result of impaired venous return during prolonged sitting.[49]

When driving on long automobile trips, prolonged immobilization of, and underthigh pressure on, the hamstring muscles can be alleviated by using automatic cruise control, which permits changing leg position, and by taking frequent "stretch" breaks.

Home Exercise Program

A basic stretch exercise that patients with hamstring TrPs should perform at home is the Long-seated Reach Exercise (Fig. 16.13). When the ankles are plantar flexed, this is primarily a hamstring and long paraspinal stretch (Fig. 16.13*A*). The sitting patient reaches as far down the shins as possible while exhaling and consciously relaxing the back muscles, allowing gravity to pull the head and shoulders down and forward. Then the patient gently presses the ankles toward the floor while slowly inhaling. The patient relaxes again, exhales fully, and slowly reaches further. This cycle is repeated until no further gains in range of motion occur.

When the ankles are simultaneously dorsiflexed by pulling the feet up with the fingers (Fig. 16.13*B*), stretch of the gastrocnemius is included. This self-stretch exercise is best performed with the patient seated in a tub of warm water; it is illustrated as the In-bathtub Stretch in Figure 48.13 of Volume 1.[98]

The seated self-stretch exercise for the gluteus maximus muscle (*see* Fig. 7.8) also helps release hamstring TrP tension. If the patient with hamstring TrPs also has weak gluteus maximus muscles (this often happens), the weak gluteal muscles must be strengthened to eliminate this factor that helps perpetuate the hamstring TrPs.

References

1. Aftimos S: Myofascial pain in children. *N Z Med J 102*:440–441, 1989.
2. Alston W, Carlson KE, Feldman DJ, *et al.*: A quantitative study of muscle factors in the chronic low back syndrome. *J Am Geriatr Soc 14*:1041–1047, 1966.
3. Anderson JE: *Grant's Atlas of Anatomy*, Ed. 8. Williams & Wilkins, Baltimore, 1983 (Figs. 4–23, 4–24, 4–39).
4. *Ibid.* (Fig. 4–26).
5. *Ibid.* (Fig. 4–30).
6. *Ibid.* (Fig. 4–31).
7. *Ibid.* (Fig. 4–34).
8. *Ibid.* (Fig. 4–53).
9. *Ibid.* (Fig. 4–62A, 4–65A).
10. *Ibid.* (Fig. 4–68).
11. Baker BA: The muscle trigger: evidence of overload injury. *J Neurol Orthop Med Surg 7*:35–44, 1986.
12. Bardeen CR: The musculature, Sect. 5. In *Morris's Human Anatomy*, edited by C.M. Jackson, Ed. 6. Blakiston's Son & Co., Philadelphia, 1921 (pp. 506–508).
13. Basmajian JV: *Grant's Method of Anatomy*, Ed. 9. Williams & Wilkins, Baltimore, 1975 (pp. 327, 328).
14. Basmajian JV, Burke MD, Burnett GW, *et al.* (Eds.): *Stedman's Medical Dictionary*. Williams & Wilkins, 1982 (p. 1288).
15. Basmajian JV, Deluca CJ: *Muscles Alive*, Ed. 5. Williams & Wilkins, Baltimore, 1985 (pp. 320, 321).
16. *Ibid.* (pp. 372, 380).
17. Bates T, Grunwaldt E: Myofascial pain in childhood. *J Pediatr 53*:198–209, 1958.
18. Baxter MP, Dulberg C: "Growing Pains" in childhood—a proposal for treatment. *J Pediatr Orthop 8*:402–406, 1988.
19. Brody DM: Running injuries. *Clin Symp 32*:1–36, 1980 (*see* pp. 24–26).
20. Broer MR, Houtz SJ: *Patterns of Muscular Activity in Selected Sports Skills*. Charles C Thomas, Springfield, 1967.
21. Carter BL, Morehead J, Wolpert SM, *et al.*: *Cross-Sectional Anatomy*. Appleton-Century-Crofts, New York, 1977 (Sects. 41–43, 46–48, 64–72).
22. Christensen E: Topography of terminal motor innervation in striated muscles from stillborn infants. *Am J Phys Med 38*:65–78, 1959.
23. Clemente CD: *Gray's Anatomy of the Human Body*, American Ed. 30. Lea & Febiger, Philadelphia, 1985 (pp. 571–573).
24. Close JR: *Motor Function in the Lower Extremity*. Charles C Thomas, Springfield, 1964 (Fig. 66, p. 79).
25. Duchenne GB: *Physiology of Motion*, translated by E.B. Kaplan. J.B. Lippincott, Philadelphia, 1949 (pp. 286, 290–292).
26. Ericson M: On the biomechanics of cycling. *Scand J Rehabil Med (Suppl) 16*:1–43, 1986.
27. Ericson MO, Nisell R, Arborelius UP, *et al.*: Muscular activity during ergometer cycling. *Scand J Rehabil Med 17*:53–61, 1985.
28. Evjenth O, Hamberg J: *Muscle Stretching in Manual Therapy, A Clinical Manual*. Alfta Rehab Førlag, Alfta, Sweden, 1984 (p. 94).
29. Ferner H, Staubesand J: *Sobotta Atlas of Human Anatomy*, Ed. 10, Vol. 2. Urban & Schwarzenberg, Baltimore, 1983 (Fig. 381).
30. *Ibid.* (Figs. 401, 403).
31. *Ibid.* (Figs. 410, 411a, 411b).
32. *Ibid.* (Fig. 412).
33. *Ibid.* (Fig. 413).
34. *Ibid.* (Figs. 417, 472)
35. *Ibid.* (Figs. 418, 419).
36. *Ibid.* (Figs. 420, 421).
37. *Ibid.* (Fig. 464).
38. *Ibid.* (p. 471).
39. Furlani J, Vitti M, Berzin F: Musculus biceps femoris, long and short head: an electromyographic study. *Electromyogr Clin Neurophysiol 17*:13–19, 1977.
40. Gantchev GN, Draganova N: Muscular synergies during different conditions of postural activity. *Acta Physiol Pharmacol Bulg 12*:58–65, 1986.
41. Garrett WE Jr, Califf JC, Bassett FH III: Histochemical correlates of hamstring injuries. *Am J Sports Med 12*:98–103, 1984.
42. Ghori GMU, Luckwill RG: Responses of the lower limb to load carrying in walking man. *Eur J Appl Physiol 54*:145–150, 1985.
43. Gray DJ: Some anomalous hamstring muscles. *Anat Rec 91*:33–38, 1945.
44. Gross D: Contralateral local anesthesia in the treatment of phantom and stump pain. *Regional-Anaesthesie 7*:65–73, 1984.
45. Gutstein M: Diagnosis and treatment of muscular rheumatism. *Br J Phys Med 1*:302–321, 1938 (Case 7).
46. Gutstein M: Common rheumatism and physiotherapy. *Br J Phys Med 3*:46–50, 1940.
47. Halperin N, Axer A: Semimembranous tenosynovitis. *Orthop Rev 9*:72–75, 1980.
48. Hellsing A-L: Tightness of hamstring- and psoas major muscles. *Ups J Med Sci 93*:267–276, 1988.
49. Homans J: Thrombosis of the deep leg veins due to prolonged sitting. *N Engl J Med 250*:148–149, 1954.
50. Joseph J, Williams PL: Electromyography of certain hip muscles. *J Anat 91*:286–294, 1957.
51. Kamon E: Electromyographic kinesiology of jumping. *Arch Phys Med Rehabil 52*:152–157, 1971.
52. Kelly M: Some rules for the employment of local analgesia in the treatment of somatic pain. *Med J Austral 1*:235–239, 1947.
53. Kelly M: The relief of facial pain by procaine (Novocain) injections. *J Am Geriatr Soc 11*:586–596, 1963 (*see* p. 589).
54. Kendall FP, McCreary EK: *Muscles, Testing and Function*, Ed. 3. Williams & Wilkins, Baltimore, 1983.
55. Lange M: *Die Muskelhärten (Myogelosen)*. J.F. Lehmanns, München, 1931 (pp. 102, 103, Fig. 35).

PART 2

56. Lewit K: *Manipulative Therapy in Rehabilitation of the Motor System*. Butterworths, London, 1985 (pp. 30, 31, 32, 154).
57. *Ibid*. (pp. 151, 156, 158, 170, 171, Fig. 4.47).
58. *Ibid*. (pp. 280, 281, Fig. 6.100).
59. *Ibid*. (pp. 309, 314, Table 7.1).
60. Lewit K: Postisometric relaxation in combination with other methods of muscular facilitation and inhibition. *Manual Med 2*:101–104, 1986.
61. Lockhart RD: *Living Anatomy*, Ed. 7. Faber & Faber, London, 1974 (p. 61).
62. Lyons K, Perry J, Gronley JK, *et al*.: Timing and relative intensity of hip extensor and abductor muscle action during level and stair ambulation. *Phys Ther 63*:1597–1605, 1983.
63. Lyu S-R, Wu J-J: Snapping syndrome caused by the semitendinosus tendon. *J Bone Joint Surg [Am] 71*:303–305, 1989.
64. Máckova J, Janda V, Máček M, *et al*.: Impaired muscle function in children and adolescents. *J Man Med 4*:157–160, 1989.
65. Maloney M: Personal Communication, 1990.
66. Mann RA, Moran GT, Dougherty SE: Comparative electromyography of the lower extremity in jogging, running, and sprinting. *Am J Sports Med 14*:501–510, 1986.
67. Manzano G, McComas AJ: Longitudinal structure and innervation of two mammalian hindlimb muscles. *Muscle Nerve 11*:1115–1122, 1988.
68. Markhede G, Stener B: Function after removal of various hip and thigh muscles for extirpation of tumors. *Acta Orthop Scand 52*:373–395, 1981.
69. McMinn RMH, Hutchings RT: *Color Atlas of Human Anatomy*. Year Book Medical Publishers, Chicago, 1977 (pp. 264, 270, 275, 277, 281, 282, 285).
70. *Ibid*. (p. 295).
71. *Ibid*. (p. 304).
72. Milner M, Basmajian JV, Quanbury AO: Multifactorial analysis of walking by electromyography and computer. *Am J Phys Med 50*:235–258, 1971.
73. Moriwaki Y: Electromyographic studies on the knee movements by means of synchronous recorder. *Nihon Univ Med J 27*:1394–1404, 1968.
74. Murray MP, Mollinger LA, Gardner GM, *et al*.: Kinematic and EMG patterns during slow, free, and fast walking. *J Orthop Res 2*:272–280, 1984.
75. Németh G, Ekholm J, Arborelius UP: Hip load moments and muscular activity during lifting. *Scand J Rehabil Med 16*:103–111, 1984.
76. Netter FH: *The Ciba Collection of Medical Illustrations*, Vol. 8, Musculoskeletal System. Part I: Anatomy, Physiology and Metabolic Disorders. Ciba-Geigy Corporation, Summit, 1987 (p. 82).
77. *Ibid*. (p. 84).
78. *Ibid*. (p. 85).
79. *Ibid*. (p. 86).
80. *Ibid*. (p. 87).
81. *Ibid*. (p. 91).
82. *Ibid*. (pp. 94, 95).
83. Oddsson L, Thorstensson A: Fast voluntary trunk flexion movements in standing: motor patterns. *Acta Physiol Scand 129*:93–106, 1987.
84. Okada M: An electromyographic estimation of the relative muscular load in different human postures. *J Human Ergol 1*:75–93, 1972.
85. Puranen J, Orava S: The hamstring syndrome: a new diagnosis of gluteal sciatic pain. *Am J Sports Med 16*:517–521, 1988.
86. Rasch PJ, Burke RK: *Kinesiology and Applied Anatomy*, Ed. 6. Lea & Febiger, Philadelphia, 1978 (pp. 279, 280, Table 15–1, Table 16–2).
87. Rask MR: "Snapping bottom": subluxation of the tendon of the long head of the biceps femoris muscle. *Muscle Nerve 3*:250–251, 1980.
88. Reynolds MD: Myofascial trigger point syndromes in the practice of rheumatology. *Arch Phys Med Rehabil 62*:111–114, 1981.
89. Rohen JW, Yokochi C: *Color Atlas of Anatomy*, Ed. 2. Igaku-Shoin, New York, 1988 (pp. 419, 420).
90. Rubin D: An approach to the management of myofascial trigger point syndromes. *Arch Phys Med Rehabil 62*:107–110, 1981.
91. Sherman RA: Published treatments of phantom limb pain. *Am J Phys Med 59*:232–244, 1980.
92. Simons DG: Myofascial pain syndrome due to trigger points, Chapter 45. In *Rehabilitation Medicine* edited by Joseph Goodgold. C.V. Mosby Co., St. Louis, 1988 (pp. 686–723, *see* pp. 710, 711, Fig. 45–8H).
93. Simons DG, Travell JG: Myofascial pain syndromes, Chapter 25. In *Textbook of Pain*, edited by P.D. Wall and R. Melzack, Ed 2. Churchill Livingstone, London, 1989 (pp. 368–385, *see* pp. 271, 272, Fig. 103A).
94. Sugar O: Charles Lasègue and his 'Considerations on Sciatica.' *JAMA 253*:1767–1768, 1985.
95. Townsend MA, Lainhart SP, Shiavi R, *et al*.: Variability and biomechanics of synergy patterns of some lower-limb muscles during ascending and descending stairs and level walking. *Med Biol Eng Comput 16*:681–688, 1978.
96. Travell J: Myofascial trigger points: clinical view. In *Advances in Pain Research and Therapy*, edited by J.J. Bonica and D. Albe-Fessard, Vol. 1. Raven Press, New York, 1976 (pp. 919–926).
97. Travell J, Rinzler SH: The myofascial genesis of pain. *Postgrad Med 11*:425–434, 1952.
98. Travell JG and Simons DG: *Myofascial Pain and Dysfunction: The Trigger Point Manual*. Williams & Wilkins, Baltimore, 1983.
99. Weber EF: Ueber die Längenverhältnisse der Fleischfasern der Muskeln in Allgemeinen. *Berichte über die Verhandlungen der Königlich Sächsischen Gesellschaft der Wissenschaften zu Leipzig 3*:63–86, 1851.
100. Weiser HI: Semimembranosus insertion syndrome: a treatable and frequent cause of persistent knee pain. *Arch Phys Med Rehabil 60*: 317–319, 1979.
101. Willer J-C, Barranquero A, Kahn M-F, *et al*.: Pain in sciatica depresses lower limb nociceptive reflexes to sural nerve stimulation. *J Neurol Neurosurg Psychiatry 50*:1–5, 1987.
102. Yang JF, Winter DA: Surface EMG profiles during different walking cadences in humans. *Electroencephalogr Clin Neurophysiol 60*:485–491, 1985.

CHAPTER 17
Popliteus Muscle

"Bent-knee Troublemaker"

HIGHLIGHTS: **REFERRED PAIN** from trigger points (TrPs) in the popliteus muscle concentrates in the back of the knee proximal to the location of the TrP. **ANATOMICAL ATTACHMENTS** of this muscle are, proximally, to the lateral aspect of the lateral condyle of the femur and, distally, to the posterior aspect of the tibia medially. The main **FUNCTION** of the popliteus muscle appears to be to "unlock" the knee at the start of weight bearing by laterally rotating the thigh on the fixed tibia. Activity of this muscle prevents forward displacement of the femur on the tibia when a person crouches, placing weight on the bent knee. Generally, the main **SYMPTOM** of which the patient complains is pain behind the knee when crouching, running or walking downhill, or going downstairs. A popliteus myofascial pain syndrome can readily be misdiagnosed as popliteus tendinitis. Other diagnoses that can appear confusingly similar include Baker's cyst, anteromedial and posterolateral instability of the knee joint, and avulsion of the popliteus tendon. **ACTIVATION OF TRIGGER POINTS** in the popliteus muscle may occur while the person plays soccer or football, runs, twists, or slides, especially when running or skiing downhill. **PATIENT EXAMINATION** reveals tenderness of the tendon and region of attachment of the tendon of the popliteus muscle to the femur. If the patient sits with the thigh fixed and the knee bent 90°, passive lateral rotation of the leg is restricted by pain. For **TRIGGER POINT EXAMINATION,** the popliteus muscle is most accessible close to the lower (medial) and upper (lateral) ends of its muscle belly. The lower, medial end of the muscle is palpated directly between the semitendinosus tendon and the medial head of the gastrocnemius muscle. The upper, lateral end is best palpated as it crosses the knee joint just above the head of the fibula between the tendon of the biceps femoris on one side and both the gastrocnemius muscle's lateral head and the plantaris muscle on the other side. For application of **INTERMITTENT COLD WITH STRETCH** to the popliteus muscle, the patient lies prone with the affected lower leg supported to bend the knee slightly. Parallel upward sweeps of ice or vapocoolant cover the muscle and its pain reference zone while the leg is laterally rotated to take up the slack that develops. A moist heating pad and then active range of motion complete this procedure. The patient continues with self-stretch exercises at home. During **INJECTION AND STRETCH** of popliteus TrPs, the clinician visualizes the course of the popliteal artery and vein and of the tibial and peroneal nerves and avoids them. The muscle belly can be approached from either its upper lateral part or its lower medial part, depending on where the TrPs are located. **CORRECTIVE ACTIONS** to be considered include use of an elastic sleeve around the knee to ameliorate symptoms and to avoid prolonged immobilization, if possible. Mechanically, excessive pronation of the foot should be corrected. Activities of walking, running, or skiing downhill should be avoided during acute flare-ups of pain due to popliteus TrPs and resumed cautiously after an episode of pain. The best corrective home exercise is postisometric relaxation, and it should be a part of the management program of every patient with this myofascial pain syndrome.

1. REFERRED PAIN
(Fig. 17.1)

Trigger points (TrPs) in the popliteus muscle refer pain primarily to the back of the knee joint (Fig. 17.1). Patients rarely present with pain in the knee due solely to TrPs in the popliteus muscle. Initially, the source of the knee pain is usually identified as coming from TrPs in other muscles, such as the gastrocnemius or biceps femoris. On first examination, the latter appears to account for the patient's pain complaint. However, after the TrPs in these other muscles have been inactivated, the patient becomes more aware of back-of-the-knee pain that examination then identifies as originating in the popliteus muscle.

2. ANATOMICAL ATTACHMENTS AND CONSIDERATIONS
(Figs. 17.2 and 17.3)

Seen from behind (Fig. 17.2), the thin flat popliteus muscle has a triangular shape. It forms the floor of the distal portion of the popliteal fossa behind the knee. ***Proximally and laterally*** (Fig. 17.3) it is anchored by a strong tendon to the lateral condyle of the femur, to the capsule of the knee joint with fibers that may include the lateral meniscus, and to the head of the fibula via the structure that is generally identified as the arcuate popliteal ligament on the outer side of the muscle.[42] Others consider this a distorted view and that this so-called ligament actually consists of the thickened condensation of fibers from the femoral, fibular, and meniscal origins of the popliteus and posterior capsule of the knee. Together, all of these fibers form a Y-shaped ligamentous attachment of the muscle.[28] From both surfaces of its proximal tendon,[30] nearly parallel fibers angle diagonally downward[45] to attach ***distally and medially*** (Fig. 17.2) to the medial two-thirds of the triangular surface on the tibia posteriorly, proximal to the soleal line.[2,12,39]

Lovejoy and Harden[28] examined in detail the proximal attachments of the popliteus muscle in 15 cadaver limbs. They concluded that, in most limbs, it formed a Y-shaped triple attachment. One part always attached to the femur. They considered the second attachment, to the head of the fibula, to be of phylogenetic origin and of uncertain purpose. Murthy[36] found the attachment to the fibular head to be missing bilaterally in four of 30 bodies.

The third attachment intimately connects the tendon with the lateral capsular ligament of the

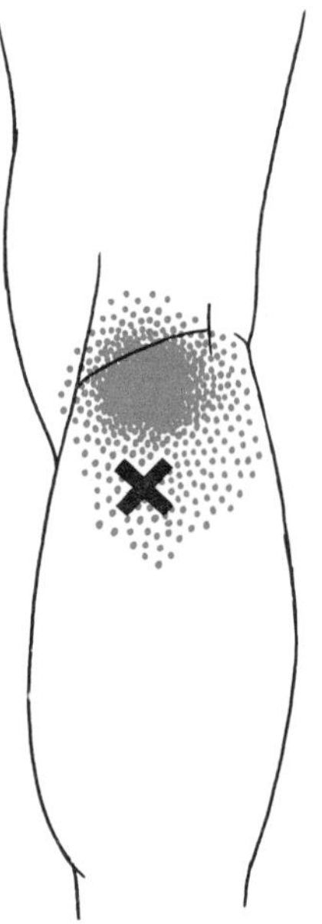

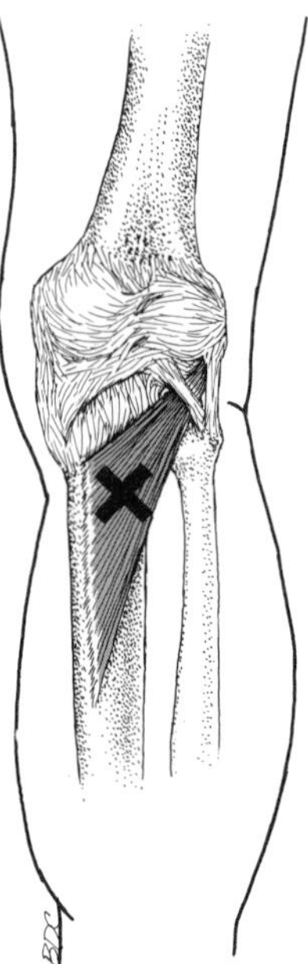

Figure 17.1. Referred pain pattern (*dark red*) of a trigger point (***X***) in the right popliteus muscle (*light red*) seen in posterior view. The essential pain pattern is *solid red*. *Red stippling* indicates occasional spillover of the essential pattern. An additional trigger point is sometimes found in the proximal end of the muscle as described in Section 13, Injection.

PART 2

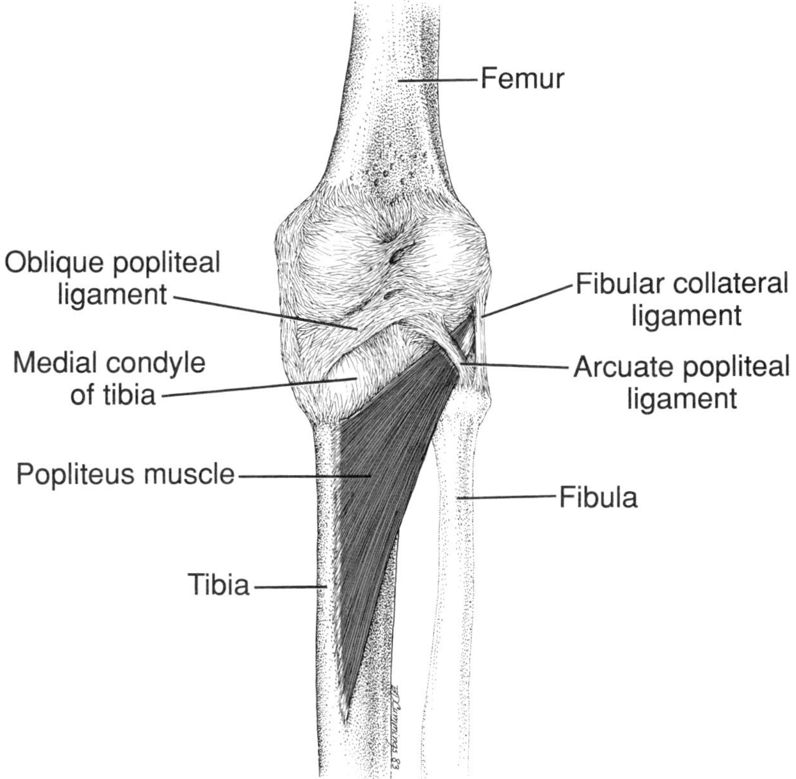

Figure 17.2. Attachments of the right popliteus muscle (*red*), from a posterior view. Its attachment to the femur is shown in Figure 17.3.

knee joint. This third part may play a role in the retraction and protection of the lateral meniscus.[30] Tendinous fibers were secured to the superior margin of the posterior horn of the lateral meniscus in 14 of 15 limbs, according to Murthy.[36] Questioning this function, Tria and associates[50] dissected 40 cadaver knees to determine the relation of the popliteus tendon to the lateral meniscus. Most (83%) of the specimens in this study demonstrated no *major* attachment to the meniscus. In another study of 60 knees,[36] the posterior aspect of the lateral meniscus was attached to the deep surface of the tendon of the popliteus muscle in every case. Unquestionably, this meniscal attachment is of importance in some, possibly in many, individuals.

The popliteus muscle is homologous to the deep portion of the pronator teres muscle in the forearm and is rarely absent.[6]

The small *fibulotibialis* (*peroneotibialis*) muscle occurred in one body of seven and extended from the medial side of the head of the fibula to the posterior surface of the tibia deep to the popliteus muscle.[6,12] Occasionally, a *popliteus minor* muscle extends from the femur underneath the plantaris muscle to the posterior capsule of the knee joint.[12,24]

The popliteus bursa[2,5,11,19] separates the popliteus tendon from the lateral condyle of the femur just above the head of the fibula. The bursa is usually an extension of the synovial membrane of the knee joint.[11]

Supplemental References

Sources depict the popliteus muscle as drawn from behind without vessels or nerves,[5,40] in relation to the arcuate popliteal ligament that holds it in place above the head of the fibula,[17] and in relation to the bursa of the popliteus muscle.[19] It is photographed in relation to the arcuate ligament,[33] and in relation to the fibular collateral ligament and soleus muscle.[35] Its structure and fiber direction are visible.[45] From behind, one can view the popliteal vessels and tibial nerve crossing over the muscle,[3] see the muscle's relation to the overlying plantaris muscle,[38] and see that it can be palpated directly between the lateral head of the gastrocnemius muscle and the tendon of the biceps

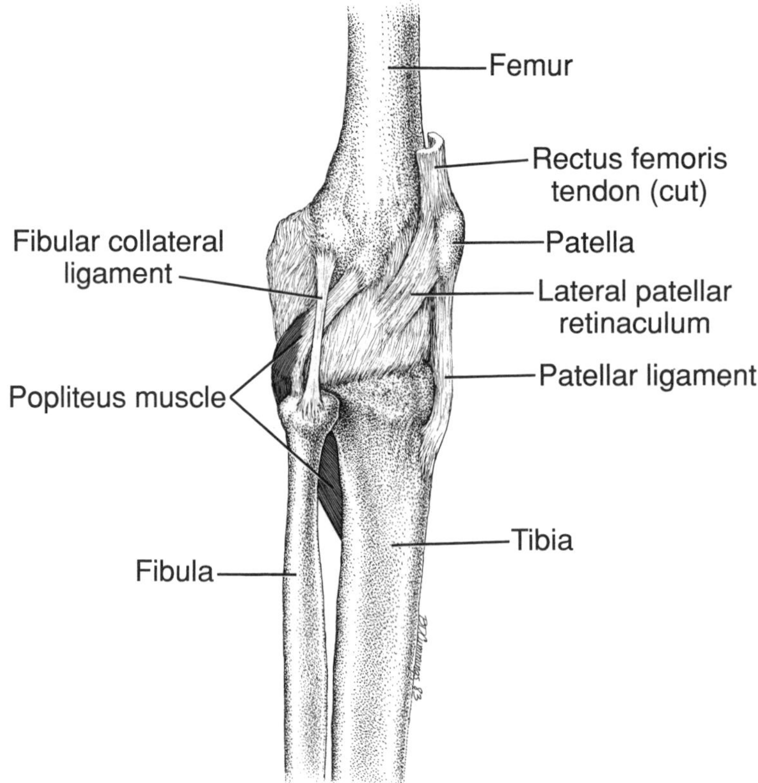

Figure 17.3. Proximal attachment of the right popliteus muscle (*red*) to the femur, from the lateral view.

femoris muscle in the posterolateral aspect of the leg near the knee.[16]

Lovejoy and Harden[28] illustrate the Y-shaped attachments to the tibia, lateral meniscus, and fibula in rear view, and the attachments to the tibia and fibula in lateral view.

The popliteus muscle is viewed and drawn from the lateral side, showing its attachment to the femur,[4,18] and is photographed also showing its relation to the fibular collateral ligament.[34]

The area of its tendinous attachment to the femur, shown in lateral view, indicates an origin within the joint capsule.[31] Also shown are the bony attachments to both the femur and tibia from behind,[39] to the tibia from behind,[2,15,32] and to the tibia from the medial view.[32]

The relation of the popliteus muscle to surrounding structures is shown in three serial cross sections,[10] and in one section below the knee.[20] A sagittal section through the middle of the knee joint visualizes the problem of localization and injection through the thick soleus muscle and the lateral head of the gastrocnemius muscle.[44]

The popliteus bursa is viewed from behind.[2,5,11,19]

3. INNERVATION

The popliteus muscle is supplied by fibers of the tibial nerve, directly from a branch of the nerve to the tibialis posterior muscle, and sometimes also by a branch from the main nerve to the knee joint. These nerve fibers to the popliteus muscle arise from the fourth and fifth lumbar and the first sacral spinal nerves.[6,12]

4. FUNCTION

Actions

The popliteus muscle rotates the tibia medially when the thigh is fixed and the leg is free to move, as when sitting erect. During weight bearing when the leg is fixed, this muscle rotates the femur laterally on the tibia to "unlock" the knee joint.[7,12,43]

The popliteus muscle is at a mechanical disadvantage for producing knee flexion by virtue of the angulation of its fibers and their proximity to the axis of rotation of the knee.

Duchenne[13] stimulated the popliteus muscle in a freshly amputated leg and found that it strongly medially rotated the leg at the knee, and weakly flexed the leg.

Basmajian and Lovejoy[8] studied this muscle electromyographically using fine-wire electrodes in 20 subjects. These investigators found that, with the leg free to move, the popliteus muscle was activated by voluntary effort to produce medial rotation of the leg at knee angles between knee straight and 90° of flexion in the sitting and prone positions.

Functions

The functional relation of this muscle to its neighboring muscles is comparable to that of the pronator teres at the elbow to its neighbors.[28,36] They both rotate the distal part of the limb and seldom present as a single-muscle myofascial syndrome.

The popliteus responds when activities require either a force that counters lateral rotation of the tibia on the femur during weight bearing,[9] or one that prevents the femur from being displaced forward on the tibial plateau. Its contraction specifically prevents the lateral femoral condyle from rotating forward off the lateral tibial plateau, as described[9,30] and illustrated.[9]

Mann and Hagy[29] studied both the electromyographic (EMG) activity of the popliteus muscle (using fine-wire electrodes) and rotation of the leg in 10 normal subjects during ambulation and other maneuvers involving rotation of the leg. The activity of the popliteus muscle corresponded to medial rotation of the tibia on the femur during gait and during the other exercises. They concluded that the basic function of the popliteus muscle is to initiate and maintain medial rotation of the tibia on the femur.

Basmajian and Lovejoy[8] observed that, when a person stood in the semicrouched bent-knee position, the popliteus muscle showed continuous motor unit activity. With the knee thus bent, the body weight tends to slide the femur downward and forward on the slope of the tibia. Then popliteal contraction assists the posterior cruciate ligament in preventing forward dislocation of the femur at the knee.[7] The muscle is inactive when the person quietly stands erect.[7]

During walking, the greatest EMG activity occurred on heel-strike to unlock the knee joint at the onset of weight bearing. The muscle was active during most of the weight-bearing phase of gait.[7]

Human fetal popliteus muscles contained many muscle spindles arranged in complex and tandem forms.[1] The author concluded that these spindles could provide a major part of the kinesthesia needed to monitor locking and unlocking of the human knee joint.

5. FUNCTIONAL (MYOTATIC) UNIT

Medial rotation of the leg by the popliteus muscle is assisted by the medial hamstrings and, to a lesser extent, by the sartorius and gracilis muscles. Although the popliteus has no comparable antagonist that is primarily a lateral rotator of the leg, the biceps femoris muscle provides some force in that direction.

6. SYMPTOMS

The chief complaint of patients with active TrPs in the popliteus muscle is pain in the back of the knee when crouching and running or walking, especially going downhill or downstairs. Patients with popliteus TrPs rarely complain of knee pain at night and are frequently not aware of their relatively slight decrease in range of motion at the knee or weakness of medial rotation of the leg at the knee.

Differential Diagnosis

Active myofascial TrPs in the popliteus muscle are easily overlooked when a diagnosis of popliteus tendinitis or tenosynovitis is the focus of attention. Other conditions to consider in the differential diagnosis of posterior knee pain include Baker's cyst, thrombosis of the popliteal vein, anteromedial and posterolateral instability of the knee, avulsion of the popliteus tendon, and tear of a meniscus or of the posterior capsule of the knee joint.

One should be wary of blaming pain in the back of the knee on a torn plantaris muscle months or years after injury. The muscle should have healed. Such residual pain is more likely to be caused by TrPs in the popliteus muscle.

Popliteus Tendinitis and Tenosynovitis

Popliteus tendinitis and popliteus tenosynovitis are closely associated with activities that would overload an inadequately conditioned popliteus muscle. Mayfield[30] reported on 30 patients seen

PART 2

with the diagnosis of tenosynovitis in a 5-year period. The findings leading to this diagnosis are apparently more common than is generally appreciated. The characteristic symptom is pain in the lateral aspect of the knee on weight bearing with the knee flexed 15–30°, as when running or walking downhill. Backpacking enthusiasts spent days ascending into the mountains without symptoms until the end of the journey; during rapid descent out of the mountains, the symptoms developed.[30] Sometimes pain was also experienced during the early part of the swing phase of gait, and on attempting to rise from the cross-legged sitting position.[30] Brody[9] also noted that symptoms were aggravated on the high side when the patient walked on a slanted surface or performed some other activity that excessively pronated the foot during weight bearing.

Mayfield[30] discussed and illustrated in detail how to distinguish by physical examination the tenderness at the origin of the popliteus tendon on the lateral femoral condyle from *meniscal tears*. For examination, the patient's knee is bent to an acute angle by having the seated patient place the ankle of the affected limb on the opposite knee so that the foot hangs down and the tibia is laterally rotated, placing gentle tension on the popliteus muscle. A length of about 2 cm of the popliteus tendon is then palpable between the well-defined landmark of the fibular collateral ligament and the tendon's attachment to the femur where maximum tenderness is found. A distinct separate area of tenderness directly over the meniscus at the joint line is present in the patient with both a meniscus tear and popliteus tenosynovitis.

Surgical management was recommended only for those patients who had a meniscus tear.[30] Conservative treatment, chiefly elimination of excessive popliteus muscle stress, was successful in most cases of tendinitis or tenosynovitis.

There were no "top flight" competitive runners in Mayfield's series of 30 patients.[30] Typically, the patients with this diagnosis of tenosynovitis were relatively sedentary individuals who stressed the knee by suddenly increasing activity. The iliotibial band friction syndrome and stress reaction of the biceps femoris tendon can be distinguished by accurately localizing tenderness over appropriate anatomical structures.[30]

Of the 20 patients on whom radiographs of the knee were taken, five showed radiopacities of apparent calcific deposits in the area of the popliteus tendon.[30] This may be another example of calcification of a tendon subjected to chronic tension due to latent or active TrPs (*see* Volume 1, Chapter 21, Supraspinatus Muscle).[49]

Remarkably, the history, symptoms, physical findings, and treatment of popliteus tendinitis and tenosynovitis are similar to what one finds in patients with TrPs in the popliteus muscle. There is no indication that the patients in Mayfield's study were examined for TrPs, which are not easy to locate because the muscle and its TrPs are so deeply buried in the popliteal region. This clinical picture points up how easily the *tenderness* produced at the musculotendinous junction by the chronic tension placed on that structure by a taut band of muscle fibers can be identified, while a TrP *origin* of the problem may be overlooked.

Baker's Cyst

The myofascial pain syndrome of the popliteus muscle mimics the symptoms of a popliteal (Baker's) cyst that produces pain in much the same posterior region of the knee joint. The cyst produces a swelling, often painful, in the popliteal space which is caused by enlargement of the bursa that lies deep to the medial head of the gastrocnemius muscle and/or enlargement of the semimembranosus bursa, both of which normally communicate with the synovial cavity of the knee joint. The swelling may be more prominent in the standing patient than in the recumbent one. Flexion of the knee increases discomfort. In adults, but not in children, the swelling (effusion) usually is due to disease or injury of the knee joint, such as rheumatoid arthritis or a meniscal tear. If appropriate treatment does not relieve the swelling and pain, the Baker's cyst should be removed surgically.[23] Although TrPs in the popliteus muscle may exhibit deep tenderness in much the same region as a Baker's cyst, the TrPs do not produce visible or palpable swelling. Ultrasonography usually visualizes these cysts well.

Rupture of a Baker's cyst may closely simulate thrombophlebitis. The diagnosis of a ruptured cyst is confirmed by an arthrogram that shows entry of dye from the knee joint into the region of the calf muscles.[26]

Anteromedial and Posterolateral Instability of the Knee

The popliteus muscle is a major contributor to rotational stability of the knee joint. Lateral rotation of the tibia on the femur in the last few degrees of extension "locks" the knee, firmly uniting the thigh and leg into a single structure.[48] In the functioning athlete, anteromedial instability results from excessive medial rotation of the femur on the fixed tibia with the knee in flexion and leads to "giving way" of the knee when the runner "cuts" away from his supporting leg.[48]

Surgically shortening the popliteus muscle-tendon unit, which was elongated or torn in eight patients, resulted in static and dynamic stability and return to full function in seven of them. None of the eight experienced any loss of power in the popliteus muscle.[48] Depending on which ligaments are lax or torn, excessive medial rotation of the femur on the tibia produces either rotary anteromedial instability[48] or rotary posterolateral instability.[21,47] In either condition, surgical relocation of the tibial attachment of the popliteus muscle in order to shorten it, increases its tension, improves its dynamic function, and corrects the problem. One report described four patients who, with the knee flexed 80–90°, could produce voluntary anterior subluxation of the lateral tibial plateau by contracting the popliteus muscle.[42]

Six of ten patients (over half of those studied with the posterolateral drawer sign)[47] were able voluntarily to evoke the posterolateral drawer sign in the knee with posterolateral instability. The remaining four patients learned to perform this maneuver. This posterior subluxation of the tibial plateau seriously interferes with descending stairs and participating in sports activities. Electromyography in three of the patients demonstrated that contraction of the biceps femoris muscle produced the subluxation, contraction of the popliteus muscle reduced it, and that neither the rectus femoris nor gastrocnemius muscles participated.[47] The authors recommended that, when this condition is suspected from the history, the patient initially should demonstrate the knee problem to the examiner. This is generally painless and, therefore, is not distorted by interfering muscle tension induced by the patient's fear of the examiner's testing.[47] Surgical relocation of the tendon attachment was considered effective because the popliteus muscle is a dynamic musculotendinous unit and not a static stabilizer like a ligament.[25]

Misdiagnosis of Popliteus Tendon

In one study,[22] magnetic resonance imaging of the normal popliteus tendon was sometimes mistaken for a tear in the posterior horn of the lateral meniscus. In another study of 200 knees,[51] the bursa of the popliteus tendon simulated a tear of the posterior horn of the lateral meniscus in 27.5% of the knees studied by magnetic resonance imaging.

Avulsion Of Popliteus Tendon

Two cases of reported avulsion or rupture of the popliteus tendon occurred when one individual was pushing a car[46] and when the other, an athlete, was running in a football game.[37] The athlete tried to stop and change direction with the weight-bearing knee in flexion. The knee was immediately painful and became swollen.[37] Arthrotomy demonstrated the retracted popliteus tendon. The lateral meniscus was intact.[37]

In another report,[46] arthroscopy, electromyography, and Cybex testing established the diagnosis of popliteus tendon rupture. Surgical repair of a ruptured popliteus tendon in these two patients followed failure of conservative therapy. Both patients returned to their preinjury levels of activity.

7. ACTIVATION AND PERPETUATION OF TRIGGER POINTS

The TrPs may be activated in the popliteus muscle while an individual plays soccer or football, runs, twists, slides, and, especially, while running or skiing downhill. This muscle is specifically overloaded by braking the forward motion of the femur on the tibia during a twisting turn with the body weight on a slightly bent knee of the side toward which the body is turning.

Overload that causes a tear of the plantaris muscle may also activate TrPs in the popliteus muscle.

A trauma or strain that tears the posterior cruciate ligament of the knee may also overload and strain the popliteus muscle.

Brody[9] reported an association between an excessively pronated foot during weight-bearing activities and aggravation of popliteus tendinitis symptoms. The added stress from excessive pronation could also perpetuate TrPs in the popliteus muscle.

8. PATIENT EXAMINATION

If the popliteus muscle harbors TrPs, the knee is painful when the patient attempts to extend it fully.

The tibial attachment and tendon of the popliteus muscle should be examined for tenderness. The position described and illustrated to examine the knee for popliteus tendinitis[9,30] may be used also for examining the femoral end of the muscle and its tendon. The seated patient places the leg of the affected limb on the opposite knee, with the foot hanging relaxed. The proximal attachment of the popliteus tendon on the lateral side of the femoral condyle is examined for tenderness and the tendon palpated along the 2-cm dis-

PART 2

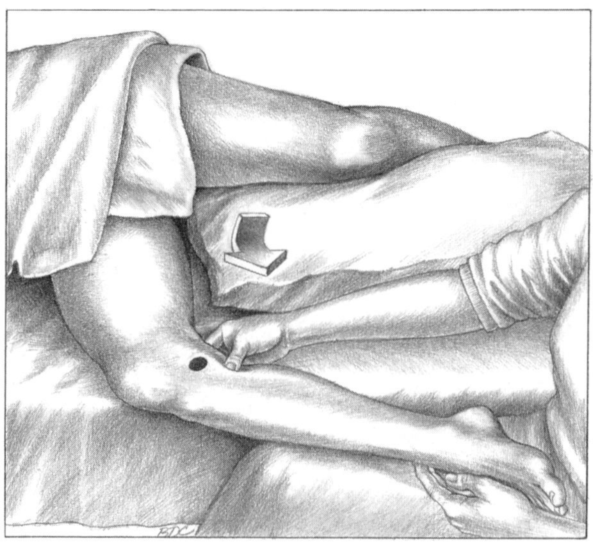

Figure 17.4. Palpation of a trigger point in the lower medial part of the right popliteus muscle. The *solid circle* marks the medial condyle of the tibia, and the *arrow* shows the direction of pressure. The knee is flexed, and the foot plantar flexed at the ankle to slacken the gastrocnemius and plantaris muscles. Lateral rotation of the leg increases tension on the popliteus muscle by placing it on a slight stretch. To explore directly the trigger point area and region of tibial attachment of the popliteus muscle, the palpating digit, in this case the examiner's thumb, pushes down and anteriorly, just medial to the laterally displaced medial head of the gastrocnemius muscle, between it and the semitendinosus tendon.

tance proximal to the point where it passes posteriorly deep to the fibular collateral ligament, which is a well-defined landmark (Fig. 17.3).[30] The TrP tightness of the popliteus muscle restricts the range of passive lateral rotation and weakens active medial rotation of the leg with the knee flexed nearly 90°.

The relatively small restriction of full knee extension (usually only 5° or possibly 10°) is often not clearly appreciated until retesting after treatment. Only then is the full range of normal extension for that patient's knee identified.

9. TRIGGER POINT EXAMINATION
(Fig. 17.4)

The popliteus muscle is palpated for TrPs with the patient lying on the affected side and the knee slightly flexed (Fig. 17.4). The leg extends over the edge of the examining table and rests on the lap of the seated operator, with the leg in slight lateral rotation and the foot in moderate plantar flexion. The slight flexion of the leg at the knee slackens the overlying gastrocnemius muscle; the plantar flexed foot further slackens the gastrocnemius and plantaris muscles; the lateral rotation of the leg places the popliteus muscle on a slight stretch and can be adjusted to increase tenderness of the popliteus TrPs for examination.

The medial side of the mid-part of the muscle, along its attachment to the tibia, is approachable between the semitendinosus tendon and the medial head of the gastrocnemius muscle.[10] The most distal portion of the tibial attachment of the popliteus is covered by the soleus muscle,[10] which can usually be displaced laterally to uncover the popliteus partially. This medial, distal end of the popliteus muscle is examined for TrPs as illustrated in Figure 17.4. It is important to displace the overlying muscles laterally when doing this part of the examination.

In the popliteal space, the upper lateral end of the popliteus muscle is covered by the plantaris muscle and the lateral head of the gastrocnemius muscle. However, as the popliteus muscle crosses the leg diagonally just above the head of the fibula (Fig. 17.2), one can reach it by palpating between the tendon of the biceps femoris laterally and the lateral head of the gastrocnemius muscle and the plantaris muscle medially.[16] With the patient in the position of Figure 17.4, one can often displace these overlying muscles to the side with one hand while palpating for TrP tenderness with the other. If the popliteus muscle has active TrPs, this spot is tender and pressure on it causes diffuse pain referred throughout the back of the knee. The region of attachment of the popliteus tendon onto the tibia is also tender.

If the popliteus TrPs are sufficiently irritable, their tenderness may be elicited by pressure exerted straight in, through the overlying muscles; these include the

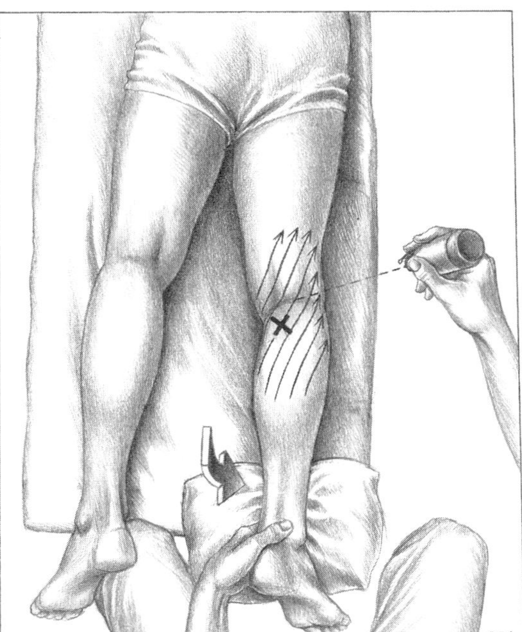

Figure 17.5. Stretch position and direction of application (*thin arrows*) of parallel sweeps of intermittent cold (ice or vapocoolant spray) for a trigger point (**X**) in the right popliteus muscle. The knee is held in slight flexion to avoid locking the knee, which would prevent rotation of the leg at that joint. *Large arrow* identifies the lateral direction of leg rotation (applied at the ankle) to lengthen the popliteus muscle passively. The thigh is fixed by its weight on the examining table.

soleus, the proximal end of which runs nearly parallel with the popliteus muscle fibers and covers the distal half of them.[38] It is difficult to distinguish TrP tenderness unambiguously in the intermediate portions of the popliteus muscle from the spot tenderness of TrPs in the intervening musculature.

10. ENTRAPMENTS

No nerve entrapments due to TrPs in this muscle are identified.

11. ASSOCIATED TRIGGER POINTS

The TrPs in the proximal portion of either or both heads of the gastrocnemius muscle are the ones most commonly associated with TrPs in the popliteus muscle. In a few patients, popliteus TrPs have been associated with a tear of the plantaris muscle and may have been activated when the plantaris was torn.

With the foot dorsiflexed, the degree of pain in the popliteal fossa and restriction of motion at the knee caused by TrPs in the lateral head of the gastrocnemius muscle is comparable to that caused by TrPs in the popliteus muscle.

12. INTERMITTENT COLD WITH STRETCH
(Fig. 17.5)

For many years, treatment of the popliteus muscle by intermittent cold with stretch produced poor results by simply extending the knee. However, results improved remarkably when the leg was rotated laterally with slightly less than full extension of the knee. Slight flexion at the knee is essential to avoid locking its rotary motion.

Techniques that augment relaxation and stretch are reviewed on page 11 and alternative treatment methods are reviewed on pages 9–11 of this volume.

The patient is placed prone with a pillow under the leg, just above the ankle (Fig. 17.5) to flex the knee slightly. Using the principles of postisometric relaxation,[27] the patient first slowly takes in a full breath and then exhales slowly and fully while consciously trying to relax the muscles. During the patient's exhalation, the clinician applies intermittent cold (ice, described in Chapter 2, page 9, or vapocoolant spray described on pages 67–74 in Volume 1[49]) in parallel lines diagonally upward across the back of the knee to cover the muscle and the referred pain zone (Fig. 17.5); simultaneously, the clinician takes up any slack in lateral rotation of the leg. The patient, while slowly taking in the next breath, then gently tries to rotate the leg medially against resistance by the operator. While exhaling slowly, the patient "lets go" and relaxes. This cycle may be repeated several times until full range of lateral rotation of the leg has been restored and the TrPs have lost their spot tenderness. Between cycles, care is taken to rewarm the skin.

After prompt application of a moist heating pad or hot pack, the seated patient actively rotates the leg slowly through full medial and lateral rotary range of motion for several cycles to restore the full functional range.

The popliteus TrPs located over the tibia are responsive to ischemic compression or deep stretching massage when compressed against the bone.[41] Pressure on the overlying midline neurovascular trunk must be avoided. Evjenth and Hamberg[14] describe and illustrate a stretch technique with the patient supine and the knee resting on a cushion and bent about 10°. The leg is laterally rotated fully and gradually brought into extension. This technique has the disadvantage that the supine positioning precludes simultaneous application of intermittent cold. Such passive stretch for releasing popliteus TrPs should be combined with postisometric relaxation techniques as described in Chapter 2 and by Lewit.[27]

The clinician should instruct the patient in a home stretch program, as described in Section 14 of this chapter.

13. INJECTION AND STRETCH
(Fig. 17.6)

When injecting popliteus TrPs, it is important to remember that the popliteal artery and vein and tibial nerve descend through the midline of the popliteal space, first between and then underneath the two heads of the gastrocnemius muscle, while resting on the underlying popliteus muscle. Laterally, the peroneal nerve courses deep to the medial edge of the biceps femoris muscle and tendon, crossing superficially over the popliteus, plantaris, and gastrocnemius (lateral head) muscles.[3,38,44]

With the patient side lying, any TrPs in the medial part of the popliteus muscle are identified by palpation as described previously in Section 9, Trigger Point Examination. The palpating hand displaces the medial head of the gastrocnemius aside laterally toward the middle of the leg. A 38-mm (1½-in) 22-gauge needle is inserted on the medial side of the back of the leg, through the skin medial to the spot tenderness so that the needle will enter deep to and medial to the neurovascular bundle in the midline of the leg (Fig. 17.6). When the needle encounters an active TrP, the clinician is likely to feel the local twitch response with the palpating hand, and the patient describes pain referred into the knee joint posteriorly. One should not expect to *see* a local twitch response in this deep muscle; it may be palpable through the needle.

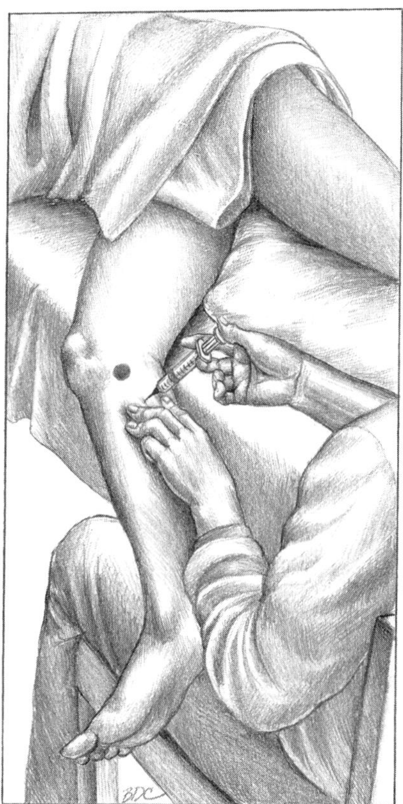

Figure 17.6. Injection of trigger points in the lower medial part of the right popliteus muscle. The *solid circle* locates the medial condyle of the tibia. The medial head of the gastrocnemius muscle is pressed aside posterolaterally to uncover the popliteus trigger point; the gastrocnemius is partially slackened by plantar flexing the foot at the ankle, while the knee is slightly flexed to permit slackening of popliteus muscle tension.

When the TrP tenderness is elicited toward the upper lateral end of the muscle, one must be careful when inserting the needle to keep the point of penetration medial to the biceps femoris muscle and tendon to avoid the peroneal nerve that courses medial or deep to them. The TrP tenderness in this upper part of the popliteus muscle is identified as described previously in Section 9, Trigger Point Examination. Unless the patient is unusually large, the same size needle is used here as for injecting the other part of the muscle.

The TrPs are injected with 0.5% procaine in isotonic saline. The injection technique is described in detail on pages 74–86 of Volume 1.[49] Immediately after injection, care is taken to maintain pressure for hemostasis at the injection site with the free palpating hand.

After injection, the clinician applies a moist heating pad over the region of the popliteus muscle for several minutes to relax the muscle further and to reduce postinjection soreness.

Then, the seated patient actively rotates the flexed leg slowly through full medial and lateral rotation for several cycles, and then through knee flexion and extension, exercising full range of motion.

Before the patient leaves, the clinician ensures that the patient understands how to perform the home exercise (*see* next section).

14. CORRECTIVE ACTIONS

The patient may wear an elastic sleeve (knee support) that extends from above the knee to below it; this elastic support can be obtained with an opening in front for the patella, and must be properly fitted. This device is consistently helpful and worth using as long as symptoms persist. It applies counter pressure over the region of the TrPs, reducing their sensitivity, and it reminds the patient that the knee should be protected.

Splinting or immobilizing the knee and leg with a brace or cast tends to aggravate popliteus TrPs. When popliteus TrPs present a problem, it is preferable that immobilization be avoided or the period of immobilization be minimized.

Corrective Posture and Activities

If one plans to go skiing and is concerned about popliteus TrPs, training should be undertaken to condition the muscle gradually; a vitamin C supplement should be taken before this strenuous activity. The lower limbs should be kept warm.

Individuals prone to popliteus TrPs should avoid a sudden major increment in the amount of running or walking downhill that is beyond the level to which they are accustomed.

High heels should be avoided because wearing them is tantamount to continuously walking downhill.

Effort should be made to limit walking or running on laterally sloped surfaces (which increases pronation of the foot and the effect of a longer lower limb on the high side). Running can be performed on a track, on the crown of an isolated road, or one can run on the same side of the road for both directions of the trip. Appropriate shoe inserts should be utilized if indicated.

Home Exercise Program

Self-stretch of the popliteus muscle may be performed in the prone or seated position. In each position, the knee is flexed 15–20°. Reciprocal inhibition can be used instead of passive stretch, if no one is available to be instructed as an assistant at home.

For the prone position, the patient assumes the position illustrated in Figure 17.5 with enough blanket roll or pillow under the distal leg to flex the knee 15–20°. The patient tries to rotate the leg laterally for several seconds (reciprocally inhibiting the popliteus), and then relaxes fully. The cycle is repeated a few times. The advantage of this position is that the thigh is stabilized so that the leg, rather than the thigh, rotates. If the blanket roll or pillow touches the foot, the friction may help to maintain lateral rotation during relaxation. Otherwise, gravity pulls the foot and leg back into neutral position.

For relaxation of the popliteus in the sitting position, the seated patient places the leg forward with the heel on the floor and the knee flexed 15–20°. A low-seated bench or chair may be required. Since thigh rotation is often substituted for leg rotation in this position, special care must be taken to ensure that the patient knows the difference and achieves lateral rotation of the leg at the knee. After a maximal lateral rotation effort for several seconds, the patient relaxes fully while gravity tends to maintain the lateral rotation. This cycle is repeated at least three times with a pause between each cycle.

Each stretching session is completed with full active range of motion through medial and lateral rotation of the leg, and then through knee flexion and extension.

References

1. Amonoo-Kuofi HS: Morphology of muscle spindles in the human popliteus muscle. Evidence of a possible monitoring role of the popliteus muscle in the locked knee joint? *Acta Anatomica 134*:48–53, 1989.
2. Anderson JE: *Grant's Atlas of Anatomy*, Ed. 8. Williams & Wilkins, Baltimore, 1983 (Figs. 4–24, 4–50).
3. *Ibid.* (Figs. 4–53, 4–86).
4. *Ibid.* (Fig. 4–67).
5. *Ibid.* (Fig. 4–68).
6. Bardeen CR: The musculature, Sect. 5. In *Morris's Human Anatomy*, edited by C.M. Jackson, Ed. 6. Blakiston's Son & Co., Philadelphia, 1921 (p. 518).
7. Basmajian JV, Deluca CJ: *Muscles Alive*, Ed. 5. Williams & Wilkins, Baltimore, 1985 (pp. 259, 332–334).
8. Basmajian JV, Lovejoy JF, Jr: Functions of the popliteus muscle in man: a multifactorial electromyographic study. *J Bone Joint Surg [Am] 53*: 557–562, 1971.
9. Brody DM: Running injuries. *Clinical Symposia 32*:1–36, 1980 (pp. 15, 16).
10. Carter BL, Morehead J, Wolpert SM, *et al.*: *Cross-Sectional Anatomy*. Appleton-Century-Crofts, New York, 1977 (Sects. 71–73).
11. Clemente CD: *Gray's Anatomy of the Human Body*, American Ed. 30. Lea & Febiger, Philadelphia, 1985 (p. 406).
12. *Ibid.* (pp. 577–578).
13. Duchenne GB: *Physiology of Motion*, translated by E.B. Kaplan. J. B. Lippincott, Philadelphia, 1949 (pp. 286, 291–292).
14. Evjenth O, Hamberg J: *Muscle Stretching in Manual Therapy, A Clinical Manual*. Alfta Rehab Førlag, Alfta, Sweden, 1984 (p. 132).
15. Ferner H, Staubesand J: *Sobotta Atlas of Human Anatomy*, Ed. 10, Vol. 2. Urban & Schwarzenberg, Baltimore, 1983 (Figs. 420, 469).
16. *Ibid.* (Fig. 436).
17. *Ibid.* (Fig. 440).
18. *Ibid.* (Fig. 443).
19. *Ibid.* (Fig. 444).
20. *Ibid.* (Fig. 472).
21. Fleming RE Jr, Blatz DJ, McCarroll JR: Posterior problems in the knee, posterior cruciate insufficiency and posterolateral rotary insufficiency. *Am J Sports Med* 9:107–113, 1981.
22. Herman LJ, Beltran J: Pitfalls in MR imaging of the knee. *Radiology 167*:775–781, 1988.
23. Hollinshead WH: *Anatomy for Surgeons*, Ed. 3, Vol. 3, *The Back and Limbs*. Harper & Row, New York, 1982 (pp. 751–752).
24. *Ibid.* (pp. 778–779).
25. Hughston JC, Jacobson KE: Chronic posterolateral rotatory instability of the knee. *J Bone Joint Surg [Am] 67*:351–359, 1985.
26. Kontos HA: Vascular diseases of the limbs due to abnormal responses of vascular smooth muscle, Chapter 54. In *Cecil Textbook of Medicine*, edited by J.B. Wyngaarden, L.H. Smith, Jr., Ed. 17. W. B. Saunders, Philadelphia, 1985 (pp. 353–364, *see* p. 364).
27. Lewit K: Postisometric relaxation in combination with other methods of muscular facilitation and inhibition. *Manual Med* 2:101–104, 1986.
28. Lovejoy JF, Jr, Harden TP: Popliteus muscle in man. *Anat Rec 169*:727–730, 1971.
29. Mann RA, Hagy JL: The popliteus muscle. *J Bone Joint Surg [Am] 59*:924–927, 1977.
30. Mayfield GW: Popliteus tendon tenosynovitis. *Am J Sports Med* 5:31–36, 1977.
31. McMinn RMH, Hutchings RT: *Color Atlas of Human Anatomy*. Year Book Medical Publishers, Chicago, 1977 (p. 277).
32. *Ibid.* (pp. 281, 282).
33. *Ibid.* (p. 307D).
34. *Ibid.* (p. 308C).
35. *Ibid.* (p. 315C).
36. Murthy CK: Origin of popliteus muscle in man. *J Ind Med Assoc 67*:97–99, 1976.
37. Naver L, Aalberg JR: Avulsion of the popliteus tendon, a rare cause of chondral fracture and hemarthrosis. *Am J Sports Med 13*:423–424, 1985.
38. Netter FH: *The Ciba Collection of Medical Illustrations*, Vol. 8, Musculoskeletal System. Part I: Anatomy, Physiology and Metabolic Disorders. Ciba-Geigy Corporation, Summit, 1987 (pp. 85, 101).
39. *Ibid.* (pp. 86, 107).
40. *Ibid.* (p. 95).
41. Nielsen AJ: Personal Communication, 1989.
42. Peterson L, Pitman MI, Gold J: The active pivot shift: the role of the popliteus muscle. *Am J Sports Med 12*:313–317, 1984.
43. Rasch PJ, Burke RK: *Kinesiology and Applied Anatomy*, Ed. 6. Lea & Febiger, Philadelphia, 1978 (pp. 292, 309, Table 16–2).
44. Rohen JW, Yokochi C: *Color Atlas of Anatomy*, Ed. 2. Igaku-Shoin, New York, 1988 (p. 412).
45. *Ibid.* (p. 424).
46. Rose DJ, Parisien JS: Popliteus tendon rupture. Case report and review of the literature. *Clin Orthop 226*:113–117, 1988.
47. Shino K, Horibe S, Ono K: The voluntarily evoked posterolateral drawer sign in the knee with posterolateral instability. *Clin Orthop 215*: 179–186, 1987.
48. Southmayd W, Quigley TB: The forgotten popliteus muscle, its usefulness in correcting anteromedial rotatory instability of the knee; a preliminary report. *Clin Orthop 130*:218–222, 1978.
49. Travell JG, Simons DG: *Myofascial Pain and Dysfunction: The Trigger Point Manual*. Williams & Wilkins, Baltimore, 1983.
50. Tria AJ Jr, Johnson CD, Zawadsky JP: The popliteus tendon. *J Bone Joint Surg [Am] 71*:714–716, 1989.
51. Watanabe AT, Carter BC, Teitelbaum GP, *et al.*: Common pitfalls in magnetic resonance imaging of the knee. *J Bone Joint Surg [Am] 71*:857–862, 1989.

PART 3

CHAPTER 18
Leg, Ankle, and Foot Pain-and-Muscle Guide

INTRODUCTION TO PART 3

This third part of THE TRIGGER POINT MANUAL includes the muscles of the leg, ankle, and foot. Differential diagnosis of an individual muscle's referred pain pattern is considered under Section 6, Symptoms, in each muscle chapter.

This chapter also includes an illustration of the bones of the foot (Fig. 18.2) for a ready reference to the relations among these bones. An understanding of these structural relations is essential for comprehending the functions of the intrinsic foot muscles that are covered in Chapters 26 and 27. The last chapter of Part 3 includes an overview of the management of chronic myofascial pain syndromes. It explains how one integrates the information from the various chapters of Volume 1[2] and Volume 2 of THE TRIGGER POINT MANUAL to solve the puzzling pain problems of the patient with chronic myofascial pain.

PAIN GUIDE TO INVOLVED MUSCLES

This guide lists the muscles that may be responsible for referred pain in each of the areas shown in Figure 18.1. These areas, which identify where patients may complain of pain, are listed alphabetically. The muscles most likely to refer pain to each designated area are listed under the name of that area. One uses this chart by locating the name of the area that hurts and then by looking under that heading for the muscles that are likely to cause the pain. Reference should then be made to the pain patterns of individual muscles, as indicated by the figure and page numbers in parentheses.

In a general way, the muscle listings follow the order of frequency in which they are likely to cause pain in that area. This order is only an approximation; the selection process by which patients reach an examiner greatly influences which of their muscles are most likely to be symptomatic. **Bold face** type indicates that the muscle refers an essential pain pattern to that pain area. Normal type indicates that the muscle may sometimes refer pain (a spillover pattern) to that pain area. TrP means trigger point.

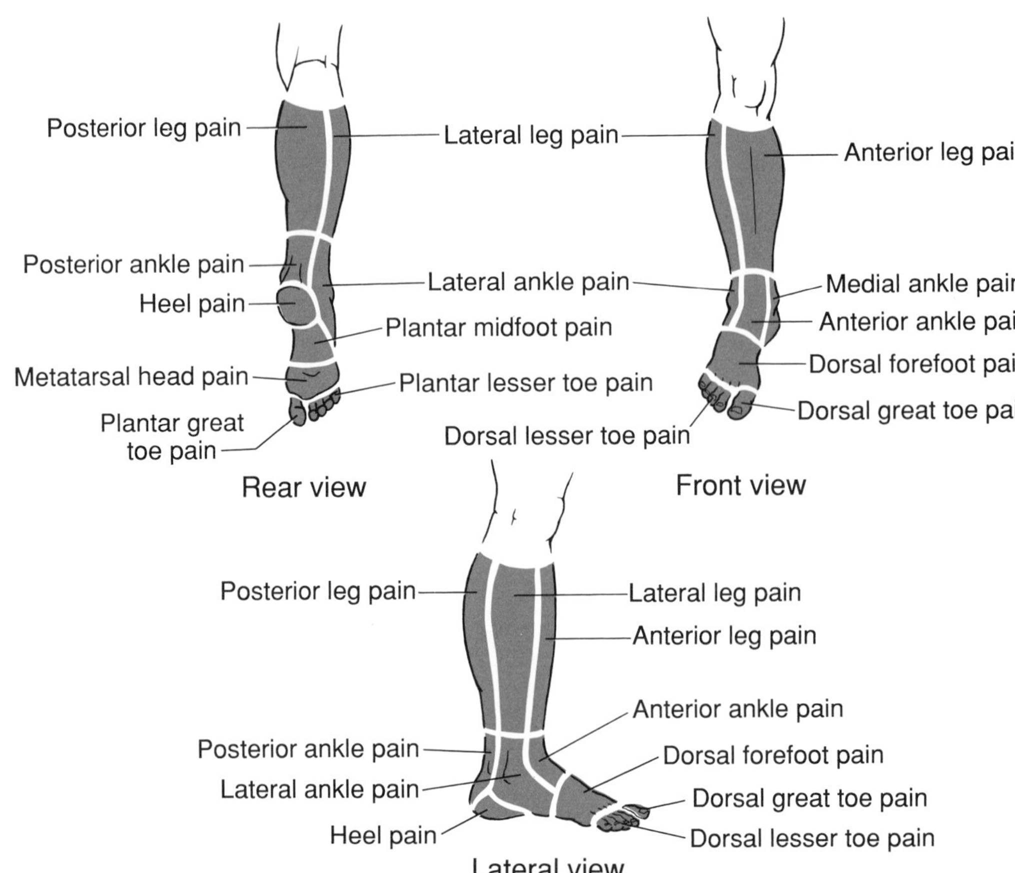

Figure 18.1. Designated areas *(red)* within the leg, ankle, and foot regions where patients may describe myofascial pain. The pain may be referred to each area from the muscles listed in the PAIN GUIDE.

PAIN GUIDE

ANTERIOR ANKLE PAIN

Tibialis anterior (19.1, p. 356)
Peroneus tertius (20.1*B*, p. 372)
Extensor digitorum longus (24.1*A*, p. 474)
Extensor hallucis longus (24.1*B*, p. 474)

ANTERIOR LEG PAIN

Tibialis anterior (19.1, p. 356)
Adductors longus and brevis (15.1, p. 291)

DORSAL FOREFOOT PAIN

Extensor digitorum brevis and extensor hallucis brevis (26.1, p. 503)
Extensor digitorum longus (24.1*A*, p. 474)
Extensor hallucis longus (24.1*B*, p. 474)
Flexor hallucis brevis (27.2*B*, p. 524)
Interossei of foot (27.3*A*, p. 525)
Tibialis anterior (19.1, p. 356)

DORSAL GREAT TOE PAIN

Tibialis anterior (19.1, p. 356)
Extensor hallucis longus (24.1*B*, p. 474)
Flexor hallucis brevis (27.2*B*, p. 524)

DORSAL LESSER TOE PAIN

Interossei of foot (27.3*A*, p. 525)
Extensor digitorum longus (24.1*A*, p. 474)

HEEL PAIN

Soleus (22.1 TrP_1, p. 429)
Quadratus plantae (27.1, p. 523)
Abductor hallucis (26.2, p. 504)
Tibialis posterior (23.1, p. 461)

LATERAL ANKLE PAIN

Peronei longus and brevis (20.1*A*, p. 372)
Peroneus tertius (20.1*B*, p. 372)

LATERAL LEG PAIN

Gastrocnemius (21.1 TrP_2, p. 399)
Gluteus minimus, anterior section (9.1, p. 169)
Peronei longus and brevis (20.1*A*, p. 372)
Vastus lateralis (14.4 TrP_2, p. 253)

MEDIAL ANKLE PAIN

Abductor hallucis (26.2, p. 504)
Flexor digitorum longus (25.1*A*, p. 490)

METATARSAL HEAD PAIN

Flexor hallucis brevis (27.2*B*, p. 524)
Flexor digitorum brevis (26.3*B*, p. 505)
Adductor hallucis (27.2*A*, p. 524)
Flexor hallucis longus (25.1*B*, p. 490)
Interossei of foot (27.3*B*, p. 525)
Abductor digiti minimi (26.3*A*, p. 505)
Flexor digitorum longus (25.1*A*, p. 490)
Tibialis posterior (23.1, p. 461)

PLANTAR GREAT TOE PAIN

Flexor hallucis longus (25.1*B*, p. 490)
Flexor hallucis brevis (27.2*B*, p. 524)
Tibialis posterior (23.1 p. 461)

PLANTAR LESSER TOE PAIN

Flexor digitorum longus (25.1*A*, p. 490)
Tibialis posterior (23.1, p. 461)

PLANTAR MIDFOOT PAIN

Gastrocnemius (21.1 TrP_1, p. 399)
Flexor digitorum longus (25.1*A*, p. 490)
Adductor hallucis (27.2*A*, p. 524)
Soleus (22.1 TrP_1, p. 429)
Interossei of foot (27.3*B*, p. 525)
Abductor hallucis (26.2, p. 504)
Tibialis posterior (23.1, p. 461)

POSTERIOR ANKLE PAIN

Soleus (22.1 TrP_1, p. 429)
Tibialis posterior (23.1, p. 461)

POSTERIOR LEG PAIN

Soleus (22.1 TrP_2, p. 429)
Gluteus minimus, posterior section (9.2, p. 169)
Gastrocnemius (21.1, p. 399)
Semitendinosus and semimembranosus (16.1, p. 317)
Soleus (22.1 TrP_1, p. 429)
Flexor digitorum longus (25.1*A*, p. 490)
Tibialis posterior (23.1, p. 461)
Plantaris (22.3, p. 430)

References

1. McMinn RMH, Hutchings RT, Logan BM: *Color Atlas of Foot and Ankle Anatomy*. Appleton-Century-Crofts, Connecticut, 1982 (p. 26).
2. Travell JG, Simons DG: *Myofascial Pain and Dysfunction: The Trigger Point Manual*. Williams & Wilkins, Baltimore, 1983.

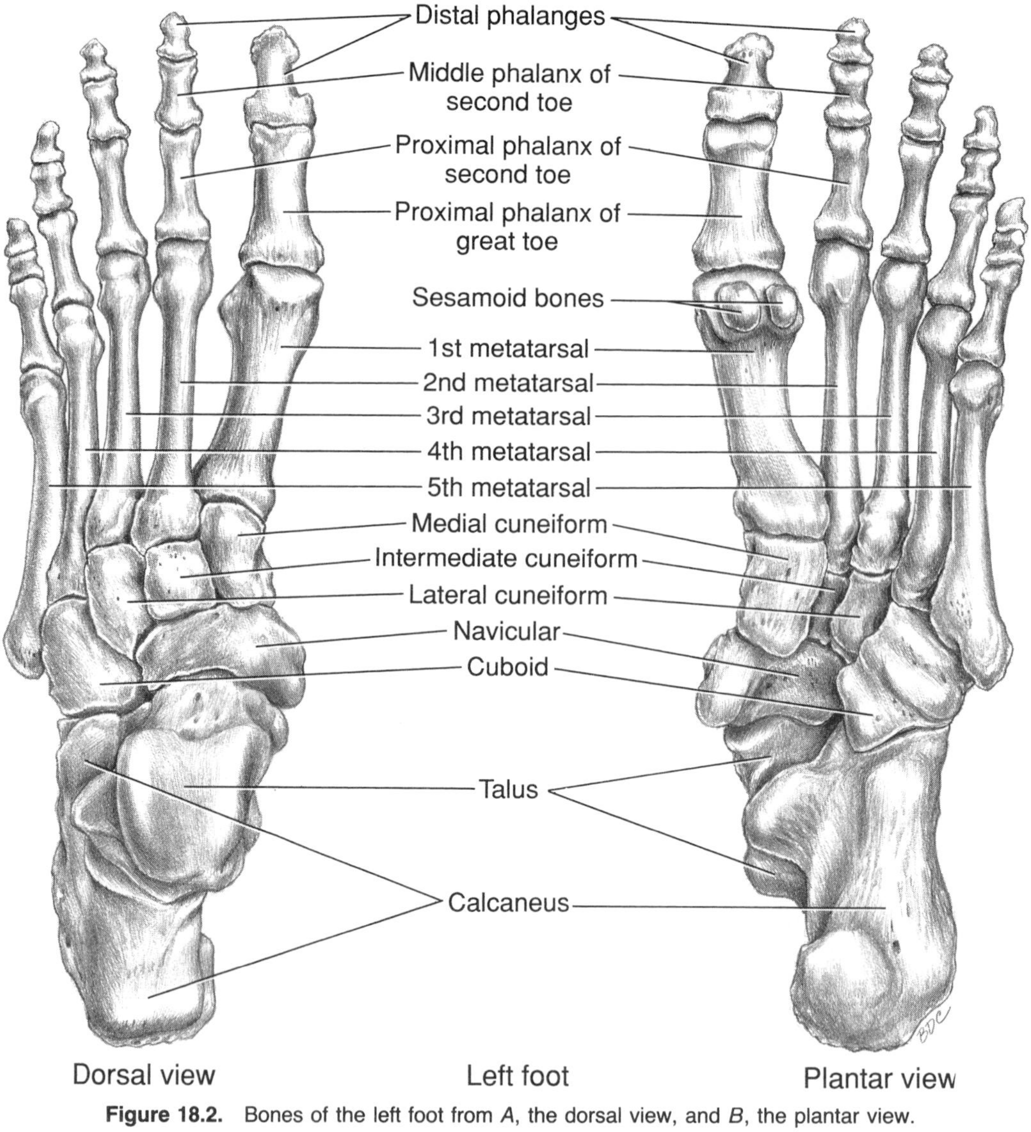

Figure 18.2. Bones of the left foot from *A*, the dorsal view, and *B*, the plantar view. Redrawn from McMinn *et al.*[1]

CHAPTER 19
Tibialis Anterior Muscle

"Foot-drop Muscle"

HIGHLIGHTS: **REFERRED PAIN** from trigger points (TrPs) in the tibialis anterior muscle concentrates on the anteromedial aspect of the ankle and on the dorsal and medial surfaces of the great toe. A spillover pattern may extend downward over the shin from the TrP to the ankle. **ANATOMICAL ATTACHMENTS** anchor proximally to the lateral condyle of the tibia, the upper half or more of the lateral surface of the body of the tibia, and to surrounding fascial structures. The muscle's tendon attaches distally to the medial and plantar surfaces of the medial cuneiform bone and to the base of the first metatarsal. **FUNCTIONS** of the tibialis anterior muscle during ambulation are to prevent foot slap at heelstrike and to help the toes clear the floor during swing phase. It is vigorously active during jogging, running, sprinting, two-leg upward jumps, and other sports activities. It acts as a dorsiflexor of the foot at the talocrural joint and acts to supinate the foot at the subtalar and transverse tarsal joints. Type 1 (slow-twitch) fibers predominate in this muscle. **SYMPTOMS** caused by TrPs in the tibialis anterior muscle include referred pain and tenderness in the ankle anteromedially and in the big toe, painful motion of the ankle, dragging of the toes or ankle weakness, and tripping or falling when walking because of the weak dorsiflexion. The referred pain pattern of the tibialis anterior may resemble the patterns of the extensor hallucis longus and the other two anterior compartment muscles, but can be distinguished from them. Symptoms of an anterior compartment syndrome must be recognized and should not be dismissed as myofascial pain. **ACTIVATION OF TRIGGER POINTS** usually results from major overload of the muscle or from an accident that causes additional skeletal injury. On **PATIENT EXAMINATION**, the clinician usually finds a tendency for foot slap and foot drop during ambulation, deep tenderness in the referred pain zone, slight weakness, and some restriction of the stretch range of motion of the tibialis anterior muscle. **TRIGGER POINT EXAMINATION** reveals taut bands parallel to the tibia with spot tenderness of TrPs in the upper one-third of the muscle. Snapping palpation at the TrP evokes highly visible local twitch responses, and digital pressure reproduces the referred pain pattern of active TrPs. To employ **INTERMITTENT COLD WITH STRETCH**, the clinician applies ice or vapocoolant spray in parallel sweeps downward over the muscle and its referred pain pattern. At the same time, passive plantar flexion and eversion of the foot lengthen the muscle. This technique can be augmented by postisometric relaxation and reciprocal inhibition. Massage can be effective for inactivating tibialis anterior TrPs. **INJECTION AND STRETCH** of this muscle employs a 21-gauge, 38-mm (1½-in) needle, and a 45° angle of skin entry aimed toward the tibia to avoid the underlying anterior tibial artery and vein and the deep peroneal nerve. A local twitch response is often observed when the needle penetrates a TrP in this muscle. Application of intermittent cold with stretch of the muscle after injection, followed by moist heat, helps ensure inactivation of any residual TrPs. Active range of motion follows in order to restore normal function of the muscle. **CORRECTIVE ACTIONS** to prevent reactivation of the TrPs in this muscle include a home self-stretch exercise program and elimination of prolonged shortening of the muscle, for instance, by leveling an acutely upward-angled accelerator pedal of a car. In addition, cruise control permits periodic relief to avoid a fixed position of the lower limb for an extended time. Release of antagonist tight calf musculature helps restore balance and reduce overload of anterior compartment muscles.

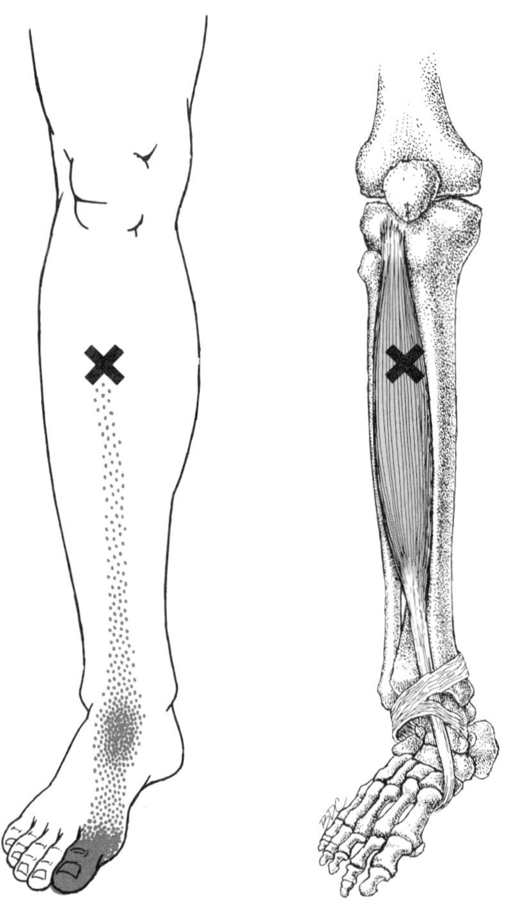

Figure 19.1. Pain pattern (*dark red*) referred from a trigger point (**X**) at its usual location in the right tibialis anterior muscle (*light red*), as seen in the anterior view with the foot slightly abducted. The essential pain pattern is *solid red*; the *red stippling* indicates occasional spillover extension of the essential pattern.

1. REFERRED PAIN
(Fig. 19.1)

Myofascial trigger points (TrPs) in the tibialis anterior muscle refer pain and tenderness primarily to the anteromedial aspect of the ankle and over the dorsal and medial surfaces of the great toe (Fig. 19.1).[95] In addition, sometimes the pain (spillover pattern) may extend from the TrP downward over the shin to the ankle and foot anteromedially.[86,87,96] The TrPs usually occur in the upper third of the muscle (Fig. 19.1).

Other authors reported that tibialis anterior TrPs referred pain to the anterior leg and dorsal ankle,[88–90] dorsal ankle and dorsal region of the great toe,[49] or to the lower leg, ankle, and foot (or specifically the dorsal surface of the great toe).[7,90]

Tibialis anterior TrPs are occasionally the source of the chief pain complaint in children. The referred pain pattern is similar to that seen in adults.[14]

Gutstein[42] described a patient with severe burning pain in the foot and knee, especially after long periods of standing. He attributed the pain to myalgic spots along the lower half of the tibialis anterior muscle. Treatment with heat followed by firm local massage at the myalgic spots relieved the pain.

In 14 subjects, Kellgren[52] injected the proximal and middle parts of the belly of the tibialis anterior muscle with 0.1 mL of hypertonic saline solution. The injection produced referred pain to the front of the ankle and in the outer and middle part of the front of the leg in most subjects. A few subjects had pain only at the ankle and a few only in the leg. This is similar to the pattern of referred pain seen clinically in patients with tibialis anterior TrPs, except that Kellgren reported no pain over the great toe. Injection of 0.05 mL of the hypertonic saline solution into the tibialis anterior tendon caused diffuse pain in a small area on the medial aspect of the instep in all subjects.[52]

2. ANATOMICAL ATTACHMENTS AND CONSIDERATIONS
(Figs. 19.2 and 19.3)

The tibialis anterior muscle is subcutaneous just lateral to the anterior sharp edge of the tibia (the shin) and becomes tendinous in the lower third of the leg (Fig. 19.2). It anchors ***proximally*** to the lateral condyle and upper half or two-thirds of the lateral surface of the tibia, the adjacent interosseous membrane, the deep surface of the crural fascia, and the intermuscular septum common to the extensor digitorum longus.[22] The muscle fibers of the tibialis anterior converge on their aponeurosis and tendon to form a pennate structure.[9] The tendon crosses in front of the tibia to the medial side of the foot where it attaches ***distally*** to the medial and plantar surfaces of the medial cuneiform bone and to the base of the first metatarsal medially.[9,22] Accessory attachments in the foot occurred in 21.7% of 64 human cadaver legs.[58]

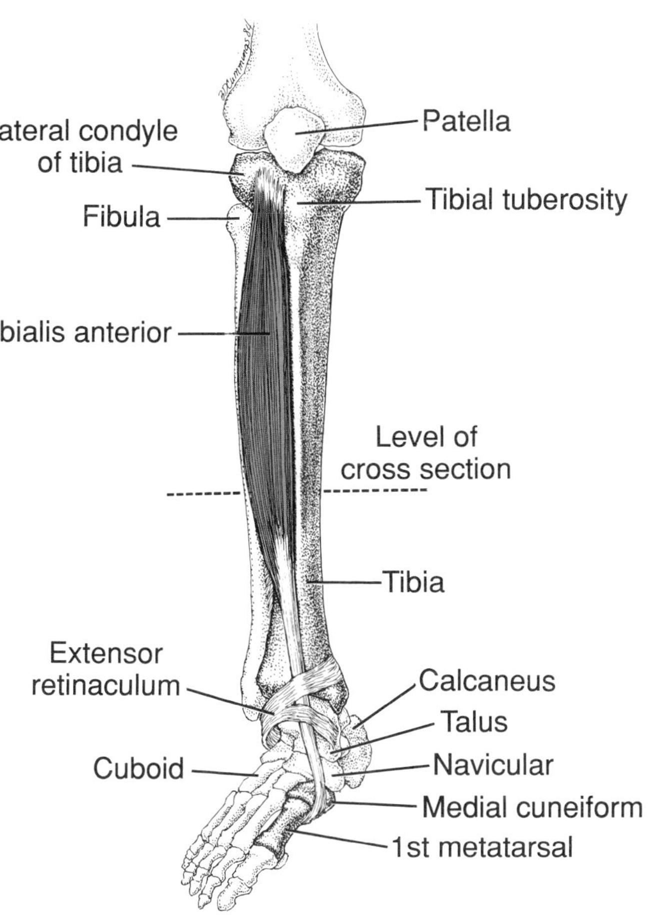

Figure 19.2. Attachments of the right tibialis anterior muscle (*red*), anterior view. The foot is turned outward to show the distal attachments to the medial cuneiform and first metatarsal bones. The cross section indicated on this figure is shown in Figure 19.3.

A cross section at the lower part of the middle third of the leg (Fig. 19.3) shows that the tibialis anterior muscle occupies a triangular space bounded by the tibia medially, by only skin and crural fascia anteriorly, and by the extensor hallucis longus muscle laterally. These structural relations continue throughout the length of the muscle belly of the tibialis anterior. The deep peroneal nerve and anterior tibial vessels lie on the interosseus membrane deep to the muscle.[17]

Unyielding fascial structures and bone that form the anterior compartment surround the tibialis anterior muscle. This muscle shares this compartment with the extensor digitorum longus, extensor hallucis longus, and the peroneus tertius muscles, and with the deep peroneal nerve and the anterior tibial artery and vein.[71]

The myoneural endplates in whole tibialis anterior muscles of three adult human subjects were diffusely distributed with the greatest concentration found toward the periphery and toward the proximal end of the muscle.[6] A similar location of endplates around the periphery of this pennate muscle appeared in the muscles of a stillborn infant.[18] The tibialis anterior has fibers of intermediate length, 8.7 cm. This length is similar to that of fibers in the extensor hallucis longus and extensor digitorum longus muscles.[98]

Supplemental References

The tibialis anterior muscle appears in front view without nerves or vessels[35,72,83] and in relation to the anterior tibial artery and vein and deep peroneal nerve.[4,32,73] The view from the medial side shows the course of its tendon[33] and the view from the lateral side demonstrates its close relation to the extensor digitorum longus muscle.[34,63,82]

Markings on the bones locate the muscle's attachments to the tibia and to the medial cuneiform and first metatarsal bones of the foot.[1,36,62,74]

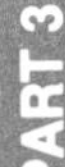

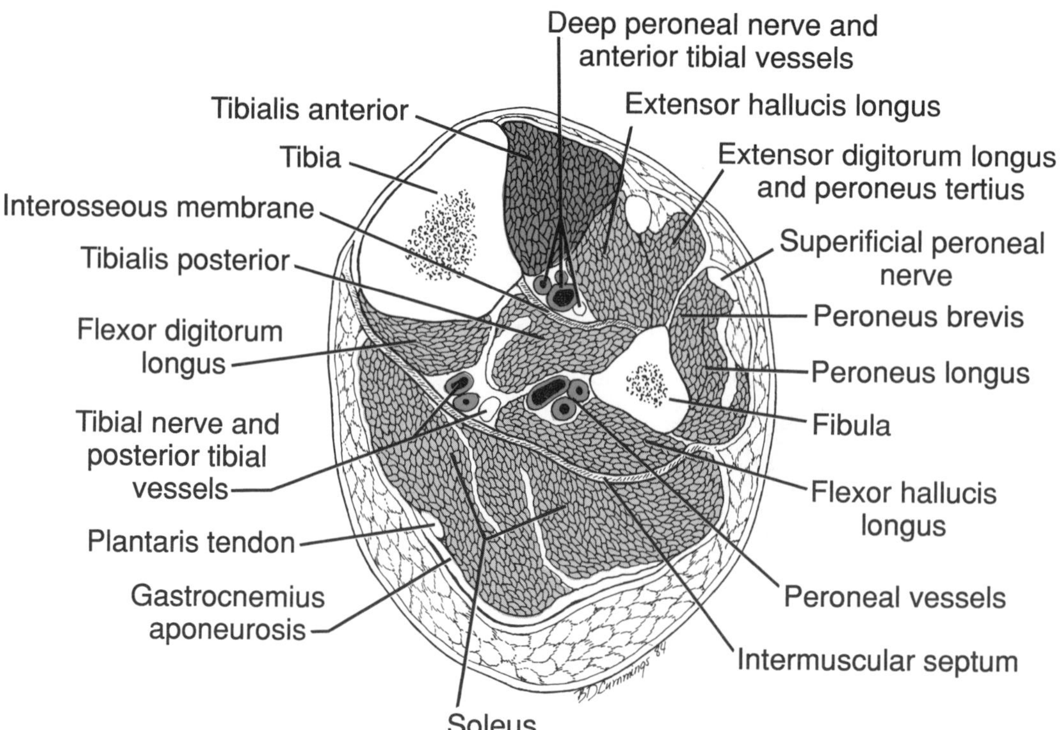

Figure 19.3. Cross section through the lower part of the middle third of the right leg, viewed from above. Major blood vessels and the tibialis anterior muscle are *dark red*; other muscles are *light red*. Level of the cross section, below the gastrocnemius muscle belly, is shown in Figure 19.2. (After Figure 4-72 in *Grant's Atlas of Anatomy*.[3])

A photograph reveals details of its tendinous attachments in the foot.[5]

Cross sections portray the relation of the tibialis anterior muscle to surrounding structures and its accessibility for injection: throughout its length in 13 serial cross sections,[17] in three cross sections of the upper, middle, and lower thirds of the leg,[37] in two cross sections of the upper and lower thirds of the leg,[20] in one cross section just above the middle of the leg,[71] and one at the lower part of the middle third of the leg.[3]

Photographs of well-muscled subjects illustrate surface contours produced by the tibialis anterior muscle.[2,21,31,57]

3. INNERVATION

The deep peroneal nerve supplies the tibialis anterior muscle with fibers from the fourth and fifth lumbar and the first sacral spinal nerves.[22]

4. FUNCTION

The tibialis anterior muscle helps maintain standing balance through lengthening contractions to control excessive sway posteriorly, and through shortening contractions as needed to pull the leg and body forward over the fixed foot. It functions to prevent foot slap following heel-strike and helps the foot clear the ground during the swing phase of gait. Loss of foot clearance greatly increases "balance problems" and the danger of falling (a common hazard in the elderly). During jogging and running, electromyographic (EMG) activity begins just after toe-off and continues through the first half of the support (stance) phase. This muscle is moderately to vigorously active during most sports activities. Its type 1 (slow-twitch) fibers predominate; type 2 (fast-twitch) fibers compose, at most, only one-third of the muscle.

The tibialis anterior muscle dorsiflexes and supinates (inverts and adducts) the foot when the distal segment is free. However, it does not contribute to inversion when the foot is plantar flexed.

Actions

In the non-weight-bearing limb, the tibialis anterior muscle dorsiflexes the foot at the talocrural joint and supinates (inverts and adducts) the foot at the subtalar and transverse tarsal joints;[12,22] it is not active as an invertor during plantar flexion.[80]

Direct electrical stimulation of the tibialis anterior muscle first produces vigorous dorsiflexion and then weak adduction[26] of the foot. Stimulation specifically elevates the head of the first metatarsal bone.[27]

Functions

Standing and Postural Changes

In normal subjects standing at ease, primarily the soleus muscle made minor forward balance adjustments.[10] In more than one-quarter of these normal barefooted subjects, the tibialis anterior remained silent. The EMG activity observed in some subjects disappeared when the subject leaned forward. Tibialis anterior motor unit activity developed or increased when the subject leaned backward,[10] as the muscle helps control this movement.

The tibialis anterior became active when subjects leaned backward, and activity ceased when they leaned forward, at any rate of movement.[39,75] It became active in response to equivalent separate or combined bilateral limb displacements standing on a double treadmill,[25] when combined with other variations of standing posture,[76] when thrown off balance by voluntary, rapid arm pushes or pulls against a fixed resistance,[23] or when standing on an oscillating platform.[24] The further a subject leaned back and the closer the center of pressure moved toward the heel, the greater became the EMG activity of the tibialis anterior.[77]

Squatting with the heels flat on the floor caused the tibialis anterior to produce 60% of its maximum voluntary contraction level of EMG activity.[76]

Ambulation

During *walking*, EMG activity in the tibialis anterior muscle reaches its primary peak at heel-strike and a secondary peak at toe-off. Paralysis of this muscle results in foot-drop[11,80] and a tendency to stub the toes on curbs or steps.[80]

More specifically, the ankle dorsiflexors (tibialis anterior and long extensors of the toes) prevent *foot slap* just after heel-strike; they undergo a lengthening contraction as they control the descent of the foot to the floor, or as they decelerate the foot at heel-strike.[79] Foot clearance (or toe clearance) during the swing phase requires a combination of hip flexion, knee flexion, and ankle dorsiflexion.

Dragging of the toes at the beginning of swing phase is due to inadequate hip and knee flexion; later in swing, as the limb moves forward, toe dragging results from inadequate dorsiflexion.[79]

The primary peak of EMG activity in this muscle occurs at heel-strike[11,40,94] at all speeds of ambulation.[101] During the 100 milliseconds around heel-strike, this activity averages 44% of a maximum voluntary contraction.[50] During full-foot contact at midstance phase, a brief period of no EMG activity occurs.[11,64] The secondary peak during walking appears at toe-off (end of stance phase)[11,94] at all speeds.[101] The continuation of EMG activity in this muscle throughout swing phase is variable from person to person. In various reports, it: *(a)* continued throughout swing phase;[94] *(b)* continued in four of seven subjects and was biphasic in the other three at all speeds;[70] *(c)* faded out during most of the swing phase;[11] and *(d)* reached zero activity at some point during swing phase in six of six subjects at a wide range of walking speeds.[64]

The tibialis anterior muscle does not contribute significantlyto *arch support* of the normal foot during weight bearing.[11,13] However, the tibialis anterior of standing subjects showed greater EMG activity in those subjects who had flat feet.[41]

Increasing the thickness of *heel lifts* in men increased tibialis anterior EMG activity during walking.[55] The opposite effect occurred in women, presumably because they had accommodated to high heels; for them, the unaccustomed flatness of the lowest heel lifts stimulated activity in this muscle.[56]

When subjects descended *stairs*, EMG activity in the tibialis anterior muscle showed a similar pattern to that seen during ambulation. Activity occurred around the beginning and end of stance phase, but in one-third of subjects, the tibialis anterior was continuously active throughout the cycle.[93] When ascending stairs, EMG activity began near the end of stance and continued throughout most of swing phase. This activity apparently serves to ensure foot clearance on its way up to the next step.[93]

Athletic Activities

The pattern of EMG activity of the tibialis anterior muscle changes between *jogging, running, and sprinting*. During jogging and running, activity is absent at toe-off but appears shortly thereafter and continues throughout the remainder of the swing phase and the first half of the support phase. During swing phase, continued activity of the muscle ensures dorsiflexion of the foot. However, during sprinting, EMG activity ceases briefly at midswing when plantar flexion of the foot begins.[59]

When the subject does a *two-leg jump upward*, EMG activity in the tibialis anterior muscle begins as the foot clears the ground. Activity ceases before the subject reaches the highest point in the jump. Vigorous EMG activity returns before landing and continues at reduced intensity during the landing itself and into the stabilization phase.[51]

During *ergometer cycling*, this muscle generated EMG activity that corresponded to only 9% of its maximum voluntary contraction as the pedal was passing its highest position. At this time, the ankle joint is in its most dorsiflexed position.[28]

Broer and Houtz[16] measured the EMG activity of the tibialis anterior muscle during 13 *right-handed sports* activities. The activities included overhand throws, underhand throws, tennis and golf swings, hitting a baseball, and single-foot jumps. The EMG activity in the right tibialis anterior muscle was equal to or greater than that of the left in every activity except the single-foot jump volleyball spike. In every right-handed sport activity, the right tibialis anterior exhibited at least moderate EMG activity, and frequently, this was as vigorous as for any of the other muscles monitored.[16]

Fiber Types

Henriksson-Larsén and associates[47] determined the fiber type distribution in a 1-mm² area every 9 mm throughout whole-muscle cross sections of the tibialis anterior muscles from six young previously healthy adult males who suffered sudden accidental death. Type 1 (slow-twitch) fibers predominated and type 2 (fast-twitch) fibers were *NOT* randomly distributed. A gradual, often dramatic, relative increase in type 2 fibers was seen from the surface of the muscle toward the deeper regions, where the number of type 2 fibers was approximately twice that near the surface. In addition, two or more major foci with a comparatively high density of type 2 fibers were sometimes present. Within a distance of only 10 mm, the proportion of type 2 fibers could vary 20%. The average value for all samples in one muscle varied from 19–33% for type 2 fibers among the six tibialis anterior muscles and the mean for the group was 28% of type 2 fibers.[47] Similar results were observed in female anterior tibialis muscles.[45]

Sandstedt[85] found that the proportion of type 2 fibers could vary from 7–30% in two biopsies from the same muscle. These studies emphasize the large sampling errors inherent in a single small-sample biopsy of this muscle. Both type 1 and type 2 fibers that lie deep in this muscle have larger diameters than those that lie in superficial areas.[46]

Other authors who took small, superficial samples of the tibialis anterior muscle found that it averaged 22% type 2 fibers among 29 healthy volunteers[84] and 77% type 1 fibers (less than 23% type 2 fibers) among seven normal male subjects.[44]

5. FUNCTIONAL (MYOTATIC) UNIT

Dorsiflexion of the foot can occur as a balanced action of two dorsiflexors: the tibialis anterior, which also inverts, and the extensor digitorum longus, which also everts the foot.[27] The third primary dorsiflexor is the peroneus tertius. These dorsiflexors are assisted by the extensor hallucis longus.[80] The chief antagonists to dorsiflexion are the gastrocnemius and soleus muscles, assisted by the peroneus longus and brevis, long flexors of the toes, and the tibialis posterior muscle.[80]

6. SYMPTOMS

The chief complaint of patients with active TrPs in the tibialis anterior is usually pain on the anteromedial aspect of the ankle and in the big toe. Other complaints may include: weakness of dorsiflexion when walking, falling, dragging of the foot that causes tripping, and general weakness of the ankle. Painful motion of the ankle may bother the patient in the absence of any evidence of joint injury.[95] Loss of function is especially evident when TrPs in the long extensor muscles of the toes cause additional dorsiflexion weakness.

Usually, patients with tibialis anterior TrPs do not complain of nocturnal pain, and a plantar flexed position of the ankle throughout the night does not bother this muscle unless its TrPs are sufficiently active to cause some degree of constant referred pain.

The tibialis anterior myofascial pain syndrome rarely presents alone as a single-muscle syndrome, but occurs in association with TrPs in other leg muscles.

Differential Diagnosis

The pain referred from TrPs in several other leg and foot muscles can have a confusingly similar distribution to that of the tibialis anterior TrPs. The pain pattern of **extensor hallucis longus** TrPs (*see* Fig. 24.1), which is the most similar, appears on the dorsum of the foot in an area between the ankle and great toe, concentrating over the first metatarsal head, not over the great toe. However, the extensor hallucis longus may refer spillover pain to the antero*medial* ankle and to the dorsum of the great toe. The TrPs of the **extensor digitorum longus** (*see* Fig. 24.1) and of the **extensor digitorum brevis** and the **extensor hallucis brevis** (*see* Fig. 26.1) also refer pain to the *mid*dorsum of the foot, but more laterally over the long extensor tendons of the lesser toes. In addition, the **extensor digitorum longus** may refer spillover pain up to the antero*lateral* ankle and down to the four lesser toes. The pain from **peroneus tertius** TrPs (*see* Fig. 20.1*B*) mimics the ankle pain of the tibialis anterior, but not the toe pain. Pain referred from **flexor hallucis longus** TrPs (*see* Fig. 25.1) appears on the plantar, not the dorsal, surface of the great toe without spillover pain to the ankle. **First dorsal interosseous** TrPs refer pain (*see* Fig. 27.3) primarily to the second toe with spillover pain to the space between the first and second metatarsals, on the dorsum of the foot lateral to the pain pattern due to tibialis anterior TrPs.

To distinguish myofascial referred pain from painful fascial and articular structures in the ankle and foot, the examiner palpates: associated muscles for taut bands and for TrP tenderness with induced referral of pain, the joints for tenderness and restricted range of motion, and the ligaments for tenderness. Referred pain and tenderness of tibialis anterior TrPs can readily be mistaken for disease of the first metatarsophalangeal joint.[81]

Other conditions deserving differential consideration include L_5 radiculopathy, anterior compartment syndrome, and herniation of the tibialis anterior muscle.

Radiculopathy

Preservation of the tendon reflex of the tibialis anterior muscle reduces the likelihood of an L_5 radicular compression as a contributing cause of the patient's pain. This reflex[91] was absent bilaterally in 11%, and missing on only one side in an additional 6%, of 70 healthy subjects. A hand-held reflex hammer elicited the reflex response and surface electrodes recorded it electromyographically. However, the reflex was absent on only the affected side in 72% of 18 patients with L_5 radicular compression.[91] Electrodiagnostic testing is indicated if a serious question of radiculopathy remains.

Anterior Compartment Syndrome

Compartment syndromes are characterized by increased pressure within a muscular compartment sufficient to compromise the circulation of the muscles within it. A compartment space is determined anatomically by an unyielding fascial (and bony) enclosure of the muscles. Four compartments are recognized in the leg: *(a)* the anterior compartment includes the tibialis anterior, extensor hallucis longus, extensor digitorum longus, and peroneus tertius. *(b)* The deep posterior compartment comprises the antagonists to the muscles of the anterior compartment: the tibialis posterior, flexor hallucis longus, and flexor digitorum longus. *(c)* The superficial posterior compartment is usually defined as including both the soleus and gastrocnemius muscles,[100] but the soleus is more vulnerable to developing a compartment syndrome. *(d)* The lateral compartment encompasses the peroneus longus and brevis muscles. Anterior compartment syndromes are recognized more commonly than are posterior compartment syndromes.[100] Consideration of the posterior compartment syndrome appears on pages 443–444 of this volume.

If the patient's leg pain is caused by an anterior compartment syndrome, it is most important that this condition be recognized immediately and managed properly to avoid possibly catastrophic consequences. Diffuse tightness and tenderness over the entire belly of the tibialis anterior suggests an anterior compartment syndrome.

The anterior (tibial) compartment syndrome is also sometimes called **anterior shin splints**, a term that is properly used to describe periosteal irritation from overuse. A compartment syndrome should be distinguished from shin splints. Shin splints are discussed on pages 443–444 of this volume. The compartment syndrome arises because of increased pressure within the unyielding anterior compartment of the leg. The pressure obstructs venous outflow, which causes further swelling and more pressure. The resultant ischemia leads to necrosis of the muscles and nerves within the compartment. The process can begin with swelling of the tibialis anterior, extensor hallucis longus, extensor digitorum longus, and/or the peroneus tertius muscles in response to strong eccentric contractions sufficient to produce post-exercise soreness.[38] Patients with the anterior compartment syndrome exhibit pain, paresthesias, and tenderness both in the ischemic muscles and in the region supplied by the deep peroneal nerve. The muscles are sensitive to passive stretch, and active contraction of the muscles increases symptoms. Among athletes, symptoms may develop progressively over a period of time.[48,66,67] Rarely, an anterior tibial compartment syndrome may present as a painless weakness of dorsiflexion. The lack of pain has been attributed to pressure-induced neurapraxia.[19]

Patients for whom surgical release of pressure is too late, and who have postnecrotic scarring of the muscles and nerves within the compartment, are prone also to develop active TrPs in muscles within the compartment. These TrPs add to the pain of direct neurological origin. Massage is often poorly tolerated because of residual allodynia and hyperesthesia. Injection of any space-occupying substance may also be poorly tolerated by the scarred, hypersensitive, poorly vascularized tissues. Owen and associates studied certain postures that are commonly assumed during drug overdose (the squat and knee-chest positions); when these postures were tested in 17 normal volunteers, anterior compartment pressures in the range of 49–100 mm Hg were produced.[78]

Tight, shortened calf muscles overload weakened anterior compartment muscles and predispose the athlete to developing an anterior compartment syndrome.[65]

The definitive diagnostic test for an anterior compartment syndrome is measurement of intramuscular pressure within the anterior compartment. Three techniques are in common use and are graphically summarized.[48] The Whitesides technique[99] employs a mercury manometer and needle, which are readily available in any emergency room, but are less accurate than a wick catheter. The wick catheter technique of Mubarak and associates[68] uses a fiber-filled polyethylene catheter inserted into the compartment and attached to a pressure transducer. It is resistant to blockage. The continuous infusion technique of Matsen[60] substitutes a low-rate infusion pump for a wick to maintain patency of the monitoring needle; using this method, the pressure can be monitored continuously for 3 days. Sustained pressures in excess of 30 mm Hg[69] or 40–50 mm Hg[60] have been considered the indication for extensive fasciotomy of the compartment.

In acute cases, a *brief* period of rest and cryotherapy to reduce pain, swelling, and metabolic demand can be tried only with *close* monitoring before more drastic measures are considered.

Elevation of the leg is contraindicated because it has been shown to reduce oxygen tension within the compartment.[61]

Among runners, anterior shin splints (periosteal irritation) may develop when the athlete changes from a flatfooted to a toe-running style, begins training on a track or hill [especially downhill running], or runs in a shoe with a sole that is too flexible.[15] A too-rigid shoe can also cause shin splints. The activities listed previously may also overload the tibialis anterior muscle and activate TrPs in it.

Herniation

Subcutaneous herniation of the tibialis anterior muscle through its investing fascia may be painful during standing and walking or it may be of cosmetic concern.[43] Magnetic resonance imaging, unlike computed tomography, unequivocally identifies the extent of fascial splitting and the size of muscle herniation because it distinguishes more clearly between these two soft-tissue structures.[102]

7. ACTIVATION AND PERPETUATION OF TRIGGER POINTS

Trigger points in the tibialis anterior muscle may be activated by the same forces that cause an ankle sprain or fracture, and by overload sufficient to induce an anterior compartment syndrome. The TrPs of this muscle seem more likely to be the result of serious gross trauma than due simply to overuse (repetitive, micromechanical trauma). Walking on rough ground or on a slanted surface, however, can precipitate myofascial problems.

A motor vehicle accident did not activate TrPs in the tibialis anterior muscle in any of the 100 patients examined, although other lower limb muscles were commonly involved.[8] Such an accident is unlikely to cause a forceful lengthening contraction of this muscle.

Catching the toe on an obstruction during early swing phase (tripping or stumbling during the contraction phase of the tibialis anterior) can cause eccentric contraction overload that activates or perpetuates TrPs in the muscle. The overload is aggravated by a proportional increase in the reflex response to sudden stretch, a response that ranges from 0–40% of maximum voluntary contraction.[92]

8. PATIENT EXAMINATION

The clinician observes the patient for foot slap and foot-drop during ambulation. Foot slap occurs when the forefoot slaps to the floor immediately following heel-strike. Foot-drop is a failure to dorsiflex the foot sufficiently to provide adequate clearance between the toes and the floor, particularly during late swing.

Active TrPs in this muscle cause some degree of weakness. This weakness is easily masked by compensatory contraction of the long extensor muscles of the toes or the peroneus tertius muscle. To test the tibialis anterior muscle for strength, the seated patient first inverts and then dorsiflexes the foot against resistance without extension of the great toe.[53]

Active or latent TrPs in the tibialis anterior muscle restrict the stretch range of motion because of pain and muscle tightness.

Deep tenderness over the ankle and great toe may be referred from TrPs of the tibialis anterior muscle.[95]

9. TRIGGER POINT EXAMINATION (Fig. 19.4)

To find tibialis anterior TrPs in the supine patient, the examiner first locates the sharp edge of the tibia at approximately the junction of the proximal and middle thirds of the leg. Flat palpation reveals taut bands and TrP spot tenderness in the muscle mass lateral to the tibia (Fig. 19.4). The taut bands in this muscle are parallel to the tibia. Snapping transverse palpation at the TrP in the taut band evokes a vigorous and highly visible twitch response in this muscle. This response appears as transient inversion and dorsiflexion of the foot if the foot is free to move (Fig. 19.4). Digital pressure applied to an active TrP will usually evoke or intensify the spontaneous pain referred to the ankle[95] and foot.

Sola[89] observed that the TrPs were most commonly located in the upper one-third of this muscle, as we have found. Lange[54] pictured myogelosis (tender taut bands [of TrPs]) as running vertically through the midportion of the muscle belly.

10. ENTRAPMENTS

To our knowledge, TrPs in this muscle do not cause nerve entrapment; however, tibialis anterior TrPs are a likely sequela to an anterior compartment syndrome.

11. ASSOCIATED TRIGGER POINTS

The peroneus longus and tibialis anterior muscles often become involved together; they operate as a pair of well-matched antagonists for stabilization and balance of the foot. The extensor hallucis longus and, to a lesser degree, the extensor digitorum longus may also develop TrPs as agonists to the tibialis anterior muscle. Tibialis posterior TrPs are not usually identified as related to TrPs in the tibialis anterior muscle.

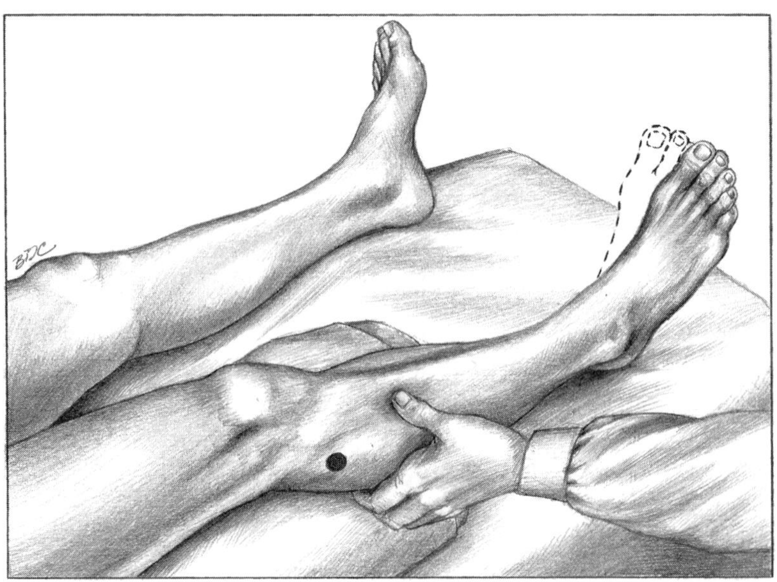

Figure 19.4. Palpation of trigger points in the right tibialis anterior muscle. The *solid circle* covers the head of the fibula. Digital pressure is exerted toward the tibia. The *dotted outline* of the foot indicates the movement (inversion and dorsiflexion at the ankle) that is characteristic of a strong local twitch response on snapping palpation at the trigger point.

12. INTERMITTENT COLD WITH STRETCH
(Fig. 19.5)

The technique for application of vapocoolant spray is discussed in Volume 1, pages 67–64.[97] Details for using ice as the vehicle for intermittent cold appear on page 9 in this volume, and reflex techniques to augment relaxation and stretch are described on pages 10–11. Avoid stretching hypermobile joints in the foot and ankle to their full range. Alternative treatment techniques are presented on pages 9–11 of this volume.

In preparation for the procedure of intermittent cold with stretch, the patient lies supine with the foot of the involved side over the end of the treatment table. A sheet or blanket covers the patient to ensure comfort and to avoid body cooling. The patient notes where passive plantar flexion stops to mark the limit of its range. The initial application of parallel sweeps of ice or vapocoolant spray follows the *thin arrows* in Figure 19.5, downward over the muscle and over the referred pain pattern.[86,87] Gentle, steady pressure is applied to the foot to increase plantar flexion and to take up any slack that develops. To enhance release of tight tibialis anterior fibers, the patient employs postisometric relaxation by first slowly inhaling while gently contracting the tibialis anterior against resistance. The patient then exhales slowly while relaxing, during the application of the intermittent cold with passive elongation of the muscle by the operator. Stretch of this muscle begins by placing the foot in the position of maximum available plantar flexion (Fig. 19.5*A*). Then, addition of passive pronation of the foot further elongates the tibialis anterior (Fig. 19.5*B*). Gentle pressure sustained in this position helps take advantage of the slack that develops during the application of intermittent cold combined with enhancement of relaxation. Several cycles of intermittent cold combined with postisometric relaxation usually suffice to lengthen the muscle fully and to achieve as much range of motion as will occur in this patient with this technique.

The patient compares the new range of motion to that noted before this procedure. The progress helps fix in the patient's mind the critical importance of full range of motion for relief of pain. It also improves compliance with the home stretch program.

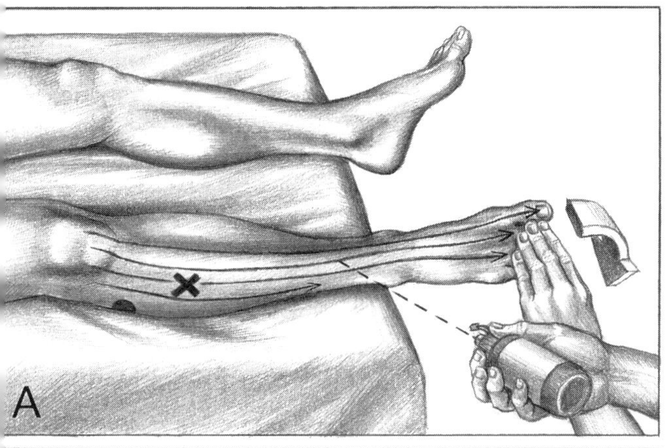

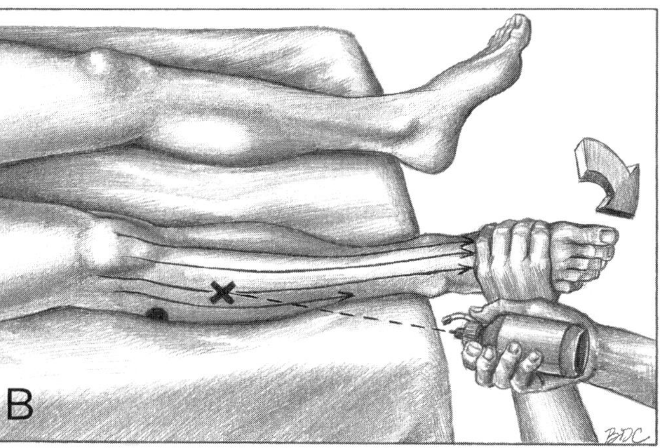

Figure 19.5. Stretch position and intermittent cold pattern (*thin arrows*) for trigger points in the right tibialis anterior muscle. The **X** marks the usual location of trigger points in this muscle. The *solid semicircles* cover the fibular head. The *thick arrow* indicates the direction of pressure that the operator exerts to stretch the muscle. *A*, icing or vapocoolant spray pattern during initial stretch to plantar flex the foot. *B*, while continuing passive plantar flexion, the foot is also pronated (everted and abducted).

Travell[95] reported that applying sweeps of spray just to the reference zone over the ankle relieves the pain only momentarily. Applying the spray over the TrP and the entire muscle can abolish pain, restriction of motion, and deep tenderness in the reference zone for long periods of time.

Following the therapy described previously, a moist, wet-proof heating pad applied promptly for several minutes rewarms the skin. Several cycles of full active range of motion (movement from full plantar flexion to full dorsiflexion) complete the procedure. Following demonstration and written instructions, the patient should then practice the home exercise program described in Section 14, Corrective Exercise.

To stretch this muscle in the supine patient, Evjenth and Hamberg[30] support the bent knee with a pillow and add a pad beneath the leg while applying passive plantar flexion to the foot. Meanwhile, the patient actively contracts the calf muscles to assist plantar flexion and reciprocally inhibit contraction of the tibialis anterior. This supplemental effort by the patient can be very effective for releasing tension in the tibialis anterior muscle.

Using implanted fine-wire electrodes, Etnyre and Abraham[29] showed the error of previous EMG studies that reported spontaneous co-contraction of the tibialis anterior while being stretched during antagonist muscle activation. The surface electrodes previously used detected volume-conducted "cross talk" from the tibialis anterior and not co-contraction activity. This later study removes any theoretical objection to this useful supplemental relaxation technique.

The TrPs in the tibialis anterior muscle are usually sufficiently superficial to respond well to slow, deep, stripping massage.

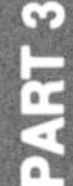

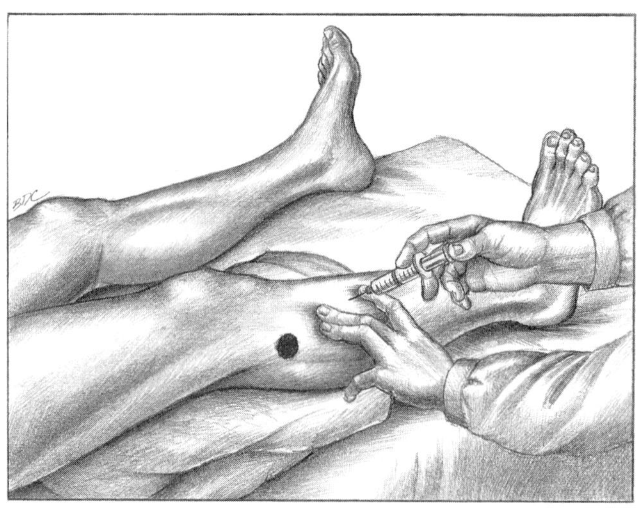

Figure 19.6. Injection of a trigger point in the right tibialis anterior muscle. The *solid circle* marks the head of the fibula. A pad that slightly flexes the knee makes the patient more comfortable.

13. INJECTION AND STRETCH
(Fig. 19.6)

The principles for injecting TrPs are presented in detail on pages 74–86 of Volume 1.[97]

The patient lies supine with the knee of the affected limb resting on a pad to flex it slightly and to make the patient more comfortable. Section 9 of this chapter describes how to locate the taut bands in this muscle. The TrP is that spot along the band which shows the greatest tenderness, the largest local twitch response, and from which the most intense pain is referred in response to the least pressure. Precise injection of the TrP is illustrated in Figure 19.6. Ten milliliters of 0.5% procaine solution are used to fill a syringe to which a 21-gauge, 38-mm (1½-in) needle has been attached.

In many patients, this length of needle can reach to the anterior tibial artery and vein and deep peroneal nerve if the needle is pointed straight down through the full depth of the muscle close to the tibia.[71] For this reason, the clinician should direct the needle toward the tibia at a 45° angle to the skin to avoid the possibility of hitting neurovascular structures. During injection, cutaneous and deep hemostasis should be supplied by spreading finger pressure against the skin astride the needle. A jump response of the patient and a local twitch response of the muscle usually accompany penetration of one of these TrPs by the needle. Inactivation of the entire cluster of TrPs in that region should be ensured by probing exploration with the needle and injection of TrPs until all local tenderness disappears. However, after injection, several sweeps of cold applied during passive stretch of the muscle help inactivate any remaining TrPs.

Prompt application of moist heat for several minutes reduces postinjection soreness and enhances the effect of several cycles of active range of motion to help restore muscle "memory" and normal function.

Before leaving the office, the patient practices the home exercise program as presented in the next section.

14. CORRECTIVE ACTIONS

A major source of overload of the tibialis anterior muscle can be tension of the calf musculature. In that situation, an essential first step of tibialis anterior therapy is to release the calf muscle tightness and inactivate any responsible TrPs.

If the anterior compartment muscles are weak, a strengthening program for the dorsiflexors of the foot is in order to restore muscular balance at the ankle.

Corrective Body Mechanics

The postural distortion caused by a Morton foot structure should be corrected, as described in Chapter 20, to normalize foot mechanics and muscle balance at the ankle.

Corrective Posture and Activities

Some automobile accelerator pedals are steeply angled and cause sustained shortening of the tibialis anterior. A block under the driver's heel reduces the excessive dorsiflexion. Use of a cruise control provides the opportunity for the driver to change foot position and obtain periodic relief from immobility.

The individual is encouraged to walk on smooth surfaces instead of uneven ground, e.g., to walk on a smooth pathway instead of a sidewalk with uneven bricks or cracks. In addition, a surface should be selected that is level from side to side and not tilted laterally, as is the edge of a crowned road or a slanted beach.

In general, the leg muscles feel better if the ankle is maintained in a neutral position throughout the night. This position is facilitated by use of a foot-bracing pillow as described and illustrated in Figure 21.11 of Chapter 21.

Home Therapeutic Program

The patient should stretch the tibialis anterior at home one to three times daily. Good control may be exerted in the sitting position by crossing the involved foot over the other thigh and using the hands to plantar flex and evert the foot passively. An alternative stretch is with the patient sitting forward on a chair so that the foot of the leg to be stretched reaches back under the chair with the *dorsal* surface of the toes and metatarsal heads solidly on the floor, placing the foot in plantar flexion. The patient presses the dorsum of the foot against the floor to further plantar flex and slightly evert the ankle. He or she learns to adjust the degree of foot eversion to optimize the feeling of tension on the tight tibialis anterior muscle.

Incorporating the principles of postisometric relaxation (*see* Chapter 2, pages 10–11) while performing the stretch markedly improves its effectiveness. Addition of calf contraction to enhance plantar flexion during the stretch phase (reciprocal inhibition) can also be helpful.

When a person is seated for a prolonged period of time, the Pedal Exercise (*see* Fig. 22.13) stretches the tibialis anterior as well as the soleus muscle and usually provides welcome relief.

References

1. Anderson JE: *Grant's Atlas of Anatomy*, Ed. 8. Williams & Wilkins, Baltimore, 1983 (Figs. 4–70B, 4–103, 4–107).
2. *Ibid.* (Fig. 4–71C).
3. *Ibid.* (Fig. 4–72).
4. *Ibid.* (Fig. 4–73).
5. *Ibid.* (Figs. 4–98, 4–117).
6. Aquilonius S-M, Askmark H, Gillberg P-G, *et al.*: Topographical localization of motor endplates in cryosections of whole human muscles. *Muscle Nerve 7*:287–293, 1984.
7. Arcangeli P, Digiesi V, Ronchi O, Dorigo B, Bartoli V: Mechanisms of ischemic pain in peripheral occlusive arterial disease. In *Advances in Pain Research and Therapy*, edited by J. J. Bonica and D. Albe-Fessard, Vol. 1. Raven Press, New York, 1976 (pp. 965–973).
8. Baker BA: The muscle trigger: evidence of overload injury. *J Neurol Orthop Med Surg 7*:35–44, 1986.
9. Bardeen CR: The musculature, Sect. 5. In *Morris's Human Anatomy*, edited by C. M. Jackson, Ed. 6. Blakiston's Son & Co., Philadelphia, 1921 (pp. 512, 515–516).
10. Basmajian JV, Deluca CJ: *Muscles Alive*, Ed. 5. Williams & Wilkins, Baltimore, 1985 (pp. 256–257).
11. *Ibid.* (pp. 374–377).
12. Basmajian JV, Slonecker CE: *Grant's Method of Anatomy. A Clinical Problem-Solving Approach*, Ed. 11. Williams & Wilkins, Baltimore, 1989 (p. 332).
13. Basmajian JV, Stecko G: The role of muscles in arch support of the foot. An electromyographic study. *J Bone Joint Surg [Am] 45*:1184–1190, 1963.
14. Bates T, Grunwaldt E: Myofascial pain in childhood. *J Pediatr 53*:198–209, 1958.
15. Brody DM: Running injuries. *Clinical Symposia 32*:1–36, 1980 (*see* pp. 19, 20).
16. Broer MR, Houtz SJ: *Patterns of Muscular Activity in Selected Sports Skills*. Charles C Thomas, Springfield, 1967.
17. Carter BL, Morehead J, Wolpert SM, *et al.*: Cross-Sectional Anatomy. Appleton-Century-Crofts, New York, 1977 (Sects. 72–84).
18. Christensen E: Topography of terminal motor innervation in striated muscles from stillborn infants. *Am J Phys Med 38*:65–78, 1959.
19. Ciacci G, Federico A, Giannini F, *et al.*: Exercise-induced bilateral anterior tibial compartment syndrome without pain. *Ital J Neurol Sci 7*:377–380, 1986.
20. Clemente CD: *Gray's Anatomy of the Human Body*, American Ed. 30. Lea & Febiger, Philadelphia, 1985 (p. 111).
21. *Ibid.* (p. 112).
22. *Ibid.* (pp. 573–574).
23. Cordo PJ, Nashner LM: Properties of postural adjustments associated with rapid arm movements. *J Neurophysiol 47*:287–302, 1982.
24. Dickstein R, Pillar T, Hocherman S: The contribution of vision and of sidedness to responses

of the ankle musculature to continuous movement of the base of support. *Int J Neurosci 40*: 101–108, 1988.
25. Dietz V, Horstmann GA, Berger W: Interlimb coordination of leg-muscle activation during perturbation of stance in humans. *J Neurophysiol 62*:680–693, 1989.
26. Duchenne GB: *Physiology of Motion*, translated by E.B. Kaplan. J. B. Lippincott, Philadelphia, 1949 (pp. 337–339).
27. *Ibid.* (pp. 341–344).
28. Ericson MO, Nisell R, Arborelius UP, *et al.*: Muscular activity during ergometer cycling. *Scand J Rehabil Med 17*:53–61, 1985.
29. Etnyre BR, Abraham LD: Antagonist muscle activity during stretching: a paradox re-assessed. *Med Sci Sports Exer 20*:285–289, 1988.
30. Evjenth O, Hamberg J: *Muscle Stretching in Manual Therapy, A Clinical Manual.* Alfta Rehab Førlag, Alfta, Sweden, 1984 (p. 135).
31. Ferner H, Staubesand J: *Sobotta Atlas of Human Anatomy*, Ed. 10, Vol. 2. Urban & Schwarzenberg, Baltimore, 1983 (Fig. 380).
32. *Ibid.* (Fig. 458).
33. *Ibid.* (Fig. 464).
34. *Ibid.* (Figs. 465, 467).
35. *Ibid.* (Fig. 466).
36. *Ibid.* (Figs. 468, 500).
37. *Ibid.* (Figs. 472–474).
38. Fridén J, Sfakianos PN, Hargens AR, *et al.*: Residual muscular swelling after repetitive eccentric contractions. *J Orthop Res 6*:493–498, 1988.
39. Gantchev GN, Draganova N: Muscular synergies during different conditions of postural activity. *Acta Physiol Pharmacol Bulg 12*:58–65, 1986.
40. Gray EG, Basmajian JV: Electromyography and cinematography of leg and foot ("normal" and flat) during walking. *Anat Rec 161*:1–16, 1968.
41. Gray ER: The role of leg muscles in variations of the arches in normal and flat feet. *Phys Ther 49*:1084–1088, 1969.
42. Gutstein M: Common rheumatism and physiotherapy. *Br J Phys Med 3*:46–50, 1940 (*see* p. 50, Case 3).
43. Harrington AC, Mellette JR, Jr: Hernias of the anterior tibialis muscle: case report and review of the literature. *J Am Acad Dermatol 22*:123–124, 1990.
44. Helliwell TR, Coakley J, Smith PEM, *et al.*: The morphology and morphometry of the normal human tibialis anterior muscle. *Neuropathol Appl Neurobiol 13*:297–307, 1987.
45. Henriksson-Larsén K: Distribution, number and size of different types of fibres in whole cross-sections of female m tibialis anterior. An enzyme histochemical study. *Acta Physiol Scand 123*:229–235, 1985.
46. Henriksson-Larsén K, Fridén J, Wretling ML: Distribution of fibre sizes in human skeletal muscle. An enzyme histochemical study in m tibialis anterior. *Acta Physiol Scand 123*:171–177, 1985.
47. Henriksson-Larsén KB, Lexell J, Sjöström M: Distribution of different fibre types in human skeletal muscles. I. Method for the preparation and analysis of cross-sections of whole tibialis anterior. *Histochem J 15*:167–178, 1983.
48. Henstorf JE, Olson S: Compartment syndrome: pathophysiology, diagnosis, and treatment. *Surg Rounds Orthop*:pp. 33–41, Feb. 1987.
49. Jacobsen S: Myofascielt smertesyndrom (Myofascial pain syndrome). *Ugeskr Laeger 149*:600–601, 1987.
50. Jakobsson F, Borg K, Edstrom L, *et al.*: Use of motor units in relation to muscle fiber type and size in man. *Muscle Nerve 11*:1211–1218, 1988.
51. Kamon E: Electromyographic kinesiology of jumping. *Arch Phys Med Rehabil 52*:152–157, 1971.
52. Kellgren JH: Observations on referred pain arising from muscle. *Clin Sci 3*:175–190, 1938 (*see* pp. 177–178, Fig. 2).
53. Kendall FP, McCreary EK: *Muscles, Testing and Function*, Ed. 3. Williams & Wilkins, Baltimore, 1983 (p. 141).
54. Lange M. *Die Muskelhärten (Myogelosen).* J.F. Lehmanns Verlag, München, 1931.
55. Lee KH, Matteliano A, Medige J, *et al.*: Electromyographic changes of leg muscles with heel lift: therapeutic implications. *Arch Phys Med Rehabil 68*:298–301, 1987.
56. Lee KH, Shieh JC, Matteliano A, *et al.*: Electromyographic changes of leg muscles with heel lifts in women: therapeutic implications. *Arch Phys Med Rehabil 71*:31–33, 1990.
57. Lockhart RD: *Living Anatomy*, Ed. 7. Faber & Faber, London, 1974 (p. 66, Fig. 136).
58. Luchansky E, Paz Z: Variations in the insertion of tibialis anterior muscle. *Anat Anz 162*:129–136, 1986.
59. Mann RA, Moran GT, Dougherty SE: Comparative electromyography of the lower extremity in jogging, running, and sprinting. *Am J Sports Med 14*:501–510, 1986.
60. Matsen FA: Monitoring of intravascular pressure. *Surgery 79*:702, 1976.
61. Matsen FA: Increased tissue pressure and its effect on muscle oxygenation in level and elevated human limbs. *Clin Orthop 144*:311–320, 1979.
62. McMinn RMH, Hutchings RT: *Color Atlas of Human Anatomy*. Year Book Medical Publishers, Chicago, 1977 (pp. 281, 282, 289).
63. *Ibid.* (p. 312).
64. Milner M, Basmajian JV, Quanbury AO: Multifactorial analysis of walking by electromyography and computer. *Am J Phys Med 50*:235–258, 1971.
65. Mirkin G: Keeping pace with new problems when your patients exercise. *Mod Med NZ*:pp. 6–14, Dec. 1980.
66. Moore MP: Shin splints. Diagnosis, management, prevention. *Postgrad Med 83*:199–210, 1988.
67. Moretz WH: The anterior compartment (anterior tibial) ischemia syndrome. *Am Surg 19*: 728–749, 1953.
68. Mubarak SJ, Hargens AR, Owen CA, *et al.*: The wick catheter technique for measurement of intramuscular pressure. *J Bone Joint Surg [Am] 58*: 1016–1020, 1976.
69. Mubarak SJ, Owen CA, Hargens AR, *et al.*: Acute compartment syndromes: diagnosis and

treatment with the aid of the wick catheter. *J Bone Joint Surg [Am] 60*:1091–1095, 1978.

70. Murray MP, Mollinger LA, Gardner GM, *et al.*: Kinematic and EMG patterns during slow, free, and fast walking. *J Orthop Res 2*:272–280, 1984.
71. Netter FH: *The Ciba Collection of Medical Illustrations*, Vol. 8, Musculoskeletal System. Part I: Anatomy, Physiology and Metabolic Disorders. Ciba-Geigy Corporation, Summit, 1987 (p. 98).
72. *Ibid.* (p. 99).
73. *Ibid.* (pp. 100, 104).
74. *Ibid.* (p. 107).
75. Oddsson L: Motor patterns of a fast voluntary postural task in man: trunk extension in standing. *Acta Physiol Scand 136*:47–58, 1989.
76. Okada M: An electromyographic estimation of the relative muscular load in different human postures. *J Human Ergol 1*:75–93, 1972.
77. Okada M, Fujiwara K: Muscle activity around the ankle joint as correlated with the center of foot pressure in an upright stance. In *Biomechanics 8A*, M. Matsui, K. Kobayashi (eds). Human Kinetics Publ., Champaign, 1983 (pp. 209–216).
78. Owen CA, Mubarak SJ, Hargens AR, *et al.*: Intramuscular pressures with limb compression. Clarification of the pathogenesis of the drug-induced muscle-compartment syndrome. *N Engl J Med 300*:1169–1172, 1979.
79. Perry J: The mechanics of walking. *Phys Ther 47*:778–801, 1967.
80. Rasch PJ, Burke RK: *Kinesiology and Applied Anatomy*, Ed. 6. Lea & Febiger, Philadelphia, 1978 (pp. 317–318, 330, Table 17–2).
81. Reynolds MD: Myofascial trigger point syndromes in the practice of rheumatology. *Arch Phys Med Rehabil 62*:111–114, 1981.
82. Rohen JW, Yokochi C: *Color Atlas of Anatomy*, Ed. 2. Igaku-Shoin, New York, 1988 (p. 423).
83. *Ibid.* (p. 426).
84. Sandstedt P, Nordell LE, Henriksson KG: Quantitative analysis of muscle biopsies from volunteers and patients with neuromuscular disorders. A comparison between estimation and measuring. *Acta Neurol Scand 66*:130–144, 1982.
85. Sandstedt PER: Representativeness of a muscle biopsy specimen for the whole muscle. *Acta Neurol Scand 64*:427–437, 1981.
86. Simons DG: Myofascial pain syndrome due to trigger points, Chapter 45. In *Rehabilitation Medicine*, edited by Joseph Goodgold. C. V. Mosby Co., St. Louis, 1988 (*see* pp. 710–711, Fig. 45–9C).
87. Simons DG, Travell JG: Myofascial pain syndromes, Chapter 25. In *Textbook of Pain*, edited by P.D. Wall and R. Melzack, Ed 2. Churchill Livingstone, London, 1989 (*see* p. 378, Fig. 25.9C).
88. Sola AE: Treatment of myofascial pain syndromes. In *Recent Advances in the Management of Pain*, edited by C. Benedetti, C. R. Chapman, G. Moricca. Raven Press, New York, 1984, Series title: *Advances in Pain Research and Therapy*, Vol. 7 (pp. 467–485, *see* p. 481).
89. Sola AE: Trigger point therapy, Chapter 47. In *Clinical Procedures in Emergency Medicine*, edited by J.R. Roberts and J.R. Hedges. W.B. Saunders, Philadelphia, 1985 (pp. 674–686, *see* p. 683, Fig. 47–14).
90. Sola AE, Williams RL: Myofascial pain syndromes. *Neurology 6*:91–95, 1956.
91. Stam J: The tibialis anterior reflex in healthy subjects and in L5 radicular compression. *J Neurol Neurosurg Psychiatry 51*:397–402, 1988.
92. Toft E, Sinkjaer R, Andreassen S: Mechanical and electromyographic responses to stretch of the human anterior tibial muscle at different levels of contraction. *Exp Brain Res 74*:213–219, 1989.
93. Townsend MA, Lainhart SP, Shiavi R: Variability and biomechanics of synergy patterns of some lower-limb muscles during ascending and descending stairs and level walking. *Med Biol Eng Comput 16*:681–688, 1978.
94. Townsend MA, Shiavi R, Lainhart SP, *et al.*: Variability in synergy patterns of leg muscles during climbing, descending and level walking of highly-trained athletes and normal males. *Electromyogr Clin Neurophysiol 18*:69–80, 1978.
95. Travell J: Ethyl chloride spray for painful muscle spasm. *Arch Phys Med Rehabil 33*:291–298, 1952.
96. Travell J, Rinzler SH: The myofascial genesis of pain. *Postgrad Med 11*:425–434, 1952.
97. Travell JG, Simons DG: *Myofascial Pain and Dysfunction: The Trigger Point Manual.* Williams & Wilkins, Baltimore, 1983.
98. Weber EF: Ueber die Längenverhältnisse der Fleischfasern der Muskeln in Allgemeinen. *Berichte über die Verhandlungen der Königlich Sächsischen Gesellschaft der Wissenschaften zu Leipzig 3*:63–86,1851.
99. Whitesides TE: Tissue pressure measurements as a determinant for the need of fasciotomy. *Clin Orthop 113*:43, 1975.
100. Wiley JP, Clement DB, Doyle DL, *et al.*: A primary care perspective of chronic compartment syndrome of the leg. *Phys Sportsmed 15*:111–120, 1987.
101. Yang JF, Winter DA: Surface EMG profiles during different walking cadences in humans. *Electroencephalogr Clin Neurophysiol 60*:485–491, 1985.
102. Zeiss J, Ebraheim NA, Woldenberg LS: Magnetic resonance imaging in the diagnosis of anterior tibialis muscle herniation. *Clin Orthop 244*:249–253, 1989.

CHAPTER 20
Peroneal Muscles
Peroneus Longus, Peroneus Brevis, Peroneus Tertius

"Weak Ankle" Muscles

HIGHLIGHTS: **REFERRED PAIN** and tenderness arising from myofascial trigger points (TrPs) in the peroneus longus and peroneus brevis muscles concentrate primarily over the lateral malleolus, above, behind, and below it, and also extend a short distance along the lateral aspect of the foot. An occasional spillover pattern may cover the lateral aspect of the middle third of the leg. Peroneus tertius TrPs refer pain and tenderness primarily over the anterolateral aspect of the ankle (anterior to the lateral malleolus) with spillover to the outer side of the heel. Proximal **ANATOMICAL ATTACHMENTS** for all three peroneal muscles are to the fibula and adjacent intermuscular septa. However, the longus and brevis form the lateral compartment while the tertius is part of the anterior compartment of the leg. Distally, the tendon of the peroneus longus passes behind the lateral malleolus, runs obliquely across the sole of the foot from lateral to medial, and ends on the first metatarsal and medial cuneiform bones. The tendon of the peroneus brevis also curves behind the lateral malleolus but ends on the tuberosity of the fifth metatarsal. The tendon of the peroneus tertius passes in front of the lateral malleolus and ends on the proximal portion of the fifth metatarsal. **INNERVATION** of the peroneus longus and peroneus brevis muscles is by the superficial peroneal nerve from spinal nerves L_4, L_5, and S_1. The peroneus tertius receives its innervation through the deep peroneal nerve from spinal nerves L_5 and S_1. The basic **FUNCTION** of the peroneus longus and peroneus brevis muscles is to prevent medial inclination of the leg over the fixed foot during the midstance phase of gait (controlling excessive relative inversion and controlling mediolateral balance in walking). The peroneus longus and peroneus brevis plantar flex and pronate (evert and abduct) the foot. The peroneus tertius also assists eversion, but dorsiflexes rather than plantar flexes the foot. **SYMPTOMS** characteristic of this myofascial pain syndrome are pain in the ankle and ankle weakness. The referred pain patterns of the peroneal muscles are different from, but might be confused with, those of the extensor muscles of the foot and toes. Lateral compartment syndromes and entrapments of the common, superficial, and deep peroneal nerves cause pain in a distribution similar to that caused by peroneal TrPs. The tendon of each peroneal muscle can rupture spontaneously. **ACTIVATION AND PERPETUATION OF TRIGGER POINTS** can result from prolonged immobilization of the leg and foot by a cast. These TrPs are also perpetuated by the Morton foot structure, crossing the legs when seated, wearing high heels, wearing tight elastic around the calf, and by flat feet. **PATIENT EXAMINATION** reveals some weakness of the involved muscle(s), and the stretch range of motion is restricted by pain. Examination of the feet for the Morton foot structure shows (when this structure is present) a relatively short first metatarsal and long second metatarsal bone. Calluses are likely to develop: under the heads of the second and, sometimes, the third metatarsal bones; on the medial side of the distal phalanx of the great toe; medially beside the head of the first metatarsal; and sometimes along the lateral border of the sole anteriorly. Thorough inspection of the shoes worn regularly includes examination of six major features. **TRIGGER POINT EXAMINATION** of the peroneus longus muscle reveals taut bands palpable against the shaft of the fibula with TrP tenderness located about 2–4 cm below the head of the fibula. The local twitch responses (LTRs) that are readily elicited in the taut bands of these TrPs cause visible eversion of the foot. **ENTRAPMENT** of the common peroneal nerve by a peroneus longus muscle that is tense because of active TrPs occurs as the nerve is compressed against the fibula by the taut muscle fibers or their tendon. Inactivation of the TrPs in this muscle relieves the related symptoms of peroneal neurapraxia. **INTERMITTENT COLD WITH STRETCH** requires application of ice or vapocoolant spray downward over the anterolateral aspect of the leg, ankle, and foot. The regions of the lateral malleolus and lateral heel must be included. During intermittent cooling, to lengthen the peroneus longus and brevis, the foot is fully inverted and adducted and then dorsiflexed (ankle and first metatarsal). To stretch the peroneus tertius, the foot is inverted and plantar flexed. A moist heating pad rewarms the skin and then the patient executes full active range of motion. Postisometric relaxation, ischemic compression, and stripping massage are also useful techniques to inactivate TrPs in these muscles. **INJECTION AND STRETCH** of the peroneus longus muscle requires consideration of the nearby peroneal nerves. The needle is aimed nearly straight toward the fibula to impale and inject the clearly identified TrP with 0.5% procaine solution. The approach to the peroneus brevis or peroneus tertius is through the posterolateral aspect of the leg. The needle passes deep to the tendon of the peroneus longus. Passive lengthening of the injected muscle, moist heat, and then full active range of motion again complete the procedure. The most important **CORRECTIVE ACTION** for the patient with a peroneus longus or brevis myofascial pain syndrome and the Morton foot structure is one of two shoe corrections. Either a first metatarsal felt pad is added to a modified sole insert that fits inside the shoe, or a "Flying Dutchman" type of correction modifies the outside of the shoe. A high heel or a spike heel of any height can perpetuate peroneal TrPs and should be avoided. All patients with peroneal TrP problems should perform the Peroneal Self-stretch Exercise regularly at home to prevent recurrence of peroneus longus and peroneus brevis TrP pain, tenderness, and weakness.

---

1. REFERRED PAIN
(Fig. 20.1)

Peroneus longus and **peroneus brevis** trigger points (TrPs) project pain and tenderness primarily to the region over the lateral malleolus of the ankle, above, behind, and below it; they also extend a short distance along the lateral aspect of the foot (Fig. 20.1*A*).[93,94,101] A spillover pattern of the peroneus longus TrPs may cover the lateral aspect of the middle third of the leg.[93,94]

Jacobsen[47] reported a pain pattern referred from peroneus longus and peroneus brevis TrPs as going around the back of the lateral malleolus. Bates and Grunwaldt[18] reported that, in children, the referred pain pattern of the peroneus longus muscle also concentrates behind the lateral malleolus, but tends to extend up the side of the leg rather than along the side of the foot. Good[43] attributed the symptoms in 15 of 100 patients with painful feet to myalgic spots in the peroneus brevis muscle. Kellgren[51] reported that the injection of 6% hypertonic saline solution into the peroneus longus muscle evoked pain referred to the ankle.

Peroneus tertius TrPs refer pain and tenderness along the anterolateral aspect of the ankle with a spillover pattern projecting downward behind the lateral malleolus to the lateral aspect of the heel (Fig. 20.1*B*).

2. ANATOMICAL ATTACHMENTS AND CONSIDERATIONS
(Figs. 20.2 and 20.3)

The peroneus longus and peroneus brevis muscles, accompanied by the superficial peroneal nerve (*see* Fig. 20.9), fill the lateral compartment of the leg. The peroneus tertius muscle lies in the anterior compartment with the tibialis anterior muscle and the deep peroneal nerve.[77] The cross section of the middle third of the leg, Figure 19.3 in the previous chapter, shows these relationships.

The **peroneus longus** muscle covers most of the peroneus brevis (Fig. 20.2*A*). ***Proximally***, the longus attaches to the head of the fibula and to the upper two-thirds of the fibula's lateral surface. The common peroneal nerve enters the ante-

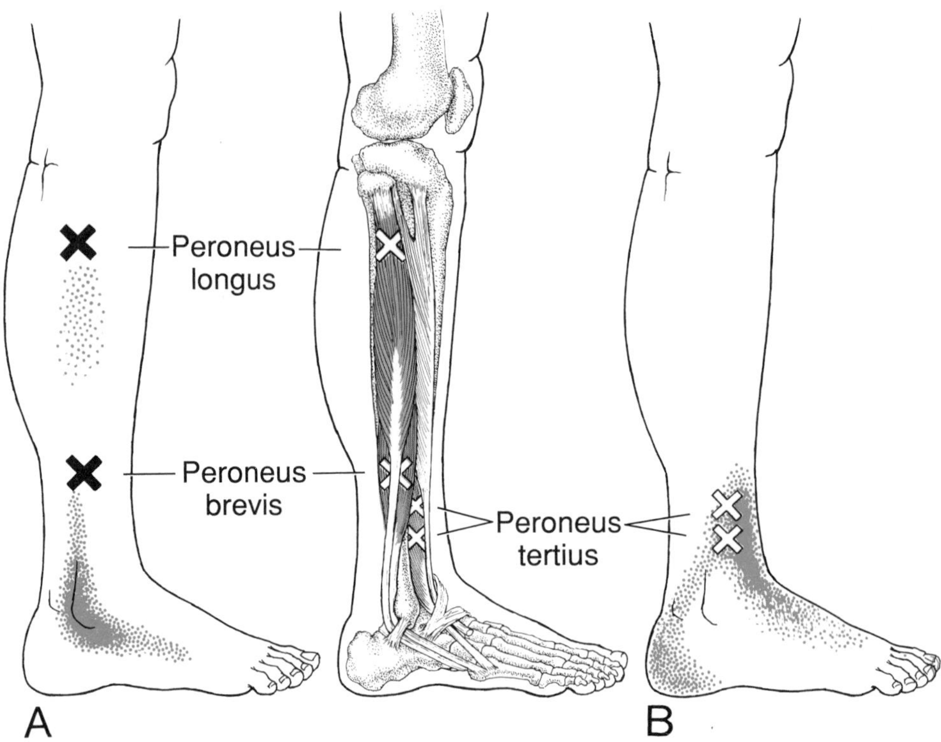

Figure 20.1. Pain patterns (*dark red*) referred from trigger points (***X**s*) at commonly observed locations in the peroneal muscles. The essential patterns of referred pain and tenderness are *solid red*, and the *red stippling* shows the less common spillover extension of pain. These trigger points all refer pain distally. *A*, composite pain pattern for the peroneus longus and peroneus brevis muscles (*medium red*). The spillover pattern between the illustrated trigger points applies only to the peroneus longus trigger point. *B*, pain pattern of the peroneus tertius muscle (*light red*).

rior leg through a gap between these two upper attachments of the peroneus longus muscle. In addition, the muscle anchors to adjacent intermuscular septa. ***Distally***, it becomes tendinous in the middle third of the leg. The tendon curves behind the lateral malleolus and passes, together with the tendon of the peroneus brevis muscle, deep to the superior peroneal retinaculum. On the lateral side of the calcaneus, these tendons occupy separate osseoaponeurotic canals. The tendon of the peroneus longus then again curves sharply, this time over the cuboid bone, and crosses the sole of the foot obliquely to attach to the ventral and lateral aspects of both the base of the first metatarsal and the medial cuneiform (Fig. 20.2*B*). This long tendon of the peroneus longus attaches opposite to the tendon of the tibialis anterior on the medial aspect of the base of the first metatarsal bone.[82]

On the underside of the cuboid bone, the tendon of the peroneus longus is thickened to form a sesamoid fibrocartilage.[26] When this fibrocartilage ossifies, it becomes the os peroneum.[62] This sesamoid bone appears in approximately 20% of mature individuals and its shape is irregular. Phylogenetically, it may be in the process of disappearing from the human race due to loss of its functional importance for hallux opposability.[62]

The **peroneus brevis** muscle is shorter and smaller than the peroneus longus and lies deep to it. Distally, the belly of the peroneus brevis extends beyond that of the peroneus longus (Figs. 20.2*A* and 20.3). ***Proximally***, the peroneus brevis attaches to the distal two-thirds of the lateral surface of the fibula deep to the peroneus longus where there is overlap, and to adjacent intermuscular septa (Fig. 20.3). The tendon of this muscle travels with that of the peroneus longus within a

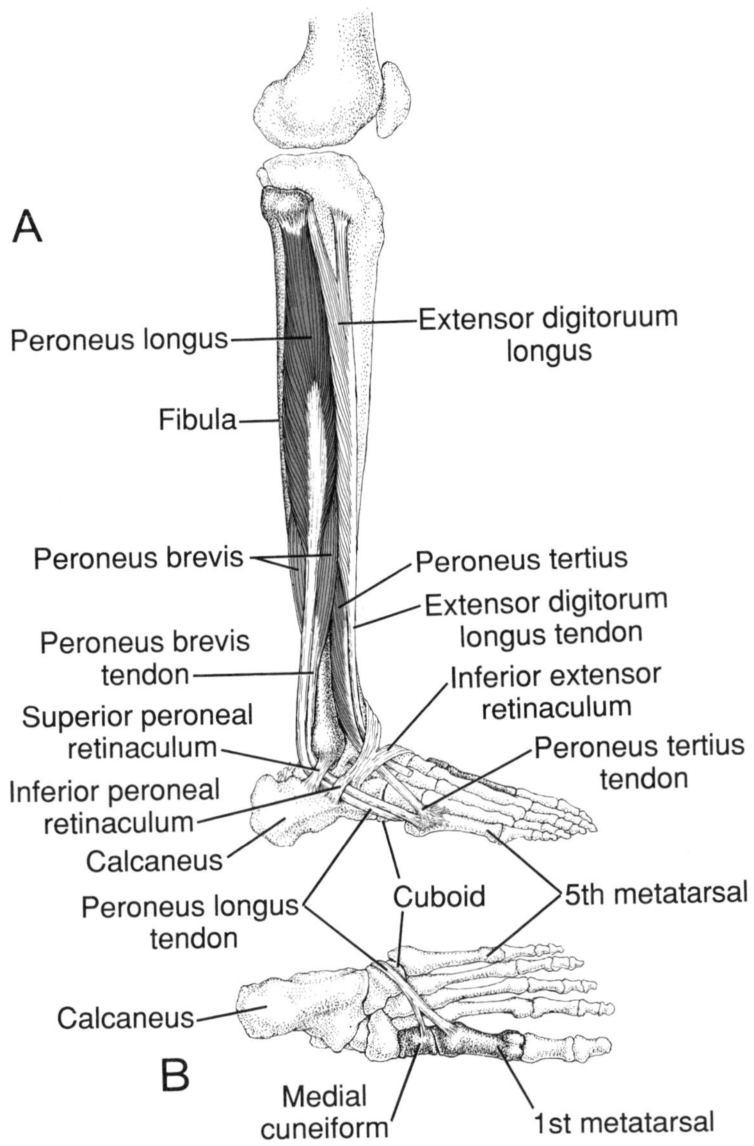

Figure 20.2. Anatomical relations and attachments of the right peroneus longus muscle (*dark red*). Deeper peroneal muscles are *light red*. *A*, lateral view. *B*, plantar view of the right foot. The bones to which the peroneus longus muscle attaches are darkened.

common synovial sheath as they curve behind the lateral malleolus under the superior peroneal retinaculum (Figs. 20.2 and 20.3). Farther distally, these tendons have separate synovial sheaths. The peroneus brevis tendon anchors ***distally*** to the tuberosity on the lateral aspect of the fifth metatarsal (Fig. 20.2*A*).[26]

The peroneus tertius muscle (Fig. 20.3) differs anatomically and functionally from the other two peroneal muscles. Although the peroneus tertius is located close to and parallel to the extensor digitorum longus muscle, the tertius is usually anatomically distinct from the extensor digitorum longus, contrary to conventional opinion.[57] ***Proximally***, it anchors to the distal one-half to two-thirds of the anterior margin of the fibula and to the adjacent anterior crural intermuscular septum. The two lateral peroneal muscles attach to the other side of this septum. The peroneus tertius is usually as large as or larger than the extensor digitorum longus.

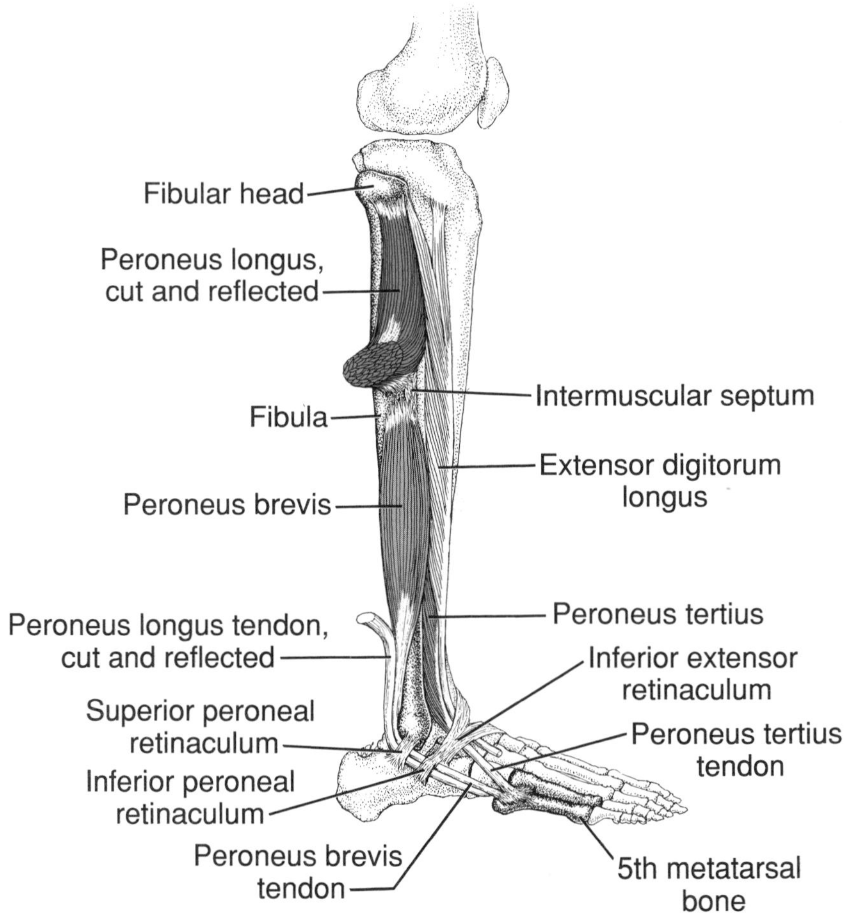

Figure 20.3. Attachments of the deeper peroneal muscles (*light red*), right side, lateral view. The more superficial peroneus longus (*dark red*) is cut and reflected. The peroneus tertius is partly covered by the peroneus brevis. The bones to which the peroneus brevis and tertius attach are darkened.

Distally, the peroneus tertius normally has a tripartite anchor: to the tubercle of the fifth metatarsal, along the mediodorsal surface of this metatarsal, and to the base of the fourth metatarsal. These tendinous projections spiral and tighten during passive inversion of the foot or straighten and relax during passive eversion.[57]

Anatomists report many variants of the three peroneal muscles. The peroneus tertius was absent in 7.1–8.2% of specimens.[57] A bifid peroneus brevis was reported as the cause of symptoms that required surgical correction.[44] A commonly noted but rare (2%)[57] muscle, the **peroneus digiti minimi**, arises from the distal quarter of the fibula and attaches to the extensor aponeurosis of the fifth toe.[15,26] A **peroneus quartus** muscle was present in about 13% of specimens. It attaches proximally onto the back of the fibula between the peroneus brevis and the flexor hallucis longus, and distally to either the calcaneus or the cuboid.[26]

Supplemental References

The *front view* of the peroneus longus and peroneus brevis shows their relations to the superficial peroneal nerve[78] and also to the deep peroneal nerve.[35,79] A front view also reveals the relation of the peroneus tertius muscle to the anterior tibial artery and deep peroneal nerve.[8] Another front view identifies the tendon of the peroneus tertius in relation to other tendons at the ankle.[90] A *rear view* that also includes the peroneal artery and tibial nerve shows the thin slice of peroneus longus and peroneus brevis visible from behind.[36,81] *Lateral views* without vessels or nerves identify all three peroneal muscles,[37] portray the peroneus longus and peroneus brevis photographically,[71] and show in detail the relations of the three peroneal tendons to other tendons at the ankle.[74] A lat-

PART 3

eral view also presents in detail the passage of the common peroneal nerve between the peroneus longus muscle and the fibular head.[70] Another lateral view[78] and an *anterolateral view*[4] show the relations between all three peroneal muscles and the superficial peroneal nerve. The *dorsal view* of the foot displays in detail the tendinous attachment of the peroneus tertius.[40,57]

Cross sections show the relation of the peroneus longus to surrounding structures in 14 serial sections,[22] of the peroneus brevis in 11 serial sections,[23] and of the peroneus tertius in five serial sections.[24] The relations of all three peroneal muscles appear in cross section at the lower part of the middle one-third of the leg[7] and above the middle of the leg.[77] Three cross sections, one through the proximal third of the leg, one through the middle third of the leg, and one above the malleoli, delineate the relations of the peroneus longus and peroneus brevis muscles to neighboring structures.[39]

Photographs of well-muscled subjects disclose the *surface contours* produced by the peroneus longus,[34] by both the peroneus longus and peroneus brevis muscles,[6,64] and by the tendons at the ankle.[72]

A schematic drawing demonstrates clearly all *bony attachments* of the peroneus longus and peroneus brevis muscles.[5] Markings on the bones indicate the attachment sites of the peroneus longus tendon to the plantar surface of the foot,[12,41] of the brevis and tertius tendons to the dorsum of the foot,[11,41] of the brevis tendon as seen from behind,[10] of the longus and brevis tendons to bones in the leg,[38] of all three peroneal muscles to bones in the leg,[3,69,82] and of all three tendons to the foot.[41]

Various views show the *synovial sheaths* surrounding the tendons of the three peroneal muscles in the ankle region.[9,42,73,83]

3. INNERVATION

Branches of the superficial peroneal nerve supply the peroneus longus and peroneus brevis muscles. This nerve contains fibers from the L_4, L_5, and S_1 spinal nerves. The deep peroneal nerve supplies the peroneus tertius in the anterior compartment with fibers from only the L_5 and S_1 spinal nerves.

4. FUNCTION

The peroneal muscles, like most other lower limb muscles, frequently function to control movement rather than to produce it; this is particularly evident when the foot is fixed during standing and walking. At this time, these muscles often function through lengthening contractions.

The peroneus longus and peroneus brevis assist the tibialis posterior and soleus in controlling (decelerating) the forward movement of the tibia over the fixed foot during the stance phase of walking.[97]

Matsusaka[67] suggests that the peroneal muscles (as well as the tibialis posterior and flexor digitorum longus) contribute to control of mediolateral balance in walking, together with the motion within the foot.

The peroneus longus, brevis, and tertius all act to evert the non-weight-bearing foot. A major difference in these muscles is that the peroneus tertius dorsiflexes the foot because its tendon crosses in front of the ankle joint, whereas the peroneus longus and peroneus brevis muscles plantar flex the foot since their tendons pass behind the ankle joint.

Actions

The peroneus longus and peroneus brevis cause the foot, when free, to abduct (toe out)[26,31] and to evert (elevate its lateral side);[26,31,97] together these two movements produce pronation.[26,31] Both muscles assist plantar flexion of the foot.[26,31,97] Static loading of the foot without arch support up to 180 kg (400 lb) did not evoke activity in the peroneus longus muscle unless the foot was inverted. Then, the activity was minimal.[17]

The peroneus tertius dorsiflexes the foot and assists eversion.[26,32,97] Duchenne observed that when there was absence or weak development of the peroneus tertius, the extensor digitorum longus substituted for the peroneus tertius in dorsiflexion, abduction, and eversion.[32]

Because they attach to opposite sides of the same bone (first metatarsal), the tibialis anterior and peroneus longus muscles form an effective sling for control of inversion and eversion of the foot.[80,82]

The peroneus longus can produce about one-tenth of the moment for plantar flexion as the gastrocnemius muscle (128 vs. 1123 kg/cm). The peroneus brevis exerts only about half of the moment that the peroneus longus exerts for plantar flexion of the foot.[97]

Functions

Standing

The peroneus longus plays a minor role during balanced standing at ease. Among 16 men and 16 women standing barefooted,[16] only one man and two women showed some degree of continuous electrical activity in this muscle. Another man and five women showed intermittent activity. When standing in high heels, all of the women exhibited some activity, and half of them generated continuous marked activity in the peroneus longus. Contrary to past speculation, the peroneus longus plays no important role in the *static* support of the long arches of the normal foot.[17] However, this muscle may provide important support for them during locomotion.[16]

Tropp and Odenrick[106] recently studied postural control in single-limb stance using surface electromyography and force plate recordings of 30 physically active men. They found that the ankle played a central role in minor corrections of postural balance. Peroneus longus electromyographic (EMG) activity and the location of the center of pressure on the force plate correlated closely with ankle position. When the body was in major disequilibrium, however, subjects made corrections at the hip. The mode of maintaining balance in these subjects changed from an inverted pendulum model to a multisegmental chain model when adjustments at the ankle were no longer adequate to maintain postural control.

Patients with ankle instability, when tested by standing on one foot following an ankle inversion injury, showed no significant inversion or eversion weakness compared with the other, uninjured, ankle.[63] The problem was apparently one of impaired muscle control and balance rather than one of muscle weakness. These subjects apparently were not examined for myofascial TrPs.

Walking

Basmajian and Deluca[16] established that, during level walking, the peroneus longus helps stabilize the leg and foot in midstance. The peroneus longus and the tibialis posterior, working in concert, control the shift from inversion during early stance to a neutral position at midstance. The peroneus brevis acts synchronously with the peroneus longus during ordinary walking. Throughout most of the stance phase, the peroneus longus generally is more active in flatfooted subjects [with more flexible feet] than in "normal" subjects.[16]

Matsusaka[67] studied the control of mediolateral balance of the foot during walking in 11 normal adults. When the force plate measured a large lateral component of ground reaction force, EMG activity of the peroneus longus was marked during midstance phase, while the amount of pronation (eversion and abduction) of the foot was small. Matsusaka[67] proposes that the peroneals control excessive inversion of the foot by preventing medial inclination of the tibia over the fixed foot during the midstance phase of gait. Conversely, when the lateral component of the ground reaction force was small, the peroneus longus remained inactive during midstance phase, and the tibialis posterior, flexor digitorum longus, and extensor hallucis longus were all active.

Krammer and associates[57] concluded that the peroneus tertius muscle evolved in bipedal posture for the purpose of shifting the line of body weight toward the medial margin of the foot. This shift from lateral to medial develops in infant standing balance and with the onset of walking, and it occurs in each walking cycle of an adult human.

Sports Activities

In a study of 15 highly trained track men,[66] fine-wire intramuscular electrodes in the peroneus longus muscle showed EMG activity during the first half of stance phase of jogging. During running, this activity shifted toward midstance and lasted for a smaller percentage of the gait cycle. When the subjects were sprinting, peroneus longus activity began shortly before stance phase and continued through most of that phase for a total of about 25% of the gait cycle.

Examination of EMG activity from fine-wire electrodes in the peroneus longus muscle during a standing vertical jump by five subjects[50] revealed that activity during the take-off phase peaked at the time of toe-off. Only occasional minimal activity appeared during the flight phase, followed by return of vigorous activity during the landing phase, with activity gradually diminishing during the stabilization phase after landing.

Surface electrodes monitored bilateral EMG activity of the peroneus longus muscle during 13 right-handed sports activities including overhand and underhand throws, tennis serve, golf swing, hitting a baseball, and one-foot jumps. Peaks of activity characteristically appeared in the right leg preceding release of, or contact with, the ball and appeared in the left leg throughout and following release of a ball or on contact during a swing. In the one-foot jump, however, peaks of activity appeared in each leg prior to clearing the ground and on landing.[20]

5. FUNCTIONAL (MYOTATIC) UNIT

All three peroneal muscles are prime movers for eversion of the "free" foot. The primary agonist to the peroneal muscles for eversion is the extensor digitorum longus.[88] This muscle is likely to be overloaded and to develop TrPs at the same time as the peroneal muscles because an involved weak peroneal muscle fails to provide the help that the extensor digitorum longus needs at times of maximum loading.

The antagonists to the eversion function of the peroneal muscles are primarily the tibialis anterior and tibialis posterior assisted by the extensor hallucis longus and flexor hallucis longus.[88] The tibialis anterior and the peroneus longus attach opposite to each other on the same bones.[82] These antagonists are likely to be chronically overloaded when they must work against the increased tension of the peroneal muscles produced by shortened taut bands associated with their TrPs.

Since the peroneus tertius, tibialis anterior, and extensor digitorum longus are prime dorsiflexors, they are strong antagonists to the plantar flexor function of the peroneus longus and peroneus brevis muscles.

6. SYMPTOMS

Weakness of any of the three peroneal muscles can contribute to "weak ankles." Patients with peroneal TrPs complain of pain and tenderness in the ankle behind and over the lateral malleolus, especially after an inversion sprain of the ankle. These patients sprain their ankles frequently. Their ankles tend to be unstable so that they cannot perform on a balance beam[14] or ice skate. They are likely to have foot drop if the deep peroneal nerve is entrapped.

Patients with peroneal TrPs, in addition to inverting and spraining their ankles because of inadequate peroneal muscle support, are also prone to ankle fractures. Treatment of the fracture by a cast on the ankle, which immobilizes the peroneal muscles, aggravates and perpetuates peroneal TrPs that cause ankle pain. In this situation, the fracture can be healing, or fully healed, and not be the cause of the ankle pain. When this ankle pain comes from myofascial TrPs, it responds well to myofascial management.

Painful feet and calluses characteristic of the Morton foot structure commonly appear on the list of symptoms because this foot configuration aggravates peroneus longus and peroneus brevis TrPs.

Differential Diagnosis

Myofascial Syndromes

Five extensor muscles of the lower limb project referred pain in patterns that might be confused with those of the peroneal muscles. They are the tibialis anterior and the long extensors and short extensors of the hallux and of the lesser toes. However, TrPs in these other muscles do not refer pain behind the lateral malleolus, to the heel, or to the lateral side of the leg.

The tibialis anterior (*see* Fig. 19.1) projects medial, not lateral, anterior ankle pain and also refers pain to the great toe. As compared to the distribution of pain referred from peroneal TrPs, the extensor digitorum longus (*see* Fig. 24.1*A*) refers pain farther distally over the dorsum of the foot. The extensor hallucis longus pain pattern (*see* Fig. 24.1*B*) covers the medial, not the lateral, side of the dorsum of the foot and extends farther distally, adjacent to the great toe. The composite pain pattern of the extensor hallucis brevis and extensor digitorum brevis (*see* Fig. 26.1) overlaps the peroneus tertius pattern on the dorsum of the foot, but does not extend as far proximally as the ankle.

The lateral heel pain referred from peroneus tertius TrPs does not include the entire Achilles tendon nor the bottom of the heel, as does the soleus referred pain pattern.

Because of the local tenderness associated with the pain referred to the ankle by TrPs in the peroneal muscles, these myofascial pain symptoms are easily mistaken for arthritis of the ankle joint.[89]

Entrapment Syndromes

Entrapment of the common peroneal nerve, the superficial peroneal nerve, or the deep peroneal nerve can produce symptoms of pain and paresthesias of the anterolateral ankle and dorsum of the foot[56] with weakness of the ankle[92] that can be suggestive of peroneal myofascial pain syndromes.

The **common peroneal nerve** leaves the popliteal space to swing around the neck of the fibula toward the front of the leg where it enters the lateral compartment and passes deep to the peroneus longus muscle along the lateral edge of the soleus and lateral head of the gastrocnemius muscle, as seen in cross sections.[22] At this level, it divides into the superficial and deep peroneal nerves (Fig. 20.9). Myofascial TrPs in the peroneus longus muscle can entrap the common peroneal nerve close to the fibular head. Section 10 of this chapter presents this anatomy of the nerve and its entrapment there in more detail. The superficial branch supplies the structures in the lateral compartment and the deep branch supplies those in the anterior compartment.[25,56]

Entrapment of the common peroneal nerve weakens both the anterior and lateral compartment muscles. Loss of sensation is most marked in a triangular patch on the dorsum of the foot distally between the first and second toes, an area that is supplied exclusively by the deep and superficial branches of the common peroneal nerve.[27]

Together, the symptoms of common peroneal nerve entrapment and the referred pain of peroneal TrPs strongly suggest a ruptured intervertebral disc which, if present, can also activate peroneal TrPs in a segmental distribution. Therefore, patients with such symptoms may have a myofascial pain syndrome with or without neurological symptoms and signs; or their symptoms may be due to a combination of radiculopathy, peroneal nerve entrapment, and referred myofascial pain.

Reported causes of peroneal nerve palsy by compression in the leg include: a popliteal (Baker's) cyst,[56,87] a ganglion (cyst) that locally replaced the peroneus longus muscle,[19] a large fabella (sesamoid bone in the lateral head of the gastrocnemius muscle) in seven cases,[98] a cystic swelling in the peroneal nerve itself,[87] and bunching of the peroneus longus muscle after its rupture.[56]

The habit of crossing the legs may lead to the uppermost leg "falling asleep" due to compression neurapraxia and a temporary peroneal nerve palsy. If this practice is continued too often and too long, it can lead to lasting nerve damage.[108] Another reported postural cause of entrapment neuropathy of the common peroneal nerve was harvesting a wheat crop in the squatting position by army personnel unaccustomed to this activity.[85]

The **superficial peroneal nerve** emerges through the deep fascia in the lower third of the leg[27] where it is vulnerable to acute or chronic trauma and subject to entrapment by the fascia.[55] The pain and altered sensation without motor deficit in the distribution of this nerve appears confusingly like a combination of tibialis anterior and peroneus tertius myofascial pain syndromes. However, this entrapment is not dependent on myofascial TrPs in these muscles.

Styf[96] made the diagnosis of superficial peroneal nerve entrapment when examination revealed: *(a)* pain and altered sensibility over the dorsum of the foot; *(b)* a positive response to at least one of three provocative tests; and *(c)* a superficial peroneal nerve conduction velocity of less than 44 m/sec or a fascial defect where the nerve emerges. The three provocative tests were positive when the patient experienced the foot pain in response to: *(a)* pressure applied where the nerve emerges from the deep fascia while the patient actively dorsiflexed and everted the foot against resistance; *(b)* passive plantar flexion and inversion without local pressure over the nerve; and *(c)* gentle percussion over the course of the nerve while maintaining passive stretch (Tinel's sign).

Using the criteria listed, Styf[96] identified three mechanisms of entrapment among 21 patients with this diagnosis. Others also reported on patients with entrapment of the superficial peroneal nerve.[53,65,68,95]

Entrapment of the **deep peroneal nerve** by the extensor hallucis longus muscle is considered in Section 10 of Chapter 24.

The **Morton foot structure** (the Dudley J. Morton foot configuration) must be distinguished from Morton's neuroma (Morton's metatarsalgia). The latter is generally thought to result from interdigital nerve entrapment in the region of the transverse metatarsal ligament.[1] The Morton foot structure is a variation in skeletal structure[75] that usually is not of itself painful, but can cause problems for the muscles and other structures. Indeed, abnormal pressures caused by the *structure* could be a factor in development of the *neuroma*. The Morton foot structure is considered in Sections 7, 8, and 14 of this chapter.

Lateral Compartment Syndrome

Chapters 19 and 22 of this volume review the diagnoses of anterior and posterior compartment syndromes on pages 361–362 and pages 443–444. The same principles apply here. The lateral compartment syndrome with pain along the lateral side of the leg that is aggravated by activity can be suggestive of peroneus longus and peroneus brevis TrP pain, but the tenderness and tension of the musculature in the compartment syndrome is diffuse, not localized as in the myofascial syndromes.[46] The lateral compartment syndrome is likely to develop in runners with excessive pronation and abnormally mobile subtalar joints.[17] It can also develop secondary to rupture of the peroneus longus muscle.[30] A measured abnormal increase in compartment pressure confirms the diagnosis.[46]

Ankle Sprain

The trauma that causes a lateral ankle sprain can also readily activate peroneal TrPs that refer pain and tenderness to the ankle. Examination of the peroneal muscles for TrPs discloses this source of the symptoms. However, other causes of the pain should be ruled out.

Usually, injury to the lateral ligaments of the ankle results from an inversion-plantar flexion strain. The first structures to tear are the anterior lateral joint capsule and the anterior talofibular ligament.[28] The immediate region of the torn ligament is tender and swollen. Tenderness referred from TrPs usually includes a larger area without such marked swelling.

Muscle and Tendon Rupture

Rupture of the peroneus longus muscle may produce a lateral compartment syndrome.[30]

The os peroneum is a sesamoid bone of the peroneus longus tendon that develops in about 10% of individuals. When it has suffered trauma and becomes painful, it can be treated successfully either surgically[107] or conservatively.[21]

The os peroneum may fracture and rupture the peroneus longus tendon[99] when the individual tries to prevent a fall[86] or imposes sudden inversion stress on the ankle, often with an audible snap.[21]

Rupture of the peroneus brevis muscle occurred in a ballet dancer in the congenital absence of the peroneus longus muscle.[29]

Degenerative lesions of the peroneus brevis tendon were reported in 13 patients,[91] and ruptures of the peroneus brevis tendon in nine patients.[59,61]

7. ACTIVATION AND PERPETUATION OF TRIGGER POINTS

Activation

A fall with twisting and inversion of the ankle can overload the peroneus longus and peroneus brevis muscles and is likely to activate TrPs in them.

Weakness induced by prolonged immobilization, as by an ankle cast, predisposes strongly to activation of these TrPs.

Active TrPs in the anterior gluteus minimus muscle, which refer pain strongly to the lateral aspect of the leg, may induce satellite TrPs in the peroneus longus and peroneus brevis muscles.

In a study of 100 patients, it was reported that a motor vehicle accident rarely activated TrPs in the peroneus longus muscle.[13]

Perpetuation

Immobilization by a cast can perpetuate latent TrPs that were activated previously by the initial trauma of a fracture or strain.

The Morton foot structure (relatively short first and long second metatarsals) with a mediolaterally rocking foot commonly perpetuates TrPs primarily in the peroneus longus[93,94,100] and also in the peroneus brevis muscles, but rarely in the peroneus tertius. Individuals may have an equally marked Morton foot structure bilaterally, but have pain only on one side, usually the side of a shorter lower limb. Similarly, bunions may appear the same on both feet, but may be painful on only one foot. Patients ask why, if they have the same foot structure bilaterally, do they have pain only on one side? The answer is that the body is tilted toward the shorter lower limb. When there is lower limb-length inequality, the shorter limb usually carries more weight in standing, receives more forceful impact during ambulation, may be more fully inverted at heel-strike, and has a delayed toe-off. The limb may be short because of low arch height caused by a hyperpronated, hypermobile foot on that side.

Chronic tension caused by active (or latent) TrPs in the antagonistic tibialis anterior or tibialis posterior muscles tends to overload the peroneus longus and peroneus brevis muscles and to perpetuate TrPs in them.

Sleeping with the foot strongly plantar flexed places the peroneus longus and peroneus brevis muscles in the shortened position for prolonged periods. This common position aggravates their TrPs.

Crossing one leg over the other to compensate for a small hemipelvis (*see* page 44, Chapter 4) can compress the common peroneal nerve in the uppermost leg against the underlying knee. The weight of the crossed leg may also traumatize the uppermost peroneus longus muscle, perpetuating TrPs in it.

Wearing high heels perpetuates peroneal TrPs by shifting the body weight forward onto the ball of the foot during standing, by reducing the base of support, and by increasing the length of the lever arm against which the muscles must operate. The resultant instability overloads the peroneus longus and peroneus brevis muscles. A shoe with a spike heel of any height provides an unstable base of support that can overload the peroneal muscles.

Patients with flat feet and unsupported arches are likely to have spot tenderness and taut bands in the peroneus longus and peroneus brevis muscles,[58] probably because these muscles are then more active during the stance phase of walking.[16]

A tight elastic top of a long sock can constrict circulation in the peroneus longus, extensor digitorum longus, and gastrocnemius muscles by direct compression, like a tourniquet, and thus perpetuate their TrPs. An indented red line or marking around the leg indicates a high probability of this constriction. The soleus muscle usually is too deep to be affected.

8. PATIENT EXAMINATION
(Figs. 20.4–20.7)

Patients with latent TrPs in the peroneus longus muscle are asymptomatic with regard to pain but, for years, these latent TrPs may cause characteristic calluses and weak ankles.[100]

Examination of the feet frequently reveals a relatively short first and long second metatarsal (Morton foot structure) with characteristic calluses. Shoes that show uneven wear and are poorly designed for comfort, or are well designed but too tight, can make a major contribution to the pain problem.

While the patient walks, the clinician observes from behind to note excessive pronation of the foot or other deviations. A mediolaterally rocking foot with associated peroneus longus TrPs can produce a sense of ankle weakness severe enough to convince some patients to use a cane.

If, while sitting in a chair, the patient crosses the legs, he or she may be attempting to compensate for a small hemipelvis on the side of the uppermost crossed leg. This seated pelvic asymmetry should be examined as described on pages 43–45 of Chapter 4 in this volume.

To examine for peroneus longus and peroneus brevis weakness, the patient lies on the side not being tested. The clinician stabilizes the uppermost leg and places the foot in plantar flexion and eversion (pronation); with the *toes relaxed*, the patient then holds the foot in that position against resistance supplied by the clinician, who presses against the lateral border of the foot in the direction of inversion and dorsiflexion.[48,52] The calf muscles and long flexors of the toes can also produce powerful plantar flexion, but these two peroneal muscles are the chief force for eversion of the foot in plantar flexion. The peroneus tertius and extensor digitorum longus also produce eversion,

PART 3

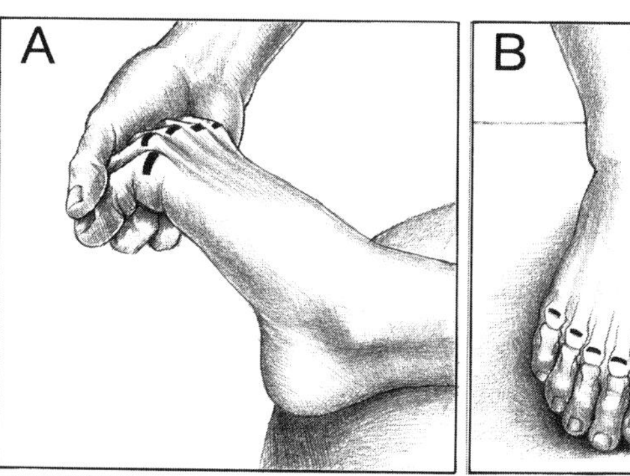

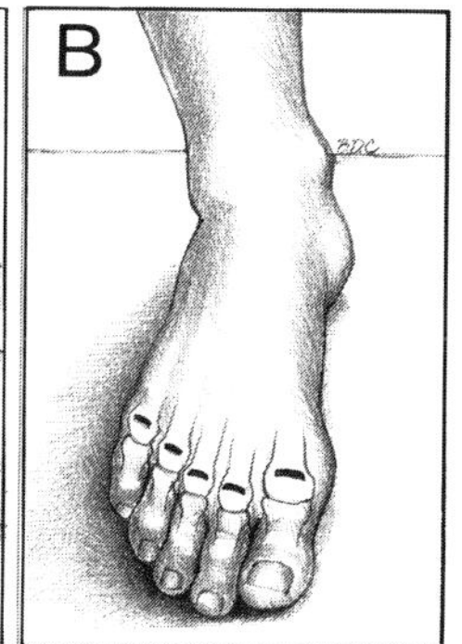

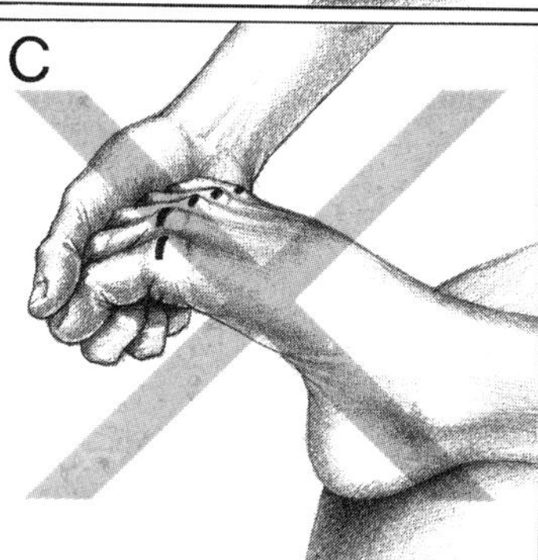

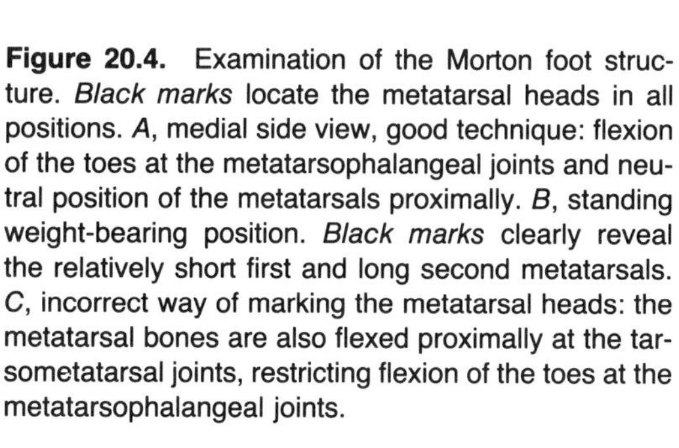

Figure 20.4. Examination of the Morton foot structure. *Black marks* locate the metatarsal heads in all positions. *A*, medial side view, good technique: flexion of the toes at the metatarsophalangeal joints and neutral position of the metatarsals proximally. *B*, standing weight-bearing position. *Black marks* clearly reveal the relatively short first and long second metatarsals. *C*, incorrect way of marking the metatarsal heads: the metatarsal bones are also flexed proximally at the tarsometatarsal joints, restricting flexion of the toes at the metatarsophalangeal joints.

but they dorsiflex, rather than plantar flex the foot. Patients with peroneus longus and peroneus brevis TrPs have difficulty holding that foot in eversion and plantar flexion against resistance as compared with the uninvolved side. Baker[14] describes this ratchety resistance to movement as "breakaway" weakness. The more active the TrPs, the more marked is this weakness.

Active *peroneus longus* and *peroneus brevis* TrPs cause pain on eversion effort with the foot already everted, and they also painfully restrict passive inversion range of motion. *Peroneus tertius* TrPs cause pain on active dorsiflexion in the dorsiflexed (shortened) position and limit passive plantar flexion.

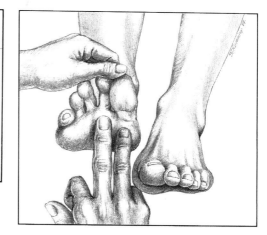

Figure 20.5. Plantar palpation of the distal ends of the first two metatarsal heads, during strong extension of the toes, demonstrates the Morton foot structure (a relatively short first and long second metatarsal).

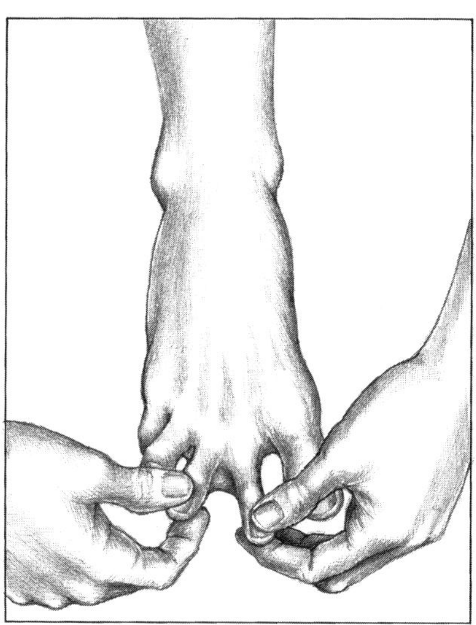

Figure 20.6. The long web between the second and third toes is characteristic of the Morton foot structure (a relatively short first and long second metatarsal).

Morton Foot Structure
(Figs. 20.4–20.7)

In 1935, Dudley J. Morton, M.D.,[75] described two structural variations in the foot, one or both of which appeared regularly among 150 patients complaining of metatarsalgia. The most common variation was hypermobility of the first metatarsal (at the tarsometatarsal articulation) with laxity of longitudinal plantar ligaments; the other, nearly as common, was a relatively short first metatarsal

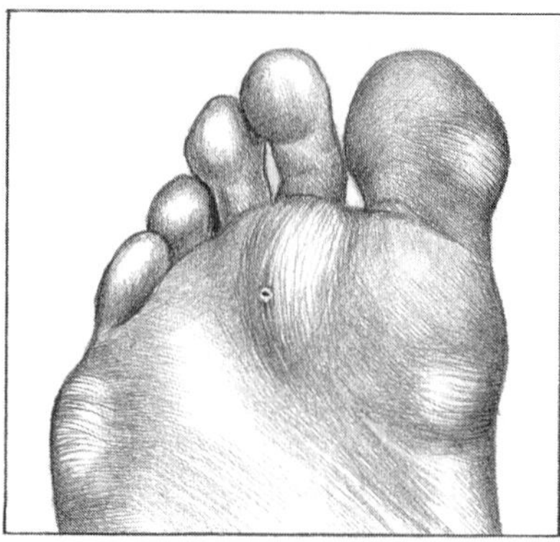

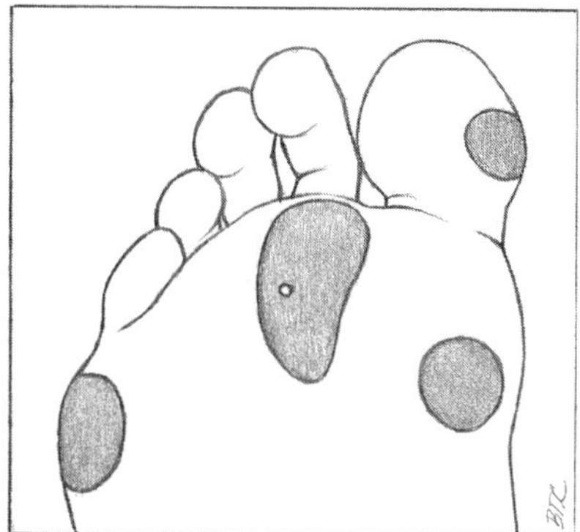

Figure 20.7. Calluses frequently associated with the Morton foot structure. The second toe usually extends farther from the foot than the first toe when the second metatarsal is longer than the first metatarsal. Thick calluses may develop under the head of the second metatarsal, and lateral to the head of the fifth metatarsal. Another callus occurs under the medial side of the head of the first metatarsal and still another usually appears on the medial side of the great toe along the interphalangeal joint.

bone. Hypermobility of the first metatarsal overloads the tibialis posterior and flexor digitorum longus muscles.[75] The short first metatarsal configuration tends to overload primarily the peroneus longus and, less frequently, the peroneus brevis muscles. The peroneus brevis tendon does not cross the sole of the foot to reach the first metatarsal bone as does the peroneus longus tendon.

A relatively short first metatarsal occurs commonly (approximately 40% of individuals).[45] In both conditions described, the mechanical fault results in a failure of the first metatarsal bone to carry its share of body weight (normally at least one-third) between heel-rise and toe-off during ambulation. Athletes with the Morton foot structure who run about 80 km (50 miles) or more per week are likely to develop painful symptoms.[84]

Chapter 4 of Volume 1[105] reviews the literature relating to the relatively short first metatarsal bone. Section 14, Corrective Actions, of this chapter describes the management of this condition. This anatomical configuration causes mediolateral rocking of the foot on the "knife edge" of a line extending from the heel through the head of the long second metatarsal bone. Travell[100] emphasized the muscular consequences of this mechanical imbalance in foot dynamics. The muscle imbalance and overload caused by the Morton foot structure can affect other muscles in addition to the peroneals. Common postural compensations associated with the Morton foot structure involve the vastus medialis, gluteus medius, and gluteus minimus (*see* Fig. 8.3).

To examine for the Morton foot structure, the clinician grasps the foot and flexes the joints of the toes by supporting the heads of the metatarsals with the fingers against the sole of the foot (Fig. 20.4*A*). The dorsal crease formed by the metatarsophalangeal joint becomes visible. By marking the prominence of each metatarsal head with a pen, the relative lengths of the five metatarsals become apparent (Fig. 20.4*B*). The second toe usually stands out as a prominent feature, as seen in Figure 20.4*B*. The locations of the metatarsal heads are more difficult to mark accurately if the metatarsal bones are bent down with the toes (Fig. 20.4*C*).

Figure 20.5 shows how to examine the plantar surface of the foot for a short first, long second metatarsal relationship. The distal end of the second metatarsal extends farther than the end of the first. Sometimes the phalanges of the second toe are so short that its tip does not extend beyond the end of the first toe, even though the second *metatarsal* is longer than the first. The length of the metatarsal is the more important factor because it bears body weight. Therefore, the clinician should examine the first two *metatarsals* for relative length, not just the toes, when the patient has peroneal TrPs.

Usually, when the first metatarsal is shorter than the second, the web of skin between the second and third toes is large compared with that between the first and second toes (Fig. 20.6). This finding alerts the examiner to look at metatarsal length.

Although some individuals have a shorter first metatarsal with *normal* distribution of body weight on the metatarsal heads, those with *abnormal* weight distribution develop calluses.[45] These calluses usually develop in conjunction with TrPs in the peroneus longus muscle. They occur under the head of the second metatarsal (Fig. 20.7) and sometimes under the third and fourth metatarsal heads, which may also carry additional weight. These calluses further aggravate abnormal weight distribution on the metatarsal heads at the end of stance phase.

Other calluses also tend to develop: on the medial side of the great toe, toward the end of this toe; medially beside the head of the first metatarsal; along the lateral border of the sole of the foot anteriorly; and, sometimes, on the lateral side of the fifth metatarsal (Fig. 20.7).

Duchenne[31] observed that patients with paralysis of only the peroneus longus muscle presented primarily with painful calluses on the lateral border of the sole of the foot. This reinforces the impression that when patients develop TrPs that inhibit the peroneus longus and weaken its function, they eventually develop calluses. The presence of these lateral calluses indicates abnormal lateral forces that rub the feet against the side of the shoe. Callus formation along both sides of the foot may also depend on shoe tightness. The callus at the medial side of the first metatarsal head indicates one source of bunions that, in its early stages, is correctable without surgery by modifying the shoes.

Shoe Examination

Inappropriate shoes aggravate the mechanical instability induced by the Morton foot structure. Even a proper correction can cause additional trouble in the wrong style of shoe. Examination of the shoes should include at least the following considerations:

1. The shoe should have a *straight last* to provide maximum support under the arch. With the shoes placed beside each other positioned as the patient wears them, the *medial sides* should touch each other from heel to near the toe. The toes should not be pointed and should not curve away from each other. Such pointed shoes forcibly abduct the great toe, cramp the metatarsal heads, exaggerate mechanical imbalance, and contribute to bunion formation in men and women.

2. The *cap* (or toe box) of the shoe covers the toes and metatarsal heads. The vertical height of the cap should provide ample room for movement of the toes and metatarsal heads with shoe inserts in place. If the cap is tight during ambulation, the patient loses normal toe movement; a pad inserted for compensation of a Morton foot structure often makes the cap tighter and aggravates symptoms by crowding the toes. For this reason, patients should take a foam insole with them when buying new shoes and slip the insole into each new shoe when trying it on the larger foot to ensure adequate room for addition of the first metatarsal pad and insole. If the patient already has favorite shoes that are too tight, a shoe repairman can often stretch a leather vamp (part covering the instep and toes) overnight.

3. The *sole* should be flexible at the heads of the metatarsals. Unless the sole of a shoe is stiff because it is new, the examiner should be able to bend it readily with hand pressure. A rigid wooden sole is obviously unsatisfactory in this respect. Ice skates pose a similar problem.

4. The *heel counter* should be firm and the shoe should fit well. Heel space that is excessively wide allows the heel of the foot to wallow loosely from side to side inside the shoe. This, in turn, lets the entire foot turn and slip sideways in the shoe, which requires additional stabilization by the muscles and can cause blisters and Achilles tendon irritation. This problem is characteristic of women's sandal-type shoes, especially if the shoes have high heels. A sufficiently thick, firm foam or felt pad added inside a shoe along the sides of the heel prevents such traumatic movement.

5. A critical observation is *excessive wear* on the outer side of the heel and on the inner edge of the sole. Some lateral heel wear is normal. The excessive wear pattern develops because of excessive inversion and then excessive eversion of the foot during stance phase (side to side rocking in the frontal plane). Patients with more severe hyperpronation may show only excessive medial heel and sole wear patterns. Shoes with a worn heel aggravate mechanical imbalance of the foot and should be replaced and the imbalance corrected. The patient may need to consult a competent podiatrist.

6. The heel of the shoe should be *flat* and not pitched in any direction as a correction for uneven wear caused by the Morton foot structure. Some practitioners add a wedge to the heel to raise its medial side, which may help when the patient is standing still, but it aggravates mechanical imbalance when the patient walks. Good arch support is needed.

9. TRIGGER POINT EXAMINATION (Fig. 20.8)

For examination of the peroneal muscles for TrPs, the patient lies supine with the foot free to move while the other limb (not being examined) is covered to prevent chilling of the patient (Fig. 20.8). The most common TrP location in the peroneus longus muscle (Fig. 20.1*A* and proximal point of palpation in Fig. 20.8)

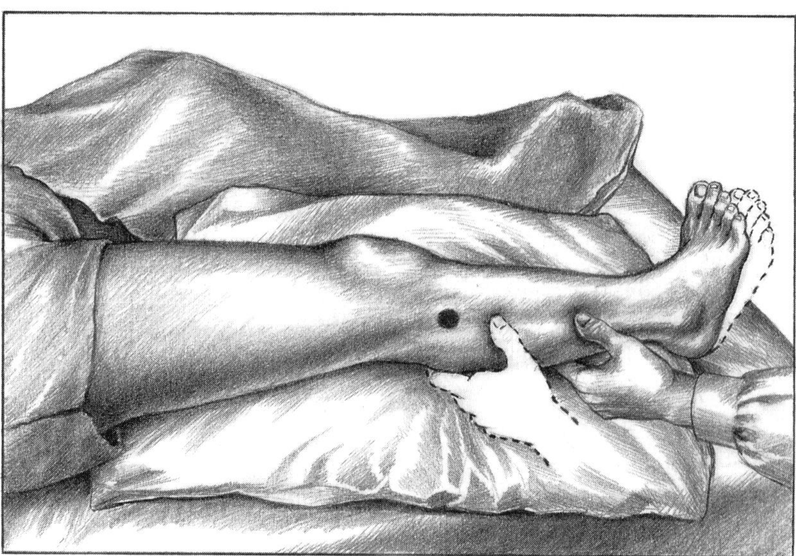

Figure 20.8. Palpation of trigger points in the right peroneus longus and brevis muscles. The *solid circle* marks the head of the fibula. The *outlined hand* illustrates palpation of a trigger point in the peroneus longus muscle against the fibula. The *dotted outline of the foot* indicates its movement due to a local twitch response elicited by snapping palpation across the trigger point in the peroneus longus muscle. The *fully rendered hand* illustrates palpation of a trigger point in the peroneus brevis muscle.

is about 2–4 cm (approximately an inch or slightly more) distal to the head of the fibula over the shaft of the fibula. Taut bands at this TrP location are clearly delineated by palpation against the underlying bone. This firm foundation makes it easy to elicit a local twitch response (LTR) in the peroneus longus muscle by snapping palpation. The transient twitch causes the foot to swing outward and down, as indicated by the outlined foot in Figure 20.8. The common peroneal nerve crosses diagonally over the neck of the fibula just below the fibular head and has a cordlike consistency. The nerve is distinguished from a taut band by its proximal position and a course running across the muscle rather than running the length of the muscle nearly parallel to the shaft of the fibula.[70] Excessive pressure on the nerve may cause painful tingling sensations over the lateral side of the leg and the foot.

This location of peroneus longus TrPs corresponds to the location where Lange[58] found myogelosis of the peroneal muscles.

TrPs in the peroneus brevis muscle (Fig. 20.1*A* and the distal point of palpation in Fig. 20.8) are usually found on either side of, and deep to, the peroneus longus tendon near the junction of the middle and lower thirds of the leg. These TrPs also are palpable against the shaft of the fibula. Obvious LTRs are more difficult to elicit from this muscle than from the peroneus longus, but the visible response of the foot is essentially the same. Pressure on active TrPs in either of these muscles characteristically elicits referred pain in, behind, and distal to the lateral malleolus, in which case this area also exhibits referred tenderness.

TrPs in the peroneus tertius muscle (*see* Fig. 20.1*B*) are palpable slightly distal and anterior to peroneus brevis TrPs, and proximal and anterior to the lateral malleolus. The tendon of this muscle stands out and is readily palpable in the anterolateral aspect of the ankle and foot (lateral to the extensor digitorum longus tendons) when the seated patient attempts to evert the foot by lifting the fifth metatarsal from the floor. Taut bands in this muscle are often difficult to delineate by palpation, but pressure on the sensitive active TrP usually refers pain to the anterolateral ankle and sometimes to the lateral side of the heel (*see* Fig. 20.1*B*).

10. ENTRAPMENTS
(Fig. 20.9)

Section 6, under **Differential Diagnosis**, reviews the symptoms caused by entrapment of the common peroneal nerve and its branches, the superficial and deep peroneal nerves.

An opening at the proximal attachment of the peroneus longus muscle provides passage for the peroneal nerves. This opening lies between the proximal fibers and tendon of the peroneus longus and the neck of the fibula. The opening is delimited by a fibrous edge that takes the form of the letter "J" on the left leg and a reversed "J" on the right. The superficial and deep peroneal nerves bend over the bottom of the "J"; the superficial peroneal nerve bends most sharply. In the anatomical specimen and at surgery, inverting and plantar flexing the foot pulled the nerves taut against this fascial edge.[56]

Neurolysis of the peroneal nerve as it passed deep to this sharp fibrous edge at the origin of the peroneus longus muscle relieved signs and symptoms of peroneal nerve compression neuropathy in seven of eight patients.[60] The symptoms were initiated by vigorous exercise, but the report did not mention whether myofascial TrPs of the peroneus longus contributed to the symptoms, particularly in the patient for whom neurolysis was ineffective.

Taut bands caused by TrPs in the peroneus longus muscle increase the tension of the muscle and can cause entrapment of the common peroneal nerve and/or the superficial and deep peroneal[100] nerves, if the nerve branches far enough proximally (Fig. 20.9*A*). The nerve compression may occur against the fibula, or it may result from strangulation of the nerve by muscle tension on the bands of fascia that surround the nerve.[49] The compression of motor fibers in the common peroneal nerve or in the deep peroneal nerve by taut bands in the peroneus longus muscle can cause significant foot drop.[93,94] Foot drop and changes in sensation caused by entrapment of the peroneal nerve may result from residual peroneal TrPs that originated during a radiculopathy that was later resolved.

Numbness and tingling caused by entrapment of the common peroneal nerve (Fig. 20.9*B*) appear on the dorsum of the foot in the triangular area between the first and second toes. This specific patch of skin area is supplied only by the deep and superficial peroneal nerves,[54] whereas the surrounding dorsum of the foot is also supplied by other nerves.

The deep peroneal nerve may also be entrapped against the fibula by the taut bands of TrPs in the extensor digitorum longus muscle (Fig. 20.9*A*). This neurological distribution of pain due to entrapment is distinguishable from the pattern of aching pain referred to the ankle region by TrPs in the peroneus longus or brevis muscles (Fig. 20.1*A*).

Another potential source of compression of the common peroneal nerve or its branches is the use of a pneumatic stocking for "mechanical anti-thrombophlebitis therapy." Symptoms of nerve impairment have been observed in several older patients following use of this pneumatic stocking.[2]

11. ASSOCIATED TRIGGER POINTS

The peroneus longus is almost always involved when either of the other two peroneal muscles harbors TrPs. Not surprisingly, the muscle that most commonly develops secondary TrPs associated with TrP-weakened peroneal muscles is their prime agonist for eversion, the extensor digitorum longus. The fact that the extensor digitorum longus also serves as a prime antagonist to the plantar flexion action of the peroneus longus can account for the likelihood of both muscles developing TrPs. The chronic tension of taut bands in the involved muscle overloads its antagonist. Peroneus longus TrPs are also likely to occur in association with tibialis posterior TrPs; these two muscles are specific antagonists in regard to inversion-eversion, but are agonistic in regard to plantar flexion and to stabilizing the weight-bearing foot.

Although the peroneus longus and peroneus brevis are weak assistants to the prime plantar flexors, TrPs in the powerful gastrocnemius and soleus muscles are not likely to induce problems in the peroneal muscles. Nor is

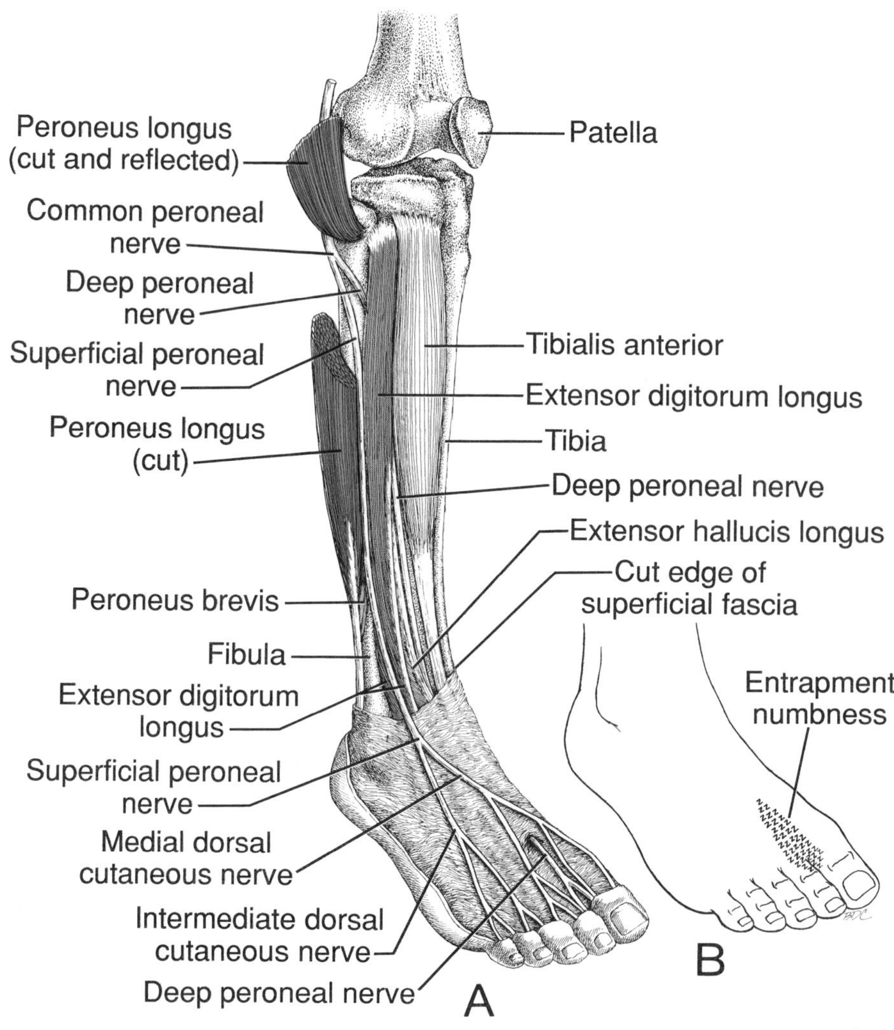

Figure 20.9. Entrapment of the common, deep or superficial peroneal nerve. *A*, by a tense peroneus longus muscle (*dark red*), which is reflected. Entrapment of the deep peroneal nerve can be caused also by a tense extensor digitorum longus muscle (*medium red*). Both the deep and superficial branches of the peroneal nerve pass between the peroneus longus muscle and the underlying fibula where taut bands associated with trigger points in the peroneus longus can compress the nerve and cause neurapraxia. *B*, the zone of entrapment numbness (*Zs*) due to taut trigger point bands in the peroneus longus muscle occupies the space between the first and second toes dorsally. The skin of this part of the foot is innervated exclusively by branches of both the deep and superficial peroneal nerves. The reversed "J" entrapment structure and the peroneus tertius are not shown here.

any function of the triceps surae likely to be compromised because of TrPs in the peroneal muscles.

Anterior gluteus minimus TrPs refer pain to the lateral aspect of the leg and can induce satellite TrPs in the peroneal muscles.

The extensor digitorum longus and peroneus tertius muscles work closely together as agonists and TrPs in one can induce secondary TrPs in the other.

12. INTERMITTENT COLD WITH STRETCH
(Fig. 20.10)

The use of ice for applying intermittent cold with stretch is explained on page 9 of this volume and the use of vapocoolant spray with stretch is detailed on pages 67–74 of Volume 1.[102] Techniques that augment relaxation and stretch are reviewed on pages 10–11 and alternative

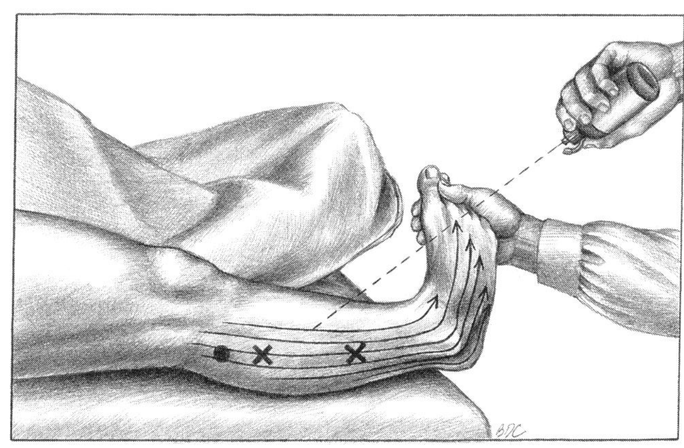

Figure 20.10. Stretch position and ice or vapocoolant spray pattern (*thin arrows*) for trigger points (**X**s) in the peroneus longus and peroneus brevis muscles. The *solid circle* marks the fibular head. The stretch movement combines full inversion and dorsiflexion to stretch these muscles. Stretch of the peroneus tertius (not shown) combines inversion and plantar flexion with an additional anterior (medial) sweep of intermittent cold over the skin covering the peroneus tertius muscle.

treatment methods on pages 9–11 of this volume. It is important to avoid stretching to their full range of motion those muscles that cross hypermobile joints.

Release of TrP tension in the peroneal muscles by intermittent cold with stretch begins by making the supine patient comfortable and fully relaxed on the treatment table. Several slow parallel sweeps of ice or vapocoolant downward over the anterolateral aspect of the leg, ankle, and foot (Fig. 20.10) help inhibit stretch reflexes prior to and during passive lengthening of the shortened muscle(s). The sweeps of coolant should cover the skin over all three peroneal muscles and their referred pain patterns.

To release TrP tightness of the **peroneus longus** and **peroneus brevis**, the clinician applies the ice or vapocoolant downward to cover those muscles and is careful to include the areas behind the lateral malleolus and on the foot laterally where pain is usually referred. After fully inverting and adducting the foot, the clinician then dorsiflexes it within the limit of comfort.[93] (Vapocoolant application is illustrated in Fig. 20.10). As the patient inhales, the clinician resists gentle isometric contraction of the peroneus longus and peroneus brevis muscles. The patient slowly exhales and relaxes as the clinician takes up any slack that develops, moving the foot gently into dorsiflexion and inversion, while again applying parallel sweeps of the coolant.

To lengthen the **peroneus tertius**, the foot is then moved from dorsiflexion to plantar flexion while maintaining inversion. Combining deep breathing with postisometric relaxation, the patient inhales and actively attempts gentle eversion and dorsiflexion against isometric resistance supplied by the clinician. As the patient then *slowly* exhales and relaxes, the clinician applies sweeps of the ice or vapocoolant spray in the pattern illustrated (Fig. 20.10) and takes up any slack that develops in the peroneus tertius muscle by maintaining a slow steady pull toward inversion and plantar flexion. In this stretch position, adding passive flexion of the toes also stretches the extensor digitorum longus, which requires sweeps of the coolant that include the dorsum of the foot and toes (*see* Chapter 24).

To prevent a reactive cramp from developing in the tibialis anterior muscle, tension in it should be released promptly by intermittent cold with stretch. The clinician passively stretches the tibialis anterior by eversion and plantar flexion of the foot (*see* Fig. 19.5).

Following the procedures described previously, a moist heating pad rewarms the skin that was exposed to intermittent cold, and the patient performs several repetitions of active range of motion *slowly* to the fully lengthened and fully shortened positions of the treated muscles. The Peroneal Self-stretch Exercise (*see* Section 14 of this chapter) performed daily at home helps to prevent recurrences.

The peroneus longus muscle and its skin representation are well suited for the use of ice instead of a vapocoolant (*see* Chapter 2), for stripping massage,[104] or for ischemic compression[103] against the fibula to release the TrPs.

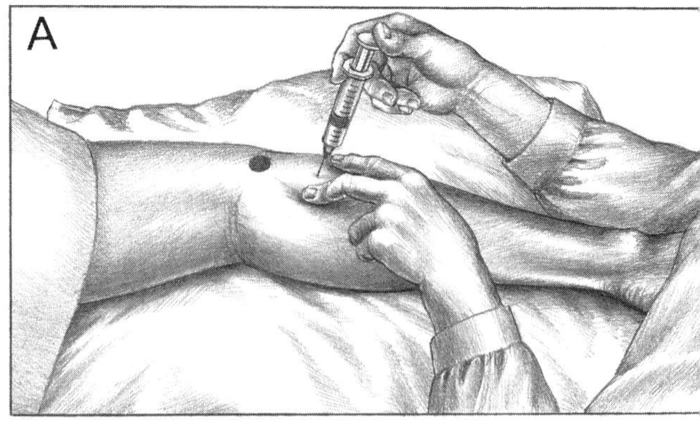

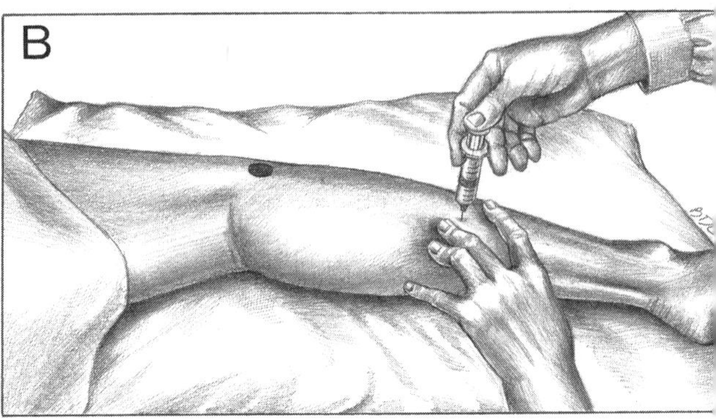

Figure 20.11. Injection of trigger points in the right peroneal muscles. The *solid circle* marks the head of the fibula. Note the pillow between the knees that extends to the ankles so that it supports the leg being injected. *A*, peroneus longus trigger-point injection near, but distal, to the course of the common peroneal nerve that crosses the fibula just below the fibular head. The needle is directed toward the underlying bone. *B*, peroneus brevis trigger-point injection, posterolateral approach, near the junction of the middle and lower thirds of the leg on either side of and deep to the tendon of the peroneus longus muscle.

Evjenth and Hamberg[33] illustrate another technique for fully inverting the foot in dorsiflexion to stretch the peroneus longus and peroneus brevis muscles and a technique for fully inverting and plantar flexing the foot to stretch the peroneus tertius.

13. INJECTION AND STRETCH (Fig. 20.11)

A detailed description of the technique for injection and stretch of any muscle appears on pages 74–86 in Volume 1.[102]

Peroneus longus TrPs usually occur about 2–4 cm distal to the head of the fibula; this TrP location may be only 1 cm (less than ½ in) from the common peroneal nerve as it crosses the fibula diagonally just below the fibular head (Fig. 20.9). Ordinarily, TrP injection does not cause a nerve block, but the TrP may be so close that sometimes the local anesthetic solution spreads as far as the nerve (Fig. 20.11*A*). It is wise to warn patients prior to injection that the foot may "go to sleep" briefly if there is any "spillover" of the anesthetic solution and to reassure them that the foot will "wake up" within 15 or 20 minutes as the anesthetic effect of the 0.5% procaine fades.

Before injecting the peroneus longus TrP, the clinician should first locate the common peroneal nerve by palpation behind the fibular head. If tapping over the nerve where it passes under the peroneus longus muscle (not on the TrP) sets off tingling of the foot in the nerve's distribution (Tinel's sign), the nerve is probably suffering entrapment at that point.

During injection of TrPs in the peroneus longus muscle, a pillow separates the knees of the patient, who lies comfortably on the side with the treatment side uppermost (Fig. 20.11*A*). In a cool room, a blanket or sheet covers exposed skin above the knee to prevent chilling of the patient. Flat palpation of the peroneus longus muscle against the fibula clearly delineates the taut band and precisely localizes the spot of maximum TrP tenderness in the band. With gloves on, a 10-mL hypodermic syringe is filled with 0.5% solution of procaine in isotonic saline. The skin is cleansed with an alcohol swab and can be sprayed with vapocoolant (*without* frosting the

PART 3

skin) to cold-anesthetize the cutaneous area of needle entry. The clinician inserts the 22-gauge, 37-mm (1½-in) needle into the TrP localized between the fingers by directing the needle nearly straight downward toward the fibula to avoid accidentally encountering the common peroneal nerve or its branches. The TrP often lies close to the bone. In addition to the usual jump sign of the patient in response to the sharp pain caused by impaling the TrP with the needle, the clinician feels the LTR and often sees movement of the foot due to the LTR (Fig. 20.8, outlined foot). At the same time, the patient usually reports pain felt in the predictable reference zone of the TrP, which concentrates over the lateral malleolus. Pain projected by the nerve, however, centers on the dorsum of the foot in the region proximal to the great toe. If palpation reveals a residual TrP close to the main one, it too must be injected. Following TrP injection, the muscle should be passively lengthened during intermittent cold application.

The procedure for injecting the peroneus brevis is similar to the one described previously, except that the TrPs are more distal, usually near the junction of the middle and distal thirds of the leg (Figs. 20.1*A* and 20.11*B*). The needle approaches the muscle from the posterolateral direction, passing deep to the peroneus longus tendon. This injection should cause no concern about producing a peroneal nerve block.

Injection of peroneus tertius TrPs, which are somewhat distal and anterior to peroneus brevis TrPs (Fig. 20.1*B*), is similar to that described for the peroneus brevis muscle. A cross section at the level of the junction of the middle and lower thirds of the leg (*see* Fig. 19.3) shows that the safest and most direct approach to the peroneus tertius is through the skin overlying the muscle, with the needle directed toward the fibula. This avoids the superficial peroneal nerve overlying the peroneus brevis muscle, and stays well clear of the deep peroneal nerve and anterior tibial vessels on the interosseous membrane.

Following injection and passive muscle lengthening, a moist heating pad applied promptly over the treated muscles helps minimize postinjection soreness. Then, several cycles of slow active range of motion to the fully shortened and to the fully lengthened positions help restore promptly the muscle's normal range and function. The Peroneal Self-stretch Exercise (*see* next section) performed daily at home helps greatly to prevent recurrences.

Baker[14] reported a 14-year-old girl with a peroneus longus TrP that produced pain and instability during local gymnastics on the balance beam. Injection of the active TrP relieved the pain and instability; she was then able to win the local balance beam competition.

14. CORRECTIVE ACTIONS (Figs. 20.12–20.15)

Body Mechanics and Corrections (Figs. 20.12–20.14)

Morton Foot Structure

If the patient with a Morton foot structure has *no* calluses and *no* peroneus longus TrPs with local twitch responses, a first metatarsal pad may not be required, but the added support might be good preventive medicine. However, in the absence of calluses, there is a possibility that the sesamoid bones in the tendon of the flexor hallucis brevis muscle under the short first metatarsal head (*see* Fig. 27.4*B*) may provide the necessary support. On the other hand, to manage a pain complaint of peroneal origin, the Morton foot structure usually requires correction.

The principle in correcting for the symptomatic Morton foot structure is to equalize the forces between the relatively long second and the short first metatarsal bones during toe-off by adding one, sometimes two, thin layers of a supporting pad of *firm* adhesive felt under the first metatarsal head.[75,76,84] A sole insert cut as illustrated in Figure 20.12*A* facilitates accurate placement of the pad. In this way, one insert can serve to correct several shoes. On the medial side of the foot, the insert should extend beneath the first metatarsal head, almost as far as the interphalangeal joint of the great toe. The end should coincide with the distal crease of the shoe (Fig. 20.13), about 1 cm

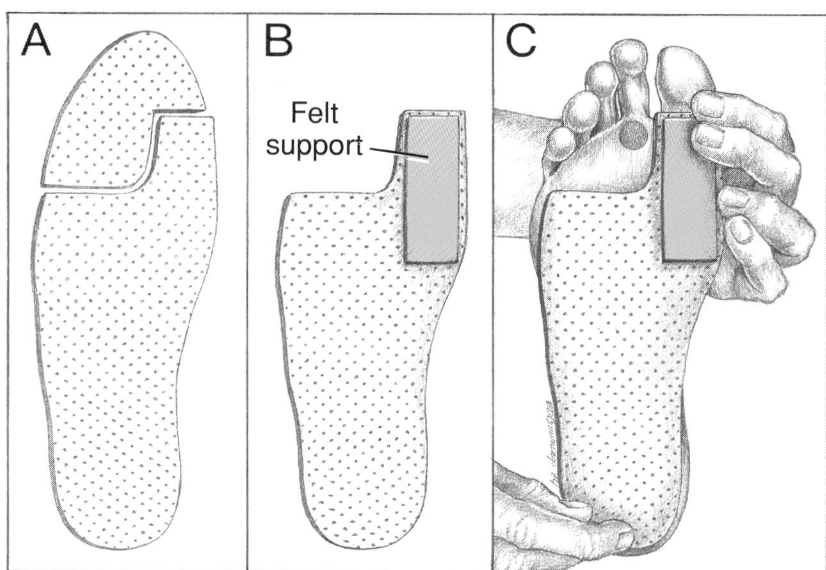

Figure 20.12. Modification of a shoe insert to correct for the Morton foot structure (short first, long second metatarsal bones) by padding under the first metatarsal head. *A*, removal of toe portion of the sole insert to extend support only under the first metatarsal head. The lateral side of the sole insert should not extend under the second metatarsal head, and the insert should reach to the end of the first metatarsal bone (crease of the big toe). *B*, addition of an adhesive felt support beneath head of the first metatarsal. *C*, proper fit of the insert against the sole of the foot; the pad is located beneath only the first metatarsal head. The *solid circle* marks the head of the second metatarsal bone in the midline of the foot, which must *not* be supported by the first metatarsal pad.

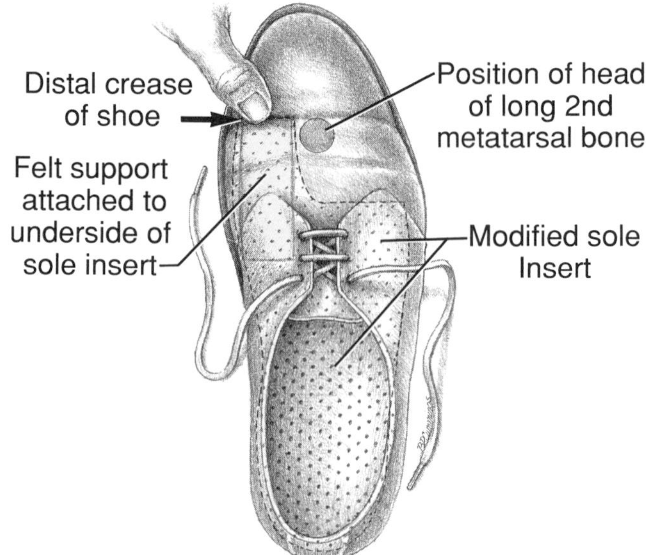

Figure 20.13. Proper placement of a modified sole insert inside the shoe to compensate for the Morton foot structure (short first, long second metatarsal bones). The end of the first metatarsal pad *reaches precisely* to the distal crease of the shoe, as identified by the *arrow and thumbnail*. The felt pad can be fixed to the underside of a foam sole insert cut as shown. The *solid circle* in the middle of the sole at the distal crease locates the head of the long second metatarsal bone. The felt pad transfers weight from the second to the first metatarsal head, placing the foot on a tripod base, instead of on a straight-line base through the second metatarsal.

(⅜ in) beyond the metatarsophalangeal joint (Fig. 20.12*C*). The lateral part of the cut insert should end just short of the lateral four metatarsal heads so that it adds no support beneath these bones when placed in the shoe.

The felt pad can be attached to the under side of the sole insert (Fig. 20.12*B*) through the use of either adhesive felt or an additional adhesive such as double-sticky carpet tape. The felt pad should cover the area under the head of the first metatar-

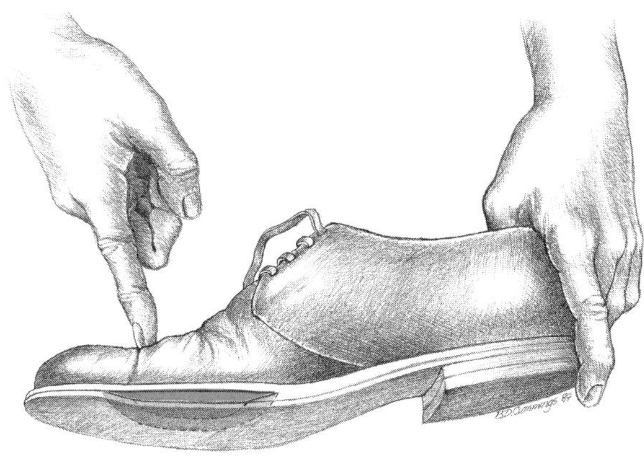

Figure 20.14. A "Flying Dutchman" wedge for lasting correction of the short first, long second metatarsal bones (Morton foot structure) is outlined in *red*. The wedge is inserted by a shoe repairman into the sole of the shoe between the layers of leather, under the head of the first metatarsal. The *dotted lines* show the wedge insert in the sole. The finger points to the distal crease of the shoe, which marks the end of the full thickness of the wedge (1/8 inch, inner edge). This permanent correction solves the problems of felt pads wearing thin and falling out, of the cap of the shoe being too tight to permit insertion of the support *inside* the shoe, and of ensuring accurate placement of the felt pad, as in a high boot.

sal, extending to the inner (medial) side of the shoe, but *not* under any part of the second metatarsal head. The pad should extend over the *end* of the first metatarsal head so that it adds support at toe-off, placing the foot on a tripod base, but it should not extend under the distal phalanx of the great toe. The insert assembly can be held against the foot (Fig. 20.12*C*) to ensure that the pad covers all of the first metatarsal head and *none* of the second metatarsal head. Lateral displacement of the metatarsal pad only a millimeter or two can make a significant difference in effectiveness. Since the Morton foot structure is usually (but not always) bilateral, ordinarily both shoes should be corrected.

The sole insert must be wide enough to prevent its slipping sideways. The insert is ineffective if it slides laterally inside the shoe, partly underneath the second metatarsal head. For adequate width, a woman should buy the male size insert. If she wears a size 10 shoe, she should purchase a man's size 10 sole insert. Similarly, a man who wears a size 10 shoe should purchase a size 12 man's insert. The excess length of the insole must be trimmed at the heel.

This assembly fits into the shoe as shown in Figure 20.13. The patient should try on the shoe and test the insert for comfort, paying special attention to any discomfort during ambulation. The head of the second metatarsal should feel completely free of pressure.

This is a relatively temporary correction. The felt becomes compressed and the insert may wear out after several months of use. Even if the foam insole does not need replacement, it may need an additional layer of felt added to it after a period of use.

With inactivation of the peroneal TrPs and restoration of the exercise tolerance of these muscles, often less padding is required, but complete elimination of the padding makes the muscles prone to reactivation of TrPs.

On return visits, the patient's shoes should be checked for the metatarsal-pad correction. The pads can fall out or slide around in the shoe and may be forgotten when the patient changes shoes or buys a new pair. Recurrence of peroneal myofascial pain symptoms after many months of relief is often due to loss of adequate shoe correction.

A permanent "Flying Dutchman" correction (Fig. 20.14) requires no maintenance and cannot be "forgotten" when shoes are changed. To make this correction, a shoe repairman inserts a leather wedge, with the thick edge medially, 3-mm (1/8-in) thick at the inner (medial) edge, between layers of the leather sole underneath the head of the first metatarsal. For women's shoes in which the sole does not have at least two layers of leather, as usually found in men's shoes, the "Flying Dutchman" can be placed between the existing sole and an added thin rubber sole. Glue-on rubber soles for home use are no longer generally available, but shoe repairmen have thin black rubber half-soles suitable for the purpose.

Badly worn shoe heels should be replaced or a metal cleat or rubber tap added over the worn part. Use of the sole insert with a corrective first metatarsal pad usually ends or greatly reduces the excessive lateral heel-medial sole pattern of shoe wear. Patients with just the Morton foot structure need both a first metatarsal pad and a *flat* heel. Addition of a pad under the shafts of the middle three[2] or all five[76] metatarsals may also be helpful.

If a patient with a short first metatarsal bone walks with the toes in rather than the usual position of slight out-toeing, the first metatarsal pads for correction of the Morton foot structure may prove ineffective. For all individuals, and for these patients especially, foot problems may be aggravated by the patient's heel fitting loosely in a shoe heel that is too wide. Adding felt padding to the inside of the shoe along the sides of the heel usually corrects the problem. Adhesive pads for this purpose can be found in some shoe stores, and the correction can be made when the shoe is bought.

Sometimes a patient with a Morton foot structure is already using a metatarsal support that seems to have helped. The support may be retained but only if it does *not* extend under the head of the second metatarsal. If the support is too short, a first metatarsal pad may be added to lengthen it. Morton[75] recommended both corrections.

Corrective orthoses can be constructed by competent podiatrists or physical therapists who are aware of the principles outlined above.

The clinician should insist that the patient bring all pairs of shoes for evaluation and correction. Each pair may present a different problem for correction. With the Morton foot structure, patients may prefer to walk in their bare feet or bedroom slippers. Bedroom slippers and sandals with rigid soles should be discarded.

Other Corrections

Patients with other foot types or structural deviations (*see* Chapters 26 and 27 of this volume) need appropriate procedures and shoe modification to provide support, comfort, and facilitation of dynamic balance.

An ischial (butt) lift (*see* Chapter 4 of this volume) corrects a small hemipelvis and eliminates or reduces at least one need to cross the legs.

Shoes with a narrow pointed toe and tight cap should be avoided. People who walk barefoot are much less likely to develop bunions than are those who wear tight shoes. Additional pertinent information regarding shoes is found in Section 8 of this chapter.

As people become older, their feet may spread and tend to swell. If old shoes that once were snug but comfortable are now too tight, they should be discarded.

Socks that have tight elastic at the top and leave an indented ring in the skin should be replaced or the elastic slackened. A hot iron can be used to release the elastic. The patient should buy hose snug enough to stay up without constricting elastic bands.

Corrective Posture and Activities

Shoes that provide good arch and foot support, such as some sneakers, jogging shoes, and boots that are snug, effectively reduce strain on the peroneal muscles, thus making specific TrP therapy more effective. High heels and spike heels should be avoided.

For correction of underthigh compression caused by too high a chair seat, possible solutions include a footstool to raise the feet, shortening of the chair legs, or tilting the seat bottom downward at the front.

The patient with TrPs and weakness of the peroneus longus and peroneus brevis muscles should avoid walking on a slanted sidewalk or running on a laterally slanted track, which contributes to overload of those muscles.

Corrective Exercises
(Fig. 20.15)

The Peroneal Self-stretch Exercise for the peroneus longus and peroneus brevis muscles is more effective if performed in a warm bath or hot tub with circulating water (Fig. 20.15). Gentle passive stretch of the peroneus longus and peroneus brevis muscles results when the patient grasps the forefoot, fully inverts and adducts it, and then pulls it upward toward dorsiflexion. Postisometric relaxation can facilitate painless stretch; the patient uses one hand to stabilize the leg just above the ankle, and uses the other hand to resist an active effort to evert and plantar flex the foot gently while slowly taking in a deep breath. Then, while exhaling slowly and fully relaxing the leg and foot, the patient takes up any slack that develops by maintaining a steady pull toward inversion and dorsiflexion. After a pause, this cycle should be repeated until no fur-

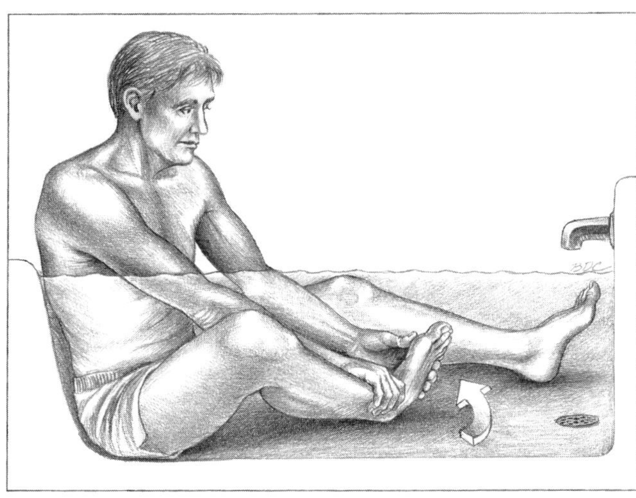

Figure 20.15. Passive self-stretch exercise of the peroneus longus and peroneus brevis muscles, patient seated in a tub of warm water. The *arrow* identifies the direction of pull: inversion first with plantar flexion, then dorsiflexion of the fully inverted foot. This stretch can be effectively combined with postisometric relaxation.

ther gain in the range of inversion and dorsiflexion occurs.

For patients able to handle the additional complexity, further gains may be realized by voluntarily trying to invert and dorsiflex the foot while using the hand to assist moving it in the same direction. This contraction activates antagonists of the peroneus longus and peroneus brevis muscles, reciprocally inhibiting them and thereby increasing their relaxation and tolerance to stretch.

The peroneus longus depresses the first metatarsal for weight bearing, and its cocontraction with the tibialis posterior helps to support the medial arch in runners who have hyperpronating feet and the Morton foot structure. In addition to a metatarsal pad for these individuals, exercises that progressively increase aerobic capacity and endurance of the peroneus longus and the tibialis posterior increase their tolerance for running.[2]

15. CASE REPORTS

Case 20.1

(Seen by J. G. Travell, M.D.)

A female pediatrician in her mid-fifties drove alone 150 miles and arrived at her destination with acute ankle pain and a mild foot drop on the right, the side of her accelerator-pedal foot. She habitually drove her car on long trips. On examination, a clearly defined, triangular patch of cutaneous hypesthesia was noted on the dorsum of the foot between the bases of the first and second toes. The sensory loss was more marked to cold than to touch. The upper part of the right peroneus longus muscle showed an active TrP that, on palpation, referred pain down to the lateral malleolus and to the adjacent lateral region of the foot. Bilaterally, the patient had the Morton foot structure and large bunions.

The active TrP in the right peroneus longus muscle was injected with 0.5% procaine solution, which evoked its referred pattern of pain with no evidence of contact with the common peroneal nerve; 24 hours later, the skin sensation was normal and weakness on extension of the great toe had markedly diminished. The shoe was corrected by insertion of a first metatarsal pad, and the accelerator pedal was lubricated.

She had no further recurrence of her peroneus longus syndrome. She kept the accelerator pedal well lubricated, and used the first metatarsal pad in all her shoes. The patient continued to live a very active life for more than 20 years.

Case 20.2

(Seen by J. G. Travell, M.D.)

Six months before he was first seen in July, the patient, a healthy middle-aged male, had severe left-sided low back pain and the classical signs of lumbar disc protrusion that included neurological deficit, complete foot drop, loss of skin sensation between the first and second toes, and constant severe pain. A myelogram revealed a defect so large that a tumor was suspected. In January, surgery had revealed a ruptured herniated disc. The surgeon reported that much disc material could have escaped among the nerve roots and into the spinal canal.

By June, 5 months following surgery, his left low back and sciatic pain was largely relieved. The power of his foot dorsiflexion had returned to a large extent, although it was still weak. Much of the impaired skin sensation had become normal, but the patient had constant pain in the leg and in the foot. This caused difficulty in sleeping at night. He had been advised to exercise and he attempted to jog. When he returned from jogging, he could hardly move his left foot. At the end of the day, he could not work.

From this preliminary history, I suspected that he had a long second metatarsal bone. When he came to see me, I did find the short first, long second metatarsal Morton foot structure and a remarkably strong local twitch response in the left peroneus longus muscle. Prickling in the foot was produced by pressing on the peroneal nerve just below the left fibular head over the point of potential entrapment by the peroneus longus muscle. Although he had the Morton foot structure in both feet, it was only the left foot that hurt, and the disc had protruded on the left side. He had a lower limb-length inequality, with the left lower limb shorter.

The history revealed further that, when he was a boy, his feet hurt. To his recollection, his feet had always hurt. I stretched and sprayed the peroneal muscles, long toe extensors, and the tibialis anterior muscles bilaterally. Then, I placed first metatarsal pads in his shoes and corrected the lower limb-length inequality with a heel lift on the left side.

Following the treatment, the patient had his first night's sleep without pain for many months. He went jogging the next morning without any pain in either foot. The following day, I again stretched and sprayed the peroneal, anterior tibial, and toe extensor muscles. Three years later, this pain had not recurred.

In summary, the patient had a lower limb-length inequality with a shorter left lower limb that caused greater impact of his weight on the symptomatic (left) side with left peroneal muscle strain due to the mediolateral rocking foot of the Morton foot structure. Permanent relief required simply correction of the shoe for the Morton foot structure, correction for lower limb-length inequality, and treatment by intermittent cold with stretch of the involved peroneal muscles and their associated extensor muscles in the leg.

References

1. Alexander IJ, Johnson KA, Parr JW: Morton's neuroma: a review of recent concepts. *Orthopedics 10*:103–106, 1987.
2. Anderson A: Personal communication, 1991.
3. Anderson JE: *Grant's Atlas of Anatomy*, Ed. 8. Williams & Wilkins, Baltimore, 1983 (Fig. 4–70).
4. *Ibid*. (Fig. 4–71A).
5. *Ibid*. (Fig. 4–71B).
6. *Ibid*. (Fig. 4–71C).
7. *Ibid*. (Fig. 4–72).
8. *Ibid*. (Fig. 4–73).
9. *Ibid*. (Fig. 4–79).
10. *Ibid*. (Fig. 4–81).
11. *Ibid*. (Fig. 4–106).
12. *Ibid*. (Fig. 4–107).
13. Baker BA: The muscle trigger: evidence of overload injury. *J Neurol Orthop Med Surg 7*:35–44, 1986.
14. Baker BA: Myofascial pain syndromes: ten single muscle cases. *J Neurol Orthop Med Surg 10*: 129–131, 1989.
15. Bardeen CR: The musculature, Sect. 5. In *Morris's Human Anatomy*, edited by C.M. Jackson, Ed. 6. Blakiston's Son & Co., Philadelphia, 1921 (pp. 512, 515–516).
16. Basmajian JV, Deluca CJ: *Muscles Alive*, Ed. 5. Williams & Wilkins, Baltimore, 1985 (pp. 334, 335, 337, 345, 378–379).
17. Basmajian JV, Stecko G: The role of muscles in arch support of the foot. An electromyographic study. *J Bone Joint Surg [Am] 45*:1184–1190, 1963.
18. Bates T, Grunwaldt E: Myofascial pain in childhood. *J Pediatr 53*:198–209, 1958.
19. Bowker JH, Olin FH: Complete replacement of the peroneus longus muscle by a ganglion with compression of the peroneal nerve: a case report. *Clin Orthop 140*:172–174, 1979.
20. Broer MR, Houtz SJ: *Patterns of Muscular Activity in Selected Sports Skills*. Charles C Thomas, Springfield, 1967.
21. Cachia VV, Grumbine NA, Santoro JP, *et al.*: Spontaneous rupture of the peroneus longus tendon with fracture of the os peroneum. *J Foot Surg 27*:328–333, 1988.
22. Carter BL, Morehead J, Wolpert SM, *et al.*: *Cross-Sectional Anatomy*. Appleton-Century-Crofts, New York, 1977 (Sects. 72–85).
23. *Ibid*. (Sects. 73–83).
24. *Ibid*. (Sects. 80–84).
25. Clemente CD: *Gray's Anatomy of the Human Body*, American Ed. 30. Lea & Febiger, Philadelphia, 1985 (p. 575).
26. *Ibid*. (pp. 579–581).
27. *Ibid*. (p. 1230, Fig. 12–59, pp. 1241–1243).
28. Cox JS, Brand RL: Evaluation and treatment of lateral ankle sprains. *Phys Sportsmed 5*:51–55, 1977.
29. Cross MJ, Crichton KJ, Gordon H, *et al.*: Peroneus brevis rupture in the absence of the peroneus longus muscle and tendon in a classical ballet dancer: a case report. *Am J Sports Med 16*: 677–678, 1988.
30. Davies JA: Peroneal compartment syndrome secondary to rupture of the peroneus longus: a case report. *J Bone Joint Surg [Am] 61*:783–784, 1979.
31. Duchenne GB: *Physiology of Motion*, translated by E.B. Kaplan. J.B. Lippincott, Philadelphia, 1949 (pp. 305–9, 313, 319, 362–363, 395, 408).
32. *Ibid*. (pp. 345–346).
33. Evjenth O, Hamberg J: *Muscle Stretching in Manual Therapy, A Clinical Manual*. Alfta Rehab Førlag, Alfta, Sweden, 1984 (pp. 140, 147).

34. Ferner H, Staubesand J: *Sobotta Atlas of Human Anatomy*, Ed. 10, Vol. 2. Urban & Schwarzenberg, Baltimore, 1983 (Fig. 380).
35. *Ibid.* (Fig. 458).
36. *Ibid.* (Fig. 462).
37. *Ibid.* (Figs. 465, 467).
38. *Ibid.* (Figs. 468, 469).
39. *Ibid.* (Figs. 472–474).
40. *Ibid.* (Fig. 488).
41. *Ibid.* (Figs. 500, 503).
42. *Ibid.* (Fig. 504).
43. Good MG: Painful feet. *Practitioner 163*:229–232, 1949.
44. Hammerschlag WA, Goldner JL: Chronic peroneal tendon subluxation produced by an anomalous peroneus brevis: case report and literature review. *Foot Ankle 10*:45–47, 1989.
45. Harris RI, Beath T: The short first metatarsal: its incidence and clinical significance. *J Bone Joint Surg [Am] 31*:553–565, 1949.
46. Henstorf JE, Olson S: Compartment syndrome: pathophysiology, diagnosis, and treatment. *Surg Rounds for Orthop*: pp. 33–41, Feb. 1987.
47. Jacobsen S: Myofascielt smertesyndrom (Myofascial pain syndrome). *Ugeskr Laeger 149*:600–601, 1987.
48. Janda V: *Muscle Function Testing*. Butterworths, London, 1983 (pp. 200–202).
49. Jeyaseelan N: Anatomical basis of compression of common peroneal nerve. *Anat Anz 169*:49–51, 1989.
50. Kamon E: Electromyographic kinesiology of jumping. *Arch Phys Med Rehabil 52*:152–157, 1971.
51. Kellgren JH: Observations on referred pain arising from muscle. *Clin Sci 3*:175–190, 1938 (pp. 179, 186).
52. Kendall FP, McCreary EK: *Muscles, Testing and Function*, Ed. 3. Williams & Wilkins, Baltimore, 1983 (pp. 138, 143).
53. Kernohan J, Levack B, Wilson JN: Entrapment of the superficial peroneal nerve. Three case reports. *J Bone Joint Surg [Br] 67*:60–61, 1985.
54. Kopell HP, Thompson WAL: *Peripheral Entrapment Neuropathies*. Robert E. Krieger Publishing Co., Huntington, New York, 1976 (pp. 34–38).
55. *Ibid.* (pp. 40–43).
56. *Ibid.* (pp. 44–50).
57. Krammer EB, Lischka MF, Gruber H: Gross anatomy and evolutionary significance of the human peroneus III. *Anat Embryol 155*:291–302, 1979.
58. Lange M: *Die Muskelhärten (Myogelosen)*. J.F. Lehmanns, München, 1931 (pp. 136, 137, Fig. 43).
59. Larsen E: Longitudinal rupture of the peroneus brevis tendon. *J Bone Joint Surg [Br] 69*:340–341, 1987.
60. Leach RE, Purnell MB, Saito A: Peroneal nerve entrapment in runners. *Am J Sports Med 17*: 287–291, 1989.
61. LeMelle DP, Janis LR: Longitudinal rupture of the peroneal brevis tendon: a study of eight cases. *J Foot Surg 28*:132–136, 1989.
62. Le Minor JM: Comparative anatomy and significance of the sesamoid bone of the peroneus longus muscle (os peroneum). *J Anat 151*:85–99, 1987.
63. Lenteil GL, Katzman LL, Walters MR: The relationship between muscle function and ankle stability. *J Sports Phys Therap 11*:605–611, 1990.
64. Lockhart RD: *Living Anatomy*, Ed. 7. Faber & Faber, London, 1974 (pp. 66–67, Figs. 136, 138, 140).
65. Lowdon IMR: Superficial peroneal nerve entrapment. A case report. *J Bone Joint Surg [Br] 67*:58–59, 1985.
66. Mann RA, Moran GT, Dougherty SE: Comparative electromyography of the lower extremity in jogging, running, and sprinting. *Am J Sports Med 14*:501–510, 1986.
67. Matsusaka N: Control of the medial-lateral balance in walking. *Acta Orthop Scand 57*:555–559, 1986.
68. McAuliffe TB, Fiddian NJ, Browett JP: Entrapment neuropathy of the superficial peroneal nerve. A bilateral case. *J Bone Joint Surg [Br] 67*: 62–63, 1985.
69. McMinn RMH, Hutchings RT: *Color Atlas of Human Anatomy*. Year Book Medical Publishers, Chicago, 1977 (pp. 282, 285, 289).
70. *Ibid.* (p. 305C).
71. *Ibid.* (p. 312).
72. *Ibid.* (p. 318).
73. *Ibid.* (p. 319).
74. *Ibid.* (p. 321).
75. Morton DJ: *The Human Foot. Its Evolution, Physiology and Functional Disorders*. Columbia University Press, New York, 1935.
76. Morton DJ: Foot disorders in women. *J Am Med Women's Assoc 10*:41–46, 1955.
77. Netter FH: *The Ciba Collection of Medical Illustrations*, Vol. 8, Musculoskeletal System. Part I: Anatomy, Physiology and Metabolic Disorders. Ciba-Geigy Corporation, Summit, 1987 (p. 98).
78. *Ibid.* (p. 99).
79. *Ibid.* (pp. 100, 104).
80. *Ibid.* (p. 102).
81. *Ibid.* (p. 103).
82. *Ibid.* (p. 107).
83. *Ibid.* (pp. 109, 111).
84. Pagliano J: The final word on the most talked-about toe in running. *Runner's World*: pp. 68–69, Sept. 1980.
85. Parashar SK, Lal HG, Krishnan NR: 'Harvesters Palsy': Common peroneal nerve entrapment neuropathy. (Report of 5 cases). *J Assoc Physicians India 24*:257–262, 1976.
86. Peacock KC, Resnick EJ, Thoder JJ: Fracture of the os peroneum with rupture of the peroneus longus tendon: a case report and review of the literature. *Clin Orthop 202*:223–226, 1986.
87. Perlmutter M, Ahronson Z, Heim M, *et al.*: A case of foot-drop and the significance of a popliteal mass. *Orthop Rev 10*:134–136, 1981.
88. Rasch PJ, Burke RK: *Kinesiology and Applied Anatomy*, Ed. 6. Lea & Febiger, Philadelphia, 1978 (pp. 318, 319–320, 330, Table 17–2).
89. Reynolds MD: Myofascial trigger point syndromes in the practice of rheumatology. *Arch Phys Med Rehabil 62*:111–114, 1981.

90. Rohen JW, Yokochi C: *Color Atlas of Anatomy*, Ed. 2. Igaku-Shoin, New York, 1988 (p. 426).
91. Sammarco GJ, DiRaimondo CV: Chronic peroneus brevis tendon lesions. *Foot Ankle 9*:163–170, 1989.
92. Sidey JD: Weak ankles. A study of common peroneal entrapment neuropathy. *Br Med J 3*: 623–626, 1969.
93. Simons DG: Myofascial pain syndrome due to trigger points, Chapter 45. In *Rehabilitation Medicine* edited by Joseph Goodgold. C.V. Mosby Co., St. Louis, 1988 (pp. 686–723, *see* pp. 711–712, Fig. 45–9E).
94. Simons DG, Travell JG: Myofascial pain syndromes, Chapter 25. In *Textbook of Pain*, edited by P.D. Wall and R. Melzack, Ed 2. Churchill Livingstone, London, 1989 (pp. 368–385, *see* p. 378, Fig. 25.9F).
95. Sridhara CR, Izzo KL: Terminal sensory branches of the superficial peroneal nerve: an entrapment syndrome. *Arch Phys Med Rehabil 66*:789–791, 1985.
96. Styf J: Entrapment of the superficial peroneal nerve. Diagnosis and results of decompression. *J Bone Joint Surg [Br] 71*:131–135, 1989.
97. Sutherland DH: An electromyographic study of the plantar flexors of the ankle in normal walking on the level. *J Bone Joint Surg [Am] 48*:66–71, 1966.
98. Takebe K, Hirohata K: Peroneal nerve palsy due to fabella. *Arch Orthop Trauma Surg 99*:91–95, 1981.
99. Thompson FM, Patterson AH: Rupture of the peroneus longus tendon: report of three cases. *J Bone Joint Surg [Am] 71*:293–295, 1989.
100. Travell J: Low back pain and the Dudley J. Morton foot (long second toe). *Arch Phys Med Rehabil 56*:566, 1975.
101. Travell J, Rinzler SH: The myofascial genesis of pain. *Postgrad Med 11*:425–434, 1952.
102. Travell JG, Simons DG: *Myofascial Pain and Dysfunction: The Trigger Point Manual*. Williams & Wilkins, Baltimore, 1983.
103. *Ibid*. (pp. 86–87).
104. *Ibid*. (p. 88).
105. *Ibid*. (p. 110–112).
106. Tropp H, Odenrick P: Postural control in single-limb stance. *J Orthop Res 6*:833–839, 1988.
107. Wilson RC, Moyles BG: Surgical treatment of the symptomatic os peroneum. *J Foot Surg 26*: 156–158, 1987.
108. Woltman HW: Crossing the legs as a factor in the production of peroneal palsy. *JAMA 93*: 670–674, 1929.

CHAPTER 21
Gastrocnemius Muscle

"Calf Cramp Muscle"

HIGHLIGHTS: **REFERRED PAIN** from myofascial trigger points (TrPs) in the gastrocnemius muscle may extend from the instep of the ipsilateral foot, over the posteromedial aspect of the ankle and over the calf and back of the knee to the lower posterior thigh. The most common TrP, TrP_1, located along the medial border of the medial head proximal to midbelly of the muscle, projects the most extensive pattern. The other three gastrocnemius TrP locations refer pain more locally around the TrP. **ANATOMICAL ATTACHMENTS** of this muscle cause it to **span** two joints, the knee and ankle. Proximally, the medial and lateral heads attach separately to the distal femur posteriorly; distally, the fibers end on an aponeurosis that joins the soleus muscle to form the tendo calcaneus. This combined tendon of the two muscles attaches to the posterior surface of the calcaneus. A third head of the gastrocnemius, when present, is an unusual variant that also attaches to the femur. **INNERVATION** of the gastrocnemius is supplied by medial popliteal and tibial nerve fibers derived from spinal segments S_1 and S_2. This muscle **FUNCTIONS** to assist other plantar flexors in controlling the forward rotation of the leg over the fixed foot during ambulation, and it contributes to stabilization of the knee. It acts in unusually vigorous plantar flexion of the foot. The **FUNCTIONAL UNIT** that includes the soleus muscle comprises a close-knit team. The chief antagonists are the tibialis anterior and the extensor digitorum longus. **SYMPTOMS** relating to gastrocnemius TrPs are nocturnal calf cramps for TrP_1 and pain in the referred patterns evoked by any active TrPs in the muscle. **ACTIVATION AND PERPETUATION OF TRIGGER POINTS** in the gastrocnemius muscle depend largely on physical overload and malpositioning of the foot. Climbing steep slopes, jogging uphill, riding a bicycle with the seat too low, and wearing a cast on the leg can activate the TrPs. Leaving the foot plantar flexed for prolonged periods is likely to perpetuate them. **PATIENT EXAMINATION** reveals primarily inability to extend the knee fully with the ankle in dorsiflexion. **TRIGGER POINT EXAMINATION** should include all four TrP locations in the gastrocnemius muscle. Proximally, tender superficial aponeurotic bands along the medial and lateral borders of the muscle can be mistaken for tender taut bands of TrPs in the muscle fibers. **ENTRAPMENT** of nerves is rarely caused by this muscle. However, some proximal configurations of its anomalous third head can cause serious vascular compression that requires surgical release. **ASSOCIATED TRIGGER POINTS** are found in the agonistic soleus and hamstring muscles and sometimes in the long flexors of the toes and in the tibialis posterior muscle. TrPs in the gastrocnemius are also sometimes associated with TrPs in the antagonistic tibialis anterior and long extensors of the toes. The **INTERMITTENT COLD-WITH-STRETCH** procedure starts with the application of ice or vapocoolant spray distalward over the muscle and the referred pain pattern to the instep. The patient is positioned prone to hold the knee straight while the ankle is passively dorsiflexed over the end of the treatment table to take up slack as muscle tension is released. **INJECTION** of TrP_1 and TrP_2 is relatively simple and free of hazard. However, when injecting TrP_3, an anomalous course of the popliteal artery can bring it within reach of the needle. The likelihood of such an aberrant course is greatly increased when a third head of the gastrocnemius muscle is present. **CORRECTIVE ACTIONS** include reducing sustained plantar flexion, e.g., by avoiding shoes with high heels and by using a footrest if the heels do not reach the floor when the individual is seated. Gastrocnemius self-stretch exercises are usually effective.

Immediate relief from calf cramps may be obtained by passively stretching the gastrocnemius muscle (dorsiflexing the foot, with the knee straight). Recurrences of cramps are usually prevented by inactivating the responsible gastrocnemius TrPs, which are perpetuated by sustained plantar flexion of the foot at night. Also, elevating the foot of the bed and taking vitamin E as a therapeutic trial help alleviate nocturnal calf cramps in some individuals.

1. REFERRED PAIN
(Fig. 21.1)

Gastrocnemius TrPs tend to cluster in four locations designated TrP_1–TrP_4 (Fig. 21.1). The first pair, TrP_1 and TrP_2, are found just proximal to the midlevel of the medial and lateral muscle bellies, respectively. The other two, TrP_3 and TrP_4, are located behind the knee near where the medial and lateral heads each attach to a femoral condyle. Thus, each head has two TrP regions, located toward its outer margin. The most common, TrP_1, occurs distal to the knee, close to the medial border of the *medial head* of the gastrocnemius muscle (TrP_1, Fig. 21.1). This TrP_1 refers pain primarily to the instep of the ipsilateral foot with a spillover zone that extends from the region of the lower posterior thigh, over the back of the knee, and down the posteromedial aspect of the leg to the ankle.

The next most common location for gastrocnemius TrPs is TrP_2, which is found slightly more distal, near the lateral border of the belly of the *lateral head*. This TrP_2 and the two remaining gastrocnemius TrPs, TrP_3 and TrP_4, all refer pain primarily locally around and near the TrP (Fig. 21.1).

Tenderness in the region of TrP_3 and TrP_4 can be caused by musculotendinous tension produced by taut bands accompanying a TrP_1 or TrP_2. Either or both of the two TrP regions behind the knee (TrP_3 and TrP_4), however, may harbor TrPs with their own palpable taut bands in the absence of the two more distal TrPs. They produce pain primarily in the popliteal fossa. Rarely, all four gastrocnemius TrPs occur together. In that case, after the more distal TrP_1 and TrP_2 have been inactivated, the patient then becomes aware of the pain in the back of the knee that is caused by TrP_3 or TrP_4.

Both TrP_1 and TrP_2 are likely to be associated with nocturnal calf cramps, but rarely are the two most proximal gastrocnemius TrPs associated with cramps. The nature of calf cramps and their relation to myofascial TrPs are considered further in Section 6.

The TrP_1 referred pain pattern has been reported previously for adults,[153,155,173] and a similar pattern has been reported in children.[23]

Good[64] illustrated four locations of "myalgic spots" in the gastrocnemius muscle that are similar to our designated TrP sites. He identified this muscle as the source of foot pain that was relieved by injecting procaine into all of these myalgic spots. Sola[156,157] illustrated pain from TrPs in the medial and lateral margins of the gastrocnemius muscle as extending around the TrPs. Kelly[83] described pain from "fibrositic lesions" in this muscle as extending anywhere from the back of the knee to the lower part of the leg; the pain was relieved by injecting the lesions with procaine. Arcangeli and associates[13] illustrated the pain from a "trigger area" located between the areas we describe as TrP_1 and TrP_2, which projected pain along the back of the lower limb from above the knee to midleg.

Kellgren[82] demonstrated experimentally the potential of gastrocnemius nociceptors to refer pain by injecting 0.2 mL of 6% saline solution into the muscle belly. Pain radiated over the posterior aspect of the lower limb from the buttock to the ankle.

The association of gastrocnemius TrPs with intermittent claudication and the fact that claudication pain may be markedly increased by the TrPs are discussed in Section 6 of this chapter.

2. ANATOMICAL ATTACHMENTS AND CONSIDERATIONS
(Fig. 21.2)

The gastrocnemius is the most superficial muscle of the calf and is primarily responsible for its contour. The muscle crosses the knee and the ankle and is divided into two clearly separated bellies, the medial and lateral heads. The medial head is thicker and extends farther distally than the lateral head. ***Proximally***,

PART 3

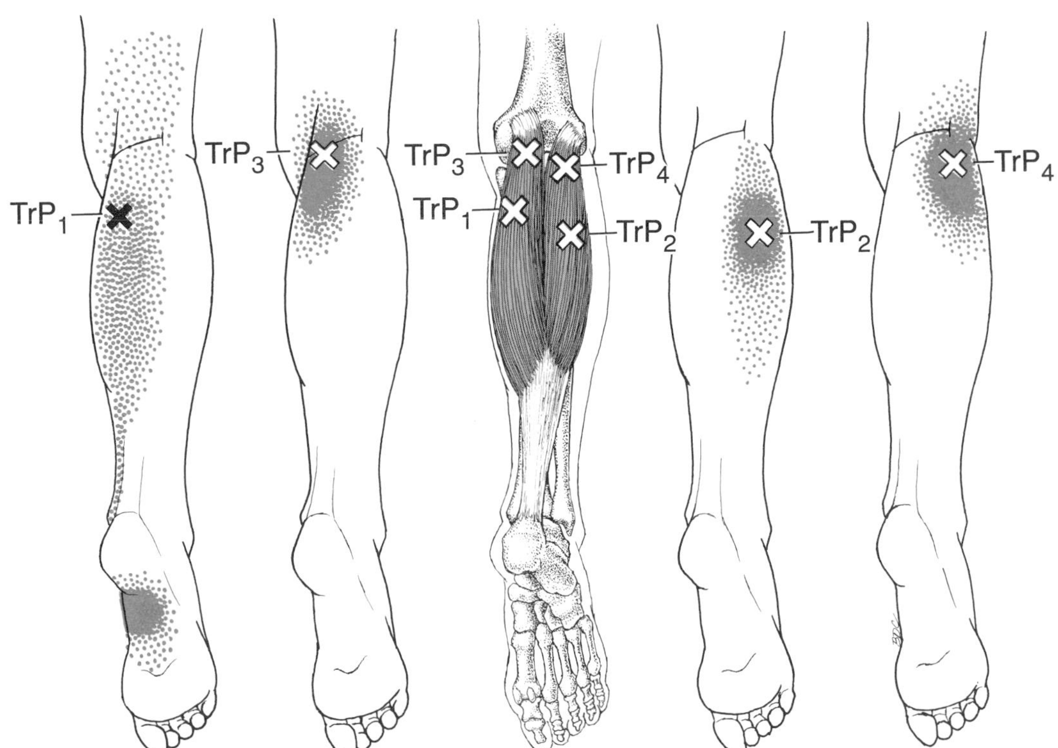

Figure 21.1. Pain (*dark red*) referred from trigger points (***X**s*) in the right gastrocnemius muscle (*light red*). The essential pain pattern is *solid red*. *Red stippling* indicates the spillover extension of the essential pattern. TrP_1 in the belly of the medial head, and to a lesser extent TrP_2 in the belly of the lateral head, are likely to be present when the patient has painful nocturnal calf cramps. The two more proximal trigger points, TrP_3 and TrP_4, project pain higher to the back of the knee.

each head attaches to the corresponding condyle of the femur[2,53,103] by a strong, flat tendon and to the underlying capsule of the knee joint. The thickest part of the tendon lies close to the outer margin of each head. ***Distally***, both heads have a common attachment to the tendo calcaneus (Achilles tendon),[6] which is fixed to the posterior surface of the calcaneus (Fig. 21.2).

The muscle belly is 15–18 cm (6–7 in) long, but individual fibers are only 5.0–6.5 cm (2–2½ in) in length.[179] The fibers are angled diagonally between their superficial and deep aponeuroses.

The aponeurosis of the tendo calcaneus extends along the under side of the muscle almost to the knee to provide attachment for these relatively short fibers. A thickening of this aponeurosis divides the two heads and serves as an intermuscular septum for attachment of muscle fibers. This aponeurosis has the shape of a "T" in cross section. The aponeuroses of the two femoral attachments cover the proximal two-thirds of the posterior surface of each head. The muscle fibers angle between this superficial aponeurosis and the deep aponeurosis of the tendo calcaneus.[18]

The details of this fiber arrangement[18] are important when palpating for taut bands in this muscle. The fiber arrangement is poorly shown in Figure 21.2 and also in the drawings of many anatomy texts. Some illustrations,[7,18,104,108,138] however, do show this diagonal fiber orientation well. In general, the most proximal fibers of the two heads of the gastrocnemius muscle are strongly angulated to form a "V" shape. As one proceeds distally, the fibers gradually become aligned with the leg. The most central fibers of both heads, however, continue to angulate toward the intermuscular septum. When palpating the proximal portion of the muscle, it is important to distinguish between tender diagonal taut bands of

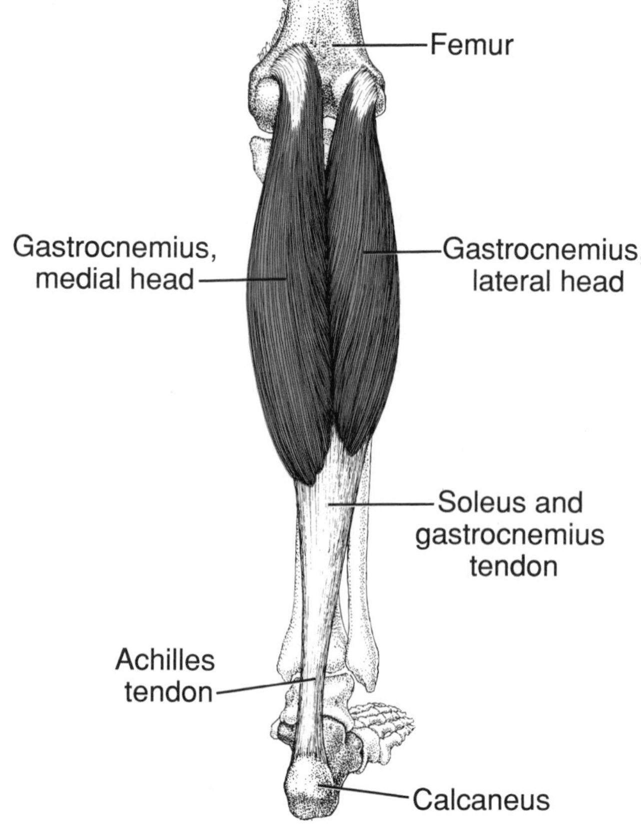

Figure 21.2. Attachments of the right gastrocnemius muscle (*red*) seen from the rear. The distal (deep) aponeurosis of the gastrocnemius merges with the superficial soleus aponeurosis to form the Achilles tendon.

muscle fibers and longitudinally oriented tendons that also feel firm and "ropy." A tendon may exhibit tenderness along the line of attachment of the fibers to the aponeurosis.

A third head of the gastrocnemius muscle is a variant that has been reported in approximately 5.5% of Japanese people and in 2.9–3.4% of people of other nationalities.[78] This head attaches proximally to the posterior surface of the femur between the attachments of the medial and lateral heads and sometimes considerably proximal to them. Distally, the third head may join either the medial or lateral head of the muscle, more often the medial head.[78] Detailed drawings of this third head show that it may cross over part or all of the neurovascular bundle containing the popliteal vessels and tibial nerve.[61]

Two bursae are associated with the gastrocnemius muscle. Illustrations of the lateral gastrocnemius bursa[2,5,34,53] show that it lies between the tendon of the lateral head of the gastrocnemius muscle and the posterior capsule of the knee joint, and that it sometimes communicates with the joint.[34]

The other bursa, the calcaneal subtendinous bursa,[6,55] is interposed between the Achilles tendon and the calcaneus.[36]

A sesamoid (the fabella) in the proximal tendon of the lateral head appeared in 27–29% of dissections. A sesamoid was found about half as often in the tendon of the medial head. Only about one-third of these sesamoids were bony; the others were cartilaginous.[74]

Khan and Khan[85] counted the proportions of red, intermediate, and white fibers (those with oxidative, combined, and glycolytic metabolism, respectively) in three autopsy samples from each of ten gastrocnemius and ten soleus muscles. They found marked variability among individuals. The mean percentages of these three fiber types in the gastrocnemius muscle were, respectively, 56%, 11%, and 33%. (As expected, the soleus muscles had an even greater proportion of red fibers.)

The average length of muscle fibers in the single-joint soleus muscle was only 3.7 cm ($1\frac{1}{2}$ in) as compared with an average length of 5.8 cm ($2\frac{5}{16}$ in) in the gastrocnemius muscle that crosses two functional joints.[179]

The myoneural junctions in the gastrocnemius muscle of a stillborn infant were found to form a horseshoe-shaped line approximately halfway between the outer margins of the muscle and the midline separation of its two heads.[30]

Supplemental References

Both heads of the gastrocnemius are illustrated from behind with clear detail of fiber direction,[7,18,104,108,138] and with a less detailed overview.[57,161,167] The tibial nerve and popliteal artery and vein are shown passing between the two heads as the heads diverge to form the popliteal fossa.[3,52,106,124]

The lateral head is presented from a lateral view with clear delineation of tendon and fibers,[105,140] and with less structural detail.[55,107,159]

The medial head is viewed from the medial aspect with clear resolution of the extent of the aponeurosis,[139] and with less structural detail.[54,107] This head can also be seen from the front,[56,160] and in cross section.[28,58]

3. INNERVATION

Both heads of the gastrocnemius muscle are supplied by branches of the tibial nerve. The nerve fibers are derived from spinal segments S_1 and S_2.[4,35,37]

4. FUNCTION

During standing and walking, the gastrocnemius frequently functions in what is sometimes called a "reverse pull"; that is, it pulls on the proximal segment. This muscle functions through lengthening contractions much of the time in the weight-bearing position.

During ambulation, the plantar flexors (including the gastrocnemius) restrain (control) the forward rotation of the tibia on the talus during stance phase,[165] contribute to knee stability, provide ankle stability, and conserve energy by minimizing vertical oscillation of the center of mass of the body.[166] Ordinarily, they do not propel the body forward,[166] and the gastrocnemius generally contributes little or no push-off even in running.[99]

The gastrocnemius muscle is inactive or minimally active during erect standing unless balance is disturbed, and becomes more active when one is leaning forward. It functions as a reserve muscle for plantar flexion in activities such as walking up steep grades, ascending and descending stairs, jumping, and bicycling.

The differences in function between the gastrocnemius and soleus muscles derive from differences in fiber length, fiber type, and anatomical attachments. The gastrocnemius is a functional two-joint muscle that is shortened by knee flexion but has improved leverage for ankle function in the extended position of the knee. However, the soleus crosses only the ankle and is mechanically unaffected by knee angle.

The chief action of the gastrocnemius muscle, when the foot is free to move, is to plantar flex the foot; it also tends to produce supination. Although both heads attach to the femur above the knee joint, this muscle exerts only a limited effect as a flexor of the leg at the knee, particularly with the knee extended. The location of this attachment serves the purposes of adjusting gastrocnemius muscle length and stabilizing the knee joint.

Actions

At the knee, the gastrocnemius muscle may assist flexion. At the ankle, the gastrocnemius and soleus muscles together, through the tendo calcaneus, are the prime plantar flexors of the foot. The gastrocnemius muscle is most effective as a plantar flexor when the knee is extended; as the knee becomes progressively more flexed, this muscle loses effectiveness and plantar flexion of the foot is accomplished increasingly by the soleus muscle.

The gastrocnemius, when contracted in the weight-bearing limb with the knee held in full extension, assists stabilization of the knee joint.[130]

The gastrocnemius also supinates the foot. Duchenne[44] observed this supination when he stimulated either head of the muscle. His explanation of this movement was that the force of plantar flexion is transmitted through the calcaneus primarily to the cuboid, and the cuboid transmits the force to only the fourth and fifth metatarsals. This mechanism is illustrated by Anderson.[8] Because the force is applied only to the lateral side of the foot, supination occurs during plantar flexion.

Although the gastrocnemius is reported to flex the leg at the knee,[35,130] Duchenne[44] points out that stimulation of the muscle produces, at most, a very weak flexion. It is fortunate that the action at the knee is weak with the knee extended, because generally, this muscle is acting most forcefully (at the ankle) when the knee needs to be stabilized, as in running and jumping. However, with the improved leverage of the gastrocnemius for knee flexion when the leg is *flexed* 90°, the muscle's effect on flexion at that joint apparently takes on a new significance.

The relative activities of the soleus and the medial head of the gastrocnemius muscle change markedly when a strong effort is required to both flex the knee and plantar flex the ankle.[65] With the knee fixed at 90° of flexion and the ankle fixed in the neutral position, sitting subjects were asked to exert effort to produce various combinations of knee flexion and ankle plantar flexion at 0, 25%, 50%, and 100% of maximum voluntary force. The gastrocnemius responded with increasing electrical activity for all combinations of effort. With increasing simultaneous effort at both the knee and ankle joints, gastrocnemius activity increased markedly while that of the soleus declined.[65] This selective activation of the gastrocnemius apparently occurs because of the greater flexion force the muscle can exert when the knee is bent than when it is straight. It takes place despite shortening of the gastrocnemius muscle when the knee is flexed.

The medial and lateral heads of the gastrocnemius muscle show some functional differences. Andriacchi and co-workers,[10] using fine-wire electrodes, tested four healthy males who exerted isometric knee-flexion effort to resist a strong knee-extension force ranging up to 32 newton-meters with the knee held at an angle of 40° of flexion. Electromyographic (EMG) activity of the *lateral* head during knee flexion effort reached only 10–20% of maximum EMG activity for all angles and all force levels tested. The force exerted ranged from 8–32 newton-meters. The only vigorous response of the gastrocnemius muscle to knee flexion effort was by the *medial* head at 40° of flexion; its EMG activity reached 70% of maximum at 32 newton-meters of force.[10]

The considerable antagonistic activity of the medial head on knee extension effort was interpreted as supplying a stabilizing force for the knee joint.[10] The vigorous graded activity of the lateral head at lesser angles of knee flexion during extension effort was interpreted as specifically countering the slight tendency of the quadriceps femoris muscles to produce an adduction-type moment of force at the knee joint.[10]

The gastrocnemius and soleus muscles have the least refined motor control of any of the muscles in the body. Instead of the usual motor unit innervation ratio of about 500 muscle fibers per motor nerve axon present in the majority of skeletal muscles, these two muscles have nearly 2,000 muscle fibers per axon.[20]

Functions

Postural Control

In the standing position, the gastrocnemius and soleus muscles are activated to maintain balance when the line of gravity is in front of the axis of the ankle joint. There is frequently a periodicity in the activity of these muscles that is apparently related to an almost imperceptible forward-and-backward sway of the body. A shift of as little as 5° produces reflex activity of the posterior or anterior leg muscles. The soleus tends to become active before the gastrocnemius under light loads.[21]

Campbell and associates[27] used fine-wire electrodes inserted into the medial and lateral heads of the gastrocnemius muscle proximally and into the medial and lateral portions of the soleus muscle distal to the gastrocnemius fibers to ensure clear separation of recorded EMG activity. They found that when the subjects stood in bare feet the two heads of the gastrocnemius were quiescent until contraction was needed to give impetus to forward motion. Inversion of the foot while standing barefoot increased activity at all four sites; however, the activity in both the medial head of the gastrocnemius and the medial portion of the soleus increased threefold as compared to that in the lateral electrode sites. Eversion of the foot produced an equal increase in activity in both heads of the gastrocnemius. The stabilizing function was tested when standing on heels of various heights and widths. Both heads of the gastrocnemius showed increased stabilizing activity when confronted with unstable heel foundations.

In another study,[21] standing on heels 6 and 7.5 cm ($2\frac{1}{2}$ and 3 in) in height increased the EMG activity observed in the lateral head of the gastrocnemius muscle.

Campbell and co-workers[27] also observed that, in movements requiring variable effort, the athletes in their study showed smoothly graded increases and decreases in muscle activity among the four sites in the gastrocnemius and soleus that were monitored. In non-athletes, there was no such smooth variation; both the degree and duration of activity fluctuated markedly and in no particular pattern. Apparently, either training or an athletic propensity imparted a synchronous blending of component muscular activities that was absent in non-athletes.

When standing subjects were required to respond to sudden forceful movements of their hands and arms, EMG activity for stabilization consistently appeared in the gastrocnemius muscle before local responses appeared in the upper extremity muscles.[39]

Okada[118] found that the postures that produced the most EMG activity in the medial and lateral heads of the gastrocnemius muscle were standing on the balls of the feet and leaning forward while standing with the feet flat on the floor. Ninety degrees of forward flexion of the trunk induced less activity. Standing straight produced negligible activity in either head of the gastrocnemius; when standing at ease, the muscle on the side bearing the most weight sometimes briefly reached 10% of maximum EMG activity.[118]

Relating EMG activity to the center of foot pressure, Okada and Fujiwara[119] used surface electrodes and found that all parts of the triceps surae were active when the center of pressure was in front of the middle of the foot, as measured from the heel to the tip of the great toe. As the center of pressure moved posterior to that midregion, the tibialis anterior became active instead of the calf muscles. The transition at this part of the foot suggests that the functional axis of the human foot for dorsi-plantar flexion while bearing body weight lies adjacent to the transverse-tarsal joint rather than within the talocrural joint.

Perry and associates[125] examined the issue of selectivity of surface electrodes for specific muscles and concluded that only 60% of the activity recorded over the gastrocnemius was attributable to that muscle, and a mere 36% of the EMG activity recorded by surface electrodes over the soleus muscle derived from it. Similar non-selectivity of surface electrodes was reported by others.[119,127] The relative advantages and disadvantages of surface versus inserted fine-wire electrodes were examined in detail and summarized by Andersson and associates.[9]

Walking

The triceps surae apparently does not contract to assist "push-off" in walking or running,[99,166] but restrains forward rotation of the tibia on the talus as the weight is shifted during stance phase from the heel to the ball of the foot.[165,166]

The two heads of the gastrocnemius muscle, and the medial and lateral portions of the soleus muscle, when monitored with surface electrodes, showed a remarkably constant timing of the EMG activity pattern with regard to the phase of gait. There was a 75% increase in activity when the walking speed was increased from 2.5 to 4.2 mph and the grade was increased from 0° to 10°. In contrast, the vasti medialis and lateralis of the quadriceps femoris showed a much greater response to these increases in load.[24] The timing of EMG activity of the two heads of the gastrocnemius coincided closely during normal level walking. However, the highest percent of maximum-effort EMG activity reached in 10 subjects was nearly 40% for the medial gastrocnemius and soleus muscles, but only about 20% for the lateral gastrocnemius.[49]

Regardless of uphill grade or speed during walking, calf muscle activity rapidly increased just before heel rise and reached its peak intensity at the transition from knee extension to knee flexion as the ankle began to plantar flex.[24] This study confirmed the earlier observation that EMG activity of the gastrocnemius muscle predominates in the middle part of the stance phase and its intensity is relatively independent of speed. In addition, the optimum pace period per gait cycle for minimum EMG activity was about 1 sec ± 0.2 sec.[110]

The EMG activity of the gastrocnemius showed a variety of patterns at self-selected walking speeds. Shiavi and Griffin[149] performed sophisticated computer analysis on the records of 25 normal individuals to identify different patterns of EMG activity during 16 segments of the gait cycle. They found five common patterns and three unusual ones. All common patterns began shortly after the beginning of stance phase and continued to, and for various periods into, swing phase. Of the recordings made at the highest speed of walking (1.6 m/sec), 5% showed a separate, additional burst of activity just before and at the onset of stance phase.

Recordings from surface electrodes on the gastrocnemius muscle showed that loads equal to 10% and 15% of body weight that were carried in one hand while walking increased the duration of EMG activity only on the ipsilateral side, but a load of 20% increased activity in this muscle bilaterally.[63]

Stair Climbing

A surface electrode study of 25 normal subjects ascending and descending stairs[168] demonstrated that during stair ascension the medial head of the gastrocnemius muscle was active in most people throughout all of the stance phase and for a part of double limb support. During stair descent, the muscle in most subjects anticipated weight bearing and remained active through stance phase until double limb support. In another analysis of the same study,[169] the authors concluded that the atypical patterns of gastrocnemius activity were not related to speed of climbing, and occurred for no apparent reason.

Running, Jumping, and Sports

Mann and co-workers[99] monitored the EMG activity of this lower limb muscle with surface electrodes during jogging, running, and sprinting. In all these activities, the amount of plantar flexion that occurred while the gastrocnemius muscle was active was a small percentage of the plantar flexion observed through the gait cycle. This is further indication that this calf muscle contributes little or nothing at push-off. Activity at this time helps knee extension by preventing dorsiflexion at the ankle. The consistent activity of the gastrocnemius prior to heel-strike, when the tibialis anterior is also active, probably contributes to stabilization of the ankle joint.[99]

Kamon,[81] using surface electrodes on the lateral head of the gastrocnemius muscle, found that when the subject performed a standing jump, an abrupt burst of EMG activity appeared at take-off and stopped suddenly at the commencement of air-borne flight. Moderate activity reappeared before landing and sometimes remained throughout the landing and stabilization period.

Bilateral EMG activity of the lateral head of the gastrocnemius was monitored with surface electrodes during the single-foot volleyball spike and basketball layup. In both situations, EMG activity was vigorous and greater on the dominant side, but not as vigorous as that recorded with equal amplification from the medial section of the soleus muscle distal to the gastrocnemius fibers.[26]

The same recording arrangement[26] was used to record the EMG activity during 11 other right-handed sports activities that included overhand throws, underhand throws, tennis and golf strokes, and hitting a baseball. In each of these, the EMG activity of the soleus was more vigorous than that of the lateral head of the gastrocnemius muscle. In this right-handed subject, activity in the right gastrocnemius was always greater than activity in the left gastrocnemius.

Bicycling

Houtz and associates[76] found that, during stationary bicycling, the medial head of the gastrocnemius muscle was active in the latter half of the power (down) stroke and activity continued into the early return stroke.

Subsequently, Ericson and co-workers[48] found that when subjects were riding an ergometer cycle, the medial head of the gastrocnemius exerted its peak effort (19% of maximum EMG activity) in the middle of the downward power stroke, but the lateral gastrocnemius did not reach its peak effort (23% of maximum EMG activity) until the beginning of the upward return stroke and maintained a high level for another 90° of pedal movement. A lesser initial peak of the lateral head was timed so that it could help move the opposite pedal forward beyond dead center preparatory to the next power stroke. The remaining activity during upward pedal movement may relate to knee stabilization or flexion. The two heads apparently performed different functions, but the nature of the difference is conjectural. Activity of the soleus muscle was synchronous with the downward power stroke and faded quickly on the return stroke. Activity of the medial gastrocnemius muscle was not affected by a change in foot position on the pedal, which changes the mean ankle load moment of force twofold.[48] Together, the plantar flexors of the foot contributed about 20% of the total muscular work on the ergometer cycle.[47]

Resection of Muscles

The effect of anatomical loss on strength and function was studied in nine patients who had lost at least one head, but not all, of the triceps surae.[100] Only two patients reported a mild symptom: unsteadiness of gait when walking on uneven ground. One had lost the lateral gastrocnemius and lateral soleus, and the other, all of the soleus and the medial head of the gastrocnemius. Among these nine patients, in whom up to 75% of the triceps surae muscle mass had been removed, the loss of plantar flexion strength never exceeded 30% with the foot in the neutral position, compared with the normal contralateral side.

In a study of one woman who was normal except for surgical excision of the gastrocnemius and soleus, Murray and associates[114] found that the subject was able to compensate for most of her gait abnormalities by excessive lateral tilt and prolonged quadriceps femoris activity. Her disability was mild and consisted of inability to increase walking speeds beyond the normal pacing.

As demonstrated earlier,[72] the gastrocnemius was more active when an effort was made to plantar flex the foot rapidly in the plantar flexed position, and the soleus was more active when that same effort was exerted in the dorsiflexed position. This conclusion was reinforced[100] by the observation that the two patients in whom parts of the gastrocnemius had been removed had greatest loss of strength in plantar flexion, and those without a soleus muscle suffered the greatest loss of strength with the foot in dorsiflexion. In those patients in whom part of the gastrocnemius had been removed, loss of strength was greatest on fast angular motion at the ankle. This observation supports the view that the gastrocnemius is of greatest importance for the rapid development of power.

Fiber Types, Contractile Properties, Blood Flow

The composition by fiber types of both heads of the gastrocnemius muscle and of the soleus was determined in 32 autopsies.[46] The gastrocnemius muscle contained approximately 50% slow-twitch fibers (type 1) and the soleus muscle contained about 70% slow-twitch fibers. The two heads of the gastrocnemius muscle showed no significant difference in the proportion of fiber types.

A study of 11 normal subjects of both sexes and of unknown athletic training[89] compared the smoothed rectified surface electromyograms of the soleus and lateral gastrocnemius muscles directly on an X-Y plot to identify the relative timing and contribution of each muscle during slow and fast contractions. As expected, the soleus muscle, with predominantly slow-twitch (type 1) fibers, initiated slow contractions. With rapid contractions (hopping on one foot), the lateral head of the gastrocnemius sometimes initiated the activity and sometimes did not. It apparently was used occasionally as a supplementary muscle.

Clarkson and co-workers[32] found that maximum isometric strength was strongly related to fatigability of the gastrocnemius muscle. They biopsied the medial gastrocnemius of eight endurance athletes (competitive long distance runners) and eight power athletes (experienced weight lifters). When the subjects lay prone with the knees straight, plantar flexion at the ankle fatigued five times faster in the relatively strong power-trained group than in the weaker endurance-trained group. Both groups performed the same effort/rest exercise schedule.[32] The same authors,[31] in a companion study, found an equally impressive, but inverse relation between strength and percentage of slow-twitch fibers. The abundance of slow-twitch fibers varied from a minimum of 40% in the strongest (power-trained) athlete to a maximum of 95% in the weakest (endurance-trained) athlete. There was no overlap in the percentage range of slow-twitch fibers in these two groups of athletes.

The contractile properties of the three parts of the triceps surae in ten volunteers[177] showed consistent differences when examined with surface electrodes. The lateral head of the gastrocnemius had the fastest twitch, the medial head had slightly slower twitch, and the soleus muscle had the slowest twitch. The contraction times were, respectively, 100, 114, and 157 ms and the half-relaxation times were 101, 111, and 152 ms. This indicates that the medial head of the gastrocnemius functionally employed a slightly lower proportion of fast-twitch fibers than the lateral head used, and that the soleus muscle had a much lower proportion of these fibers than did either head of the gastrocnemius muscle.

To determine the nature of the shortening of gastrocnemius muscles in stroke patients, Halar and associates[66] compared the resting length and extensibility of the muscle bellies and their tendons in stroke patients with those of normal controls; resting length of the muscle belly was shortened in stroke patients, but not that of its tendon. The spastic muscle fibers appeared to have normal *passive* elongational characteristics; the cause of the shortening was in the contractile tissue of the muscle, not in the tendon.

Examining the force of contraction required to interrupt blood flow in the triceps surae as determined by clearance of ^{133}Xe, Sadamoto and associates[146] found that the mean values for force of contraction that would stop intramuscular blood flow varied between 50% and 64% of the force of maximum voluntary contraction. Interestingly, with increasing fatigue, the muscle "softened" and its contraction more readily obstructed blood flow. As fatigue developed, the mean rectified electromyogram increased and/or the force of contraction decreased, although the intramuscular pressure increased, which further compromised blood flow. Apparently because of the greater angulation of its fibers, the soleus muscle developed lower levels of intramuscular pressure than the gastrocnemius muscle did at the same percentage of maximum voluntary contraction. This study establishes a lower limit to the strength of contraction that causes onset of ischemia in brief contractions, but does not answer the question of how much contraction-induced ischemia can be tolerated for a prolonged period of continuous contraction.

5. FUNCTIONAL (MYOTATIC) UNIT

The gastrocnemius and soleus muscles form a close-knit team. They share the same Achilles tendon that attaches to the calcaneus. Differences in function between the two muscles relate to knee flexion and are described in the preceding section.

At the *knee*, the gastrocnemius assists the hamstrings in flexion, as do also the plantaris, gracilis, and sartorius muscles[129] and the popliteus. At the *ankle*, the gastrocnemius and soleus muscles are the primary plantar flexors. There, they are assisted by the plantaris, peroneus longus and brevis, flexor hallucis longus, flexor digitorum longus, and tibialis posterior muscles.[80,131]

Antagonists to the gastrocnemius at the knee are the four parts of the quadriceps femoris muscle; antagonists at the ankle are the extensors of the toes and the tibialis anterior muscle.

6. SYMPTOMS

This section first presents the symptoms to be expected in a patient with active myofascial TrPs in the gastrocnemius muscle. The differential diagnosis follows. Finally, two associated conditions are reviewed, nocturnal calf cramps and intermittent claudication.

The patient with only *latent* TrPs in the medial head (sometimes in the lateral head) of the gastrocnemius muscle may complain chiefly of calf cramps. When the TrPs become active, the patient is aware of pain in the calf, and sometimes in the back of the knee or instep of the foot, as described and illustrated in Section 1 of this chapter.

The patient may complain of pain in the back of the knee on effort, as when climbing up steep slopes, over rocks, or when walking along a slanted surface, such as a beach or the side of a domed street. Patients with gastrocnemius TrPs are rarely concerned about weakness or restricted range of motion.

Differential Diagnosis

The pain referred from gastrocnemius TrPs can easily be mistakenly attributed to other conditions. The posterior knee, calf, and plantar foot pain from these TrPs can be misinterpreted as an S_1 radiculopathy.[134] However, it is not unusual to see the activation of gastrocnemius TrPs as a complication of this radiculopathy. In this situation, examination of the muscle for TrPs will demonstrate the myofascial component. Electrodiagnostic testing for neuropathy and imaging of the lumbosacral spine helps identify a radiculopathy. The ankle jerk is not affected by TrPs in the gastrocnemius (although it can be suppressed by strongly active TrPs in the soleus). In the case of piriformis entrapment of the sciatic nerve (Chapter 10), imaging is normal but appropriate electrodiagnostic studies show nerve conduction abnormality.

Pain in the lower limbs due to myofascial TrPs in children under 5 years of age often is passed off as "growing pains."[22,23] Martin-du-Pan[101] found that growing pains of the legs in 56 of 60 children were caused by "gelo-myose" of the proximal insertion of the gastrocnemius muscle. The description of "gelo-myose" (myogelosis to other authors[151]) was compatible with myofascial TrPs.

Patients who have undergone a successful laminectomy for lumbar radiculopathy may continue to complain of referred pain that is misinterpreted as the pain for which they had received the surgery. Residual TrPs in posterior muscles of the lower limb, including the gastrocnemius muscle,[145] are likely to be causing this postlaminectomy syndrome. Inactivation of these TrPs often relieves them of the pain completely.

Unfortunately, some laminectomy patients develop postoperative arachnoradiculitis.[132] In many of these cases, a part of the pain is caused by myofascial TrPs, some of which may be in the gastrocnemius muscle. Inactivation of the TrPs is recommended as part of the management program for this condition.[132] Like others, we have found that a search for active TrPs is often rewarded in patients with postlaminectomy pain.

In contrast to the previously mentioned situations in which symptoms caused by myofascial TrPs are ascribed to other causes, there is a group of conditions that should be recognized and whose symptoms should not be misinterpreted as myofascial in origin. Some of these conditions are: tennis leg, posterior compartment syndrome, phlebitis, popliteal synovial (Baker's) cyst, Achilles tendinitis, and retrocalcaneal bursitis.

"**Tennis leg**" is a partial tearing of the medial belly of the gastrocnemius muscle, which is caused by suddenly resisting dorsiflexion of a foot held in marked plantar flexion with the knee in full extension, often with a degree of supination of the foot.[14,62] Serving at tennis is the archetype of such an activity. Immediately after hitting the ball, the back foot, which is supinated in strong plantar flexion, is brought forward as the knee is extended. The foot then takes the force of the full body weight and the gastrocnemius is subjected to a vigorous lengthening contraction. Patients with "tennis leg" experience a sudden intense pain in the calf, as if kicked, followed by circumscribed tenderness and swelling of the medial aspect of the midcalf.

In some cases of this musculotendinous rupture of the gastrocnemius, the location of swelling and tenderness is sufficiently proximal to be confused with thrombophlebitis.[102] A few days following rupture, a hematoma becomes evident in the calf and discoloration extends toward the medial malleolus.[14] The symptoms are sometimes attributed to rupture of the plantaris muscle, but careful examination reveals sharply localized tenderness and, frequently, a palpable defect in the medial belly of the gastrocnemius close to the distal end of its muscle fibers.[62,102]

Failure to recognize rupture of the medial head of the gastrocnemius muscle can lead to a serious complication, **posterior compartment syndrome**.[11,122] This causes more diffuse pain and tenderness. It is best diagnosed by intracompartmental pressure measurements employing continuous infusion or a wick catheter. Treatment should be a prompt and thorough decompression fasciotomy.[71]

Phlebitis can be distinguished from myofascial TrPs by the relatively constant pain regardless of muscular activity and the diffuse warmth, redness, swelling, and tenderness of the foot and leg. Thrombophlebitis is confirmed by Doppler ultrasound and venographic studies.

A **popliteal synovial cyst** (Baker's cyst) causes a palpable swelling in the popliteal space that is best appreciated when the knee is extended,[115] and is confirmed by sonography. This may cause knee pain that should be distinguishable from myofascial TrPs by the lack of muscular involvement. A ruptured Baker's cyst may produce severe pain and tenderness that simulates thrombophlebitis, which can occur with (probably as a result of) a ruptured cyst. The rupture of the Baker's cyst is confirmed by an arthrogram that shows the passage of dye from the joint to the calf muscles; the venogram is negative.[86,128] Aspiration of cyst fluid from the swollen area may be helpful diagnostically and therapeutically.

Achilles tendinitis[25,33] and **retrocalcaneal bursitis**[25,74,123] are more likely to be confused with the referred pain and tenderness from soleus than from gastrocnemius TrPs, and are discussed in Chapter 22 of this volume.

Calf Cramps

The most frequent symptom clearly associated with TrPs in the gastrocnemius muscle is nocturnal calf cramps.

Such cramps (systremma) are common. Estimates of occurrence range from 40% among unselected patients in New York[97] to 49% of the men, 75% of the women, and 16% of healthy children in Germany.[113] Among 121 college students, 115 (95%) had experienced spontaneous muscle cramps at least once, and 18 of these 115 (16%) were awakened from sleep more often than twice per month by cramps, usually of the calf muscles.[116]

Cramps often develop when the subject has been sitting or lying too long without movement and with the foot held in plantar flexion with the gastrocnemius shortened. Usually the affected individual is awakened by intense pain in one calf after several hours of sleep with the foot strongly plantar flexed. The gastrocnemius muscle feels hard due to its vigorous sustained contraction. Many patients seek relief by getting out of bed and standing or walking. Walking tends to stretch the gastrocnemius, but also requires its active contraction, and voluntary contraction in the fully shortened position is a reliable way to reactivate the cramp.

The most effective relief is obtained by stretching the cramped muscle, either by passively or actively dorsiflexing the foot. If effective relief measures are not taken, the cramp may last for half an hour or longer. The muscle may then be sore for a day or two afterward. Other lower limb muscles, including the tibialis anterior and intrinsic foot muscles, can be similarly affected, either separately or with the gastrocnemius.

Recently, the topic of muscle cramps was reviewed by Eaton.[45]

Calf cramps are associated with, and may be induced by, many medical conditions including dehydration (as during hemodialysis),[93,109,142] electrolyte disturbance and metabolic alkalosis (from persistent vomiting),[182] low serum magnesium,[163,182,183] hypokalemia (from diarrhea),[73] hypocalcemia,[182] hypoparathyroidism,[182] heat stress with myoglobinuria,[144] Parkinson's disease with dystonia, and, possibly, diabetes.[97,137] They are not related to occlusive vascular disease.[97] Calf cramps in 64% of 50 cancer patients were not benign idiopathic occurrences but were, often ominously, of neurological origin.[163] Rish[135] noted that 20–30% of 1500 patients with lumbar disc disease and radiculopathy complained of night cramps in the compartment supplied by the compressed nerve root: L_5 compression produced cramps of anterior compartment muscles; S_1 compression produced cramps of posterior compartment muscles. The complaint was likely to persist despite surgical decompression of the nerve root. Although the author[135] made no reference to examining the muscles for TrPs, this observation reinforces the previous conclusion that nerve compression can initiate TrPs in muscles supplied by that nerve. In these patients, the TrPs could have persisted following surgery and then could have become major contributors to the leg cramps. Certain drugs (phenothiazines, vincristine, lithium, cimetidine, and bumetanide) can cause cramps.[109]

Sleep studies for two or three consecutive nights on seven people who complained of painful leg cramps revealed two individuals with nocturnal myoclonus, one with obstructive sleep apnea, and two who were awakened by cramps but showed no sleep abnormality. The timing of the cramps had no relation to the stage of sleep. Nocturnal leg cramps were not related to electroencephalographic changes during sleep and no disturbances characteristic of sleep pathology were noted.[147]

Cramps in the calf have been associated with blockage of movement of the proximal tibiofibular joint.[96]

PART 3

Myofascial TrPs as a Cause of Nocturnal Calf Cramps

When TrPs are present in the medial head of the gastrocnemius muscle, intermittent calf cramps often result.[170] Sometimes, TrPs in the lateral head cause calf cramps. Elimination of the TrPs, when present, usually relieves the calf-cramp syndrome. The fact that calf cramps are so commonly associated with TrPs has not been widely recognized.

Both calf cramps and myofascial TrPs are provoked when the muscle is placed in the shortened position for a period of time, especially when sleeping at night,[164] and by forceful contraction in the shortened position.[92] Calf cramps and TrPs are prone to occur in fatigued (or chilled) muscles[97] and are relieved by passive stretch.[92]

Another type of cramp is *painless* and does not seem to be related to myofascial TrPs. It occurs in hand muscles as well as in lower limb muscles and develops in response to voluntary contraction of the muscle(s) involved. Although painless, it usually is temporarily disabling because it is so strong that the antagonist muscles cannot overpower it. This cramp also can be relieved by steady passive stretch of the contracted muscle. Patients with this type of cramp and hypokalemia may obtain relief by taking supplemental potassium.

Treatment of Nocturnal Calf Cramps

The management of nocturnal calf cramps is reviewed at the end of Section 14 in this chapter.

Etiology of Nocturnal Calf Cramps

Quinine and many of the other drugs recommended for treatment of calf cramps reduce cell membrane excitability. Quinine increases the refractory period of muscle and decreases excitability of the motor endplate region.[141] Chloroquine, a similar drug, may have a similar action. Phenytoin reduces abnormally increased excitability of cell membranes. Carbamazepine apparently decreases nerve excitability, and procainamide primarily decreases muscle fiber membrane responsiveness. This suggests that increased excitability of the myoneural junction or the sarcolemma of the muscle fibers is a major factor causing calf cramps. (Although the mechanism for the sustained contracture of muscle fibers in the taut band of a TrP is not yet established, it would not be surprising if electrical instability of the muscle fiber membrane were a significant contributory factor. These considerations suggest further experimental studies to resolve questions concerning the pathophysiology of both TrPs and calf cramps.)

A different mechanism is suggested by the effectiveness of drugs, such as theophylline and procainamide, that tend to increase vascular perfusion in the muscle. Hirsch[73] remarked that the muscle pump in the legs "sleeps" at night, which contributes to venous stasis and circulatory insufficiency in the calf muscles. Simmons[150] emphasized the probable importance of ischemia in the pain of calf cramps.

EMG recordings of calf cramps have been published.[42,109,148] The cramps are characterized by high-voltage, high-frequency, irregular bursts of motor unit action potentials.[93] Norris and coworkers[116] conducted an extensive EMG study of five healthy volunteers and four patients who experienced episodic muscle cramps. They studied both induced and spontaneous cramps, primarily in the quadriceps femoris muscle, using surface, concentric, or microtip electrodes in multiple locations. Their detailed report makes a number of valuable observations. No EMG or clinical difference existed between spontaneous cramps and those induced by maximally contracting the muscle in the shortened position (as also observed by Basmajian[19]). During cramping, some motor unit potentials were as much as twice the amplitude of, and were polyphasic as compared with, potentials previously recorded at the same site with the same needle during a voluntary contraction. During a cramp, the firing rate of individual motor units greatly increased, sometimes to double the rate (from 34 to 60 discharges per second) observed during voluntary contraction.[116]

The authors[116] also observed that the more intense the EMG activity recorded, the harder (more tense) the muscle felt, and the more pain the subject experienced. When a muscle cramp was left alone, the involuntary electrical activity (and pain) gradually subsided. This spontaneous resolution could result from local metabolic depletion in the muscle or by neural "fatigue" at the spinal level.

The following observations from this study[116] suggest that central nervous system control, at least at the spinal level, plays a role in nocturnal cramps. During a cramp, the electrical activity was spotty throughout the muscle, unlike the more uniform distribution of motor unit activity during normal voluntary muscular contractions. The locations of electrical activity in the muscle shifted from place to place during the cramp. Voluntary contraction of the corresponding contralateral muscle increased the painfulness of the cramp and the amount of EMG activity recorded. As others also found,[19,38,59] voluntary contraction of the ipsilateral antagonist quieted the cramp.

In persons with Schwartz-Jampel syndrome, voluntary contraction of an involved muscle induces a cramp with complex repetitive discharges attributed to ephaptic transmission.[79] This mechanism might account for the appearance of polyphasic potentials during nocturnal cramps. Single-fiber electromyography[162] should make it possible to determine whether ephaptic transmission among the muscle fibers makes a local contribution to the cramps.

Basmajian[19] observed that the cramp induced in calf muscles produced very active electrically normal motor units while the antagonist tibialis anterior was electrically silent. Immediately following recovery with a variety of treatment maneuvers, recruitment of both groups of muscles was normal. It is his impression that there is a reflex inhibition of the antagonist muscle (tibialis anterior in this case) and that an external mechanical assist (passive stretch of cramping muscle) is required to overcome the inhibition. Thus, both the voluntary effort and external assistance to stretch the muscles that are cramping are essential components to optimal treatment. The reason for this needs to be investigated.

Relation to Myofascial Trigger Points

Most of the clinical features of nocturnal calf cramps are compatible with their being causally related to myofascial TrPs. The local twitch response (LTR) of TrPs is likely to have a close relation to calf cramps; to our knowledge, this relationship has not been explored experimentally. TrPs are not the sole cause of cramps, however, and a full understanding of nocturnal muscle cramps awaits further research.

Intermittent Claudication

The term intermittent claudication applies when an individual experiences calf pain after walking a fixed distance. It is generally assumed that the pain is either caused by exercising ischemic leg muscles or is of neurogenic origin caused by spinal stenosis. However, in many patients, myofascial TrPs are a major contributor to the pain. The TrPs are apparently induced, at least in part, by the impaired circulation.

Arcangeli and associates[12] examined 27 patients with intermittent claudication for spot tenderness in the gastrocnemius, soleus, and anterior tibialis muscles. Using a pressure algometer, they found hyperalgesic areas in one or more of these muscles in 12 (44%) of the patients. No diffuse tenderness of muscles was found. The pain threshold in these myalgic areas was below 800 gm; it was above 1200 gm in the homologous region of the normal leg or, if that contralateral area had been amputated, in the biceps femoris. In eight of the 27 patients (30%), pressure on a tender spot induced referred pain in a distribution that was similar to the pain patterns referred from TrPs in these muscles.[173] Arcangeli *et al.*[12] also found that muscles subject to claudication became painful following injection of lower concentrations of sodium chloride solution than did the uninvolved contralateral muscles. The ischemic muscles were diffusely more reactive to this noxious stimulus; this may relate to their tendency to develop TrPs.

In a subsequent study of intermittent claudication, Arcangeli and other co-workers[13] found that the pain and other discomforts that occurred during walking were mainly localized in the calf (81% of 58 patients). Myalgic spots that referred pain on pressure were identified (as in the earlier study) and were often located in the triceps surae and tibialis anterior muscles. In seven of these patients, the walking distance was related more to the sensitivity of myalgic spots than to the reduction of calf blood flow.

Travell and associates[172] reported that seven of eight patients with advanced arteriosclerosis obliterans and intermittent claudication, four of whom were also diabetic, experienced marked improvement of their claudication pain by injection or spray and stretch of TrPs in their calf muscles. Improvement was measured by ergometer tests, walking tolerance, or toe-standing tests.

Subsequently, Dorigo and associates[43] studied TrPs in the calf muscles of 15 patients with intermittent claudication. They identified a TrP when digital pressure on a circumscribed tender spot in the muscle caused a jump response of the patient. In some muscles, pressure on this spot also evoked referred pain. These TrPs were injected with 10 mL of procaine solution. Any remaining TrPs were similarly injected on subsequent visits, up to a total of 10 injections. Following this treatment, workload and work duration of the calf muscles increased significantly. However, the peak blood flow and duration of exercise hyperemia in the muscles did not change.

TrPs can be present in the skin as well as in the muscle of the calf. Trommer and Gellman[176] described a patient who had cutaneous TrPs associated with intermittent claudication that restricted walking to 46 meters (50 yards). Three TrPs were located in the *skin* overlying the belly of the right calf muscle. Infiltrating them with anesthetic caused excruciating pain down to the outer malleolus, but afterward the patient could walk 366 meters (400 yards) and resumed playing 18 holes of golf.

In summary, a major component responsible for the pain of intermittent claudication in many patients may be myofascial TrPs in the gastrocnemius and soleus muscles. The TrPs appear to develop as a result of the ischemia. Inactivation of the TrPs improves performance because of pain relief, but does not improve circulation.

7. ACTIVATION AND PERPETUATION OF TRIGGER POINTS

Gastrocnemius TrPs are often activated by chilling of the muscle and by mechanical overload. Perpetuating factors include sustained contraction, sustained shortening, immobility, and compromised circulation. Some of these factors may contribute both to initial activation and to perpetuation of gastrocnemius TrPs.

Activation of Trigger Points

Myofascial TrPs in the gastrocnemius muscle are likely to be activated by climbing up steep slopes and over rocks, by jogging uphill, or by riding a bicycle with the seat set too low. These situations require forceful plantar flexion at the ankle with the knee bent.

Another source of TrPs in the gastrocnemius muscle is an accident that causes a fracture of the ankle or leg, which requires the subject to wear a walking cast. Myofascial TrPs may be initiated or activated by muscular reaction to the same stress that caused the fracture. A walking cast fixes the ankle, and thus immobilizes and deconditions the gastrocnemius muscle, which promotes development of TrPs. These TrPs often remain latent until the cast is removed and the patient starts loading the deconditioned, stiff muscle. The TrPs then become active and cause pain.

Walking along a slanted surface, such as a beach beside the ocean or the side of a domed street or road, can activate TrPs in the medial head of the gastrocnemius muscle on the lower side of the slant and produce pain in the back of the knee with each step. This pain is likely to feel as if it arises in the knee joint. The patient tends to be tilted toward the low side so that limb becomes effectively shortened, requiring the gastrocnemius muscle and the pelvis to compensate.

Standing in one position while leaning forward for a prolonged period places the gastrocnemius muscle under sustained tension and aggravates its TrPs, causing a cramplike pain. This can occur, for instance, when one must lean forward to reach a microphone at a lectern or to work at a kitchen sink that has no toe room.

All of these stress factors are aggravated by cooling of the muscle, which seems to be more vulnerable to TrPs when it is chilled.

Baker[16] evaluated 100 patients for myofascial TrP involvement in 24 muscles bilaterally following each patient's first motor vehicle accident. No TrPs were found in the lateral head of the gastrocnemius muscle in any of these patients. He[16] found that the medial head of the gastrocnemius muscle only occasionally developed TrPs. In 16 broadside accidents with the impact on the driver's side, four patients developed TrPs in the medial head of the left gastrocnemius muscle. However, in 16 broadside accidents on the passenger's side, the medial head was unaffected. Impacts from in front were four times more likely to involve the medial head of the gastrocnemius on either side of the body than impacts from behind.[16]

Perpetuation of Trigger Points

Long socks with a tight elastic band at the top, or garters that compress the leg just below the knee and produce a red line with a skin indentation, can strongly perpetuate and aggravate TrPs in the gastrocnemius and peroneus longus muscles. (The resultant impairment of circulation is similar to that caused by a tight shoulder strap compressing the upper trapezius muscle.) The soleus is generally too deep to be troubled by this kind of superficial pressure.

Walking straight up a long steep hill repeatedly can perpetuate gastrocnemius TrPs. Relief is obtained by zigzagging back and forth, in effect reducing the steepness of the grade.

As noted previously, any situation that markedly shortens the gastrocnemius muscle for a prolonged period aggravates and perpetuates its TrPs. This shortening occurs when the knee is bent and the foot is plantar flexed. Such situations include: wearing high heels, hooking the heel on the rung of a high stool with the foot pointed down, driving long distances in a car with an accelerator pedal that is angled too nearly horizontal, and sleeping at night with the foot plantar flexed at the ankle.

Any situation that impairs circulation in the gastrocnemius muscle encourages myofascial TrPs. The effect of ischemia was covered in the preceding section. A chair seat with a high front edge can produce compression of the thighs. When mild, this compromises venous return from the legs; when severe, it may reduce arterial flow. This effect can occur also when the chair seat is pitched downward at the back, raising the knees, or when the seat is too high for a person of short stature (*see* Fig. 16.6); both situations tend to lift the feet off the floor.

Reclining chairs can also reduce blood flow in the calf muscles, particularly the gastrocnemius, when the leg rest has a high edge at calf level and provides inadequate heel support. This arrangement places the weight of the leg on the calf muscles. Some ottomans and some dental chairs cause this problem.

Viral infections are generally myotoxic, sometimes severely so, and usually increase the irritability of myofascial TrPs.[175]

Farrell and associates[50] observed a myopathy in 24 children following influenza B infection as the respiratory symptoms waned. It preferentially involved the gastrocnemius and soleus muscles, and caused severe pain and difficulty in walking. These muscles were exquisitely tender to palpation. The foot was held in plantar flexion; dorsiflexion was painful and actively resisted. Biopsies showed segmental necrosis of muscle fibers.[50]

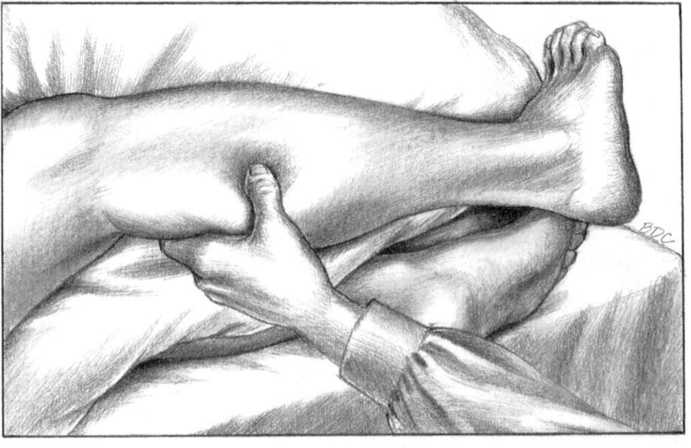

Figure 21.3. Pincer palpation of the lateral head of the right gastrocnemius muscle where its trigger points are most commonly located. Patient is lying on the left side with a pillow between the knees and legs for comfort.

8. PATIENT EXAMINATION (Fig. 21.3)

There is no reliable clinical technique for detecting a moderate degree of gastrocnemius weakness in the presence of competent soleus function.[80,84]

Patients with gastrocnemius and soleus muscle TrPs are likely to have a flat-footed, stiff-legged gait; they have difficulty walking fast and walking on uneven ground.

The patient who has TrP shortening of a gastrocnemius muscle usually cannot fully extend that knee when standing if the heel is kept flat on the floor.

The examiner should look for high heels on the patient's shoes and for the indentation caused by a tight elastic band of the stocking around the leg below the knee. Either one is likely to aggravate TrPs in the gastrocnemius muscles. Varicose veins over the calf, which dilate when the person stands, suggest compromised venous circulation at or above that level. Dilatation of these veins may not be evident when the patient is lying down.

TrPs in the gastrocnemius muscle do not inhibit the Achilles tendon reflex. (However, strongly active TrPs in the soleus characteristically do inhibit this reflex.) The ankle jerks are conveniently tested while the patient kneels as shown in Figure 21.4*A*.[67] This tendon reflex is augmented by any strong muscular contraction, such as clenching the teeth or pulling the clasped hands against each other.

The addition of dorsiflexion of the foot to hip flexion with the knee straight (LaSégue maneuver, *see* Fig. 16.7*B*) is usually considered positive for sciatic nerve or spinal nerve root irritation when it causes pain or cramping in the posterior thigh. A tight gastrocnemius muscle produces pain in the calf or back of the knee.

The dorsalis pedis and posterior tibial arteries are palpated for amplitude of pulsation to uncover evidence of arterial disease or entrapment.

9. TRIGGER POINT EXAMINATION (Figs. 21.3 and 21.4)

The gastrocnemius muscle can often be delineated by inspection if the foot is plantar flexed and the muscle is contracted.[51,98]

In many patients, one can examine the gastrocnemius muscle by pincer palpation, if the subcutaneous tissues are sufficiently slack and the adipose layer is not too thick.

The patient may be examined while either recumbent or kneeling on a chair seat. When recumbent, the patient lies on the side that places the head of the gastrocnemius muscle to be examined uppermost. The lateral head is smaller and usually easier to grasp for pincer palpation (Fig. 21.3) than is the medial head (Fig. 21.4*B*). The lateral head is grasped by inserting the thumb between its lateral border and the fibula with the fingers in the midline groove between the two bellies of the gastrocnemius. Pincer palpation is more informative if the patient's foot is placed in a neutral position or is slightly plantar flexed to slacken the muscle partially. If the intervening tissues are too thick or tight for pincer palpation of the muscle, then flat palpation (Fig. 21.4*A*) is performed by compressing the muscle against the underlying bone to identify taut bands that harbor TrPs. Flat palpation is best done with any slack in the muscle taken up by gentle dorsiflexion of the foot.

The most common TrPs, TrP_1 and TrP_2 (Fig. 21.1), are found proximal to the midpoint of the bellies of the muscle along its medial (Fig. 21.4) or lateral (Fig. 21.3)

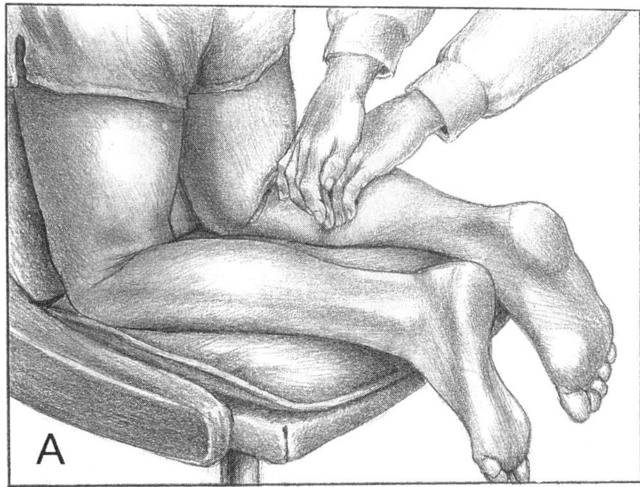

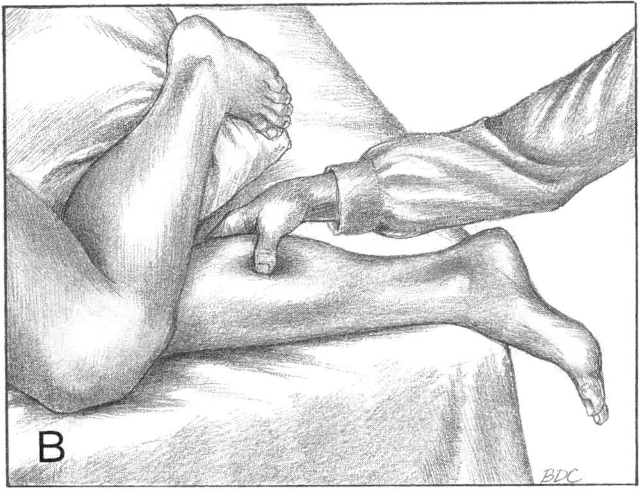

Figure 21.4. Palpation of the medial head of the right gastrocnemius muscle for trigger points. *A*, examination using flat palpation while the patient kneels on a chair seat and holds onto the back of the chair. (This position can also be used to test the ankle reflexes.) The foot may need to be slightly dorsiflexed to place optimal tension on the muscle. *B*, pincer palpation of the medial head (grasping the muscle between the fingertips and thumb) with the patient recumbent, lying on the affected (right) side; the right knee should be flexed about 35° with the ankle in a neutral position that takes up the slack in the muscle without causing excessive tension. Either pincer or flat palpation may be used in both positions.

borders. Frequently local twitch responses (LTRs) can be elicited from these TrPs by snapping palpation.

The proximal TrPs, TrP_3 in the medial head and TrP_4 in the lateral head (Fig. 21.1), may be palpated in the popliteal space. Only flat palpation can be used to palpate these proximal TrPs. Here LTRs are rarely observed because of the greater depth of these TrPs (but they often can be felt when the needle penetrates the TrP during injection).

Proximally, the aponeurosis of the gastrocnemius is superficial to the muscle fibers and has a ropy consistency along the medial and lateral margins of the muscle.[7,18,104,108,138] Tenderness of the musculotendinous junctions along these margins should not be confused with tenderness of taut bands of muscle fibers. Often, tenderness in both is present.

Lange[90] illustrated the location of palpable myogelosis in the medial head of the gastrocnemius muscle along its medial border near the midlevel of the muscle belly. This location was just slightly distal to where we find TrP_1. His sclerometric (tissue compliance) measurements[91] of one of these palpable hardenings in the gastrocnemius muscle permitted only 16–18 mm of skin indentation compared with adjacent control muscle tissue that allowed 24 mm of indentation.

Popelianskii and co-workers[126] studied 12 patients with osteochondrosis, 11 of whom had involvement of the calf muscles. These patients also had variable findings of L_5 and S_1 radiculopathy. To illustrate typical muscular findings in the gastrocnemius muscle, they described a patient with a tense band and painful thickening within the medial head of the muscle. Vibration of this nodular trigger zone caused pain referred to the inside surface of the thigh. Stretch of the calf muscle sharply increased the pain, while massage softened the nodule and decreased the pain. Electromyographic evidence of an early stage of denervation was observed in three of the 12 cases. This EMG finding in the gastrocnemius muscle was related to pathomorphologic changes in the biopsy of two patients and to clinical symptoms of S_1 root compression in a third patient who

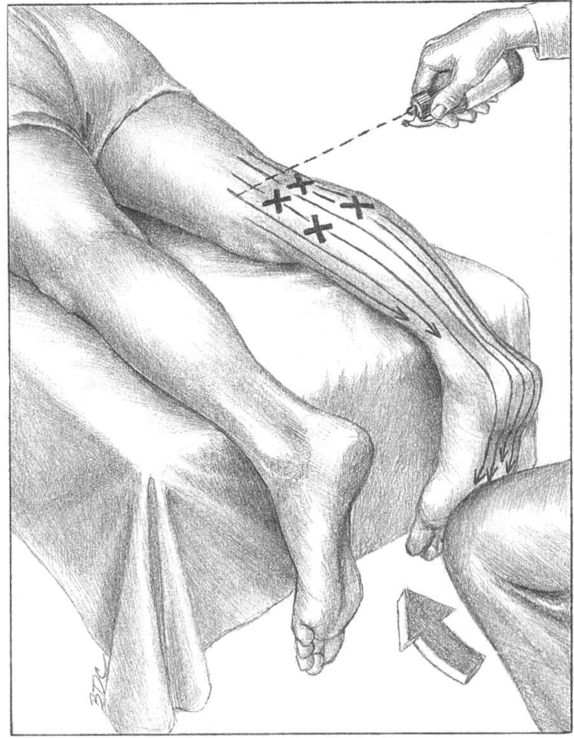

Figure 21.5. Stretch position and ice or vapocoolant spray pattern (*thin arrows*) for trigger points (**X**s) in the right gastrocnemius muscle. To take up slack in the muscle, gentle pressure in a cephalad direction is applied by the operator's knee against the patient's forefoot, as indicated by the *thick arrow*. The patient's knee should be kept straight. Starting above the knee, the intermittent cold covers the entire posterior aspect of the leg and ankle (including the medial and lateral sides) and also the sole of the foot. A small pad may be used to soften the edge of the examining table where the ankle hangs over it in the neutral position. Active range of motion and application of a moist heating pad over the gastrocnemius follow intermittent cold with stretch.

showed normal biopsy findings. No clear-cut relationship emerged among the conditions observed in this study.

10. ENTRAPMENTS

No nerve entrapment due to TrPs in the gastrocnemius muscle has been identified.

When the popliteal artery lies more medial than usual, it can be entrapped by the medial head of the gastrocnemius. This can cause intermittent claudication.[41,77] Symptoms are relieved by dividing the medial head of the muscle. Iwai and associates[78] reported three cases in which a third head of the gastrocnemius muscle (described in Section 2 of this chapter) caused symptomatic entrapment of the popliteal vein; the symptoms were relieved by partial resection of the third head.

11. ASSOCIATED TRIGGER POINTS

The soleus and hamstring muscles are likely to harbor active myofascial TrPs when TrPs have developed in the gastrocnemius muscle. Also, when the pain from medial gastrocnemius TrPs has been relieved, the distribution of pain may shift distally because of remaining active TrPs in the long flexors of the toes or in the tibialis posterior muscle.

TrPs in the posterior portion of the gluteus minimus muscle refer pain and tenderness to the upper calf region and are likely to cause satellite TrPs in the gastrocnemius.

It is interesting to note that TrPs do not seem to develop in the antagonist quadriceps femoris in association with TrPs in the gastrocnemius.

However, the tibialis anterior and long extensors of the toes are antagonists that may become involved as part of the functional unit.

12. INTERMITTENT COLD WITH STRETCH

(Fig. 21.5)

Before releasing the tight gastrocnemius muscle, showing the patient the limited range of dorsiflexion helps him or her appreciate later the results achieved by treatment.

The use of ice for applying intermittent cold with stretch is explained on page 9 of this volume and the use of vapocoolant spray with stretch is detailed on pages 63–74 of Volume 1.[174] Techniques that augment relaxation and stretch are described on pages 10–11 and alternative treatment methods are reviewed on pages 9–11 of this volume.

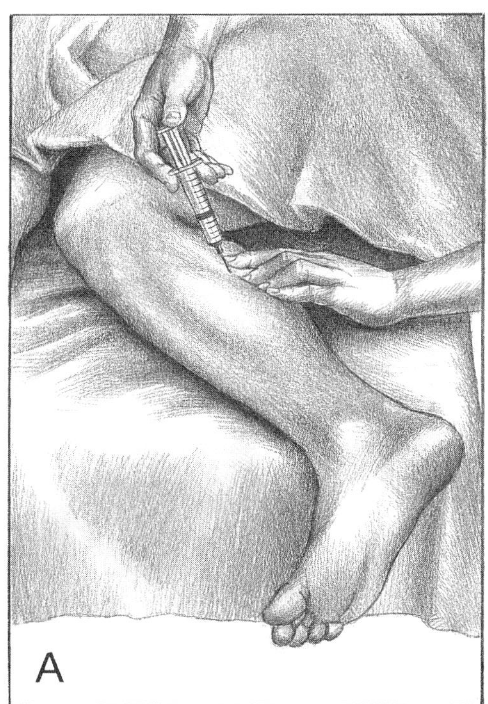

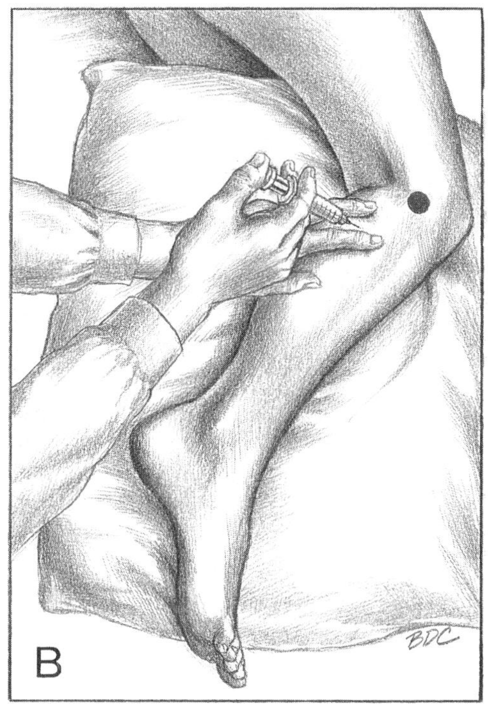

Figure 21.6. Injection of the more distal trigger points (TrP_1 and TrP_2) in the right gastrocnemius muscle. *A*, injecting TrP_1 in the medial head of the muscle with the patient lying on the involved (right) side. *B*, injecting TrP_2 in the lateral head with the patient lying on the uninvolved (left) side. The *solid circle* marks the head of the fibula.

When treating patients with gastrocnemius TrPs, it is important to keep this muscle warm by applying a dry heating pad over the abdomen to warm the core of the body. This warmth induces reflex vasodilatation that progressively warms the lower limbs from proximal to distal. Covering the body and opposite limb with a blanket helps to conserve body heat.

For intermittent cold with stretch of the gastrocnemius muscle, the patient lies prone with the feet extending off the end of the examining table so that the knee remains straight as the operator applies firm pressure to the ball of the foot to take up slack while dorsiflexing the foot at the ankle (Fig. 21.5). At the same time, parallel sweeps of ice or vapocoolant spray are applied distalward starting just above the knee to cover the entire muscle and the referred pain zone.

Immediately following intermittent cold with stretch, the patient slowly performs, several times, full active plantar flexion and dorsiflexion of the foot, keeping the knee straight. Then the calf is wrapped in a moist hot pack or wet-proof heating pad to rewarm the skin and to relax the muscle fully. The patient's body is covered with a blanket to help restore heat lost by exposure of the skin to room air and to the intermittent cold.

Muscular reflexes produced by TrPs can cross from one lower limb to the other. Therefore, it is wise to release gastrocnemius muscle tightness on both sides of the body even if only one muscle has active TrPs. (This principle also applies to the hamstring and adductor magnus muscles.)

To include the gastrocnemius muscle when treating the hamstring muscles (*see* Fig. 16.11), one applies the coolant distally over the calf with the patient supine, the hip flexed 90°, and the knee straight. Then, the gastrocnemius is passively stretched by dorsiflexing the foot during brief application of intermittent cold.

13. INJECTION AND STRETCH (Figs. 21.6 and 21.7)

A detailed description of the procedure for TrP injection and stretch of any muscle appears in Volume 1, pages 74–86.[174] For injection, the physician should wear gloves.

The gastrocnemius is very prone to postinjection soreness. The medial head

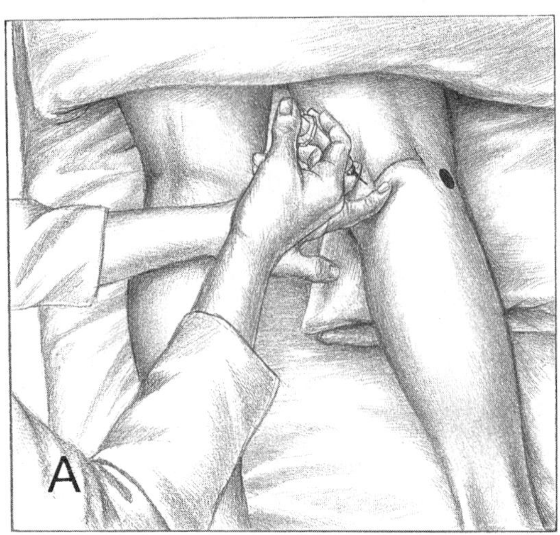

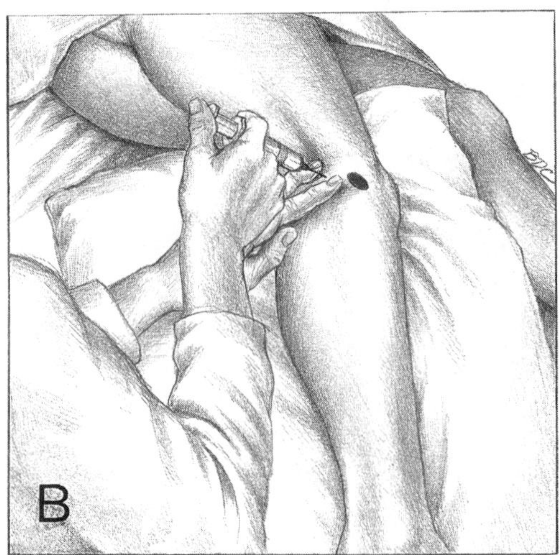

Figure 21.7. Injection of the more proximal trigger points (TrP_3 and TrP_4) in the popliteal portion of the right gastrocnemius muscle. The *solid circle* locates the fibular head. *A*, injecting TrP_3 in the medial head with the patient prone. The transverse *solid line* marks the popliteal crease. *B*, injecting TrP_4 in the lateral head with the patient in the semi-side-lying position.

is more vulnerable to this than the lateral head, perhaps because the TrPs in the medial head are more tender and are usually more numerous. The muscle may remain sore for as long as 5 or 6 days following TrP injection and, for the first day or two, the patient may experience marked discomfort while walking or standing. For this reason, one should avoid injecting TrPs in both the right and left gastrocnemius muscles at the same visit; doing so might immobilize the patient.

It is especially important, prior to injecting TrPs in this muscle, to ensure that the patient's tissues are well supplied with vitamin C. If there is doubt, a supplement of 1,000 mg of time-release ascorbic acid twice daily for 2 days prior to injection is recommended. Smokers are particularly likely to have low tissue reserves of vitamin C and to experience marked postinjection soreness.

To inject the most common TrPs in the medial head (TrP_1 area, Fig. 21.6*A*), the patient lies on the same side as the leg to be injected. After cleansing of the skin, the TrP within a taut band is fixed between the fingers by pincer or flat palpation. The TrP is injected with 0.5% procaine solution, usually employing a 37-mm (1½-inch), 22-gauge needle. There are no major neurovascular structures within or near this portion of the muscle that would prohibit the use of a probing injection technique. The frequent presence of multiple TrPs requires widespread probing with the needle to ensure inactivation of as many TrPs in the cluster as possible.

For injection of the more distal TrPs in the belly of the lateral head of the gastrocnemius muscle (TrP_2), the patient lies on the side opposite the leg to be injected (Fig. 21.6*B*). Otherwise, the same technique is employed as for the medial head.

Injection of TrPs in the proximal popliteal portion of the ***medial*** head is performed with the patient lying prone (Fig. 21.7*A*), and injection of the popliteal portion of the ***lateral*** head of this muscle is performed with the patient either prone or lying partly on the opposite side (Fig. 21.7*B*). One should aim the needle away from the midline to avoid the neurovascular bundle that passes through the popliteal space. When injecting TrP_3 in the popliteal portion of the medial head, the possibility of a displaced popliteal artery must be considered; the pulsating artery can be located by palpation before injection so that it can be avoided. A test that may indicate an anomalous medial course of the artery is to determine whether the pedal arterial pulses are reduced by passive dorsiflexion of the foot with the knee straight, which

Table 21.1
Check List of Gastrocnemius Corrective Actions

POSTURE
- Avoid shoes with high heels
- Avoid excessive resistance of accelerator pedal in car
- Avoid too flat an accelerator pedal in car
- Provide adequate foot support when seated
- Avoid hooking heels on rung of high stool

ACTIVITIES
- Avoid smooth leather shoe soles on slippery floor
- Avoid vigorous kick with toes pointed in crawl stroke
- Keep calves and body warm
- Avoid tight elastic at top of socks
- Avoid excessive uphill walking
- Avoid walking on surfaces slanted sideways

HOME THERAPY
- Sit in an appropriate rocking chair
- Do gastrocnemius/soleus pedal exercise
- Do gastrocnemius standing self-stretch
- Do Lewit postisometric self-stretch for gastrocnemius

CALF CRAMPS
- Inactivate gastrocnemius TrP_1
- Passively stretch cramping muscle
- Avoid prolonged plantar flexion of foot (in bed)
- Try vitamin E supplementation

would further tighten the muscle and compress the artery.

Following TrP injection, a few parallel sweeps of intermittent cold are applied as the muscle is passively lengthened fully. Then the patient actively moves the foot slowly through full plantar flexion and dorsiflexion; quick jerky movements should be avoided. Finally, a moist heating pad is applied to the calf.

14. CORRECTIVE ACTIONS (Figs. 21.8–21.11)

Table 21.1 provides a summary of the main corrective actions considered in this section.

Corrective Posture and Activities

Posture

Heels in excess of 7.5 cm (3 in) are likely to cause sore toes, gastrocnemius TrPs, knee problems, and backache. Heels less than 5 cm (2 in) in height can also shorten the gastrocnemius. In addition, high heels reduce the normal activity of the gastrocnemius during walking.[94] Every effort should be made to discourage the wearing of high heels, especially by patients with myofascial problems in the back or lower limbs.

If the automobile accelerator pedal is too flat and positions the foot nearly parallel to the floor in plantar flexion, it maintains the calf muscles in the shortened position. A wedge can be added to the pedal surface to position the ankle more nearly at a right angle. During a long trip, drivers should get out of the car and walk around at least every hour or take turns at the wheel. Cruise control is very helpful on long trips.

Individuals of short stature are likely to experience persistent plantar flexion of the feet that causes calf-muscle TrPs when the seat is too high for the heels to reach the floor. This situation can be corrected by a footrest that lifts the legs and thighs sufficiently to position the ankles at nearly a right angle. A *slanted* footstool is ideal; a flexible sand bag or bean bag can serve as a foot support that is readily adaptable to the most comfortable position, even at the dining room table.

When sitting on a high (bar- or kitchen-type) stool, one should avoid hooking the heels over the rung and allowing the feet to hang down fully plantar flexed. The feet should be pushed back far enough on the rung to balance them in a neutral position.

Activities

When working on a slippery tile or well-waxed floor, one should avoid hard, smooth leather soles that provide poor traction and easily overload the calf muscles. Adding half-soles of rubber or other high-traction material solves this problem.

When swimming, a vigorous crawl kick with the toes pointed backward should be avoided if calf TrPs are a problem; such a kick overloads the calf muscles in the shortened position.

The gastrocnemius muscle is readily subject to excessive cooling that can aggravate its TrPs. When the patient works at a desk in a cool room, a heater that

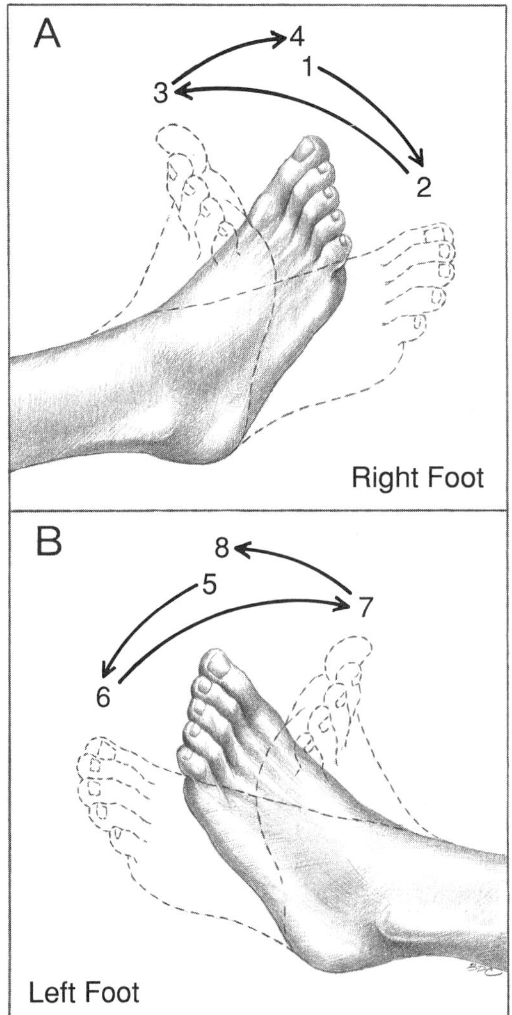

Figure 21.8. Pedal Exercise using dorsiflexion and plantar flexion to ensure the normal range of motion of the gastrocnemius muscle and to enhance the venous pumping action of the soleus muscle. The knees are extended with the patient either seated or supine. One foot moves in a cycle (*dotted lines*) to full plantar flexion, then to full dorsiflexion, with a slow rhythmic movement, while the other foot rests. Then the cycle is repeated with the opposite foot. The exercise continues with cycles of activity alternating between the feet. The *numbers* indicate the sequence of movements. (For seated version of this exercise, *see* Soleus Muscle, Fig. 22.13) *A*, right foot, full plantar flexion, full dorsiflexion, and pause in midposition. *B*, left foot, exercise as in *A*.

warms the space underneath the desk protects the muscle. In a number of patients, frequent exposure to this cold work space proved to be a critical perpetuating factor, correction of which permitted lasting inactivation of gastrocnemius TrPs.

The patient with gastrocnemius TrPs must avoid tight elastic in socks and tight garters that constrict circulation. The elastic top in socks can be loosened by pressing it with a hot iron. It is wise to buy socks that have elasticity distributed uniformly throughout their whole length and are snug enough to stay up without a tight elastic band at the top. This uniformity of pressure supports rather than constricts the circulation.

Home Therapeutic Program
(Fig. 21.8–21.10)

Patients with gastrocnemius (and soleus) TrPs are strongly encouraged to sit in a suitable rocking chair and to rock when engaged in sedentary activity, such as watching TV. The movement prevents prolonged immobility of the calf muscles and increases their blood flow.

A more specific and more vigorous form of gastrocnemius isotonic movement is provided by the Pedal Exercise illustrated in Figure 21.8. The patient, either sitting or lying supine, moves one foot rhythmically from neutral to plantar flexion, to dorsiflexion, to neutral, and then pauses. The same cycle is performed with the other foot, and then repeated, alternating feet. This exercise helps to maintain the full functional range of motion of the gastrocnemius muscle and when used at night in bed, may prevent night cramps.

An excellent way to prevent reactivation of TrPs in the gastrocnemius muscles following treatment is to have the standing patient perform a passive stretching exercise for this muscle (Fig. 21.9). For the most effective stretch, the patient must keep the knee on that side extended, the heel on the floor, and the foot aligned straight forward (rear foot in Fig. 21.9*A*), not turned outward (Fig. 21.9*B*). A magazine or small book can be placed under the forefoot (Fig. 21.9*C*) to increase dorsiflexion of the foot and stretch of the muscle. Attempting to stretch both gastrocnemius muscles simultaneously by leaning against a wall can be hazardous if the feet slip and should be avoided (Fig. 21.9*D*). However, bilateral stretching can be done safely and effectively in the seated position (*see* Fig. 16.13*B*).

A sports medicine study of intercollegiate athletes[95] revealed that the plantar flexors of the foot were among the most neglected muscles in the athletes' stretching routines. The authors comment on how unfortunate it is that soccer players do not stretch their plantar flexors because, in this sport, players with gastroc-

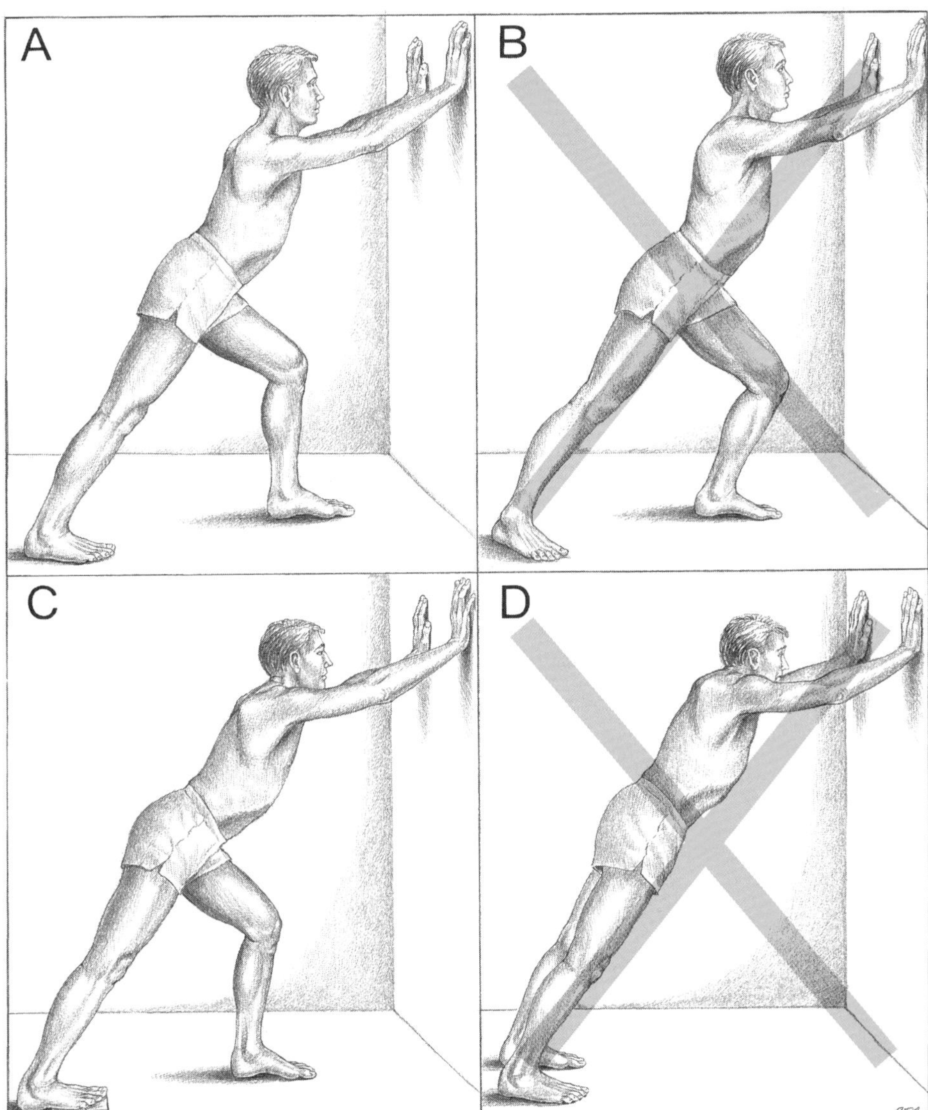

Figure 21.9. Standing passive self-stretch exercise for the right gastrocnemius muscle. The heel on the side of the muscle to be stretched *must* remain solidly on the floor as the patient shifts the pelvis forward with the knee straight, dorsiflexing the right foot. *A*, effective position for stretch with the foot pointed straight forward; stretch is increased by bending the opposite knee to lower the body, which further dorsiflexes the foot at the ankle. *B*, less effective technique because the right lower limb is laterally rotated. *C*, addition of a lift under the right *forefoot* to provide additional stretch by increasing dorsiflexion at the ankle. *D*, hazardous bilateral self-stretch: the patient can readily lose control of balance and cause jerky overstretching of the gastrocnemius muscles, especially if the feet slip backward on the floor.

nemius tightness are particularly liable to injuries [and developing TrPs].

Patients can often inactivate their own gastrocnemius TrPs by applying Lewit's postisometric relaxation technique[96] as a self-stretch exercise (Fig. 21.10). Starting in the long sitting position, the patient uses a towel to dorsiflex the foot passively while keeping the knee extended (Fig. 21.10*A*). The standard Lewit technique is applied: *(a)* gently contract the tight muscle isometrically against resistance (Fig. 21.10*A*); *(b)* relax and take a deep breath; *(c)* then *slowly* let the breath out and at the same time, gently passively dorsiflex the foot, taking up all of the slack that develops while exhaling (Fig. 21.10*B*). Repeat the sequence until no further range of dorsiflexion is obtained at the ankle. One can employ this procedure regularly to maintain the full range of motion and prevent recurrences of gastrocnemius TrPs.

PART 3

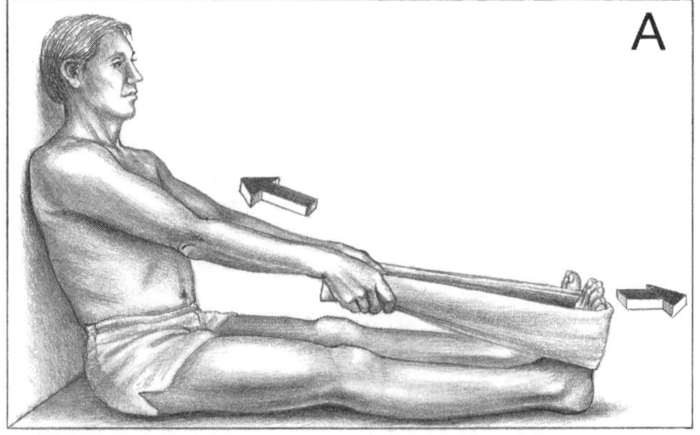

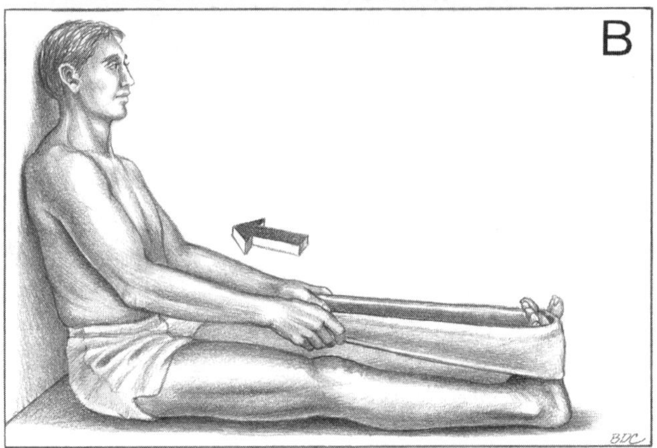

Figure 21.10. Seated self-stretch with postisometric relaxation of the right gastrocnemius muscle. The knee must remain straight. *Arrows* indicate the directions of the forces applied. *A*, initial position for a 5-second, minimal-strength, gentle isometric contraction of the right gastrocnemius against resistance during slow deep inhalation. Contraction is followed by relaxation facilitated by slow full exhalation. *B*, as relaxation occurs, the foot is passively dorsiflexed by pulling slowly on the towel, with just enough force to take up the slack that has developed. The cycle may be repeated three or four times, or until the full stretch-length of the muscle is achieved.

Nocturnal Calf Cramps
(Fig. 21.11)

Several kinds of treatments have been recommended for calf cramps: inactivation of myofascial TrPs in afflicted muscles, stretching the calf muscles, positioning of the feet, electrolyte replacement, vitamins, drugs that stabilize excitable membranes, drugs that improve circulation in the muscles, and electrical stimulation.

Stretching of the Muscle

Passively stretching the gastrocnemius muscle by standing with the knee extended and moving the hips forward to slowly dorsiflex the ankle (*see* Fig. 21.9*A*) has repeatedly been reported to terminate calf cramps in a minute or two.[40,45,70,88,92,97,116,180] Travell[111] suggested that application of vapocoolant spray combined with passive stretch may be more effective than passive stretch alone. Fowler[59,60] and Conchubhair[38] emphasized that active stretch of the calf muscles by contraction of their antagonist, the tibialis anterior, had the advantage of invoking reciprocal inhibition to quiet the calf muscle contractions more effectively. One must be careful, however, not to impose a prolonged contraction on the fully shortened antagonist muscle, or it may develop cramps of its own. Should this occur, those cramps are also relieved by passively stretching the muscle. Many patients have learned to get up and walk to relieve an acute nocturnal calf cramp. Passively stretching the afflicted muscle usually provides relief much faster than does walking. The combination of reciprocal inhibition supplemented with passive stretch is the most effective.[19]

Sontag and Wanner[158] were so successful using stretching exercises in the treatment of leg cramps (and knee pains) among more than 100 patients that they considered stiff, shortened muscles to be

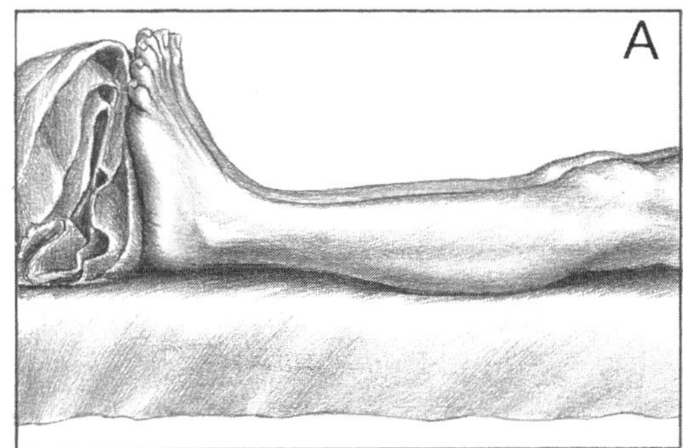

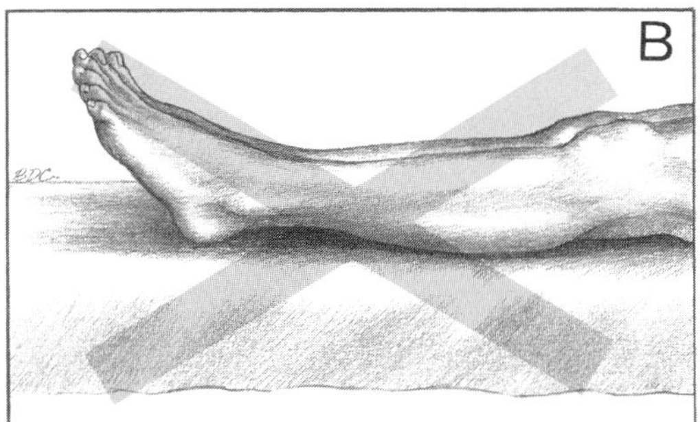

Figure 21.11. Foot support in bed to prevent nocturnal calf cramps and to reduce trigger-point irritability of the gastrocnemius muscle. *A*, correct support under the sheet, which maintains the feet in a neutral position at the ankle. This correction is effective in both the supine and side-lying positions. *B*, incorrect position (*red* ***X***) with lack of foot support.

the cause of the symptoms. The authors[158] do not mention myofascial pain or TrPs, but their findings and treatment are consistent with what we find in patients with recurrent calf cramps caused by intermittent aggravation of latent myofascial TrPs in the gastrocnemius.

Norris and associates[116] used fine-wire electromyograms of the gastrocnemius and quadriceps muscles in a study of five healthy volunteers and four patients who complained of calf cramps. They induced cramps by having the subject contract the muscle in the shortened position and inactivated the cramps by passively stretching the cramped muscle. Voluntary activation of the antagonist muscle also rapidly reduced the intensity of the cramp and its electrical activity. This response was also observed electromyographically by Schimrigk[148] and by Basmajian.[19] However, Schimrigk noted that the effectiveness of antagonist activation waned and disappeared with repetition.

Warmth

Sleeping under an electric blanket or warming the calves with a heating pad at night generally reduces TrP irritability and the tendency of the muscle to cramp. The heating pad may also be placed on the abdomen for reflex heating. For individuals who prefer not to sleep under an electric blanket or pad, effective neutral warmth (conservation of body heat) can be provided by wrapping the legs in a wool blanket or large wool scarf.

Positioning of the Feet

An effective way to prevent nocturnal calf cramps is simply to prevent the feet from remaining in the plantar flexed position during sleep. Plantar flexion of the foot is increased by the weight of heavy bedcovers (as suggested in Fig. 21.11*B* and also as illustrated by Weiner and Weiner[180]). Simply lying on an electric warmer and using a lighter bedcover may help.[69] A firm pillow or blanket roll placed against the feet under the top sheet provides a "footrest" that holds the foot in the neutral position and elevates the covers to provide a space for the feet (Fig. 21.11*A*). Lying on the side makes it easier to maintain a neutral foot position during sleep. Side lying alone does not ensure relief unless the individual develops an awareness of foot position during arousal and consciously returns the foot angle to neutral whenever it strays into plantar flexion. If the patient insists on sleeping prone, he or she can place a pillow under the lower legs or slide down on the bed until the feet hang over its end in order to maintain a neutral position of the foot. It usually takes many nights of persistent effort to develop new sleeping habits; therefore, the patient should not expect speedy relief. Uninterrupted restful sleep is an important part of therapy for patients with myofascial pain.

Elevating the foot of the bed with lifts under it also was effective in reducing nocturnal calf cramps.[181] An elevation of 23 cm (9 in) was recommended by one author.[136] This procedure was thought to improve circulation by reducing venous pooling, but it also may have reduced plantar flexion of the feet.

Electrolyte Replacement

Electrolyte imbalance can increase the excitability of muscle and nerve cell membranes. Low potassium or calcium reserves are recognized as predisposing to chronicity of myofascial TrPs.[152,154,171]

An increased incidence of nocturnal leg cramps is observed in pregnant women[97] for reasons that are not clear.[69] Since quinine is contraindicated in pregnancy, supplemental calcium is often prescribed and has been reported to be effective.[69,97,121] Hammar and coinvestigators[68] compared treatment with calcium to an ascorbic acid placebo in a controlled double-blind trial of 60 pregnant patients with leg cramps. A good response was seen in 75% of those taking calcium and in 77% of those taking ascorbic acid as a "placebo." No differences in blood Ca^{++} or Mg^{++} levels were observed in patients with and without leg cramps, and no differences in these levels were observed in the calcium-treated patients before and during treatment. The authors concluded that either the symptom of leg cramps in pregnancy responds unusually well to placebo, or else vitamin C had an unexpected salutary effect on leg cramps. In a similar, earlier study of 129 pregnant patients in Africa, Odendaal[117] also found that 75% of calcium-treated patients and 77% of the patients given ascorbic acid reported a good response.

Vitamins

Several reports strongly recommend vitamin E, 300 international units daily, as an effective treatment for leg cramps[1,15] and one author considered it more effective and safer than quinine,[29] although no reports of controlled studies were found.

Our own experience is that supplemental oral vitamin E (400 I.U. daily) for a maximum of 2 weeks may eliminate the cramps. Any vitamin E taken in a multivitamin preparation should be included in this total dose. Vitamin E is a fat-soluble vitamin, is well stored in the body, and should be discontinued when the calf cramps disappear. The course of supplementation may be repeated if the cramps recur. Some patients are remarkably responsive to this supplementation. With it, TrPs respond well to local therapy and the patient remains free of cramps and TrPs.

Vitamin B_2 (riboflavin or lactoflavin) has been recommended[87] for this complaint during pregnancy.

Membrane-Stabilizing Drugs

The most common medical therapy for nocturnal calf cramps has been quinine sulfate, 300 mg orally, at bedtime.[97,143,182] A dose of only 60 mg of quinine was reported to be just as effective as 300 mg.[75] However, two studies found quinine ineffective in the elderly,[17,178] and a recent controlled study also found it ineffective in younger people as well.[45] In two studies, investigators found the combination of quinine, 240 mg, and aminophylline, 180 mg, more effective than quinine alone.[112,133] The aminophylline was thought to improve circulation in the lower extremities.

Chloroquine often provided prolonged relief that lasted weeks after treatment.[120] Procainamide HCl was reported to be useful.[182] Phenytoin, diazepam, diphenhydramine,[143,182] and carbamazepine[92] have also been tried.

Circulatory Drugs

Papaverine HCl provided significant relief to geriatric diabetic patients with calf cramps in a double blind cross-over study.[164]

Electrical Stimulation

Mills and co-workers[109] confirmed electromyographically the resolution of calf cramps by treatment with transcutaneous nerve stimulation. The calf cramp was induced by voluntary plantar flexion in an atypical patient who had resting EMG activity in the muscle and muscle hypertrophy.

Electrical stimulation of sensory nerves during stretching was reported to be helpful in achieving stretch of muscles subject to cramps.[88]

References

1. Aitchison WR: Nocturnal cramps. *NZ Med J* 2: 137, 1974.
2. Anderson JE: *Grant's Atlas of Anatomy*, Ed. 8. Williams & Wilkins, Baltimore, 1983 (Fig. 4–50).
3. *Ibid.* (Figs. 4–51, 4–53).
4. *Ibid.* (Fig. 4–52).

PART 3

5. *Ibid.* (Fig. 4–68).
6. *Ibid.* (Fig. 4–81).
7. *Ibid.* (Fig. 4–82).
8. *Ibid.* (Fig. 4–120).
9. Andersson JG, Jonsson B, Örtengren R: Myoelectric activity in individual lumbar erector spinae muscles in sitting. A study with surface and wire electrodes. *Scand J Rehabil Med (Suppl.) 3*:91–108, 1974.
10. Andriacchi TP, Andersson GBJ, Örtengren R, *et al.*: A study of factors influencing muscle activity about the knee joint. *J Orthop Res 1*:266–275, 1984.
11. Anouchi YS, Parker RD, Seitz WH Jr: Posterior compartment syndrome of the calf resulting from misdiagnosis of a rupture of the medial head of the gastrocnemius. *J Trauma 27*:678–680, 1987.
12. Arcangeli P, Corradi F, D'Ayala-Valva: Alterations of skin and muscle sensibility in chronic obliterating arteriopathy of the lower limbs and their importance in determining intermittent claudication. *Acta Neurovegetativa 27*:511–545, 1965.
13. Arcangeli P, Digiesi V, Ronchi O, Dorigo B, Bartoli V: Mechanisms of ischemic pain in peripheral occlusive arterial disease. In *Advances in Pain Research and Therapy*, edited by J. J. Bonica and D. Albe-Fessard, Vol. I. Raven Press, New York, 1976 (pp. 965–973).
14. Arner O, Lindholm Å: What is tennis leg? *Acta Chir Scand 116*:73–77, 1958.
15. Ayres S Jr., Mihan R: Nocturnal leg cramps (systremma). *South Med J 67*:1308–1312, 1974.
16. Baker BA: The muscle trigger: evidence of overload injury. *J Neurol Orthop Med Surg 7*:35–43, 1986.
17. Baltodano N, Gallo BV, Weidler DJ: Verapamil vs quinine in recumbent nocturnal leg cramps in the elderly. *Arch Intern Med 148*:1969–1970, 1988.
18. Bardeen CR: The musculature, Sect. 5. In *Morris's Human Anatomy*, edited by C.M. Jackson, Ed. 6. Blakiston's Son & Co., Philadelphia, 1921 (Fig. 444, pp. 516–517).
19. Basmajian JV: Personal communication, 1990.
20. Basmajian JV, Deluca CJ: *Muscles Alive*, Ed. 5. Williams & Wilkins, Baltimore, 1985 (p.14).
21. *Ibid.* (pp. 256–257, 335–340).
22. Bates T: Myofascial pain, Chapter 14. In *Ambulatory Pediatrics II*, edited by M. Green and R.J. Haggerty. W.B. Saunders, Philadelphia, 1977 (pp. 147, 148).
23. Bates T, Grunwaldt E: Myofascial pain in childhood. *J Pediatr 53*:198–209, 1958.
24. Brandell BR: Functional roles of the calf and vastus muscles in locomotion. *Am J Phys Med 56*:59–74, 1977.
25. Brody DM: Running injuries. *Clin Symp 32*:2–36, 1980 (*see* p. 21).
26. Broer MR, Houtz SJ: *Patterns of Muscular Activity in Selected Sports Skills*. Charles C Thomas, Springfield, 1967.
27. Campbell KM, Biggs NL, Blanton PL, *et al.*: Electromyographic investigation of the relative activity among four components of the triceps surae. *Am J Phys Med 52*:30–41, 1973.
28. Carter BL, Morehead J, Wolpert SM, *et al.*: *Cross-Sectional Anatomy*. Appleton-Century-Crofts, New York, 1977 (Sects. 68–75).
29. Cathcart RF III: Leg cramps and vitamin E. *JAMA 219*:51–52, 1972.
30. Christensen E: Topography of terminal motor innervation in striated muscles from stillborn infants. *Am J Phys Med 38*:65–78, 1959.
31. Clarkson PM, Kroll W, McBride TC: Maximal isometric strength and fiber type composition in power and endurance athletes. *Eur J Appl Physiol 44*:35–42, 1980.
32. Clarkson PM, Kroll W, McBride TC: Plantar flexion fatigue and muscle fiber type in power and endurance athletes. *Med Sci Sports Exerc 12*:262–267, 1980.
33. Clement DB, Taunton JE, Smart GW: Achilles tendinitis and peritendinitis: etiology and treatment. *Am J Sports Med 12*:179–184, 1984.
34. Clemente CD: *Gray's Anatomy of the Human Body*, American Ed. 30. Lea & Febiger, Philadelphia, 1985 (p. 406).
35. *Ibid.* (p. 576).
36. *Ibid.* (p. 577).
37. *Ibid.* (p. 1239).
38. Conchubhair SU: Nocturnal calf cramp. *Lancet 1*:203–204, 1973.
39. Cordo PJ, Nashner LM: Properties of postural adjustments associated with rapid arm movements. *J Neurophysiol 47*:287–382, 1982.
40. Daniell HW: Simple cure for nocturnal leg cramps. *N Engl J Med 301*:216, 1979.
41. Darling RC, Buckley CJ, Abbott WM, *et al.*: Intermittent claudication in young athletes: popliteal artery entrapment syndrome. *J Trauma 14*: 543–552, 1974.
42. Denny-Brown D: Clinical problems in neuromuscular physiology. *Am J Med 15*:368–390, 1953.
43. Dorigo B, Bartoli V, Grisillo D, *et al.*: Fibrositic myofascial pain in intermittent claudication. Effect of anesthetic block of trigger points on exercise tolerance. *Pain 6*:183–190, 1979.
44. Duchenne GB: *Physiology of Motion*, translated by E.B. Kaplan. J.B. Lippincott, Philadelphia, 1949 (pp. 308–310).
45. Eaton JM: Is this really a muscle cramp? *Postgrad Med 86*:227–232, 1989.
46. Edgerton VR, Smith JL, Simpson DR: Muscle fibre type populations of human leg muscles. *Histochem J 7*:259–266, 1975.
47. Ericson M: On the biomechanics of cycling: a study of joint and muscle load during exercise on the bicycle ergometer. *Scand J Rehabil Med (Suppl.)16*:1–43, 1986.
48. Ericson MO, Nisell R, Arborelius UP, *et al.*: Muscular activity during ergometer cycling. *Scand J Rehabil Med 17*:53–61, 1985.
49. Ericson MO, Nisell R, Ekholm J: Quantified electromyography of lower-limb muscles during level walking. *Scand J Rehabil Med 18*:159–163, 1986.
50. Farrell MK, Partin JC, Bove KE: Epidemic influenza myopathy in Cincinnati in 1977. *J Pediatr 96*:545–551, 1980.
51. Ferner H, Staubesand J: *Sobotta Atlas of Human Anatomy*, Ed. 10, Vol. 2. Urban & Schwarzenberg, Baltimore, 1983 (Figs. 380, 381).

52. *Ibid.* (Figs. 401, 412, 435).
53. *Ibid.* (Fig. 420).
54. *Ibid.* (Fig. 464).
55. *Ibid.* (Figs. 465, 467).
56. *Ibid.* (Fig. 466).
57. *Ibid.* (Fig. 470).
58. *Ibid.* (Fig. 472).
59. Fowler AW: Relief of cramp. *Lancet 1*:99, 1973.
60. Fowler AW: Night cramp. *Br Med J 2*:1563, 1976.
61. Frey H: Musculus gastrocnemius tertius. *Gegenbaurs Morphol Jahrb 50*:517–530, 1919.
62. Froimson AI: Tennis leg. *JAMA 209*:415–416, 1969.
63. Ghori GMU, Luckwill RG: Responses of the lower limb to load carrying in walking man. *Eur J Appl Physiol 54*:145–150, 1985.
64. Good MG: Painful feet. *Practitioner 163*:229–232, 1949.
65. Gravel D, Arsenault AB, Lambert J: Soleus-gastrocnemius synergies in controlled contractions produced around the ankle and knee joints: an EMG study. *Electromyogr Clin Neurophysiol* 27:405–413, 1987.
66. Halar EM, Stolov WC, Venkatesh B, *et al.*: Gastrocnemius muscle belly and tendon length in stroke patients and able-bodied persons. *Arch Phys Med Rehabil 59*:476–484, 1978.
67. Hall H: Examination of the patient with low back pain. *Bulletin on the Rheumatic Diseases 33* No. 4:1–8, 1983.
68. Hammar M, Berg G, Solheim F, *et al.*: Calcium and magnesium status in pregnant women. *Int J Vitam Nutr Res 57*:179–183, 1987.
69. Hammar M, Larsson L, Tegler L: Calcium treatment of leg cramps in pregnancy. *Acta Obstet Gynaecol Scand 60*:345–347, 1981.
70. Harnack G-A von: Nächtliche Wadenkrämpfe bei Kindern. *Dtsch Med Wochenschr 95*:2394, 1970.
71. Henstorf JE, Olson S: Compartment syndrome: pathophysiology, diagnosis, and treatment. *Surg Rounds Orthop*:33–41, Feb. 1987.
72. Herman R, Bragin J: Function of the gastrocnemius and soleus muscles. *Phys Ther 47*:105–113, 1967.
73. Hirsch W, Malsy-Mink O: Ursache von Wadenkrämpfen. *Med Klin 71*:168, 1976.
74. Hollinshead WH: *Anatomy for Surgeons*, Ed. 3., Vol. 3, *The Back and Limbs*. Harper & Row, New York, 1982 (pp. 773–777).
75. Hope-Simpson RE: Night cramp. *Br Med J 2*: 1563, 1976.
76. Houtz SJ, Fischer FJ: An analysis of muscle action and joint excursion during exercise on a stationary bicycle. *J Bone Joint Surg 41[Am]*: 123–131, 1959.
77. Insua JA, Young JR, Humphries AW: Popliteal artery entrapment syndrome. *Arch Surg 101*: 771–775, 1970.
78. Iwai T, Sato S, Yamada T, *et al.*: Popliteal vein entrapment caused by the third head of the gastrocnemius muscle. *Br J Surg 74*:1006–1008, 1987.
79. Jablecki C, Schultz P: Single muscle fiber recordings in the Schwartz-Jampel syndrome. *Muscle Nerve 5*:S64–S69, 1982.
80. Janda V: *Muscle Function Testing*. Butterworths, London, 1983 (pp. 188–190).
81. Kamon E: Electromyographic kinesiology of jumping. *Arch Phys Med Rehabil 52*:152–157, 1971.
82. Kellgren JH: Observations on referred pain arising from muscle. *Clin Sci 3*:175–190, 1938 (p. 186).
83. Kelly M: Some rules for the employment of local analgesic in the treatment of somatic pain. *Med J Austral 1*:235–239, 1947.
84. Kendall FP, McCreary EK: *Muscles, Testing and Function*, Ed. 3. Williams & Wilkins, Baltimore, 1983 (pp. 145–146).
85. Khan MA, Khan N: Statistical analysis of muscle fibre types from four human skeletal muscles. *Anat Anz 144*:246–256, 1978.
86. Kilcoyne RF, Imray TJ, Stewart ET: Ruptured Baker's cyst simulating acute thrombophlebitis. *JAMA 240*:1517–1518, 1978.
87. Kleine HO: Laktoflavintherapie der Wadenkrämpfe in der Schwangerschaft [Lactoflavin therapy for calf cramps during pregnancy]. *Zentralbl Gynakol 76*:344–356, 1954.
88. Kunze K: Muskelkrämpfe. *Dtsch Med Wochenschr 102*:1929, 1977.
89. Kuo KHM, Clamann HP: Coactivation of synergistic muscles of different fiber types in fast and slow contractions. *Am J Phys Med 60*:219–238, 1981.
90. Lange M: *Die Muskelhärten (Myogelosen)*. J.F. Lehmanns, München, 1931 (p. 33, Fig. 6).
91. *Ibid.* (p. 137, Fig. 43; p. 139, Fig. 44).
92. Layzer RB: Muscle pain, cramps, and fatigue, Chapter 66. In *Myology: Basic and Clinical*, edited by A.G. Engel, B.Q. Banker. McGraw-Hill Book Company, New York, 1986 (pp. 1907–1922).
93. Layzer RB, Rowland LP: Cramps. *N Engl J Med 285*:31–40, 1971.
94. Lee KH, Matteliano A, Medige J, *et al.*: Electromyographic changes of leg muscles with heel lift: therapeutic implications. *Arch Phys Med Rehabil 68*:298–301, 1987.
95. Levine M, Lombardo J, McNeeley J, *et al.*: An analysis of individual stretching programs of intercollegiate athletes. *Phys Sportsmed 15*: 130–138, 1987.
96. Lewit K: *Manipulative Therapy in Rehabilitation of the Motor System*. Butterworths, London, 1985 (pp. 256–257, 315).
97. Lippmann HI, Perchuk E: Nocturnal cramps of the legs. *NY State J Med 54*:2976–2979, 1954.
98. Lockhart RD: *Living Anatomy*, Ed. 7. Faber & Faber, London, 1974 (Fig. 118).
99. Mann RA, Moran GT, Dougherty SE: Comparative electromyography of the lower extremity in jogging, running, and sprinting. *Am J Sports Med 14*:501–510, 1986.
100. Markhede G, Nistor L: Strength of plantar flexion and function after resection of various parts of the triceps surae muscle. *Acta Orthop Scand 50*:693–697, 1979.
101. Martin-du-Pan R: Cause et traitement des prétendues «douleurs de croissance» chez-l'enfant. [Origin and treatment of the socalled growing pains in children]. *Praxis 65*:1503–1505, 1976.

102. McClure JG: Gastrocnemius musculotendinous rupture: a condition confused with thrombophlebitis. *South Med J 77*:1143–1145, 1984.
103. McMinn RMH, Hutchings RT: *Color Atlas of Human Anatomy*. Year Book Medical Publishers, Chicago, 1977 (p. 277B).
104. *Ibid*. (p. 294B).
105. *Ibid*. (p. 305C).
106. *Ibid*. (p. 306A).
107. *Ibid*. (p. 312 *A* & *B*).
108. *Ibid*. (p. 313).
109. Mills KR, Newham DJ, Edwards RHT: Severe muscle cramps relieved by transcutaneous nerve stimulation: a case report. *J Neurol Neurosurg Psychiatry 45*:539–542, 1982.
110. Milner M, Basmajian JV, Quanbury AO: Multifactorial analysis of walking by electromyography and computer. *Am J Phys Med 50*:235–258, 1971.
111. Modell W, Travell J, Kraus H, *et al.*: Relief of pain by ethyl chloride spray. *NY State J Med 52*: 1550–1558, 1952 (*see* pp. 1556, 1557).
112. Mörl H, Dieterich HA: Nächtliche Wadenkrämpfe–Ursachen und Behandlung. *Med Klin 75*:264–267, 1980.
113. Mumenthaler M: Nächtliche Wadenkrämpfe. *Dtsch Med Wochenschr 105*:467–468, 1980.
114. Murray MP, Guten GN, Sepic SB, *et al.*: Function of the triceps surae during gait. Compensatory mechanisms for unilateral loss. *J Bone Joint Surg [Am] 60*:473–476, 1978.
115. Nakano KK: Entrapment neuropathies, Chapter 111. In *Textbook of Rheumatology*, Vol. 2, edited by W.N. Kelley, E.D. Harris, Jr., S. Ruddy, *et al.* W.B. Saunders, Philadelphia, 1981 (pp. 1829–1846, *see* pp. 1841–1843).
116. Norris FH Jr, Gasteiger EL, Chatfield PO: An electromyographic study of induced and spontaneous muscle cramps. *EEG Clin Neurophysiol 9*:139–147, 1957.
117. Odendaal HJ: Kalsium vir die Behandeling van Beenkrampe tydens Swangerskap. *S Afr Med J 48*:780–781, 1974.
118. Okada M: An electromyographic estimation of the relative muscular load in different human postures. *J Hum Ergol 1*:75–93, 1972.
119. Okada M, Fujiwara K: Muscle activity around the ankle joint as correlated with the center of foot pressure in an upright stance. In *Biomechanics VIIIA*, edited by H. Matsui, K. Kobayashi. Human Kinetics Publ., Champaign, IL, 1983 (pp. 209–216).
120. Parrow A, Samuelsson S-M: Use of chloroquine phosphate—a new treatment for spontaneous leg cramps. *Acta Med Scand 181*:237–244, 1967.
121. Patterson MA: Treatment of cramps. Letter to the Editor. *J R Soc Med 75*:988, 1982.
122. Patton GW, Parker RJ: Rupture of the lateral head of the gastrocnemius muscle at the musculotendinous junction mimicking a compartment syndrome. *J Foot Surg 28*:433–437, 1989.
123. Pavlov H, Heneghan MA, Hersh A, *et al.*: The Haglund syndrome: initial and differential diagnosis. *Radiology 144*:83–88, 1982.
124. Pernkopf E: *Atlas of Topographical and Applied Human Anatomy*, Vol. 2. W.B. Saunders, Philadelphia, 1964 (Fig. 352).
125. Perry J, Easterday CS, Antonelli DJ: Surface versus intramuscular electrodes for electromyography of superficial and deep muscles. *Phys Ther 61*:7–15, 1981.
126. Popelianskii Ia Iu, Bogdanov EI, Khabirov FA: [Algesic trigger zones of the gastrocnemius muscle in lumbar osteochondrosis] (clinicopathomorphological and electromyographic analysis). *Zh Nevropatol Psikhiatr 84*:1055–1061, 1984.
127. Portnoy H, Morin F: Electromyographic study of postural muscles in various positions and movements. *Am J Physiol 186*:122–126, 1956.
128. Ramchandani P, Soulen RL, Fedullo LM, *et al.*: Deep vein thrombosis: significant limitations of noninvasive tests. *Radiology 156*:47–49, 1985.
129. Rasch PJ, Burke RK: *Kinesiology and Applied Anatomy*, Ed. 6. Lea & Febiger, Philadelphia, 1978 (p. 309).
130. *Ibid*. (pp. 318–319).
131. *Ibid*. (p. 330).
132. Rask MR: Postoperative archnoradiculitis: report of 24 patients and the conservative therapy therefore. *J Neurol Orthop Surg 1*:157–166, 1980.
133. Rawls WB: Management of nocturnal leg cramps. *West J Med 7*:152–157, 1966.
134. Reynolds MD: Myofascial trigger point syndromes in the practice of rheumatology. *Arch Phys Med Rehabil 62*:111–114, 1981.
135. Rish BL: Nerve root compression and night cramps. *JAMA 254*:361, 1985.
136. Rivlin S: Nocturnal calf cramp. *Lancet 1*:203, 1973.
137. Roberts HJ: Spontaneous leg cramps and "restless legs" due to diabetogenic (functional) hyperinsulinism. *J Fla Med Assoc 60*:29–31, 1973.
138. Rohen JW, Yokochi C: *Color Atlas of Anatomy*, Ed. 2. Igaku-Shoin, New York, 1988 (pp. 420, 421).
139. *Ibid*. (p. 422).
140. *Ibid*. (p. 423).
141. Rollo IM: Drugs used in the chemotherapy of malaria, Chapter 45. In *The Pharmacological Basis of Therapeutics*, edited by Goodman and Gilman, Ed. 6. MacMillan Publishing Co., Inc., New York, 1980 (pp. 1038–1060, see p. 1056).
142. Rowland LP: Cramps, spasms and muscle stiffness. *Rev Neurol (Paris) 141*:261–273, 1985.
143. Rowland LP: Diseases of muscle and neuromuscular junction, Section 16, Chapter 537. In *Cecil Textbook of Medicine*, edited by J.B. Wyngaarden, L.H. Smith, Jr, Ed. 17. W. B. Saunders, Philadelphia, 1985 (pp. 2198–2216, *see* pp. 2215–2216).
144. Rowland LP, Penn AS: Heat-related muscle cramps. *Arch Intern Med 134*:1133, 1974.
145. Rubin D: An approach to the management of myofascial trigger point syndromes. *Arch Phys Med Rehabil 62*:107–110, 1981.
146. Sadamoto T, Bonde-Petersen F, Suzuki Y: Skeletal muscle tension, flow, pressure, and EMG during sustained isometric contractions in humans. *Eur J Appl Physiol 51*:395–408, 1983.
147. Saskin P, Whelton C, Moldofsky H, *et al.*: Sleep and nocturnal leg cramps (letter). *Sleep 11*: 307–308, 1988.

148. Schimrigk K: Muskelkater und Muskelkrampf. *Med Welt 30*:780–788, 1979.
149. Shiavi R, Griffin P: Changes in electromyographic gait patterns of calf muscles with walking speed. *IEEE Trans Biomed Eng 30*:73–76, 1983.
150. Simmons VP: Muscle spasm—why does it hurt? *Philadelphia Med 78*:307–308, 1982.
151. Simons DG: Muscle pain syndromes—Parts I and II. *Am J Phys Med 54*:289–311, 1975, and 55:15–42, 1976.
152. Simons DG: Myofascial pain syndrome due to trigger points, Chapter 45. In *Rehabilitation Medicine*, edited by Joseph Goodgold. C. V. Mosby Co., St. Louis, 1988 (pp. 686–723, *see* pp. 691, 719).
153. *Ibid.* (p. 712, Fig. 45–9B).
154. Simons DG: Myofascial Pain Syndromes. In *Current Therapy of Pain*, edited by K.M. Foley, R.M. Payne. B.C. Decker Inc., Philadelphia, 1989 (pp. 251–266, *see* Table 4).
155. Simons DG, Travell JG: Myofascial pain syndromes, Chapter 25. In *Textbook of Pain*, edited by P.D. Wall and R. Melzack, Ed 2. Churchill Livingstone, London, 1989 (pp. 368–385, *see* p. 378).
156. Sola AE: Treatment of myofascial pain syndromes. In *Recent Advances in the Management of Pain*, edited by Costantino Benedetti, C. Richard Chapman, Guido Moricca. Raven Press, New York, 1984, Series title: *Advances in Pain Research and Therapy*, Vol. 7 (pp. 467–485, *see* pp. 480–481).
157. Sola AE: Trigger point therapy, Chapter 47. In *Clinical Procedures in Emergency Medicine*, edited by J.R. Roberts and J.R. Hedges. W.B. Saunders, Philadelphia, 1985 (pp. 683–685).
158. Sontag SJ, Wanner JN: The cause of leg cramps and knee pains: an hypothesis and effective treatment. *Med Hypotheses 25*:35–41, 1988.
159. Spalteholz W: *Handatlas der Anatomie des Menschen*, Ed. 11, Vol. 2. S. Hirzel, Leipzig, 1922 (p. 363).
160. *Ibid.* (p. 364).
161. *Ibid.* (p. 366).
162. Stålberg E, Trontelj JV: *Single Fibre Electromyography*. Miravalle Press Ltd., Surrey, 1979 (pp. 99–107).
163. Steiner I, Siegal T: Muscle cramps in cancer patients. *Cancer 63*:574–577, 1989.
164. Stern FH: Leg cramps in geriatric diabetics with peripheral vascular ischemia: Treatment. *J Am Geriatr Soc 14*:609–616, 1966.
165. Sutherland DH: An electromyographic study of the plantar flexors of the ankle in normal walking on the level. *J Bone Joint Surg [Am] 48*:66–71, 1966.
166. Sutherland DH, Cooper L, Daniel D: The role of the ankle plantar flexors in normal walking. *J Bone Joint Surg [Am] 62*:354–363, 1980.
167. Toldt C: *An Atlas of Human Anatomy*, translated by M.E. Paul, Ed. 2, Vol. 1. Macmillan, New York, 1919 (p. 368).
168. Townsend MA, Lainhart SP, Shiavi R: Variability and biomechanics of synergy patterns of some lower–limb muscles during ascending and descending stairs and level walking. *Med Biol Eng Comput 16*:681–688, 1978.
169. Townsend MA, Shiavi R, Lainhart SP, *et al.*: Variability in synergy patterns of leg muscles during climbing, descending and level walking of highly-trained athletes and normal males. *Electromyogr Clin Neurophysiol 18*:69–80, 1978.
170. Travell J: Symposium on mechanism and management of pain syndromes. *Proc Rudolf Virchow Med Soc 16*:126–136, 1957.
171. Travell J: Myofascial trigger points: clinical view. In *Advances in Pain Research and Therapy*, edited by J.J. Bonica and D. Albe-Fessard, Vol. 1. Raven Press, New York, 1976 (pp. 919–926).
172. Travell J, Baker SJ, Hirsch BB, *et al.*: Myofascial component of intermittent claudication. *Fed Proc 11*:164, 1952.
173. Travell J, Rinzler SH: The myofascial genesis of pain. *Postgrad Med 11*:425–434, 1952.
174. Travell JG, Simons DG: *Myofascial Pain and Dysfunction: The Trigger Point Manual*. Williams & Wilkins, Baltimore, 1983.
175. *Ibid.* (pp. 151–152).
176. Trommer PR, Gellman MB: Trigger point syndrome. *Rheumatism 8*:67–72, 1952.
177. Vandervoort AA, McComas AJ: A comparison of the contractile properties of the human gastrocnemius and soleus muscles. *Eur J Appl Physiol 51*:435–440, 1983.
178. Warburton A, Royston JP, O'Neill CJ, et al.: A quinine a day keeps the leg cramps away? *Br J Clin Pharmacol 23*:459–465, 1987.
179. Weber EF: Ueber die Längenverhältnisse der Fleischfasern der Muskeln in Allgemeinen. *Berichte über die Verhandlungen der Königlich Sächsischen Gesellschaft der Wissenschaften zu Leipzig 3*:63–86, 1851.
180. Weiner IH, Weiner HL: Nocturnal leg muscle cramps. *JAMA 244*:2332–2333, 1980.
181. Weller M: Nocturnal calf cramp. *Lancet 1*:203, 1973.
182. Whiteley AM: Cramps, stiffness and restless legs. *Practitioner 226*:1085–1087, 1982.
183. Zumkley H: Nächtliche Wadenkrämpfe. *Dtsch Med Wochenschr 104*:1128, 1979.

CHAPTER 22
Soleus Muscle
and
Plantaris Muscle

"Jogger's Heel"

HIGHLIGHTS: **REFERRED PAIN** and tenderness from myofascial trigger points (TrPs) in the distal portion of the *soleus* muscle usually appear primarily in the posterior aspect and plantar surface of the heel and often include the distal end of the Achilles tendon. Pain may also project to an area over the sacroiliac joint on the same side of the body. The TrPs in the proximal portion of the soleus usually refer pain and tenderness over the back of the calf. The *plantaris* muscle refers pain and tenderness primarily to the back of the knee; pain may extend down the back of the calf to the middle of the leg. **ANATOMICAL ATTACHMENTS** of the *soleus* muscle proximally are to the posterior surface of the head of the fibula and along the middle third of this bone's posterior border, to the middle third of the medial border of the tibia, and to the tendinous arch that spans the two bones. Distally, the soleus and gastrocnemius muscles join to form the Achilles tendon. The soleus portion of the tendon attaches to the medial one-third of the calcaneus. An accessory soleus sometimes appears as an additional belly of the soleus muscle; this *accessory soleus* is found anterior to the Achilles tendon just above the ankle, usually chiefly on the medial side of the ankle. The soleus muscle has short fibers that are predominantly slow-twitch type 1. The frail, variable *plantaris* muscle attaches proximally to the femur deep and medial to the lateral head of the gastrocnemius; it has a long tendon that passes between the soleus and gastrocnemius muscles to attach to the medial side of the posterior part of the calcaneus. The **FUNCTION** of the *soleus* during gait is to contribute to knee stability, provide ankle stability, and restrain the forward rotation of the tibia over the fixed foot. When a person walks at an easy pace, the soleus together with the gastrocnemius stabilizes (prevents further flexion of) the knee through its action at the ankle. The soleus becomes of critical importance during running and jumping. Because of large venous sinuses, a tough fascial covering, and competent veins above, it is an effective musculovenous pump that serves as a "second heart." Both the *soleus* and *plantaris* muscles plantar flex and assist inversion of the foot. The *plantaris* weakly assists the gastrocnemius muscle in flexion of the knee. The **FUNCTIONAL UNIT** consists primarily of the soleus and the gastrocnemius muscles, which are assisted chiefly by the long flexors of the toes and the posterior tibial muscle; chief antagonists are the tibialis anterior and the long extensors of the toes. **SYMPTOMS** caused by *soleus* TrPs are primarily referred heel pain and tenderness, and restricted dorsiflexion at the ankle. Pain and tenderness may be so severe that walking is difficult or impossible, especially walking uphill or up and down stairs. Soleus TrPs are one cause of growing pains in children. An accessory soleus muscle is readily mistaken for a soft-tissue tumor. A rupture of the *plantaris* tendon should be distinguished from a tear of the gastrocnemius or soleus muscle. Soleus TrPs are easily misdiagnosed as Achilles tendinitis, thrombophlebitis, or a popliteal (Baker's) cyst. A discussion of the relation of *shin splints* to soleus TrPs completes this section, and an extensive review of *postexercise muscle soreness* appears in the Appendix of this volume. **ACTIVATION AND PERPETUATION OF TRIGGER POINTS** are caused by overload of the soleus when the individual walks in shoes with smooth leather soles on a slippery surface, or walks on soft sand, or on a laterally slanted surface, such as a beach. Jogging and running are also often responsible, as is the sudden overload from slipping or almost falling. Leaving the muscle in the shortened position for prolonged periods, during the day by foot positioning, during sitting, by wearing high heels, and at night by improper foot positioning in bed, strongly perpetuates soleus TrPs. Circulation impairment by a leg rest can be an important contributing factor. Systemic perpetuating factors must also be considered. **PATIENT EXAMINATION** when *soleus* TrPs are suspected includes testing for restriction of dorsiflexion at the ankle with the knee bent. The ankle jerk in response to an Achilles tendon tap may be reduced in amplitude. A tap with the percussion hammer on the *belly* of the muscle over the TrP may then induce a local twitch response that appears similar to, but is *NOT*, a tendon tap response. **TRIGGER POINT EXAMINATION** of *soleus* TrPs can be conducted with the patient kneeling on a chair seat or side lying with the knee bent. The distal soleus TrPs on the inner side of the Achilles tendon may be overlooked if pincer palpation does not include both sides of the Achilles tendon in the grasp. The proximal TrPs require flat palpation against the underlying bone. **ENTRAPMENTS** of the blood vessels and tibial nerve at the soleus canal can be aggravated, if not caused, by TrPs in the proximal portion of the soleus muscle. An anomalous fibrous band of the soleus muscle, when present, is another possible source of entrapment. The plantaris tendon can entrap the popliteal artery. **INTERMITTENT COLD WITH STRETCH** of the soleus may be accomplished with the patient kneeling on a chair seat or lying prone with the knee flexed 90°. Sweeps of vapocoolant spray or ice are applied distalward over the calf, heel, and instep, and should also include the sacroiliac joint area when that is painful. Simple stretch techniques, such as contract-relax, are even more effective when augmented with sychronized respiration (Lewit's postisometric relaxation) or with simultaneous antagonist contraction during the stretch phase. These techniques can be effectively incorporated in the application of intermittent cold with stretch. This procedure should always be followed promptly by moist heat applied over the muscle and then by active full range of motion. **INJECTION** of soleus TrPs is performed with the patient side lying. Care is exercised to avoid the tibial nerve, posterior tibial artery, and posterior tibial veins on those unusual occasions when TrPs need to be injected deep in the midline of the muscle. Postinjection soreness of the soleus muscle is often severe and can be reduced by having the patient apply moist heat to the muscle twice daily and avoid strenuous activity for a few days. **CORRECTIVE ACTIONS** include modification of posture and activities of daily living that overload the soleus muscle or maintain it in a fixed, shortened position for prolonged periods. Such modifications include maintaining the feet in the neutral position by pillows at night, by reducing excessive height of a chair seat or by adding a footrest, and by not wearing high heels. Slippery soles of shoes are corrected with a rubber half-sole. Leg rests should support *both* heels and calf. Walking in soft sand and on slanted surfaces should be avoided by patients with soleus TrPs, and lower limb-length inequality should be corrected. Patients are taught how to angle the body and feet when going up and down stairs, and how to pick things up from the floor without overstretching a sore, tense soleus muscle and without excessive forward bending. Following treatment by TrP injection, or by intermittent cold with stretch, the patient is given a home self-stretch program to maintain and improve on the gains made. The Soleus Pedal Exercise is useful for preventing recurrence of TrPs.

---

1. REFERRED PAIN
(Figs. 22.1 and 22.2)

Soleus
(Figs. 22.1 and 22.2)

The most common soleus trigger point, TrP_1, (Fig. 22.1) refers pain and tenderness primarily to the posterior aspect and plantar surface of the heel and also to the distal end of the Achilles tendon.[136,150] Many runners complain of this heel pain.[149] Spillover pain may be reported in the region of the trigger point (TrP) and sometimes slightly forward from the heel in the instep. This soleus TrP_1 is generally located 2 or 3 cm distal to the end of the gastrocnemius muscle belly and slightly medial to the midline.

The less common and more proximal TrP_2 (Fig. 22.1) is found high on the lateral side of the calf. This soleus TrP causes diffuse pain in the upper half of the calf.

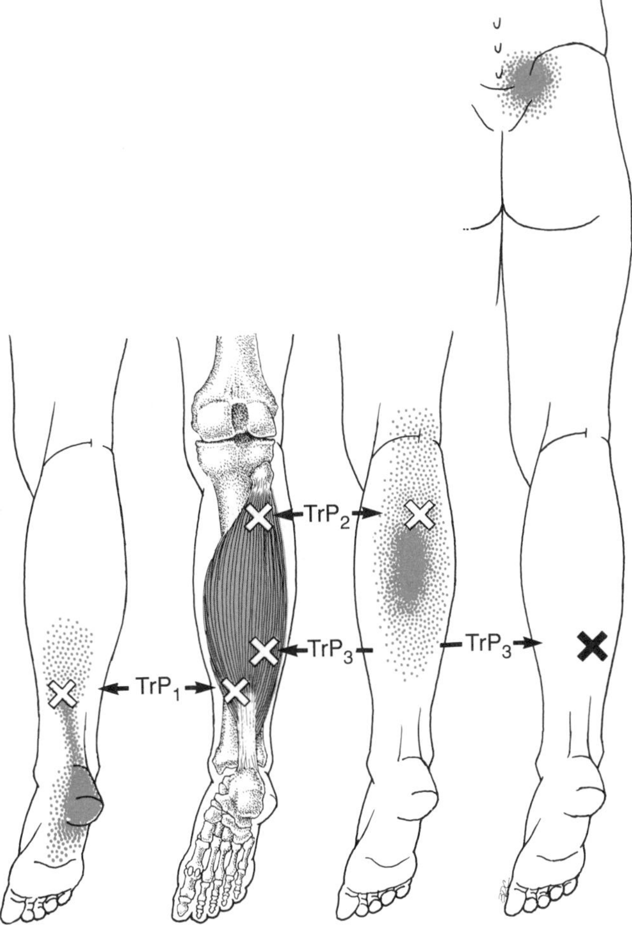

Figure 22.1. Pain patterns (*dark red*) referred from trigger points (***X**s*) commonly observed in the right soleus muscle (*light red*). The essential pain pattern (*solid red*) denotes the pain experienced by nearly everyone in whom these trigger points are active. *Red stippling* indicates the occasional spillover pain pattern. The most distal trigger point, TrP_1, causes heel pain and tenderness. The most proximal trigger point, TrP_2, is associated with calf pain (but not with nocturnal calf cramps). An intermediate and less common trigger point, TrP_3, slightly proximal and lateral to TrP_1, refers pain mainly to the region of the ipsilateral sacroiliac joint.

The very rare soleus TrP_3 (Fig. 22.1) is slightly more proximal and more lateral than TrP_1 and refers deep pain in the ipsilateral sacroiliac joint in an area about 2.5 cm (1 in) in diameter.[135] Less frequently, this TrP_3 may cause less intense spillover pain in the region of the TrP itself and over the posterior and plantar surfaces of the heel, mimicking the pattern of TrP_1.

An exceptional pain pattern referred to the jaw from the TrP_3 region has been observed twice (Fig. 22.2). In one patient, this TrP referred severe pain to the ipsilateral face deep in the jaws and temporomandibular joint with malocclusion ("Now my teeth don't meet," she said) whenever the ankle on that side was actively or passively dorsiflexed, but with no pain that is usually characteristic of the soleus muscle. The jaw pain and spasm were eliminated immediately by injecting soleus TrP_3. Occasionally, one sees such totally unexpected patterns of pain referred from TrPs in other muscles, which emphasizes the importance of obtaining a detailed and comprehensive pain history.

Other authors reported that TrPs in the soleus muscle cause heel pain[9] or pain in the heel and sole of the foot.[7]

The TrPs in the soleus muscle do *not* cause calf cramps, as do TrPs in the gastrocnemius muscle.

Plantaris
(Fig. 22.3)

Trigger points in the plantaris muscle (Fig. 22.3) refer pain behind the knee and downward over the calf as far as the midleg level. In some patients, a TrP in the vicinity of the plantaris refers pain to the ball of the foot and base of the big toe. However, it is not clear whether this pain arises from TrPs in the plantaris muscle

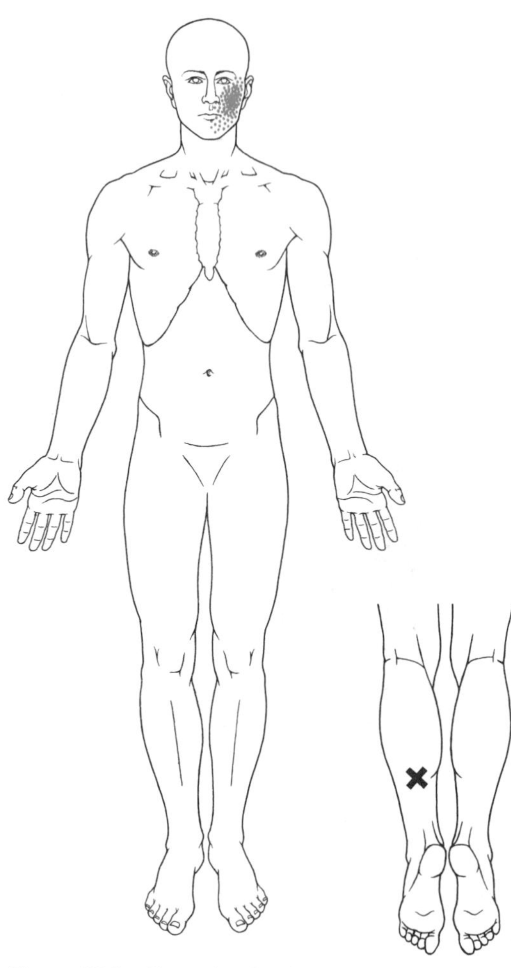

Figure 22.2. Exceptional pain pattern (*red*) referred to the left face and jaw from a rare trigger point (***X***) in the ipsilateral (left) soleus muscle.

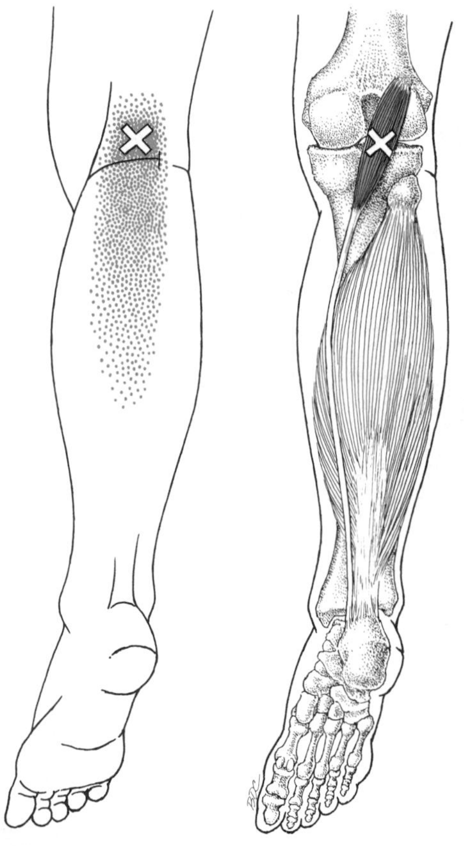

Figure 22.3. Pain pattern (*bright red*) referred from a trigger point (***X***) in the right plantaris muscle (*dark red*). The pain pattern back of the knee and usually extending down to midcalf locates the superficial diffuse pain experienced when this trigger point is active.

or in the fibers of the lateral head of the gastrocnemius.

2. ANATOMICAL ATTACHMENTS AND CONSIDERATIONS

(Figs. 22.4–22.7)

Soleus

(Figs. 22.4–22.7)

The soleus muscle crosses only the ankle joint region and not the knee joint, unlike the gastrocnemius. The soleus acts across the talocrural ('ankle') and the talocalcaneal (subtalar) joints.

The soleus muscle attaches ***proximally*** to the posterior surface of the head of the fibula and along the proximal third of the posterior surface of that bone (Fig. 22.4), to the middle third of the medial border of the tibia, and to the tendinous arch (Figs. 22.5 and 22.6) between the proximal tibia and fibula. This arch forms the roof of the soleus canal. The canal encloses the posterior tibial artery, veins, and tibial nerve. It is unusual that a tendinous arch for nerve and vessels should serve as a major attachment site for a muscle. ***Distally***, the soleus fibers attach to the underside of the aponeurosis that also provides an anchor for the gastrocnemius muscle. This aponeurosis forms the tendo calcaneus (Achilles tendon) that attaches to the posterior part of the calcaneus.

The soleus muscle is enclosed between two layers of unyielding fascia: the aponeurosis of the Achilles tendon superficially and a layer of tough fascia deep to the soleus, which is distinct from the thinner fascia that covers the deep poste-

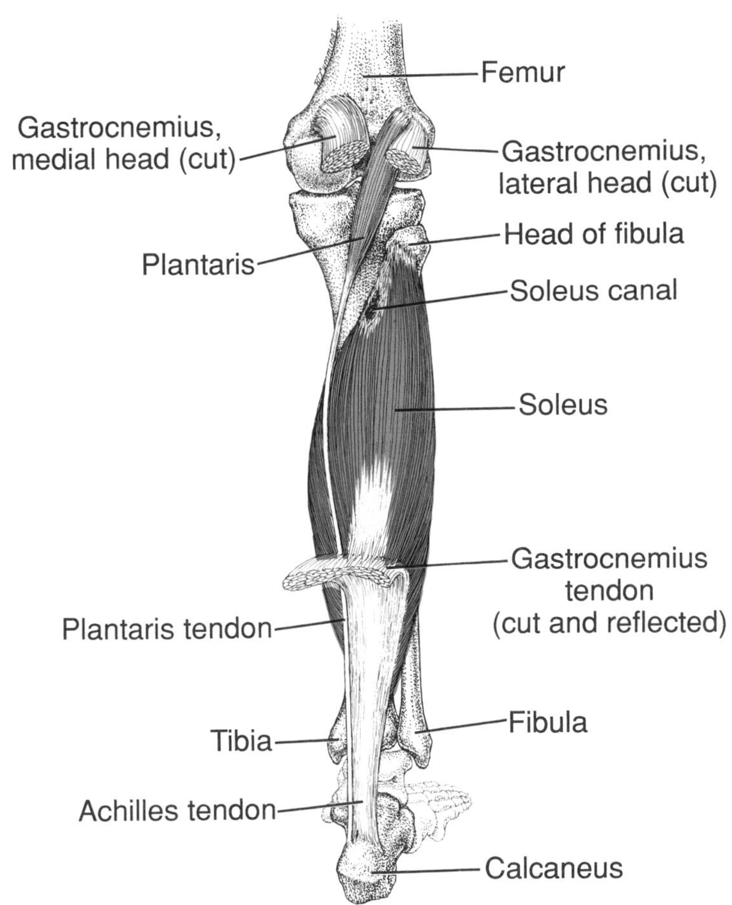

Figure 22.4. Attachments of the soleus (*dark red*) and plantaris (*light red*) muscles of the right leg. The gastrocnemius muscle (*not colored*) has been cut and most of the muscle removed.

rior compartment muscles. These thick layers of fascia on the front and back of the soleus muscle fuse together beyond the medial edge of the muscle to form an impressively tough attachment to the medial border of the tibia.[96] In this way, the soleus muscle and its fascia form an unyielding "soleus bridge" over the deep compartment, a fact that is important in the understanding and management of deep posterior compartment syndromes of the leg.[96] This unusually rigid encasement of the soleus muscle may also help to explain some of its unique hemodynamic characteristics.

The fibular side of the soleus muscle sometimes has a fibrous band (Fig. 22.5) extending across the soleus canal to the medial condyle of the tibia. This band is not usually shown in anatomy texts. It was observed by the senior author and was drawn from a photograph of one of several cadaver dissections that showed this structure. When present, it may contribute to entrapment of the neurovascular bundle at the proximal edge where the bundle enters the soleus canal.

The view showing the deep surface of the soleus muscle (Fig. 22.6) depicts its attachment to the tendinous arch of the soleus canal and also shows the neurovascular bundle leaving the canal.[29]

This same view illustrates the complexity of the soleus muscle. The most superficial fibers overlap like shingles angling down and outward. The deepest, more proximal fibers have a bipennate arrangement (Fig. 22.6). These fibers originate proximally from the tibia and fibula and attach distally to a tendinous septum that is part of the Achilles tendon.

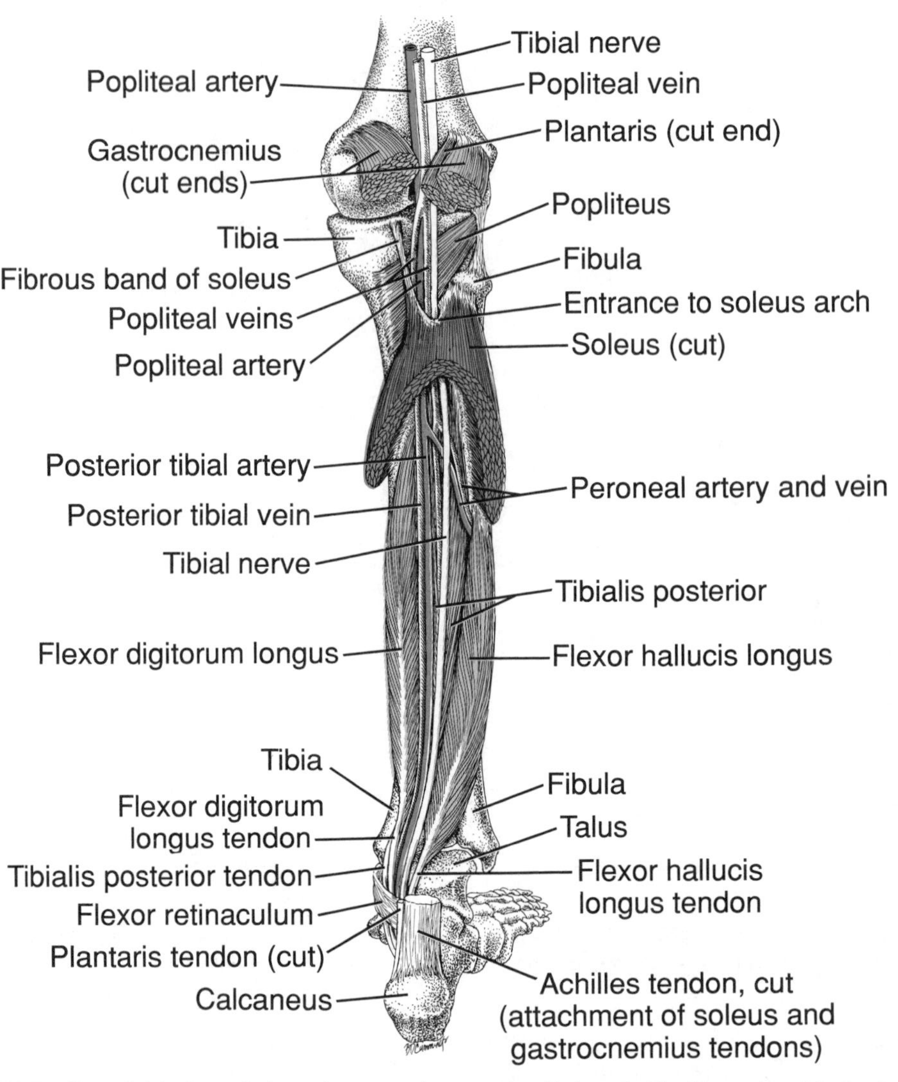

Figure 22.5. Superficial view of the soleus canal with the major portion of the right soleus muscle (*dark red*) cut and removed. This shows the relations of the soleus tendinous arch and the muscle to the posterior tibial artery (*bright red*), posterior tibial veins (*black cross hatching*), tibial nerve (*white*), and neighboring muscles (*light red*). The fibrous band that extends upward from the medial side of the arch that forms the soleus canal is drawn from a photograph of an anatomical specimen in which the band was unusually well developed.

The fibers of the Achilles tendon twist approximately 90°. The tendinous fibers from the soleus attach to the medial one-third of the calcaneus (Fig. 22.7)[96] and the fibers from the gastrocnemius attach to the lateral two-thirds of the bone.

Figure 19.3 in Chapter 19 of this volume presents a cross-sectional view of the soleus muscle at the level of the lower portion of the middle third of the leg, well below the soleus canal.

Anatomical variations in the soleus muscle include doubling (two layers),[10,160] partial deficiency,[160] or absence of the medial head.[10]

Accessory Soleus

Occasionally, an accessory soleus muscle is identified. It appears as an additional belly of the soleus muscle that extends distally from the deep surface of the soleus to the calcaneus[10] and usually lies more on the medial than on the lateral side of the tendon. The bulk

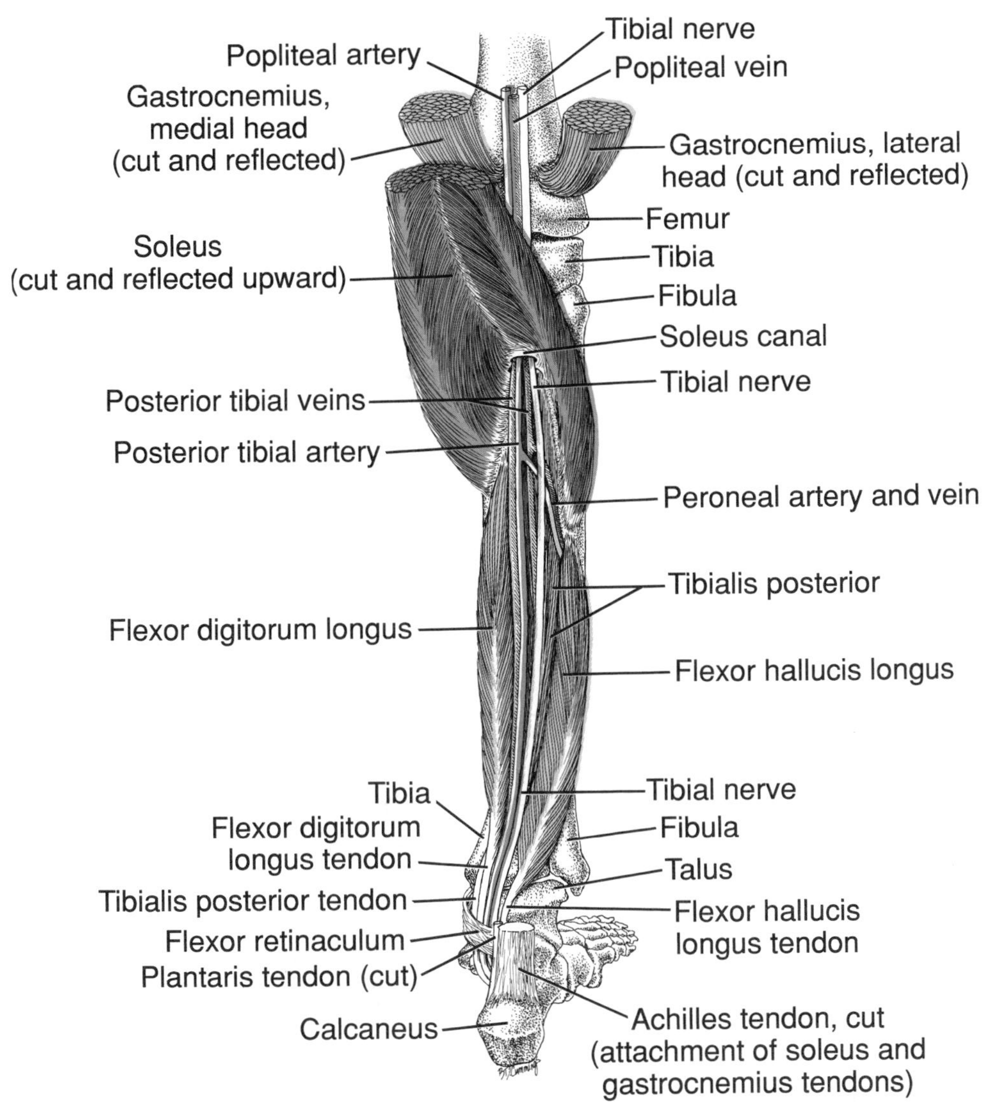

Figure 22.6. The soleus muscle (*dark red*) has been reflected upward showing the distal opening of the soleus canal and its relation to the tibial nerve (*white*), to the posterior tibial artery (*bright red*), to the posterior tibial veins, (*black cross hatching*), and to the adjacent musculature (*light red*). This is an artist's reconstruction of what the canal would look like if it were possible to reflect the muscle without cutting its proximal attachments to the tibia and fibula. The gastrocnemius muscle is cut and reflected.

of the accessory muscle is found in Karger's triangle and replaces the fibrofatty tissue that usually occupies this space above the ankle joint between the Achilles tendon and the tibia. The accessory soleus muscle has been described as covered with fascia that is separate from the soleus muscle.[130]

Proximally, the accessory muscle fibers merge with the soleus muscle at about midleg. Distally, it sometimes attaches to the anterior (deep) surface of the Achilles tendon and sometimes directly to the calcaneus.[42,80,81,113,130,153]

The accessory soleus is of special clinical importance because it may be mistaken for a tumor, as discussed in Section 6 of this chapter.

Fiber Types and Size

The proportion of slow-twitch, type 1 muscle fibers that depend on oxidative metabolism is higher in the soleus (70–75%) than in other muscles of the lower limb.[36] Two other studies observed a similar relationship between the soleus muscle and the vastus lateralis.[37,140] The soleus comprised about 75% type 1 (slow-twitch) fibers

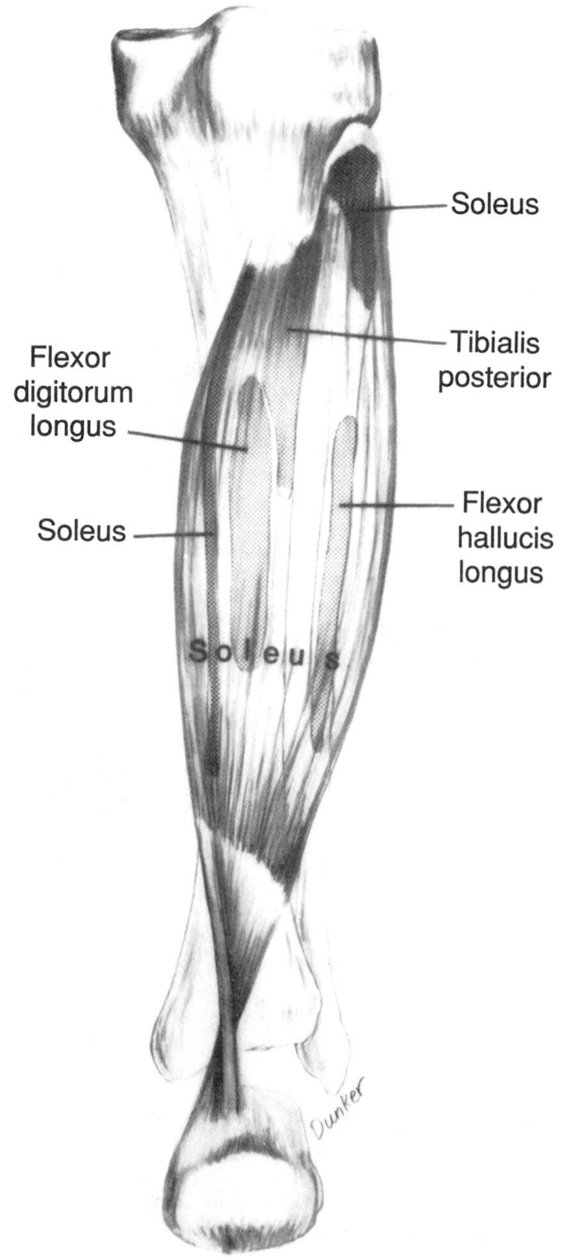

Figure 22.7. Attachment of the soleus portion of the right Achilles tendon to the os calcis, posterior view. Note the tendon's rotation of 90° and attachment to the medial one-third of the calcaneus. The gastrocnemius portion of the tendon (not shown) attaches to the lateral two-thirds of the os calcis. [Reproduced with permission.[96]]

and the vastus lateralis about 50%. The percentage of type 1 fibers in the soleus muscle was higher in six athletic young adult men (79%) than in six comparable women (67%).[140]

Elder and associates[37] found that the variability in the distribution of fiber types was so large that five sites must be sampled from the same muscle to keep the standard deviation below 5%.

Weber[157] reported that the muscle fibers of the soleus muscle weighed 335 g, about one-fourth the weight of the gluteus maximus muscle and nearly the same weight as the gastrocnemius muscle. The average fiber length of both the soleus and gastrocnemius muscles was quite short, 3.7 and 3.5 cm (1.5 in).

Plantaris
(Fig. 22.4)

Because it attaches proximally beside the lateral head of the gastrocnemius muscle, the plantaris can be thought of as an accessory lateral head of that muscle. The plantaris is a small, frail muscle, the fibers of which angle across the capsule of the knee joint in the popliteal space (Fig. 22.4). Its ***proximal*** attachment is on the femur along the lateral prolongation of the linea aspera proximal to the attachment of the lateral head of the gastrocnemius muscle.[86] The muscle then crosses to the medial aspect of the popliteal space where it becomes a thin tendon that lies between the gastrocnemius and soleus muscles. ***Distally***, the plantaris tendon runs along the medial border of the tendo calcaneus[29] (Fig. 22.4) and attaches with it to the calcaneus. Most of the muscle belly is covered by the lateral head of the gastrocnemius.

The plantaris is a rudimentary muscle that is analogous to the palmaris longus of the upper extremity.[64] Like the palmaris longus, it is exceedingly variable in origin, structure, and insertion,[10] and has been reported as absent in 6.2–7.5% of lower extremities.[64]

Supplemental References

The surface contour of the soleus muscle is shown from in front[43] and from the lateral side.[28,78] The edges of the muscle can be seen from in front in a dissection.[128,142]

The superficial upper half of the soleus is presented from behind without vessels or nerve, alone,[3] and with the plantaris muscle.[48,147] Rear views of the plantaris and upper portion of the superficial soleus muscle include the posterior tibial vessels and tibial nerve entering the soleus canal.[64,104,114,126] The plantaris muscle belly is shown in detail.[92] The entire plantaris muscle and the superficial surface of the soleus muscle, including the Achilles tendon, are seen from behind.[143] Partial removal of the soleus reveals the posterior tibial vessels and tibial nerve penetrating the soleus canal.[4,45,65,91,105] An illustration with the edges of the soleus arch cut portrays clearly the short extent of the soleus canal, approximately 2.5 cm (1 in).[90]

The Achilles tendon is viewed from the medial side,[5,46,106,127] and from the medial side and below.[93] The soleus muscle is viewed from the medial side.[46,127] As seen from the lateral side, the muscle is illustrated alone[47,89,103,141] and with the Achilles tendon.[30] The lateral view of the tendon appears in detail.[94,106]

The subcutaneous calcaneal bursa provides a cushion between the attachment of the Achilles tendon at the heel and the overlying skin.[106] The subtendinous calcaneal bursa reduces friction between the Achilles tendon and the calcaneus near the tendon's attachment.[46,47,106]

A complete series of cross sections is available for the soleus muscle and Achilles tendon[24] and for the plantaris muscle and its tendon.[23] Selected cross sections can be seen of the soleus and plantaris muscles at the upper third of the leg,[26,49,115] at the middle third of the leg,[1,116] and at the lower third of the leg.[27,117] The distal sections show the relations of the plantaris and Achilles tendons to the space in Karger's triangle that lies between the tendons and the posterior surface of the tibia. This space is occupied by the accessory soleus muscle, when present.

A sagittal section through the knee joint shows the soleus muscle.[125] The proximal bony attachments are marked for the plantaris muscle[2,44,86] and for the soleus muscle.[2,44,87] The attachments of the Achilles tendon[88,127] and of the plantaris tendon[88] are marked on the calcaneus.

3. INNERVATION

The soleus muscle is supplied by a branch of the tibial nerve that contains fibers from the first and second sacral spinal nerves. The branch of the tibial nerve that supplies the plantaris muscle contains fibers from the fourth and fifth lumbar and first sacral spinal nerves.[29]

4. FUNCTION

During normal walking, electrical activity of the soleus begins with toe-off of the opposite foot and ends as the opposite heel strikes the ground. The function of the muscle appears to be that of resisting the kinetic force of forward movement.[144] The plantar flexors (including the soleus) first produce a lengthening contraction and, later, a shortening contraction during stance. This muscle activity contributes to knee stability, provides ankle stability, restrains the forward rotation of the tibia on the talus, and conserves energy by minimizing vertical oscillation of the body's center of mass; this activity does not ordinarily propel the body forward.[145] According to Perry,[118] the soleus helps restrain the valgus thrust on the ankle that occurs during single-limb balance.

Together, the soleus and gastrocnemius muscles compose the triceps surae, the primary plantar flexor of the foot. Of these two muscles, only for the soleus muscle is the forcefulness of plantar flexion almost independent of knee angle. Because of the 90° rotation of the Achilles tendon[64,96] and its attachment to the medial one-third of the calcaneus (Fig. 22.7),[96] the soleus also helps invert the foot.

Soleus

Action

The soleus muscle is a primary plantar flexor of the "free" foot. Janda[68] regards the soleus muscle as an assistant to supination of the foot.

Although a number of authors have not recognized an inversion function of the soleus,[29,71,123] a recent study by Michael and Holder[96] substantiated that the soleus muscle selectively assists inversion of the foot. They found in all of 28 dissections that the soleus portion of the Achilles tendon attached only to the medial one-third of the calcaneus; hence, it would be expected to produce inversion of the heel. In all of the 10 subjects tested, stimulation of the medial part of the soleus muscle produced plantar flexion and heel inversion, never eversion. The lateral portion of the muscle was not tested in this way.[96]

The work of Campbell and associates,[22] recording electromyographic (EMG) activity of the soleus using fine-wire electrodes, established that there is no simple relation between inversion or eversion of the foot and the motor unit activity of medial or lateral portions of the muscle. Surprisingly, they found in untrained subjects that the medial part of the soleus was more active in foot eversion but, in trained subjects, the expected EMG activity of the lateral part during eversion was predominant. This difference may be due to athletic training enabling people to use their muscles more efficiently.[22]

Comparing soleus and gastrocnemius activity during ankle plantar flexion effort against varying loads, Herman and Bragin[61] reported that the soleus EMG activity seemed to predominate in minimal contractions, particularly in dorsiflexed positions. The slope of the relation comparing EMG activity and tension was nearly constant for the soleus muscle regardless of its length. On the other hand, the gastrocnemius was most active electromyographically when the ankle was plantar flexed, in strong contraction, and rapidly developing tension.

Soleus Contractile Properties

The soleus muscle is remarkable among human muscles for its resistance to fatigue. Kukulka *et al.*[72] found the soleus much more fatigue resistant than intrinsic hand and foot muscles. Its contraction time was about 50% slower and its half-relaxation time was 50% longer than that of either head of the gastrocnemius muscle.[154] Van Hinsbergh *et al.*[155] found that the soleus muscle had the highest oxidative enzyme activity of all the lower extremity muscles examined (gluteal, quadriceps femoris, and gastrocnemius). Soleus muscle biopsy samples[155] oxidized more palmitate and showed more cytochrome c oxidase activity per milligram of homogenate than did the other lower extremity muscles, probably because of its higher percentage of type 1 (slow-twitch) fibers that depend on oxidative rather than on glycolytic metabolism.

The degree to which the soleus is composed of fatigue-resistant slow-twitch fibers correlates with how the muscle is used. Nardone and Schieppati[101] found that, during lengthening contractions of the triceps surae, the lateral head of the gastrocnemius was activated in subjects with long soleus half-relaxation times (more slow-twitch fibers), whereas the soleus was activated preferentially in subjects with short soleus half-relaxation times.

The responsiveness of the soleus muscle interacts with conditions in other parts of the body. Hufschmidt and Sell[67] stimulated the tibial nerve and interpreted changes in the latency of the silent period in the *contralateral* soleus muscle as indicative of crossed motor reflexes in 17 of 30 subjects.

Traccis and associates[148] found that head rotation influenced the excitability of soleus motor neurons as measured by the amplitude of Hoffman (H) reflexes. Response progressively increased with contralateral rotations from 0–16° and progressively decreased with ipsilateral rotations.

Using the same H reflex measure, Romano and Schieppati[129] showed that soleus motoneurone excitability increased during concentric (shortening) contractions of the soleus muscle and that the more rapid the movement, the greater the increase. Conversely, excitability was decreased during eccentric (lengthening) contractions to less than the control values observed during rest, and the more rapid the movement, the greater the reduction in excitability. Passive dorsiflexion of the foot contributed to H-reflex inhibition. These modulations would help prevent overload of the soleus during sudden lengthening contractions.

Functions

The soleus muscle is active during walking, bicycling, running, and jumping. Its pumping action increases the venous flow of blood from the feet and legs.

Surface electrode EMG studies of soleus function must be regarded with caution. Perry and associates[119] found that only 36% of the data obtained by soleus surface electrodes was related to activity of the soleus muscle. The bulk of the recorded activity came from other muscles.

Walking. Computer analysis of soleus muscle EMG activity among 25 normal individuals walking at a variety of self-selected speeds identified 10 different patterns of EMG activity.[134] Activity always began either at or shortly before heel-strike. As walking speed increased, it began earlier in the gait cycle. At higher walking speeds, 5.3% of all patterns showed a second phase of soleus activity around toe-off, suggesting that some individuals were using the soleus, at times, to help impart forward momentum. This study substantiated the marked variability in the way normal individuals use their soleus muscles.

Brandell[18] found that, regardless of grade or speed during walking, calf muscle activity rapidly increased just before heel-rise and reached its peak intensity at the transition from knee extension to knee flexion as the ankle began to plantar flex. Yang and Winter[161] found that the timing of the EMG activity was closely coupled to the percentage of stride time that had elapsed, regardless of the cadence of walking. This is consistent with the previous conclusion that the primary role of the triceps surae in walking is to stabilize (prevent further flexion of) the knee during the stance phase of gait.[11,12]

Campbell and associates[22] showed with fine-wire electrodes that the medial and lateral portions of the soleus muscle can have distinctly different functions in some subjects. The medial part is a strong plantar flexor of the foot at the ankle, and a strong stabilizer of the leg on the foot. The lateral part adds little power to moving the foot at the ankle, but is largely a stabilizer, especially when the base of support is rendered unstable by wearing high heels.

Bicycling. Ericson and associates[38] recorded EMG activity in each of 11 young men during ergometer cycling. The soleus muscle averaged 37% of its maximum-effort EMG activity just beyond the forward position of the pedal on the down stroke. This activation was slightly more than that of the gastrocnemius, but less than that of the vastus medialis and lateralis muscles. The soleus was the only one of the lower limb muscles monitored that increased its activity when the pedal was shifted from the instep to the toe position. An increase in pedalling rate increased soleus activity; an increase in seat height did not. Among the 10 subjects tested, the soleus muscle EMG activity showed no significant difference in mean peak amplitude between cycling and walking.

Sports and Falls. Bilateral EMG activity of the soleus and lateral head of the gastrocnemius muscle was recorded from surface electrodes with equal amplification during a single-foot volleyball spike and a basketball layup. Activity was greatest on the dominant side and appeared more vigorous in the soleus than in the lateral head of the gastrocnemius. Likewise, during right-handed sports activities, including overhand throws, underhand throws, tennis, golf, and hitting a baseball, the right soleus was more active than the left and appeared to be responding more vigorously than the gastrocnemius.[20]

Greenwood and Hopkins[59] recorded EMG activity in the soleus during sudden falls. When the fall was unexpected, two peaks of activity appeared. One was present immediately after loss of support and appeared in muscles throughout the body. No such initial soleus EMG activity was found in two patients with absent labyrinthine function. The other peak appeared only in falls of sufficient height, exclusively in lower extremity muscles, and was related to the time of landing. The first peak was interpreted as a startle reaction to an unexpected fall and the second to voluntary preparation for landing.

Venous Pump. **As military people know well, raw recruits in the army who stand immobile at attention may suddenly faint when venous blood pools in the lower limbs because it is not being pumped upward by the soleus muscle. Trained recruits rhythmically contract and relax the calf muscles isometrically and thus avoid fainting while they stand at attention.**

The soleus provides a major pumping action to return blood from the lower limb toward the heart. Venous sinuses in the soleus muscle are compressed by the muscle's strong contractions so that its venous blood is forced upward toward the heart. This pumping action (the body's second heart) depends on compe-

tent valves in the popliteal veins. Valves in the veins to prevent reflux of the blood are most numerous in the veins of the lower limbs where the vessels must return blood against high hydrostatic pressure. The popliteal vein usually contains four valves.[31] Deeper veins that are subject to the pumping action of muscle contraction are more richly provided with valves.[79]

Ludbrook[82] compared the soleus to other lower extremity muscles for its effectiveness as a musculovenous pump. On maximal contraction, the soleus generated the most intramuscular pressure, 250 mm Hg, as compared to 230 mm Hg by the gastrocnemius and only 140 mm Hg and 60 mm Hg by the vastus lateralis and an adductor muscle, respectively. A single contraction of the calf ejected about 60% of the blood that had entered it while standing, whereas thigh contraction ejected only about 20%. Ludbrook estimated that a single contraction reduces the blood volume of the calf by 60–95 mL and of the thigh by 35 mL. The intramuscular sinuses that are so prominent in the calf are absent in the musculature of the thigh. An additional factor enhancing the soleus pump is the much greater competence of the valves in the popliteal veins in response to postural changes. The thigh veins refilled with reflux of blood from above; the calf veins did not.

Unlike most muscles, which show cessation of arterial flow (^{133}Xe clearance) at nearly 50% of maximum voluntary contraction for only a brief period, in two of four subjects,[133] arterial flow continued in the soleus despite an 80% maximal contraction sustained for 2 minutes or until fatigue intervened.

McLachlin and McLachlin[85] pioneered an understanding of the value of the soleus as a musculovenous pump in clinical practice. They demonstrated by contrast venography the pooling of blood in the soleus muscle in a relaxed recumbent subject and the effectiveness of calf contraction in emptying the soleus venous system. Venography of six patients under anesthesia for surgery[74] demonstrated that contrast dye cleared the soleus muscle in one-third of the time when the patient was placed in the Trendelenburg position (ankles placed 20 cm (8 in) above heart level) as compared to clearance in the supine position.[74]

Sabri and co-workers[132] surgically attached electromagnetic flowmeters to the femoral vein and artery to evaluate the pumping action of a motor-driven pedal that passively dorsiflexed the foot 15° and stretched the soleus muscle. Mean blood flow increased progressively and doubled as the pedal rate was increased from 24 to 50 cycles per minute.

Frazier[51] trained his surgical patients to plantar flex the foot actively against a foam pad placed at the foot of the bed pre- and postoperatively. He demonstrated radiographically with contrast medium that this resisted isometric plantar flexion effort was remarkably more effective in emptying the veins within the soleus muscle than unresisted plantar flexion.

The value of electrical stimulation to contract the calf muscles under general anesthesia was reported in 1972 by Nicolaides and associates.[108] They found that a pulse duration of 50 ms at the rate of 12–15 pulses/min was optimal and effective in preventing deep vein thrombosis.

Since these studies were reported, the use of anticoagulants, such as heparin, have become popular to prevent venous thrombosis. In a recent study, the combination of heparin and electrical activation of the tibialis anterior and gastrocnemius-soleus muscles proved significantly more effective than heparin alone in preventing deep vein thrombosis.[95]

"Spontaneous" thrombosis of the deep leg veins can occur due to prolonged sitting when travelling in a car or airplane, especially in susceptible individuals.[66] This can be prevented by activating the soleus pump sufficiently often. The danger of sitting immobilized for prolonged periods in chairs that produce underthigh compression was demonstrated in air raid shelters by the frequency with which pulmonary embolism followed immediately after air raids on London during World War II.[137]

Winkel and Bendix[159] found that subjects who were seated, either typing or doing desk work, activated the soleus muscle only occasionally and then merely to 6% of maximum voluntary contraction.

Postures. When an individual tries to stand quietly, a slight forward and backward sway develops that is controlled by alternate contraction of the anterior tibial and soleus muscles.[11,70] When the person voluntarily tries to sway forward and backward either slowly or rapidly, the same pattern of muscle activity becomes very marked. The soleus is active while the center of gravity is anterior, and the anterior tibial muscle becomes active

PART 3

when the center of gravity swings posterior to the relaxed position.[53,109,110] Standing upright at military attention nearly doubles soleus activity, as compared with standing at ease. Standing with weight mainly on the balls of the feet activates the soleus muscle vigorously.[109] Wearing high heels usually increases the load on the soleus muscle.[70] A high heel also causes ankle instability that requires additional bursts of soleus activity to maintain equilibrium.[22]

Specific and consistent stabilizing adjustments (inhibition and excitation) appear in the lower limbs *preparatory* to vigorous movement of an upper extremity in standing subjects.[16] Repeated tests of 11 subjects established that the soleus muscle was the first muscle to show EMG changes in this situation.

Resection of Soleus. Markhede and Nistor[83] studied seven patients in whom part or all of the soleus muscle had been removed surgically. All seven patients could stand and walk on tiptoe. The only two patients reporting unsteadiness of gait when walking on uneven ground were the two who had either the left or right half of all calf musculature removed. Just the soleus muscle was completely removed in three patients. Only one of the seven patients had a mean isometric plantar flexion strength less than 80% of the normal side and that was the one who had lost all of the soleus and half of the gastrocnemius muscle.

Plantaris

The plantaris weakly assists the gastrocnemius muscle in flexion of the knee and plantar flexion of the foot at the ankle.[12,29,64,123] Basmajian[12] found, using fine-wire electrodes, that its primary action is plantar flexion and inversion of the foot. Only in a loading situation does the plantaris assist in knee flexion.[12]

5. FUNCTIONAL (MYOTATIC) UNIT

Together, the soleus and gastrocnemius muscles (triceps surae) are the prime plantar flexors of the foot. This function of the triceps surae is assisted by the peroneus longus and brevis, flexor hallucis longus, flexor digitorum longus, tibialis posterior,[68,123] and by the plantaris muscle.[123] Compared to all of these muscles (except the relatively insignificant plantaris), the triceps surae has a marked mechanical advantage due to the longer lever arm created by its calcaneal attachment. Many individuals do not use the peroneus longus and brevis as plantar flexors, although if necessary, they can learn to do so.[63]

Antagonists to plantar flexion by the soleus muscle include primarily the tibialis anterior, extensor digitorum longus, and peroneus tertius muscles, which are assisted by the extensor hallucis longus.[123]

6. SYMPTOMS

This section first summarizes the symptoms that patients experience as a result of soleus and plantaris TrPs. Then it addresses major differential diagnostic concerns, and finally it summarizes postexercise muscle soreness (covered in detail in the Appendix of this volume) and considers how shin splints may relate to myofascial TrPs.

Symptoms due to Trigger Points

Soleus

An active TrP_1 is, by far, the most common of the soleus TrPs. Patients with this TrP complain of tenderness referred to the heel in addition to pain in the distribution described in Section 1 of this chapter. It may hurt unbearably to place weight on the heel. The heel may ache at night. However, nocturnal calf pain is more likely to be caused by gastrocnemius than soleus TrPs. One of the most frequent complaints by recreational runners is heel pain.[15]

An active TrP_2 or TrP_3 causes pain referred in the patterns described in Section 1 of this chapter. These upper soleus TrPs are more likely to interfere with the soleus musculovenous pump, causing symptoms of calf and foot pain together with edema of the foot and ankle.

Soleus TrPs restrict ankle dorsiflexion. This limitation makes it difficult or impossible for many patients to pick things up from the floor by employing safe body mechanics to keep the trunk erect, which requires knee flexion and unrestricted ankle dorsiflexion. Individuals with soleus TrPs are prone to develop low back pain because the restriction of ankle dorsiflexion leads them to lean over and lift improperly.

A person with a very active soleus TrP can be severely immobilized. Walking becomes difficult and painful, especially walking uphill, or up and down stairs. Some patients complain of low back pain when getting up from a chair without the assistance of armrests.

"Growing pains" were studied in 54 children between the ages of 5 and 14 years.[14] One of the four stretch techniques used to provide lasting relief of the symptoms was a stretch specifically for the soleus muscle. This beneficial result suggests that active soleus TrPs may have been a contributing cause of "growing pains" in these children, which matches our experience and that of Bates and Grunwaldt.[13]

Accessory Soleus

A 1986 review[130] found this variant reported in only 15 patients, suggesting that symptoms caused by an accessory soleus muscle occur rarely.

Physical examination reveals a firm mass between the medial malleolus and the Achilles tendon. The mass may or may not be tender. Traction on the muscular mass plantar flexes the foot.[6] The mass becomes hard (tense) when the foot is forcefully actively plantar flexed,[42,130,153] or when standing on tiptoe.[58] The mass appears more prominent when the foot is dorsiflexed, which causes the accessory muscle to bulge out from between the Achilles tendon and the distal tibia.

If pain develops, it is located in the region of the accessory muscle belly posterior to the medial malleolus. The pain frequently starts after a conditioning program that requires running, and then is aggravated by running or just by walking.

Diagnostic testing can help distinguish an accessory soleus muscle from a neoplasm. Plain soft tissue radiography shows the extent of the mass,[6,58,130] but does not confirm that it is muscle. A computerized tomography scan more clearly delineates the mass and can confirm that its density is similar to that of muscle.[35,102,120,130] However, Pettersson et al.[120] emphasize that uncertainty as to whether the mass is muscle or not can be resolved if, on magnetic resonance imaging, the T1 and T2 relaxation times of the mass are the same as in neighboring muscles.

The diagnosis was sometimes made when normal muscle tissue was found on biopsy or at operation.[33] Several authors[35,54] established the muscular nature of the mass when they recorded normal motor units by needle electromyography. They and Graham[58] observed the same motor latency as for the soleus muscle in response to tibial nerve stimulation. Other authors reported the use of xeroradiography[6,153] and sonography[102] to help establish the diagnosis.

Pain due to an accessory soleus muscle was relieved by total or subtotal resection of the muscle,[80,102,107,130,153] by fasciotomy,[80,113,130] and by reattaching the accessory tendon from the calcaneus to the Achilles tendon.[81] Painful accessory soleus muscles were generally described as tender. The painfulness of some of these accessory muscles may have been caused by TrPs. No reports were found that specifically examined the muscle for them. Since fasciotomy was repeatedly successful, some of the painful muscles may have suffered from a compartment syndrome, but no intramuscular pressure measurements were mentioned.

Plantaris

An active TrP in the plantaris muscle refers pain to the back of the knee and upper calf, as illustrated in Figure 22.3.

Differential Diagnosis

Differential diagnoses to be considered in patients with pain in a distribution characteristic of common soleus TrPs include TrP syndromes of other muscles, rupture of a calf muscle, S_1 radiculopathy, Achilles tendinitis, thrombophlebitis, a ruptured popliteal cyst, or possibly a systemic viral infection. Patients with peripheral occlusive arterial disease and intermittent claudication often also develop myofascial TrPs in the ischemic muscles. These TrPs can contribute significantly to the patient's pain.[7]

Other Trigger Points

Another myofascial TrP source of heel pain and tenderness is the quadratus plantae muscle of the sole of the foot (*see* Fig. 27.1). The tenderness caused by TrPs in the quadratus plantae muscle is located in front of the heel and can be elicited by pressing on the medial side of this muscle and backward toward the heel deep in the instep. Myofascial TrPs in this muscle, like those in the soleus, also cause the bottom of the heel to be hypersensitive and the patient complains that it hurts to bear weight on the heel.

Abductor hallucis TrPs also refer pain to the heel, but to its medial side only (*see* Fig. 26.2).

Rupture

The plantaris muscle belly lies between the two heads of the gastrocnemius muscle in the popliteal space and its tendon passes distally between the soleus and gastrocnemius muscles. It is important to distinguish between rupture of the plantaris muscle or tendon, which is temporarily painful but does not impair the power of plantar flexion, and rupture of the soleus muscle, which can cause plantar flexion weakness.

The same stresses are likely to cause rupture of either the plantaris or soleus muscles. However, the plantaris muscle is more likely to be torn during a forceful lengthening contraction with the knee straight; the soleus is more vulnerable when the knee is bent to some degree and is not protected by the gastrocnemius. Plantaris muscle rupture causes a sudden sharp pain at the moment of tearing and may produce a snapping sound with a sense of injury in the calf. The patient may describe an overload lengthening contraction caused by a fall, near-fall, or one caused by slipping while walking up a steep hill. Plantaris muscle rupture immediately produces acute pain up and down the center of the calf followed later by ecchymosis as low as the ankle.

Plantaris rupture should also be distinguished from a tear of the gastrocnemius muscle ("Tennis leg," *see* Chapter 21, page 407), which is now thought to be more common than rupture of the plantaris tendon.[52] A rupture of the belly of the gastrocnemius muscle (usually medial head) is palpable near its distal musculotendinous junction and is also likely to cause ecchymosis that appears a day or two later in the region of the lower calf and ankle. Ultrasonography, magnetic resonance imaging, and computed tomography scans can identify the source of the symptoms and extent of injury if these are not apparent from careful palpation of the muscles and from the location of tenderness.

Heel Spur

If the patient happens to have a bone spur on the plantar surface of the calcaneus, the spur is frequently thought to be the cause of heel tenderness. However, if one looks at a radiograph of the other heel, it, too, may show an equally large spur that is symptom free. The heel spur in such a patient is usually coincidental and has no causal relation to the pain or tenderness. A soleus muscle TrP_1 is often a major source of tenderness referred to the heel. As pointed out by Singer,[139] an elevated serum uric acid level may render a heel spur painful, and is likely to aggravate TrPs in the soleus (and many other muscles).

Other causes of heel pain include plantar fasciitis, Achilles tendinitis, calcaneal stress fractures, entrapment of the calcaneal branch of the posterior tibial nerve, and a fat pad syndrome.[15]

Achilles Tendinitis

Some cases of Achilles tendinitis, or peritendinitis, may be due to shortening of the soleus and gastrocnemius muscles caused by TrPs in those muscles with chronically increased tension on the Achilles tendon. Patients with tendinitis are likely to complain of diffuse pain in or about the Achilles tendon that is aggravated by activity.[25] Runners experience burning pain early in the run which eases off during the run, but then worsens afterward.[19] Tenderness is most severe 4–5 cm (1½–2 in) proximal to the tendon attachment on the calcaneus, but may be diffuse along the entire Achilles tendon. When tendinitis is severe, swelling, crepitus, and a tender nodule in the tendon may be present.[19] Sonography can demonstrate thickening of the peritendinous connective tissue, and structural disturbance of the tendon including rupture with hematoma.[97]

In a study of 109 runners with Achilles tendinitis, Clement and associates[25] found the most common cause to be overtraining or injudicious training. Nearly half of their cases showed gastrocnemius/soleus weakness and loss of flexibility, both of which are also caused by myofascial TrPs in these muscles. Excessive training is also likely to activate myofascial TrPs, a cause of pain which was apparently not considered in this study. Another common cause of Achilles tendinitis, functional overpronation, is well illustrated and described by these authors and can be corrected with shoe inserts. One easily correctable cause of tendinitis, footwear with an inflexible sole, overloads and may activate TrPs in the soleus muscle.

If the pain and tenderness are referred to the tendon by an active soleus TrP, they can be distinguished from the symptoms of tendinitis. Inactivation of the soleus TrP relieves the pain and tenderness immediately if these symptoms are referred and not due to tendinitis.

Posterior heel pain of the Haglund Syndrome is associated with a visible and palpable "pump-bump."[112] In this syndrome, there is a thickening of the soft tissues at the insertion of the Achilles tendon. It is seen in those who wear stiff shoes with a shallow heel while engaging in strenuous activity; it is characterized by a radiographically prominent calcaneal enlargement at the insertion of the Achilles tendon, retrocalcaneal bursitis, thickening of the Achilles tendon, and a convexity of the superficial soft tissues at the level of the Achilles tendon insertion. The degree of enlargement is measurable by radiography.[112]

Thrombophlebitis

The calf tenderness of deep vein thrombosis, particularly of veins within the soleus muscle, could mimic an acute myofascial syndrome. In thrombophlebitis, the relatively constant pain regardless of muscular activity, and the presence of warmth and redness, are helpful in the diagnosis. However, these signs may be absent, and clinical examination alone is unreliable for detection of thrombophlebitis.[124] Diagnostic techniques include Doppler ultrasonography,[17] impedance plethysmography, and fibrinogen uptake.[17,124] None of these is satisfactory for a definitive diagnosis, so contrast venography remains the standard.[122,124]

Treatment of acute thrombophlebitis usually includes anticoagulant medication and bed rest. If the patient has active TrPs in the soleus (or other lower-limb muscles), the immobility of bed rest will likely aggravate them. When assessing clinical progress, it is important to distinguish the pain and tenderness of thrombophlebitis from that of TrPs. There are no convincing data that strict bed rest is necessary or even desirable for patients with thrombophlebitis.[138]

Popliteal (Baker's) Cyst

The effusion within the knee joint of a popliteal (Baker's) cyst greatly increases intra-articular pressure when the knee is flexed. This pressure can cause a cystic enlargement of the articular capsule posteriorly, or enlargement of the gastrocnemius-semimembranous bursa if it communicates with the knee joint. (This communication is seen in about half of cadaver specimens.[55]) Effusion producing a popliteal cyst is likely to occur in patients with arthritis (especially rheumatoid arthritis) of the knee and with internal derangements of the knee joint (especially tears of the posterior aspect of the medial meniscus).[100] An unruptured popliteal cyst may extend down the leg deep to the gastrocnemius muscle nearly to the ankle, and it may be asymptomatic or may cause pain and swelling.[55] When the patient stands with knees straight, the visible mass in the popliteal space may be fluctuant on palpation.

A Baker's cyst may cause sufficient pressure, pain, and tenderness to be readily confused with thrombophlebitis or with soleus TrPs.[55] The pain and swelling of the cyst tend to be more medial in the calf, whereas thrombophlebitis pain is more frequently lateral. When an enlarging cyst dissects soft tissue, bleeding may cause a crescent-shaped ecchymotic area around the malleoli, the so-called "crescent sign."[55] Rupture of a cyst can cause acute pain, tenderness, heat, and erythema strongly suggestive of thrombophlebitis.[55,100]

Thrombophlebitis and Baker's cyst may occur at the same time.[55,57,121] The distinction is important, since their management is vastly different. Thrombophlebitis requires anticoagulation therapy. A ruptured Baker's cyst is treated with elevation of the leg and bed rest.[55] A Baker's cyst is reliably diagnosed by ultrasonography.[56] Arthrography reveals the popliteal cyst and demonstrates its rupture.

Postexercise Muscle Soreness

Delayed-onset muscle soreness, which appears a day or two following unaccustomed exercise that demands lengthening contractions, and which clears up in a week or so, is not a myofascial TrP phenomenon. It has features that suggest the soreness may be related in some ways to myofascial TrPs. A comprehensive review of a large amount of experimental data reported on the topic of delayed-onset muscle soreness appears in the Appendix of this volume for those who are interested in understanding more about it and its possible relation to myofascial TrPs.

Shin Splints

The term shin splints is used to describe pain in the anterior or medial leg associated with exercise. This pain is now recognized to have a number of specific causes that should be distinguished from referred pain caused by myofascial TrPs. The topic is reviewed here. Similar stress reactions are fully summarized for the adductor muscles on page 301 of this volume.

In the past, the term "shin splint" denoted any chronic exercise-related leg pain. In recent years, it has acquired a much more specific meaning: *periostalgia along the line of attachment of a repeatedly overloaded muscle*.

Used in the general sense, shin splints manifested by chronic pain and tenderness in the *anterior* portion of the leg often represent an anterior compartment syndrome (discussed in Chapter 19). Shin splints in the *medial* regions of the leg are usually caused by one of three identifiable conditions, or some combination of them: *(a)* stress fractures of the tibia; *(b)* chronic periostalgia (the soleus syndrome, also called the medial tibial stress syndrome); and *(c)* a deep posterior compartment syndrome. (As noted previously, some authors now reserve the term shin splints exclusively for periostalgia.) The anatomical, diagnostic, and therapeutic distinctions among these three conditions were well described and illustrated by Detmer[34] under the term medial tibial stress syndrome. The differential diagnosis and treatment of shin splints were recently reviewed by Brown and Braly.[21]

Stress Fracture

The stress fracture and its pain and tenderness occur along the medial aspect of the lower third of the tibia, solely in the bone; it may be focal or a band of varying length of microfracture where the fused fascial coverings of the *soleus* muscle attach to the tibia.[34,131] Athletes with stress fractures are unable to "run through" the pain.[62]

Radionuclide scan reveals this fracture within a few days. Radiographic changes may not appear until weeks later. Radionuclide scans may image the fracture for as long as 10 months.[131] Patients with stress fractures require 6–10 weeks of rest from sports activities followed by a gradual reconditioning program.[34]

The reason why some athletes develop this problem and others do not has not been established. The prevalence of soleus TrPs among patients with stress fractures is unknown. TrPs in the medial portion of the muscle could account for the focal decompensation of the osteoblastic repair process where the taut band could impose chronic tension on its bony attachment site.

Soleus Syndrome (Periostalgia, Medial Tibial Stress Syndrome)

The pain of the soleus periostalgia syndrome is likely to occur during repetitive rhythmic exercise, such as aerobic dancing or running. Initially, mild pain develops during the later stages of exercise and is relieved by rest. Successive episodes of pain progressively increase in intensity, occur earlier during exercise, and may persist after exercise.[99]

In 1985, Michael and Holder[96] attributed shin splints of the medial tibia to stress overload of the attachments of the soleus muscle (medial tibial stress syndrome[69]). A year later, Detmer[34] showed histologically that the medial tibial stress syndrome (soleus syndrome) was caused by loosening and sometimes separation of the periosteum from the tibial cortex. He attributed this to rupture of Sharpey's fibers that extend from muscle through periosteum into the cortical bone structure. For these reasons, he called this condition chronic periostalgia.

On examination, the distal one-third to one-half of the medial side of the tibia is exquisitely tender; this is also the site of the pain. This tenderness is parallel and slightly posterior to the location of tibial stress fractures.[34] The lesions demonstrated by the third phase of three-phase radionuclide studies were longitudinally oriented, often involving a third of the length of the tibia, and usually showed varying intensity of tracer activity along their length.[62] This radiographic technique is now established as a reliable and prompt way of identifying periostalgia (the soleus syndrome) and of distinguishing it from stress fractures.[62,77,96,99,111,131,156]

The strong relation of periostalgic shin splints to the kind and amount of exercise, and the localization of pain and tenderness to the insertion of the overstressed muscle, distinguish this condition clinically from myofascial TrP syndromes.

Compartment Syndrome

Although anterior compartment syndromes are recognized more often than posterior compartment syndromes,[158] the two posterior compartments are of special interest in this chapter. The superficial posterior compartment contains the

PART 3

soleus and gastrocnemius muscle bellies. The deep posterior compartment encloses the flexor digitorum longus, flexor hallucis longus, popliteus, and posterior tibial muscle bellies.[103] Compartment syndromes of the leg are also discussed in Chapters 19, 20, and 23.

Compartment syndromes of the leg are usually induced by exercise and are of gradual onset. They produce a sense of tightness and dull aching of the involved muscles. As the condition intensifies, pain persists for longer periods following exercise. Posterior compartment syndromes are commonly bilateral, usually fail to respond to conservative therapy, and often require fasciotomy.[158] On examination, tenderness is not located along the tibia laterally but is located in the muscle tissue itself, deep in the calf. The diagnosis of superficial posterior compartment syndrome is confirmed by finding an elevated pressure within the soleus muscle.[34,60,158]

The precise etiology of the posterior compartment syndromes is not yet established.[34] An initiating trauma or hypertrophy of the muscle has been postulated.[158] The role of TrPs as part of this process is unknown, but there is a strong possibility that, in muscles prone to developing a compartment syndrome, TrPs may make a significant contribution.

7. ACTIVATION AND PERPETUATION OF TRIGGER POINTS

Activation of Trigger Points

The mechanical stresses that activate TrPs in the soleus muscle include overuse caused by the foot slipping at toe-off and overloading the muscle, especially during forceful quick lengthening contractions. Additional stresses include direct trauma to the muscle, development of satellite TrPs in the muscle, and chilling of the muscle. When a lower limb-length inequality is present, soleus TrPs are more likely to be activated and perpetuated in the shorter limb, toward which the body weight is shifted.

Muscle Overload

Individuals wearing shoes with smooth leather soles while walking on a hard slippery surface, such as wet pavement, waxed tile, or marble floor, usually experience slipping of the forefoot on push-off. This slippage imposes an overload on the soleus muscles if the person proceeds at more than a slow pace.

A common complaint of joggers is heel pain,[15] which often represents referred tenderness from soleus TrPs. These TrPs are more likely to be activated when the jogger lands on the forefoot with the soleus shortened, which induces a vigorous eccentric contraction (*see* Appendix to this volume). The soleus muscle is also vulnerable to overload when an individual is skiing or ice skating without adequate ankle support.

Prolonged unaccustomed activity, such as playing shuffleboard during a vacation or hiking up a long steep hill, can overload the soleus muscle sufficiently to induce TrPs in it.

The soleus and other muscles that cross the ankle region can be overloaded when an individual walks along the beach or on other laterally slanted surfaces. Muscles on either side may become overloaded, depending on how each individual uses these muscles to compensate for the slant. In most cases, the soleus on the downward side (comparable to a shorter lower limb) must work harder. This situation is aggravated if that is also the side of an uncorrected shorter lower limb.

A somewhat similar overload occurs when an individual wears inflexible shoes with rigid soles that allow only ankle and no toe movement. The stiff sole greatly increases the lever arm against which the soleus must work. Shoes must be examined specifically for flexibility of the sole.

Other Causes

Slipping or losing balance in a situation that requires an unexpectedly vigorous lengthening contraction of the soleus muscle[59] can activate TrPs in the muscle. An example is that of a foot unexpectedly slipping on the stairs, throwing the entire body weight and recovery efforts on the other (weight-bearing) soleus muscle, particularly when only the forefoot of that limb is on the step.

Sustained pressure on the soleus can initiate TrPs in it. In one case, a woman had been standing on the steps of a crowded bus, facing the door, for nearly an hour with her soleus muscle pressed against the next higher step to maintain her balance. The painful, tender heel that resulted had been treated with injection of a steroid into the Achilles tendon without relief of pain, and with partial rupture of the tendon. Examination of the soleus muscle revealed multiple active TrPs. Inactivating them by local procaine injection relieved her heel pain and tenderness.

Myofascial TrPs of the soleus muscle can develop as satellites to primary TrPs in the posterior part of the gluteus minimus muscle, which often refer pain into the calf in the region of the soleus.

Prolonged cooling of tired, immobile legs, as by an air conditioner in a car on a long trip on a hot day, can activate soleus TrPs. It is important to take frequent breaks and walk around for a few minutes when on a long auto trip.

Perpetuation of Trigger Points

In addition to the systemic factors that perpetuate TrPs, which are covered in Chapter 4 of Volume 1,[152] several mechanical factors can perpetuate soleus TrPs. Three common ones are keeping the muscle in the shortened position for a prolonged period, chronic overuse, and compression ischemia of the muscle.

The soleus muscles are obviously placed in a shortened position when one wears high heels. No treatment for active soleus TrPs is likely to provide lasting relief as long as the individual continues to wear high heels regularly. The same effect as wearing a high heel can be produced unilaterally when a thick heel lift is placed inside the heel of one shoe to correct a lower limb-length discrepancy.

During sitting, sustained plantar flexion is produced if the chair seat is too high for the heels to rest firmly flat on the floor. Prolonged soleus shortening results during sleep if the ankles are allowed to remain immobilized in the strongly plantar flexed position at night. This position can activate latent soleus TrPs.

Any of the postural situations described previously that are capable of activating TrPs in the soleus muscle can perpetuate them as long as the situation remains uncorrected.

Compromise of circulation by compression of the calf can perpetuate soleus TrPs. Resting the weight of the calf on the high edge of an ottoman, or on the footrest of some dental chairs, directly compresses the soleus muscle causing local ischemia, which aggravates TrPs. Sitting on a chair seat that is too high for the feet to reach the floor fully usually causes a degree of underthigh compression of the neurovascular trunk. If the seat has a high front edge, and especially if the seat is pitched backward (lower behind than in front), blood flow to the soleus muscle can be compromised. Underthigh compression should be avoided. Tight elastic at the top of a sock below the knee can act like a tourniquet, limiting blood flow in the calf muscles. Arcangeli and coauthors[7] found that the occurrence of myalgic spots (TrPs) and the severity of limb ischemia were often parallel in patients with peripheral vascular disease.

8. PATIENT EXAMINATION

Figs. 22.8 and 22.9

The soleus muscle should be tested for the Achilles tendon reflex (ankle jerk) and for range of ankle dorsiflexion. This response to the calcaneal tendon tap is best examined with the patient kneeling on a chair seat (Fig. 22.8). Flexing the knee to 90° in this way isolates the soleus response by slackening the gastrocnemius at the knee joint and reducing its response. To ensure maximum relaxation, the patient should be positioned with the torso erect and stabilized by holding onto the backrest of the chair. The patient should also be encouraged to breathe naturally and to feel comfortable and relaxed. This test is performed with the patient in this position because the amplitude of the Achilles tendon reflex is likely to be reduced if the patient lies in the prone position with the knees straight; it is also likely to be reduced if the patient has a sensory neuropathy from a vitamin B_1 (thiamine) inadequacy, diabetic neuropathy, or other neurological impairment.

With a moderately active TrP in the soleus muscle, the ankle jerk is usually reduced in amplitude and may fatigue after six or eight taps. When there is more

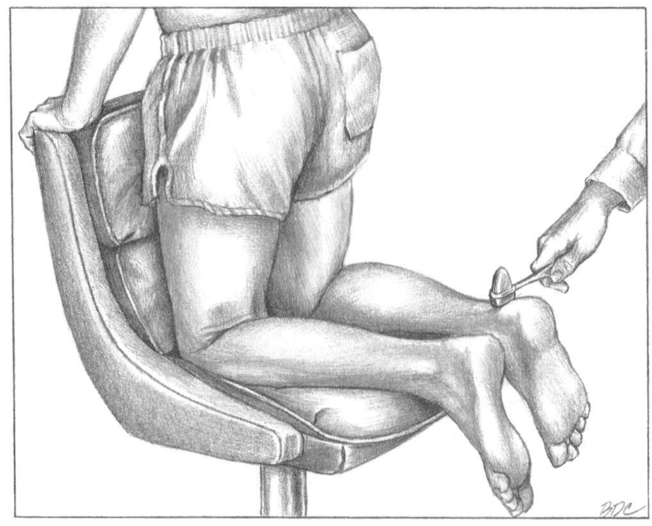

Figure 22.8. Optimal position, kneeling on a chair seat, for tapping the Achilles tendon to test the tendon reflex (ankle jerk) of the soleus muscle, and for comparing the response bilaterally.

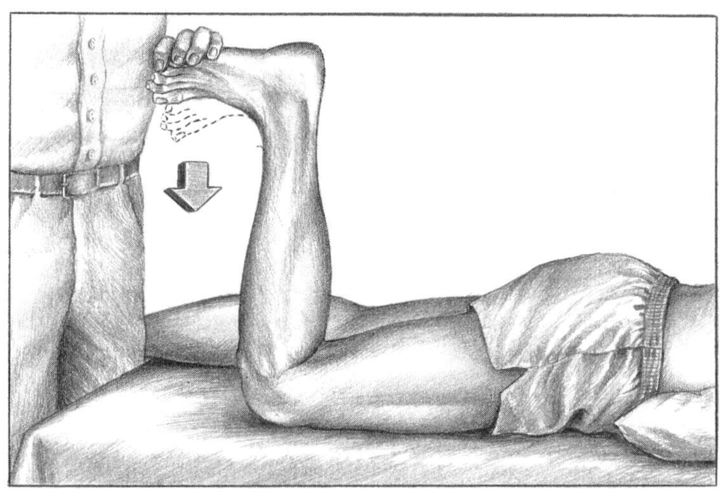

Figure 22.9. Testing the right soleus muscle for range of motion at the ankle with the knee flexed to 90°, patient prone. The *dotted outline of the foot* approaches the full normal dorsiflexion range. The *arrow* shows the downward direction of pressure.

marked TrP activity, the reflex may be nearly or completely inhibited. In such a case, intermittent cold with stretch may be applied to the soleus muscle while the patient kneels on the chair seat.

A blow of the percussion hammer on the *belly* of the soleus muscle *directly on a TrP* distal to the gastrocnemius muscle produces a soleus local twitch response and an ankle movement that is not a tendon tap response. Tapping a soleus muscle belly that is free of TrPs does not elicit this twitch response. The more active the soleus TrP, the more vigorous is the local twitch response, but the less vigorous is the Achilles tendon tap response. Following inactivation of the responsible soleus TrPs, the local twitch response (that is restricted to the muscle fibers associated with taut bands) disappears and the Achilles tendon tap response (of the entire muscle) returns at once.

When TrPs in the soleus muscle refer pain proximally to the region of the posterior superior iliac spine, exploration of that referral area by palpation reveals a very sore, but circumscribed tender region corresponding to the area of pain complaint.

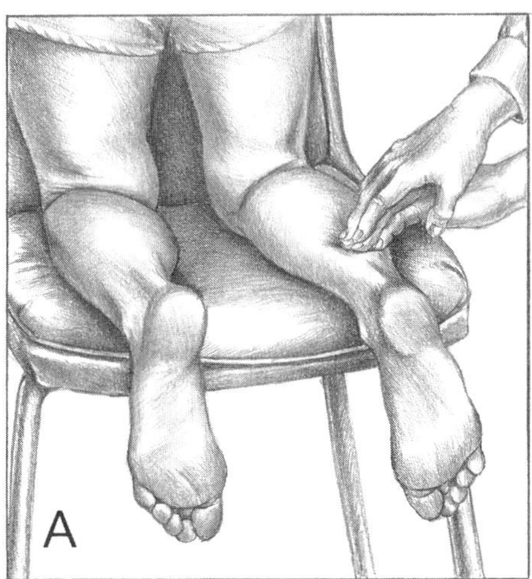

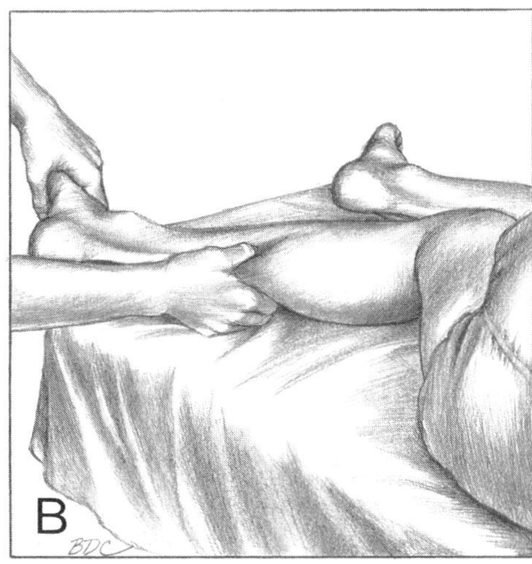

Figure 22.10. Palpation for trigger points in the right soleus muscle. The ankle is in the neutral position. *A*, initial flat palpation of TrP_1 after testing the ankle jerks bilaterally while the patient kneels on a chair seat. *B*, pincer palpation of TrP_3, patient recumbent, lying on the right side.

A convenient screening test of soleus range of motion is the ability to squat with the heels flat on the floor. Patients with active soleus TrPs are either unable to squat at all or to do so only on the toes.[75] This test can be damaging to the knee ligaments if the knee is flexed too acutely while weight bearing. For manual testing of the soleus range of motion (Fig. 22.9), the patient is best positioned lying prone with the knee bent 90°. The range of ankle dorsiflexion is then tested by pushing downward on the ball of the foot toward the examining table. Any TrP tension of the soleus muscle restricts ankle dorsiflexion, which should have a range of 20°.

Soleus weakness is tested by having the patient stand on the ball of one foot with adequate stabilization. During this test, a strong tendency for the foot to invert indicates substitution by the tibialis posterior and/or the long flexors of the toes, whereas a strong tendency for it to evert indicates substitution by the peroneus longus and brevis muscles.[71] These substitutions suggest soleus weakness. With normal triceps surae strength, the subject should be able to jump at least 10 times on the ball of the foot without heel contact on the floor.

The Laségue test (straight-leg raising with ankle dorsiflexion) is less likely to produce calf pain because of soleus TrPs than because of TrPs in the gastrocnemius muscle.

Active TrPs in the soleus that cause shortening of the muscle can lead to the false conclusion that the lower limb on that side is longer than the other limb when the patient bears body weight on the toes instead of the heel, holding the heel off the floor slightly.

9. TRIGGER POINT EXAMINATION (Fig. 22.10)

All **soleus** TrPs can be examined by flat palpation (Fig. 22.10*A*), and the distal TrP_1 and TrP_3 also by pincer palpation from side to side deep to the tendo calcaneus (Fig. 22.10*B*). The kneeling position is convenient for testing the ankle jerk, for testing the local twitch response using the percussion hammer, and for screening all three TrP locations by palpation (Fig. 22.10*A*).

When examining a recumbent patient for soleus TrPs (Fig. 22.10*B*), the knee is flexed to slacken the gastrocnemius muscle.

Soleus TrP_1 is usually located approximately 3 cm (1¼ in) below the end of the bulge that marks the lower border of the gastrocnemius fibers, or about 14 cm (5½ in) above the heel. TrP_3 is located proximal and lateral to TrP_1 close to the lower end of the gastrocnemius fibers (Fig. 22.1). These distal TrPs may also be conveniently examined with the involved leg of the side-lying patient placed on the examining table with the calf facing the examiner (Fig. 22.10*B*). The tenderness due to these distal soleus TrPs is localized deep to the aponeurosis of the Achilles tendon. Taut bands are located by holding the muscle between the fingers and thumb using pincer palpation (Fig. 22.10*B*) and then rolling the muscle between the digits. These taut bands and their TrPs are difficult to locate unless the palpation is done skillfully; they are easily missed. One must insert the fingers distal to the gastrocnemius muscle and posterior to the underlying tibia and fibula, lift up, and examine the underside for TrPs by rolling the muscle fibers under the fingers, holding the thumb in place. Or, the fingers can be kept in place and the thumb used for palpation. The medial and lateral sides of the muscle may require separate examinations. If one is considering injecting these TrPs, such precise localization is necessary.

Active TrPs in the proximal portion of the muscle, the TrP_2 area, are rarely found in isolation; they usually occur in conjunction with the more distal TrPs in the soleus muscle. With severe involvement, TrPs may be found also in other parts of the muscle. It is important to examine the proximal TrP_2 by flat palpation against the underlying bone with the knee bent to about 90° in order to release tension in the gastrocnemius muscle. This minimizes the likelihood of mistaking a TrP in the overlying gastrocnemius for a soleus TrP. Only a gastrocnemius TrP should increase its sensitivity to palpation with a change in knee angle to greater extension. With the patient in the kneeling position, additional stretch may be applied to the soleus muscle by gently dorsiflexing the foot with the hand, assisted by the operator's knee, to increase sensitivity of the soleus TrPs (Fig. 22.11*A*).

Taut bands in the **plantaris** muscle are not likely to be palpable and the spot tenderness of its TrPs is difficult to identify because of the overlying thick lateral head of the gastrocnemius muscle, which also may have TrPs.

10. ENTRAPMENTS

Soleus

Figures 22.5 and 22.6 illustrate the soleus canal through which the posterior tibial veins, posterior tibial artery, and tibial nerve pass. Arkoff *et al.*[8] noted during surgical exposure of the popliteal veins that, when the leg was extended and the foot dorsiflexed, the vein was compressed as it entered the soleus canal under the tendinous arch. Mastaglia and associates[84] reported five cases of compression of the tibial nerve at the tendinous arch of the soleus muscle. Three were simply entrapment of the tibial nerve by the arch and were relieved by surgical sectioning of the arch. Although the histories of these patients were compatible with myofascial TrPs of the soleus muscle, no mention was made of examination for TrPs. In one case, the nerve was entrapped by swelling associated with thrombosis of a tributary of the popliteal vein.

Figure 22.5 shows a fibrous band of the soleus muscle which, when well developed, also has the potential for entrapping this popliteal neurovascular bundle. Obstruction affects mainly the soft-walled veins, causing edema of the foot and ankle.

The authors have seen several patients with compromised circulation of posterior tibial veins that was relieved by inactivating TrPs deep in the soleus TrP_3 region. One patient had severe heel pain and tingling in the lateral portion of the foot suggestive of nerve entrapment; these symptoms, too, were relieved by inactivating a very irritable TrP_2 in the soleus muscle.

Plantaris

Taunton and Maxwell[146] found occlusion of the popliteal artery by the plantaris tendon in a 26-year-old female athlete who was limited to a walking distance of three blocks because of calf pain that had been diagnosed as shin splints. After sectioning of the plantaris tendon and endarterectomy with patch graft angioplasty, she resumed full activity.

11. ASSOCIATED TRIGGER POINTS

Associated TrPs are most likely to occur in the gastrocnemius and posterior tibial

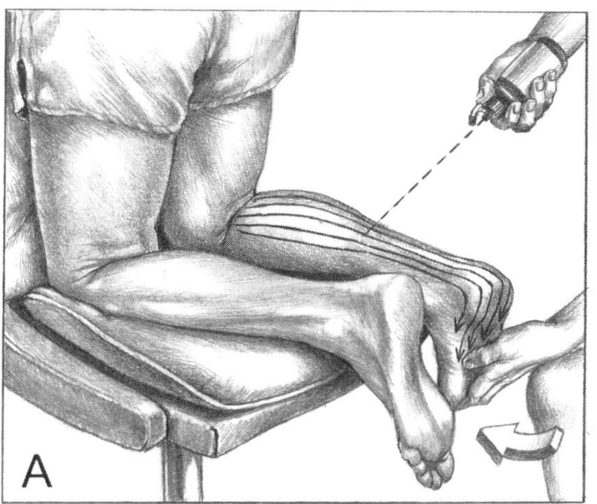

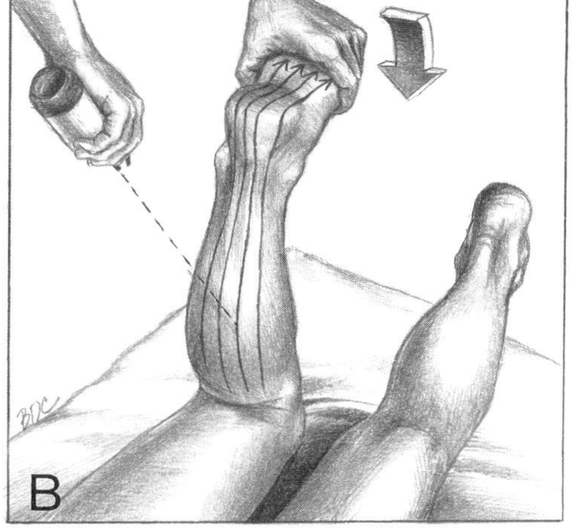

Figure 22.11. Stretch position and intermittent cold pattern (*thin arrows*) for trigger points in the right soleus muscle. *Thick arrows* indicate the direction in which gradually increasing pressure is applied in order to dorsiflex the ankle, passively lengthening the muscle. *A*, preliminary treatment while the patient is kneeling on a chair seat. Operator's knee assists by applying pressure through the hand. *B*, more effective, relaxed position, patient lying prone.

muscles and, not infrequently, in the long flexors of the toes, all of which are agonists of the soleus. When there is extensive involvement of these plantar flexor muscles, their antagonists (the tibialis anterior, extensor digitorum longus, peroneus tertius, and extensor hallucis longus) may also become involved. The ankle should be checked for restriction of plantar flexion and these anterior leg muscles should be examined for TrPs.

When the patient with an active soleus TrP complains of knee pain, a likely place to look for TrPs is in the ipsilateral quadriceps femoris muscle. Impairment of soleus function places increased demands on the quadriceps femoris.

Since patients with soleus TrPs cannot squat comfortably, they usually lean over to pick up an object from the floor and are thus likely to overload their back muscles and activate a new group of TrPs.

12. INTERMITTENT COLD WITH STRETCH
(Fig. 22.11)

The use of ice for applying intermittent cold with stretch is explained on page 9 of this volume and the use of vapocoolant spray with stretch is detailed on pages 67–74 of Volume 1.[151] Techniques that augment relaxation and stretch are reviewed on page 11 and alternative treatment methods are reviewed on pages 9–10 of this volume.

Soleus
(Fig. 22.11)

Intermittent Cold with Stretch

During examination of the calf muscles with the patient kneeling on a chair seat, as illustrated in Figure 22.10*A*, one can also test the response of soleus TrPs to intermittent cold with stretch (Fig. 22.11*A*). For inactivation of less responsive TrPs, this procedure is more effective with the patient lying prone (Fig. 22.11*B*). In either position, an initial sweep of ice or vapocoolant spray is applied distalward over the calf, heel, and instep. Then, during parallel sweeps of the intermittent cold, increasing pressure is exerted *gently* to dorsiflex the foot fully. This is always done with the knee flexed to release any tightness of the gastrocnemius that would block ankle dorsiflexion and prevent full stretch of the soleus muscle. When soleus TrPs refer pain to the sacroiliac region, that referral area should also be included as part of the intermittent cold pattern.

With the patient recumbent, a moist heating pad or hot pack should be applied to the calf at once after intermittent cold with stretch, and then a few active pedal movements are performed through plantar flexion and dorsiflexion to reestablish full active range of motion of the muscle.

Other Modalities

Other stretch techniques and the application of transcutaneous electrical nerve stimulation (TENS) have been found helpful in alleviating the pain caused by soleus TrPS.

Stretch Techniques. Lewit[75] described and illustrated the use of postisometric relaxation for releasing a tight soleus muscle, using the positioning of Figure 22.11*B*. We find this postisometric relaxation technique often effective when used alone and particularly effective when used as a stretch component of intermittent cold with stretch.

Evjenth and Hamberg[41] describe and illustrate soleus stretch in one limb for the standing patient who leans forward against a wall. Simultaneous knee flexion and ankle dorsiflexion are controlled by manual pressure of the clinician to stabilize the heel on the floor with one hand while applying pressure to the calf below the knee with the other.

Möller and associates[98] investigated the effect of the sequence of contract-relax-stretch on dorsiflexion at the ankle with the knee bent (soleus stretch) in eight *normal* subjects with no history of musculoskeletal disorder. This technique required maximal isometric contraction of the soleus muscle in the lengthened position for 4–6 seconds, then complete relaxation for at least 2 seconds, and passive dorsiflexion as far as possible without causing pain, with this lengthened position maintained for eight seconds. This cycle was repeated five times. Immediately afterward, dorsiflexion at the ankle had increased 18% and maintained an increase of more than 12% of the prestretch range 1½ hours later. One would expect the gain in range of motion to be greater in muscles shortened by active TrPs than in normal muscles.

A revealing study of soleus stretch by Etnyre and Abraham[39] employed three methods, each on *separate* days, in 12 subjects. *(a)* Static stretch alone for 9 seconds with a force of 7.4 kg was ineffective. *(b)* A contract-relax technique was significantly more effective ($p<0.001$) and increased the range of motion 2.2°. In this method, passive lengthening of the soleus was followed by isometric plantar flexion for 6 seconds, then followed by 3 seconds more of passive stretch. *(c)* Even more effective was a combined technique of contract-relax and antagonist contraction that improved the average range another 1.6°. The contract-relax method was assisted by active dorsiflexion effort during the last 3 seconds of passive stretch. This study shows the additive effects of static stretch, postisometric relaxation, and reciprocal inhibition.

The soleus/tibialis anterior pair of muscles presents a classic example of reciprocal inhibition,[32] which should be employed liberally for release of soleus tightness.

Transcutaneous Electrical Nerve Stimulation (TENS). Francini and coinvestigators[50] measured pain threshold, amplitude of responses to Achilles tendon taps, and amplitude of H reflexes before, during, and after application of 50-Hz pulses of TENS stimulation. Responses were measured on the stimulated and unstimulated sides in 40 healthy subjects and in 25 patients with pain caused by TrPs in the triceps surae. The reported location of these TrPs at the junction of the triceps surae and the Achilles tendon makes it likely that the TrPs were located in the soleus, rather than in the gastrocnemius muscle. These authors[50] found that, in the patients with pain, both facilitation and inhibition of the sensorimotor system during and after TENS were more marked than in normal subjects. Also, in the patients with pain, the initial pain threshold of the painful limb was either notably higher or lower than that of the other limb. This asymmetry was reduced by TENS. The investigators concluded that TENS induced a normalization of the sensory and muscular functions, both of which outlasted the period of TENS application. Pain relief was concomitant with this reset effect of TENS. The authors gave no indication that the TENS inactivated the TrPs, only that it temporarily relieved the pain from them.

Plantaris

Intermittent cold with stretch of the plantaris muscle is performed as for the gastrocnemius muscle (*see* Fig. 21.5), since these two muscles have nearly identical attachments (Fig. 22.4).

In their description and illustration of a stretch technique for the plantaris muscle, Evjenth and Hamberg[40] apply the same method used to stretch the medial head of the gastrocnemius muscle, since

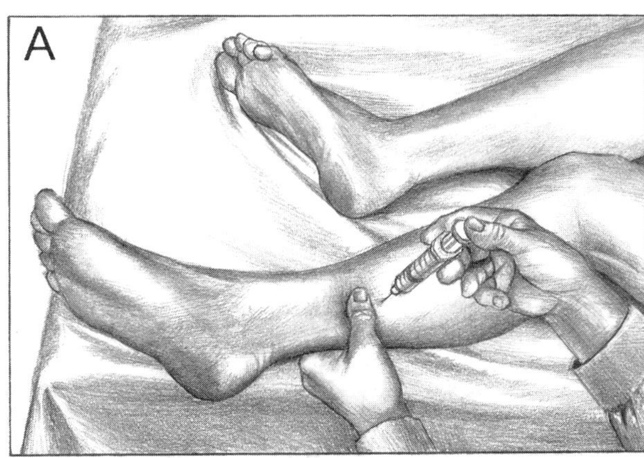

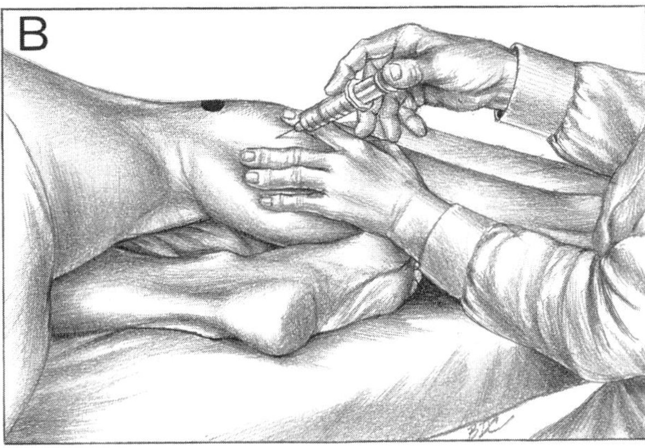

Figure 22.12. Injection of trigger points in the right soleus muscle. *A*, medial approach to the most common location, distal TrP_1, with the patient lying on the same (right) side. *B*, lateral approach to the less common and most proximal TrP_2. The patient is lying on the opposite side. *Solid circle* locates the fibular head.

the tendon of the plantaris muscle attaches to the medial side of the Achilles tendon. These authors press the heel against a lateral wedge to evert the heel while dorsiflexing the foot and keeping the knee straight.

13. INJECTION AND STRETCH (Fig. 22.12)

A full description of the procedure for TrP injection and stretch of any muscle appears in Volume 1, pages 74–86.[151] For injection, the physician should wear gloves. A solution of 0.5% procaine in isotonic saline is used for injection.

Soleus (Fig. 22.12)

Steroids are to be avoided when injecting the distal part of this muscle because of the danger of causing rupture of the Achilles tendon. In many patients, a 37-mm (1½-in) 22-gauge needle is sufficient, but a 50-mm (2-in) 21-gauge needle may be required for injection of soleus TrPs when the calf muscles are unusually large.

The distal soleus TrP_1 is usually most accurately localized by pincer palpation from both sides of the muscle, anterior to the Achilles tendon. For injection, TrP_1 is easily approached from the medial side at the point of maximum tenderness, distal to the bulge that marks the lower end of the gastrocnemius muscle fibers. The patient lies on the right side for injection of the right soleus, with the uppermost (left) leg in front of the involved one (Fig. 22.12*A*). The operator applies counter pressure to the tender spot with one finger pressing directly on the TrP from the lateral side of the muscle, while the needle is inserted on the medial side and aimed directly at the center of that finger. Probing of the area may be necessary to inactivate a cluster of TrPs.

To inject proximal TrP_2, the patient lies on the opposite side so that the soleus can be approached laterally. The needle is di-

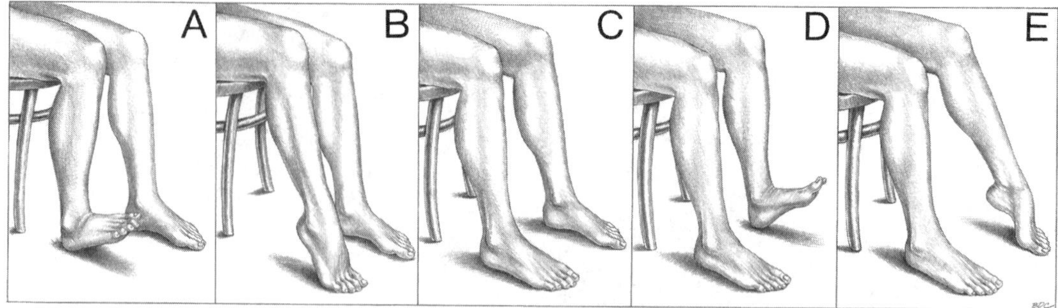

Figure 22.13. Soleus Pedal Exercise for active stretch of the soleus muscle and to enhance its vascular pumping action. One foot completes a rhythmic cycle of full dorsiflexion, full plantar flexion, and a rest pause. The other foot then completes a similar cycle. *A*, first foot, full dorsiflexion; *B*, full plantar flexion; *C*, pause and rest position; *D*, other foot, full dorsiflexion; *E*, full plantar flexion, followed by a pause and rest as in *C*.

rected toward the fibula at the spot of maximum tenderness, which is encountered deep, close to the bone (Fig. 22.12*B*).

Soleus TrP_3 is injected with a technique similar to that used for TrP_1, except that it is approached from the lateral side.

Occasionally, a soleus TrP is located deep in the middle portion of the muscle. When the needle must penetrate deeply near the midline of the muscle, one must consider the tibial nerve and posterior tibial veins and artery (Fig. 22.6). In this case, it is better to start with a midline skin penetration of the needle and angle the needle away from the neurovascular bundle.

Postinjection soreness may be severe, so it is wise never to inject the soleus muscles in both legs at one visit. The patient is directed to use moist heat on the calf twice daily for several days during this period of soreness, to take acetaminophen (Tylenol) for relief of pain, and to avoid strenuous exercise or activities that may overload this muscle. The patient may find it beneficial to wear long, loose wool socks to provide warmth for the calf by conserving body heat.

Plantaris

A plantaris TrP, when present, is usually located between the two heads of the gastrocnemius muscle and slightly lateral to the midline at the level of the tibial plateau. On examination, it appears similar to a TrP in the popliteal portion of the gastrocnemius muscle. If it is injected, the needle should approach the TrP through the lateral head of the gastrocnemius to avoid the popliteal neurovascular bundle in the midline (Figs. 22.3–22.5).

14. CORRECTIVE ACTIONS (Figs. 22.13–22.17)

Corrective Posture and Activities (Figs. 22.13–22.16)

Active soleus TrPs often will not resolve if the soleus muscle remains shortened at night. When a person sleeps either supine or prone, the feet usually are strongly plantar flexed (*see* Fig. 21.11*B*); this may occur also when lying on the side. As illustrated in Figure 21.11*A*, a firm pillow or other support can be placed against the feet under the bed sheet to maintain a neutral position at the ankles. Instead of using a pillow, the bed can be positioned against a piece of furniture or wall at the end of the bed to provide such foot support, or for prone lying, the feet may be allowed to hang down over the end of the bed.

For those who sleep on the back, a small pillow under the knees may be helpful. Full extension of the knee tends to occlude the popliteal veins in some individuals. However, too much knee and hip flexion caused by a large pillow under the knees can result in undesirable prolonged shortening of the knee and hip flexors.

For patients who are prone to chilliness, long loose socks worn at night to cover the calves conserve body warmth and prevent cooling of the calf muscles.

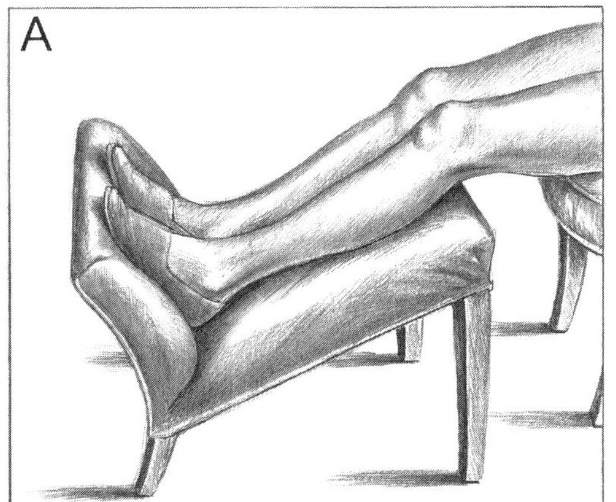

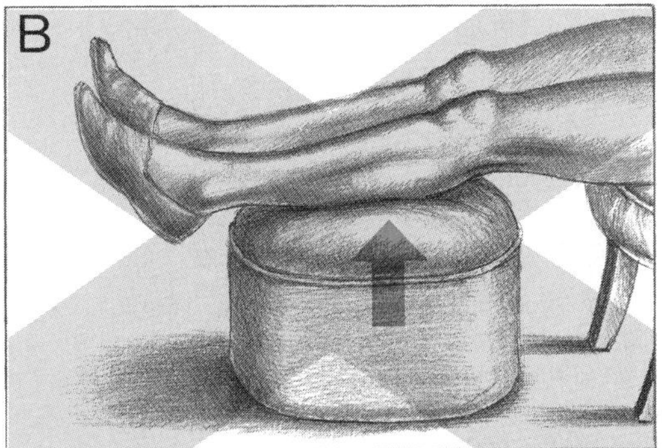

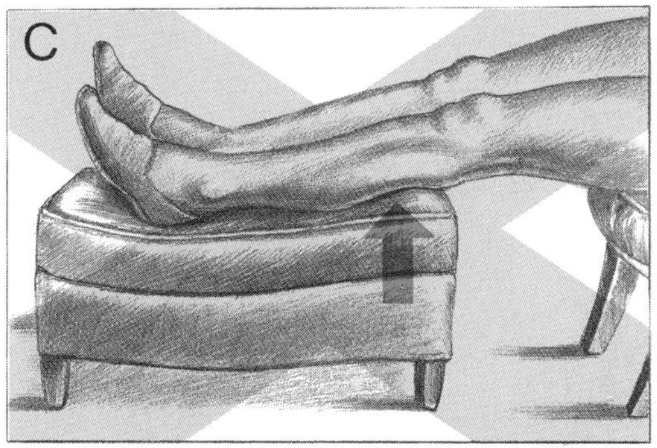

Figure 22.14. Correct and incorrect (*red* **X**) footrests. The *arrows* indicate excessive pressure. *A*, correct footrest distributes the weight of the lower limb evenly on the sole, heel, and calf. It also holds the foot in a neutral position at the ankle. *B*, incorrect footrest with a domed shape compresses the calf muscles and obstructs their circulation. It also encourages plantar flexion of the foot and prolonged shortening of the calf muscles. *C*, incorrect footrest with a soft center and a hard edge compresses the neurovascular bundle in the soleus canal and obstructs circulation in the gastrocnemius and soleus muscles. It also favors plantar flexion at the ankle and shortening of these muscles.

An activity that helps reduce the irritability of TrPs in this muscle is the Soleus Pedal Exercise (Fig. 22.13). It can be performed regularly while a person sits for a prolonged period, as on a long airplane trip. This active stretching exercise is executed in an alternating fashion: first, raising the toes and then the heel of one foot, and then after a pause raising the toes and heel of the other foot (Fig. 22.13). This pedal exercise also activates the "soleus pump" and improves the venous return from the lower limbs. A half-dozen such pedalling cycles should be performed at least every half hour when sitting.

For anyone prone to syncope when standing still, activation of the soleus pump by alternately contracting the soleus muscles, or by bearing weight on the toes alternately on right and left sides, helps prevent pooling of blood in the legs and can prevent syncope. Those who are prone to soleus TrPs and syncope should avoid tight garters or tight elastic cuffs on socks that can act like a tourniquet and compromise venous return from the calf.

Application of thin rubber half-soles to substitute for slippery leather shoe soles can help, especially if the patient with soleus TrP problems walks on hard, slippery floors. The shoes should be examined for flexibility. The toe of the shoe should bend easily. If the sole is so rigid that it fails to bend fully during ambulation, the soleus is forced to work against an extended lever arm. This chronic overload may cause the muscle to respond poorly to specific TrP treatment. Shoe traction and flexibility are impressively important to soleus function, and wearing proper shoes may be essential for lasting relief of calf and heel pain.

When a chair seat is too high and only the toes reach the floor, either the chair seat must be lowered, or an adequate footrest must be provided. A cone-shaped footstool provides a variety of heights for different degrees of knee flexion and for supporting the ankle in a neutral position.

High heels not only place the soleus in a chronically shortened position, but provide an unstable base of support. In some patients, changing to low heels is a critical factor in the recovery of the calf muscles from myofascial pain syndrome. The unilateral "high heel" effect of placing a heel lift in one shoe can be minimized if

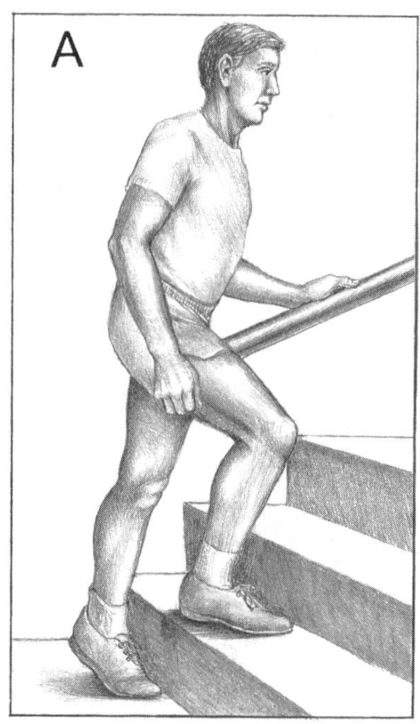

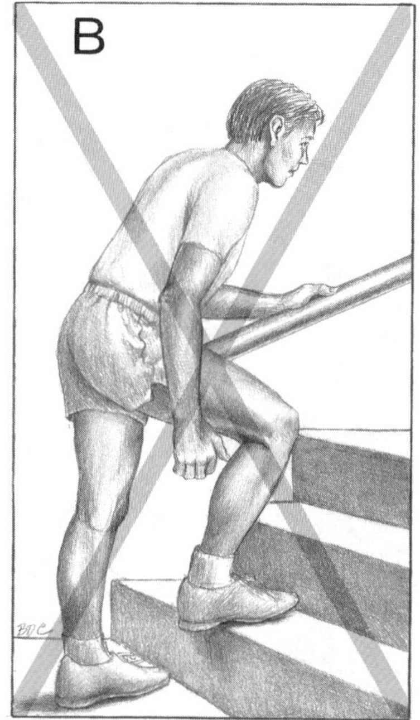

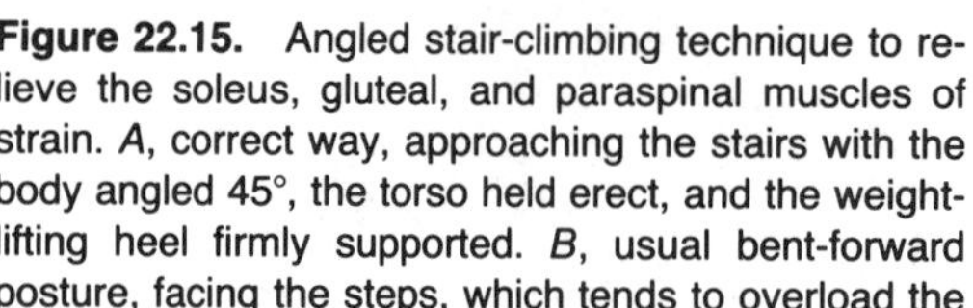

Figure 22.15. Angled stair-climbing technique to relieve the soleus, gluteal, and paraspinal muscles of strain. *A*, correct way, approaching the stairs with the body angled 45°, the torso held erect, and the weight-lifting heel firmly supported. *B*, usual bent-forward posture, facing the steps, which tends to overload the soleus, paraspinal, and posterior hip muscles. Climbing the stairs in this posture is analogous to leaning over a low sink. That posture also can markedly dorsiflex the leading ankle, overloading the soleus in its fully lengthened position.

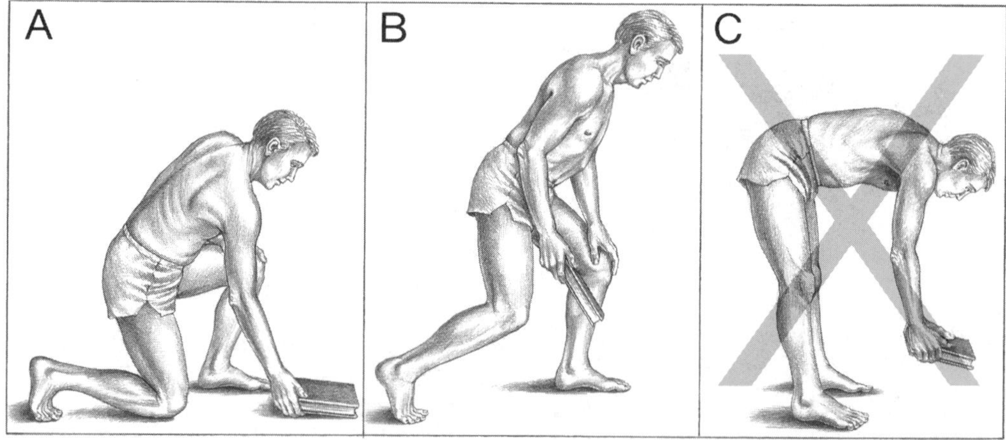

Figure 22.16. Correct and incorrect solutions to the problem of safely bending down to pick up an object on the floor when trigger points in the soleus muscle restrict ankle dorsiflexion and prevent the commonly recommended technique using knee flexion. *A*, correct pick-up position. Bending down on one knee does not require full dorsiflexion of either ankle. The left hand presses down on the left knee to divide the load and prevent back strain. *B*, correct way of returning to the standing position with the feet and left arm in essentially the same position as when reaching down to the floor. *C*, incorrect way of bending over and reaching to the floor to pick up an object.

part or all of the total correction is made by cutting down the heel height of the shoe worn on the longer limb. However, if the shoe has no heel to cut down, it may be necessary to add a half-sole as well as a heel lift on the shorter side.

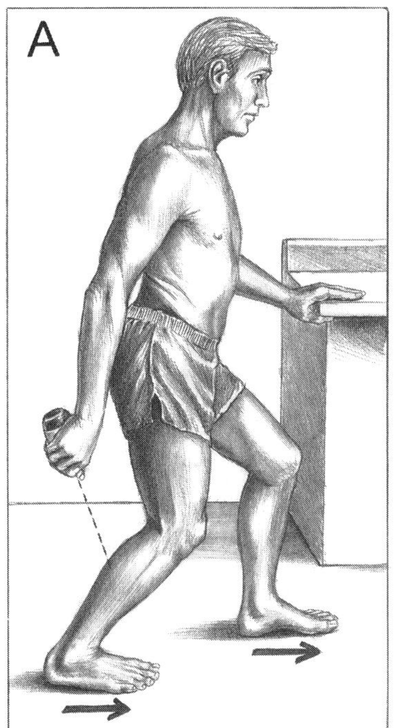

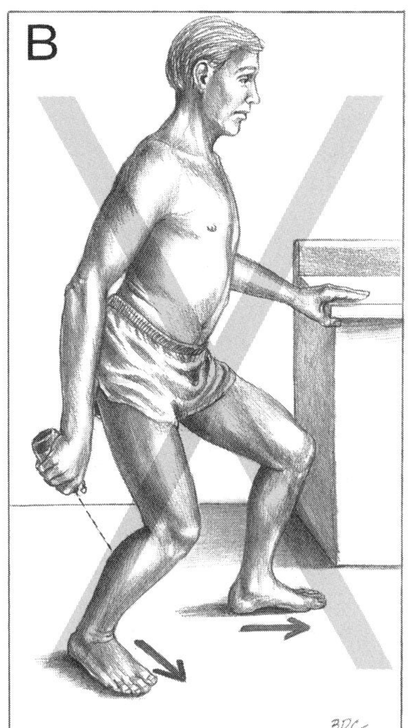

Figure 22.17. Standing self-spray and self-stretch technique for the right soleus muscle, bending the right knee to dorsiflex the right ankle passively. The heel of the stretched muscle must remain flat on the floor. The spray is applied in the same pattern of downward sweeps over the muscle to the heel as in Figure 22.11. *A*, correct position of feet. *B*, ineffective positioning (*red* **X**) of the rear (right) foot on the side of the muscle being sprayed and stretched. The right lower limb is laterally rotated and the foot is turned outward, which prevents full dorsiflexion at the ankle and thus lessens the stretch on the right soleus muscle.

When driving on a long trip, one should make frequent stops and walk around for a few minutes to restore circulation; cruise control also provides an opportunity to change positions.

A common perpetuating cause of TrPs in the soleus muscle is an improperly designed or improperly used leg rest that causes calf compression. People who sit in reclining chairs with built-in leg rests that concentrate weight on a portion of the calf may require additional pillows or may need to restrict elevation of the leg rest. If an ottoman is used for leg support, it should be designed and arranged so that part of the weight is carried by the heels. Figure 22.14*A* shows such a good position with lower limb weight evenly distributed and the ankles in a neutral position.

Figure 22.14*B* demonstrates use of a domed, firm ottoman that compresses calf muscles and obstructs venous circulation. This should be avoided. Figure 22.14*C* shows another type of ottoman that should be avoided. This demonstrates how a soft-centered leg rest with a hard edge can produce soleus compression.

One solution is a slanted footrest that places the ankles at nearly 90° when the feet rest on it (*see* Fig. 16.6*C* in the Hamstring chapter). With such a footrest, from time to time the forefoot can be placed against the footrest with the heels on the floor to provide additional ankle dorsiflexion (*see* Fig. 16.6*B*).

Soleus overload can be avoided by limiting walking in soft sand, unless the calf muscles are conditioned for it, and by not walking long distances on a sidewalk or beach slanted to one side. Lower limb-length inequality should be corrected by an appropriate lift (Chapter 4).

Patients with active soleus TrPs often experience pain when walking up stairs facing forward as usual (Fig. 22.15*B*). The problem is corrected by approaching the stairway with the body erect and angled

45°, placing the entire foot flat on the step above without markedly dorsiflexing it (Fig. 22.15*A*). This technique avoids painful strain and stretch of the soleus muscle by minimizing ankle plantar flexion and dorsiflexion. Keeping the body erect minimizes strain on the back muscles and gives the strong quadriceps femoris muscle a larger share of the load. This angling technique works equally well on a ladder. It can also be used when ascending a steep slope, by turning the body and feet to one side and climbing sideways, or by following a zigzag course up the hill.

When patients have active soleus TrPs, painful restriction of dorsiflexion limits the ability to bend the knees and keep the back erect as recommended for picking an object up from the floor (*see* Volume 1, Fig. 48.11). The individual should be taught to reach an object safely by kneeling on one knee to avoid painful dorsiflexion of either foot at the ankle (Fig. 22.16*A* and *B*).

Home Therapeutic Program (Fig. 22.17)

The soleus is one muscle that can easily be treated by the patients themselves using intermittent cold with stretch (Fig. 22.17*A*). The patient stands, keeping the involved knee bent to slacken the gastrocnemius muscle, and gradually transfers weight onto the posteriorly placed affected leg. With the knee straight, a tight gastrocnemius may block full passive stretch of the soleus. Support by the contralateral arm is important for stability. The foot of the leg being stretched must point straight ahead. If the foot is allowed to turn outward, stretch on the soleus muscle is reduced (Fig. 22.17*B*). The patient is taught to apply a safe vapocoolant spray downward over the calf in slow parallel sweeps, starting with the muscle under comfortable tension. The muscle is gradually lengthened by further bending the knee, taking up the slack that develops as the soleus muscle tension releases. For added stretch, a wedge can be placed under the heel laterally to evert the heel slightly while the foot is being dorsiflexed.

Addition of postisometric relaxation augments the effectiveness of intermittent cold with stretch, or postisometric relaxation alone may be used. Lewit[76] describes and illustrates a seated version of soleus self-stretch that employs postisometric relaxation.

Patients with soleus TrPs are benefitted by first soaking in a tub of warm water or taking a moderately hot shower, and then performing the soleus self-stretch.

A valuable exercise for the home program is the Soleus Pedal Exercise described on page 453 (Fig. 22.13).

Stretching of the calf muscles is important to athletes who participate in running sports, such as soccer and basketball, yet it is surprisingly neglected in practice.[73]

PART 3

References

1. Anderson JE: *Grant's Atlas of Anatomy*, Ed. 8. Williams & Wilkins, Baltimore, 1983 (Fig. 4–72).
2. *Ibid.* (Fig. 4–81).
3. *Ibid.* (Fig. 4–83).
4. *Ibid.* (Fig. 4–84).
5. *Ibid.* (Fig. 4–98).
6. Apple JS, Martinez S, Khoury MB, *et al.*: Case report 376. *Skel Radiol* 15:398–400, 1986.
7. Arcangeli P, Digiesi V, Ronchi O, Dorigo B, Bartoli V: Mechanisms of ischemic pain in peripheral occlusive arterial disease. In *Advances in Pain Research and Therapy*, edited by J. J. Bonica and D. Albe-Fessard, Vol. I. Raven Press, New York, 1976 (pp. 965–973, see p. 966 and Fig. 2).
8. Arkoff RS, Gilfillan RS, Burhenne HJ: A simple method for lower extremity phlebography–Pseudo-obstruction of the popliteal vein. *Radiology 90*:66–69, 1968.
9. Baker BA: Myofascial pain syndromes: ten single muscle cases. *J Neurol Orthop Med Surg 10*: 129–131, 1989.
10. Bardeen CR: The musculature, Sect. 5. In *Morris's Human Anatomy*, edited by C.M. Jackson, Ed. 6. Blakiston's Son & Co., Philadelphia, 1921 (pp. 517, 523).
11. Basmajian JV, Deluca CJ: *Muscles Alive*, Ed. 5. Williams & Wilkins, Baltimore, 1985 (pp. 256–257, 337–340, 370).
12. *Ibid.* (pp. 338, 345–347).
13. Bates T, Grunwaldt E: Myofascial pain in childhood. *J Pediatr 53*:198–209, 1958 (p. 202, Fig. 3).
14. Baxter MP, Dulberg C: "Growing pains" in childhood—a proposal for treatment. *J Pediatr Orthop 8*:402–406, 1988.
15. Bazzoli AS, Pollina FS: Heel pain in recreational runners. *Phys Sportsmed* 17:55–61, 1989.
16. Bouisset S, Zattara M: A sequence of postural movements precedes voluntary movement. *Neurosci Lett 22*:263–270, 1981.
17. Bradford JA, Lewis RJ, Giordano JM, *et al.*: Detection of deep vein thrombosis with Doppler ultrasound techniques in patients undergoing

total knee replacement. *Orthopedics* 5:305–308, 1982.
18. Brandell BR: Functional roles of the calf and vastus muscles in locomotion. *Am J Phys Med* 56:59–74, 1977.
19. Brody DM: Running injuries. *Clin Symp* 32:2–36, 1980 (see p. 21).
20. Broer MR, Houtz SJ: *Patterns of Muscular Activity in Selected Sports Skills*. Charles C Thomas, Springfield, 1967.
21. Brown MR, Braly WG: Differential diagnosis and treatment of shin splints. *Surg Rounds Orthop* pp. 27–32, Sept, 1989.
22. Campbell KM, Biggs, NL, Blanton PL, *et al.*: Electromyographic investigation of the relative activity among four components of the triceps surae. *Am J Phys Med* 52:30–41, 1973.
23. Carter BL, Morehead J, Wolpert SM, *et al.*: *Cross-Sectional Anatomy*. Appleton-Century-Crofts, New York, 1977 (Sects. 68–80).
24. *Ibid.* (Sects. 71–80).
25. Clement DB, Taunton JE, Smart GW: Achilles tendinitis and peritendinitis: etiology and treatment. *Am J Sports Med* 12:179–184, 1984.
26. Clemente CD: *Gray's Anatomy of the Human Body*, American Ed. 30. Lea & Febiger, Philadelphia, 1985 (p. 111, Fig. 3–46).
27. *Ibid.* (p. 111, Fig. 3–47).
28. *Ibid.* (p. 112, Fig. 3–48).
29. *Ibid.* (pp. 576–577).
30. *Ibid.* (p. 582, Fig. 6–79).
31. *Ibid.* (pp. 850, 861).
32. Crone C, Nielsen J: Spinal mechanisms in man contributing to reciprocal inhibition during voluntary dorsiflexion of the foot. *J Physiol* 416: 255–272, 1989.
33. Danielsson L, Theander G: Supernumerary soleus muscle. *Acta Radiol Diagn* 22:365–368, 1981.
34. Detmer DE: Chronic shin splints. Classification and management of medial tibial stress syndrome. *Sports Med* 3:436–446, 1986.
35. Dokter G, Linclau LA: Case Report. The accessory soleus muscle: symptomatic soft tissue tumour or accidental finding. *Neth J Surg* 33:146–149, 1981.
36. Edgerton VR, Smith JL, Simpson DR: Muscle fibre type populations of human leg muscles. *Histochem J* 7:259–266, 1975.
37. Elder GCB, Bradbury K, Roberts R: Variability of fiber type distributions within human muscles. *J Appl Physiol* 53:1473–1480, 1982.
38. Ericson MO, Nisell R, Arborelius UP, *et al.*: Muscular activity during ergometer cycling. *Scand J Rehabil Med* 17:53–61, 1985.
39. Etnyre BR, Abraham LD: Gains in range of ankle dorsiflexion using three popular stretching techniques. *Am J Phys Med* 65:189–196, 1986.
40. Evjenth O, Hamberg J: *Muscle Stretching in Manual Therapy, A Clinical Manual*, Vol. 1, *The Extremities*. Alfta Rehab Førlag, Alfta, Sweden, 1984 (p. 143).
41. *Ibid.* (pp. 144–145).
42. Fasel J, Dick W: Akzessorische Muskeln in der Regio retromalleolaris medialis. *Z Orthop* 122: 835–837, 1984.
43. Ferner H, Staubesand J: *Sobotta Atlas of Human Anatomy*, Ed. 10, Vol. 2. Urban & Schwarzenberg, Baltimore, 1983 (Fig. 380).
44. *Ibid.* (Figs. 420, 469).
45. *Ibid.* (Fig. 461).
46. *Ibid.* (Fig. 464).
47. *Ibid.* (p. 465).
48. *Ibid.* (p. 471).
49. *Ibid.* (p. 472).
50. Francini F, Maresca M, Procacci P, *et al.*: The effects of non-painful transcutaneous electrical nerve stimulation on cutaneous pain threshold and muscular reflexes in normal men and in subjects with chronic pain. *Pain* 11:49–63, 1981.
51. Frazier CH: Improving venous flow and leg muscle activity in postoperative patients: an experimental method. *Orthop Rev* 4:45–47, 1975.
52. Froimson AI: Tennis leg. *JAMA* 209:415–416, 1969.
53. Gantchev GN, Draganova N: Muscular synergies during different conditions of postural activity. *Acta Physiol Pharmacol Bulg* 12:58–65, 1986.
54. Ger R, Sedlin E: The accessory soleus muscle. *Clin Orthop* 116:200–202, 1976.
55. Gordon GV: Baker's cyst and thrombophlebitis: a problem in differential diagnosis. *Internal Medicine* (Oct) 1980 (pp. 39–45).
56. Gordon GV, Edell S: Ultrasonic evaluation of popliteal cysts. *Arch Intern Med* 140:1453–1455, 1980.
57. Gordon GV, Edell S, Brogadir SP, *et al.*: Baker's cysts and true thrombophlebitis. Report of two cases and review of the literature. *Arch Intern Med* 139:40–42, 1979.
58. Graham CE: Accessory soleus muscle. *Med J Austral* 2:574–576, 1980.
59. Greenwood R, Hopkins A: Muscle responses during sudden falls in man. *J Physiol* 254:507–518, 1976.
60. Henstorf JE, Olson S: Compartment syndrome: pathophysiology, diagnosis, and treatment. *Surg Rounds Orthop* 33–41, (Feb) 1987.
61. Herman R, Bragin J: Function of the gastrocnemius and soleus muscles. *Phys Ther* 47:105–113, 1967.
62. Holder LE, Michael RH: The specific scintigraphic pattern of "shin splints in the lower leg": concise communication. *J Nucl Med* 25: 865–869, 1984.
63. Hollinshead WH: *Functional Anatomy of the Limbs and Back*, Ed. 4. W.B. Saunders, Philadelphia, 1976 (pp. 329–330).
64. Hollinshead WH: *Anatomy for Surgeons*, Ed. 3., Vol. 3, *The Back and Limbs*. Harper & Row, New York, 1982 (pp. 775–778, Fig. 9–36).
65. *Ibid.* (p. 783, Fig. 9–45).
66. Homans J: Thrombosis of the deep leg veins due to prolonged sitting. *N Engl J Med* 250:148–149, 1954.
67. Hufschmidt HJ, Sell G: Über gekreuzte Reflexe in Beinmotorik des Menschen. *Z Orthop* 116: 60–65, 1978.
68. Janda V: *Muscle Function Testing*. Butterworths, London, Boston, 1983 (pp. 189, 191–193, 198, 229).

69. Jones DC, James SL: Overuse injuries of the lower extremity: shin splints, iliotibial band friction syndrome, and exertional compartment syndromes. *Clin Sports Med 6*:273–290, 1987.
70. Joseph J, Nightingale A: Electromyography of muscles of posture: leg and thigh muscles in women, including the effects of high heels. *J Physiol 132*:465–468, 1956.
71. Kendall FP, McCreary EK: *Muscles, Testing and Function*, Ed. 3. Williams & Wilkins, Baltimore, 1983 (pp. 145–146).
72. Kukulka CG, Russell AG, Moore MA: Electrical and mechanical changes in human soleus muscle during sustained maximum isometric contractions. *Brain Res 362*:47–54, 1986.
73. Levine M, Lombardo J, McNeeley J, *et al.*: An analysis of individual stretching programs of intercollegiate athletes. *Phys Sportsmed 15*: 130–138, 1987.
74. Lewis CE Jr, Mueller C, Edwards WS: Venous stasis on the operating table. *Am J Surg 124*: 780–784, 1972.
75. Lewit K: *Manipulative Therapy in Rehabilitation of the Motor System*. Butterworths, London, 1985 (pp. 151, 152, Figs. 4.40, 4.41).
76. *Ibid*. (pp. 282–283, Fig. 6.104).
77. Lieberman CM, Hemingway DL: Scintigraphy of shin splints. *Clin Nucl Med 5*:31, 1980.
78. Lockhart RD: *Living Anatomy*, Ed. 7. Faber & Faber, London, 1974 (Fig. 118).
79. Lockhart RD, Hamilton GF, Fyfe FW: *Anatomy of the Human Body*, Ed. 2. J.B. Lippincott Co., Philadelphia, 1969 (p. 650).
80. Lorentzon R, Wirell S: Anatomic variations of the accessory soleus muscle. *Acta Radiol 28*: 627–629, 1987.
81. Lozach P, Conard JP, Delarue P, *et al.*: [A case of an accessory soleus muscle.] *Rev Chir Orthop 68*:391–393, 1982.
82. Ludbrook J: The musculovenous pumps of the human lower limb. *Am Heart J 71*:635–641, 1966.
83. Markhede G, Nistor L: Strength of plantar flexion and function after resection of various parts of the triceps surae muscle. *Acta Orthop Scand 50*:693–697, 1979.
84. Mastaglia FL, Venerys J, Stokes BA, *et al.*: Compression of the tibial nerve by the tendinous arch of origin of the soleus muscle. *Clin Exp Neurol 18*:81–85, 1981.
85. McLachlin J, McLachlin AD: The soleus pump in the prevention of venous stasis during surgery. *Arch Surg 77*:568–575, 1958.
86. McMinn RMH, Hutchings RT: *Color Atlas of Human Anatomy*. Year Book Medical Publishers, Chicago, 1977 (p. 277B).
87. *Ibid*. (pp. 281, 282, 285).
88. *Ibid*. (p. 289).
89. *Ibid*. (p. 312B).
90. *Ibid*. (p. 315C, No. 11).
91. *Ibid*. (p. 316).
92. *Ibid*. (p. 317).
93. *Ibid*. (p. 320).
94. *Ibid*. (p. 321).
95. Merli GJ, Herbison GJ, Ditunno JF, *et al.*: Deep vein thrombosis: prophylaxis in acute spinal cord injured patients. *Arch Phys Med Rehabil 69*:661–664, 1988.
96. Michael RH, Holder LE: The soleus syndrome. A cause of medial tibial stress (shin splints). *Am J Sports Med 13*:87–94 1985.
97. Milbradt H, Reimer P, Thermann H: [Ultrasonic morphology of the normal Achilles tendon and pattern of pathological changes.] *Radiologe 28*:330–333, 1988.
98. Möller M, Ekstrand J, Oberg B, *et al.*: Duration of stretching effect on range of motion in lower extremities. *Arch Phys Med Rehabil 66*:171–173, 1985.
99. Moore MP: Shin splints: diagnosis, management, prevention. *Postgrad Med 83*:199–210, 1988.
100. Nance EP Jr, Heller RM, Kirchner SG, *et al.*: *Advanced Exercises in Diagnostic Radiology*. 17. Emergency Radiology of the Pelvis and Lower Extremity. W.B. Saunders Co., Philadelphia, 1983 (pp. 28–29).
101. Nardone A, Schieppati M: Shift of activity from slow to fast muscle during voluntary lengthening contractions of the triceps surae muscles in humans. *J Physiol 395*:363–381, 1988.
102. Nelimarkka O, Lehto M, Järvinen M: Soleus muscle anomaly in a patient with exertion pain in the ankle. A case report. *Arch Orthop Trauma Surg 107*:120–121, 1988.
103. Netter FH: *The Ciba Collection of Medical Illustrations*, Vol. 8, Musculoskeletal System. Part I: Anatomy, Physiology and Metabolic Disorders. Ciba-Geigy Corporation, Summit, 1987 (pp. 98, 99).
104. *Ibid*. (p. 101).
105. *Ibid*. (pp. 103, 105).
106. *Ibid*. (p. 109).
107. Nichols GW, Kalenak A: The accessory soleus muscle. *Clin Orthop 190*:279–280, 1984.
108. Nicolaides AN, Kakkar VV, Field ES, *et al.*: Optimal electrical stimulus for prevention of deep vein thrombosis. *Br Med J 3*:756–758, 1972.
109. Okada M: An electromyographic estimation of the relative muscular load in different human postures. *J Hum Ergol 1*:75–93, 1972.
110. Okada M, Fujiwara K: Muscle activity around the ankle joint as correlated with the center of foot pressure in an upright stance. In *Biomechanics VIIIA*, edited by H. Matsui, K. Kobayashi. Human Kinetics Publ., Champaign, IL, 1983 (pp. 209–216).
111. Ozburn MS, Nichols JW: Pubic ramus and adductor insertion stress fractures in female basic trainees. *Milit Med 146*:332–333, 1981.
112. Pavlov H, Heneghan MA, Hersh A, *et al*: The Haglund syndrome: initial and differential diagnosis. *Radiology 144*:83–88, 1982.
113. Percy EC, Telep GN: Anomalous muscle in the leg: soleus accessorium. *Am J Sports Med 12*: 447–450, 1984.
114. Pernkopf E: *Atlas of Topographical and Applied Human Anatomy*, Vol.2. W.B. Saunders, Philadelphia, 1964 (Figs. 347, 381).
115. *Ibid*. (Fig. 356).
116. *Ibid*. (Fig. 357).
117. *Ibid*. (Fig. 358).

118. Perry J: The mechanics of walking. *Phys Ther 47*:778–801, 1967.
119. Perry J, Easterday CS, Antonelli DJ: Surface versus intramuscular electrodes for electromyography of superficial and deep muscles. *Phys Ther 61*:7–15, 1981.
120. Pettersson H, Giovannetti M, Gillespy T III, *et al.*: Magnetic resonance imaging appearance of supernumerary soleus muscle. *Eur J Radiol 7*: 149–150, 1987.
121. Prescott SM, Pearl JE, Tikoff G: "Pseudo-pseudothrombophlebitis": ruptured popliteal cyst with deep venous thrombosis. *N Engl J Med 299*:1193, 1978.
122. Ramchandani P, Soulen RL, Fedullo LM, *et al.*: Deep vein thrombosis: significant limitations of noninvasive tests. *Radiology 156*:47–49, 1985.
123. Rasch PJ, Burke RK: *Kinesiology and Applied Anatomy*, Ed. 6. Lea & Febiger, Philadelphia, 1978 (pp. 318–319).
124. Ricci MA: Deep venous thrombosis in orthopaedic patients. Current techniques in precise diagnosis. *Orthop Rev 13*:185–196, 1984.
125. Rohen JW, Yokochi C: *Color Atlas of Anatomy*, Ed. 2. Igaku-Shoin, New York, 1988 (p. 412).
126. *Ibid.* (pp. 421, 446).
127. *Ibid.* (p. 422).
128. *Ibid.* (p. 426).
129. Romano C, Schieppati M: Reflex excitability of human soleus motoneurones during voluntary shortening or lengthening contractions. *J Physiol 90*:271–281, 1987.
130. Romanus B, Lindahl S, Stener B: Accessory soleus muscle. *J Bone Joint Surg [Am] 68*:731–734, 1986.
131. Rupani HD, Holder LE, Espinola DA, *et al.*: Three-phase radionuclide bone imaging in sports medicine. *Radiology 156*:187–196, 1985.
132. Sabri S, Roberts VC, Cotton LT: Measurement of the effects of limb exercise on femoral arterial and venous flow during surgery. *Cardiovasc Res 6*:391–397, 1971.
133. Sadamoto T, Bonde-Petersen F, Suzuki Y: Skeletal muscle tension, flow, pressure, and EMG during sustained isometric contractions in humans. *Eur J Appl Physiol 51*:395–408, 1983.
134. Shiavi R, Griffin P: Changes in electromyographic gait patterns of calf muscles with walking speed. *AIEEE Trans Biomed Eng 30*:73–76, 1983.
135. Simons DG, Travell JG: Myofascial origins of low back pain. 3. Pelvic and lower extremity muscles. *Postgrad Med 73*:99–108, 1983 (see pp. 104, 105).
136. Simons DG, Travell JG: Myofascial pain syndromes, Chapter 25. In *Textbook of Pain*, edited by P.D. Wall and R. Melzack, Ed 2. Churchill Livingstone, London, 1989 (pp. 368–385, see p. 378).
137. Simpson K: Shelter deaths from pulmonary embolism. *Lancet* 2:744, 1940.
138. Singer A: Bed rest, deep-vein thrombosis, and pulmonary embolism. *JAMA 250*:3162, 1983.
139. Singer AE: Management of heel pain. *JAMA 239*:1131–1132, 1978.
140. Sjøgaard G: Capillary supply and cross-sectional area of slow and fast twitch muscle fibres in man. *Histochemistry 76*:547–555, 1982.
141. Spalteholz W: *Handatlas der Anatomie des Menschen*, Ed. 11, Vol.2. S. Hirzel, Leipzig, 1922 (p. 441).
142. *Ibid.* (p. 442).
143. *Ibid.* (p. 445).
144. Sutherland DH: An electromyographic study of the plantar flexors of the ankle in normal walking on the level. *J Bone Joint Surg [Am] 48*:66–71, 1966.
145. Sutherland DH, Cooper L, Daniel D: The role of the ankle plantar flexors in normal walking. *J Bone Joint Surg [Am] 62*:354–363, 1980.
146. Taunton JE, Maxwell TM: Intermittent claudication in an athlete—popliteal artery entrapment: a case report. *Can J Appl Sport Sci* 7:161–163, 1982.
147. Toldt C: *An Atlas of Human Anatomy*, translated by M.E. Paul, Ed. 2, Vol. 1. Macmillan, New York, 1919.
148. Traccis S, Rosati G, Patraskakis S, *et al.*: Influences of neck receptors on soleus motoneuron excitability in man. *Exp Neurol* 95:76–84, 1987.
149. Travell J: Symposium on mechanism and management of pain syndromes. *Proc Rudolf Virchow Med Soc* 16:126–136, 1957.
150. Travell J, Rinzler SH: The myofascial genesis of pain. *Postgrad Med 11*:425–434, 1952.
151. Travell JG, Simons DG: *Myofascial Pain and Dysfunction: The Trigger Point Manual*. Williams & Wilkins, Baltimore, 1983.
152. *Ibid.* (pp. 114–164).
153. Trosko JJ: Accessory soleus: a clinical perspective and report of three cases. *J Foot Surg 25*: 296–300, 1986.
154. Vandervoort AA, McComas AJ: A comparison of the contractile properties of the human gastrocnemius and soleus muscles. *Eur J Appl Physiol 51*:435–440, 1983.
155. Van Hinsbergh VW, Veerkamp JH, Van Moerkark HT: Cytochrome c oxidase activity and fatty acid oxidation in various types of human muscle. *J Neurol Sci* 47:79–91, 1980.
156. Walz D, Craig BM, McGinnis KD: Bone imaging showing shin splints and stress fractures. *Clin Nucl Med 12*:822, 1987.
157. Weber EF: Ueber die Längenverhältnisse der Fleischfasern der Muskeln in Allgemeinen. *Berichte über die Verhandlungen der Königlich Sächsischen Gesellschaft der Wissenschaften zu Leipzig 3*:63–86,1851.
158. Wiley JP, Clement DB, Doyle DL, *et al.*: A primary care perspective of chronic compartment syndrome of the leg. *Phys Sportsmed 15*:111–120, 1987.
159. Winkel J, Bendix T: Muscular performance during seated work evaluated by two different EMG methods. *Eur J Appl Physiol 55*:167–173, 1986.
160. Wood J: On some varieties in human myology. *Proc R Soc Lond 13*:299–303, 1864.
161. Yang JF, Winter DA: Surface EMG profiles during different walking cadences in humans. *Electroencephalogr Clin Neurophysiol 60*:485–491, 1985.

CHAPTER 23
Tibialis Posterior Muscle

"Runner's Nemesis"

HIGHLIGHTS: **REFERRED PAIN** from myofascial trigger points (TrPs) in the tibialis posterior muscle concentrates proximally over the Achilles tendon above the heel. A spillover pattern extends from the TrP down over the calf, the entire heel, and the plantar surface of the foot and toes. **ANATOMICAL ATTACHMENTS** of the tibialis posterior are, proximally, chiefly to the interosseous membrane and fibula and also to the tibia and intermuscular septa. Distally, the tendon passes behind the medial malleolus and anchors to the navicular, the calcaneus, each cuneiform, the cuboid, and the second, third, and fourth metatarsals. **FUNCTION** of the tibialis posterior muscle is to prevent excessive pronation of the foot during midstance of the walking cycle, to prevent excessive weight bearing on the medial side of the foot, and to distribute body weight among the heads of the metatarsals. It acts primarily as a supinator (invertor and adductor) of the foot and, to a lesser degree, as an assistant to plantar flexion of the foot. Weakness or absence of the muscle causes a pronated foot with severe flexible pes valgus deformity that must be corrected within months of the loss to avoid permanent damage to the foot structure. **SYMPTOMS** caused by active TrPs in the tibialis posterior muscle include pain in the sole of the foot when running or walking, especially on an uneven surface. The pain is felt severely in the arch of the foot, Achilles tendon, and, to a lesser degree, in the heel, toes, and calf. Other conditions that need to be considered in relation to tibialis posterior TrPs include shin splints, a deep posterior compartment syndrome, chronic tenosynovitis of the posterior tibial tendon, and tendon rupture. **ACTIVATION** of TrPs in the tibialis posterior muscle results from chronic postural overload (such as jogging on uneven surfaces) or as secondary TrPs to other muscles in its functional unit. **PATIENT EXAMINATION** includes testing this muscle for functional weakness, restricted range of motion, and for aching pain in the muscle when it is actively contracted in the fully shortened position. It also includes examining the patient for the Morton foot structure and for other causes of a hyperpronating foot. **ASSOCIATED TRIGGER POINTS** of the tibialis posterior usually develop in the flexor digitorum longus, flexor hallucis longus, and peroneal muscles. **INTERMITTENT COLD WITH STRETCH** of this muscle should incorporate augmented postisometric relaxation to maximize effectiveness. The application of reciprocal inhibition also facilitates muscle lengthening. The procedure concludes with rewarming of the skin and several cycles of active motion, moving the tibialis posterior through its fully shortened and its fully lengthened range. **INJECTION** of TrPs in this muscle is generally not recommended. **CORRECTIVE ACTIONS** include running or jogging with full arch support only on a smooth flat surface, but *not* on the sides of a crowned road or similar slanted surface. The shoe needs correction when the patient has the Morton foot structure or has a hypermobile midfoot. Augmented postisometric relaxation in a home program maintains full range of motion of the tibialis posterior muscle.

1. REFERRED PAIN
(Fig. 23.1)

Pain due to myofascial trigger points (TrPs) in the tibialis posterior muscle (Fig. 23.1) is not likely to present as a single-muscle syndrome. The pain concentrates primarily over the Achilles tendon above the heel and has a spillover pattern that spreads from the TrP distally through the midcalf down to the heel and over the entire plantar surface of the foot and toes.

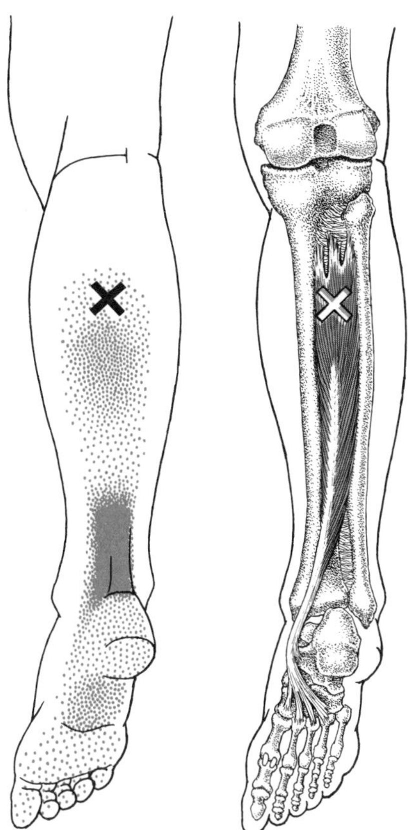

Figure 23.1. Composite pain pattern (*bright red*) referred from trigger points (***X**s*) at their common location in the right tibialis posterior muscle (*darker red*). The essential pain pattern (*solid dark red*) denotes where pain is usually experienced when these trigger points are active. *Red stippling* indicates the occasional extension of the essential pain pattern.

2. ANATOMICAL ATTACHMENTS AND CONSIDERATIONS
(Fig. 23.2)

The tibialis posterior is the most deeply located muscle in the calf. It lies between the interosseus membrane anteriorly and the soleus muscle posteriorly (*see* Fig. 23.5). ***Proximally*** it attaches primarily to the interosseous membrane and to the medial surface of the fibula (Fig. 23.2); it also attaches to the lateral portion of the posterior surface of the body of the tibia, the deep transverse fascia, and to intermuscular septa of adjacent muscles.[15,19] The tibial attachment of the muscle commonly continues into the distal third of the leg as far as, or more distal than, the crossing of the tibialis posterior tendon with that of the flexor digitorum longus.[65] The attachment to the fibula usually includes an intramuscular septum, in which case the muscle is multipennate.[52] In the lower fourth of the leg, its tendon passes deep (anterior) to that of the flexor digitorum longus.[18,61] The two tendons pass behind the medial malleolus together but in separate sheaths. The tibialis posterior tendon then passes deep to the flexor retinaculum and superficial to the deltoid ligament. The tendon usually contains a sesamoid fibrocartilage near where it passes superficial to the plantar calcaneonavicular ligament.[10,19]

Distally it anchors to the plantar surface of most of the bones that form the arch of the foot (Fig. 23.2), primarily to the navicular, but also to the calcaneus, each cuneiform, the cuboid, and the base of the second, third, and fourth metatarsals.[19]

The fibular portion of the muscle is more extensive than the tibial portion.[10,52]

Occasionally, the tibialis posterior muscle may be doubled,[10] or it may have an anomalous insertion of its tendon to an enlarged navicular tuberosity.[66]

Supplemental References

Netter[15] drew the tibialis posterior, including all attachments in phantom, from the front view.

The view from behind without blood vessels shows the arrangement of the tendons at the ankle,[5] the attachments of the tibialis posterior tendon to bones in the foot,[5,8,15] the relation of the tibialis posterior muscle to the adjacent flexor digitorum longus and flexor hallucis longus deep to the soleus muscle,[27,45] and the crossing of the tendon of the tibialis posterior deep to that of the flexor digitorum longus.[61] The posterior view portrays the relation of the tibialis posterior muscle to the tibial and peroneal arteries and the tibial nerve,[4,55] and to only the tibial nerve.[56]

Views from the medial side of the ankle region also show the relation of the tendon to other tendons and to the ligaments and bones.[6,24,47]

An uninterrupted series of 12 cross sections[17] clarifies this muscle's relation to other muscles and to neurovascular structures throughout its length. A series of four cross sections provides this information for the fleshy part of the muscle (*see* Fig. 23.5). Other authors present a cross section through the middle third of the leg.[3,26]

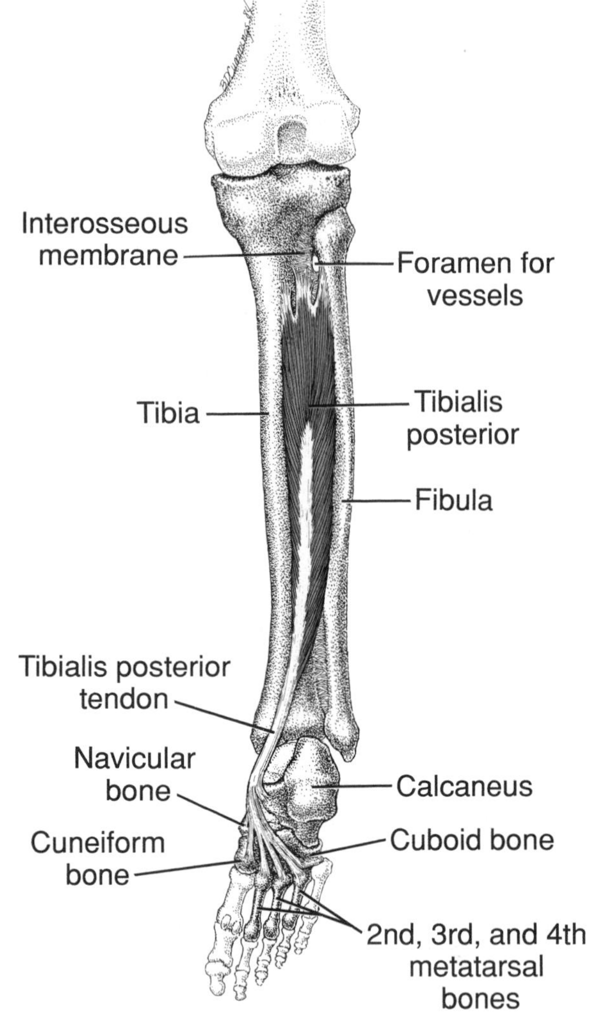

Figure 23.2. Attachments of the right tibialis posterior muscle (*red*). The bones to which this muscle attaches are *darkened*. Note the Morton foot (short first, long second metatarsal) structure.

A posterior view[2,25] and a posterolateral view[43] locate where the posterior tibial muscle attaches to the bones of the leg. A plantar view shows where its tendon attaches to the bones of the foot.[7,15,28,44] One figure shows all bony attachments.[57]

Photographs depict the surface contours produced by the tibialis posterior tendon at the ankle.[37,40,46]

3. INNERVATION

The tibial nerve supplies the tibialis posterior muscle with fibers from the fifth lumbar and first sacral spinal nerves.[19]

4. FUNCTION

For weight bearing, the tibialis posterior muscle functions to distribute body weight among the heads of the metatarsals, helping shift weight toward the lateral side of the foot. This muscle appears to restrain the valgus thrust on the ankle that occurs during the early stance phase of walking. During midstance, it prevents excessive lateral inclination of the leg and provides transverse plane balance. It prevents excessive pronation of the foot, thereby preventing excessive medial rotation (spiraling) of the leg. It has been suggested that during stance, the tibialis posterior assists other plantar flexors in controlling (decelerating) the forward movement of the tibia over the fixed foot. When the foot is free (not weight bearing), the tibialis posterior acts to invert and adduct the foot and to assist in plantar flexion.

Actions

The tibialis posterior muscle supinates (inverts and adducts) the foot.[10,19,35,60] Some authors consider it a major plantar flexor also,[10,35,60] but others do not consider plantar flexion one of its primary actions.[19,21]

In electrical stimulation studies of the muscle, Duchenne[21] found that the foot adducted with great force, but, when plantar flexed or dorsiflexed, returned weakly to neutral. Sutherland[68] calculated that the tibialis posterior potentially is the third most powerful plantar flexor; however, it could exert only 6% of the moment of force contributed by the gastrocnemius and soleus muscles combined.

Functions

Walking

The tibialis posterior muscle prevents eversion of the foot beyond the neutral position during midstance of the walking cycle.[29] It distributes body weight on the heads of the metatarsals, helping shift weight toward the lateral side of the foot which has the strong plantar ligaments that equip it well to bear body weight.[12,54] Perry[58] suggested that the tibialis posterior appears to restrain the valgus thrust on the ankle that occurs during the early stance phase of walking. Sutherland[68] concluded that the plantar flexors, including the tibialis posterior, control (decelerate) the forward movement of the tibia over the fixed foot during stance, indirectly providing knee stabilization. During level walking in normal subjects, it is not active at heel-off (or shortly after) when this would be required if it were functioning as a plantar flexor.[12] In flat-footed subjects, this muscle is active throughout stance phase and maintains inversion of the foot, which keeps the body weight on the lateral border of the sole.[29]

In a study of 11 normal adults, Matsusaka[41] tested gait by measuring ground reaction forces, myoelectric activity, and the degree of pronation-supination of the foot. He found that when the lateral component of ground reaction force was large, the degree of pronation of the foot was small, and activity in the tibialis posterior disappeared early. *Conversely*, when the lateral component of force was small, the degree of pronation was larger and the tibialis posterior (also flexor digitorum longus and extensor hallucis longus) showed extended myoelectric activity.[41] This suggests that the force necessary to throw the weight onto the lateral sole can be supplied largely by the motion of the body or by the tibialis posterior and other invertor muscles. Matsusaka suggested that the tibialis posterior functions by preventing excessive lateral inclination of the leg over the fixed foot.[41]

Perry and coauthors[59] compared the myoelectric activity of the tibialis posterior muscle during slow, free, and fast gait with the amount of activity generated by various degrees of voluntary effort graded according to muscle testing criteria. Results showed that EMG activity increased directly as more muscular force was required during the different manual muscle test levels and with increased walking speeds.

Based on its myoelectric activity, the tibialis posterior does not contribute significantly to arch support under static load conditions.[11,13] However, the changes in the foot that occur in the absence of the force exerted by this muscle show that it is essential for maintenance of normal foot configuration and posture. Co-contractions of the tibialis posterior with the peroneus longus may help support the medial arch and prevent hyperpronation of the foot, especially in runners.[1]

Weakness or Absence

Duchenne noted that, in patients with tibialis posterior deficit, the foot turned outward when they were walking or standing.[22] Weakness of this muscle can lead to an excessively pronated foot, unlocking of the midtarsal joint that allows plantar subluxation of the hindfoot on the forefoot, and development of a severe pes valgus deformity.[30] Tendon rupture or weakness of the tibialis posterior caused by slippage of the tendon around the medial malleolus will quickly cause a flexible pes valgus deformity.[42] Loss of tibialis posterior function may result in progressive and dramatic collapsing pes valgo planus deformity with a marked abduction component. If uncorrected within months of loss, tendon transfer alone will no longer suffice and arthrodesis will be required.[50]

Rupture of the tibialis posterior tendon due to rheumatoid arthritis caused a sag in the medial longitudinal arch on weight bearing within 10 days. In another patient, examination 2½ years after rupture revealed a collapsed, but mobile, longitudinal arch. Radiographs of the foot showed marked osteopenia, a valgus heel calcaneal angle, and anterior and inferior displacement of the talar head.[20]

5. FUNCTIONAL (MYOTATIC) UNIT

The flexor digitorum longus and flexor hallucis longus muscles are agonists for the primary non-weight-bearing action of the tibialis posterior, inversion of the foot, and also for the weaker action of plantar flexion. These toe flexors are agonists also for the weight-bearing function of assisting transverse plane balance. Other muscles that also assist inversion are the tibialis anterior and extensor hallucis longus. Other agonists for plantar flexion include the gastrocnemius, soleus, plantaris, and the peroneus longus and brevis muscles.

The chief muscular antagonists to the tibialis posterior's strong inversion action are the peroneal muscles; gravity is the primary antagonist when the individual is weight bearing.

6. SYMPTOMS

An individual with active TrPs in the tibialis posterior muscle is likely to complain of pain in the foot when running or walking. The pain is felt severely in the sole of the foot and Achilles tendon, and also to a lesser degree in the midcalf and heel. It is especially bothersome during walking or running on uneven surfaces, e.g., on gravel or over old bricks or cobblestones that are sufficiently irregular to require additional stabilization of the foot.

Differential Diagnosis

Serious dysfunction of the tibialis posterior muscle/tendon complex is not unusual and deserves careful consideration in the differential diagnosis of ankle and foot pain.

Shin Splints and Deep Posterior Compartment Syndrome

Chapters 19, 20, and 22 of this volume make note of relevant compartment syndromes and shin splints. Most authors identify four muscular compartments in the leg: the anterior, lateral, superficial posterior, and deep posterior compartments.[51,53] The deep posterior compartment contains the tibialis posterior muscle, the flexor digitorum longus, and the flexor hallucis longus. Surgically, the tibialis posterior behaves as if it has an additional compartment of its own.[62,63]

Some authors consider the term "shin splints" to apply only to pain along the inner (medial) distal two-thirds of the tibial shaft.[15,16,70] It is considered to be an overuse syndrome that usually develops during exercise in poorly conditioned athletes or novice runners, and it is specifically attributed to the posterior tibial muscle by these authors. In those individuals whose tibialis posterior attachment to the tibia extends well into the lower third of the leg, as far as or distal to the crossing of its tendon with that of the flexor digitorum longus, excessive pronation would severely strain this region of distal attachment.[65] This condition requires only conservative treatment, not surgery.[15] On the other hand, a deep posterior compartment syndrome can require surgery.

A female aerobic dancer abruptly developed pain bilaterally in the mid-distal tibias, posteromedially (shin splints). Radionuclide bone scan revealed hyperconcentration of activity in the areas of pain, which corresponded to the attachments of the tibialis posterior muscles. The patient recovered within a few days with rest.[14] She apparently had suffered overload stress along the tibial attachment of this muscle.

How to tell whether these symptoms are caused by a chronic compartment syndrome requiring surgery is controversial. One group of surgeons reported an 88% success rate on 26 leg compartment syndromes, performing the operation only after conservative measures failed, but without measuring intramuscular pressures.[70] Other surgeons who performed fasciotomy of the deep posterior compartment based on intramuscular pressure criteria did not achieve results that were as good as those obtained when treating the anterior compartment syndrome surgically.[63] In this series of eight patients, a deep posterior compartment syndrome was diagnosed if intramuscular pressure was more than 15 mm Hg at rest, if it increased during exercise, and if it showed a delayed return to the pre-exercise level.[63]

However, using stringent intramuscular pressure criteria, Melberg and Styf[48] were unable to find anyone among 25 patients with exercise-induced posteromedial pain in the lower leg who qualified for the diagnosis of deep posterior compartment syndrome. The authors made no suggestion as to what was causing the patients' pain. Apparently, they did not consider the possibility of myofascial TrPs in the deep posterior compartment musculature. Myofascial TrPs could cause pain on exertion without producing a true compartment syndrome.

PART 3

Tibialis Posterior Tendon Dysfunction

Johnson and Strom[36] clearly explain and diagram three successive stages of tibialis posterior tendon dysfunction: *(a) tendon length normal* with minimal pain and dysfunction; *(b) tendon elongated, hindfoot mobile* with medial foot pain during and after weight bearing, serious dysfunction, and displacement of bones of the foot; and *(c) tendon elongated, hindfoot deformed and stiff* with lateral foot pain and marked eversion of the foot when bearing weight.

Stage 1 shows weakness of tibialis posterior function when the patient tries to perform the ***single-heel-rise test*** while standing on one foot. Normally, the tibialis posterior muscle first inverts and locks the hindfoot to provide a rigid structure that permits transfer of weight to the forefoot. In stage 1, initial heel inversion is weak and the patient either raises the heel incompletely without locking the hindfoot, or fails to rise onto the ball of the foot. Pain and tenderness are found along the path of the tendon, chiefly just before it passes behind the medial malleolus and medial to its primary navicular insertion. Unfortunately, patients do not usually present with this dysfunction as a chief complaint, but it is at this early stage that the condition should be fully correctable, often with conservative measures. The examiner must look for this condition.[36] The authors offered no suggestions as to why patients develop this condition and gave no indication that the patients were examined for myofascial TrPs that could make a significant contribution to their dysfunction.

Hirsh and coauthors[33] divide chronic tenosynovitis of the tibialis posterior into three descriptive categories: peritendinitis crepitans, stenosing tenosynovitis, and chronic tenosynovitis with effusion. Apparently all of these would fall within stage 1 as described by Johnson and Strom.[36]

With progression to stage 2, pain increases in severity and distribution and the patient has serious difficulty in walking. The single-heel-rise test is more abnormal and the patient stands with the foot everted and abducted sufficiently to display "too many toes" when viewed from behind. This is a simple, reproducible, and recordable measure of posture. Routine radiographs from the anteroposterior view show the forefoot abducted in relation to the hindfoot because the calcaneus and navicular are subluxed laterally off the head of the talus. In lateral view, the talus is tipped forward in relation to the calcaneus. A tomogram is rarely helpful but magnetic resonance imaging of the tendon is valuable. This stage requires surgical repair of the tendon.[36]

In stage 3, damage to the static supports of the foot have resulted in fixed flatfoot and requires realignment of the foot structures and arthrodesis. An isolated subtalar arthrodesis suffices in most cases.[36]

As noted repeatedly in both this volume and in Volume 1,[69] muscles with myofascial TrPs are weakened without atrophy. They also are under continuous increased tension because of taut bands. Thus, myofascial dysfunction in the tibialis posterior muscle is one condition that could possibly account for Johnson and Strom's stage 1 findings: a detectable muscle weakness under high-load conditions, and degenerative changes of the tendon exposed to abnormal sustained tension caused by taut bands. Subsequent stages could follow failure to correct the condition in its initial stage.

A number of authors discuss rupture of the tibialis posterior tendon as a separate entity (stages 2 and 3 of Johnson and Strom),[9,20,32,39,49,64,66,67] including a comprehensive review.[34] The patient presents with a complaint that "my foot is becoming flat," "my shoe is running over," "I can't walk like I used to," or "I have trouble going up and down stairs." Frequently, the absence of the displaced tendon is noted on palpation when compared with the normal side. The discontinuity of the tendon has been imaged by ultrasound and by magnetic resonance imaging.[20]

7. ACTIVATION AND PERPETUATION OF TRIGGER POINTS

Running and jogging, especially on uneven ground or on laterally slanted surfaces, may activate and will perpetuate TrPs in this muscle. Interestingly, tibialis posterior TrPs are not commonly observed in tennis players who characteristically work out on smooth level surfaces and wear shoes that provide ample foot support. Conversely, footwear that is badly worn and that encourages eversion and rocking of the foot promotes TrPs in this muscle.

Although some pronation in early stance is normal, hyperpronation can overload the tibialis posterior muscle and may contribute to the activation, and certainly to the perpetuation, of TrPs in it. The foot may excessively pronate due to a hypermobile midfoot, ankle equinus, muscular imbalance, a Morton foot structure, or some other cause. Chapter 20 of this volume reviews imbalance due to the Morton foot structure in detail.

A systemic perpetuating factor is hyperuricemia with or without signs and symptoms of gout in the big toe. Polymyalgia rheumatica, like hyperuricemia, markedly increases the irritability and susceptibility of the muscles to the development and perpetuation of myofascial TrPs. Chapter 4 of Volume 1[69] reviews these and other perpetuating factors.

8. PATIENT EXAMINATION

If the tibialis posterior TrPs are active and have been present for some time, the patient walks with the foot partly everted and abducted, in a flatfooted gait. The patient should be observed walking barefoot, with the clinician looking particularly for a hyperpronating foot.

The usual method of manually testing the tibialis posterior muscle for strength[37] is unsatisfactory to identify relatively slight weakness. Manual testing of this muscle poorly discriminates its function from force substituted by agonist muscles.[36,59] If manual testing is used, the examiner should watch for curling of any toes, indicating an effort to substitute the long flexors of the toes for the weak tibialis posterior. Instead, the authors recommend the single-heel-rise test,[36] described previously on page 465; it specifically detects the instability associated with weakness of the tibialis posterior. Active TrPs in this muscle cause a perceptible degree of functional weakness.

To test this muscle for restricted range of motion, the patient may be supine or seated. The clinician first fully everts and abducts the foot and then attempts to place it in dorsiflexion. Tibialis posterior TrPs painfully restrict this movement. Restriction of this movement can also be caused by tightness of the flexor digitorum longus and flexor hallucis longus, but not by the other major invertor, the tibialis anterior, because it is a dorsiflexor. If, at the limit of the restricted range of motion, the clinician can extend all five toes without pain, the restriction is caused by the tibialis posterior and not by either of the long toe flexors.

Muscles with active TrPs are likely to develop cramplike pain when contracted in the shortened position. If the tibialis posterior is involved and the patient tries to invert, adduct, and plantar flex the foot fully, pain is likely to occur deep in the calf, where the muscle is located.

The ankle and foot should be examined for joint hypermobility or hypomobility.

The clinician identifies a Morton foot structure by examining the patient's feet and shoes (*see* Section 8 in Chapter 20 of this volume). By the time patients with tibialis posterior TrPs and this foot structure are seen for their persistent foot pain, they usually have tried one or more corrective devices. The device frequently used is an insert that adds support to the foot but often ends short of the head of the first metatarsal, and needs only to be extended with an adhesive felt pad to provide adequate support under the great toe's metatarsal head. However, people with tibialis posterior TrPs frequently find that wearing a corrective orthotic device is painful because it presses on the region of tenderness referred from the TrPs to the sole of the foot. This referred tenderness disappears promptly with inactivation of the responsible TrPs.

If hyperuricemia is suspected, the clinician should check for tophi in the upper rim of the patient's ears. If a systemic condition is suspected of perpetuating these TrPs, the clinician should obtain an erythrocyte sedimentation rate to rule out many possibilities, including polymyalgia rheumatica or other collagen disease.

9. TRIGGER POINT EXAMINATION (Fig. 23.3)

The TrPs in the tibialis posterior muscle lie deep in the leg and are accessible to examination by palpation only indirectly through other muscles. At most, one can only determine a direction of deep tenderness. Interpreting this tenderness as due to tibialis posterior TrPs depends on the preceding examination having established evidence of this muscle's involvement and on having reason to believe that the intervening muscles are free of TrPs. As shown in Figures 19.3 and 23.5, the tibialis posterior is inaccessible to digital

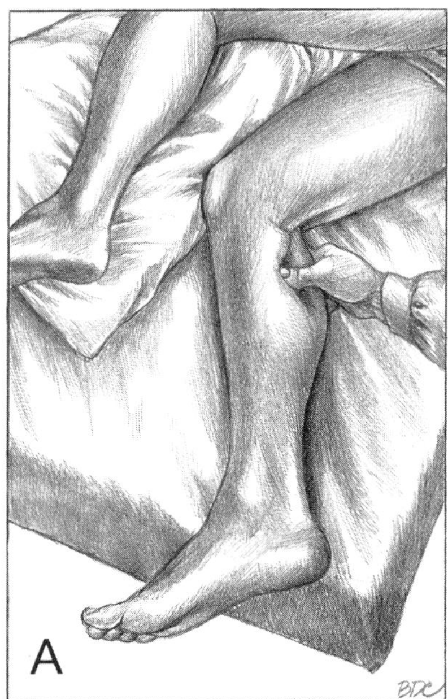

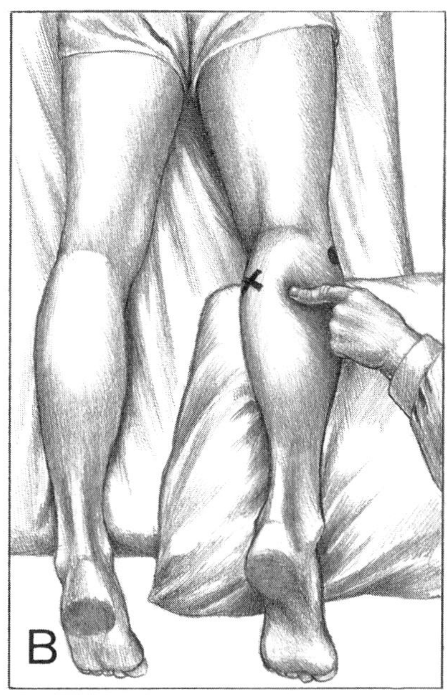

Figure 23.3. Application of strong pressure beside the gastrocnemius and through the soleus muscle to detect deep trigger-point tenderness in the right tibialis posterior muscle. The ***X*** marks the usual medial location for palpating this tenderness. *A*, examination using the medial approach. Tenderness of the tibial attachment of this muscle is palpable in the middle third of the leg, also deep along the posterior border of the tibia. *B*, examination using the lateral approach, pressing medially. The *solid circle* (partial view) marks the head of the fibula.

examination from in front because of the intervening interosseous membrane.

From behind, one can usually elicit tenderness of tibialis posterior TrPs and tenderness of that muscle's tibial attachment by pressing deeply between the posterior border of the tibia and the soleus muscle, which can be partially displaced posteriorly (Fig. 23.5). The muscle should be examined for tenderness as illustrated in Figure 23.3*A* proximal to the midleg. As one palpates distalward from the location illustrated, the flexor digitorum longus will also be encountered behind the tibia. This more distal location on the medial border of the tibia is the same as that of "shin-splint" tenderness attributed to overstress of the tibialis posterior as noted in Section 6, Differential Diagnosis.

Occasionally, on the lateral side (Fig. 23.3*B*), one can elicit tenderness of the tibialis posterior muscle through the soleus and the flexor hallucis longus muscles (*see* Fig. 19.3).[53]

Gutstein[31] included the tibialis posterior among those muscles in which he found myalgic spots [probably TrPs] that referred pain and responded to conservative therapy.

10. ENTRAPMENTS

No neural or vascular entrapments by this muscle have been observed, nor are any expected since it lies deep to the vessels and nerves.

11. ASSOCIATED TRIGGER POINTS

The two toe muscles that also invert and plantar flex the foot, the flexor digitorum longus and flexor hallucis longus, are commonly involved with the tibialis posterior muscle. However, the primary foot plantar flexors, the gastrocnemius and soleus muscles, are not prone to develop TrPs in association with the tibialis posterior.

Active TrPs in the peroneal muscles, especially in patients with the Morton foot structure, are also commonly associated with TrPs in the tibialis posterior muscle. The peroneus longus and peroneus brevis muscles are prime antago-

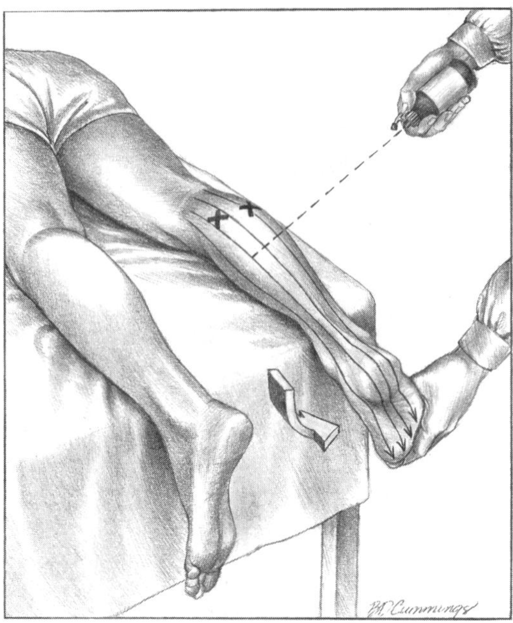

Figure 23.4. Stretch position and vapocoolant spray pattern (*thin arrows*) for the right tibialis posterior muscle. The **X**s mark locations that are usually most effective for palpation using a medial or lateral approach. Trigger points actually lie centrally between the two sets of **X**s. The foot should be moved into dorsiflexion and then eversion (*thick arrow*) to stretch this muscle passively.

nists to the inversion action of the tibialis posterior, but are agonists to its plantar flexion and stabilization of the foot.

12. INTERMITTENT COLD WITH STRETCH
(Fig. 23.4)

Since injection of TrPs in the tibialis posterior muscle is difficult and not recommended, it is especially important to utilize effective noninvasive techniques for releasing this muscle's tightness.

The use of ice for applying intermittent cold with stretch is explained on page 9 of this volume and the use of vapocoolant spray with stretch is detailed on pages 67–74 of Volume 1.[69] Techniques that augment relaxation and stretch are reviewed on pages 10–11 of this volume.

Stretching through full range should not be performed if either the hindfoot or the midfoot is hy*per*mobile. In this case, alternative treatment methods should be used (*see* pages 9–10 of this volume). On the other hand, if the joints of the foot are hy*po*mobile, they should be mobilized.

For intermittent cold with stretch, the patient lies prone and relaxed in a comfortable position on the examining table with the feet extending beyond the end (Fig. 23.4). Pillows support the patient as necessary for comfort, and a blanket covers the patient for warmth, if needed. The clinician demonstrates use of ice or suitable vapocoolant, and warns that it may feel startlingly cold. Then downward parallel sweeps of intermittent cold cover the back of the leg, the heel, and the plantar surface of the foot (Fig. 23.4), while the clinician simultaneously grasps the ball of the foot and gently but firmly everts and dorsiflexes the foot to take up any slack in the tibialis posterior muscle. Any tension in the flexor digitorum longus and flexor hallucis longus can be released by simultaneously passively extending all five toes.

The patient then initiates an augmented postisometric relaxation procedure by *slowly* taking in a *full* breath and, at the same time, *gently* contracting the tibialis posterior muscle isometrically against resistance supplied by the clinician. At the beginning of a *slow* exhalation, the patient concentrates on relaxing the whole body, particularly the limb under treatment. The clinician applies parallel sweeps of the stream of vapocoolant or applies parallel strokes with ice in the pattern shown in Figure 23.4, while maintaining gentle but firm pressure into eversion and dorsiflexion to take up any slack that develops in the tibialis posterior and associated muscles. The first cycle concludes when the patient completes the *total* exhalation and must take another breath. The treatment cycle is repeated in rhythm to the patient's slow, full respiratory cycle with careful attention to synchronization between the patient and the clinician.

When no further gain in range of motion occurs, the patient can then substitute relaxation during the exhalation phase with a voluntary effort to assist the clinician in placing the foot in eversion and dorsiflexion. This activation of antagonists to the tibialis posterior weakens its stretch reflexes by reciprocal inhibition, thus increasing the effectiveness of intermittent cold with stretch.

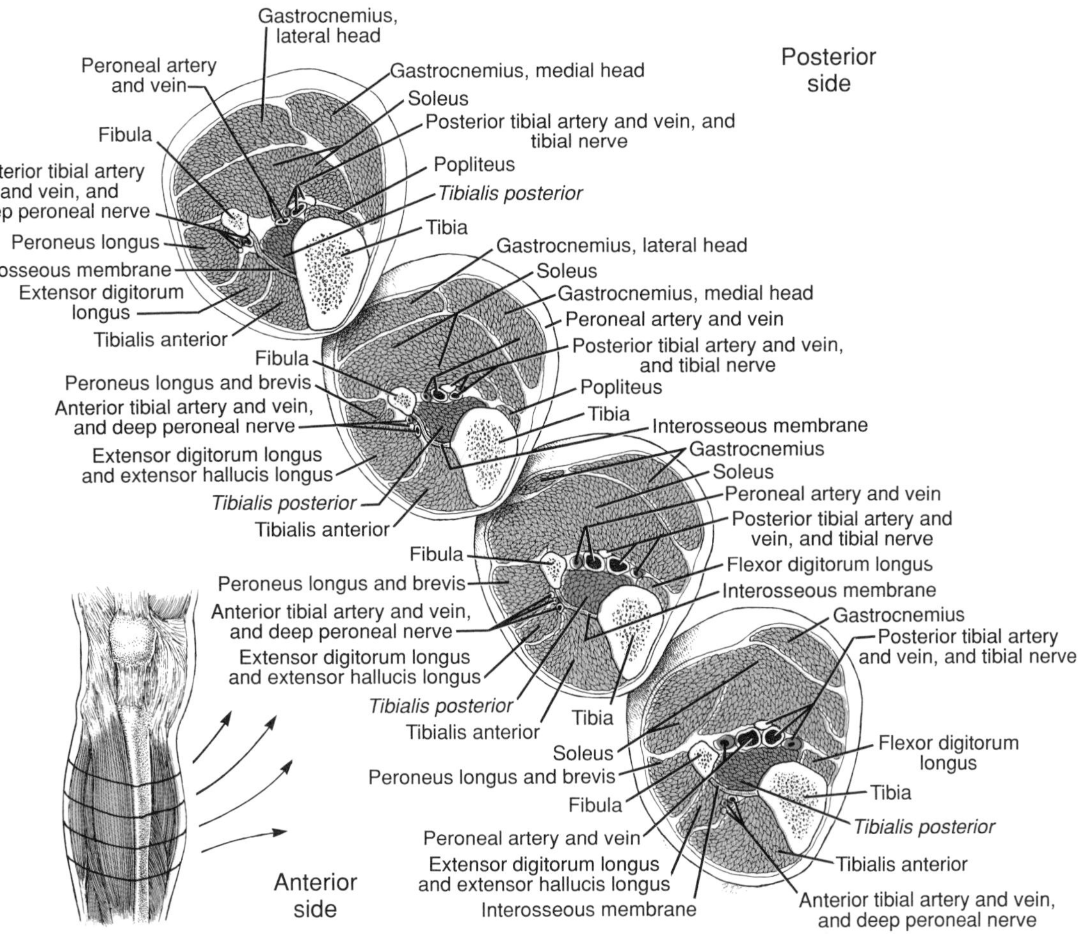

Figure 23.5. Four serial cross sections of the right tibialis posterior muscle (*medium red*), in relation to other muscles of the leg (*light red*), viewed from above. Arteries are *bright red*, veins are *black* surrounded by uncolored walls, and nerves are uncolored. These sections are oriented as one palpates the calf of the prone patient. The levels of the cross section are identified in the lower left corner. The flexor hallucis longus is not distinguished from the soleus muscle in the distal section. Adapted from *A Cross-Section Anatomy*, by Eycleshymer and Schoemaker, published by D. Appleton Company, 1911.

Following use of the stretch procedures described previously, the clinician applies a moist heating pad to the skin over the treated muscle to rewarm the skin and to further release muscle tension as the patient relaxes in comfort. The patient then performs several *slowly* and *smoothly* executed cycles of *full* active range of motion, placing the tibialis posterior successively in the fully lengthened and fully shortened positions.

Finally, the patient learns how to perform the postisometric relaxation technique at home on a daily basis to maintain the muscle's full stretch range of motion and to keep its sarcomere lengths equalized. This helps prevent or inactivate a recurrence of TrPs in this muscle.

The tibialis posterior lies under too many layers of other muscles to be readily accessible to massage therapy. Ultrasound does reach it and can be used in conjunction with stretch.

Evjenth and Hamberg[23] describe and illustrate a bimanual method of stretching the tibialis posterior muscle.

PART 3

13. INJECTION AND STRETCH (Fig. 23.5)

The authors do not recommend injection of the tibialis posterior muscle, especially from behind. Examination of Figure 23.5

shows that there is no access to the muscle without passing close to nerves, arteries, and veins. Since the muscle lies so deep, localization of the TrPs will be imprecise. Figure 19.3 shows more clearly the details of this problem. The poor localization of the TrPs in this muscle would require considerable probing for the TrPs with the needle, which would increase the danger of its encountering a nerve or an artery. If arterial bleeding resulted, it might be difficult to know promptly that it was occurring, and even more difficult to apply counter pressure effectively to stop the bleeding.

An injection approach to this muscle was described and illustrated in detail by Rorabeck.[62] He used an *anterior* approach through the interosseous membrane to insert a wick catheter into the tibialis posterior muscle. This procedure provided a measure of the muscle's intramuscular pressure in order to diagnose a suspected posterior compartment syndrome that would require surgical intervention. Lee *et al.*[38] also described an anterior approach for performing needle electromyography on this muscle.

14. CORRECTIVE ACTIONS

Corrective Body Mechanics

A patient with active tibialis posterior TrPs who is a runner or jogger should exercise on a smooth surface and wear shoes with adequate arch support. Pads should be added to the shoe beneath the head of the first metatarsal to correct for a Morton foot structure, if present (*see* Chapter 20, Figs. 20.4–20.7 and 20.12–20.14). If there is hyperpronation due to a hypermobile midfoot, a good arch support should be used. If muscle imbalances are present, they should be corrected.

Corrective Posture and Activities

In patients with painful hyperpronating "runners' feet," the problem may be corrected by exercises to increase the endurance and aerobic capacity of both the tibialis posterior and peroneus longus muscles.[1]

Walking and running should be confined to smooth, level surfaces.

If the TrP activity responds poorly to treatment, jogging or running as a form of exercise should be replaced by swimming or bicycling. Initially, corrections made to the insert of the shoe may be uncomfortable due to referred tenderness from the TrPs, but with resolution of the tibialis posterior TrPs, this related tenderness of the sole of the foot disappears.

Whether or not the individual runs or jogs, he or she should always wear a well-fitted shoe that is high enough to enhance lateral stability of the foot. If the heel counter of the shoe is too wide and loose (when a finger will slide in between the patient's heel and the shoe), the heel of the shoe should be made snug by adding pads inside the shoe beside the person's heel.

High heels and spike heels must be avoided. High top shoes may be necessary if other measures do not suffice.

Home Therapeutic Program

The patient needs to perform an augmented postisometric relaxation exercise daily, as described previously in Section 12. Properly performed, this should keep the muscle free of recurrent TrPs unless the patient has significant unresolved perpetuating factors, which may be not only mechanical, but systemic, as discussed on pages 114–155 in Volume 1.[69]

References

1. Anderson A: Personal communication, 1991.
2. Anderson JE: *Grant's Atlas of Anatomy*, Ed. 8. Williams & Wilkins, Baltimore, 1983 (Figs. 4–70, 4–81).
3. *Ibid.* (Fig. 4–72).
4. *Ibid.* (Fig. 4–86).
5. *Ibid.* (Fig. 4–95).
6. *Ibid.* (Fig. 4–98).
7. *Ibid.* (Fig. 4–107).
8. *Ibid.* (Fig. 4–117).
9. Banks AS, McGlamry ED: Tibialis posterior tendon rupture. *J Am Podiatr Med Assoc 77*:170–176, 1987.
10. Bardeen CR: The musculature, Sect. 5. In *Morris's Human Anatomy*, edited by C.M. Jackson, Ed. 6. Blakiston's Son & Co., Philadelphia, 1921 (pp. 522, 523).
11. Basmajian JV, Deluca CJ: *Muscles Alive*, Ed. 5. Williams & Wilkins, Baltimore, 1985 (pp. 342–345).
12. *Ibid.* (pp. 377–378).
13. Basmajian JV, Stecko G: The role of muscles in arch support of the foot. An electromyographic

PART 3

study. *J Bone Joint Surg [Am] 45*:1184–1190, 1963.
14. Brill DR: Sports nuclear medicine bone imaging for lower extremity pain in athletes. *Clin Nucl Med 8*:101–106, 1983.
15. Brody DM: Running injuries. *Clin Symp 32*:1–36, 1980 (pp. 15, 18–19).
16. Bryk E, Grantham SA: Shin splints. *Orthop Rev 12*:29–40, 1983.
17. Carter BL, Morehead J, Wolpert SM, *et al.*: *Cross-Sectional Anatomy*. Appleton-Century-Crofts, New York, 1977 (sects. 72–83).
18. Clemente CD: *Gray's Anatomy of the Human Body*, American Ed. 30. Lea & Febiger, Philadelphia, 1985 (p. 578, Fig. 6–78).
19. *Ibid*. (p. 579).
20. Downey DJ, Simkin PA, Mack LA, *et al.*: Tibialis posterior tendon rupture: a cause of rheumatoid flat foot. *Arthritis Rheum 31*:441–446, 1988.
21. Duchenne GB: *Physiology of Motion*, translated by E.B. Kaplan. J. B. Lippincott, Philadelphia, 1949 (pp. 362–363).
22. *Ibid*. (p. 368).
23. Evjenth O, Hamberg J: *Muscle Stretching in Manual Therapy, A Clinical Manual*. Alfta Rehab Førlag, Alfta, Sweden, 1984 (p. 146).
24. Ferner H, Staubesand J: *Sobotta Atlas of Human Anatomy*, Ed. 10, Vol. 2. Urban & Schwarzenberg, Baltimore, 1983 (Fig. 464).
25. *Ibid*. (Fig. 469).
26. *Ibid*. (Fig. 473).
27. *Ibid*. (Figs. 475, 476).
28. *Ibid*. (Fig. 500).
29. Gray EG, Basmajian JV: Electromyography and cinematography of leg and foot ("normal" and flat) during walking. *Anat Rec 161*:1–16, 1968.
30. Green DR, Lepow GM, Smith TF: Pes cavus, Chapter 8. In *Comprehensive Textbook of Foot Surgery*, edited by E.D. McGlamry, Vol. 1. Williams & Wilkins, Baltimore, 1987 (pp. 287–323, *see* p. 287).
31. Gutstein M: Diagnosis and treatment of muscular rheumatism. *Br J Phys Med 1*:302–321, 1938.
32. Helal B: Tibialis posterior tendon synovitis and rupture. *Acta Orthop Belg 55*:457–460, 1989.
33. Hirsh S, Healey K, Feldman M: Chronic tenosynovitis of the tibialis posterior tendon and the use of tenography. *J Foot Surg 27*:306–309, 1988.
34. Holmes GB Jr, Cracchiolo A III, Goldner JL, *et al.*: Current practices in the management of posterior tibial tendon rupture. *Contemp Orthop 20*: 79–108, 1990.
35. Janda V: *Muscle Function Testing*. Butterworths, London, 1983 (pp. 197–199).
36. Johnson KA, Strom DE: Tibialis posterior tendon dysfunction. *Clin Orthop 239*:196–206, 1989.
37. Kendall FP, McCreary EK: *Muscles, Testing and Function*, Ed. 3. Williams & Wilkins, Baltimore, 1983 (p. 142).
38. Lee HJ, Bach JR, DeLisa JA: Needle electrode insertion into tibialis posterior: a new approach. *Am J Phys Med Rehabil 69*:126–127, 1990.
39. Lipsman S, Frankel JP, Count GW: Spontaneous rupture of the tibialis posterior tendon. *J Am Podiatr Assoc 70*:34–39, 1980.
40. Lockhart RD: *Living Anatomy*, Ed. 7. Faber & Faber, London, 1974 (Figs. 136, 141).
41. Matsusaka N: Control of the medial-lateral balance in walking. *Acta Orthop Scand 57*:555–559, 1986.
42. McGlamry ED, Mahan KT, Green DR: Pes valgo planus deformity, Chapter 12. In *Comprehensive Textbook of Foot Surgery*, edited by E.D. McGlamry, Vol. 1. Williams & Wilkins, Baltimore, 1987 (pp. 403–465, *see* p. 411).
43. McMinn RMH, Hutchings RT: *Color Atlas of Human Anatomy*. Year Book Medical Publishers, Chicago, 1977 (pp. 282, 285).
44. *Ibid*. (p. 289).
45. *Ibid*. (p. 315).
46. *Ibid*. (p. 318).
47. *Ibid*. (p. 320).
48. Melberg P-E, Styf J: Posteromedial pain in the lower leg. *Am J Sports Med 17*:747–750, 1989.
49. Mendicino SS, Quinn M: Tibialis posterior dysfunction: an overview with a surgical case report using a flexor tendon transfer. *J Foot Surg 28*:154–157, 1989.
50. Miller SJ: Principles of muscle–tendon surgery and tendon transfers, Chapter 23. In *Comprehensive Textbook of Foot Surgery*, edited by E.D. McGlamry, Vol. 2. Williams & Wilkins, Baltimore, 1987 (pp. 714–752, *see* p. 739).
51. Moore MP: Shin splints: diagnosis, management, prevention. *Postgrad Med 83*:199–210, 1988.
52. Morimoto I: Notes on architecture of tibialis posterior muscle in man. *Kaibogaku Zasshi 58*: 74–80, 1983.
53. Netter FH: *The Ciba Collection of Medical Illustrations*, Vol. 8, Musculoskeletal System. Part I: Anatomy, Physiology and Metabolic Disorders. Ciba-Geigy Corporation, Summit, 1987 (p. 98).
54. *Ibid*. (p. 102).
55. *Ibid*. (p. 103).
56. *Ibid*. (p. 105).
57. *Ibid*. (p. 107).
58. Perry J: The mechanics of walking. A clinical interpretation. *Phys Ther 47*:778–801, 1967.
59. Perry J, Ireland ML, Gronley J, *et al.*: Predictive value of manual muscle testing and gait analysis in normal ankles by dynamic electromyography. *Foot Ankle 6*:254–259, 1986.
60. Rasch PJ, Burke RK: *Kinesiology and Applied Anatomy*, Ed. 6. Lea & Febiger, Philadelphia, 1978 (pp. 321–323, 330, Table 17–2).
61. Rohen JW, Yokochi C: *Color Atlas of Anatomy*, Ed. 2. Igaku-Shoin, New York, 1988 (p. 424).
62. Rorabeck CH: Exertional tibialis posterior compartment syndrome. *Clin Orthop 208*:61–64, 1986.
63. Rorabeck CH, Fowler PJ, Nott L: The results of fasciotomy in the management of chronic exertional compartment syndrome. *Am J Sports Med 16*:224–227, 1988.
64. Sammarco GJ, DiRaimondo CV: Surgical treatment of lateral ankle instability syndrome. *Am J Sports Med 16*:501–511, 1988.
65. Saxena A, O'Brien T, Bunce D: Anatomic dissection of the tibialis posterior muscle and its correlation to medial tibial stress syndrome. *J Foot Surg 29*:105–108, 1990.
66. Smith TF: Common pedal prominences, Chapter 6. In *Comprehensive Textbook of Foot Surgery*, edited by E.D. McGlamry, Vol. 1. Williams &

Wilkins, Baltimore, 1987 (pp. 252–263, *see* pp. 252, 253).

67. Soballe K, Kjaersgaard–Anderson P: Ruptured tibialis posterior tendon in a closed ankle fracture. *Clin Orthop 231*:140–143, 1988.
68. Sutherland DH: An electromyographic study of the plantar flexors of the ankle in normal walking on the level. *J Bone Joint Surg [Am] 48*:66–71, 1966.
69. Travell JG and Simons DG: *Myofascial Pain and Dysfunction: The Trigger Point Manual*. Williams & Wilkins, Baltimore, 1983.
70. Wiley JP, Clement DB, Doyle DL, *et al.*: A primary care perspective of chronic compartment syndrome of the leg. *Phys Sportsmed 15*:111–120, 1987.

CHAPTER 24
Long Extensors of Toes
Extensor Digitorum Longus and Extensor Hallucis Longus

"Muscles of Classic Hammer Toes"

HIGHLIGHTS: **REFERRED PAIN** from both long extensor muscles of the toes (extrinsic extensors) projects primarily to the dorsum of the foot. Pain referred from trigger points (TrPs) in the extensor digitorum longus concentrates on the dorsolateral aspect of the foot and may extend nearly to the tips of the middle three toes. Pain referred from TrPs in the extensor hallucis longus muscle concentrates over the region of the first metatarsophalangeal joint and may extend nearly to the tip of the great toe. **ANATOMICAL ATTACHMENTS** of the extensor digitorum longus are, proximally, to the lateral condyle of the tibia, to the fibula and the interosseus membrane, and to intermuscular septa. Distally, it anchors to the middle and distal phalanges of the four lesser toes. The extensor hallucis longus muscle attaches, proximally, only to the fibula and interosseus membrane. Distally, it ends on the distal phalanx of the great toe. **FUNCTION**: Both long extensors of the toes assist in preventing foot slap immediately following heel-strike, and they help the foot clear the floor during the swing phase. Function of the extensor digitorum longus is critical for normal foot mechanics. The extensor digitorum longus acts primarily as a powerful extensor of the proximal phalanx of the four lesser toes and also assists dorsiflexion and *eversion* of the foot. The extensor hallucis longus acts primarily to extend the proximal phalanx of the great toe powerfully and also to assist dorsiflexion and *inversion* of the foot. **SYMPTOMS** produced by myofascial TrPs in the long extensors of the toes include persistent pain over the dorsum of the foot, sometimes foot slap during ambulation, night cramps in the long extensors of the toes, and "growing pains" in children. Differential diagnoses include other myofascial pain syndromes with overlapping pain patterns, and hammer or clawtoes caused by muscle imbalance. **ACTIVATION AND PERPETUATION OF TRIGGER POINTS** may result from an L_4-L_5 radiculopathy, an anterior compartment syndrome, habitually using the muscle in the lengthened position, and from an acute stress overload. **PATIENT EXAMINATION** includes looking for evidence of and testing for dorsiflexor weakness at the ankle and then, specifically, for extension weakness of the great toe and of the four lesser toes. Active resisted or unresisted dorsiflexion causes pain when the long extensor muscles of the toes harbor active TrPs. Passive plantar flexion to full range is painful, as also is resisted extension effort of the corresponding toes and passive flexion of the toes. The foot should be examined for abnormalities in joint play. **TRIGGER POINT EXAMINATION** of the extensor digitorum longus requires digital palpation of the muscle several centimeters distal to the head of the fibula between the tibialis anterior and peroneus longus muscles. Examination of the extensor hallucis longus employs digital palpation just distal to the junction of the middle and distal thirds of the leg anterior to the fibula. Examination of active TrPs characteristically elicits local spot tenderness and referred pain from both muscles, but rarely elicits a perceptible local twitch response. **ENTRAPMENT** of the deep branch of the peroneal nerve can occur by its impingement against the fibula as it passes deep to the taut bands associated with TrPs in the extensor digitorum longus muscle. **INTERMITTENT COLD WITH STRETCH** of all extensors of the toes, both short and long, can be accomplished simultaneously. The clinician applies vapocoolant or ice stroking in downward parallel sweeps over the anterior leg and dorsum of the foot, including the toes, while plantar flexing the foot and flexing all toes. Prompt application of moist heat and full active range of motion complete the procedure. **INJECTION** of the long extensors of the toes requires full knowledge of the location of the anterior tibial vessels and deep peroneal nerve and careful orientation of the needle. Generally, alternative treatment techniques are recommended instead of TrP injection of the extensor hallucis longus muscle. **CORRECTIVE ACTIONS** include avoidance of prolonged severe dorsiflexion or plantar flexion when driving a car or sleeping. Activities that overload the long extensors of the toes, such as wearing spike or high heels or excessive running and jogging, should be avoided. The body and legs must be kept warm, especially in a cold or drafty environment.

1. REFERRED PAIN
(Fig. 24.1)

Active myofascial trigger points (TrPs) are not unusual in the long extensor muscles of the toes, which include the extensor digitorum longus and extensor hallucis longus muscles. The referred pain patterns of TrPs in these muscles are analogous to the referred pain patterns of the extensor digitorum muscle of the hand.

Extensor digitorum longus TrPs refer pain primarily over the dorsum of the foot and toes, nearly to the tips of the middle three toes (Fig. 24.1*A*), as previously reported.[62,66] Children present a similar pattern of pain referred from this muscle.[10] Sometimes the pain referred from extensor digitorum longus TrPs concentrates more strongly at the ankle than over the dorsum of the foot.[65] A spillover pattern may extend halfway up the leg from the

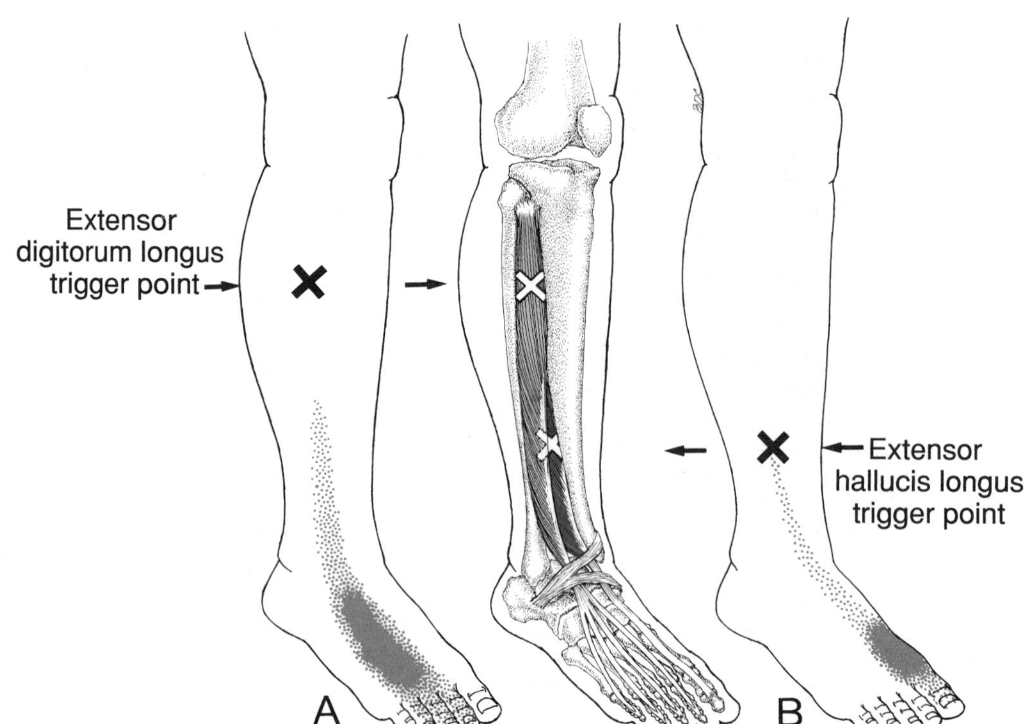

Figure 24.1. Pain patterns (*bright red*) referred from trigger points (***X**s*) commonly observed in the right long extensor muscles of the toes. The essential pain pattern (*solid bright red*) denotes the pain experienced by nearly everyone when this trigger point is active. *Red stippling* indicates occasional spillover of the essential pattern. *A*, extensor digitorum longus muscle (*light red*). *B*, extensor hallucis longus muscle (*dark red*).

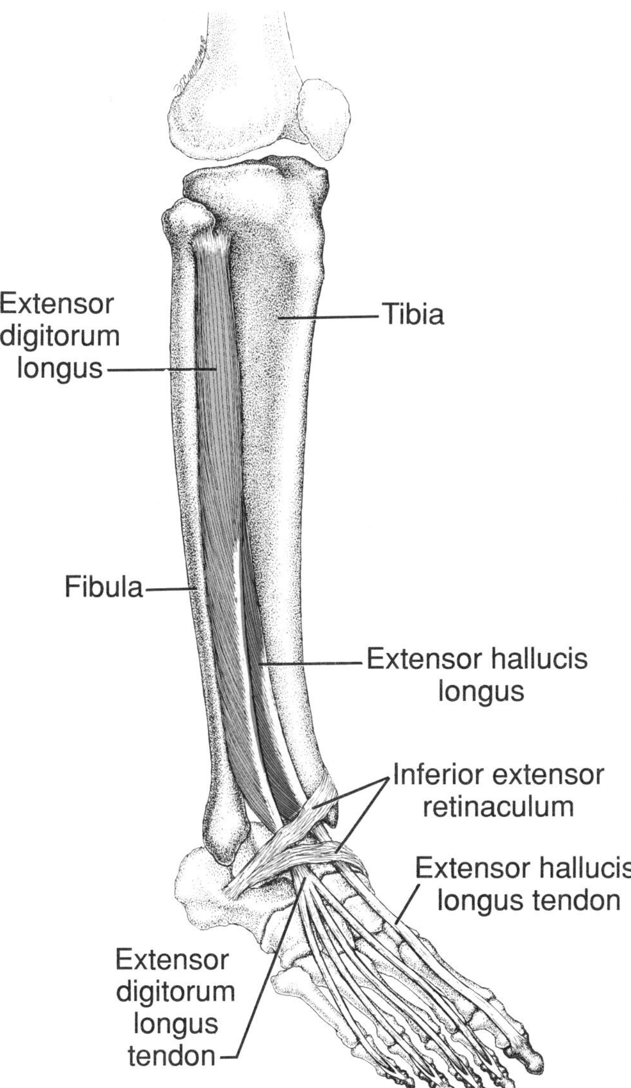

Figure 24.2. Attachments of the right long extensor muscles of the toes, anterolateral view. The extensor digitorum longus is *medium red*, and the extensor hallucis longus is *dark* red. The superior extensor retinaculum is not pictured.

ankle toward the TrP (Fig. 24.1*A*). Jacobsen[31] reported pain radiating to the anterolateral region of the ankle from TrPs in this muscle.

Extensor hallucis longus TrPs refer pain primarily to the dorsum of the foot over the distal aspect of the first metatarsal and the base of the great toe with spillover patterns extending downward to the tip of the great toe and upward over the dorsum of the foot and leg, sometimes as far as the TrP (Fig. 24.1*B*).

Lewit[35] reported that patients with increased tension of the long extensors of the toes experience pain on the anterior aspect of the tibia.

2. ANATOMICAL ATTACHMENTS AND CONSIDERATIONS
(Fig. 24.2)

The extensor digitorum longus and extensor hallucis longus muscles (the extrinsic extensors of the toes) share the anterior compartment of the leg with the tibialis anterior and peroneus tertius muscles.[49]

Extensor Digitorum Longus
(Fig. 24.2)

The extensor digitorum longus is a penniform muscle that attaches ***proximally*** to the lateral condyle of the tibia (Fig. 24.2), to the upper three-fourths of the anterior surface of the body of the fibula, to the proximal portion of the interosseus membrane (above the extensor hallucis longus) and to intermuscular septa shared with adjacent muscles in the anterior compartment.[15] The part of the muscle that anchors to the tibial condyle and head of the fibula covers the deep peroneal nerve as it courses around the neck of the fibula to reach the intermuscular septum. At the ankle, the tendon passes deep to the superior and inferior extensor retinacula and then divides into four tendinous slips that attach ***distally*** to the middle and distal phalanges of the four lesser toes. Each tendon receives a fibrous expansion from the interossei and lumbricals. The tendon then spreads into an aponeurosis called the extensor hood, which covers the dorsal surface of the proximal phalanx. It sends one slip to the base of the middle phalanx; two collateral slips unite and continue on to attach to the dorsal base of the distal phalanx.[15] Duchenne[18] describes an extensor digitorum longus attachment (by means of fibrous expansions from the plantar surface of the tendons) also to the dorsal surface of the *proximal* phalanges of the four lesser toes. Bardeen[8] also describes this attachment to the proximal phalanges; however, not all anatomists mention it.[15]

The part of the extensor digitorum longus that ends in a tendon to the second toe often forms a distinctly separate muscle belly from the semipennate part of the muscle that supplies the remaining lesser toes.[34] The belly of the entire muscle may be more or less completely divided to correspond with the tendons to individual toes.[8]

The arrangement of its tendinous attachment to the toes varies considerably. Additional slips may span from a tendon to its corresponding metatarsal bone, to the short extensor of the toe, or to one of the interosseus muscles.[8,15]

PART 3

Extensor Hallucis Longus

The extensor hallucis longus lies between, and is largely covered by, the tibialis anterior and the extensor digitorum longus muscles. Its tendon emerges to a superficial position in the lower third of the leg. ***Proximally***, it attaches along the middle two-fourths of the medial surface of the fibula, medial to the extensor digitorum longus, and to the interosseus membrane. At the ankle, it passes deep to the superior extensor retinaculum and through a separate compartment of the inferior extensor retinaculum. ***Distally***, it anchors to the base of the distal phalanx of the great toe. An expansion from the medial side of the tendon is usually inserted into the base of the proximal phalanx.[15]

The proximal attachment of the extensor hallucis longus is occasionally united with that of the extensor digitorum longus.[15] Occasionally, a small *extensor ossis metatarsi hallucis* may run from the extensor hallucis longus (or from the extensor digitorum longus or tibialis anterior) through the same compartment deep to the inferior extensor retinaculum as the extensor hallucis longus.[15] It ends on the first metatarsal bone. Rarely, a separate *long extensor of the first phalanx* of the great toe may originate on the tibia or interosseous membrane.[68]

Supplemental References

The front view portrays both the extensor digitorum longus and extensor hallucis longus in their entirety without associated nerves or vessels.[25,50,61] A similar view shows their tendons and synovial sheaths at the ankle.[6,30,45,54,60] Other figures show their attachments to the toes in detail.[5,28,46,54]

Front views portray the relations of the two muscles to the deep peroneal nerve and to the anterior tibial artery throughout the leg.[4,51] Deep dissections with the proximal end of the extensor digitorum longus reflected reveal how sustained tension in that muscle could entrap the deep peroneal nerve against the tibia.[23,43,52]

The extensor digitorum longus[16] and both long extensors of the toes[24,60] appear in lateral view.

Cross sections show the relations of these two muscles to neighboring muscles and to major vessels and nerve trunks in 16 serial sections,[12] in three sections through the upper, middle, and lower thirds of the leg,[27] in two sections through the upper and lower thirds of the leg,[13] in one section just above the middle of the leg,[49] and in one section through the lower part of the middle third of the leg.[3]

Markings on the bones locate the osseous attachments of both muscles in the leg,[1,26,41,53] and of the extensor hallucis longus to the distal phalanx of the great toe.[7,29,42,53]

Photographs reveal the surface skin contours produced by the extensor digitorum longus muscle,[14,37] by that muscle's tendon at the ankle,[2,37] and by the tendons of both muscles at the ankle and on the dorsum of the foot.[44]

3. INNERVATION

Both the extensor digitorum longus and extensor hallucis longus muscles receive their innervation via deep peroneal nerve branches, which contain fibers from the fourth and fifth lumbar and first sacral spinal nerves.[15]

4. FUNCTION

The extensor digitorum longus and the extensor hallucis longus muscles function as assistants in controlling (decelerating) the descent of the forefoot to the floor immediately following heel-strike, thereby preventing foot slap. During the swing phase of gait, they assist in providing foot-floor clearance. The extensor digitorum longus helps provide pure dorsiflexion of the foot by balancing the inversion pull of the tibialis anterior muscle. The long extensors of the toes also assist in preventing excessive postural sway in a posterior direction.

The extensor hallucis longus is thought to help the foot adapt to the ground in walking.

The extensor digitorum longus acts to dorsiflex and evert the foot and to extend the four lesser toes. The extensor hallucis longus assists in dorsiflexion and inversion of the foot and extends the great toe.

Actions

The extensor digitorum longus powerfully extends the proximal phalanx of the four lesser toes, and extends the middle and distal phalanges less vigorously.[18] It also dorsiflexes and everts the foot.[8,15,58] Electrical stimulation of this muscle caused extension of the proximal phalanx of each of the lesser four toes with dorsiflexion, abduction of the foot, and elevation of its lateral border (eversion).[18] Simultaneous electrical stimulation of the tibialis anterior muscle resulted in more vigorous pure dorsiflexion at the ankle; normally, any tendency for abduction or adduction of the foot was balanced out in this test.[20]

Although the extensor hallucis longus attaches to the distal phalanx of the great toe with a tendinous slip to the proximal phalanx, it extends the proximal phalanx most powerfully.[8,21,32] It also assists dorsiflexion and inversion of the foot.[8,15,58] Stimulation of this muscle produced vigorous extension of the proximal phalanx of the great toe with weak dorsiflexion and inversion of the foot.[19,21] For the extensor hallucis longus to produce strong extension of the distal phalanx of the great toe, synergistic action of the first dorsal interosseus muscle is required for firm fixation of its proximal phalanx.[19]

Functions

Standing and Ambulation

The extensor hallucis longus was electrically silent during quiet stance, but became active when subjects swayed backwards and also during dorsiflexion of the ankle.[9]

During ambulation, the extensor hallucis longus showed a spike of activity immediately after heel-strike, apparently to help control (decelerate) plantar flexion and prevent foot slap. Motor unit activity in this muscle and in the extensor digitorum longus began shortly before swing phase and continued throughout swing phase, apparently to assist in lifting the forefoot clear of the floor.[17,56] Measurement of ground reaction force, myoelectric activity, and motion in pronation-supination of the foot in 11 normal adults revealed that, when the lateral component of ground reaction force was small, the extensor hallucis longus, the tibialis posterior, and the flexor digitorum longus were active.[40] The extensor hallucis longus was considered to be active during the midstance phase in order to allow the foot to adapt to the ground.

Among seven normal subjects, the intensity of myoelectric activity in the extensor digitorum longus and the extensor hallucis longus muscles during slow gait corresponded to manual muscle testing levels of mostly fair, occasionally fair −, in those muscles. During free gait, the myoelectric activity increased slightly to a level corresponding to manual testing of mostly fair, occasionally fair +. During fast gait, the myoelectric activity usually corresponded to a manual testing level of fair +.[57]

Jumping and Sports Activities

During a standing two-leg vertical jump, the extensor digitorum longus of five normal adults showed a strong peak of EMG activity at the beginning of the upward spring and another at the time of take-off from the ground. Activity resumed shortly before landing and persisted until both feet were again solidly on the ground and stability was achieved.[33]

The extensor digitorum longus muscle consistently showed more surface myoelectric activity on the left side than on the right during 13 right-handed sports activities that included overhand throws, underhand throws, tennis strokes, golf swings, and hitting a baseball. Generally, this muscle on the right side exhibited a prolonged burst of moderate activity shortly before release of, or contact with, the ball. The muscle on the left side sometimes showed a burst of activity preceding contact or release, and always produced a vigorous burst following contact or release. The left muscle also exhibited a crescendo of activity throughout the golf swing.[11] No report was located that described the activity of the extensor hallucis longus during these activities.

Weakness

Weakness of the extensor digitorum longus allows the foot to assume a more inverted (varus) position as the tibialis anterior muscle overpowers the compensatory effect of the extensor digitorum longus. In addition, a mild foot drop may develop with inversion, forefoot equinus, and a flexed position of the toes.[48]

Abnormal Extensor Reflex Response

The abnormal extensor reflex response of the great toe, or Babinski response, is associated with abnormally vigorous activity, primarily of the extensor hallucis longus muscle.[9]

5. FUNCTIONAL (MYOTATIC) UNIT

The agonists to the long extensors of the toes for their primary function of toe extension are the corresponding two short extensors (intrinsic extensors), namely, the extensors hallucis brevis and digitorum brevis. The chief antagonists to toe extension are all of the toe flexors, both short and long (intrinsic and extrinsic).

For dorsiflexion of the foot, the primary agonists to the long extensors of the toes are the tibialis anterior and peroneus tertius muscles. Antagonists to the foot dorsiflexion action of these two toe extensor muscles are chiefly the gastrocnemius and soleus muscles.

For eversion of the foot, the agonists of the extensor digitorum longus are all three peroneal muscles. For inversion of the foot, the extensor hallucis longus is assisted by the tibialis anterior, tibialis posterior, and the two long flexor muscles of the toes.[58]

6. SYMPTOMS

The chief complaint of patients with TrPs in the long extensors of the toes is usually pain on the top of the foot extending to the "knuckles" (metatarsophalangeal joints). If asked, the patient often merely says that the feet hurt. Frequently, however, patients do not complain spontaneously about painful feet and when queried will respond, "But don't everybody's feet hurt?". Inquiry is essential because these individuals have become so accustomed to the referred pain and tenderness in their feet that they think such pain is a normal part of everyone's life.

The patient also may complain of foot slap or weakness of the foot during walking because of a compromised ability to control the descent of the forefoot to the floor following heel-strike. This is likely to happen if the extensor digitorum longus muscle harbors TrPs. When, in addition, the TrPs in this muscle cause entrapment of the deep peroneal nerve (see Section 10 in this chapter and page 386 of this volume), symptoms may include complete foot-drop due to neurapraxia and weakness of all anterior compartment muscles.

An intermediate severity of dorsiflexion weakness of the foot occurs with TrP activity in the extensor hallucis longus muscle also, but without nerve entrapment.

Night cramps of the long extensors of the toes are commonly encountered when the muscles have active TrPs. (Chapter 21 of this volume includes an extensive review of nocturnal leg cramps.) These extrinsic extensor muscles of the toes are vulnerable to similar cramping when fatigued and placed in the shortened position for a long time.

Children and adolescents are likely to complain of "growing pains" caused by TrPs that were activated by the stresses of their excessively vigorous locomotor activity.

Differential Diagnosis

Pain referred from TrPs in the extensor digitorum longus muscle can easily be mistaken for pain arising in synovial joints of the tarsal bones.[59]

Other Myofascial Pain Syndromes

The TrPs in five other muscles refer pain in patterns that could be confused with the pattern referred by the **extensor digitorum longus** muscle (Fig. 24.1*A*). It may be necessary to examine these muscles for TrPs to determine which one or ones are responsible for the pain. The pain referred by the *peroneus longus and brevis* muscles appears over the lateral malleolus and more laterally on the dorsum of the foot (*see* Fig. 20.1.*A*). The pain referred by TrPs in the third muscle, the *peroneus tertius*, concentrates at and above the ankle; pain also often extends to the lateral side of the heel below the lateral malleolus (*see* Fig. 20.1*B*), an area outside the pattern of the extensor digitorum longus. Pain caused by the fourth muscle, the *extensor digitorum brevis* (*see* Fig. 26.1), is the most difficult to distinguish based only on the pain distribution. Pain referred from the extensor digitorum brevis centers more proximally on the dorsum of the foot and does not extend into the toes, the latter projection being much more characteristic of the extensor digitorum longus TrPs. Lastly, TrPs of the *interossei* can also produce toe pain, but the pain is specific to one toe or adjacent portions of two toes; this TrP pain of interossei concentrates in the toes rather than the dorsum of the foot, although considerable overlap may occur (*see* Fig. 27.3*A*).

The referred pain from TrPs in two other muscles can easily be confused with the referred pain pattern of the **extensor hallucis longus** (Fig. 24.1*B*). The pattern referred from the tibialis anterior muscle (*see* Fig. 19.1) concentrates farther distally on the great toe itself, and not so much on the region of the metatarsophalangeal joint at the base of the great toe. The *tibialis anterior* pain pattern also concentrates more in the ankle region rather than distally over the dorsum of the foot. Pain referred from the *extensor hallucis brevis* (*see* Fig. 26.1) is felt more in the tarsal region and near the lateral aspect of the first metatarsal than on the dorsal aspect of the *base* of the great toe. Both the extensor hallucis longus and the tibialis anterior referred pain patterns may involve the dorsal aspect of the great toe itself.

Hammer Toes and Clawtoes

The hammer toe can manifest itself in different ways, including the classic hammer toe, clawtoe, or mallet toe.[32] In the classic hammer toe (of the four lesser toes), the metatarsophalangeal (MP) joint is extended, the proximal interphalangeal (IP) joint is flexed, and the distal IP joint is extended, producing a flat "hammer head" at the end. In clawtoes, the MP joints are markedly extended and the proximal and distal IP joints are fixed in flexion, producing a claw curvature. In the mallet toe, only the distal IP joint is flexed. True clawtoe deformity is often associated with cavus foot deformity and neuromuscular conditions. The clawtoe deformity tends to create a more severe functional disability than the hammer toe.[32]

These conditions usually develop because of muscle imbalance initiated by compensatory mechanisms. Three mechanisms are identified: flexor stabilization, flexor substitution, and extensor substitution. The first two mechanisms concern the long flexor muscles of the toes and are covered in the next chapter. Extensor substitution concerns the extensor digitorum longus muscle.[32]

Extensor substitution can produce both clawtoes and classic hammer toes. This mechanism is more common than flexor substitution, but less common than flexor stabilization.[32] Extensor substitution produces excessive digital contraction during the swing phase of gait. Because the extensor digitorum longus has a mechanical advantage, this overactivity causes a functional imbalance with the lumbrical muscles. The MP joints are hyperextended during swing phase and heel-strike, and, as the condition progresses, may remain in that position during weight bearing.

Extensor substitution occurs when the extensor digitorum longus attempts to provide more than its fair share of dorsiflexion effort. This muscle does not become effective as a dorsiflexor of the foot until it has completed its easier function of extending the MP joint; if the latter movement is unopposed by adequate lumbrical action, this extended toe positioning occurs with every step. Any condition that plantar flexes the forefoot, such as anterior pes cavus or ankle equinus, can initiate a vicious cycle of increasing distortion of toe position. Primary lumbrical weakness, or chronically increased tension of the flexor digitorum longus muscle (due to spasticity or to shortening of the muscle by taut bands of TrPs) can be responsible. A painful forefoot that causes the individual to lift the foot in a flat manner and avoid forefoot pressure at the end of stance phase disproportionately loads the extensor digitorum longus.[32] Wearing shoes (especially tight ones) appears to be a major contributing factor to disuse atrophy of the lumbrical muscles, or to failure of their normal development in childhood.

A case[64] of an individual presenting with the symptoms of acute shin splints and loss of strength of only the extensor digitorum longus, with evidence of denervation of the muscle, was presented as an example of a partial anterior compartment syndrome due to acute overuse of toe extensors on a motorcycle trip. The severe neural impairment of only one of the four muscles in the anterior compartment raises the question of a possible entrapment syndrome (see Section 10, following). The possibility that the muscular overload activated TrPs in the extensor digitorum longus was apparently not considered.

Tendinitis and Rupture of Tendon

Hypertrophy or exostosis at the first metatarsocuneiform joint, due to osteoarthritis or other causes, may cause foot irritation by a shoe and hypertrophy of the extensor hallucis longus tendon as it crosses this region. Such chronic microtrauma to the tendon may also produce tendinitis, pain, thinning of the tendon, and possibly rupture.[63]

A 28-year-old female suffered rupture of the anterior talofibular ligament with partial involvement of the calcaneofibular ligament as the result of an acute right foot-inversion injury. Following immobilization, the patient had constant pain over the dorsal aspect of the midfoot aggravated by resistance to contraction of the extensor digitorum longus. Tenogram demonstrated a filling defect of the extensor digitorum longus tendon sheath distal to the head of the talus. At operation, the inferior extensor retinaculum was adherent to the extensor digitorum longus tendon. Lysis and excision of the adhesions provided relief of the pain and restored normal muscle function.[55]

A 16-year-old male experienced a closed rupture at the musculotendinous junction of the extensor hallucis longus muscle during a powerful forced flexion of the great toe against fixed resistance while attempting to kick a football. This may have been a late complication of fracture of the distal tibial shaft with associated compromise of blood supply to the tendon in the region of the tear.[47]

7. ACTIVATION AND PERPETUATION OF TRIGGER POINTS

Activation

Radiculopathy at the L_4-L_5 level can, but does not always, activate and perpetuate TrPs in these long extensor muscles of the toes. The TrPs may also result from tripping or falling. They are likely to appear following an anterior compartment syndrome and the associated ischemia of the muscles in that compartment.

For the driver of a car, a steep accelerator pedal that maintains the ankle at an acute angle in dorsiflexion can place the long extensors of the toes in a shortened position for an extended time. This situation favors the activation of latent TrPs. Similarly, sitting for long periods with the feet back under a chair with the ankles in an extreme dorsiflexed position can activate TrPs in these long extensors.

On the other hand, excessively stretched-out muscle fibers at a long sarcomere length are weaker than at mid-length; thus, the stretched-out muscle must work harder to do the same job. For this reason, these extensor muscles are chronically overloaded and, therefore, susceptible to developing TrPs in people who wear high heels. Placing the ankle in a strongly plantar flexed position for long periods, as when the accelerator of the car is nearly parallel to the floor, can have this same weakening effect. Shortened triceps surae musculature that produces a "tight" Achilles tendon and restricts active dorsiflexion to less than 10° can chronically overload the long extensors of

PART 3

the toes, inciting the development of TrPs in them.[39]

In addition, TrPs may be activated by excessive jogging or running, unaccustomed walking on uneven ground or in soft sand, and catching the toes on the ground when kicking a ball.

Direct gross trauma to the muscle, stress fractures of the tibia or fibula, and immobilization after an ankle fracture or sprain are other causes of TrP activation. The TrPs that result from these acute overload conditions usually respond well to myofascial therapy.

Perpetuation

Any factor that activates TrPs, when continued, also perpetuates them. More commonly, however, one stress activates the TrPs and other factors perpetuate them.

Mechanical factors, such as the prolonged plantar flexed position of the ankle during sleep, and systemic factors, such as nutritional inadequacies, may be responsible for the fact that good initial results with myofascial therapy provide only temporary relief (*see* Chapter 4 in Volume 1).[67]

8. PATIENT EXAMINATION

During ambulation of the patient, the clinician should look and listen for foot slap and should examine heel walking for evidence of dorsiflexor weakness. The extensors of the great toe, of the lesser toes, and the tibialis anterior muscle are tested separately to identify the muscle(s) responsible for weakness in dorsiflexion. Marked weakness of all five toes suggests entrapment of the deep peroneal nerve by the extensor digitorum longus; mild-to-moderate, ratchety, or "breakaway" weakness suggests only TrP involvement without significant neurapraxia due to nerve entrapment.

Macdonald demonstrated experimentally[38] in patients with tenderness of the extensor hallucis longus muscle that voluntary extension of the great toe against resistance (forceful contraction of the muscle) was painful, but resisted flexion effort was not. Also, passive stretching of this extensor muscle was painful, but passive shortening (passive toe extension) was not painful. We observe these same findings in patients with TrPs in this muscle. These same tests apply equally well for identifying TrP involvement of the extensor digitorum longus muscle by similarly testing these movements of the four lesser toes.

The clinician should examine the patient's foot for abnormalities in joint play.

9. TRIGGER POINT EXAMINATION (Fig. 24.3)

Usually, digital examination of active TrPs in the **extensor digitorum longus** (Fig. 24.3*A*) elicits local spot tenderness and referred pain in the foot and ankle (pain distribution shown in Fig. 24.1*A*). Pressure is applied approximately 8 cm (3 in) distal to the level of the fibular head between the tibialis anterior and peroneus longus muscles. At this level, the most proximal part of the extensor hallucis longus is deep to and between the extensor digitorum longus and the tibialis anterior muscles.[49] Contraction of the extensor digitorum longus usually is distinguishable by palpation when the patient selectively extends the lesser toes against resistance *without* exerting dorsiflexion effort at the ankle.

Similarly, palpation of active TrPs in the **extensor hallucis longus** (Fig. 24.3*B*) elicits local tenderness and pain that is referred over the dorsum of the forefoot medially in the vicinity of the first MP joint (Fig. 24.1*B*). The examiner usually finds these TrPs slightly distal to the junction of the middle and distal thirds of the leg anterior to the fibula. In this region, the extensor hallucis longus may be emerging from between the tibialis anterior and the extensor digitorum longus, as the latter becomes tendinous. As the extensor hallucis longus becomes subcutaneous, it lies anterior and adjacent to the fibula.[27] Contraction of this muscle can usually be distinguished by palpation distal to the TrP region when the patient selectively extends the great toe against resistance *without* exerting dorsiflexion effort at the ankle.

Placing either of the long extensor muscles of the toes on slight stretch increases the sensitivity of TrP tenderness, makes the taut band stand out with maximum contrast to surrounding

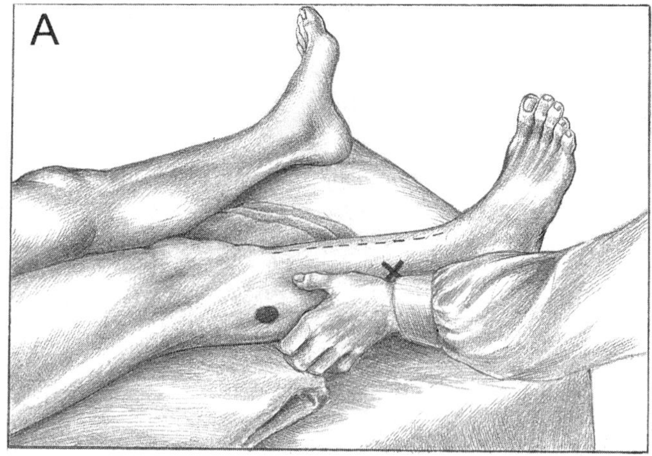

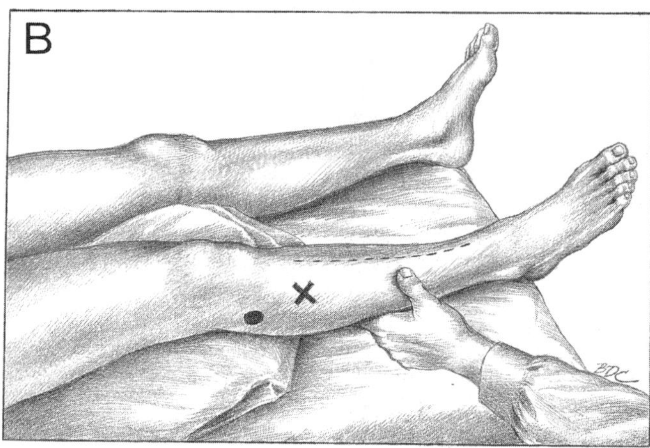

Figure 24.3. Palpation of trigger points in the right long extensor muscles of the toes. The proximal ***X*** locates the usual region of extensor digitorum longus trigger points, and the distal ***X*** shows the usual region of extensor hallucis longus trigger points. The *dashed line* locates the anterior crest of the tibia. The *solid circle* marks the head of the fibula. *A*, extensor digitorum longus trigger point. The operator exerts pressure deep in the anterior compartment of the leg lateral to the tibialis anterior muscle. *B*, extensor hallucis longus trigger point. Examination by flat palpation, slightly distal to the junction of the middle and distal thirds of the leg anterior to the fibula.

slack muscle fibers, and enhances the local twitch response. Local twitch responses are much less readily elicited in the long extensors of the toes than in the peroneus longus and tibialis anterior muscles and are less easily elicited in the toe extensors than in the long extensors of the fingers.

10. ENTRAPMENTS

The deep peroneal nerve enters the anterior compartment of the leg by passing first deep to the peroneus longus in the company of the superficial peroneal nerve and then continues alone deep to the extensor digitorum longus muscle (*see* Fig. 20.9).[52] Here, only the deep peroneal nerve is subject to impingement against the fibula by the taut bands of TrPs in the extensor digitorum longus muscle. Similar taut bands in the peroneus longus muscle can entrap both superficial and deep branches of this nerve, as described in Section 10 of Chapter 20 in this volume. When the responsible TrPs in the extensor digitorum longus are inactivated, the neurapraxia due to entrapment of the deep peroneal nerve may disappear within 5 or 10 minutes with return of strength of all four of the anterior compartment muscles that it innervates; namely, the tibialis anterior, extensor hallucis longus, extensor digitorum longus, and peroneus tertius.

The patient is often mystified by this method of producing recovery, especially when entrapment has caused severe neurapraxia of the anterior compartment muscles with serious foot-drop. The patient wonders how an injection of a local anesthetic like procaine can cause the muscle to become stronger, and instead expects the anesthetic to "put the nerve to sleep" and cause weakness. The clinician then explains to the patient the mechan-

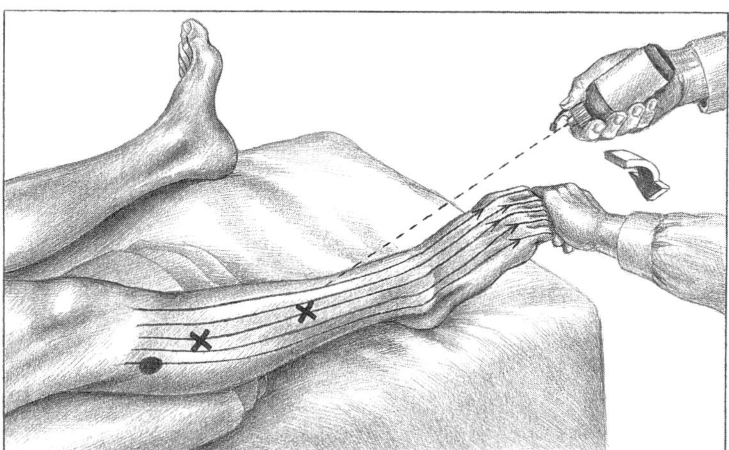

Figure 24.4. Stretch position and spray or icing pattern (*thin arrows*) for the long extensors of the toes. The *solid circle* covers the head of the fibula. The *proximal* ***X*** marks the common location of trigger points in the extensor digitorum longus muscle, and the *distal* ***X*** marks the common location of those in the extensor hallucis longus. The *thick arrow* indicates the downward pressure exerted on the toes and foot to stretch both muscles simultaneously.

ism of relief of symptoms that were due to peripheral nerve entrapment by the muscle.

11. ASSOCIATED TRIGGER POINTS

The TrPs often appear independently in the long extensors of the toes, but also may develop in conjunction with TrPs in neighboring muscles. Not surprisingly, the peroneus longus and brevis muscles are likely to develop TrPs associated with those in the extensor digitorum longus since all three muscles are prime agonists for eversion of the foot. The extensor hallucis longus and, to a lesser extent, the extensor digitorum longus may develop TrPs in association with TrPs in the tibialis anterior muscle.

The extensor digitorum longus and peroneus tertius work closely together as a team in both dorsiflexion and eversion of the foot. Existence of active TrPs in one apparently can induce TrPs in the other as a result of compensatory overload of the parallel unimpaired muscle.

At times, particularly with severe perpetuating factors, the entire anterior compartment musculature harbors TrPs. Thus, it is important to check the long extensors of the toes for TrPs if the other anterior compartment muscles are involved.

12. INTERMITTENT COLD WITH STRETCH
(Fig. 24.4)

These two long extensor muscles of the toes respond well to intermittent cold with stretch. To apply this treatment to inactivate TrPs in either of the muscles, one must plantar flex the foot at the ankle and also flex the corresponding toes (Fig. 24.4).[62] In addition, the foot should be *inverted* to achieve full lengthening of the extensor *digitorum* longus and everted for full lengthening of the extensor *hallucis* longus. For each muscle, parallel downsweeps of vapocoolant spray or ice should cover both the full length of the muscle and its referred pain pattern (Fig. 24.4).

In the presence of hypermobility in the tarsometatarsal region, a two-handed stretch approach is needed so that this midfoot region can be stabilized. In such cases, intermittent cold could *precede* the stretch rather than being applied simultaneously with it.

The use of ice for applying intermittent cold with stretch is explained on page 9 of this volume and the use of vapocoolant spray and stretch is detailed on pages 67–74 of Volume 1.[67]

Simply applying sweeps of spray or stroking with ice over the reference zone where the patient complains of pain, with-

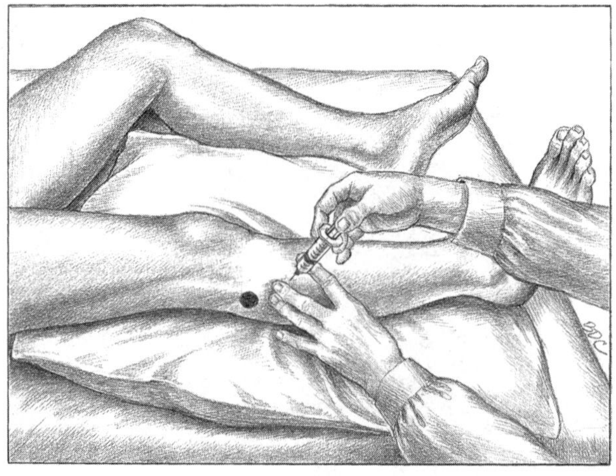

Figure 24.5. Injection of trigger points in the right extensor digitorum longus muscle. The *solid circle* marks the head of the fibula. See text for description of the course of the deep peroneal nerve and anterior tibial vessels, and how to avoid them. Injection of the extensor hallucis longus is not generally recommended.

out including the skin overlying the muscle and its TrPs, usually relieves the pain only momentarily. Including the muscle and its TrPs is much more likely to abolish the pain, the restricted range of motion, and the referred deep tenderness for a long period of time, even permanently.[65]

The application of intermittent cold with passive stretch should include coverage of four agonistic muscles, the short and long extensors of both the great and lesser toes, effectively releasing TrP tightness in those muscles. The antagonist toe flexors may also need to be treated in a similar manner to prevent activating their TrPs by unaccustomed shortening.

The effectiveness of this procedure is augmented by incorporating Lewit's postisometric relaxation[35] with reflex augmentation,[36] as described on pages 10–11 of this volume.

Following intermittent cold with stretch, moist heat applied promptly over the muscles that have been treated rewarms the skin (and muscles if they were unintentionally cooled) and reduces posttreatment soreness. Slow active range of motion from the *fully* shortened to the *fully* lengthened positions of these muscles (to the limits of toe flexion and extension) helps further increase range of motion and incorporate *full* range of motion into daily activities.

Evjenth and Hamberg[22] describe techniques that are specific for stretching the extensor digitorum longus or the extensor hallucis longus muscles. These techniques would be awkward to combine with vapocoolant spray or ice stroking. However, the advantage of their method is that it includes stabilization of the tarsometatarsal region.

Ischemic compression and deep massage, two valuable techniques, are followed immediately by full passive and active lengthening of the muscle except when such stretching exercises are contraindicated by hypermobility. Additional techniques for releasing myofascial TrPs are discussed in Chapter 2 of this volume.

13. INJECTION AND STRETCH (Fig. 24.5)

If it is considered necessary to inject TrPs in the long extensors of the toes, one should take care to avoid the deep peroneal nerve and anterior tibial vessels. This is less difficult for TrPs in the extensor digitorum longus muscle than in the extensor hallucis longus. The deep peroneal nerve passes across the fibula deep to the extensor digitorum longus proximal to the region where one usually finds TrPs in that muscle (Fig. 24.1). The nerve then accompanies the anterior tibial vessels that together lie on the interosseus membrane deep to the extensor hallucis longus (*see* Fig. 19.3).[27] Thus, when injecting TrPs in the extensor digitorum longus muscle (Fig. 24.5), one inserts the needle close to the lateral border of the tibialis anterior muscle and angles the needle posteriorly toward the fibula.[27]

Injection of TrPs in the extensor hallucis longus muscle is generally not recommended, and should be considered only if the taut band and TrP tenderness have been clearly localized and their depth determined. In this case, one must be especially careful of the depth of needle penetration. One may have to pass the needle through the lateral portion of the tibialis anterior to direct the needle toward the fibula at an angle deep enough to reach the TrPs in the extensor hallucis longus, but sufficiently superficial to avoid the underlying deep peroneal nerve and anterior tibial vessels (*see* Fig. 19.3).[27]

If TrPs are to be injected in these muscles, one should warn the patient in advance that he or she may feel some numbness and that the muscle may become "lazy" following the injection. If this happens, there is no need to worry. When 0.5% procaine solution is used, even if some procaine seeps around the nerve, nerve conduction will recover in 15 or 20 minutes; it is not uncommon for this transient nerve block to occur. It is better to warn the patient ahead of time than to confront him or her with an unexpected event. It is important to use ***0.5% procaine***; if 1% or 2% procaine is injected, or a longer-acting local anesthetic is selected, the patient may be unable to walk out of the office for an hour or longer.

Following injection of these TrPs, active range of motion is performed slowly and repeatedly to the limits of toe flexion and extension. Application of several sweeps of ice or vapocoolant in the muscle's lengthened position helps ensure inactivation of any residual TrPs and helps normalize muscle function. Prompt application of moist heat for several minutes minimizes postinjection soreness. This may be applied prior to active range of motion if it is painful.

14. CORRECTIVE ACTIONS

In addition to correction of systemic perpetuating factors, such as those described in Chapter 4 of Volume 1,[67] corrective actions are recommended for the following specific physical stresses on these long extensor muscles of the toes.

If there is hypomobility in the joints of the ankle and foot, these areas should be mobilized. If there is hypermobility, appropriate support should be added to the shoes.

Corrective Posture and Activities

If the automobile accelerator pedal places the foot in a markedly dorsiflexed or plantar flexed position, the slope of the pedal should be adjusted by adding an appropriately shaped wedge pad to it in order to produce a more neutral angulation of the foot at the ankle. The patient should be advised to stop and walk around the car every 30–60 minutes on a long drive to prevent the adverse effects of prolonged immobilization of the leg muscles.

The patient should wear low heels with a full base (not spike heels) to provide a neutral angle at the ankle and a stable base for walking, and should walk on even surfaces.

If excessive jogging or sports activity that involved running was responsible for the development of the TrPs in these toe extensors, such strenuous weight-bearing activities should be avoided for a period immediately after specific TrP treatment. It is best if the patient rows, swims, or bicycles for exercise. If the patient insists on returning to the previous activity, a graded program of progressively increasing levels of exercise helps avoid re-exposure to overload beyond tolerance.

One should avoid both the plantar flexed position and an extreme dorsiflexed position of the foot during sleep; the angle of the foot at the ankle should be in the neutral position. A pillow placed against the feet beneath the sheet helps avoid excessive plantar flexion caused by heavy or tight covers, as shown for the gastrocnemius muscle in Figure 21.11. Care should be taken in the placement of the pillow, however, to avoid excessive dorsiflexion (shortened position of the muscle).

Home Therapeutic Program

Since cooling a muscle aggravates its TrPs, the patient should wear warm socks or stockings and slacks to keep the legs warm. Cold, drafty locations should be warmed, possibly by a space heater under the desk. A blanket may be needed over the legs when sitting. An electrically heated floor pad protects from a cold floor. An electric blanket at night is helpful in maintaining body warmth and muscular relaxation.

The patient should be instructed in an exercise to lengthen these long extensors of the toes passively. The patient can sit in a comfortable position, use one hand to stabilize the leg (or to support the midfoot if there is hypermobility), and use the other hand to plantar flex the ankle and flex the toes. This can be done while the patient sits with the back supported in a bathtub of warm water.

An active pedal exercise that combines toe flexion and extension with ankle movement (*see* Fig. 22.13) should be performed every 20–30 minutes when a person sits or reclines for long periods.

References

1. Anderson JE: *Grant's Atlas of Anatomy*, Ed. 8. Williams & Wilkins, Baltimore, 1983 (Fig. 4–70).
2. *Ibid.* (Fig. 4–71).
3. *Ibid.* (Fig. 4–72).
4. *Ibid.* (Fig. 4–73).
5. *Ibid.* (Fig. 4–77).
6. *Ibid.* (Fig. 4–79).
7. *Ibid.* (Fig. 4–106).
8. Bardeen CR: The musculature, Sect. 5. In *Morris's Human Anatomy*, edited by C.M. Jackson, Ed. 6. Blakiston's Son & Co., Philadelphia, 1921 (pp. 512–514).
9. Basmajian JV, Deluca CJ: *Muscles Alive*, Ed. 5. Williams & Wilkins, Baltimore, 1985 (pp. 351, 353).
10. Bates T, Grunwaldt E: Myofascial pain in childhood. *J Pediatr 53*:198–209, 1958.
11. Broer MR, Houtz SJ: *Patterns of Muscular Activity in Selected Sports Skills*. Charles C Thomas, Springfield, 1967.
12. Carter BL, Morehead J, Wolpert SM, *et al.*: *Cross-Sectional Anatomy*. Appleton-Century-Crofts, New York, 1977 (Sects. 72–87).
13. Clemente CD: *Gray's Anatomy of the Human Body*, American Ed. 30. Lea & Febiger, Philadelphia, 1985 (p. 111).
14. *Ibid.* (p. 112).
15. *Ibid.* (pp. 574–575).
16. *Ibid.* (p. 582).
17. Close JR: *Motor Function in the Lower Extremity*. Charles C Thomas, Springfield, 1964 (p. 78).
18. Duchenne GB: *Physiology of Motion*, translated by E.B. Kaplan. J.B. Lippincott, Philadelphia, 1949 (pp. 338, 340, 341, 346, 370–371, 412).
19. *Ibid.* (pp. 343–344, 371, 381, 416–417, 421).
20. *Ibid.* (p. 345).
21. *Ibid.* (pp. 371, 381, 416–417).
22. Evjenth O, Hamberg J: *Muscle Stretching in Manual Therapy, A Clinical Manual*. Alfta Rehab Förlag, Alfta, Sweden, 1984 (pp. 136–139).
23. Ferner H, Staubesand J: *Sobotta Atlas of Human Anatomy*, Ed. 10, Vol. 1. Urban & Schwarzenberg, Baltimore, 1983 (Fig. 458).
24. *Ibid.* (Figs. 465, 467).
25. *Ibid.* (Fig. 466).
26. *Ibid.* (Fig. 468).
27. *Ibid.* (Figs. 472–474).
28. *Ibid.* (Fig. 488).
29. *Ibid.* (Fig. 503).
30. *Ibid.* (Fig. 504).
31. Jacobsen S: Myofascielt smertesyndrom (Myofascial pain syndrome). *Ugeskr Laeger 149*:600–601, 1987.
32. Jimenez L, McGlamry ED, Green DR: Lesser ray deformities, Chapter 3. In *Comprehensive Textbook of Foot Surgery*, edited by E. Dalton McGlamry, Vol. 1. Williams & Wilkins, Baltimore, 1987 (pp. 57–113, *see* pp. 57–58, 66–71).
33. Kamon E: Electromyographic kinesiology of jumping. *Arch Phys Med Rehabil 52*:152–157, 1971.
34. Krammer EB, Lischka MF, Gruber H: Gross anatomy and evolutionary significance of the human peroneus III. *Anat Embryol 155*:291–302, 1979.
35. Lewit K: *Manipulative Therapy in Rehabilitation of the Motor System*. Butterworths, London, 1985 (p. 282).
36. Lewit K: Postisometric relaxation in combination with other methods of muscular facilitation and inhibition. *Manual Med 2*:101–104, 1986.
37. Lockhart RD: *Living Anatomy*, Ed. 7. Faber & Faber, London, 1974 (Figs. 136, 138).
38. Macdonald AJR: Abnormally tender muscle regions and associated painful movements. *Pain 8*: 197–205, 1980.
39. Maloney M: Personal communication, 1991.
40. Matsusaka N: Control of the medial-lateral balance in walking. *Acta Orthop Scand 57*:555–559, 1986.
41. McMinn RMH, Hutchings RT: *Color Atlas of Human Anatomy*. Year Book Medical Publishers, Chicago, 1977 (pp. 282, 285).
42. *Ibid.* (p. 289).
43. *Ibid.* (p. 314).
44. *Ibid.* (p. 318).
45. *Ibid.* (p. 319).
46. *Ibid.* (p. 321).
47. Menz P, Nettle WJS: Closed rupture of the musculotendinous junction of extensor hallucis longus. *Injury 20*:378–381, 1989.
48. Miller SJ: Principles of muscle-tendon surgery and tendon transfers, Chapter 23. In *Comprehensive Textbook of Foot Surgery*, edited by E. Dalton McGlamry, Vol. 2. Williams & Wilkins, Baltimore, 1987 (pp. 714–755, *see* p. 737).
49. Netter FH: *The Ciba Collection of Medical Illustrations*, Vol. 8, Musculoskeletal System. Part I: Anatomy, Physiology and Metabolic Disorders. Ciba-Geigy Corporation, Summit, 1987 (p. 98).
50. *Ibid.* (p. 99).
51. *Ibid.* (p. 100).
52. *Ibid.* (p. 104).
53. *Ibid.* (p. 107).
54. *Ibid.* (p. 111).
55. Perlman MD, Leveille D: Extensor digitorum longus stenosing tenosynovitis. *J Am Podiatr Med Assoc 78*:198–199, 1988.

56. Perry J: The mechanics of walking. *Phys Ther 47*: 778–801, 1967.
57. Perry J, Ireland ML, Gronley J, *et al.*: Predictive value of manual muscle testing and gait analysis in normal ankles by dynamic electromyography. *Foot Ankle 6*:254–259, 1986.
58. Rasch PJ, Burke RK: *Kinesiology and Applied Anatomy*, Ed. 6. Lea & Febiger, Philadelphia, 1978 (pp. 318, 330, Table 17–2).
59. Reynolds MD: Myofascial trigger point syndromes in the practice of rheumatology. *Arch Phys Med Rehabil 62*:111–114, 1981.
60. Rohen JW, Yokochi C: *Color Atlas of Anatomy*, Ed. 2. Igaku-Shoin, New York, 1983 (p. 423).
61. *Ibid.* (p. 426).
62. Simons DG, Travell JG: Myofascial pain syndromes, Chapter 25. In *Textbook of Pain*, edited by P.D. Wall and R. Melzack, Ed. 2. Churchill Livingstone, London, 1989 (pp. 368–385, *see* p. 378, Fig. 25.9*G*).
63. Smith TF: Common pedal prominences, Chapter 6. In *Comprehensive Textbook of Foot Surgery*, edited by E. Dalton McGlamry, Vol. 1. Williams & Wilkins, Baltimore, 1987 (pp. 252–263, *see* p. 260).
64. Streib EW, Sun SF, Pfeiffer RF: Toe extensor weakness resulting from trivial athletic trauma. Report of three unusual cases. *Am J Sports Med 10*:311–313, 1982.
65. Travell J: Ethyl chloride spray for painful muscle spasm. *Arch Phys Med Rehabil 33*:291–298, 1952.
66. Travell J, Rinzler SH: The myofascial genesis of pain. *Postgrad Med 11*:425–434, 1952.
67. Travell JG, Simons DG: *Myofascial Pain and Dysfunction: The Trigger Point Manual.* Williams & Wilkins, Baltimore, 1983.
68. Wood J: On some varieties in human myology. *Proc R Soc Lond 13*:299–303, 1864.

CHAPTER 25
Long Flexor Muscles of Toes
Flexor Digitorum Longus and Flexor Hallucis Longus

"Clawtoe Muscles"

HIGHLIGHTS: **REFERRED PAIN** from trigger points (TrPs) in the *flexor digitorum longus* muscle is felt primarily in the middle of the plantar forefoot proximal to the four lesser toes, with a spillover pattern over the plantar surface of these toes. The TrPs in the *flexor hallucis longus* refer pain strongly to the plantar surface of the great toe and head of the first metatarsal. **ANATOMICAL ATTACHMENTS** of the *flexor digitorum longus* are proximally, to the posterior surface of the tibia and distally, to the base of the distal phalanx of each of the four lesser toes. The *flexor hallucis longus* attaches proximally to the posterior surface of the fibula and distally to the distal phalanx of the great toe. Its tendon crosses deep to that of the flexor digitorum longus distal to the medial malleolus, behind which both tendons pass. **INNERVATION** of both long flexor muscles of the toes is via branches of the tibial nerve. These extrinsic toe flexors **FUNCTION** to help maintain equilibrium when body weight is on the forefoot and to help stabilize the foot and ankle during the midstance to late stance phase of walking. The flexor digitorum longus is generally more active than the flexor hallucis longus during vigorous sports activities. The primary action of both of these long flexor muscles in a "free" lower limb is vigorous flexion of the distal phalanx of the related toes and weak flexion of the other joints of the toes. For both muscles, their assistance in controlling movements of the foot in the sagittal plane and in the frontal plane becomes more important when the position of the foot is fixed. The chief **SYMPTOM** of TrPs in the long flexors of the toes is painful feet, especially when weight bearing. Differential diagnoses include other myofascial pain syndromes, shin splints, chronic compartment syndrome, and rupture of the flexor hallucis longus tendon. Differential diagnosis requires an understanding of toe deformities. **ACTIVATION AND PERPETUATION** of flexor digitorum longus and flexor hallucis longus TrPs can result from running on uneven ground, particularly in badly worn footgear. Walking and running barefoot on soft sand tend to perpetuate these TrPs, as does a Morton foot structure or other deviation that produces hyperpronation or an unstable foot. **PATIENT EXAMINATION** includes evaluation of gait, foot configuration, toe extension range, toe flexor strength, and footgear. **TRIGGER POINT EXAMINATION** of the *flexor digitorum longus* requires the clinician to exert pressure on the muscle between the back of the tibia and the medial edge of the gastrocnemius muscle. The examiner locates *flexor hallucis longus* TrP tenderness by compressing the muscle against the fibula with pressure through the overlying gastrocnemius aponeurosis and the soleus muscle. **INTERMITTENT COLD WITH STRETCH** of these long flexor muscles of the toes requires application of vapocoolant spray or ice stroking over the muscles, the sole of the foot, and the plantar surface of the toes. Simultaneously, the foot is passively dorsiflexed and everted and the distal phalanges of all toes are extended. The procedure is completed with application of moist heat and slow active range of motion. The patient is taught a passive self-stretch home program. **INJECTION** of flexor digitorum longus TrPs requires consideration of the location of the posterior tibial vessels and nerve, and also of the anterior tibial vessels and deep peroneal nerve on the other side of the interosseus membrane. Injection of the flexor hallucis longus is more difficult and requires consideration of the peroneal vessels. **CORRECTIVE ACTIONS** include replacement of badly worn shoes, installation of first metatarsal pads or arch supports, if indicated, and limitation of running or jogging (at first only on smooth level surfaces). The patient should perform a self-stretch exercise program regularly at home and progress to strengthening exercises for these muscles.

1. REFERRED PAIN
(Fig. 25.1)

Trigger points (TrPs) in the **flexor digitorum longus** muscle refer pain and tenderness primarily to the middle of the plantar forefoot proximal to the four lesser toes and sometimes with spillover pain to these toes (Fig. 25.1*A*). Only occasionally do these TrPs refer pain to the medial side of the ankle and calf, and they do not refer pain to the heel. Thus, when patients complain that the sole of the forefoot is painful and tender, few clinicians think to examine the calf for the source of the pain.

Myofascial TrPs in the **flexor hallucis longus** muscle refer pain strongly to the plantar surface of the great toe and head of the first metatarsal (Fig. 25.1*B*). The pain may occasionally radiate proximally for a short distance on the plantar surface, but does not extend to the heel or leg.

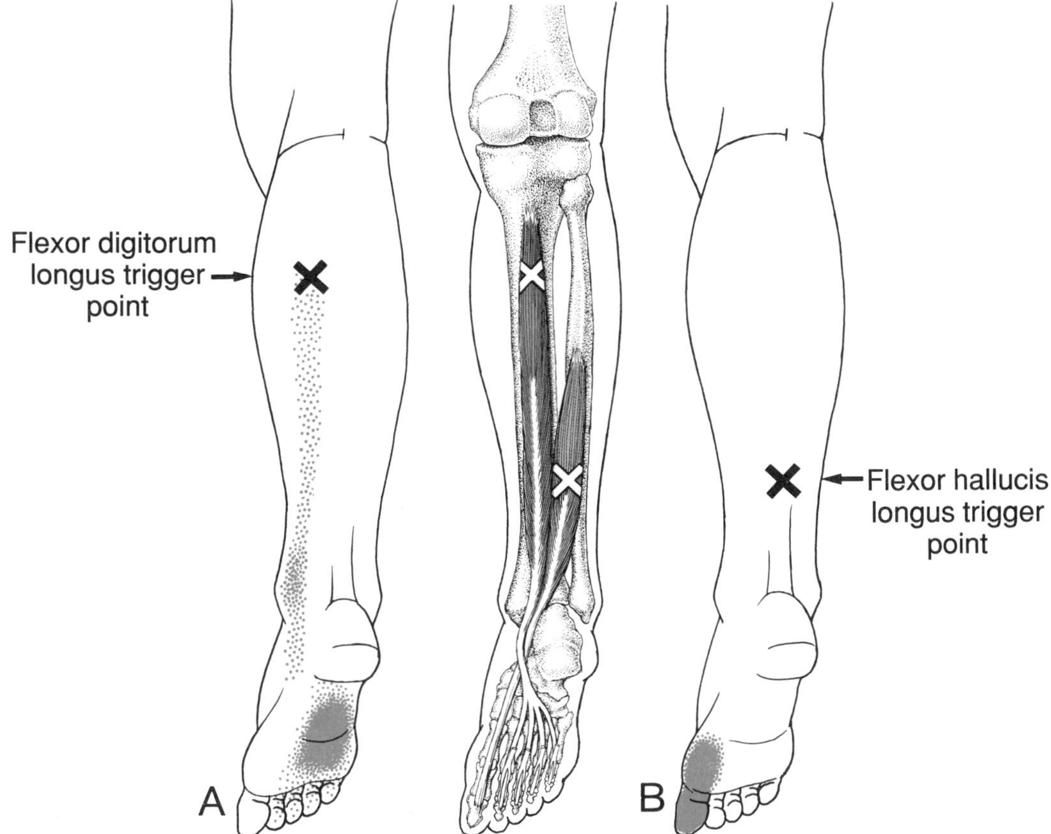

Figure 25.1. Pain patterns (*bright red*) referred from trigger points (**X***s*) in the long flexors of the toes (right side, posterior view). The essential pain pattern (*solid red*) shows the pain distribution characteristically referred by these trigger points. *Red stippling* illustrates the occasional extension of the essential pain pattern. *A*, for flexor digitorum longus muscle (*dark red*). *B*, for flexor hallucis longus muscle (*light red*).

2. ANATOMICAL ATTACHMENTS AND CONSIDERATIONS
(Fig. 25.2)

The two long (extrinsic) flexor muscles of the toes share the deep posterior compartment of the leg with the tibialis posterior and the popliteus muscles.[41]

The **flexor digitorum longus** muscle lies on the back of the tibia deep to the soleus and gastrocnemius and medial to the tibialis posterior. ***Proximally*** it attaches to the posterior surface of the middle two-quarters of the tibia,[43] beginning distal to the soleus attachment (Fig. 25.2) and including the intermuscular septum that is shared with the tibialis posterior muscle. The fibers of this pennate muscle converge on the tendon that passes behind the medial malleolus in a groove shared with the tendon of the tibialis posterior muscle, but in a separate compartment and in a separate synovial sheath. As its tendon approaches the navicular bone and passes into the sole of the foot, it crosses superficial to the flexor hallucis longus tendon from which it receives a strong tendinous slip. At approximately midsole, the quadratus plantae muscle joins the flexor digitorum longus tendon, which then divides into four tendons, each of which passes through an opening in the corresponding tendon of the flexor digitorum brevis. ***Distally*** each of the four tendons attaches to the base of the distal phalanx of its corresponding lesser toe.[12,16]

Variations are not uncommon. The flexor digitorum longus muscle may be more or less divided into separate fasciculi for the individual toes.[12] One of the more common anomalous muscles of the leg is the *flexor accessorius longus digitorum*, which spans from the fibula or tibia to the tendon of the flexor digitorum longus or to the quadratus plantae.[16,30,49,55]

The **flexor hallucis longus** muscle lies distal and lateral to the flexor digitorum longus (Fig. 25.2) and the tibialis posterior. It also lies deep to the soleus and gastrocnemius muscles. This pennate muscle attaches ***proximally*** to the inferior two-thirds of the body of the fibula, to the interosseous membrane, and to intermuscular septa shared with muscles on both sides of it. The fibers of this muscle continue to converge on its tendon as it crosses the posterior surface of the lower end of the tibia. The tendon then crosses the posterior surface of the talus and the inferior surface of the sustentaculum tali of the calcaneus—deep to the tendon of the flexor digitorum longus muscle. In the sole of the foot, the tendon of the flexor hallucis longus courses forward between the two heads of the flexor hallucis brevis muscle to attach ***distally*** to the base of the terminal phalanx of the great (first) toe.[16]

Occasionally, the *peroneocalcaneus internus* muscle runs from the posterior aspect of the fibula under the sustentaculum tali together with the flexor hallucis longus tendon and inserts on the calcaneus.[16,49] A sesamoid bone may develop in the tendon of the flexor hallucis longus where it passes over the talus and calcaneus.[12]

Supplemental References

Photographs present the flexor digitorum longus and the flexor hallucis longus from behind,[39,47] and drawings show the tendons at the ankle from behind,[6] and from a posteromedial view.[7] Views from behind portray both muscles in relation to the posterior tibial artery and nerve,[4,21,42] and in relation to only the posterior tibial artery.[40] Other posterior views include the peroneal artery,[21,40,42] the tibialis posterior muscle,[4,42] and the tendon crossover in the foot.[40,42] A schematic drawing in a posterior view of the leg and a plantar view of the foot portray the muscles, the tendon crossover, and tendinous attachments to the toes.[8]

A photograph from a medial and plantar view shows both the flexor digitorum longus and the flexor hallucis longus muscles.[48] Drawings present the tendons at the ankle from the medial view[5] and with tendon sheaths.[17,22] The plantar view reveals the course of the tendons in the foot and their attachments to the toes.[7,9,25,48]

The entire length of the flexor digitorum longus is presented in 14 cross sections,[15] and the flexor hallucis longus is presented in 13 cross sections.[14] Both muscles are presented in three cross sections through the proximal, middle, and distal thirds of the leg,[24] in a single cross section at the lower part of the middle third of the leg,[2] and in one cross section just above the middle of the leg.[41] The latter cross section portrays the relation of the deep posterior compartment to the other compartments of the leg.[41]

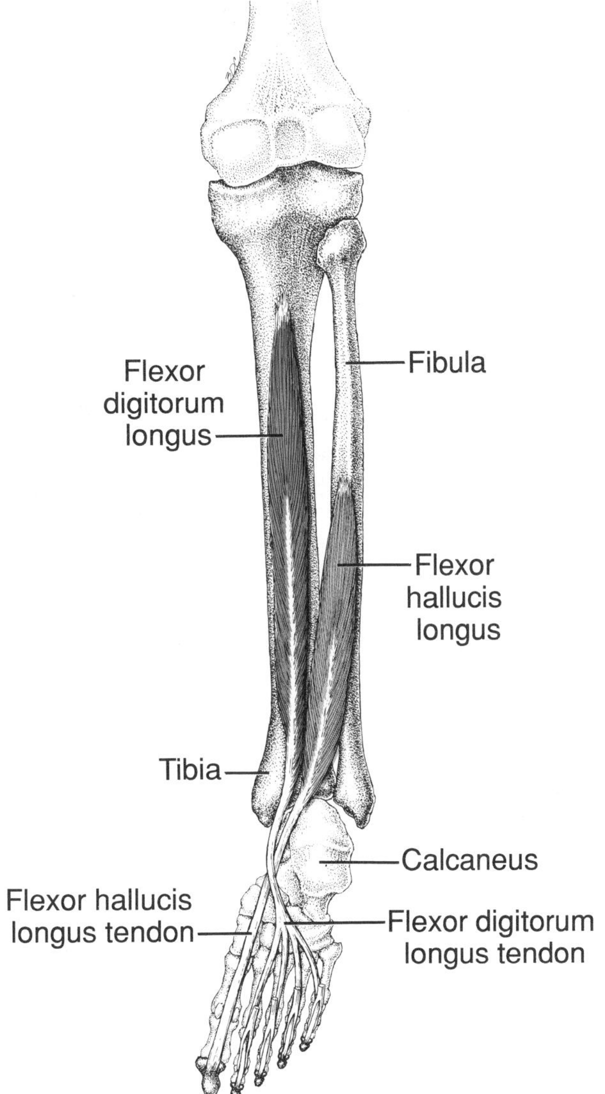

Figure 25.2. Attachments of the long flexors of the toes, right side, seen from behind. The flexor digitorum longus is *dark red*, and the flexor hallucis longus is *medium red*.

Posterior views locate the bony attachments of both long flexor muscles of the toes to the fibula and tibia.[3,23,37,43] Plantar views of the foot locate the tendinous attachments on the toes.[10,26,38,43]

3. INNERVATION

The flexor digitorum longus receives fibers from a branch of the tibial nerve that contains fibers from the L_5 and S_1 spinal nerves. The flexor hallucis longus is innervated by a branch of the tibial nerve that contains fibers from the L_5, S_1, and S_2 spinal nerves.[16]

4. FUNCTION

The flexor digitorum longus and the flexor hallucis longus muscles function during walking to stabilize the foot and ankle in midstance to late stance, playing a role in mediolateral balance. They assist other plantar flexors in enabling the individual to transfer weight to the forefoot, and they help in the maintenance of equilibrium when weight is on the forefoot.

The flexor digitorum longus flexes the distal phalanx of each of the four lesser toes; the flexor hallucis longus flexes the distal phalanx of the great toe. They both assist in plantar flexion and inversion of the foot when the foot is free to move.

Actions

The flexor digitorum longus and the flexor hallucis longus act primarily as flexors of the distal phalanges of their respective toes with important additional actions of assisting plantar flexion and inversion of the foot.[16,45]

Direct electrical stimulation of the flexor digitorum longus muscle with the limb free caused forceful flexion only of the distal phalanges of the four lesser toes; the middle and proximal phalanges could easily be extended. Stimulation of the flexor hallucis longus muscle similarly caused powerful flexion of the distal phalanx and relatively weak flexion of the proximal phalanx of the great toe.[19]

Functions

Standing

Without flexor hallucis longus function, it is difficult for the individual to maintain equilibrium when standing on the toes.[27]

Walking

Electromyographic studies showed that, during ambulation, the flexor hallucis longus[13,18,51] and flexor digitorum longus[18,51] muscles were active primarily when body weight was concentrated on that same limb, at the time when these muscles could position and stabilize the foot and ankle during midstance to late stance. The flexor hallucis longus muscle was slightly active in flatfooted subjects at heel-off but negligibly so in normal subjects. Flexor hallucis longus activity at that time in the flatfooted subjects could help prevent excessive dorsiflexion of the great toe.[13,29]

Perry and associates[44] found that, among seven normal subjects, the peak intensity of electrical activity of the long flexor muscles of the toes during fast gait, free gait, and slow gait approximated the activity elicited by a manual muscle testing effort of fair+, fair+, and fair, respectively, for most subjects.

Following tibial nerve block and loss of motor function in the plantar flexors (including the flexor digitorum longus and the flexor hallucis longus) subjects noted inability to transfer weight to the forward part of the foot, making it difficult to lean forward with the weight solely on one limb.[52]

Running and Sports Activities

The flexor digitorum longus is important in "drive" for sports. For instance, Kamon[32] found it to be vigorously active during the take-off and landing of an upward two-leg jump. Running in soft sand calls for powerful toe-curling action.[45]

5. FUNCTIONAL (MYOTATIC) UNIT

The agonists for these long flexors of the toes are the short flexors of the toes, the flexors digitorum and hallucis brevis. The antagonists of these flexors are the long (extrinsic) and short (intrinsic) extensors of the toes.

The prime ankle plantar flexors are the gastrocnemius and soleus muscles, which are assisted by these long flexors of the toes, the tibialis posterior, peroneus longus, and peroneus brevis. The prime muscles for inversion of the foot are the tibialis anterior and tibialis posterior, which these extrinsic toe flexors can also assist.

6. SYMPTOMS

Patients complain that their feet hurt when they walk. The pain occurs in the sole of the forefoot and on the plantar surfaces of the toes. These people have frequently obtained custom-made inserts (orthoses) to reduce stress on the foot. Most patients like the inserts and retain them even after the TrPs causing the pain have been inactivated.

The TrPs in these long extrinsic flexors of the toes may occasionally cause painful contraction of these muscles similar to the calf cramps of gastrocnemius TrPs. However, toe flexor "cramping" is more likely to be caused by TrPs of the *intrinsic* flexors of the toes.

Differential Diagnosis

The medial ankle pain sometimes referred by flexor digitorum longus TrPs can present symptoms easily mistaken for a tarsal tunnel syndrome if the clinician is not aware of this referred pain pattern and fails to examine the muscle for TrPs.

Other Myofascial Pain Syndromes

The referred pain patterns of the flexor digitorum longus (Fig. 25.1*A*) and tibialis posterior (*see* Fig. 23.1) both appear on the sole of the foot and plantar surface of the toes. However, TrP pain from the flexor digitorum longus concentrates on the sole, whereas pain referred from the tibialis posterior concentrates over the Achilles tendon and its pain distribution on the sole is only a spillover, not an essential, pattern. The pain patterns of the flexor digitorum longus and the abductor digiti minimi (*see* Fig. 26.3*A*) both appear on the lateral side of the sole, but that of the abductor digiti minimi is usually restricted to the region of the head of the fifth metatarsal and does not cause pain in the toes. The essential patterns of the flexor digitorum longus and the adductor hallucis (*see* Fig. 27.2*A*) are quite similar, but the adductor hallucis pattern does not include spillover patterns to the toes or leg. The pain syndromes of the flexor digitorum longus and the interossei (*see* Fig. 27.3) could be confusingly similar if several interosseous muscles were involved. An interosseous TrP refers pain primarily to the corresponding toe and in a longitudinal band at the base of the toe, especially on the plantar surface.

Pain referred from flexor digitorum brevis TrPs (*see* Fig. 26.3*B*) runs transversely across the sole of the foot in the region of the metatarsal heads. The pain from neither the flexor hallucis longus nor the flexor digitorum longus has this transverse orientation.

The essential pain patterns of both the flexor hallucis longus (Fig. 25.1*B*) and the flexor hallucis brevis (*see* Fig. 27.2*B*) involve the plantar surface of the great toe, but the pattern of the flexor hallucis brevis extends around the medial side of the foot and has a spillover pattern across the dorsal surface of the great toe.

These ambiguities should be resolved by palpating all suspected muscles for taut bands, TrP spot tenderness, and reproduction of the patient's pain complaint.

Toe Deformities

Hammer toes and clawtoes. Hammer toe and clawtoe deformities (described in Chapter 24 of this volume) may result from overactivity of the long flexor muscles of the toes by either of two mechanisms, flexor stabilization or flexor substitution.[31]

Flexor stabilization most commonly occurs when the long flexors of the toes attempt to stabilize the osseous structures of the foot in the presence of a flexible pes valgus deformity (flat foot). Pronation of the subtalar joint allows hypermobility and unlocking of the midtarsal joint, which, in turn, leads to hypermobility of the forefoot.[31] The long flexors of the toes then act earlier and longer than in normal gait.[29] Instead of stabilizing the forefoot, this abnormal activity usually overpowers the smaller intrinsic lumbrical and interosseous muscles, as well as the quadratus plantae. Loss of quadratus plantae function allows adducto varus deviation of the fifth toe and possibly of the fourth toe. Flexor stabilization is the most common etiology of hammer toes.[31]

Flexor substitution develops when the triceps surae muscles are weak and the deep posterior and lateral leg muscles try to substitute for this weakness. This substitution occurs in a high-arched and supinated foot in the *late stance* phase of gait when the flexors have gained mechanical advantage over the interossei; it usually produces total flexion (clawing) of all toes without adducto varus of the fourth and fifth toes. If triceps surae strength is inadequate for *heel lift*, this action readily leads to a hammer-toe syndrome. Flexor substitution is the least common of the three mechanisms (flexor stabilization, flexor substitution, and extensor substitution) that can produce clawtoes and hammer toes.[31] Extensor substitution is reviewed under Section 6 in Chapter 24.

Toe curling may result from spasticity following traumatic brain injury or any cerebrovascular accident. Simply releasing the flexor hallucis longus and flexor digitorum longus tendons provided satisfactory relief in only about one-fourth of 41 feet. Additional release of the flexor digitorum brevis often achieved a more functional result.[33]

Hallux valgus. Snijders and co-workers[50] used a force plate to study the biomechanical effects of an increased valgus angle of the great toe (hallux valgus) and of an increased varus angle of the first metatarsal bone (spread foot) during standing and push-off. They found that the greater the valgus angle of the great toe, the more the force exerted by the flexor hallucis longus tended to further increase the abnormal angle. This matched the observation that if a woman succeeded in reaching the age of 20 years with a valgus angle of 10° or less, she was unlikely to develop bunions later.[50] This finding strongly reinforces the importance of wearing, from early childhood through adulthood, footwear that exerts no pressure directed laterally on the great toe.

Shin Splints and Chronic Compartment Syndrome

Garth and Miller[28] examined 17 athletes who presented for treatment of incapacitating pain and soreness located posteromedially along the middle third of the tibia (over the attachment and belly of the flexor digitorum longus muscle). Symptoms were provoked and aggravated by repetitive weight bearing. Similar symptoms are referred to as *shin splints*,[28] *medial tibial stress syndrome*,[28] and *chronic compartment syndrome*.[54] Seventeen asymptomatic athletes served as controls. The symptomatic athletes consistently had a mild claw deformity of the second toe with abnormal displacement of its arc of motion toward extension of the metatarsophalangeal (MP) joint. Examiners found weakness of the lumbrical muscles.[28] It appears as if the relatively stronger flexor digitorum longus muscle became overloaded because of inadequate MP joint stabilization caused by the lumbrical weakness, which resulted in clawing of the lesser toes rather than in effective stabilization. Symptoms were relieved by a treatment regimen consisting of toe flexion exercises, reduced athletic activity, and metatarsal and arch pads to compensate for the weak lumbrical action. The athletes apparently were not examined for TrPs in the sore muscle to assess their contribution to the athletes' conditions.

Tendon Rupture

Spontaneous rupture of the flexor hallucis longus tendon can occur during overload without evidence of previous disease or injury.[46] Even though surgical repair does not always restore function of the great toe, the authors[46] concluded that, in cases of laceration or rupture, surgical repair seems justified.

7. ACTIVATION AND PERPETUATION OF TRIGGER POINTS

Activation

The TrPs in the flexor digitorum longus and flexor hallucis longus muscles can be activated, and are then perpetuated, by running or jogging on uneven ground or on laterally slanted surfaces. The problem is aggravated by the presence of a Morton (mediolateral rocking) foot structure (*see* Chapter 20, pages 381–383 for details.)

When the foot excessively pronates (due to a hypermobile midfoot, flexible pes valgus deformity, muscular imbalance, or some other cause), the flexor digitorum longus and flexor hallucis longus can become overloaded and develop TrPs. These muscles may also become overloaded in a high-arched supinated foot with triceps surae weakness.

In a study of 100 patients who had incurred a motor vehicle accident that activated TrPs in numerous muscles, the flexor hallucis longus was rarely involved.[11]

Perpetuation

Impaired mobility of the joints of the foot can perpetuate TrPs in these muscles.

A common error among joggers and runners is to continue to use a shoe after it has developed excessive wear on the sole and heel. Loss of cushioning and flexibility produces excessive strain on the joints and muscles, including the long flexors of the toes. Walking and running on soft sand, especially barefoot, heavily loads the flexor digitorum longus; this activity can perpetuate, or activate, TrPs in this muscle.

An inflexible shoe sole prevents normal extension of the MP joints during walking and running. This stiffness of the sole effectively lengthens the lever arm against which these two long flexor muscles of the toes function, and thus overloads them.

8. PATIENT EXAMINATION

While the patient is walking, the examiner should look for a hyperpronating ankle or foot. One should also examine the feet for a long second, short first metatarsal (Morton foot structure). The patient's shoe may show a wear pattern characteristic of this foot structure (*see* Chapter 20, page 383), or evidence of excessive wear. Indications of excessive wear include: asymmetry between the two shoes, cracks between the midsole and edge of the shoe, a definite lean of the shoe either inward or outward when set on a level surface, loss of the sole pattern in sports

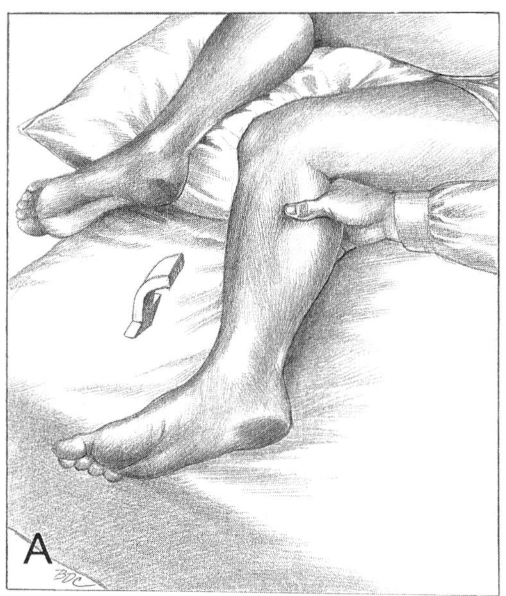

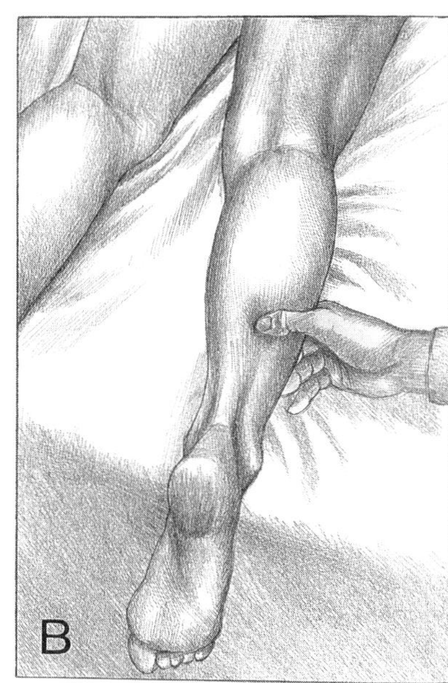

Figure 25.3. Palpation of trigger points in the long flexors of the toes on the right. *A*, flexor digitorum longus, patient in side-lying position. *Large arrow* shows the direction of pressure. This muscle is located between the posterior face of the tibia and the soleus/gastrocnemius muscles. With the knee bent and the foot plantar flexed, the gastrocnemius muscle can be pushed posteriorly away from the tibia to expose the flexor digitorum longus more fully. Pressure is first directed anteriorly to encounter the back of the tibia solidly and then laterally between the tibia and gastrocnemius to exert pressure on the flexor digitorum longus. *B*, palpation of trigger point tenderness in the flexor hallucis longus in an anterior direction through the soleus muscle and through the aponeurosis between the soleus and gastrocnemius, patient in prone position.

shoes, and a flattened or expanded heel pattern of the shoe.

The patient's feet should be examined for muscular imbalances, for restriction of motion (including joint play), and for hypermobility, as well as for the presence of deviations, such as ankle equinus, flat foot, or a high-arched rigid foot.

The clinician examines the foot for toe configuration and tenderness. The examination includes the distal phalanges of all toes for flexion weakness, as described by Kendall and McCreary.[34] Weakness of the flexor digitorum longus and the flexor hallucis longus affects flexion of the distal phalanx of the corresponding toes, and weakness of the flexor digitorum brevis affects flexion of the middle phalanx in the four lesser toes. In addition, the involved muscle often exhibits a ratchety or breakaway weakness when the examiner tests its strength during a lengthening contraction. Maximum flexion effort of the great toe or four lesser toes with the foot in the plantar-flexed position is likely to be particularly painful in the presence of TrPs in the corresponding flexor muscle. Passive extension range of motion of the great toe is restricted in the presence of flexor hallucis longus involvement,[36] and passive extension of the four lesser toes is restricted when the flexor digitorum longus harbors TrPs.

9. TRIGGER POINT EXAMINATION (Fig. 25.3)

For palpation of TrPs in the **flexor digitorum longus** muscle, the patient lies on the involved side and the clinician uses flat palpation (Fig. 25.3*A*) to exert pressure between the tibia and the soleus/gastrocnemius muscles on the medial side of the leg (*see* Fig. 19.3, cross section). With the knee bent to 90° and the foot plantar flexed, the gastrocnemius muscle can be pressed posteriorly away from the tibia to expose the flexor digitorum longus to more effective palpation. The clinician first exerts pressure toward the back of the tibia and then laterally against the flexor digitorum longus. It is difficult to elicit local twitch responses from this deep muscle, but spot tenderness is readily identified by the patient's reaction, and the expected pattern of referred pain may be evoked.

For examination of TrPs in the **flexor hallucis longus** muscle, the patient lies prone and the clinician uses flat palpation, applying deep pressure at the junction of the middle and lower thirds of the calf, just lateral to the mid-line, against the posterior face of the fibula (Fig. 25.3*B*). The pressure of palpation must be projected through the soleus muscle, as well as through the thick aponeurosis that becomes the Achilles tendon. Tenderness can be attributed to the flexor hallucis longus only if the examiner is sure the overlying muscles are free of tender TrPs.

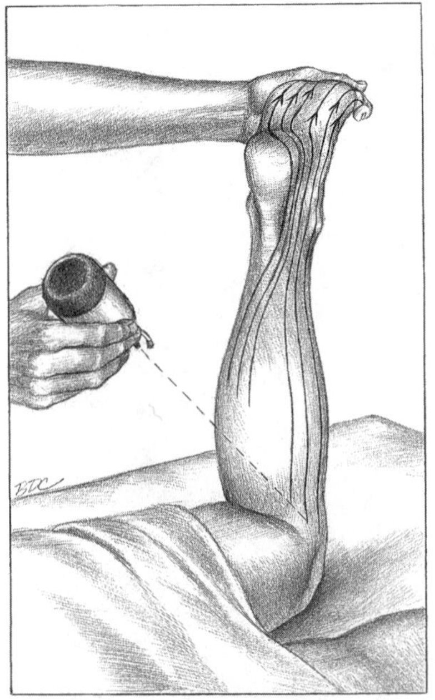

Figure 25.4. Intermittent cold with stretch of the right flexor digitorum longus and flexor hallucis longus, patient prone and knee flexed to 90°. Parallel sweeps of the vapocoolant or ice follow the direction of the *arrows*. All five toes are extended together with dorsiflexion of the ankle. As a final stretch, the foot is also everted. If the tarsometatarsal joints are hypermobile, intermittent cold is applied first, and then one hand is used to stabilize these intermediate joints while the other extends the toes. This stretch can be effectively augmented with postisometric relaxation.

10. ENTRAPMENTS

No nerve entrapment has been identified as due to TrPs in the flexor digitorum longus or the flexor hallucis longus. However, the anomalous flexor digitorum accessorius longus can cause a tarsal tunnel syndrome.[49]

11. ASSOCIATED TRIGGER POINTS

The associated muscles most likely to harbor active TrPs, when one finds them in the long flexors of the toes, are: the *tibialis posterior*, also a primary invertor and accessory plantar flexor of the foot, and the *long and short extensors of the toes*, antagonists to the toe-flexion function of the flexor digitorum longus and flexor hallucis longus.

The *short (intrinsic) flexors of the toes* may also develop TrPs as part of the functional unit.

12. INTERMITTENT COLD WITH STRETCH
(Fig. 25.4)

To inactivate TrPs in the **flexor hallucis longus** and **flexor digitorum longus** muscles, simultaneous intermittent cold with stretch of both muscles (Fig. 25.4) can be combined with postisometric relaxation as described by Lewit and Simons.[35] The patient lies prone with the knee flexed to 90° as the clinician passively dorsiflexes and everts the foot and extends the distal phalanges of all five toes, only as far as the onset of resistance. The patient breathes in deeply and, at the same time, gently attempts to flex the toes against the resistance provided by the clinician's hand. Then, the patient slowly exhales and concentrates on relaxing while the clinician applies the ice or vapocoolant spray in parallel sweeps distally over both sides of the calf, the sole of the foot, and the plantar surface of all toes. The clinician then gently presses the foot toward dorsiflexion and eversion, and the toes into extension, to take up any slack that develops in the muscles, without causing pain. This sequence is repeated until no further range of motion is gained.

The use of ice for applying intermittent cold with stretch is explained on page 9

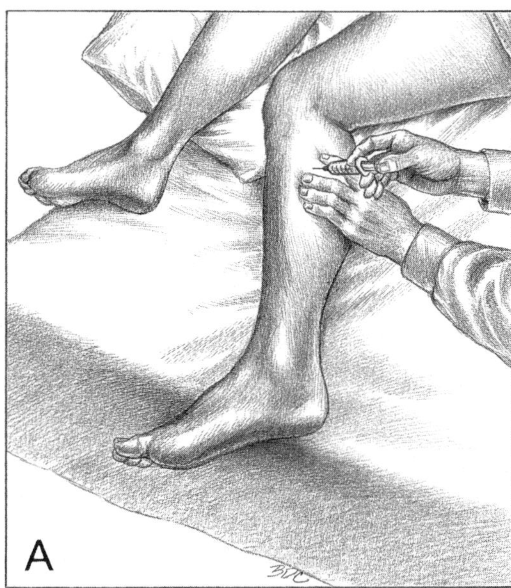

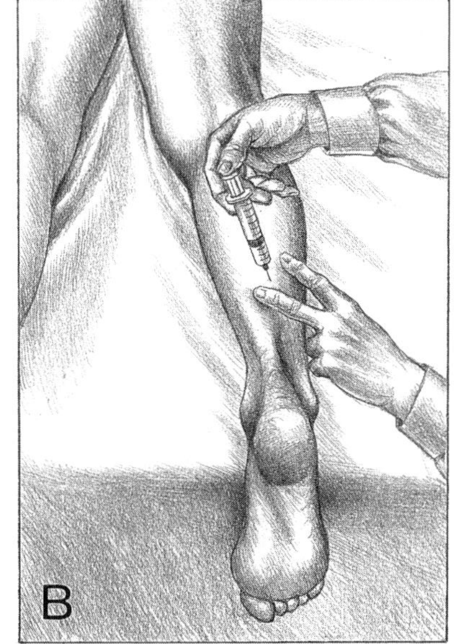

Figure 25.5. Injection of trigger points in the long flexors of the toes, right side. *A*, in the flexor digitorum longus muscle. The trigger point is spanned and fixed by the fingers of the operator's left hand. The needle is angled anteriorly toward the back of the tibia. *B*, in the flexor hallucis longus muscle. The needle is angled laterally toward the back of the fibula. *See* Figure 19.3 for a cross-sectional view of this region.

of this volume and the use of vapocoolant spray and stretch is detailed on pages 67–74 of Volume 1.[53] Techniques that augment relaxation and stretch are reviewed on pages 10–11 of this volume.

In the presence of hypermobility in the tarsometatarsal region, a two-handed stretch approach is needed so that this midfoot region can be stabilized. In such cases, the application of intermittent cold in parallel sweeps can *precede* the stretch rather than being applied simultaneously with it.

Following application of vapocoolant spray or ice stroking with stretch, the clinician applies moist heat over the treated muscles to rewarm the cooled skin while the patient relaxes. After several minutes of heat application, the patient performs slow *active* range of motion from full plantar flexion to full dorsiflexion of the ankle with full flexion and extension of the toes for several cycles, to take advantage of reciprocal inhibition and to normalize sarcomere length and restore full functional range of motion.

To maintain the gains achieved, the patient then learns and practices how to self-stretch the affected muscles passively as a home exercise. This exercise is described in Section 14 of this chapter.

Evjenth and Hamberg[20] describe and illustrate a stretch technique for each of the long flexor muscles of the toes, but it is not convenient to use with ice or vapocoolant spray, since the stretch requires two hands. However, the advantage of their method is that it includes stabilization of the tarsometatarsal region. The Lewit technique, described previously in this chapter and in Chapter 2 of this volume, is sometimes remarkably effective by itself without cooling. The combination is usually very effective.

13. INJECTION AND STRETCH
(Fig. 25.5)

The flexor digitorum longus frequently harbors multiple TrPs (like the long finger flexors) and these may separately involve individual digitations for the toes. Therefore, one can easily overlook some TrPs in this muscle. Injection requires precise localization of the TrPs and full knowledge of relevant anatomy. The cross-sectional view in Figure 19.3 shows clearly how the flexor digitorum longus lies between the tibia in front and the tibial nerve with the posterior tibial vessels behind. The anterior tibial vessels and the deep peroneal nerve also travel deep to the flexor digitorum longus and are shielded by the interosseous membrane and in some parts of the leg by the tibialis posterior muscle.

For injection of TrPs in the **flexor digitorum longus** muscle, the patient lies on the involved side (as for palpation) and the clinician carefully localizes the spots of TrP tenderness between the examining fingers (Fig. 25.5*A*). By angling the needle toward the posterior surface of the tibia through the medial edge of the soleus muscle, the clinician minimizes the danger of penetrating the tibial nerve and posterior tibial vessels. Because of this oblique approach, a needle as long as 63 mm (2½ in) may be needed. Needle penetration of a TrP is confirmed by a pain response (jump sign) of the patient. With probing movements, the clinician infiltrates the cluster of TrPs with approximately 1 mL of 0.5% procaine in isotonic saline.

The TrPs in the **flexor hallucis longus** are even more difficult to inject precisely than those in the flexor digitorum longus, and alternative non-invasive methods of therapy should be tried before injecting this muscle. Figure 19.3 illustrates the intimate association between the peroneal blood vessels and the medial portion of this muscle. To inject TrPs in the flexor hallucis longus muscle, the patient lies prone (Fig. 25.5*B*) and the clinician localizes the TrP tenderness as closely as possible by deep palpation through the gastrocnemius and soleus muscles. A needle 63 mm (2½ in) long may sometimes be required. When injecting, it is advisable to angle the needle somewhat laterally away from the peroneal vessels toward the posterior surface of the fibula. It may be necessary to contact the fibula gently to confirm the location of the needle and to ensure sufficient depth of penetration to reach the TrPs in this muscle. The clinician infiltrates each TrP with 1 mL or less of 0.5% procaine in isotonic saline.

Promptly following injection, moist heat is applied over the calf for several minutes to minimize postinjection soreness. The patient then actively contracts and stretches the muscle slowly through its fully shortened and fully lengthened positions for several cycles.

Before leaving the clinic, the patient learns and practices as a home program the passive self-stretch exercise described in the next section.

14. CORRECTIVE ACTIONS

Corrective first metatarsal pads are added to the shoe if the patient has a Morton (mediolateral rocking) foot structure (*see* Chapter 20, Peroneus Longus, pages 389–392). Arch supports may also be needed for an excessively pronated foot or for a hypermobile foot.

If hypomobility of the foot is a factor, normal joint play and motion should be restored.

Corrective Posture and Activities

The patient should wear comfortable shoes that have adequate shock absorption (a rubber sole or a foam insert inside the shoe) and adequate flexibility of the distal sole. New shoes should be tested at the time of purchase to ensure adequate space in the vamp for the addition of an insert without cramping the toes. One should replace worn-out shoes and those with poor flexibility of the distal sole. An extremely stiff sole that prevents extension of the metatarsophalangeal joint of the great toe should be avoided. The patient's heel should fit snugly inside the shoe to provide mediolateral stability; if needed, lateral pads should be added inside until the heel of the shoe fits well. High heels and spike heels should be avoided completely.

If patients with active TrPs in the flexor digitorum longus or the flexor hallucis longus are runners or joggers, initial management concentrates on inactivating the TrPs, correcting anatomical and biomechanical imbalances, and improving the stamina of deconditioned muscles. If these measures are inadequate, the runners should be encouraged to substitute non-weight-bearing activities, such as rowing, swimming, or bicycling. Running should first resume on a flat, even surface, initially with limited distance that progresses by increments that are within tolerance. If the only running surface available is slanted from side-to-side, then equal time should be allotted to running on a medial and a lateral slant during one exercise session.[1]

Running on soft sand should be avoided until TrPs are inactivated and muscles are conditioned.

Home Therapeutic Program

For passive self-stretch, the patient is instructed to rest the heel on the floor or on a stool, then to grasp the toes with the ankle dorsiflexed, and gradually to extend the toes. If there is hypermobility in the tarsometatarsal region, the patient should use the other hand to stabilize this region. Alternating periods of actively flexing the toes against resistance, relaxing, and picking up the slack (Lewit technique) facilitate full stretch. Figure 16.13*B* in the Hamstring chapter illustrates self-stretch of the long flexor muscles of the toes in combination with hamstring stretch. The Lewit technique is described in detail in Chapter 2 of this volume.

The patient will benefit by walking in a swimming pool, taking long strides, with the body submerged to approximately waist level. This requires use of these stabilizer muscles in a slowed time frame and does not overstress them because of the buoyant effect of the water. A mild exercise for toe flexor strengthening is that of picking up objects (marbles or Kleenex) with the toes. One should follow this exercise with lengthening of the muscles. More vigorous strengthening is obtained by having the patient walk slowly with a long stride on dry sand, if the soleus and other plantar flexor muscles can tolerate this stress.

References

1. Anderson A: Personal communication, 1991.
2. Anderson JE: *Grant's Atlas of Anatomy*, Ed. 8. Williams & Wilkins, Baltimore, 1983 (Fig. 4–72).
3. *Ibid.* (Fig. 4–81).
4. *Ibid.* (Figs. 4–84, 4–86).
5. *Ibid.* (Fig. 4–87).
6. *Ibid.* (Fig. 4–89).
7. *Ibid.* (Fig. 4–95).
8. *Ibid.* (Fig. 4–99B).
9. *Ibid.* (Fig. 4–102).
10. *Ibid.* (Fig. 4–107).
11. Baker BA: The muscle trigger: evidence of overload injury. *J Neurol Orthop Med Surg 7*:35–44, 1986.
12. Bardeen CR: The musculature, Sect. 5. In *Morris's Human Anatomy*, edited by C.M. Jackson, Ed. 6. Blakiston's Son & Co., Philadelphia, 1921 (pp. 521–523).
13. Basmajian JV, Deluca CJ: *Muscles Alive*, Ed. 5. Williams & Wilkins, Baltimore, 1985 (p. 378).
14. Carter BL, Morehead J, Wolpert SM, et al.: *Cross-Sectional Anatomy*. Appleton-Century-Crofts, New York, 1977 (Sects. 74–86).
15. *Ibid.* (Sects. 74–87).
16. Clemente CD: *Gray's Anatomy of the Human Body*, American Ed. 30. Lea & Febiger, Philadelphia, 1985 (pp. 578–579).
17. *Ibid.* (p. 583, Fig. 6–81).
18. Close JR: *Motor Function in the Lower Extremity*. Charles C Thomas, Springfield, 1964 (Fig. 65, p. 78).
19. Duchenne GB: *Physiology of Motion*, translated by E.B. Kaplan. J.B. Lippincott, Philadelphia, 1949 (pp. 372–374).
20. Evjenth O, Hamberg J: *Muscle Stretching in Manual Therapy, A Clinical Manual*. Alfta Rehab Førlag, Alfta, Sweden, 1984 (pp. 154, 156).
21. Ferner H, Staubesand J: *Sobotta Atlas of Human Anatomy*, Ed. 10, Vol. 2. Urban & Schwarzenberg, Baltimore, 1983 (Figs. 461, 462).
22. *Ibid.* (Fig. 464).
23. *Ibid.* (Fig. 469).
24. *Ibid.* (Figs. 472–474).
25. *Ibid.* (Fig. 499).
26. *Ibid.* (Fig. 500).
27. Frenette JP, Jackson DW: Lacerations of the flexor hallucis longus in the young athlete. *J Bone Joint Surg [Am] 59*:673–676, 1977.
28. Garth WP Jr, Miller ST: Evaluation of claw toe deformity, weakness of the foot intrinsics, and posteromedial shin pain. *Am J Sports Med 17*: 821–827, 1989.
29. Gray EG, Basmajian JV: Electromyography and cinematography of leg and foot ("normal" and flat) during walking. *Anat Rec 161*:1–16, 1968.
30. Hollinshead WH: *Anatomy for Surgeons*, Ed. 3., Vol. 3, *The Back and Limbs*. Harper & Row, New York, 1982 (p. 783).
31. Jimenez L, McGlamry ED, Green DR: Lesser ray deformities, Chapter 3. In *Comprehensive Textbook of Foot Surgery*, edited by E. Dalton McGlamry, Vol. 1. Williams & Wilkins, Baltimore, 1987 (pp. 57–113, *see* pp. 66–68).
32. Kamon E: Electromyographic kinesiology of jumping. *Arch Phys Med Rehabil 52*:152–157, 1971.
33. Keenan MA, Gorsi AP, Smith CW, *et al.*: Intrinsic toe flexion deformity following correction of spastic equinovarus deformity in adults. *Foot Ankle 7*:333–337, 1987.
34. Kendall FP, McCreary EK: *Muscles, Testing and Function*, Ed. 3. Williams & Wilkins, Baltimore, 1983 (pp. 134, 135).
35. Lewit K, Simons DG: Myofascial pain: relief by post-isometric relaxation. *Arch Phys Med Rehabil 65*:452–456, 1984.
36. Macdonald AJR: Abnormally tender muscle regions and associated painful movements. *Pain 8*: 197–205, 1980.
37. McMinn RMH, Hutchings RT: *Color Atlas of Human Anatomy*. Year Book Medical Publishers, Chicago, 1977 (pp. 281, 285).
38. *Ibid.* (p. 289).
39. *Ibid.* (p. 315).

40. *Ibid.* (p. 316).
41. Netter FH: *The Ciba Collection of Medical Illustrations*, Vol. 8, Musculoskeletal System. Part I: Anatomy, Physiology and Metabolic Disorders. Ciba-Geigy Corporation, Summit, 1987 (p. 98).
42. *Ibid.* (p. 103).
43. *Ibid.* (p. 107).
44. Perry J, Ireland ML, Gronley J, *et al.*: Predictive value of manual muscle testing and gait analysis in normal ankles by dynamic electromyography. *Foot Ankle 6*:254–259, 1986.
45. Rasch PJ, Burke RK: *Kinesiology and Applied Anatomy*, Ed. 6. Lea & Febiger, Philadelphia, 1978 (pp. 320–321, 330, Table 17.2).
46. Rasmussen RB, Thyssen EP: Rupture of the flexor hallucis longus tendon: case report. *Foot Ankle 10*:288–289, 1990.
47. Rohen JW, Yokochi C: *Color Atlas of Anatomy*, Ed. 2. Igaku-Shoin, New York, 1988 (p. 424).
48. *Ibid.* (p. 425).
49. Sammarco GJ, Stephens MM: Tarsal tunnel syndrome caused by the flexor digitorum accessorius longus. *J Bone Joint Surg [Am] 72*:453–454, 1990.
50. Snijders CJ, Snijder JGN, Philippens MMGM: Biomechanics of hallux valgus and spread foot. *Foot Ankle 7*:26–39, 1986.
51. Sutherland DH: An electromyographic study of the plantar flexors of the ankle in normal walking on the level. *J Bone Joint Surg [Am] 48*:66–71, 1966.
52. Sutherland DH, Cooper L, Daniel D: The role of the ankle plantar flexors in normal walking. *J Bone Joint Surg [Am] 62*:354–363, 1980.
53. Travell JG, Simons DG: *Myofascial Pain and Dysfunction: The Trigger Point Manual.* Williams & Wilkins, Baltimore, 1983.
54. Wiley JP, Clement DB, Doyle DL, *et al.*: A primary care perspective of chronic compartment syndrome of the leg. *Phys Sportsmed 15*:111–120, 1987.
55. Wood J: On some varieties in human myology. *Proc R Soc Lond 13*:299–303, 1864.

CHAPTER 26
Superficial Intrinsic Foot Muscles

Extensor Digitorum Brevis, Extensor Hallucis Brevis, Abductor Hallucis, Flexor Digitorum Brevis, Abductor Digiti Minimi

"Sore Foot Muscles"

HIGHLIGHTS: **REFERRED PAIN** and tenderness from trigger points (TrPs) in either of the short extensor muscles of the toes, the extensor digitorum brevis or the extensor hallucis brevis, project locally over the dorsum of the foot. Pain and tenderness referred from TrPs in the abductor hallucis muscle center along the medial side of the heel with spillover to the instep and to the back of the heel. Pain and tenderness referred from TrPs in the abductor digiti minimi concentrate along the plantar aspect of the fifth metatarsal head and may spill over onto the sole nearby and onto the distal lateral side of the forefoot. Both pain and tenderness from the flexor digitorum brevis center over the heads of the second to fourth metatarsals. **ANATOMICAL ATTACHMENTS** of the three digitations of the extensor digitorum brevis are, proximally, to the calcaneus and, distally, to the lateral surfaces of the corresponding tendons of the extensor digitorum longus muscle and via the extensor apparatus to the intermediate and distal phalanges of the second, third, and fourth toes. The extensor hallucis brevis also anchors proximally to the calcaneus, and distally, directly to the dorsal surface of the proximal phalanx of the great toe. Proximal attachments of both the abductor hallucis and the abductor digiti minimi are to the tuberosity of the calcaneus. The distal attachment of the abductor hallucis is either to the medial side or to the plantar aspect of the proximal phalanx of the great toe; the distal attachment of the abductor digiti minimi is to the lateral side of the proximal phalanx of the fifth toe. The flexor digitorum brevis also attaches, proximally, to the tuberosity of the calcaneus and, distally, by separate tendons, to the middle phalanx of each of the four lesser toes. **FUNCTION:** The abductor hallucis and the flexor digitorum brevis are active from midstance through toe-off in walking. These and other intrinsic muscles stabilize the foot for single-limb balance and for propulsion. The extensor digitorum brevis, through its attachments to the tendons of the extensor digitorum longus, acts to extend the phalanges of the second, third, and fourth toes. The extensor hallucis brevis extends the proximal phalanx of the great toe. The abductor hallucis usually flexes and may abduct the proximal phalanx of the great toe. Tension of the abductor hallucis aggravates hallux valgus after it has developed. The flexor digitorum brevis flexes the second (middle) phalanges of the four lesser toes. The abductor digiti minimi abducts and assists flexion of the proximal phalanx of the fifth toe. **SYMPTOMS** of patients with TrPs in the short flexors of the toes include sore feet and pain on walking and, if the TrPs are severe, deep aching pain at rest. The differential diagnosis should include identification of similar referred pain patterns of other myofascial pain syndromes, plantar fasciitis, congenital muscular hypertrophy, and avulsion fracture at the muscular attachment. **PATIENT EXAMINATION** entails looking for an antalgic gait, painfully restricted stretch range of motion, and diffuse deep tenderness of the plantar aponeurosis. **ENTRAPMENT** of the posterior tibial nerve and/or its branches may be caused by the abductor hallucis muscle itself, by fascial bands associated with it, or by an accessory abductor hallucis. For **INTERMITTENT COLD WITH STRETCH** to inactivate TrPs in the two short extensors of the toes, the operator applies sweeps of ice or vapocoolant spray downward over the anterolateral leg and dorsum of the foot to the toes and simultaneously flexes all five toes. Application of parallel sweeps of intermittent cold over the medial side and plantar surface of the foot during passive extension of the great toe releases TrP tightness of the abductor hallucis muscle. Parallel sweeps of ice or vapocoolant spray over the sole of the foot from the heel to the toes with passive extension of the lesser toes releases tightness of the flexor digitorum brevis. The ankle may be held in the neutral position for all of these procedures, which are concluded with prompt application of moist heat and active full range of motion. **INJECTION AND STRETCH** of these superficial foot muscles should be preceded by hydrogen peroxide cleansing of the foot. Effective injection depends on precise localization of the taut band and its TrP by flat or pincer palpation and then on penetration of the TrP with the needle. Only the abductor hallucis is so thick as to require deep palpation to locate the tenderness of its TrPs close to the bone. The posterior tibial artery and nerve and their branches pass deep to the abductor hallucis muscle below the medial malleolus and must be considered. Intermittent cold with stretch followed by a moist hot pack and then full range of motion complete the TrP injection procedure. **CORRECTIVE ACTIONS** include encouraging the patient to buy shoes that fit and to use cushioned soles when standing or walking on hard surfaces. Learning to use the Toe Flexor Self-stretch Exercise in a home program is important for TrPs in the long or short flexors of the toes. Patients with TrPs in the superficial plantar muscles of the foot can benefit by using the Golf-ball Technique and the Rolling-pin Technique as an integral part of their home treatment program.

---

1. REFERRED PAIN
(Figs. 26.1–26.3)

The superficial intrinsic foot muscles refer pain and tenderness to the foot but not to the ankle or above it. When patients say they "sprained" an ankle and complain of foot but not ankle pain, one should look for trigger points (TrPs) in the intrinsic foot muscles as a cause of the pain. Krout[63] pointed out that the myofascial TrPs in foot muscles that refer pain and tenderness to weight-bearing areas on the sole of the foot are most troublesome to patients.

Short Extensors of Toes (Intrinsic Extensors)

The composite referred pain pattern of TrPs in the **extensor digitorum brevis and extensor hallucis brevis** muscles covers the mid-dorsum of the foot (Fig. 26.1).[101]

In children, TrPs are occasionally found in these short extensors of the toes. The referred pain pattern in children is similar to that seen in adults.[18] Kelly[55] observed that a myalgic lesion in the extensor digitorum brevis muscle produced cramps in the foot and later reported,[56] more specifically, that it referred pain to the instep.

Abductors of First and Fifth Toes

The pain and tenderness referred from TrPs in the **abductor hallucis** muscle (Fig. 26.2) center along the medial side of the heel with spillover to the instep and additional extension to the back of the heel medially. This contrasts with the pain and tenderness usually referred by soleus TrPs (*see* Fig. 22.1 on page 429), which covers all of the back and bottom of the heel.

Myofascial TrPs sometimes occur in the abductor hallucis muscle in children and were identified as the source of their heel pain.[18] In a study of painful feet caused by myalgic spots in muscles, Good[47] found the abductor hallucis to be responsible for heel pain in 10 of 100 cases. Kelly[54,55] reported that a myalgic lesion in the abductor hallucis muscle produced cramps in the foot.

The chief pain pattern referred from TrPs in the **abductor digiti minimi** concentrates along the plantar aspect of the fifth metatarsal head and may spill over

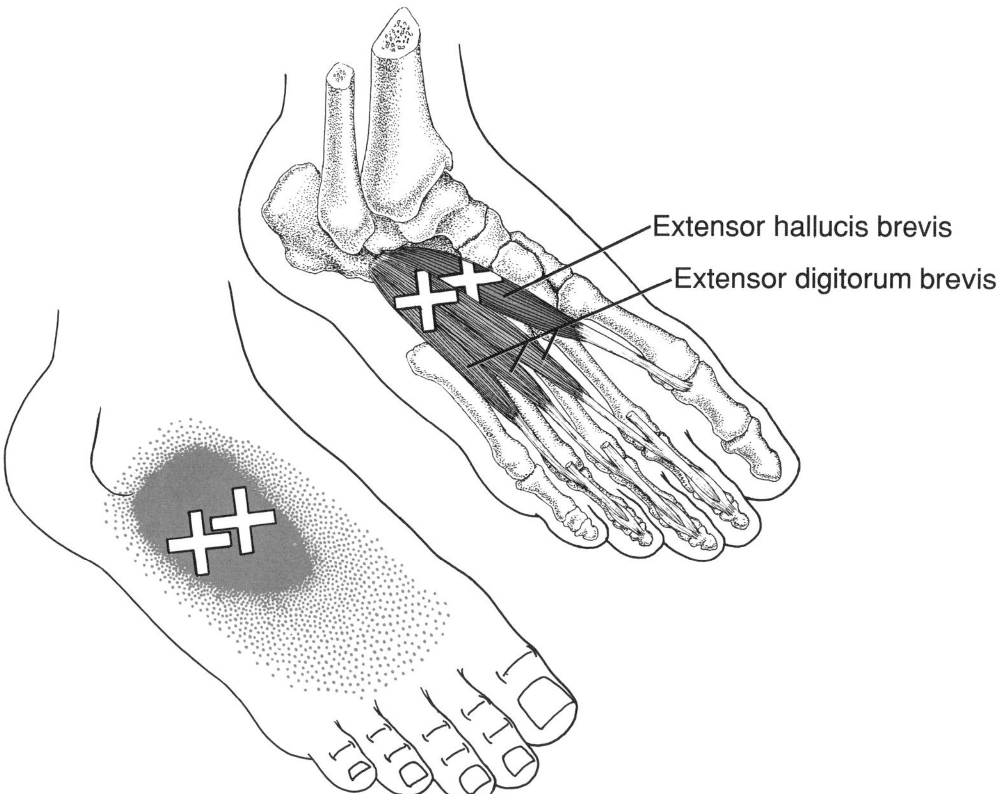

Figure 26.1. Pain and tenderness referral pattern (*bright red*) of trigger points (**X**s) in the extensor hallucis brevis (*darker red*) and in the extensor digitorum brevis (*light red*) muscles of the right foot. *Solid bright red* locates the essential pain pattern nearly always experienced when these trigger points are active. *Red stippling* indicates occasional extension of the essential referred pain pattern of these muscles.

onto the adjacent sole. The plantar spillover pattern may also include some of the distal lateral side of the forefoot (Fig. 26.3*A*).

Superficial Short Flexor of Toes

Pain and tenderness are projected from TrPs in the **flexor digitorum brevis** to the sole over the heads of the second to fourth metatarsal bones with occasional extension over the head of the fifth metatarsal (Fig. 26.3*B*). The referred pain does not extend back as far as the center of the sole, nor forward onto the toes. The bony portion of the plantar forefoot is "sore" and tender, leading to the complaint of "sore foot."

In his study of 100 patients complaining of painful feet caused by myalgic spots in foot muscles, Good[47] found the short flexors of the toes to be responsible for this complaint in more than half of the subjects. The flexor hallucis brevis (a deep intrinsic muscle) accounted for 40, and the flexor digitorum brevis for 12, of the 100 cases.

2. ANATOMICAL ATTACHMENTS AND CONSIDERATIONS
(Fig. 26.4)

The reader is referred to Figure 18.2 in this volume for a drawing of the bones of the foot. Review of this figure and of the ligamentous and other soft tissue structures of the foot should facilitate an understanding of the relationship between structure and function.

Short Extensors of Toes

The **extensor digitorum brevis and the extensor hallucis brevis** lie on the dorsum of the foot deep to the tendons of the extensor digitorum longus.[87] They attach ***proximally*** to the superior surface of the

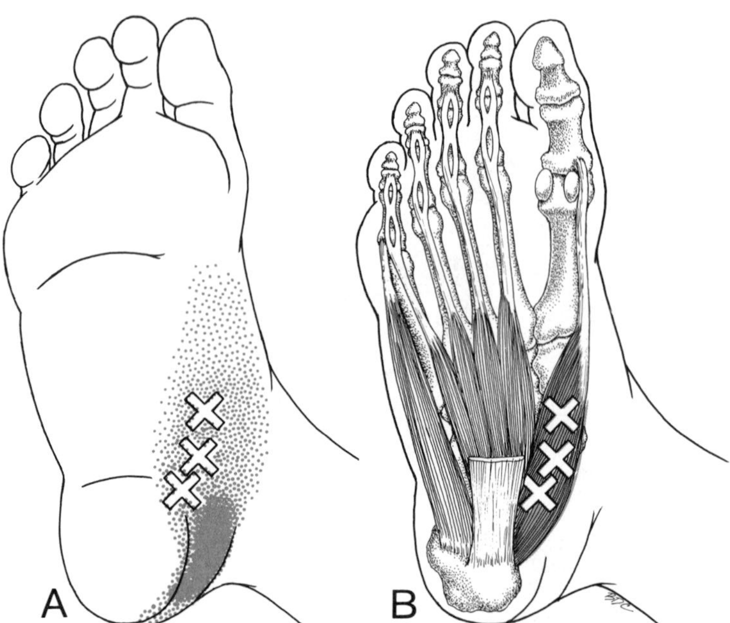

Figure 26.2. Pattern of pain and tenderness (*bright red*) referred from trigger points (***X**s*) in the abductor hallucis muscle (*darker red*) of the right foot. *A*, the essential referred pain pattern to the medial side of the heel is *solid red* and the spillover pattern to the instep is *stippled* red. *B*, attachments of the abductor hallucis.

calcaneus (Fig. 26.4*A*) distal to the groove for the peroneus brevis tendon and they attach also to adjacent ligamentous structures. Together, these muscles form four bellies. The most medial, the extensor hallucis brevis, presents the most distinct belly. The medial tendon anchors ***distally*** to the dorsal surface of the proximal phalanx of the great toe and often unites with the tendon of the extensor hallucis longus. The remaining three tendons unite with the lateral surfaces of the extensor digitorum longus tendons to form the extensor apparatus of the second, third, and fourth toes, but rarely of the fifth toe (Fig. 26.4*A*).[12,27] This extensor apparatus anchors to the intermediate and distal phalanges. Not all sources mention an attachment of the extensor apparatus to the ***proximal*** phalanges of the lesser toes;[27] however, some authors[12,32] describe specific fibrous attachments (from the margins of the long extensor tendons) to the dorsum of the proximal phalanges.

PART 3

An additional slip of the extensor digitorum brevis muscle occasionally attaches to a metatarsophalangeal articulation, to the fifth toe, or to a dorsal interosseous muscle.[27] One or more tendons may be absent, and rarely the whole extensor digitorum brevis muscle is missing.[12] Examination of the extensor digitorum brevis muscle of a stillborn infant for terminal motor innervation revealed a multipennate muscle with an oval endplate band around each central tendon.[25]

Abductors of First and Fifth Toes

The **abductor hallucis** muscle is subcutaneous along the posterior half of the medial border of the foot,[88] covering the entrance of the plantar vessels and nerves into the sole. It anchors ***proximally*** to the medial process of the tuberosity of the calcaneus (Fig. 26.4*B*), to the flexor retinaculum of the ankle, to the plantar aponeurosis, and to the intermuscular septum shared with the flexor digitorum brevis. Its tendon joins with that of the medial head of the flexor hallucis brevis and is usually said to attach ***distally*** to the medial side of the base of the proximal phalanx of the great toe (Fig. 26.4*B*).[27] However, a study of just this issue showed that in only one-fifth of 22 specimens was the attachment to the medial side of the first phalanx. In the others, the

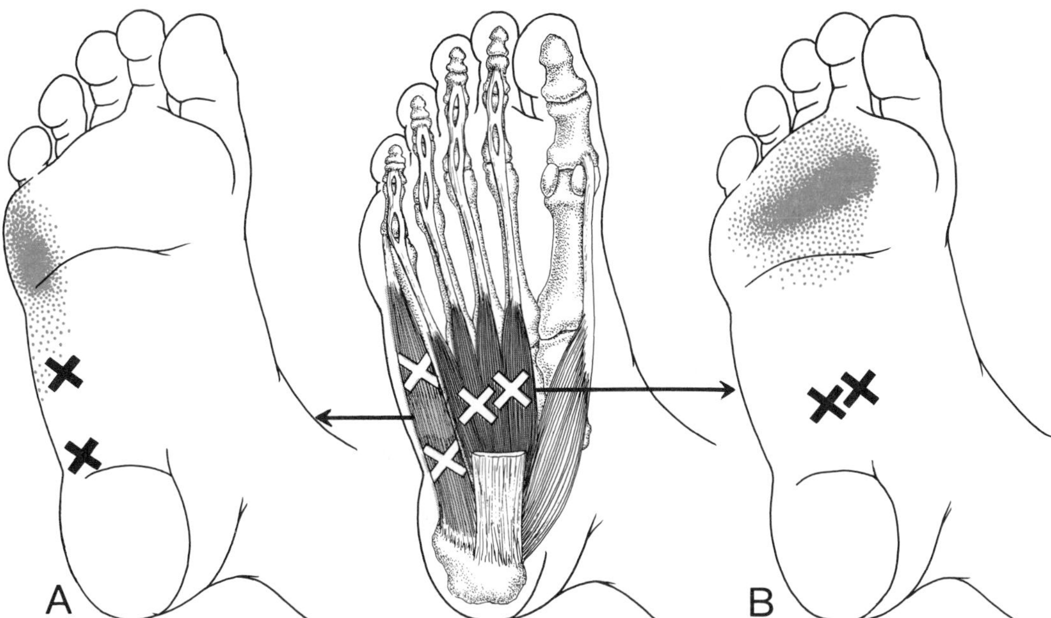

Figure 26.3. Patterns of referred pain and tenderness (*bright red*) and location of trigger points (**X**s) in two superficial intrinsic muscles of the right foot: *A*, abductor digiti minimi (*light red*). *B*, flexor digitorum brevis (*darker red*).

tendon attached directly or indirectly to its plantar surface.[17]

An accessory abductor hallucis may extend from the fascia superficial to the posterior tibial nerve above the medial malleolus to attach to the middle of the main abductor hallucis muscle.[19,50]

The **abductor digiti minimi** is subcutaneous along the length of the lateral border of the foot (Fig. 26.4*B*). It anchors ***proximally*** to the width of the tuberosity of the calcaneus[26] between the medial and lateral processes of that tuberosity, to the deep surface of the lateral plantar fascia, and to the fibrous band that extends from the calcaneus to the lateral side of the base of the fifth metatarsal.[12,27] ***Distally***, it joins the flexor digiti minimi brevis to attach to the lateral aspect of the base of the proximal phalanx of the fifth toe. Sometimes fibers of this abductor muscle attach to the base of the fifth metatarsal[44] in such large numbers that the proximal half of the muscle appears much bulkier than the distal half.

A patient with gross congenital hypertrophy of one abductor digiti minimi muscle obtained relief from pain by surgical excision of the muscle.[35] The authors[35] described the muscle as non-tender preoperatively.

Superficial Short Flexor of Toes

The **flexor digitorum brevis** muscle lies in the middle of the sole of the foot and is covered only by skin and the central part of the plantar aponeurosis (Fig. 26.4*B*). The flexor hallucis brevis muscle, more deeply situated, is a topic in the next chapter. The flexor digitorum brevis covers the lateral plantar vessels and nerves. It anchors ***proximally*** to the medial process of the tuberosity of the calcaneus, to the plantar aponeurosis, and to contiguous intermuscular septa. This muscle divides into four tendons, one to each of the lesser toes.[27] ***Distally***, each tendon splits at the base of the proximal phalanx to allow passage of the corresponding tendon of the flexor digitorum longus, then reunites, splits again, and attaches to both sides of the middle phalanx.[27]

The tendon of the flexor digitorum brevis of the fifth toe may be absent (38%), or replaced by a small muscle attached to the long flexor tendon

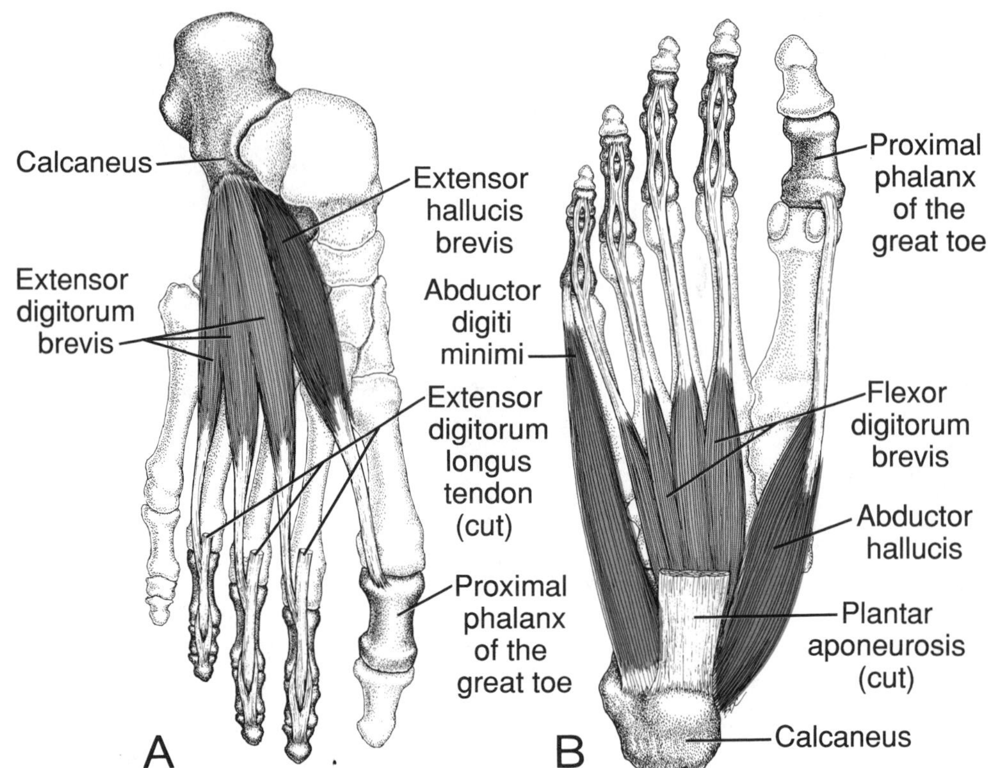

Figure 26.4. Dorsal and plantar views: superficial intrinsic muscles of the right foot and their skeletal attachments. *A*, dorsal muscles. The extensor hallucis brevis is *dark red* and the extensor digitorum brevis is *light red*. *B*, plantar muscles, most superficial layer. The abductor hallucis is *dark red*; the flexor digitorum brevis is *light red*; and the abductor digiti minimi is *medium red*.

(33%), or may be represented by a muscle coming from the quadratus plantae.[27]

Supplemental References

Plantar View. Drawings present the abductor digiti minimi and abductor hallucis muscles from the plantar view[8,28,39,43] and some include the flexor digitorum brevis muscle.[28,39] A photograph of a dissection also presents the plantar aspect of these three muscles.[93] Drawings portray, in plantar view, the three plantar muscles of this chapter (namely, the abductor digiti minimi, abductor hallucis, and flexor digitorum brevis) with the plantar digital nerves and arteries,[6] with the medial and lateral plantar nerves,[88] and with just the two toe abductors (but not the short flexor of the toes) and the medial and lateral plantar nerves.[7] A drawing shows the path of the posterior tibial artery, medial and lateral plantar arteries, and medial and lateral plantar nerves deep to the abductor hallucis muscle as they enter the sole.[42] A photograph of a dissection includes the abductor hallucis and abductor digiti minimi with nerves and arteries[79] and with nerves.[74]

Dorsal View. The extensor digitorum brevis and extensor hallucis brevis are seen from the dorsal view in drawings[2,38] and in pictures of dissections.[77,92] The extensor digitorum brevis appears in a drawing,[4] and the abductor digiti minimi and extensor digitorum brevis appear in a photograph of a dissection[76] from the dorsal view.

The two short extensors of the toes, drawn from the dorsal view, appear with the dorsalis pedis artery and with the medial branch of the peroneal nerve.[87] A photograph of a dissection shows the same structures.[73]

Lateral View. Drawings present the abductor digiti minimi and extensor digitorum brevis from the lateral[86] and dorsolateral[76] views. A photograph of a dissection shows the same muscles and the extensor hallucis brevis from the lateral view.[72]

Medial View. A photograph of a dissection shows the abductor hallucis from the medial view.[78] A drawing shows the nerves and vessels that pass deep to the abductor hallucis as they enter the sole of the foot.[5]

Cross Sections. The relation of the abductor hallucis and extensor digitorum brevis muscles to adjacent structures can be seen in a series of six serial cross sections of the foot,[21] the extensor hallucis brevis in five serial sections,[20] the abductor digiti minimi in four sections,[23] and the flexor digitorum brevis in three sections.[22] Photographs of all five muscles of this chapter appear in four cross sections through the foot.[83] Drawings of all five muscles appear in a cross section through the head of the talus,[40] and drawings of the abductor digiti minimi and abductor hallucis with tendons of the other three appear in a cross section through the metatarsal bones,[41] similar to Figure 27.9 in the next chapter of this volume.

Sagittal Sections. A photograph of a sagittal section through the medial part of the talus presents the abductor hallucis.[80] One through the second toe shows the flexor digitorum brevis.[81] One through the fifth toe includes the abductor digiti minimi and the extensor digitorum brevis muscles.[82]

Skeletal Attachments. The skeletal attachments of all five muscles of this chapter are marked on the bones of the foot as seen from the dorsal and plantar views.[10,11,70,75] The dorsal view shows the attachments of the abductor digiti minimi, abductor hallucis, extensor digitorum brevis, and the extensor hallucis brevis.[45] A medial view presents the attachments of the abductor hallucis.[9] A schematic drawing of the plantar view portrays attachments and the course of the abductor digiti minimi, abductor hallucis, and flexor digitorum brevis.[44]

Surface Contours. Photographs reveal the skin contours produced by the underlying extensor digitorum brevis muscle from a lateral view[3,66] and from the lateral and anteromedial views.[71] Photographs show the presence of the abductor digiti minimi and abductor hallucis muscles from the plantar view,[37] and the extensor digitorum brevis from the lateral view.[66]

3. INNERVATION

The extensor digitorum brevis and the extensor hallucis brevis receive their innervation via branches of the deep peroneal nerve by fibers from the fifth lumbar and first sacral spinal nerves. The abductor hallucis and the flexor digitorum brevis are innervated via branches of the medial plantar nerve by fibers also from the fifth lumbar and first sacral spinal nerves.[27] The laterally placed abductor digiti minimi is supplied through the first branch of the lateral plantar nerve[94] by fibers from the second and third sacral spinal nerves.[27]

4. FUNCTION

During ambulation, muscles of the foot function to permit flexibility for shock absorption and balance, and to provide rigidity and stability for propulsion.

In general, the intrinsic muscles of the foot function as a unit. The electromyographic (EMG) activity of these muscles closely parallels the progressive supination at the subtalar joint during level, uphill, and downhill walking. These muscles stabilize the foot at the subtalar and transverse tarsal joints during propulsion.[68]

The abductor hallucis and flexor digitorum brevis muscles are generally more active and may contribute to static arch support in *flatfooted* persons; however, intrinsic foot muscle activity is not required for static support of the arches in the normal foot.[49] These muscles are recruited during the walking cycle to compensate for lax ligaments and special stresses.[49]

The abductor hallucis acts as a flexor and abductor of the proximal phalanx of the great toe. The flexor digitorum brevis flexes the middle phalanx of each of the four lesser toes. The abductor digiti minimi abducts and assists flexion of the proximal phalanx of the fifth toe. The extensor digitorum brevis extends the second, third, and fourth toes. The extensor hallucis brevis extends the proximal phalanx of the great toe.

Actions

The **extensor digitorum brevis**, through its attachments to the tendons of the extensor digitorum longus, extends all three phalanges of the second, third, and fourth toes. The **extensor hallucis brevis** extends only the proximal phalanx of the great toe.[27]

The **abductor hallucis** may flex and/or abduct the proximal phalanx of the great toe.[27,51] In only one-fifth of 22 specimens was the attachment of the abductor hallucis found to be in a position for abduction of the great toe; in the others, it acted primarily as a flexor.[17] Electrical stimulation of this muscle produced primarily flexion and some abduction of the proximal phalanx with compensatory extension of the distal phalanx of the great toe.[31]

The **flexor digitorum brevis** flexes the second (middle) phalanx of the four lesser toes.[27] Electrical stimulation of this muscle confirmed that it forcefully flexes only the second phalanx and that simultaneous stimulation of the extensor digitorum longus produced extension of the proximal phalanges with strong clawing of the toes.[31]

The **abductor digiti minimi** abducts and assists flexion of the proximal phalanx of the fifth toe.[27] Electrical stimulation produced lateral deviation with some flexion of this toe.[31]

Functions

Electromyographic activity was generally negligible in the abductor hallucis, flexor digitorum brevis, and the abductor digiti minimi in 14 normal subjects while standing, but activity was marked when the subjects rose on tiptoes.[14] Marked activity in the abductor hallucis of a few subjects was associated with an unnecessary habit of "digging in" with the great toe. The activity was immediately abolished when the subject straightened the toe.[14] In five other normal subjects, the additional stress of standing on only one foot failed to activate the abductor hallucis muscle.[33]

Neither the abductor hallucis nor the flexor digitorum brevis contributes to static support of the arch of the normal foot, even under a load of 180 kg (400 lbs).[13] In another study, all six subjects with *flat feet* evidenced EMG activity of the abductor hallucis that showed a marked increase unilaterally when they stood on that foot and ceased when they stood on the other foot.[33]

In the normal walking subject, the abductor hallucis and flexor digitorum brevis muscles become active at midstance and continue activity to toe-off in normal subjects. In subjects with flat feet, EMG activity of these muscles is more intense and usually appears from heel-strike to toe-off.[16]

Basmajian[15] conducted an EMG study of 10 subjects with hallux valgus and found that there was no EMG activity of the abductor hallucis during abduction effort. He explained in detail how the lateral deviation of the first phalanx caused increased leverage of the abductor hallucis for further lateral deviation when activated as a flexor. Duranti and associates[33] found that the abductor hallucis in patients with hallux valgus was more active during weight bearing than in normal subjects, but this might only aggravate the problem considering its displaced line of pull. Those individuals in whom the abductor hallucis functions only as a flexor, and in whom it is not attached in a position to produce abduction, are more vulnerable to the effects of valgus deviation of the first toe by footwear and, therefore, are more vulnerable to bunion formation.

Based on a review of the literature and on their own experience, Reinherz and Gastwirth[91] concluded that radical excision of the abductor hallucis should be avoided whenever possible because of its large size, importance in first ray stabilization, and the potential for deformation of foot structure in absence of the muscle.

5. FUNCTIONAL (MYOTATIC) UNIT

The long and short extensors and flexors of the toes work together as a functional unit in conjunction with the lumbricals and interossei. Since a major action of the abductor hallucis is flexion, it forms a functional unit with the flexors hallucis brevis and longus and also with the deep adductor hallucis.

6. SYMPTOMS

Patients with active TrPs in any of the three superficial muscles in the sole of the foot (the two abductors and the flexor digitorum brevis) complain primarily of intolerably sore feet and are determined to find relief. They usually have tried all sorts of shoes and insert devices. The orthoses are often uncomfortable and quickly discarded because of the tenderness of the muscles against which they press. Many of these patients are said to have "fallen arches." The patients have a limited walking range and their friends may note that they tend to limp. After inactivation of the TrPs, appropriate arch supports are usually tolerated and often helpful in relieving perpetuating stresses on the muscles.

The deep aching pain at rest is a distressing symptom that often drives the patient to seek relief by surgical procedures.

Differential Diagnosis

For detailed descriptions and discussions of foot problems, the reader is referred to McGlamry's comprehensive two-volume textbook.[69]

Other Myofascial Pain Syndromes

Two other myofascial pain syndromes might be mistaken for TrPs in the **extensor hallucis brevis** and **extensor digitorum brevis** muscles (Fig. 26.1) that re-

PART 3

fer pain and tenderness to the proximal part of the dorsum of the foot in front of the lateral malleolus. The referred pain pattern of the extensor digitorum longus (*see* Fig. 24.1*A*) is quite similar but extends farther distally and may spill over to include the toes and the lower leg. The pattern referred by TrPs in the peroneus longus and peroneus brevis muscles (*see* Fig. 20.1*A*) differs in that it appears more on, and behind, the lateral malleolus than in front of it.

Three other myofascial pain syndromes may be mistaken for that of the **flexor digitorum brevis** muscle (Fig. 26.3*B*). This transverse plantar pattern covers the heads of the second, third, and fourth metatarsals. The most similar pattern is that of the adductor hallucis (*see* Fig. 27.2*A*), which covers the same region but also extends proximally to the instep. The flexor digitorum longus pain pattern (*see* Fig. 25.1*A*) is more longitudinal than transverse in orientation, is located more laterally on the sole, and extends farther proximally than that of the flexor digitorum brevis. The plantar pain referred from TrPs in an interosseous muscle (*see* Fig. 27.3) is more longitudinally oriented and involves the corresponding toe to a major degree. The toe pain helps distinguish the involvement of multiple interosseus muscles from active TrPs in the flexor digitorum brevis muscle.

Plantar Fasciitis

Symptoms: The patient complains of pain in the region of the plantar aponeurosis and/or of pain in the heel,[29,99,100] which has led to the term "policeman's heel."[53] The patient is likely to say, "the undersurface of my foot hurts, near the middle."[52] The pain is insidious in onset[29,99] and not associated with a specific movement or event, but often is felt after a sudden increase in an athlete's level of activity.[99] Pain is most marked on arising in the morning. The first 10–12 steps are severely painful until the plantar fascia and the muscles have been stretched.[29,96,99] The pain worsens again toward evening[96] and after sports activities that require running or jumping.[29,99,100]

Signs: Examination reveals tenderness over the medial insertion of the plantar fascia on the calcaneus[29,99] and/or diffuse tenderness along the entire medial plantar aspect of the foot.[99] The patient experiences plantar pain on passive extension of the great toe.[95,99] A calcaneal spur is usually an incidental finding that correlates poorly with pain. One treats the fasciitis without regard to the spur.[95,96] Sudden complete rupture of the plantar aponeurosis usually occurs only after a number of local steroid injections.[29,99]

Treatment: The one treatment for plantar fasciitis most strongly emphasized is rest for the foot in the form of reduced activity[29,95,99]—to the point of using crutches for a few days[29]—and lessening of stress on the plantar fascia by using stiff-soled wooden shoes temporarily[95] or by adhesive strapping of the foot.[100] An essential part of several treatment programs is stretching the heel cord (gastrocnemius/soleus muscles).[29,99,100] Orthotic corrections include a low soft (or hard) medial longitudinal arch support, heel wedges, and a Steindler heel that replaces with sponge rubber the part of the shoe under the tender area of the heel.[96,100] Several authors recommend oral anti-inflammatory medication.[96,99,100] Local injection of steroids gives inconsistent results and may be associated with rupture of the plantar aponeurosis.[29,99] Ultrasound applied with 10% cortisone, when combined with passive stretching of the triceps surae and rest, can be effective conservative therapy.[67] Surgical release of the plantar fascia is a last resort and rarely used.[29,53,96,99,100]

Cause: Plantar fasciitis is generally attributed to repeated traction with microtears of the plantar aponeurosis,[100] which produce an inflammatory degeneration of the plantar aponeurosis at its site of attachment on the medial tubercle of the calcaneus.[53,96] Tension overload is caused by a tight Achilles tendon that increases tension on the aponeurosis,[99,100] excessive walking, running, or jumping,[96,99] and pes planus with pronation of the foot on weight bearing.[99] Lewit[65] points out that tightness of the plantar aponeurosis may result from tension of the muscles that anchor to it. These are intrinsic muscles that function as flexors of the toes: the abductor hallucis, flexor digitorum brevis, and abductor digiti minimi. Myofascial TrPs cause chronic shortening of muscles that harbor them.

The fact that many of the symptoms and signs of plantar fasciitis are also characteristic of several myofascial pain syndromes raises the question as to whether TrPs may be contributing significantly to the chronic overload of the plantar aponeurosis in many of these patients. The muscles most likely to be involved are the intrinsic flexors of the toes, the gastrocnemius, and the soleus. The area of heel pain and tenderness of plantar fasciitis matches partly the referred patterns of the soleus (*see* Fig. 22.1), quadratus plantae (*see* Fig. 27.1), and abductor hallucis muscles (*see* Fig. 26.2*A*). The distribution of pain and tenderness along the plantar fascia fits the pattern produced by TrPs in the flexor digitorum longus muscle (*see* Fig. 25.1*A*). The intrinsic flexors of the toes can be overloaded by a sudden increase in running and jumping activities. The pain produced on passive extension of the great toe in plantar fasciitis is also characteristic of TrPs in the abductor hallucis muscle.

Structural Problems

Flat Feet: It is important to distinguish between a fixed flat foot due to tarsal coalition and a relaxed pronated flat foot. The former generally requires surgery. The latter usually responds to conservative therapy. In either case, surgical correction is indicated only if necessary to relieve pain.[46] Out-toeing (walking with the foot abducted and everted) is often considered so undesirable that the foot posture should be straightened. However, in case of flat feet, Lapidus[64] makes the point that the out-toeing serves a useful purpose and is best left uncorrected.

Bunions: The prevalence of bunions and hallux valgus is highly variable among different ethnic groups and apparently has a significant, if not predominant, hereditary component. The bunion protrusion may be accentuated by a combination of varus deviation of the first metatarsal and valgus deviation of the great toe. This combination may require surgery for correction when it has developed.[62] The muscle imbalance produced by the deviation tends to aggravate the condition further.[15,98]

Congenital Hypertrophy: One case of congenital hypertrophy of the abductor digiti minimi[35] and three cases of congenital hypertrophy of the abductor hallucis muscle[34] are reported. In each case, the enlarged muscle caused pain and considerable difficulty in finding suitable footwear; it was identified at surgery and resected with no adverse results reported. The nature of the mass should be readily identifiable by palpation during voluntary flexion of the great toe or abduction of the fifth toe and by EMG evaluation.

Avulsion Fracture: An avulsion fracture of the dorsolateral aspect of the calcaneus secondary to a pull-off mechanism by the extensor digitorum brevis muscle is not rare. A 10% incidence was found in a 1-year review of all emergency room cases of ankle trauma.[24] Such fracture is likely to result from an inversion injury of the foot and is treated with supportive bandages, elevation, and early range of motion exercises.[84]

Compartment Syndromes

Myerson[85] reviewed the anatomy of the four compartments of the forefoot: the central (plantar), medial, lateral, and interosseous (dorsal) compartments. He noted a dearth of literature and lack of recognition of these syndromes, which may result when a cast is applied to an injured foot.

Other Problems

Articular dysfunction in the foot can disturb mechanics and produce imbalances that cause pain at many sites.

7. ACTIVATION AND PERPETUATION OF TRIGGER POINTS

Activation

A shoe with a tight cap or vamp (a tight fit between the shoe and the forefoot) restricts toe movement. This constriction can overload the superficial intrinsic foot muscles and activate TrPs in them. Once it has initiated the TrPs, the same condition also perpetuates them. The muscle overload associated with a fracture of the ankle or other bones of the foot, especially when a cast has immobilized the foot for some time, can also activate TrPs in the short flexors of the toes.

Injuries to these muscles caused by bruising, banging, stubbing the toes, falling, and other traumas short of fracture can initiate TrPs in them.

Patients who have a (mediolateral) rocking foot because of a Morton foot structure may develop TrPs in the abductor digiti minimi and in the abductor hallucis muscles.

Perpetuation

Although some pronation of the foot during the stance phase of gait is normal, *hyper*pronation, when uncorrected, can contribute to perpetuation of TrPs in the intrinsic foot muscles.

Either hypermobility or hypomobility of the joints of the foot can perpetuate TrPs in these superficial intrinsic muscles of the foot.

Shoes with an inflexible sole (wooden sole or shoes with a steel bar along the length of the sole) can immobilize the foot sufficiently to perpetuate TrPs in the superficial intrinsic foot muscles.

A hard slippery surface under a desk chair with wheels can overload the toe flexors that must repeatedly help pull the chair close to the desk.

Walking or running on uneven terrain and on surfaces that slope transversely can perpetuate TrPs in the intrinsic muscles of the feet.

Systemic factors that can be responsible for perpetuating these TrPs are presented on pages 115–155 of Volume 1.[102]

8. PATIENT EXAMINATION

Observation of the patient's gait may reveal an antalgic limp that alerts one to ask about sore feet if the patient has not already volunteered this complaint. While the patient walks without shoes, the clinician should look for excessive supination or excessive pronation.

If plantar flexion of the lesser toes and/or the great toe is limited by pain, the extensor digitorum brevis[59] or extensor hallucis brevis[60] may be shortened by taut bands associated with TrPs. If passive extension of the fifth toe applied at the middle phalanx is painfully limited, the abductor digiti minimi may be shortened by TrPs. The same passive extension testing applies to the second, third, and fourth toes for TrPs in the flexor digitorum brevis.[58] Pressing the proximal phalanx of the great toe toward extension[57] similarly tests for painfully restricted range of motion and serves as a sign of TrP involvement of the abductor hallucis and flexor hallucis brevis. Asking the patient to press down hard against the examining finger tests for significant weakness.

Palpation of the painful areas establishes whether these areas also exhibit tenderness that may be referred from TrPs. Since chronic TrP tension in a muscle induces tenderness at the attachment of the muscle, patients with TrPs in the intrinsic flexors of the toes are likely to be tender in front of the calcaneus where the plantar aponeurosis attaches.

The patient's feet should be examined for restricted motion (including restriction of joint play) and for hypermobility. They should also be examined for structural deviations, such as hindfoot varus or valgus, forefoot varus or valgus, equinus, hypermobility or malposition of the first ray, short first (relatively long second) metatarsal, excessively high arch, hallux valgus, and hammer toes.

The dorsalis pedis and posterior tibial pulses should be palpated to assess the status of arterial circulation. The skin and nails should be examined for lesions. Edema should be noted.

The clinician should examine the patient's shoes for a tight cap, a rigid sole, a pointed front of the shoe, and for a negative heel height.

9. TRIGGER POINT EXAMINATION (Fig. 26.5)

Myofascial TrPs in the superficial intrinsic muscles of the foot are examined by flat palpation against underlying structures (Fig. 26.5). The TrPs are identified primarily by the patient's jump response to exquisite spot tenderness in a taut band. These muscles rarely exhibit local twitch responses to snapping palpation. The overlying tendons complicate palpation of the short extensors of the toes; the flexor digitorum brevis lies deep to the

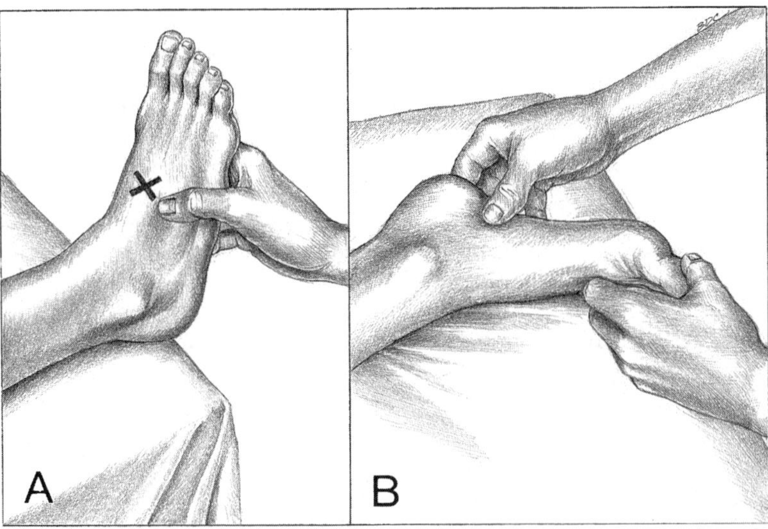

Figure 26.5. Examination to locate trigger points in the superficial intrinsic muscles of the right foot. *A*, the thumb palpates the most distal location of trigger points in the extensor digitorum brevis muscle; the ***X*** locates the most distal location of trigger points in the extensor hallucis brevis muscle. *B*, palpation of the abductor hallucis muscle for trigger points.

thick plantar aponeurosis, and the abductor hallucis is a surprisingly thick muscle. The thickness renders its deeper fibers relatively inaccessible and may require strong deep palpation rather than gentler flat palpation to elicit tenderness from its deep TrPs.

The abductor digiti minimi is usually most effectively examined by pincer palpation along the lateral edge of the sole of the foot. The examiner should explore both distal to and proximal to the base of the fifth metatarsal for taut bands and TrP tenderness.

10. ENTRAPMENTS

The posterior tibial nerve and its two branches, the medial and lateral plantar nerves, may become entrapped against the medial tarsal bones by the abductor hallucis muscle as the nerves pass deep to the muscle.[42] These nerves pass deep to the abductor hallucis just below the medial malleolus, immediately distal to the flexor retinaculum of the tarsal tunnel. Entrapment of the nerves in that area by the taut bands of TrPs in the abductor hallucis muscle may be responsible for a tarsal tunnel syndrome.

In two cases, a congenitally hypertrophied abductor hallucis muscle and, in another, an accessory muscle belly attached to the abductor hallucis caused entrapment symptoms.[34] Goodgold and associates[48] demonstrated the value of electrodiagnosis in establishing the diagnosis of nerve entrapment in tarsal tunnel syndrome and cited a case in which a fibrotic edge of the abductor hallucis muscle was responsible. Wilemon[103] reported two patients in whom fibrous bands of the abductor hallucis constricted all or parts of the posterior tibial nerve. Rask[90] relieved entrapment symptoms by injecting a TrP where the medial plantar nerve passes between the abductor hallucis muscle and the tuberosity of the navicular.

The symptom of a painful heel has been attributed to entrapment of the branch of the lateral plantar nerve to the abductor digiti minimi muscle as the nerve passes deep to the abductor hallucis muscle. Kenzora[61] reported relief of six patients obtained by following the course of the nerve through its fibrovascular tunnel deep to the abductor hallucis muscle with a curved hemostat and gently spreading it a few times to release constrictions of the nerve. Rondhuis and Huson[94] identified entrapment of the branch of the lateral plantar nerve that supplies the flexor digitorum brevis where the nerve passes between the abductor hallucis muscle and the medial head of the quadratus plantae muscle. These authors[94] found no evidence for entrapment in the region of the plantar fascia that would have been needed to substantiate the usual explanation offered for entrapment of this nerve. On the other hand, surgical release of the tibial nerve and the medial and lateral plantar nerves as they passed through and deep to the abductor hallucis muscle relieved symptoms of entrapment in 9 of 10 patients.[1] The possible [likely] role of myofascial TrPs in the abductor hallucis was apparently not considered in these patients with heel pain.

An accessory abductor hallucis attached, proximally, to the fascia superficial to the posterior tibial nerve about 4 cm proximal to the tip of the medial malleolus, passed deep to the nerve and partially encircled it to end, distally, in the middle of the main abductor hallucis muscle.[19] In this patient, at age 24 years, the muscle suddenly and inexplicably caused painful neurapraxic entrapment of the posterior tibial nerve. Symptoms were relieved by surgical excision of the accessory abductor hallucis muscle. The authors[19] did not report on the presence or absence of preoperative tenderness in the muscle. In another case,[50] the muscle did cause aching pain, which was relieved surgically. Examination for a TrP component of the pain was not reported.

Edwards and coauthors[34] reported that three patients—aged 7, 14, and 20 years, respectively—complained of painful feet, could not find shoes that would fit, and had a palpable mass that obliterated the longitudinal arch. At surgery, two patients were found to have a three times normal sized abductor hallucis, and the third was found to have an accessory muscle belly of the same muscle, which compressed the posterior tibial nerve.

11. ASSOCIATED TRIGGER POINTS

The TrPs in the extensor digitorum brevis and extensor hallucis brevis muscles are often associated with TrPs in the corresponding long (extrinsic) extensor muscles of the toes. One usually finds that, with involvement of the abductor hallucis, TrPs also appear in the neighboring deep intrinsic muscles. The whole foot is sore, especially the distal plantar surface including the midsole region.

Flexor digitorum brevis TrPs are likely to be associated with similar involvement of the long (extrinsic) flexors of the toes and sometimes of the deeper flexor hallucis brevis. On the other hand, the abductor digiti minimi is more likely to present as a single-muscle syndrome due largely to a tight shoe of inadequate width.

12. INTERMITTENT COLD WITH STRETCH
(Fig. 26.6)

In all the intermittent cold-with-stretch procedures described later in this chapter, the process will be facilitated if the operator incorporates the Lewit postisometric relaxation technique with augmentation, as described in Chapter 2, pages 10–11. Other treatment techniques are also described in Chapter 2. The use of ice for applying intermittent cold with stretch is explained on page 9 of this volume and the use of vapocoolant spray and stretch is detailed on pages 67–74 of Volume 1.[102]

If the patient has hypermobility in the tarsometatarsal region, that region needs to be stabilized during the stretch of the intrinsic muscles of the toes. In such cases, the intermittent cold can be applied prior to, rather than during, the stretch.

Since some patients have cold feet to begin with, it is critical to feel the warmth of the skin before applying intermittent cold. The skin must be warmed either reflexly with a dry hot pad on the abdomen or by direct application of heat to the feet. Skin temperature should be rechecked after several cycles of intermittent cold application.

After each of the procedures described in this chapter, the operator should rewarm the skin of the patient's foot with a moist heating pad and then have the patient actively exercise the treated muscle through several slow cycles of the com-

PART 3

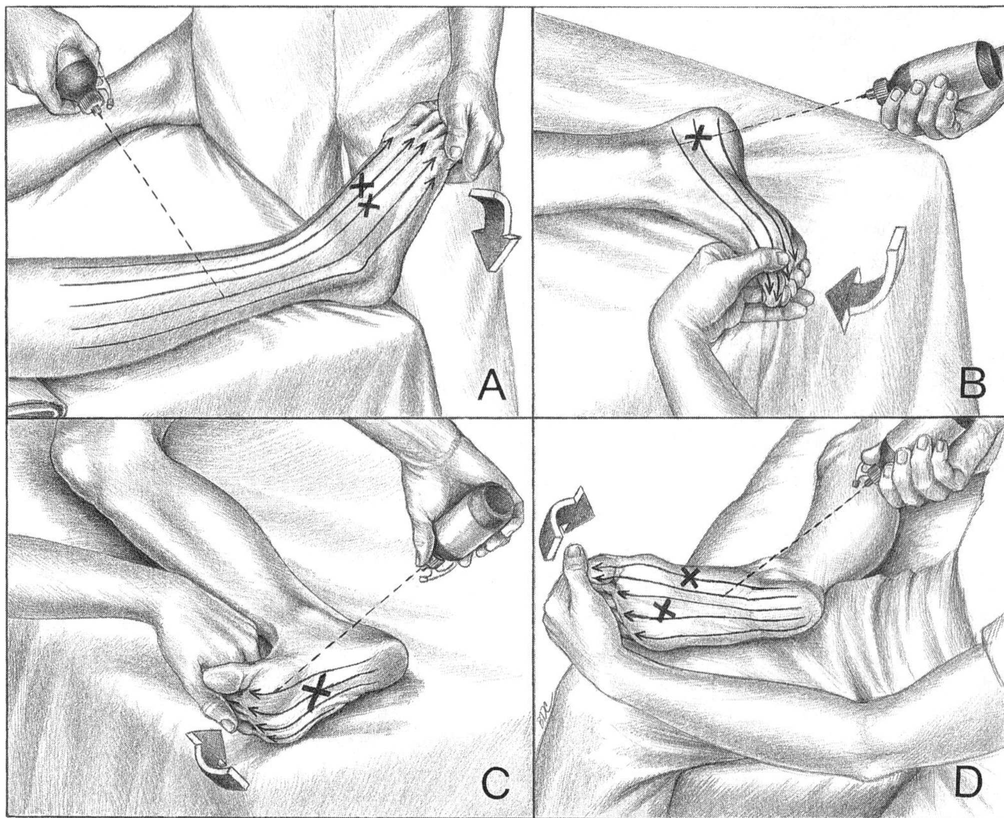

Figure 26.6. Intermittent cold patterns (*thin arrows*) and stretch positions for trigger points in the superficial foot muscles. The *thick arrows* show the direction in which pressure is exerted to stretch the muscle passively. The **X**s mark the location of trigger points in the muscles being stretched. *A*, flexion of all toes to stretch the **extensor digitorum brevis** and **extensor hallucis brevis**, with plantar flexion of the foot to stretch the long extensors of the toes also. When only the toes are flexed (without ankle plantar flexion), application of intermittent cold above the ankle is unnecessary. *B*, extension of the great toe to stretch the **abductor hallucis**. *C*, extension of the four lesser toes to stretch the **flexor digitorum brevis** (and quadratus plantae). Only the toes need be extended, while the foot remains in the neutral position at the ankle. The ice or spray pattern includes the pain reference zone on the plantar surface of the toes. *D*, if one wishes to combine intermittent cold with stretch of the **flexor digitorum brevis** and the **flexor hallucis brevis** (Fig. 27.7), the operator should also extend the great toe. When the tarsometatarsal region is hypermobile, intermittent cold should be applied prior to the passive stretch so that one hand can stabilize the midfoot while the other hand moves the toes.

plete range of shortening and lengthening of that muscle.

Short Extensors of Toes

To release TrP tightness of the **extensor digitorum brevis** and **extensor hallucis brevis** muscles using intermittent cold with stretch, the patient lies supine with pillows as needed for comfort and with the foot at the end of the table (Fig. 26.6*A*). The clinician applies a few parallel sweeps of ice or vapocoolant spray down the anterolateral aspect of the ankle and over the dorsum of the foot before taking up the slack by pressing gently on all five toes to flex them. The operator continues the cycle of applying cold in parallel sweeps, and then taking up any slack that develops in the short extensors of the toes, until no further gains occur. The skin should be covered no more than two or three times and then rewarmed to avoid chilling of the underlying muscle.

To release tension in the short extensors of the toes, the ankle can be left in a neutral position. Adding plantar flexion of the ankle, as in Figure 26.6*A*, also stretches and releases TrPs in the long extensors of the toes and requires additional downward application of cold in a pattern that includes all of the anterolateral leg.

Abductors of Toes

To inactivate TrPs in the **abductor hallucis** muscle by intermittent cold with stretch, the patient lies on the affected side or prone with the foot hanging over the end of the treatment table and with the ankle in a neutral position (neither plantar flexed nor dorsiflexed). The operator applies the vapocoolant spray or ice in parallel sweeps distally over the medial side of the foot and medial portion of the sole from the back of the heel to the tip of the great toe (Fig. 26.6*B*). Then the operator presses the proximal phalanx of the great toe into extension and repeats the application of intermittent cold while taking up any slack that develops. The process may be repeated until no further gains are realized; however, it is important after two or three cycles to rewarm the skin (and, possibly, the muscle) with a moist heating pad. Because the abductor hallucis often acts only as a flexor and not as an abductor, and because hallux valgus is such a common problem, extension without adduction is applied to the proximal phalanx. It is helpful to combine extension of the toe with deep slow massage of the muscle in a distal direction to help stretch its fibers.

Inactivation of TrPs in the **abductor digiti minimi** follows closely this same procedure except that the ice or vapocoolant spray covers the lateral rather than the medial side of the foot, and adduction of the fifth toe is emphasized as much as extension.

Inactivation of TrPs in these superficial intrinsic abductors may also be effectively accomplished with deep stripping massage or with postisometric relaxation.

Short Flexors of Toes

To release tension caused by TrPs in the **flexor digitorum brevis** muscle, the patient lies *comfortably* on the affected side with the ankle in the neutral position, as in Figure 26.6*C*. The operator applies several parallel sweeps of ice or vapocoolant spray over the sole of the foot from the heel to the toes while gently extending the lesser toes to take up any slack in the muscle. With a repeat application of intermittent cold, the operator takes up any further slack that develops in the muscle. The operator immediately applies a moist heating pad for rewarming.

One can easily modify this procedure for the flexor digitorum brevis to include both the abductor hallucis and **flexor hallucis brevis** muscles (Fig. 26.6*D*). Sweeps of intermittent cold cover the entire plantar surface of the foot including the great toe and the medial border of the foot. All five toes are passively extended together.

Evjenth and Hamberg[36] describe and illustrate stretch techniques for the abductor hallucis, extensor hallucis brevis, and the flexor digitorum brevis muscles, none of which is readily combined with application of intermittent cold because the hand covers the essential pain patterns where intermittent cold should be applied. These techniques, however, do provide stabilization of the foot and are useful when using postisometric relaxation alone.

13. INJECTION AND STRETCH (Fig. 26.7)

If less invasive procedures (for example, intermittent cold with stretch, Lewit postisometric relaxation, and ischemic compression) are not sufficiently effective, TrP injection should be considered. The basic procedure for injecting TrPs in any muscle is found on pages 74–86 in Volume 1.[102]

When injecting any TrPs in the foot, the injection site should be scrubbed carefully with alcohol or a more powerful iodine antiseptic. If the individual works on a farm or has a garden where there may be exposure to animal feces, the feet should be thoroughly scrubbed with hydrogen peroxide, which kills tetanus spores. After injection, pressure is applied promptly for hemostasis and the needle puncture site is covered with a snug adhesive bandage to ensure sealing of the wound. These extra precautions of hydrogen peroxide and the bandage are not generally used when injecting TrPs in other regions of the body, but are impor-

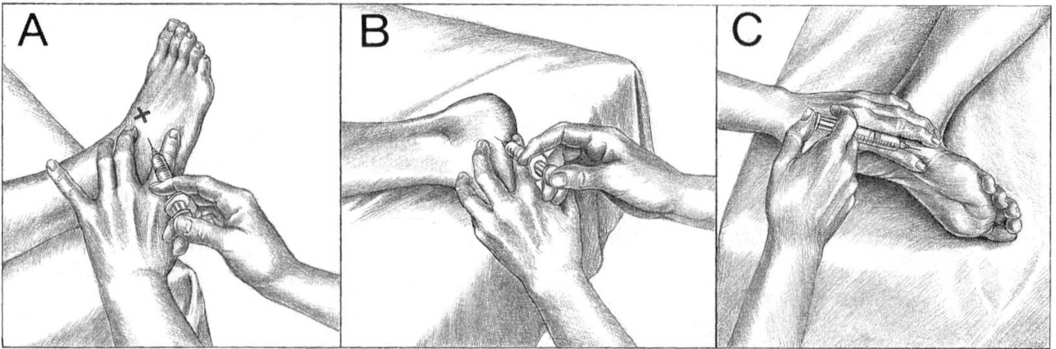

Figure 26.7. Injection of trigger points in superficial muscles of the right foot. *A*, most distal site for extensor digitorum brevis trigger points. The ***X*** locates the most distal site for injection of trigger points in the extensor hallucis brevis. *B*, in the abductor hallucis on the medial side of the foot. *C*, in the abductor digiti minimi on the lateral side of the foot.

tant when injecting through the skin of the foot.

After the injection of TrPs in any of the following muscles, the clinician applies intermittent cold with passive stretch, as described for each muscle in the previous section, and follows this promptly by application of moist heat for a few minutes to reduce the likelihood or the severity of postinjection soreness. The patient then performs several cycles of slow active range of motion through the fully shortened and fully lengthened positions of the injected muscle in order to equalize sarcomere lengths and to normalize muscle function.

Short Extensors of Toes
(Fig. 26.7)

For injection of TrPs in the **extensor digitorum brevis** muscle, the patient lies supine with pillows and a blanket as needed for comfort (Fig. 26.7*A*). The operator locates the taut band and TrP by flat palpation, marks its location, and stretches the skin for hemostasis by spreading apart the fingers on both sides of the TrP. A 37-mm (1½-in) long 22-gauge needle will reach any of these superficial TrPs; a 25-mm (1-in) needle may suffice. When the patient exhibits a jump sign and/or the toes extend, which indicates a local twitch response, the operator injects the TrP with 0.5% procaine solution prepared by dilution with isotonic saline. Before completely withdrawing the needle, by sliding the skin, the operator palpates for any TrP tenderness remaining in the muscle and similarly injects any residual TrPs.

The ***X*** in Figure 26.7*A* locates the region of TrPs in the **extensor hallucis brevis**. The injection procedure is the same as for the extensor digitorum brevis described previously, except for the location of needle penetration.

Abductors of Toes

For injection of TrPs in the **abductor hallucis** muscle, the patient lies on the involved side (Fig. 26.7*B*). The clinician cleanses the foot as described previously, locates precisely the taut band and TrP by flat palpation, and inserts the 37-mm (1½-in) long 22-gauge needle that is usually used on a 10-mL syringe. Although one might expect the TrPs in the abductor hallucis to be close to the surface, this is a surprisingly thick muscle. The main TrPs often lie close to the bone, so it is usually necessary to advance the needle to the periosteal level and then to explore the muscle for active TrPs just short of that depth. These deep TrPs in the muscle are easily overlooked. Needle encounter with the TrP usually gives the operator a feeling of penetrating hard rubber and evokes a pain response on the part of the patient; in this muscle, a local twitch response, when it occurs, is indicated by flexion of the great toe. The clinician then injects the 0.5% procaine solution into the TrP and, on probing further, may find a cluster of TrPs to be injected.

When injecting this muscle, one must know the location of the posterior tibial artery and nerve and their branches that pass behind the medial malleolus and then deep to the abductor hallucis muscle near where it attaches to the calcaneus.[5]

For injection of TrPs in the **abductor digiti minimi** muscle, the patient lies on the uninvolved side and is made comfortable (Fig. 26.7*C*). After cleansing the foot, the clinician locates the taut band and its TrPs by either flat or pincer palpation of this muscle. It is not very thick, unlike the abductor hallucis, and its taut bands and TrPs are generally easily localized. They may be either in front of, or behind, the base of the fifth metatarsal, which is palpable as a bony protuberance along the lateral border of the foot. The TrPs are injected with 0.5% procaine solution wherever they are found in the muscle. Needle penetration of TrPs in this muscle is likely to cause a local twitch response as shown by a variable combination of abduction and flexion of the fifth toe.

14. CORRECTIVE ACTIONS
(Figs. 26.8 and 26.9)

Corrective pads are installed inside the shoe under the first metatarsal head to compensate for a Morton foot structure (*see* Chapter 20, pages 389–391), especially for patients with TrPs in the abductor digiti minimi muscle. Arch supports may be needed for a hypermobile foot. Other structural deviations of the foot should be corrected or shoes must be modified to provide good overall support for dynamic balance and comfort.

If hypomobility is a factor, normal joint play and range of motion should be restored.

Corrective Body Mechanics

Many patients find that, as they age, their feet become larger. Shoes that did fit years before are too tight and no longer comfortable. Old shoes should be replaced with new ones that do not cramp and squeeze the foot and do not limit toe movement. Feet not only increase in length, but the forefoot tends to widen with age.[97] This change may relate to increased laxity of ligaments and/or loss of intrinsic muscle tone.

Patients should ensure, when buying new shoes, that the shoes are large enough. They should take a foam sole insert to the store and place it in the shoe when trying the shoe on for size. The shoes should provide snug heel support and preferably some ankle support, a flexible sole, a cap (vamp) that is high enough, a toe that is not sharply pointed, and a moderate-height (not negative, high, or spike) heel. Athletic shoes designed to fit and support the feet and ankles are now widely accepted as stylish for more general use. Shoes designed for specific activities should be selected on that basis. High-quality athletic shoes are worth the price.[30]

Corrective Posture and Activities

Walking on a hard surface with stiff, slippery, leather-soled shoes overloads the muscles of the feet. This problem is aggravated in persons with flat arches.[97] It is much better either to wear shoes with resilient heels and soles, such as running shoes, or to add a foam sole insert inside the shoe. The addition must not cramp the foot and prevent normal toe movement. Wearing crepe soles that are too flexible to support the metatarsal area, however, can be troublesome, possibly injurious.[97]

Adequate space in the shoe is an important consideration when buying new shoes. Since few people have perfectly matched feet, new shoes should be fitted on the larger foot.

Unless the patient has structural deformities, orthoses are usually unnecessary after the TrPs causing the foot soreness have been inactivated. The patients need soft cushioning, not hard orthoses. The cushioning is ineffective if the added material makes the shoe too tight and restricts normal movement.

Corrective Exercises

Walking in dry sand is vigorous exercise for intrinsic foot muscles and can easily be overdone. Walking in wet sand with special attention to "toe-off" provides a milder strengthening exercise.

Picking up marbles with the toes improves strength and coordination of the toe muscles.[89]

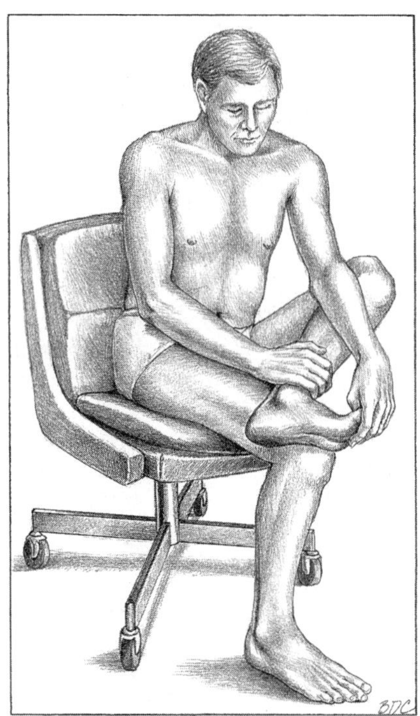

Figure 26.8. Passive Toe Flexor Self-stretch Exercise for use at home by the patient with trigger points in the short (and long) flexors of the toes. The patient pulls all five toes into extension with one hand. If the patient has any hypermobility in the tarsometatarsal region, that region should be stabilized by the patient's other hand.

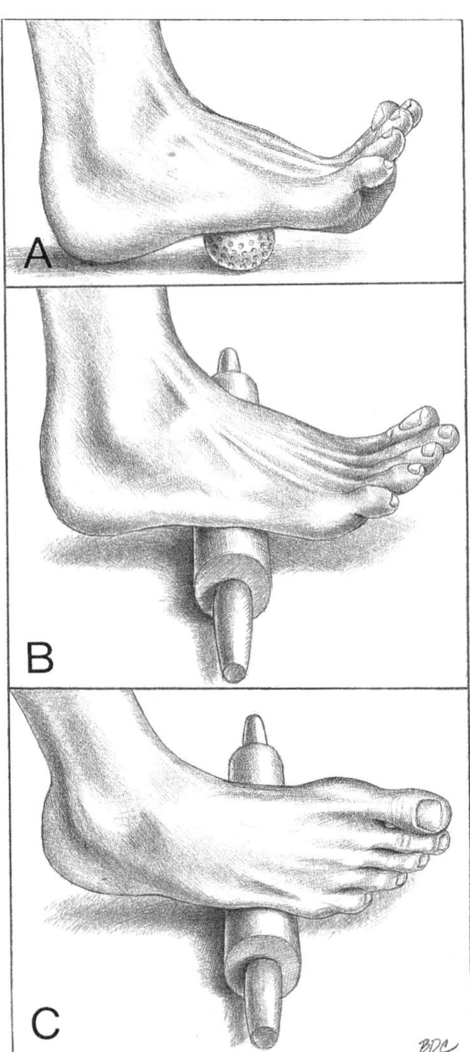

Figure 26.9. Self-application of ischemic compression and massage of plantar intrinsic foot muscles. *A*, using the Golf-ball Technique, rolling the golf ball back and forth under the foot while applying pressure with the body weight, positioned to treat the flexor digitorum brevis and sometimes the quadratus plantae muscles. *B*, using the Rolling Pin Technique with the foot flat to massage the toe flexors. *C*, using the Rolling Pin Technique to treat the abductor digiti minimi muscle with the foot inverted.

Home Treatment Program
(Figs. 26.8 and 26.9)

The Toe Flexor Self-stretch Exercise for use at home by the patient with TrPs in the short or long flexors of the toes is pictured in Figure 26.8. In its simplest form, the patient simply relaxes the leg and foot muscles as much as possible, grasps the toes, and gently pulls them into extension and the foot into dorsiflexion. By coordinating contraction and relaxation with respiration in accordance with Lewit's postisometric relaxation technique (Chapter 2, page 11), the effectiveness of the stretch is markedly improved. The patient should be instructed to stabilize the midfoot if there is any hypermobility in that region. In addition, it may be helpful for the patient to perform the passive stretch while seated in a bathtub or Jacuzzi® with the leg and foot immersed in warm water.

The addition by the patient of active toe extension and ankle dorsiflexion contributes the effect of reciprocal inhibition to further release the flexor muscle being stretched. The patient can achieve a similar effect by *slowly* performing *full* active range of motion through several cycles.

Figure 26.9 illustrates home versions of self-administered ischemic compression and deep stripping massage of the superficial plantar muscles. When using the Golf-ball Technique of Figure 26.9*A*, the patient places sufficient body weight on the golf ball to locate the tender spots in the muscles. Then the patient can either apply steady ischemic compression or roll the ball over the tender spot (TrP) along the taut band to perform a modification of stripping massage, as described in detail in Chapter 2, page 9. With this golf-ball technique, the patients can apply as much pressure as desired, for as long as desired, without overloading the hand muscles. This technique is especially useful for applying effective pressure to the flexor digitorum brevis and to that part of the abductor digiti minimi that lies deep to the plantar aponeurosis.

Figure 26.9*B* shows how to use the Rolling-pin Technique in a similar manner. This is less specific as to the location of the applied pressure, but is probably easier to apply. Foot flat, as shown in this drawing, applies pressure to the flexor digitorum brevis, flexor hallucis brevis, and the abductor hallucis.

Figure 26.9*C* shows the advantage of rolling the foot to one side to treat muscles along the sides of the foot more effectively; namely, the abductor digiti minimi when inverting the foot, and the abductor hallucis when everting the foot. Both versions of the Rolling-pin Technique can be used for self-administered ischemic compression or modified stripping massage. For the latter, the pin is rolled very slowly throughout the length of the tender part of the muscle.

The active Toe-stretch Exercise provides a general purpose flexion-extension stretch for the toe muscles in the same way that the Artisan's Finger-stretch Exercise (Fig. 35.8, Volume 1)[102] provides a general purpose active flexion-extension stretch exercise for the finger muscles. The patient sits on a chair and extends the legs, feet on the floor in front, then actively fully inverts and plantar flexes the foot while strongly curling the toes, and then slowly transitions to everting and dorsiflexing the foot fully while strongly extending the toes. This should be repeated at least five times, with a pause between each cycle.

Pagliano and Wischnia[89] illustrate a set of foot-strengthening exercises, several of which can be applied to both extrinsic and intrinsic flexors and extensors of the toes.

References

1. Albrektsson B, Rydholm A, Rydholm U: The tarsal tunnel syndrome in children. *J Bone Joint Surg [Br] 64*:215–217, 1982.
2. Anderson JE: *Grant's Atlas of Anatomy*, Ed. 8. Williams & Wilkins, Baltimore, 1983 (Fig. 4–77).
3. *Ibid*. (Fig. 4–78B).
4. *Ibid*. (Fig. 4–79).
5. *Ibid*. (Fig. 4–87).
6. *Ibid*. (Fig. 4–93).
7. *Ibid*. (Fig. 4–100).
8. *Ibid*. (Fig. 4–102).
9. *Ibid*. (Fig. 4–103).
10. *Ibid*. (Fig. 4–106).
11. *Ibid*. (Fig. 4–107).
12. Bardeen CR: The musculature, Sect. 5. In *Morris's Human Anatomy*, edited by C.M. Jackson, Ed. 6. Blakiston's Son & Co., Philadelphia, 1921 (pp. 514, 524–528, 530).
13. Basmajian JV, Deluca CJ: *Muscles Alive*, Ed. 5. Williams & Wilkins, Baltimore, 1985 (pp. 342–345).
14. *Ibid*. (p. 349).
15. *Ibid*. (pp. 351, 352).
16. *Ibid*. (pp. 351, 379).
17. *Ibid*. (pp. 353, 354).
18. Bates T, Grunwaldt E: Myofascial pain in childhood. *J Pediatr 53*:198–209, 1958.
19. Bhansali RM, Bhansali RR: Accessory abductor hallucis causing entrapment of the posterior tibial nerve. *J Bone Joint Surg [Br] 69*:479–480, 1987.
20. Carter BL, Morehead J, Wolpert SM, et al.: *Cross-Sectional Anatomy*. Appleton-Century-Crofts, New York, 1977, (Sects. 82–86).
21. *Ibid*. (Sects. 82–87).
22. *Ibid*. (Sects. 83–85).
23. *Ibid*. (Sects. 83–86).
24. Cavaliere RG: Ankle and rearfoot—calcaneal fractures, Chapter 28, Part 3. In *Comprehensive Textbook of Foot Surgery*, edited by E. Dalton McGlamry, Vol. 2. Williams & Wilkins, Baltimore, 1987 (pp. 873–903, *see* pp. 881, 885).
25. Christensen E: Topography of terminal motor innervation in striated muscles from stillborn infants. *Am J Phys Med 38*:65–78, 1959.
26. Clemente CD: *Gray's Anatomy of the Human Body*, American Ed. 30. Lea & Febiger, Philadelphia, 1985 (p. 293, Fig. 4–220).
27. *Ibid*. (pp. 575, 584–587).
28. *Ibid*. (p. 585, Fig. 6–82).
29. Coker TP Jr, Arnold JA: Sports injuries to the foot and ankle, Chapter 57. In *Disorders of the Foot*, edited by M.H. Jahss, Vol. 2. W.B. Saunders Co., London, 1982, (pp. 1573–1606, *see* pp. 1604–1605).
30. Drez D: Running footwear: examination of the training shoe, the foot, and functional orthotic devices. *Am J Sports Med 8*:140–141, 1980.

31. Duchenne GB: *Physiology of Motion*, translated by E.B. Kaplan. J.B. Lippincott, Philadelphia, 1949 (pp. 373–374, 376).
32. *Ibid*. (p. 412).
33. Duranti R, Galletti R, Pantaleo T: Electromyographic observations in patients with foot syndromes. *Am J Phys Med 64*:295–304, 1985.
34. Edwards WG, Lincoln CR, Bassett FH, *et al*.: The tarsal tunnel syndrome: diagnosis and treatment. *JAMA 207*:716–720, 1969.
35. Estersohn HS, Agins SW, Ridenour J: Congenital hypertrophy of an intrinsic muscle of the foot. *J Foot Surg 26*:501–503, 1987.
36. Evjenth O, Hamberg J: *Muscle Stretching in Manual Therapy, A Clinical Manual*. Alfta Rehab Förlag, Alfta, Sweden, 1984 (pp. 150, 155, 159).
37. Ferner H, Staubesand J: *Sobotta Atlas of Human Anatomy*, Ed. 10, Vol. 2. Urban & Schwarzenberg, Baltimore, 1983 (Fig. 381).
38. *Ibid*. (Fig. 489).
39. *Ibid*. (Fig. 491).
40. *Ibid*. (Fig. 492).
41. *Ibid*. (Fig. 493).
42. *Ibid*. (Fig. 497).
43. *Ibid*. (Fig. 498).
44. *Ibid*. (Fig. 500).
45. *Ibid*. (Fig. 503).
46. Goldner JL: Advances in care of the foot: 1800 to 1987. *Orthopedics 10*:1817–1836, 1987.
47. Good MG: Painful feet. *Practitioner 163*:229–232, 1949.
48. Goodgold J, Kopell HP, Spielholz NI: The tarsal–tunnel syndrome: objective diagnostic criteria. *N Engl J Med 273*:742–745, 1965.
49. Gray EG, Basmajian JV: Electromyography and cinematography of leg and foot ("normal" and flat) during walking. *Anat Rec 181*:1–16, 1968.
50. Haber JA, Sollitto RJ: Accessory abductor hallucis: a case report. *J Foot Surg 18*:74, 1979.
51. Hollinshead WH: *Functional Anatomy of the Limbs and Back*, Ed. 4. W.B. Saunders, Philadelphia, 1976, (p. 358, Table 20–1).
52. Hoppenfeld S: Physical examination of the foot by complaint, Chapter 5. In *Disorders of the Foot*, edited by M.H. Jahss, Vol. 1. W.B. Saunders Co., Philadelphia, 1982 (pp. 103–115, *see* pp. 108–110).
53. Hoppenfeld S, deBoer P: *Surgical Exposures in Orthopaedics: The Anatomic Approach*. J. B. Lippincott Co., Philadelphia, 1984 (p. 528).
54. Kelly M: The nature of fibrositis. II. A study of the causation of the myalgic lesion (rheumatic, traumatic, infective). *Ann Rheum Dis 5*:69–77, 1946.
55. Kelly M: Some rules for the employment of local analgesic in the treatment of somatic pain. *Med J Austral 1*:235–239, 1947.
56. Kelly M: The relief of facial pain by procaine (Novocaine) injections. *J Am Geriatr Soc 11*: 586–596, 1963.
57. Kendall FP, McCreary EK: *Muscles, Testing and Function*, Ed. 3. Williams & Wilkins, Baltimore, 1983 (p. 131).
58. *Ibid*. (p. 133).
59. *Ibid*. (p. 139).
60. *Ibid*. (p. 140).
61. Kenzora JE: The painful heel syndrome: an entrapment neuropathy. *Bull Hosp Jt Dis Orthop Inst 47*:178–189, 1987.
62. Kenzora JE: A rationale for the surgical treatment of bunions. *Orthopedics 11*:777–789, 1988.
63. Krout RR: Trigger points [letter]. *J Am Podiatr Med Assoc 77*:269, 1987.
64. Lapidus PW: Some fallacies about intoeing and outtoeing. *Orthop Rev 10*:73–79, 1981.
65. Lewit K: *Manipulative Therapy in Rehabilitation of the Motor System*. Butterworths, London, 1985 (p. 284).
66. Lockhart RD: *Living Anatomy*, Ed. 7. Faber & Faber, London, 1974 (Fig. 138).
67. Maloney M: Personal communication, 1991.
68. Mann R, Inman VT: Phasic activity of intrinsic muscles of the foot. *J Bone Joint Surg [Am] 46*: 469–481, 1964.
69. McGlamry ED (Ed): *Comprehensive Textbook of Foot Surgery*, Vols. I & II. Williams & Wilkins, Baltimore, 1987.
70. McMinn RMH, Hutchings RT: *Color Atlas of Human Anatomy*. Year Book Medical Publishers, Chicago, 1977 (p. 289).
71. *Ibid*. (p. 318).
72. *Ibid*. (p. 321).
73. *Ibid*. (p. 322).
74. *Ibid*. (p. 325B).
75. McMinn RMH, Hutchings RT, Logan BM: *Color Atlas of Foot and Ankle Anatomy*. Appleton–Century–Crofts, Connecticut, 1982 (p. 28).
76. *Ibid*. (p. 54).
77. *Ibid*. (p. 56).
78. *Ibid*. (p. 58).
79. *Ibid*. (p. 64).
80. *Ibid*. (pp. 72–73).
81. *Ibid*. (p. 74).
82. *Ibid*. (p. 75).
83. *Ibid*. (pp. 82–83).
84. Morse HH, Lambert L, Basch D, *et al*.: Avulsion fracture by the extensor digitorum brevis muscle. *J Am Podiatr Med Assoc 79*:514–516, 1989.
85. Myerson M: Diagnosis and treatment of compartment syndrome of the foot. *Orthopedics 13*: 711–717, 1990.
86. Netter FH: *The Ciba Collection of Medical Illustrations*, Vol. 8, Musculoskeletal System. Part I: Anatomy, Physiology and Metabolic Disorders. Ciba-Geigy Corporation, Summit, 1987 (p. 109).
87. *Ibid*. (p. 111).
88. *Ibid*. (p. 113).
89. Pagliano J, Wischnia B: Fabulous feet: the foundation of good running. *Runner's World* pp: 39–41, Aug. 1984.
90. Rask MR: Medial plantar neurapraxia (jogger's foot). *Clin Orthop 134*:193–195, 1978.
91. Reinherz RP, Gastwirth CM: The abductor hallucis muscle [Editorial]. *J Foot Surg 26*:93–94, 1987.
92. Rohen JW, Yokochi C: *Color Atlas of Anatomy*, Ed. 2. Igaku-Shoin, New York, 1988 (p. 426).
93. *Ibid*. (pp. 427, 428).
94. Rondhuis JJ, Huson A: The first branch of the lateral plantar nerve and heel pain. *Acta Morphol Neerl–Scand 24*:269–279, 1986.

95. Sammarco GJ: The foot and ankle in classical ballet and modern dance, Chapter 59. In *Disorders of the Foot*, edited by M.H. Jahss, Vol. 2. W.B. Saunders Co., Philadelphia, 1982 (pp. 1626–1659, *see* pp. 1654–1655).
96. Seder JI: How I manage heel spur syndrome. *Phys Sportsmed 15*:83–85, 1987.
97. Sheon RP: A joint-protection guide for nonarticular rheumatic disorders. *Postgrad Med 77*: 329–338, 1985.
98. Shimazaki K, Takebe K: Investigations on the origin of hallux valgus by electromyographic analysis. *Kobe J Med Sci 27*:139–158, 1981.
99. Tanner SM, Harvey JS: How we manage plantar fasciitis. *Phys Sportsmed 16*:39–47, 1988.
100. Torg JS, Pavlov H, Torg E: Overuse injuries in sports: the foot. *Clin Sports Med 6*:291–320, 1987.
101. Travell J, Rinzler SH: The myofascial genesis of pain. *Postgrad Med 11*:425–434, 1952.
102. Travell JG, Simons DG: *Myofascial Pain and Dysfunction: The Trigger Point Manual*. Williams & Wilkins, Baltimore, 1983.
103. Wilemon WK: Tarsal tunnel syndrome: a 50–year survey of the world literature and a report of two new cases. *Orthop Rev 8*:111–117, 1979.

CHAPTER 27

Deep Intrinsic Foot Muscles

Quadratus Plantae and Lumbricals, Flexor Hallucis Brevis, Adductor Hallucis, Flexor Digiti Minimi Brevis, and Interossei

"Vipers' Nest"

HIGHLIGHTS: **REFERRED PAIN** and tenderness induced by trigger points (TrPs) in the quadratus plantae muscle project to the plantar surface of the heel. The oblique and transverse heads of the adductor hallucis refer to the plantar surface of the forefoot in the region of the metatarsal heads. Referral from the flexor hallucis brevis covers the region of the head of the first metatarsal bone on its plantar and medial aspects, and may spill over to include all of the first toe and much of the second toe. The TrPs in the interossei refer pain and tenderness primarily along that side of the toe to which each muscle attaches and to the plantar surface of the corresponding metatarsal head. **ANATOMICAL ATTACHMENTS** of the quadratus plantae are to the calcaneus proximally and to the tendon of the flexor digitorum longus distally. The lumbricals extend from the digitations of the flexor digitorum longus tendon to the extensor hood of each of the four lesser toes. The flexor digiti minimi brevis extends from the base of the fifth metatarsal to the proximal phalanx of the fifth toe. The two parts of the flexor hallucis brevis extend from a common proximal attachment onto the adjacent surfaces of the cuboid and lateral cuneiform bones to distal attachments by two tendons, one to each side of the proximal phalanx of the large toe. Each distal tendon of the flexor hallucis brevis muscle contains a sesamoid bone. The oblique head of the adductor hallucis anchors to the bases of the second, third, and fourth metatarsals. The transverse head of this muscle attaches to the plantar metatarsophalangeal (MP) ligaments of the third, fourth, and fifth toes. Medially, both heads of this muscle join where they attach to the lateral aspect of the base of the proximal phalanx of the large toe. The four bipennate dorsal interossei anchor, proximally, to the shafts of adjacent metatarsal bones. Distally, the first dorsal interosseous attaches to the medial side and the second attaches to the lateral side of the base of the proximal phalanx of the second toe; both join the dorsal aponeurosis of the extensor digitorum longus tendon of that toe. The third and fourth dorsal interossei attach distally to only the lateral side of the third and fourth toes in a similar fashion. The three plantar interossei extend from the bases of the third, fourth, and fifth metatarsal bones to the medial aspect of the bases of the proximal phalanges of the third, fourth, and fifth toes. **FUNCTION** of the intrinsic muscles of the foot is primarily related to stabilizing the foot for propulsion. The quadratus plantae aligns the pull of the flexor digitorum longus into pure flexion and assists it in flexing the four lesser toes. The lumbricals flex the proximal phalanges of the four lesser toes and extend the two distal phalanges. The flexor digiti minimi brevis flexes the proximal phalanx of the small toe. Similarly, the flexor hallucis brevis flexes the proximal phalanx of the great toe. The adductor hallucis adducts and assists flexion of the great toe and assists in maintaining transverse plane stability. The dorsal and plantar interossei, respectively, abduct and adduct the lesser toes and stabilize the forefoot. **SYMPTOMS** caused by TrPs in the deep intrinsic muscles of the foot include impaired walking because of pain and often intolerance to corrective orthoses inserted in the shoe. The clinician may need to distinguish symptoms of the deep intrinsic muscles from those of other myofascial pain syndromes, plantar fasciitis, articular dysfunction of the foot, and an injured sesamoid bone. **PATIENT EXAMINATION** includes looking for an antalgic gait; for excessive supination or pronation; for restricted range of motion or hypermobility of the toes, forefoot, and hindfoot; for weakness of the toes; for a Morton foot structure; for the location and thickness of calluses; and for improperly designed and fitted shoes. **INTERMITTENT COLD WITH STRETCH** generally works well for TrPs in the quadratus plantae, flexor hallucis brevis, flexor digiti minimi brevis, and adductor hallucis muscles. However, TrPs in the interossei and lumbricals may be inactivated more readily by deep massage or injection. **INJECTION AND STRETCH** of the quadratus plantae, flexor hallucis brevis, and adductor hallucis are performed with the patient lying on the same (affected) side; the quadratus plantae and the flexor hallucis brevis muscles are approached with the needle from the medial aspect of the foot. The adductor hallucis is approached through the sole of the foot. Both the dorsal and plantar interossei are injected through the dorsum of the foot. **CORRECTIVE ACTIONS** include restoration of normal joint play and range of motion of articulations in the foot. Only well-designed, well-fitted shoes of high quality are recommended. Appropriate supports are added to the shoes to correct for structural problems of the foot. A self-stretch exercise program and the Golf-ball or Rolling-pin Technique are recommended to the patient.

1. REFERRED PAIN
(Figs. 27.1–27.3)

Myofascial trigger points (TrPs) in the **quadratus plantae** muscle usually refer pain and tenderness only to the plantar surface of the heel (Fig. 27.1).

Pain and tenderness referred from TrPs in either the oblique or transverse head of the **adductor hallucis** muscle (Fig. 27.2*A*) are felt in the distal portion of the sole of the foot, primarily in the region of the first through fourth metatarsal heads. The TrPs in the transverse head of the adductor hallucis are likely to cause a strange "fluffy" feeling of numbness and a sense of swelling of the skin over the region of the metatarsal heads.

Medial to the oblique head of the adductor hallucis, TrPs in the **flexor hallucis brevis** muscle refer pain and tenderness primarily to the region of the head of the first metatarsal on both its plantar and medial aspects (Fig. 27.2*B*), with a spillover pattern that may include all of the great toe and much of the second toe. Kelly[38] described pain radiating from a "fibrositic" lesion [TrP] in the flexor hallucis brevis muscle as causing cramps in the foot.

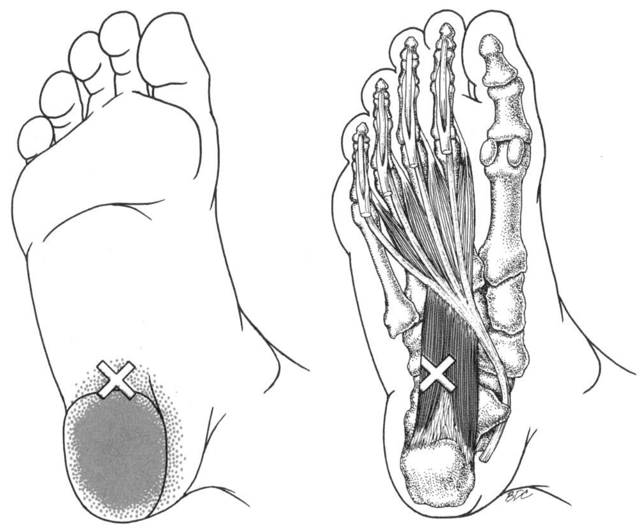

Figure 27.1. Pain pattern (*bright red*) referred from a trigger point (***X***) in the deeply placed quadratus plantae muscle (*darker red*) of the right foot. *Solid red* portrays the essential referred pain pattern; *red stippling* shows the spillover of the essential pattern. The lumbrical muscles are not colored.

PART 3

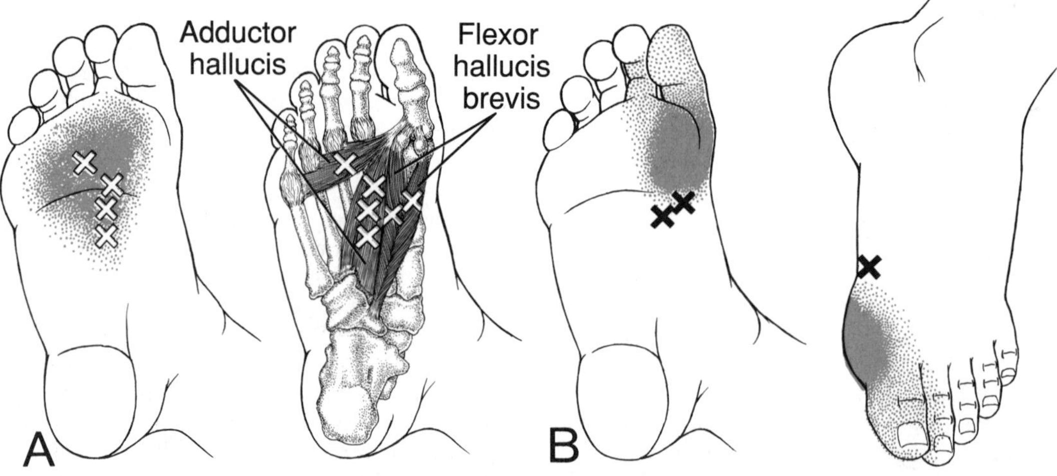

Figure 27.2. Pain patterns (*bright red*) referred from trigger points (**X***s*) in two deep intrinsic muscles of the right foot, as viewed during examination. Essential referred pain patterns are *solid red* and a spillover of the essential pattern appears as *red stippling*. *A*, adductor hallucis muscle, oblique and transverse heads (*light red*). *B*, flexor hallucis brevis muscle (*dark red*).

An isolated pain pattern for the **flexor digiti minimi brevis** is not established; it appears to be similar to that of the abductor digiti minimi muscle (*see* Fig. 26.3*A*).

As in the interossei of the hand, TrPs in **interosseous muscles of the foot** refer pain and tenderness largely to the side of the digit to which the tendon attaches; however, in the case of the foot, these TrPs also refer pain both to the dorsum and to the sole of the foot along the distal portion of the corresponding metatarsal. Figure 27.3*A* illustrates this pattern for the first dorsal interosseous muscle from the dorsal view and Figure 27.3*B* shows it from the plantar view.[70,71] In addition, TrPs in the first dorsal interosseus muscle may produce tingling in the great toe; the disturbance of sensation can include the dorsum of the foot and lower shin. The plantar interossei produce a pattern comparable to that of the dorsal interossei. The separate pain patterns of the **lumbricals** are not confirmed, but it is likely that their patterns are similar to that of corresponding interossei.

Kellgren[36] reported a patient who complained of pain in and under the metatarsal heads and in the outside of the foot and ankle; the patient experienced pain with each step and walked with a limp. When the tender region in the third interosseous space was infiltrated with 3 mL of procaine solution, the pain was reproduced momentarily and then was abolished so that he could again walk normally. Kellgren also reported[37] that injection of approximately 0.2 mL of a 6% hypertonic solution of sodium chloride into the first dorsal interosseous muscle caused pain in the lateral half of the foot and in the calf of the leg.

2. ANATOMICAL ATTACHMENTS AND CONSIDERATIONS
(Figs. 27.4 and 27.5)

The reader is referred to Figure 18.2 in this volume for a drawing of the bones of the foot. Careful review of this figure along with anatomical considerations of muscles and ligaments may help the reader understand the relationship between the structure and function of the foot.

The quadratus plantae and the lumbricals, both muscles of the second muscular layer on the plantar aspect of the foot, attach to tendon slips of the flexor digitorum longus (Fig. 27.4*A*). The **quadratus plantae** (flexor accessorius) muscle has two heads. Its larger, medial head attaches ***proximally*** to the medial side of the calcaneus, and the flat tendinous lateral head attaches ***proximally*** to the lateral side of that bone and to the long plantar ligament. The two heads are separated by the long plantar ligament and converge ***distally*** at an acute angle to join the lateral margin of the tendon and the tendon

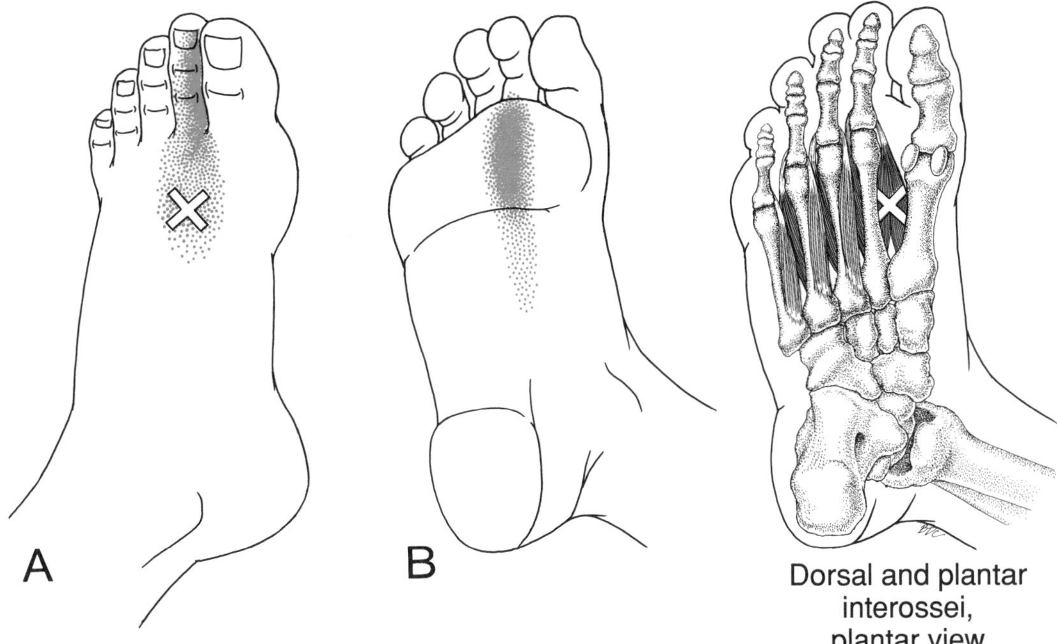

Figure 27.3. Typical pain pattern (*bright red*) referred from a trigger point (**X**) in the right first dorsal interosseous muscle. The dorsal interosseous muscles are *medium red* and the plantar interosseous muscles are *light red*. *A*, dorsal view. *B*, plantar view.

slips of the flexor digitorum longus.[14,52] The lateral plantar vessels and nerve lie between this muscle and the superficial layer of intrinsic muscles.

Sometimes the lateral head of the quadratus plantae, or even the entire muscle, is missing. The muscle also varies as to the number of digital flexor tendons that receive its muscular slips.[14]

Starting at a ***proximal*** attachment to the flexor digitorum longus tendon near the midplantar region, the **lumbricals** extend ***distally*** to the expansion of the extensor digitorum longus tendon of each of the four lesser toes (Fig. 27.4*A*).[14,52] Each lumbrical arises from two adjacent tendons except the first, which arises along the medial surface of the flexor digitorum longus tendon to the second toe. The lumbrical tendons pass on the plantar side of the deep transverse metatarsal ligaments to reach their distal attachments on the medial surface of the extensor expansion. At times, they may be attached to the bone of the first phalanx. One or more lumbricals may be absent.[14]

The third layer of muscles on the plantar aspect of the foot includes the longitudinally oriented short flexors of the great and fifth toes, the transverse head of the adductor hallucis and the more longitudinally oriented oblique head of this adductor muscle (Fig. 27.4*B*).[14]

The **flexor digiti minimi brevis** attaches ***proximally*** to the base of the fifth metatarsal and ***distally*** to the lateral side of the base of the proximal phalanx of the fifth toe (Fig. 27.4*B*).[14,30]

When the deeper fibers of the human flexor digiti minimi brevis attach to the ligament that joins the fifth metatarsal and cuboid, and then extend distally to the lateral part of the distal half of the fifth metatarsal, they are sometimes identified as the **opponens digiti minimi**,[14,30,76] an arrangement that is characteristic in apes.

The **adductor hallucis** muscle has two heads (Fig. 27.4*B*). The *oblique head* slants diagonally across the first four metatarsal bones. It anchors ***proximally*** onto the bases of the second, third, and fourth metatarsal bones and onto the sheath of the tendon of the peroneus longus; it at-

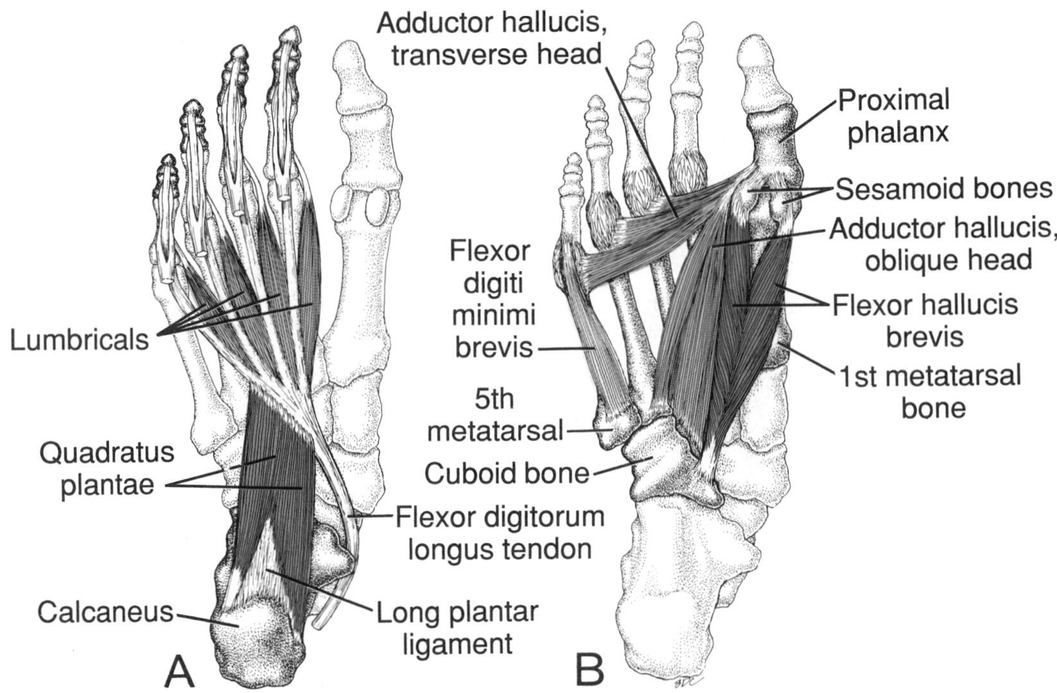

Figure 27.4. Anatomical attachments of intermediate-depth plantar muscles of the right foot, plantar view. *A*, in second muscular layer: quadratus plantae (*dark red*) and lumbricals (*medium red*). *B*, in third muscular layer: flexor hallucis brevis (*dark red*), oblique and transverse heads of the adductor hallucis (*medium red*), and flexor digiti minimi brevis (*light red*).

taches ***distally*** to the lateral aspect of the base of the proximal phalanx of the large toe together with the lateral part of the flexor hallucis brevis. The *transverse head* spans the space superficial to the second through fourth metatarsal heads. Its fasciculi attach ***laterally*** to the plantar metatarsophalangeal (MP) ligaments of the third, fourth, and fifth toes and to the transverse metatarsal ligaments of the same digits. ***Medially***, fasciculi of the transverse head join to attach to the lateral aspect of the base of the proximal phalanx of the large toe, blending with the tendon of the oblique head.[14,29]

Valvo *et al.*[75] found that the conjoined tendon of the two heads of the adductor hallucis muscle consistently passed through the bifurcation in the most medial deep transverse metatarsal ligament. At times, a portion of the muscle may attach to the first metatarsal bone, forming an **opponens hallucis** muscle.[14]

The two heads of the **flexor hallucis brevis** anchor ***proximally*** by a common tendon to adjacent surfaces of the cuboid and lateral cuneiform bones (Fig. 27.4*B*) and to the adjacent part of the attachment of the tibialis posterior tendon. ***Distally***, the two heads attach to the medial and lateral aspects of the base of the proximal phalanx of the large toe. A sesamoid bone is present in each tendon at its distal attachment. An additional slip of the flexor hallucis brevis may attach to the proximal phalanx of the second toe.[14]

The interossei are located in the fourth muscular layer on the plantar aspect of the foot. Figure 27.5*A* shows attachments of the **dorsal interossei**. Their action is relative to the midline of the second toe. The four dorsal interossei are each bipennate muscles located between two metatarsal bones. Each dorsal interosseous anchors ***proximally*** to the two adjacent metatarsal bones and attaches ***distally*** to the base of the proximal phalanx and to the aponeurosis of the tendon of the extensor digitorum longus on the side of the toe toward which it pulls.[14] (The first dorsal interosseous attaches to the medial side of the proximal phalanx of the second toe; the remaining three tendons are

PART 3

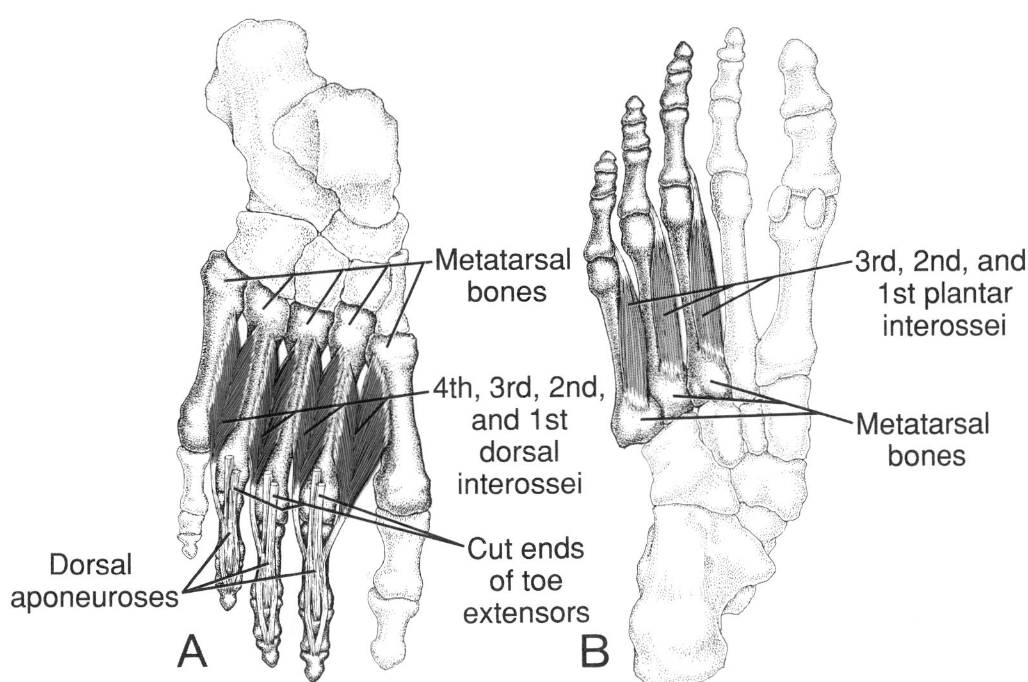

Figure 27.5. Anatomical attachments of the interossei in the deep (fourth) layer on the plantar aspect of the right foot. *A*, dorsal view of the dorsal interossei (*dark red*). *B*, plantar view of the plantar interossei (*light red*).

attached to the lateral sides of the second, third, and fourth toes.) Manter[44] contends that the dorsal interossei rarely continue dorsally into the extensor aponeurosis.

The three **plantar interossei** appear in Figure 27.5*B*. Each muscle anchors ***proximally*** to the base of the related metatarsal and attaches ***distally*** to the medial side of the base of the proximal phalanx of the corresponding toe and usually to the dorsal aponeurosis of that extensor digitorum longus tendon.[14] The pennate belly of each plantar interosseous muscle lies along the plantar surface of its corresponding metatarsal, as seen in Figure 27.5*B* and in the cross-sectional view of Figure 27.9.

Kalin and Hirsch[35] point out that, although most current anatomy texts make no mention of the fact, the interossei characteristically have extensive soft tissue origins that should significantly influence their function across the tarsometatarsal joints and ensure that the interossei contract in a coordinated manner to perform their role as stabilizers of the forefoot. These authors reported a detailed study of 69 interosseous muscles in ten feet of ten different subjects and made additional observations on 115 feet. They[35] found that 88% of the dorsal interossei and 93% of the plantar interossei originated not only from bone but also from soft tissue, including the epimysium of other muscles, a slip of the peroneus longus tendon, or the ligamentous network. This ligamentous network comprises intertwining fibers of the tarsometatarsal joint capsules, the intermediate and long plantar ligaments, and the peroneal sheath. The medial head of the first dorsal interosseous in all ten subjects received a slip of the peroneus longus tendon. In other studies, 64.3% of 115 feet[35] and 63.5% of 149 feet[44] exhibited this structure. Consistently, the muscles of the fourth ray (the second plantar and the fourth dorsal interossei) were the largest of the interossei, extended the furthest proximally, and had the most extensive areas of origin.[35] Most noteworthy, 73% of the individual muscles studied arose partly from another muscle or muscles, usually a crossover between dorsal and plantar interosseus muscles. This interweaving of origins was least common among interossei along the sides of the foot and most common among the more centrally located interossei. In apes, the longitudinal axis of the foot passes through the third digit as in the human hand. In man, the axis of the foot now passes through the second toe. This recent evolutionary change probably contributes to the large variety of anatomical variations.[44]

Supplemental References

The quadratus plantae, as listed here, was sometimes indexed and labeled as the **flexor accessorius** muscle.

Plantar View Without Major Vessels or Nerves. Drawings portray the quadratus plantae,[2,14] the lumbricals,[2,14] the flexor digiti minimi brevis,[5,15] the adductor hallucis,[15] the flexor hallucis brevis,[5,15] and both the dorsal and plantar interossei[5,16,25,60] without vessels or nerves. Photographs record the quadratus plantae,[47,52,65] the lumbricals,[47,51,52,64,65,67] the flexor digiti minimi brevis,[51-53,64-66] the adductor hallucis,[47,48,53,66] the flexor hallucis brevis,[47,48,53,66] and both the dorsal and plantar interossei[47,48,54] without major vessels or nerves.

Plantar View With Vessels or Nerves. Drawings show the medial and lateral plantar nerves in relation to the quadratus plantae,[4,23,57,59] the lumbricals,[23,57,59] the flexor digiti minimi brevis,[4,59] the adductor hallucis,[4,59] the flexor hallucis brevis,[4,57,59] and plantar interosseous muscles.[59] One drawing[59] also shows the medial and lateral plantar arteries; this drawing includes the sesamoid bones in the flexor hallucis brevis tendons at the first MP joint.

Dorsal View. Dorsal view drawings present the dorsal interossei without vessels or nerves[16,25,60] and with the deep peroneal veins and artery.[58] A photograph shows the dorsal interossei very clearly.[50]

Medial View. Seen from the medial view without blood vessels or nerves, the quadratus plantae and flexor hallucis brevis appear in a drawing[3] and the quadratus plantae appears in a photograph.[63]

Cross Sections. A series of cross sections identifies the relations to surrounding structures of the quadratus plantae,[10] lumbricals, flexor digiti minimi brevis, dorsal and plantar interossei,[12] adductor hallucis,[13] and the flexor hallucis brevis.[11] A section through the metatarsals identifies the flexor digiti minimi brevis, flexor hallucis brevis, adductor hallucis, and the dorsal and plantar interossei.[22]

Sagittal Sections. A sagittal section through the second toe shows the surroundings of the adductor hallucis,[55] and one through the fifth toe shows those of the flexor digiti minimi brevis.[56]

Skeletal Attachments. Marks on the bones identify the skeletal attachments of the quadratus plantae,[6,7,24,49] the flexor digiti minimi brevis,[7,24,49] the adductor hallucis,[7,24,46,49] the flexor hallucis brevis,[7,24,46,49] and the dorsal and plantar interossei.[46,49]

3. INNERVATION

Of the muscles covered in this chapter, only the flexor hallucis brevis and the first lumbrical are supplied by the medial plantar nerve, which contains fibers from the fifth lumbar and first sacral spinal nerves. The other muscles of this chapter are supplied by the lateral plantar nerve that carries fibers from the second and third sacral spinal nerves.[14] These muscles include the quadratus plantae, the second, third, and fourth lumbricals, the flexor digiti minimi brevis, the adductor hallucis, and all interossei.

4. FUNCTION

During upright activities, muscles of the foot provide flexibility for shock absorption and balance, and rigidity for the stability needed during propulsion. In general, the intrinsic muscles of the foot function as a unit. The electromyographic (EMG) activity of these muscles closely parallels the progressive supination at the subtalar joint during level, uphill, and downhill walking. These muscles stabilize the foot at the subtalar and transverse tarsal joints during propulsion.[42] It has been suggested that the interossei help the toes adjust to variations in terrain, and that through their extensive soft tissue origins they may serve a role as stabilizers of the forefoot, "rendering the tarsometatarsal joints rigid when weight is carried on the ball of the foot."[35]

Actions

The **quadratus plantae** muscle assists the flexor digitorum longus in flexion of the terminal phalanges of the four lesser toes.[14,27,28,61] Because of the angle at which it attaches to the flexor digitorum longus tendon, the quadratus plantae centers the line of pull of the flexor digitorum longus on the fifth and, to a lesser extent, on the fourth and third toes. The line of pull by the flexor digitorum longus on the second toe is relatively straight and needs no correction.[28,34] The quadratus plantae produces flexion of the four lesser toes even in the absence of flexor digitorum longus activity. The quadratus plantae also provides proximal stability to the lumbrical muscles of the foot.[34]

The four **lumbricals** in the foot flex the proximal phalanges at the MP joints and extend the two distal phalanges at the interphalangeal (IP) joints of the four lesser toes.[14,28,61] This action is analogous to the actions of the lumbricals in the hand.[14]

The **flexor digiti minimi brevis** muscle flexes the proximal phalanx of the small toe at the MP joint.[14,61]

The **adductor hallucis** adducts the great toe (draws it toward the second toe).[27,61] It also assists in flexion of the proximal phalanx of the great toe and in maintaining transverse plane stability.[14] The oblique head of this muscle, on stimulation, produced adduction that was more forceful than that of the lateral head of the flexor hallucis brevis.[17]

The **flexor hallucis brevis** flexes the proximal phalanx of the great toe at the MP joint.[14,61] On stimulation, the medial head of this muscle abducted the proximal phalanx and the lateral head adducted it toward the second toe.[17]

The actions of the dorsal and plantar **interossei** are in relation to the longitudinal axis of the second toe. The dorsal interossei abduct the second, third, and fourth toes (they abduct the second toe in each direction away from its own long axis, and they abduct the third and fourth toes away from the second toe). The dorsal interossei also flex the proximal phalanges and weakly extend the two distal phalanges through the extensor mechanism of the second, third, and fourth toes.[14,17,27,31,61] Some authors have noted an *absence* of interosseus attachment to the extensor mechanism, which would leave only the lumbricals to extend the IP joints.[33]

The plantar interossei adduct the third, fourth, and fifth toes toward the second toe and also are flexors of the proximal phalanges.[14,27,61] They may act as extensors of the distal phalanges of the third, fourth, and fifth toes, but only if they insert into the extensor mechanism.[31]

Functions

Muscle activity is not necessary to support the arches of the fully loaded foot at rest.[42]

According to Basmajian and Deluca,[9] an important role of the intrinsic muscles is stabilization of the foot during propulsion, acting mainly at the subtalar and transverse tarsal joints. The excessively pronated foot requires greater intrinsic muscle activity for stabilization than does the normal foot.[42]

The **quadratus plantae** changes the posteromedial pull of the flexor digitorum longus into that of pure flexion of the toes and may be especially valuable in flexing the toes when the weight-bearing foot is dorsiflexing at the ankle.[28]

Normal function of the **flexor hallucis brevis** apparently helps prevent clawing of the great toe. Clawing of the great toe with hallux varus may result from severance of the lateral tendon of the flexor hallucis brevis when the lateral sesamoid bone is removed during a McBride surgical procedure.[74]

The **lumbricals** add leverage for the toes to dig in more effectively when walking on soft sand, and they apparently function in conjunction with the interossei to provide stabilization of the forefoot. Although the lumbricals do not cross the tarsometatarsal joints, they influence the stability of those joints (in conjunction with contraction of the quadratus plantae) when weight is carried on the ball of the foot, as during push-off at the end of stance phase.[35] The lumbricals may also function during the swing phase of gait to prevent excessive extension of the MP joints that would otherwise be created by the extensor digitorum longus.[33]

The **interossei** show vigorous electrical activity from midstance to toe-off;[32,42] they contribute to stabilization of the forefoot when the heel is off the ground and the foot is subject to extension at the tarsometatarsal joints late in stance phase and during push-off. In addition, the interossei help the toes adjust to variations in terrain.[35] Jarrett and associates[33] suggest that the interossei function during the stance phase of gait to check the pull of the flexor digitorum longus and brevis, thereby allowing straight toe function for stabilization against the ground.

The **adductor hallucis** helps stabilize the forefoot (metatarsal head region) in the transverse plane.

PART 3

5. FUNCTIONAL (MYOTATIC) UNIT

The **quadratus plantae**, **flexors digitorum longus and brevis**, **lumbricals**, and **interossei** function as a team to flex the four lesser toes and to control their extension. Their antagonists are the extensors digitorum longus and brevis.

The **flexor digiti minimi brevis**, abductor digiti minimi, the **fourth lumbrical**, and the **third plantar interosseus** muscles function together to flex the fifth toe. They are opposed by the tendon slips of the extensors digitorum longus and brevis that attach to the fifth toe.

The **adductor hallucis** and **flexor hallucis brevis** form a functional unit to control the positioning of, and the force exerted by, the great toe.

The dorsal and plantar interossei together with the lumbricals control abduction and adduction efforts of the four lesser toes.

6. SYMPTOMS

Patients with TrPs in the deep intrinsic foot muscles are likely to present with marked limitation of walking due to pain, and they may complain of numbness of the foot and a feeling that it is swollen. The altered sensation usually includes the entire distal end of the foot and is not limited to only one toe. This altered sensation is especially likely to arise from TrPs in the flexor digiti minimi brevis, flexor hallucis brevis, or adductor hallucis muscles. Patients with TrPs in these muscles often have tried orthoses inserted in the shoes, but usually quickly remove them because of intolerably greater pain from the increased pressure on the TrPs and tender reference zones.

Muscular imbalances and articular dysfunctions of the foot may lead to problems in any proximal segment of the body, including the knee, hip, pelvis, and spine.

The pain complaints of patients with involvement of the deep foot intrinsic muscles are often combined with myofascial patterns of TrPs in other muscles that refer pain to the foot.

Active or latent TrPs in the dorsal interosseus muscles can be associated with **hammer toes**. The deformation of the toes may disappear after inactivation of these TrPs, especially in younger patients.

DIFFERENTIAL DIAGNOSIS

Other Myofascial Pain Syndromes

Because patients often have active TrPs in several foot and leg muscles at the same time, one sees many combinations of pain referral patterns.

Quadratus Plantae. The quadratus plantae TrPs refer pain and tenderness to the bottom of the heel (Fig. 27.1), whereas both the gastrocnemius TrP_1 (*see* Fig. 21.1) and flexor digitorum longus TrPs (*see* Fig. 25.1) refer pain and tenderness to the instep, anterior to the heel. The heel referral pattern of soleus TrP_1 (*see* Fig. 22.1) is more extensive than that of the quadratus plantae. The soleus TrP referral covers not only the plantar surface of the heel, but usually extends over the back of the heel and part of the way up the Achilles tendon. The pattern of the tibialis posterior TrPs (*see* Fig. 23.1) may spill over to the heel, but focuses primarily on the Achilles tendon above the heel. Pain and tenderness referred from the abductor hallucis muscle (*see* Fig. 26.2) concentrates along only the medial border of the heel, whereas the quadratus plantae referral pattern covers the plantar surface of the heel.

Adductor Hallucis. The adductor hallucis refers pain and tenderness to the plantar surface of much of the forefoot (Fig. 27.2*A*), but gastrocnemius TrP_1 (*see* Fig. 21.1) usually refers more proximally to the instep. Distinguishing the more restricted pain and tenderness of interosseous TrPs (that usually include a strong pattern to one toe) ordinarily is not much of a problem. Both the flexor digitorum longus (*see* Fig. 25.1) and the flexor digitorum brevis (*see* Fig. 26.3*B*) refer pain and tenderness to the plantar surface of the forefoot in an area that could easily be confused with the pattern of the adductor hallucis. When the pain complaint includes the plantar surface of the forefoot, the former two muscles and the adductor hallucis should be examined.

Flexor Hallucis Brevis. Flexor hallucis brevis TrPs refer pain and tenderness mainly to the region of the head of the first metatarsal with only a spillover pattern to the great toe (Fig. 27.2*B*), whereas TrPs in the tibialis anterior muscle refer primarily to the great toe itself (*see* Fig. 19.1). The extensor hallucis longus TrPs refer only to the dorsal side of the head of the first metatarsal bone (*see* Fig. 24.1*B*), and not to the medial and plantar sides as does the flexor hallucis brevis. The referred pain pattern of the flexor hallucis longus TrPs (*see* Fig. 25.1*B*) usually includes only the plantar surface of both the first metatarsal head and the great toe.

Interossei. The ray-specific pain pattern of TrPs in an interosseous muscle (Fig. 27.3*A* and *B*), which includes both the plantar region of the corresponding metatarsal head and the adjacent side of the corresponding toe, is not likely to be confused with the pain pattern discussed previously under the adductor hallucis muscle, unless several adjacent interossei harbor active TrPs.

Myofascial TrPs in a dorsal interosseous muscle can contribute to a hammer toe deformity, apparently by weakening the muscle.

Other Conditions

The reader is referred to McGlamry's two-volume textbook for comprehensive information on conditions that affect the foot.[45] Other conditions deserving consideration include plantar fasciitis, hallux valgus, stress fractures, calcaneal compartment syndrome, nerve entrapment, articular dysfunction, and an injured sesamoid bone.

The pain and tenderness caused by TrPs of the quadratus plantae muscle may masquerade as **plantar fasciitis**. Chapter 26 reviews this condition on pages 509–510.

Hallux valgus is a progressive deformity that can relate to contracture of numerous periarticular structures of the first MP joint. These structures include (but are not limited to) the lateral collateral ligament and the joint capsule, the *adductor hallucis* muscle and tendons, the *lateral head of the flexor hallucis brevis*, and its fibular sesamoid.[69] An EMG study revealed that in subjects with hallux valgus, while the adductor hallucis activity was markedly decreased, the abductor hallucis activity was *nil*, and so a weak adductor force was operative.[9] Adductor hallucis tenotomy has been reported to be effective in relieving hallux valgus.[74] To our knowledge, the possible contribution to hallux valgus by TrPs in the adductor hallucis (which could shorten the muscle without increased EMG activity) has not been investigated.

Alfred and Bergfeld[1] reviewed **stress fractures of the foot**. Stress fracture of the calcaneus can occur at any age and cause chronic heel pain that eludes diagnosis because it usually requires a bone scan for diagnosis. Stress fracture of the navicular is rare and is easily disregarded because arch pain is so common in adults. Usually the patient with the latter stress fracture has pain and swelling along both the dorsum of the foot and the medial arch that are worse after activity and at the end of the day. Metatarsal stress fractures cause aching pain in the forefoot and are found often among military recruits and ballet dancers. The key to diagnosis is spot tenderness over the affected metatarsal.[1]

Manoli and Weber[43] investigated why three patients with calcaneal fractures developed clawing of the lesser toes as a late sequela. Examination of 17 lower limb specimens revealed a previously unidentified separate compartment of the hindfoot, a calcaneal compartment that contains the *quadratus plantae* muscle. The authors concluded that the clawtoe deformities were late sequelae to an unrecognized **calcaneal compartment syndrome** that led to contracture of the quadratus plantae muscle. The authors proposed a surgical technique for release of this compartment in case such a compartment syndrome developed in association with a calcaneal fracture.

The pattern of heel pain characteristic of TrPs in the quadratus plantae may also be caused by **entrapment** of the first branch of the lateral plantar nerve. An extensive anatomical study showed that the most likely location of entrapment was where the nerve coursed between the *abductor hallucis* muscle and the medial head of the *quadratus plantae* muscle.[68] The mechanism of entrapment was not clear.

Articular dysfunction (either hypermobility or hypomobility) of the foot can seriously disturb foot mechanics and produce imbalances that may cause pain in many locations, ranging from the feet to the head and neck.

Other **structural deviations** can be a source of disturbed foot mechanics. Such deviations include: hindfoot varus or valgus, forefoot varus or valgus, equinus, hypermobility or malposition of the first ray, and an excessively high arch.

Injury of a **sesamoid bone** in the flexor hallucis brevis tendon can disable an athlete.[62] A specific single injury rarely initiates the pain; it appears to result from repetitive stress. The pain is usually poorly localized about the MP joint of the great toe. With gentle pressure, the examiner can elicit local tenderness over the sesamoid bone and can usually elicit pain about the joint with passive extension of the great toe. The symptoms may be caused by sesamoiditis, osteochondritis, simple stress fracture of the sesamoid, or a displaced sesamoid fracture, and are ordinarily responsive to conservative therapy.[62]

Deviation of the second toe so that it overlapped the great toe resulted from **traumatic rupture** of both the dorsal lateral MP collateral ligament and the second interosseous tendon in two cases.[26] Surgical repair was required in both cases.

7. ACTIVATION AND PERPETUATION OF TRIGGER POINTS

Activation

The factors that activate and perpetuate TrPs in the superficial intrinsic muscles of the foot, discussed in Chapter 26 on pages 510–511, are also likely to do the same to these deep intrinsic muscles. A tight shoe cap (vamp) that has an inadequate vertical dimension of the shoe covering the forefoot restricts toe movement and can be a major activator and perpetuator of TrPs in most of the deep intrinsic toe muscles. The TrPs in the interossei are more likely to be activated and perpetuated by a shoe that is too short than by a tight vamp.

TrPs can be activated in these muscles at the time of a fracture of the ankle or other bones of the foot. The TrPs are then aggravated by a cast that immobilizes the foot for some time.

Other traumas to these deep intrinsic foot muscles, such as bruising, banging, stubbing toes, and falling, can also activate TrPs in them.

Perpetuation

Walking in soft sand, walking or running on uneven or sloped surfaces, chilling the feet in cold water, or wearing wet socks in cold weather can aggravate and perpetuate these TrPs, especially when the muscles are fatigued.

Impaired mobility of the joints of the foot can perpetuate TrPs in the intrinsic foot muscles that cross those joints. Blockage of motion in the second, third, and fourth tarsometatarsal joints is common and easily determined.[41]

The Morton foot structure and other causes of a *hyper*pronated foot, when uncorrected, may contribute significantly to the perpetuation of TrPs in the intrinsic foot muscles. Pronation during early stance is normal; it is *hyper*pronation that becomes a problem.

An inflexible sole of the shoe (a wooden sole or shoe with a steel bar placed the length of the sole) limits movement of the forefoot sufficiently to perpetuate TrPs in deep intrinsic muscles.

Systemic conditions including gout of the great toe (podagra) that may perpetuate TrPs in the intrinsic foot muscles are considered on pages 115–155 of Volume 1.[73]

8. PATIENT EXAMINATION

The status of arterial circulation is examined by palpating for the dorsalis pedis and posterior tibial pulses. The skin and nails are examined for lesions, and the skin is examined for color, temperature, and edema.

The clinician should observe the patient walking barefoot, noting particularly excessive supination or pronation of the foot. An antalgic gait alerts one to ask about sore feet, if the patient has not already volunteered this complaint. The patient may respond, "Yes, of course, but don't everyone's feet hurt?" He or she cannot remember when the feet did not hurt; it has become an accepted part of life.[72]

The patient with active TrPs in the deep muscles of the forefoot is unable to hop on the sore foot.

The clinician examines the feet for configuration and for restricted range of motion of the toes in flexion and extension. Myofascial TrPs painfully restrict the stretch range of motion; strength and active contraction in the shortened position are also usually limited by pain.

The two-part screening test described by Lewit[41] for detection of restricted joint movement in the feet is simple and effective. In the first part, the patient rests the heel of the relaxed foot on the examining table and the clinician grasps a side of the forefoot in each hand, then tries to rotate the forefoot around the long axis of the foot. The center of rotation passes through the head of the talus. Blockage of tarsometatarsal joint movement may restrict rotation in either or both directions. The second part tests pronation and supination by swinging the forefoot back and forth around the subtalar joint. Restriction of this motion indicates blockage of joints proximal to the tarsometatarsal joints. If this screening test is positive, then the individual joints should be examined for restriction of mobility.[41]

Any patient with sore intrinsic foot muscles, particularly if associated with inflammation of the first MP joint (podagra), should be checked for crystal deposition disease.

The feet should be examined for structural deviations such as a Morton foot structure (Chapter 20), hindfoot varus or valgus, forefoot varus or valgus, equinus, hypermobility or malposition of the first ray, excessively high arch, hallux valgus, and hammer toes. The presence and thickness of calluses are important. The patient's shoes should be examined for a tight vamp, a rigid distal sole, and abnormal wear that indicates distorted foot mechanics.

The strength of MP flexion of the great toe tests the flexor hallucis brevis and, to some extent, the abductor hallucis and adductor hallucis muscles. This test is performed by stabilizing the forefoot and resisting flexion of the great toe at the proximal phalanx.[39] Some examiners test the strength of the interossei by resisting the patient's attempt to extend the IP joints[40] of the four lesser toes, while stabilizing the MP joints with the foot held in 20-30° plantar flexion. This test may be more an indication of lumbrical strength than of interosseus strength.[33] Interosseus strength may be estimated by springing the proximal phalanges of the toes both medially and laterally while the subject attempts to hold the toes spread apart. The examiner must keep in mind, however, that many individuals cannot perform these toe movements well.

9. TRIGGER POINT EXAMINATION (Fig. 27.6)

Quadratus Plantae. To examine the quadratus plantae for TrPs, the clinician must use deep palpation (Fig. 27.6*A*) and exert sufficient pressure to penetrate deep to the plantar aponeurosis with the toes slightly extended. Spot tenderness is usually clearly definable, but one should not expect to feel a taut band in this muscle.

Flexor Hallucis Brevis. Because the plantar aponeurosis covers much of the flexor hallucis brevis, the medial head of this muscle is most effectively palpated using flat palpation through the thinner skin along the medial margin of the sole of the foot (Fig. 27.6*B*). Lateral head TrPs must be examined for spot tenderness by deep palpation through the plantar surface of the foot. The tendon of the abductor hallucis should not be mistaken for a taut band in the flexor hallucis brevis. Occasionally, the taut band of a TrP is palpable in the medial head of the flexor hallucis brevis against the underlying first metatarsal bone.

Adductor Hallucis. To create a moderate stretch on the muscle, the great toe is gently abducted passively during examination. The adductor hallucis must be palpated through the plantar aponeurosis in the distal forefoot proximal to the heads of the four lesser metatarsals. The transverse head of the muscle extends across the foot just proximal to the metatarsal heads (Fig. 27.6*C*, *fully rendered finger*) and the oblique head angles slightly across the instep from the bases of the second, third, and fourth metatarsals (Figs. 27.4*B* and 27.6*C*, *outlined finger*). Only rarely is a taut band of either head palpable; however, one can detect TrP tenderness.

Interossei. The interossei and lumbricals may be palpated between adjacent metatarsal bones using a bimanual technique as illustrated in Figure 27.6*D*. This technique tends to separate these bones and to increase the stretch on the muscles. The dorsal interossei are palpated by the finger of one hand with precise counter pressure applied on the plantar surface by a finger of the other hand. Then tenderness in the lumbricals and plantar interossei can be elicited by deep palpation through the plantar aponeurosis against counter pressure applied to the dorsal surface by the other hand. One often can palpate the taut bands of active TrPs in a *dorsal* interosseus muscle against the adjacent metatarsal bone to which it attaches. In that case, one may

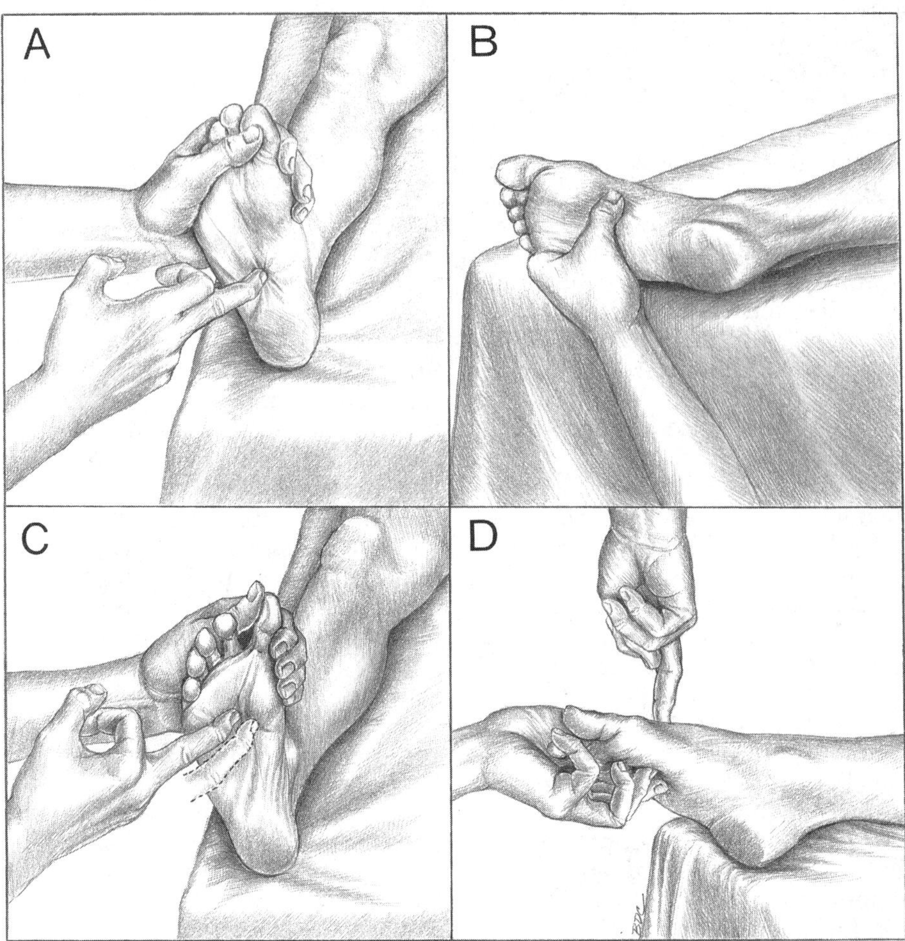

Figure 27.6. Examination of deep intrinsic muscles of the right foot for active trigger points. *A*, quadratus plantae using deep palpation. *B*, flexor hallucis brevis using flat palpation, *C*, adductor hallucis, transverse head (*fully rendered finger*) and oblique head (*finger with dashed outline*) using flat or deep palpation. *D*, interossei and lumbricals, bimanual technique that uses the finger of one hand for palpation while the finger of the other hand provides counter pressure.

elicit a local twitch response by snapping palpation of an active TrP. However, one cannot distinguish between the lumbricals and *plantar* interossei by palpation through the plantar aponeurosis and/or the oblique head of the adductor hallucis muscle.

Flexor Digiti Minimi Brevis. It is rarely possible to distinguish by palpation the flexor digiti minimi brevis from the abductor digiti minimi that lies beside it laterally. Usually, making the distinction is not important. Both are palpated by pincer palpation along the lateral border of the foot beside and plantar to the fifth metatarsal. Sometimes, the abductor digiti minimi is essentially tendinous in this region and the only muscle being palpated is the flexor digiti minimi brevis. In some patients, taut bands are palpable and local twitch responses can be elicited in this fifth toe flexor.

10. ENTRAPMENTS

No nerve entrapments have been identified that were due to TrP tension in these deep intrinsic foot muscles.

11. ASSOCIATED TRIGGER POINTS

Single-muscle myofascial pain syndromes are sometimes seen in the feet (for example, in the interossei). However, in the complex chronic cases seen in the au-

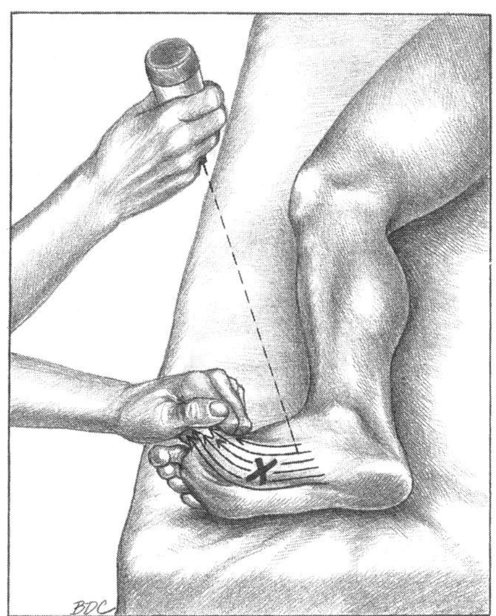

Figure 27.7. Stretch position and intermittent cold pattern (*thin arrows*) for a trigger point (**X**) in the right flexor hallucis brevis muscle. The great toe is extended at the metatarsophalangeal joint (ankle position neutral). Intermittent cold with passive stretch of all short flexors of the toes may be combined (*see* Fig. 26.6*D*) by simultaneously extending all five toes and applying parallel sweeps of the coolant to the plantar surface of the entire forefoot. If hypermobility of the tarsometatarsal region is present, the intermittent cold can be applied prior to the stretch, then the clinician's other hand can be used to stabilize the midfoot.

thors' practices, when one of these deep intrinsic muscles of the foot is involved, several others are usually involved also.

12. INTERMITTENT COLD WITH STRETCH

(Fig. 27.7)

For lasting relief, any *hypo*mobile joints in the foot should be mobilized, either prior to or following inactivation of TrPs.

The use of ice for applying intermittent cold with stretch is explained on page 9 of this volume and the use of vapocoolant spray with stretch is detailed on pages 67–74 of Volume 1.[73] Techniques that augment relaxation and stretch are reviewed on pages 10–11 of this volume.

Myofascial TrPs in the **flexor hallucis brevis** muscle respond to intermittent cold with stretch applied as illustrated in Figure 27.7. With the patient in the side-lying position, parallel applications of vapocoolant spray or ice (using the dry edge of a plastic-covered ice cube) cover the medial half of the plantar surface of the forefoot as the operator extends the great toe. The ankle in this case remains in the neutral position. If one wishes also to include release of **adductor hallucis** TrPs, the intermittent cold pattern is extended to include all of the plantar surface of the forefoot and the great toe is passively abducted as well as extended.

If the tarsometatarsal region of the foot is *hyper*mobile, that region should be stabilized by one hand while the other hand takes up slack in the muscles being lengthened. In this case, the intermittent cold can be applied prior to, rather than during, the stretch.

The remaining deep intrinsic muscles of the foot are not readily amenable to intermittent cold with stretch as individual muscles, but can be managed as a group. The technique illustrated in Figure 26.6*C* (of the previous chapter) for releasing TrPs in the flexor digitorum brevis also releases TrPs in the **quadratus plantae** and **flexor digiti minimi brevis**. The ankle should *not* be dorsiflexed at the same time, because tension in the flexor digitorum longus would then block full stretch of the quadratus plantae.

It is important when treating groups of muscles in this way to devote a few minutes to their antagonists to prevent reactive cramping. In this case, one must consider the extensor digitorum brevis and the extensor hallucis brevis muscles. The concept and prevention of reactive cramping (shortening activation) are reviewed on page 19 of this volume.

The complex actions of the interossei and lumbricals and their frequent interconnections complicate efforts to release their TrPs by intermittent cold with stretch. It is possible to stretch a dorsal interosseous muscle between its two adjacent metatarsals by moving one metatarsal dorsally while moving the other in a plantar direction and, at the same time, separating the heads of the two metatarsals transversely. Techniques of deep massage and injection may be more effective for these muscles. Alternative methods of treatment are reviewed on pages 9–10 of this volume.

Evjenth and Hamberg[18] illustrate and describe clearly how to stretch each head of the flexor hallucis brevis by extending the MP joint of the great toe. Using that technique, an assistant could apply sweeps of the intermittent cold distalward over the muscle and its referred pain pattern. Similarly, they present the technique for stretching the lumbricals,[19] for simultaneously stretching the second, third, and fourth dorsal interossei, for stretching the flexor digiti minimi brevis with the abductor digiti minimi,[21] and for stretching the adductor hallucis.[20]

13. INJECTION AND STRETCH
(Figs. 27.8 and 27.9)

Before injection, the skin of the foot is carefully cleansed, as described in Chapter 26, page 515. Injection of these deep muscles can readily result in a transient block of the plantar nerve, which lasts only 15 or 20 minutes when 0.5% procaine solution has been injected. The patient should be warned of this possibility before injection of the TrPs.

For injection of these muscles, a 10-mL syringe is filled with 0.5% procaine solution that has been prepared by dilution with isotonic saline. A 38–mm (1½-in) 22-gauge needle should be long enough to reach these deep intrinsic muscles.

For injection of the **quadratus plantae** muscle, the patient lies on the side of the involved muscle and the clinician localizes the spot of tenderness in the quadratus plantae by deep palpation through the plantar aponeurosis and from the medial border of the foot. The needle enters at the medial border of the sole (Fig. 27.8*A*), angled laterally to reach the quadratus plantae, between the medial and lateral plantar nerves.[4]

The **lumbricals** are small muscles and are indistinguishable from the plantar interossei by palpation. Their TrPs would probably be included when injecting TrPs in the plantar interossei as described later in this section.

The **flexor digiti minimi brevis** may be indistinguishable from a distal belly of the abductor digiti minimi. Its TrPs are located and injected essentially like those of the abductor digiti minimi as described in Chapter 26, on page 517.

For injection of TrPs in the **flexor hallucis brevis** muscle, the patient again lies on the side of the involved muscle and the TrP tenderness is localized in this muscle (Fig. 27.8*B*). Since the proper digital nerve lies superficial to this muscle, the needle enters the medial side of the foot to pass deep to the nerve and superficial to the first metatarsal bone into the flexor hallucis brevis.[4]

To inject TrPs in the **adductor hallucis** muscle with the patient side lying as previously described, the clinician localizes the point of maximum TrP tenderness by deep palpation. After skin preparation, the clinician inserts the needle lateral to the TrP (Fig. 27.8*C*, *syringe free*) so that the needle will angle medially in the direction of the first metatarsal to reach the oblique head of the adductor hallucis (Fig. 27.9). To inject the transverse head of this muscle, the operator inserts the needle distally, close to the heads of the metatarsal bones (Fig. 27.8*C*, *syringe in hand*).

All **interossei (dorsal and plantar) are** approached for injection through the dorsal surface of the foot (Figs. 27.8*D* and 27.9). The patient lies supine with the knee bent to place the foot nearly flat on the examining table. After localizing TrP spot tenderness in the *dorsal* interossei by palpation, the clinician injects the muscle between the metatarsal bones. The fingers of one hand press upward from the plantar surface of the foot into the interosseous space being injected (as shown in Figs. 27.6*D* and 27.8*D*). One must be careful to explore both bellies of a dorsal interosseous muscle in order to locate all of the TrPs on each side of the interosseous space (Fig. 27.5*A*).

To reach a TrP in a *plantar* interosseous muscle that is localized by tenderness to deep bimanual pressure from the plantar side of the foot, the spot of tenderness is fixed by the finger of one hand while the other hand manages the syringe. Figure 27.9 shows why, in order to reach the first plantar interosseus muscle through a dorsal approach, the needle must angle laterally between the second and third metatarsal bones to probe the muscle that lies on the medioplantar aspect of the third metatarsal.

After injecting TrPs in one of these muscles, the clinician applies a few parallel sweeps of intermittent cold while gently stretching the muscle, as

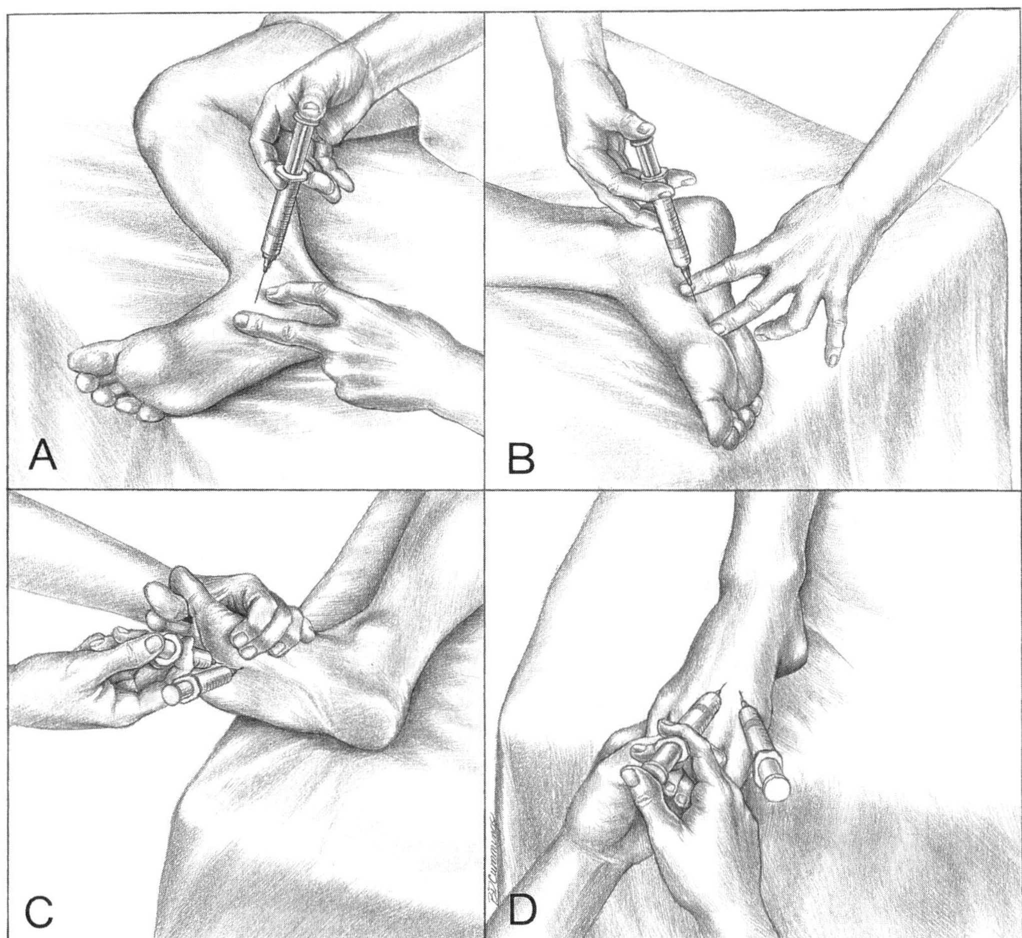

Figure 27.8. Injection of trigger points in the deep intrinsic foot muscles. *A*, quadratus plantae. *B*, flexor hallucis brevis. *C*, adductor hallucis, transverse head (*syringe in hand*) and oblique head (*syringe free*). *D*, first and second dorsal interossei. The free syringe shows the direction that must be probed to locate trigger points in the first dorsal interosseous muscle along the second metatarsal bone. The needle of the syringe in hand is directed into the second dorsal interosseous muscle between the second and third metatarsals. To reach the first plantar interosseous muscle, the needle must angle laterally and penetrate between the second and third metatarsal bones and reach deep to the third metatarsal (*see* Fig. 27.9).

described in the previous section, to release any residual TrPs that were missed by injection. The prompt application of moist heat reduces the likelihood of severe postinjection soreness. Several *slow* cycles of active range of motion to the fully shortened and fully lengthened positions help equalize sarcomere length and restore the full range of muscle function.

14. CORRECTIVE ACTIONS

Crystal deposition disease, such as gout, and other systemic conditions perpetuating the TrPs must be diagnosed and managed. Then TrPs that developed secondarily can be inactivated, whereas they had previously been refractory to local treatment.

Normal joint play and range of motion should be restored.[41]

Appropriate supports should be used in the shoes to compensate for structural and mechanical problems of the foot that cannot be otherwise corrected. This is especially important in patients who are accustomed to running and jogging, who do extensive walking for exercise, or who must stand for long periods of time.

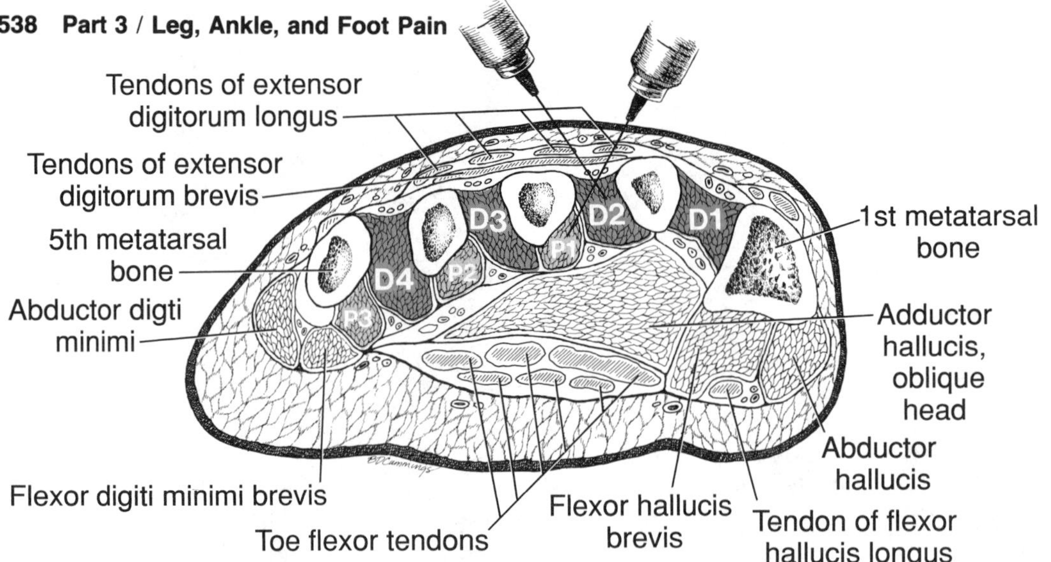

Figure 27.9. Cross section through the foot just proximal to the metatarsal heads, viewed from the front. The dorsal interosseous muscles (*D*) are *dark red*; the plantar interossei (*P*) are *light red*; other muscles, *uncolored*. Adapted from Ferner and Staubesand.[22]

Corrective Posture and Activities

Walking and running should be done on even and level surfaces until TrP activity has been resolved and the patient is ready to start conditioning of the muscles.

Shoes should fit well and should have a firm heel counter and good arch support. The shoe should have a flexible sole, particularly in the metatarsal head region. The patient should avoid shoes with high or spike heels and pointed toes. He or she should be encouraged to buy shoes with good shock absorption, including rubber heels, rubber soles, and resilient foam insoles.

Basford and Smith[8] evaluated the effect of viscoelastic polyurethane insoles in reducing back, leg, and foot pain in 96 adult women. These subjects spent most of the workday on their feet and were not under medical care. Twenty-five of the women found that the insole made their shoes too tight for comfort and they discarded it. The remaining subjects found the insoles comfortable and reported that their pain in all three regions was reduced significantly.[8]

Corrective Exercises

Conditioning and strengthening exercises described in Section 14 of Chapter 26 are also applicable to these deep intrinsic muscles.

Home Therapeutic Program

The self-stretch techniques described and illustrated in Chapter 26, pages 518–519 are equally useful for patients with involvement of the quadratus plantae, lumbricals, flexor hallucis brevis, and the short flexors of the toes. Stretching may be effectively done with the foot immersed in warm water, for example, when taking a tub bath. The methods described are the Toe Flexor Self-stretch Exercise (*see* Fig. 26.8) and the Golf-ball and Rolling-pin Techniques (*see* Fig. 26.9).

References

1. Alfred RH, Bergfeld JA: Diagnosis and management of stress fractures of the foot. *Phys Sportsmed 15*:83–89. 1987.
2. Anderson JE: *Grant's Atlas of Anatomy*, Ed. 8. Williams & Wilkins, Baltimore, 1983 (Fig. 4–95).
3. *Ibid.* (Fig. 4–98).
4. *Ibid.* (Fig. 4–100).
5. *Ibid.* (Fig. 4–102).
6. *Ibid.* (Fig. 4–103).
7. *Ibid.* (Fig. 4–107).
8. Basford JR, Smith MA: Shoe insoles in the workplace. *Orthopedics 11*:285–288, 1988.
9. Basmajian JV, Deluca CJ: *Muscles Alive*, Ed. 5. Williams & Wilkins, Baltimore, 1985 (p. 351–352).

PART 3

10. Carter BL, Morehead J, Wolpert SM, et al.: *Cross-Sectional Anatomy*. Appleton-Century-Crofts, New York, 1977 (Sects. 82–84).
11. *Ibid*. (Sects. 83–87).
12. *Ibid*. (Sects. 85,86).
13. *Ibid*. (Sects. 85–87).
14. Clemente CD: *Gray's Anatomy of the Human Body*, American Ed. 30. Lea & Febiger, Philadelphia, 1985 (pp. 587–590, Fig. 6–83).
15. *Ibid*. (p. 588, Fig. 6–89).
16. *Ibid*. (pp. 889–890, Figs. 6–85, 6–86).
17. Duchenne GB: *Physiology of Motion*, translated by E.B. Kaplan. J.B. Lippincott, Philadelphia, 1949 (pp. 375–377).
18. Evjenth O, Hamberg J: *Muscle Stretching in Manual Therapy, A Clinical Manual*. Alfta Rehab Førlag, Alfta, Sweden, 1984 (pp. 153, 158, 159).
19. *Ibid*. (p. 157).
20. *Ibid*. (p. 158).
21. *Ibid*. (p. 162).
22. Ferner H, Staubesand J: *Sobotta Atlas of Human Anatomy*, Ed. 10, Vol. 2. Urban & Schwarzenberg, Baltimore, 1983 (Fig. 493).
23. *Ibid*. (Fig. 497).
24. *Ibid*. (Fig. 500).
25. *Ibid*. (Figs. 501, 502).
26. Goldner JL, Ward WG: Traumatic horizontal deviation of the second toe: mechanism of deformity, diagnosis, and treatment. *Bull Hosp Jt Dis Orthop Inst 47*:123–135, 1987.
27. Hollinshead WH: *Functional Anatomy of the Limbs and Back*, Ed. 4. W.B. Saunders, Philadelphia, 1976 (p. 358, Table 20–1).
28. Hollinshead WH: *Anatomy for Surgeons*, Ed. 3., Vol. 3, *The Back and Limbs*. Harper & Row, New York, 1982 (pp. 840–841).
29. *Ibid*. (pp. 841–842).
30. *Ibid*. (pp. 842–843).
31. *Ibid*. (pp. 843–846).
32. Inman VT, Ralston HJ, Todd F: *Human Walking*. Williams & Wilkins, Baltimore, 1981 (p. 116).
33. Jarret BA, Manzi JA, Green DR: Interossei and lumbricales muscles of the foot: an anatomical and function study. *J Am Podiatr Assoc 70*:1–13, 1980.
34. Jimenez AL, McGlamry ED, Green DR: Lesser ray deformities, Chapter 3. In *Comprehensive Textbook of Foot Surgery*, edited by E.D. McGlamry, Vol. 1. Williams & Wilkins, Baltimore, 1987 (pp. 57–113, *see* pp. 65–67).
35. Kalin PJ, Hirsch BE: The origins and function of the interosseous muscles of the foot. *J Anat 152*: 83–91, 1987.
36. Kellgren JH: A preliminary account of referred pains arising from muscle. *Br Med J 1*:325–327, 1938.
37. Kellgren JH: Observations on referred pain arising from muscle. *Clin Sci 3*:175–190, 1938 (*see* Fig. 8).
38. Kelly M: The relief of facial pain by procaine (novocaine) injections. *J Am Geriatr Soc 11*:586–596, 1963.
39. Kendall FP, McCreary EK: *Muscles, Testing and Function*, Ed. 3. Williams & Wilkins, Baltimore, 1983 (p. 132).
40. *Ibid*. (pp. 136–137).
41. Lewit K: *Manipulative Therapy in Rehabilitation of the Motor System*. Butterworths, London, 1985 (pp. 136–137, 207–210).
42. Mann R, Inman VT: Phasic activity of intrinsic muscles of the foot. *J Bone Joint Surg [Am]) 46*: 469–481, 1964.
43. Manoli A II, Weber TG: Fasciotomy of the foot: an anatomical study with special reference to release of the calcaneal compartment. *Foot Ankle 10*:267–275, 1990.
44. Manter JT: Variations of the interosseous muscles of the human foot. *Anat Rec 93*:117–124, 1945.
45. McGlamry ED (Ed.): *Comprehensive Textbook of Foot Surgery*, Vols. I and II. Williams & Wilkins, Baltimore, 1987.
46. McMinn RMH, Hutchings RT: *Color Atlas of Human Anatomy*. Year Book Medical Publishers, Chicago, 1977 (p. 289).
47. *Ibid*. (p. 325).
48. *Ibid*. (p. 326).
49. McMinn RMH, Hutchings RT, Logan BM: *Color Atlas of Foot and Ankle Anatomy*. Appleton–Century–Crofts, Connecticut, 1982 (p. 29).
50. *Ibid*. (p. 56).
51. *Ibid*. (p. 64).
52. *Ibid*. (p. 65).
53. *Ibid*. (p. 66).
54. *Ibid*. (p. 67).
55. *Ibid*. (p. 74).
56. *Ibid*. (p. 75).
57. Netter FH: *The Ciba Collection of Medical Illustrations*, Vol. 8, Musculoskeletal System. Part I: Anatomy, Physiology and Metabolic Disorders. Ciba-Geigy Corporation, Summit, 1987 (p. 105).
58. *Ibid*. (p. 112).
59. *Ibid*. (p. 115).
60. *Ibid*. (p. 116).
61. Rasch PJ, Burke RK: *Kinesiology and Applied Anatomy*, Ed. 6. Lea & Febiger, Philadelphia, 1978 (pp. 324–325, 330, Table 17–2).
62. Richardson EG: Injuries to the hallucal sesamoids in the athlete. *Foot Ankle 7*:229–244, 1987.
63. Rohen JW, Yokochi C: *Color Atlas of Anatomy*, Ed. 2. Igaku-Shoin, New York, 1988 (p. 425).
64. *Ibid*. (p. 427).
65. *Ibid*. (p. 428).
66. *Ibid*. (p. 429).
67. *Ibid*. (p. 456).
68. Rondhuis JJ, Huson A: The first branch of the lateral plantar nerve and heel pain. *Acta Morphol Neerl–Scand 24*:269–279, 1986.
69. Ruch JA, Banks AS: Anatomical dissection of the first metatarsophalangeal joint, Chapter 5, Part 3. In *Comprehensive Textbook of Foot Surgery*, edited by E.D. McGlamry, Vol. 1. Williams & Wilkins, Baltimore, 1987 (pp. 151–172, *see* p. 159).
70. Simons DG: Myofascial pain syndrome due to trigger points, Chapter 45. In *Rehabilitation Medicine* edited by J. Goodgold. C. V. Mosby Co., St. Louis, 1988 (pp. 686–723, *see* p. 712, Fig. 45–9F).
71. Simons DG, Travell JG: Myofascial pain syndromes, Chapter 25. In *Textbook of Pain*, edited by P.D. Wall and R. Melzack, Ed 2. Churchill Livingstone, London, 1989 (pp. 368–385, *see* p. 378, Fig. 25.9H).

72. Travell JG: Chronic Myofascial Pain Syndromes. Mysteries of the History, Chapter 6. In *Myofascial Pain and Fibromyalgia*, Vol. 17 of *Advances in Pain Research and Therapy*, edited by J.R. Fricton and E.A. Awad, Raven Press, New York, 1990 (pp. 129–137).
73. Travell JG, Simons DG: *Myofascial Pain and Dysfunction: The Trigger Point Manual*. Williams & Wilkins, Baltimore, 1983.
74. Turner RS: Dynamic post-surgical hallux varus after lateral sesamoidectomy: treatment and prevention. *Orthopedics* 9:963–969, 1986.
75. Valvo P, Hochman D, Reilly C: Anatomic and clinical significance of the first and most medial deep transverse metatarsal ligament. *J Foot Surg 26*:194–203, 1987.
76. Wood J: On some varieties in human myology. *Proc R Soc Lond 13*:299–303, 1864.

CHAPTER 28
Management of Chronic Myofascial Pain Syndrome

HIGHLIGHTS: In **OVERVIEW**, pain caused by myofascial trigger points (TrPs) may present as an acute, recurrent, or chronic pain syndrome. In the presence of sufficiently severe perpetuating factors, an acute syndrome persists to become a chronic myofascial pain syndrome. For the complete **DIAGNOSIS** of a chronic myofascial pain syndrome, the clinician must conduct a *thorough* general medical history, complete a detailed trauma and pain history of each distinguishable pain area, and check for specific symptoms that would identify systemic perpetuating factors. The history also examines the total life situation and the patient's orientation toward function or pain. In addition to a *complete* general physical examination, the clinician performs a myofascial examination of each muscle suspected of harboring active or latent TrPs and a thorough evaluation for postural and structural dysfunction that could perpetuate the patient's TrPs. The object of this examination is to locate the individual active TrPs responsible for a specific part of the composite pain problem. **DIFFERENTIAL DIAGNOSIS** considers: the myofascial pain modulation disorder, in which the pain and tenderness referred from TrPs in any of the muscles in a region focus on one location; the post-traumatic hyperirritability syndrome, in which nociception and TrP irritability are greatly enhanced following central nervous system trauma; fibromyalgia, which has characteristics that distinguish it from the chronic myofascial pain syndrome; and articular dysfunction, which can interact strongly with myofascial TrPs. **TREATMENT**, besides specific TrP inactivation, concentrates on teaching patients how to recognize and stretch the muscles responsible for their myofascial pain, and on the management of muscle stress factors. Mechanical and systemic perpetuating factors that are responsible for the chronicity must be corrected. If patients are pain oriented rather than function oriented, the reasons must be identified and addressed, thus enabling them to take responsibility for the health of their muscles, including carrying out a self-treatment program. Inadequate coping skills and depression require correction. Patients may have concomitant articular dysfunction or fibromyalgia, either of which also requires attention.

---

1. OVERVIEW

Recent studies indicate that myofascial pain is the most common single source of musculoskeletal pain, and that myofascial pain compares in severity with other painful conditions that cause the patient to seek medical assistance.[10,15,39,51]

Myofascial pain due to active trigger points (TrPs) can present as acute, recurrent, or chronic. The patient with an acute-onset myofascial pain syndrome usually associates the onset of pain with a specific overload of the muscles and, therefore, expects it to be self-limiting, like postexercise soreness. In the absence of mechanical or systemic perpetuating factors, a newly activated TrP sometimes spontaneously regresses to a latent TrP, if the muscle remains moderately active but is not overloaded. This residual myofascial syndrome due to latent TrPs continues to cause some degree of dysfunction, but no pain.[55] The individual muscle chapters of Volumes 1 and 2 of THE TRIGGER POINT MANUAL deal primarily with single-muscle myofascial pain syndromes.

Active TrPs that spontaneously regress to the latent stage are readily susceptible to reactivation, and the patient may experience recurrent episodes of the same pain problem. Again, the individual expects each episode to be limited in duration and, therefore, tolerates it until relief becomes overdue.

However, in the presence of sufficiently severe perpetuating factors, the active TrPs persist and may propagate as secondary and satellite TrPs, leading to a progressively severe and widespread chronic myofascial pain syndrome. Chronic enigmatic pain, for which health care providers have been unable to find an organic cause, is a major unsolved problem of the health care system in this country.[23] Fields[9] observed, "The most common persistent and disabling pains are those of musculoskeletal origin." Many times, this chronic pain of enigmatic origin is caused by myofascial TrPs, by fibromyalgia, by articular dysfunction, or by some combination of the three that has been overlooked. This chapter deals primarily with TrP-induced chronic pain, which is both diagnosable and treatable.

When undiagnosed, interminable pain has, psychologically, a totally different impact than pain of limited duration. As emphasized by Hendler,[21] chronic pain creates psychological problems in a previously well-adjusted individual, and therefore, "if the patient's response to pain is appropriate, but there are no objective physical findings, it is incumbent upon the physician to keep looking for the source of the patient's pain complaint."[21] Gamsa[16] concluded that emotional disturbance in patients with chronic pain is more likely to be the consequence than the cause of the pain.

Since secondary and satellite TrPs usually develop in functionally related muscles of the same region of the body as the primary TrP, the term *chronic regional myofascial pain syndrome* may help distinguish the *regional* distribution of the chronic myofascial pain syndrome from the total-body painfulness of fibromyalgia. Because mechanical and systemic perpetuating factors also increase the susceptibility of the muscles to the activation of primary TrPs, patients with severe perpetuating factors are likely to develop clusters of myofascial syndromes in several regions of the body.

PART 3

2. DIAGNOSIS

Patients with chronic myofascial pain are people who have suffered more than just pain for many months or longer. The severity and chronicity of their "untreatable" pain has often reduced their physical activity, limited participation in social activities, impaired sleep, induced a major or minor degree of depression, caused loss of role in the family, led to loss of employment, and deprived them of control of their lives. Many have been depersonalized by the ultimate indignity—the conviction that their pain is not "real," but psychogenic. Well-meaning practitioners sometimes have also convinced the patients' families and friends that the pain is not real, leaving many patients nowhere to turn for help. Several of the resulting conditions listed previously may cause or augment pain; all of them cause suffering. The patients come to the clinician seeking relief from their suffering, which they may present only in terms of pain.

When examining the patient who has presented with chronic enigmatic pain, the diagnostician must first conduct a thorough, time-consuming *history* and *physical examination* to identify what conditions are contributing to the patient's pain and to determine whether there is a significant myofascial component. Materson[34] presents a clearly written, insightful, and detailed description of the examination required. Hendler[21] emphasizes how frequently a thorough examination is bypassed once the patient has been labeled a "chronic pain patient." If it appears likely that the patient does have chronic myofascial pain syndrome, the diagnostic task becomes twofold. In addition to identifying which TrPs, in which muscles, are causing what portion of the patient's total pain complaint, the examiner must determine what perpetuating factors converted the initial acute myofascial pain syndrome to a chronic one. Myofascial TrPs may be perpetuated by mechanical (structural or postural) factors, by systemic factors, by associated medical conditions, and by psychological stress. What we call perpetuating factors,

Fricton refers to as contributing factors[12] or associated problems;[13] he lists those commonly found in chronic myofascial pain syndromes of the head and neck.[13]

Myofascial Pain History

Above all, **clinicians must believe that their patients hurt as much and in the way that they say they do**. The patients are describing their suffering. The first author discovered and mapped the referred pain patterns by believing her patients, even though they described pain in areas that were originally unexplainable. We now know that the central nervous system powerfully modulates pain input from the muscles in ways that can explain referred pain and altered sensation from TrPs.[35,42] Referral of pain, tenderness, and other altered sensation from muscles is no longer the enigma that it was in the past.[35,42,48]

The examiner begins locating the active TrPs by taking a thorough pain history, precisely drawing on a body form each area of pain that the patient identifies. Each pain area can be numbered on the form in the chronological order of its first appearance, and its course and characteristics recorded, as its pattern is drawn. The technique for doing this is described in Volume 1, pages 46–50.[56] One patient may have many distinguishable areas of pain (some of which may be caused not by TrPs but by other conditions, such as peripheral nerve entrapment). The distribution of pain referred from myofascial TrPs in these patients generally corresponds to areas published in this and in the first Volume[56] of THE TRIGGER POINT MANUAL. Several active TrPs may contribute to the pain reported in one region if the referred pain patterns of the TrPs overlap.

It is critically important to delineate clearly the margins of each pain area and to identify its time of onset, any strain or trauma associated with its onset, events that aggravate it, and what relieves it. The latter two observations are influenced by the phase of that myofascial pain syndrome.[55] In phase 1 (constant pain from severely active TrPs), patients may already have such intense pain that they do not perceive an increase and cannot distinguish what makes it worse. Phase 2 (pain from less irritable TrPs that is perceived only on movement and not at rest) is ideal for educating the patient as to which muscles and movements are responsible for the pain, and how to manage it. In phase 3 (latent TrPs that are causing no pain), the patient still has some residual dysfunction and is vulnerable to reactivation of the latent TrPs.

The first author has reviewed[55] many pitfalls in taking a myofascial pain history and emphasized the importance of understanding the patient's daily routine in detail, such as sleep positions, customary diet, and posture and movements in the work situation. A recent review[49] included a sample patient information questionnaire that is useful both as a preliminary review instrument and as a check list when taking the initial and interval histories.

Specific systemic perpetuating factors that need to be considered in taking the history are listed in a recent review[47] and are considered in depth on pages 114–155 in Volume 1.[56]

The specific functional losses in the patient's life need to be identified as to kind and degree. Whether the patient's orientation is toward function or toward pain should be clarified promptly; if the orientation is not toward function, the therapy team should explore why it is not. Most patients are function oriented and want nothing more than to obtain enough understanding to control their pain so that they can return to a normal life-style. Patients with poor coping skills learn to depend on pain to survive in life and need counseling to deal with this additional suffering. Often, patients' involvement in litigation regarding their pain is based either on their conviction that the medical community has nothing more to offer them by way of pain relief and improved function, or on the hope of receiving payment for accumulated medical bills.

Myofascial Physical Examination

Specific myofascial examination of the muscles is undertaken following a complete general physical examination.

When searching for active TrPs that are responsible for the patient's pain, it is essential to know the precise location of the pain and to know which specific muscles can refer pain to that location. Muscles that could be causing the pain are tested for restriction of *passive* stretch range of motion and for pain at the shortened end of *active* range of motion, as compared with uninvolved contralateral muscles. Suspected muscles are also tested for mild to moderate weakness either by conventional isometric strength testing or during a lengthening contraction. Such weakness is not associated with atrophy of the muscle.

The muscles showing abnormalities in these tests are the ones most likely to have the taut bands and spot tenderness of the TrP. The taut bands are located by palpation and then tested for a local twitch response and reproduction of the patient's pain complaint by digital pressure on the TrP. One must try to distinguish active TrPs from latent ones, which can also respond positively to the tests described but are not responsible for a pain complaint. Active TrPs are more irritable than latent TrPs and show greater responses on examination. If inactivation of the suspected TrP does not relieve the pain, it may either have been a latent TrP or it may *not* have been the *only* active TrP referring pain to that area.

Examination for mechanical perpetuating factors requires careful observation of the patient's postures, body symmetry, and movement patterns. A recent review[47] lists many of these factors that need to be considered; they are discussed in detail on pages 104–114 in Volume 1[56] and in Section 7 (**Activation and Perpetuation of Trigger Points**) of the muscle chapters in both volumes of THE TRIGGER POINT MANUAL. Common mechanical factors that can influence many muscles are the round-shouldered, head-forward posture with loss of normal lumbar lordosis, and body asymmetries including a lower limb-length inequality and a small hemipelvis. The postural factors are discussed in the following section on treatment, in Chapter 2 of this volume, and, as appropriate, in individual muscle chapters. Body asymmetries are presented in detail in Chapter 4 of this volume. Tightness of the iliopsoas and hamstring muscles can also seriously disrupt balanced posture.

3. DIFFERENTIAL DIAGNOSIS

Two variants of myofascial pain syndromes should be recognized: the myofascial pain modulation disorder, which leads to diagnostic confusion, and the post-traumatic hyperirritability syndrome, which complicates management. In addition, either fibromyalgia or articular dysfunction can confusingly mimic a chronic myofascial pain syndrome. Each requires an additional specific examination technique and its own treatment approach.

To help a patient with chronic enigmatic pain, the examiner must find sources of pain that have been overlooked, and that means conducting examinations that were not previously performed. After the history, the first order of business is to conduct a time-consuming, detailed, complete physical examination looking for well-known causes of pain that were missed.[21,34] Such an examination is rarely performed when the examiner expects to find that the patient's pain is "all in the head."

Myofascial Pain Modulation Disorder

The term "myofascial pain modulation disorder",[45] adapted from a term used by Moldofsky,[36] identifies a relatively small group of myofascial pain patients who show a remarkable distortion of their pain referral patterns. Instead of each active TrP projecting pain to its expected location (reference zone), the referred pain and tenderness from all TrPs in a region converge on one common location. This location may not be the expected zone of pain reference for any of the involved muscles. Characteristically, the convergent focus is the site of previous trauma or intense pain prior to onset of the pain modulation disorder. These features resemble the experimental observations of Reynolds and Hutchins.[38]

It appears that the aberrant referral patterns are caused by a distortion of sensory modulation in the central nervous system. Many of these patients had previously experienced trauma or painful impact at the focus of pain, but often not of such severity that it would be expected to cause structural damage to the central nervous system. The mechanism behind this sensory nervous system dysfunction is not clear, but possible mechanisms are being explored in current neurosensory research.

Post-traumatic Hyperirritability Syndrome

The term "post-traumatic hyperirritability syndrome" was introduced[24,46] to identify a limited number of patients with myofascial pain who exhibit marked hyperirritability of the sensory nervous system and of existing TrPs. This syndrome follows a major trauma, such as an automobile accident, a fall, or a severe blow to the body that is apparently sufficient to injure the sensory modulation mechanisms of the spinal cord or brain stem. The patients have constant pain, which may be exacerbated by the vibration of a moving vehicle, by the slamming of a door, by a loud noise (a firecracker at close range), by jarring (bumping into something or being jostled), by mild thumps (a pat on the back), by severe pain (a TrP injection), by prolonged physical activity, and by emotional stress (such as anger). Recovery from such stimulation is slow. Even with mild exacerbations, it may take the patient many minutes or hours to return to the baseline pain level. Severe exacerbation of pain may require days, weeks, or longer to return to baseline.

These patients almost always give a history of having coped well in life prior to their injury, having paid no more attention to pain than did their friends and family. They were no more sensitive to these stimuli than other persons. From the moment of the initial trauma, however, pain suddenly became the focus of life. They must pay close attention to the avoidance of strong sensory stimuli; they must limit activity because even mild to moderate muscular stress or fatigue intensifies the pain. Efforts to increase exercise tolerance may be self-defeating. Such patients, who suffer greatly, are poorly understood and, through no fault of their own, are difficult to help.

In these patients, the sensory nervous system behaves much as the motor system does when the spinal cord has lost supraspinal inhibition. In the latter, a strong sensory input of almost any kind can activate non-specific motor activity for an extended period of time. Similarly, in these patients, a strong sensory input can increase the excitability of the nociceptive system for long periods. In addition, these patients may show lability of the autonomic nervous system with skin temperature changes and swelling that resolve with inactivation of regional TrPs. Since routine medical examination of these suffering patients fails to show any organic cause for their symptoms, they are often relegated to "crock" status.

Any additional fall or motor vehicle accident that would ordinarily be considered minor can severely exacerbate the hyperirritability syndrome for years. Unfortunately, with successive traumas, the individual may become increasingly vulnerable to subsequent trauma. A frequent finding is a series of motor vehicle accidents over a period of several years.

Similar phenomena have been described as the *cumulative trauma disorder*,[5] the *stress neuromyelopathic pain syndrome*,[33] and as the *jolt syndrome*.[8]

Fibromyalgia

Fibromyalgia, previously called fibrositis, is officially defined as causing WIDESPREAD pain for at least 3 months. Digital palpation of the patient must elicit pain at 11 or more of 18 prescribed tender point sites.[59] An older term, *fibrositis,* has been used in many ways,[37] and anyone who delves into that literature can easily be confused by it. Throughout this century, prior to 1977, the published descriptions of fibrositis had a closer resemblance to myofascial pain syndromes than to what is now known as fibromyalgia.[45] In 1977, Smythe and Moldofsky[52] redefined fibrositis in terms that were similar to what is now called fibromyalgia. The term *fibrositis* (in the sense that Smythe and Moldofsky used it) has now been officially replaced[59] by the term *fibromyalgia*, which was introduced in 1981.[61]

Many authors,[3,6,20,41,44,57,60] including the authors of this volume, consider myofascial pain syndrome and fibromyalgia as two separate conditions that need to be distinguished clinically. Others believe that a myofascial pain syndrome and

PART 3

fibromyalgia are different aspects of basically the same condition, with each diagnosis representing the ends of a spectrum of signs and symptoms. An *acute* single-muscle myofascial pain syndrome is easily distinguished from fibromyalgia. However, it can be difficult to distinguish *chronic* myofascial pain syndromes from fibromyalgia. The distinctions are particularly blurred if the patient has both fibromyalgia and *chronic widespread* myofascial pain that involves multiple regions.

A number of characteristics may be helpful in distinguishing one condition from the other. Patients with fibromyalgia are predominantly female (73–88% in six studies).[57] Men and women are nearly equally likely to have myofascial pain syndromes, as the senior author and other authors[51,53] have found. The patient with an *acute* myofascial pain syndrome typically can identify the onset precisely as to time and place. Usually the muscle was subjected to momentary overload, e.g. an automobile accident, a near fall, a sudden and vigorous movement (sports activity), moving a heavy box, reaching over to pick something up from the floor, or getting into an automobile, although there may be a lag of several hours to a day after the initiating event before pain appears. Patients with *chronic* myofascial pain may have difficulty identifying the onset so clearly. These patients are likely to have more than a single myofascial pain syndrome. In contrast, the symptoms of fibromyalgia typically develop insidiously; these patients usually can identify no specific moment in time when their symptoms began. Thus, the onset of myofascial pain characteristically relates much more strongly to muscular activity and specific movements than does fibromyalgia.

The orientation of the patient examination is quite different for the two conditions. For the diagnosis of myofascial pain, the clinician painstakingly identifies precisely the distribution of each pain complaint, looks for dysfunctional postures and asymmetries, and examines the muscles to determine which ones show a restricted stretch range of motion. Restriction of motion is not a part of the diagnosis of fibromyalgia.

The myofascial examination includes palpation of the suspected muscles for tender spots in taut bands, which, when compressed, refer pain to the area of the patient's pain complaint and, when snapped transversely, produce a local twitch response. To examine for fibromyalgia, the prescribed tender point locations are examined only for tenderness; a relationship between the location of the tender points and the distribution of the patient's pain is not an issue.

On palpation, the diffusely tender muscles of patients with fibromyalgia feel soft and doughy (except in specific areas, if they *also* have TrPs in taut bands[32,50]), whereas the muscles of patients with myofascial pain feel tense and are non-tender *except* at TrPs and in reference zones.

Muscles that exhibit TrPs also exhibit some weakness without atrophy, but they are not particularly fatigable. Generalized severe fatigue, rather than weakness, is characteristic of fibromyalgia.[3]

The chronicity of myofascial pain syndromes is caused by perpetuating factors that usually are correctable; the chronicity of fibromyalgia is inherent to the disease. This distinction is not evident at initial evaluation.

Some features are confusingly common to both conditions. Disturbed, non-restful sleep may occur in either, but is not required for diagnosis. Over half of the designated tender point locations are also common muscle TrP sites.[45] By definition, a latent or an active TrP at one of those tender point sites would be counted as a tender point. Recent studies indicate that taut bands may be found not only in patients with myofascial pain and in patients with fibromyalgia, but also in "normal" subjects.[14,58] This finding may have unexplored implications as to the relationship between the taut band and its TrP. Many patients with fibromyalgia also have active myofascial TrPs.[58]

At this time, no specific cause of either fibromyalgia or myofascial TrPs has been established. However, clinically, myofascial pain caused by TrPs is primarily a focal dysfunction of muscle, whereas fibromyalgia is a systemic disease[7,40,45] that also affects the muscles.[2,25]

Articular Dysfunction

We think of articular dysfunction either as joint hypomobility (including loss of joint play) that requires manual movement, mobilization, or manipulation to restore normal function, or as hypermobility that requires stabilization. The term *somatic dysfunction* is now commonly used and includes skeletal dysfunctions that are often treated by mobilization and manipulation, as well as myofascial dysfunctions that are frequently treated with myofascial release techniques.[19]

An understanding of the interface between myofascial pain syndrome and articular dysfunction is one of the great voids in our current knowledge of manual medicine. The early work of Korr *et al.*[29,30] on segmental facilitation describes modulation of referred tenderness, motor activity, and skin conductance changes more than it describes modulation of pain. The facilitation of motor responsiveness caused by articular dysfunction is especially pertinent to the myofascial pain syndrome, but remains essentially unexplored with modern instrumentation. Janda,[26] in association with others,[27] has examined distortion of the normal sequence of coordinated motor activity associated with skeletal asymmetries and muscular imbalance. Lewit[31] has emphasized the close clinical relationship between myofascial pain syndromes and articular dysfunction.

4. TREATMENT

A chronic myofascial pain syndrome became chronic because of perpetuating factors that were unrecognized or were inadequately managed. An identifying characteristic of a *chronic* myofascial pain syndrome is the initially unsatisfactory response to specific myofascial therapy. Relief is usually only temporary, lasting a few hours or days. However, *with correction of the perpetuating factors, the involved muscles become increasingly responsive to therapy*. Occasionally, severe perpetuating factors render the TrPs so irritable that even the most gentle attempts at therapy cause more distress than relief. *As progress is made in resolving the perpetuating factors, the involved muscles become increasingly treatable*.

If one starts by correcting obvious mechanical perpetuating factors, myofascial TrP therapies that were previously ineffective are then likely to provide significant relief and to encourage the patient. Each component myofascial pain syndrome should be analyzed and managed as a single-muscle syndrome in the context of other TrPs in the same region. For patients with chronic pain, a home program of stretch exercises is extremely important, probably even more so than for patients with a myofascial pain syndrome of only one or two muscles.

Setting specific goals as described by Materson[34] is critical for patients with chronic myofascial pain. The primary goal is to teach patients how to recognize specific TrP syndromes, how to employ appropriate body positioning, and which stretch techniques to use for relief. This puts the patients in control. If they want more relief, they know how to obtain it. If they prefer to trade a given level of pain for the time and effort required to relieve it, that is their decision. They learn that control of the pain is in their hands. They come to understand what constitutes abuse of their muscles (that will aggravate the pain) and what measures will reduce unnecessary overload of the muscles. They learn to converse with and listen to their muscles.

Travell[55] emphasized the importance of having the *patients*, at the end of the office visit, recollect and write down the recommendations given them. Before leaving the office, they must perform their corrective stretching exercises under supervision according to the instructions *in hand*.

Mechanical Perpetuating Factors

If the clinician selects for initial treatment a myofascial pain syndrome that is a major source of pain, is likely to respond to TrP therapy, and has a mechanical perpetuating factor that is readily correctable (such as sitting posture or lower limb-length inequality), the patient will see immediate benefits and will develop confidence in the treatment. Additional mechanical perpetuating factors relevant to the patient's pain should also be corrected promptly.

Many mechanical factors have been reviewed in detail on pages 104–114 in Volume 1[56] and in another publication.[49] Each muscle chapter in THE TRIGGER POINT MANUAL discusses relevant perpetuating factors in Section 7 (**Activation and Perpetuation of TrPs**). Faulty posture is a mechanical perpetuating factor that is becoming increasingly common and serious with the proliferation of computer terminals and computerized work stations.

Postural training should be one of the first parts, if not *the* first part, of the treatment program. Kendall and McCreary[28] described ideal standing postural alignment, identified several types of faulty standing posture, and suggested therapeutic procedures for correction of the malalignments.

The common round-shouldered, head-forward posture is discussed briefly in Chapter 2, pages 19–20. Faulty posture can aggravate TrPs in many regions of the body and can also increase the tenderness of fibromyalgia tender points.[22] Its importance has been emphasized and re-emphasized by Brügger.[4]

In the *seated* individual, the "slumped posture," or fatigue posture, is characterized by a flattened lumbar spine (loss of normal lordosis), sometimes by an increased dorsal kyphosis, by protracted scapulae, and usually by a flattened cervical spine with the head forward. This posture leads to multiple muscle and joint problems in the trunk, upper limbs, neck, and head, as well as limited respiratory function.

For the seated slumped position, the patient can improve postural alignment by consciously raising the top of the head *upward*, keeping it *slightly* forward.[1] This simple maneuver lifts the chest to an optimum position for respiratory function. A comparable alignment can be accomplished by "putting a hollow" in the low back. Since this erect posture (sitting "tall") cannot be actively held for long periods, the individual can achieve this without effort by positioning the buttocks against the back of the chair and then placing a small roll behind the lumbar spine (waist level). "Reaching" upward with the top of the head can be done several times a day as an exercise. The principle of raising the top of the head away from the shoulders should also be applied when leaning forward to bathe or eat, thereby avoiding rolling the shoulder up and forward and dropping the head.

For good seated posture, one's feet must reach the floor; when a person's legs are short or a seat is too high, a flexible footrest (small firm pillow, bean bag, or sand bag) may be used to support the feet. A hard telephone book is less desirable, but can be temporarily useful. The arms should be supported on armrests that are high enough to allow the individual to sit erect with the elbows supported. Forearm support extensions can be adapted for desk work when typing. When one sits on a sofa or at a desk, arm support can be provided by using a lap board placed on a pillow.

An alternate sitting position is one of sitting toward the front *edge* of a chair seat, placing one foot back under the chair and the other foot forward. This balanced position promotes an erect posture with a natural, but not excessive, lumbar curve. Another way to promote good sitting alignment with little effort is to place a pad at the back of the chair seat, directly under the ischial tuberosities (*not* under the thighs). The padding tilts the pelvis forward slightly to induce normal lumbar lordosis, which, in turn, facilitates good upper body alignment. Having two ways of sitting with good posture can be particularly useful for someone working at a desk. Frequent changes of position are needed to promote health of the muscles and intervertebral discs.

Most important is patient awareness of the problem, understanding of its significance, and willingness to practice sitting and standing erect. Following appropriate postural training (both "static" and dynamic), the patient can take responsibility for the management of the pain that results from chronic postural strain and many activities of daily living. As patients exercise increasing control, they improve both physically and emotionally.

Systemic Perpetuating Factors

Systemic perpetuating factors should be corrected as they are identified when laboratory test results become available.

These multiple factors are discussed in detail on pages 114–156 in Volume 1[56] and summarized in later publication.[49] Systemic factors are commonly overlooked, can be difficult to manage, and often make the difference between a successful and unsuccessful therapeutic outcome for the patient.

Vitamin inadequacy is probably the most common systemic perpetuating factor, and it has been experimentally demonstrated as important in patients with chronic pain.[43]

Another frequently overlooked systemic factor is marginal or subclinical hypothyroidism. Like vitamin inadequacies, it is correctable.[54]

Psychological Aspects

If the patient is function oriented and has developed few pain behaviors, the program described previously can be successful. If the patient has lost self-esteem, is pain oriented, and has developed pain behaviors, the clinician is faced with a complex web of problems that often requires an interdisciplinary team that includes a professional counselor in order to restore the patient to function. Elimination of the original myofascial TrP cause of the patient's pain is an essential part of the program. However, the pain is often perpetuated by poor sleep, inactivity, and hesitancy to undertake the necessary home-stretching program. Teaching the patient improved coping skills may be a necessary first step to eliminate reinforcement of pain behaviors by well-meaning, but over-protective, significant others. The principles for accomplishing this are clearly presented by Fordyce.[11]

The effectiveness of this multi-pronged approach with emphasis on patient education and on elimination of their TrPs was eloquently demonstrated experimentally by Graff-Radford *et al.*[18]

If patients with chronic pain are depressed, it is necessary to relieve their depression. Inactivity aggravates it and activity that gives them a sense of accomplishment improves it. A regular exercise program is very important. Antidepressant medication may be necessary, especially if sleep is impaired. Treatments that are done ***to*** the patient should be minimized, and effort should be concentrated on teaching what can be done ***by*** the patient.

Associated Conditions

Articular dysfunction and TrP tension in related muscles can perpetuate each other; in which case, both conditions must be corrected to obtain lasting benefit.

Addressing the myofascial pain syndrome in patients who also have fibromyalgia can significantly improve their condition; they will still have fibromyalgia and should receive therapy for it, too.[17] The extent to which these two conditions adversely affect each other is not yet clearly established.

References

1. Barker S: *The Alexander Technique*. Bantam Books, New York, 1978.
2. Bennett RM: Muscle physiology and cold reactivity in the fibromyalgia syndrome. In *The Fibromyalgia Syndrome, Rheumatic Disease Clinics of North America*, Vol. 15, edited by R.M. Bennett, D.L. Goldenberg. W.B. Saunders, Philadelphia, 1989 (pp. 135–147).
3. Bennett RM: Myofascial pain syndromes and the fibromyalgia syndrome: a comparative analysis, Chap. 2. In *Myofascial Pain and Fibromyalgia, Advances in Pain Research and Therapy*, Vol. 17, edited by J.R. Fricton, E.A. Awad. Raven Press, New York, 1990 (pp. 43–65).
4. Brügger A: *Die Erkrankungen des Bewegungsapparates und seines Nervensystems*. Gustav Fischer Verlag, New York, 1980.
5. Burnette JT, Ayoub MA: Cumulative trauma disorders. Part I. The problem. *Pain Management 2*: 196–209, 1989.
6. Campbell SM: Regional myofascial pain syndromes. In *The Fibromyalgia Syndrome, Rheumatic Disease Clinics of North America*, Vol. 15, edited by R.M. Bennett, D.L. Goldenberg. W.B. Saunders, Philadelphia, 1989 (pp. 31–44).
7. Caro XJ: Is there an immunologic component to the fibrositis syndrome? In *The Fibromyalgia Syndrome, Rheumatic Disease Clinics of North America*, Vol. 15, edited by R.M. Bennett, D.L. Goldenberg. W.B. Saunders, Philadelphia, 1989 (pp. 169–186).
8. Elson LM: The jolt syndrome. Muscle dysfunction following low-velocity impact. *Pain Management 3*:317–326, 1990.
9. Fields HL: *Pain*. McGraw-Hill, New York, 1987 (pp. 209–214).
10. Fishbain DA, Goldberg M, Meagher BR, *et al.*: Male and female chronic pain patients categorized by DSM-III psychiatric diagnostic criteria. *Pain 26*:181–197, 1986.
11. Fordyce WE: *Behavioral Methods for Chronic Pain and Illness*. C.V. Mosby, St. Louis, 1976.

PART 3

12. Fricton JR: Myofascial pain syndrome. *Neurol Clin 7*:413–427, 1989.
13. Fricton JR: Myofascial pain syndrome. Characteristics and epidemiology, Chapter 5. In Myofascial Pain and Fibromyalgia, *Advances in Pain Research and Therapy*, Vol. 17, edited by J.R. Fricton, E.A. Awad. Raven Press, New York, 1990 (pp. 107–127, *see* pp. 118–121).
14. Fricton JR: Personal communication, 1991.
15. Fricton JR, Kroening R, Haley D, Siegert R: Myofascial pain syndrome of the head and neck: A review of clinical characteristics of 164 patients. *Oral Surg 60*:615–623, 1985.
16. Gamsa A: Is emotional disturbance a precipitator or a consequence of chronic pain? *Pain 42*: 183–195, 1990.
17. Goldenberg DL: Treatment of fibromyalgia syndrome. In *The Fibromyalgia Syndrome, Rheumatic Disease Clinics of North America*, Vol. 15, edited by R.M. Bennett, D.L. Goldenberg. W.B. Saunders, Philadelphia, 1989 (pp. 61–71).
18. Graff-Radford SB, Reeves JL, Jaeger B: Management of chronic headache and neck pain: the effectiveness of altering factors perpetuating myofascial pain. *Headache 27*:186–190, 1987.
19. Greenman PE: *Principles of Manual Medicine*. Williams & Wilkins, Baltimore, 1989 (pp. 106–112).
20. Hench PK: Evaluation and differential diagnosis of fibromyalgia. Approach to diagnosis and management. In *The Fibromyalgia Syndrome, Rheumatic Disease Clinics of North America*, Vol. 15, edited by R.M. Bennett, D.L. Goldenberg. W.B. Saunders Company, Philadelphia, 1989 (pp. 19–29).
21. Hendler N: The psychiatrist's role in pain management, Chapter 6. In *Innovations in Pain Management*, Vol. 1, edited by R.S. Weiner. Paul M. Deutsch Press, Orlando, 1990 (pp. 6–1 to 6–36, *see* pp. 6–7, 6–20 to 6–23).
22. Hiemeyer K, Lutz R, Menninger H: Dependence of tender points upon posture—key to the understanding of fibromyalgia syndrome. *J Man Med 5*:169–174, 1990.
23. Institute of Medicine: *Pain and Disability: Clinical, Behavioral and Public Policy Perspectives*. National Academy Press, Washington, D.C., May 1987.
24. *Ibid*. (p. 288).
25. Jacobsen S, Danneskiold-Samsøe B: Muscle function in patients with primary fibromyalgia syndrome—an overview. *J Man Med 5*:155–157, 1990.
26. Janda V: *Muscle Function Testing*. Butterworths, London, 1983.
27. Jull GA, Janda V: Muscles and motor control in low back pain: assessment and management, Chapter 10. In *Physical Therapy of the Low Back*, edited by L.T. Twomey and J.R. Taylor. Churchill Livingstone, New York, 1987 (pp. 253–278).
28. Kendall FP, McCreary EK: *Muscles, Testing and Function*, Ed. 3. Williams & Wilkins, Baltimore, 1983.
29. Korr IM, Thomas PE, Wright HM: Symposium on the functional implications of segmental facilitation. *J Am Osteopath Assoc 54*:265–282, 1955.
30. Korr IM, Wright HM, Chace JA: Cutaneous patterns of sympathetic activity in clinical abnormalities of the musculoskeletal system. *Acta Neurovegetativa 25*:589–606, 1964.
31. Lewit K: *Manipulative Therapy in Rehabilitation of the Motor System*. Butterworths, London, 1985.
32. Lewit K: Personal communication, 1989.
33. Margoles MS: Stress neuromyelopathic pain syndrome (SNPS): report of 333 patients. *J Neurol Orthop Surg 4*:317–322, 1983.
34. Materson RS: Assessment and diagnostic techniques, Chapter 5. In *Innovations in Pain Management*, edited by R.S. Weiner, Vol. 1. Paul M. Deutsch Press, 1990 (pp. 5–3 to 5–25).
35. Mense S: Physiology of nociception in muscles, Chapter 3. In *Myofascial Pain and Fibromyalgia, Advances in Pain Research and Therapy*, Vol. 17, edited by J.R. Fricton, E.A. Awad. Raven Press, New York, 1990 (pp. 67–85).
36. Moldofsky H, Tullis C, Lue FA: Sleep related myoclonus in rheumatic pain modulation disorder (fibrositis syndrome). *J Rheumatol 13*:614–617, 1986.
37. Reynolds MD: The development of the concept of fibrositis. *J Hist Med Allied Sci 38*:5–35, 1983.
38. Reynolds OE, Hutchins HC: Reduction of central hyper-irritability following block anesthesia of peripheral nerve. *Am J Physiol 152*:658–662, 1948.
39. Rosomoff HL, Fishbain DA, Goldberg M, *et al.*: Physical findings in patients with chronic intractable benign pain of the neck and/or back. *Pain 37*:279–287, 1989.
40. Russell IJ: Neurohormonal aspects of fibromyalgia syndrome. In *The Fibromyalgia Syndrome, Rheumatic Disease Clinics of North America*, Vol. 15, edited by R.M. Bennett, D.L. Goldenberg. W.B. Saunders, Philadelphia, 1989 (pp. 149–168).
41. Scudds RA, Trachsel LC, Luckhurst BJ, Percy JS: A comparative study of pain, sleep quality and pain responsiveness in fibrositis and myofascial pain syndrome. *J Rheumatol Suppl 19*:120–126, 1989.
42. Sessle BJ: Central nervous system mechanisms of muscular pain, Chapter 4. In *Myofascial Pain and Fibromyalgia, Advances in Pain Research and Therapy*, Vol. 17, edited by J.R. Fricton, E.A. Awad. Raven Press, New York, 1990 (pp. 87–105).
43. Shealy CN: Vitamin B6 and other vitamin levels in chronic pain patients. *Clin J Pain 2*:203–204, 1987.
44. Sheon RP, Moskowitz RW, Goldberg VM: *Soft Tissue Rheumatic Pain*, Ed. 2. Lea & Febiger, Philadelphia, 1987.
45. Simons D: Muscular Pain Syndromes, Chapter 1. In *Myofascial Pain and Fibromyalgia, Advances in Pain Research and Therapy*, Vol. 17, edited by J.R. Fricton and E.A. Awad. Raven Press, New York, 1990 (pp. 1–41).
46. Simons DG: Myofascial pain syndrome due to trigger points, Chapter 45. In *Rehabilitation Medicine*, edited by J. Goodgold. C.V. Mosby Co., St. Louis, 1988 (pp. 686–723).
47. Simons DG: Myofascial pain syndromes. In *Current Therapy of Pain*, edited by K.M. Foley, R.M. Payne. B.C. Decker Inc., Philadelphia, 1989 (pp. 251–266).

48. Simons DG: Symptomatology and clinical pathophysiology of myofascial pain. *Rheuma und Schmerz, State of the Art Lectures*, edited by M. Zimmermann, H. Zeidler, H. Ehlers. Verlag: Gesellschaft zum Studium des Schmerzes, Heidelberg, pp. 29–37, 1990. (ISBN: 3–980 1528–1–2). Also, *Der Schmerz 5[Suppl. 1]*:S29–S37, 1991.
49. Simons DG, Simons LS: Chronic myofascial pain syndrome, Chapter 42. In *Handbook of Chronic Pain Management*, edited by C. D. Tollison. Williams & Wilkins, Baltimore, 1989 (pp. 509–529).
50. Simons L: Personal communication, 1989.
51. Skootsky SA, Jaeger B, Oye RK: Prevalence of myofascial pain in general internal medicine practice. *West J Med 151*:157–160, 1989.
52. Smythe HA, Moldofsky H: Two contributions to understanding of the "fibrositis" syndrome. *Bull Rheum Dis 28*:928–931, 1977.
53. Sola AE, Rodenberger ML, Gettys BB: Incidence of hypersensitive areas in posterior shoulder muscles. *Am J Phys Med 34*:585–590, 1955.
54. Sonkin LS: Endocrine disorders, locomotor and temporomandibular joint dysfunction, Chapter 6. In *Clinical Management of Head, Neck and TMJ Pain and Dysfunction*, edited by H. Gelb. W.B. Saunders Company, Philadelphia, 1977 (pp. 158–164).
55. Travell JG: Chronic myofascial pain syndromes. Mysteries of the history, Chapter 6. In *Myofascial Pain and Fibromyalgia, Advances in Pain Research and Therapy*, Vol. 17, edited by J.R. Fricton, E.A. Awad. Raven Press, New York, 1990 (pp. 129–137).
56. Travell JG, Simons DG: *Myofascial Pain and Dysfunction: The Trigger Point Manual*. Williams & Wilkins, Baltimore, 1983.
57. Wolfe F: Fibrositis, fibromyalgia, and musculoskeletal disease: the current status of the fibrositis syndrome. *Arch Phys Med Rehabil 69*:527–531, 1988.
58. Wolfe F, Simons D, Fricton J, *et al.*: The fibromyalgia and myofascial pain syndromes: a study of tender points and trigger points in persons with fibromyalgia, myofascial pain syndromes and no disease. *Arthritis Rheum 33* (Sup):S137, Abst. No. D22, 1990.
59. Wolfe F, Smythe HA, Yunus MB, *et al.*: American College of Rheumatology 1990 Criteria for the Classification of Fibromyalgia: Report of the Multicenter Criteria Committee. *Arth Rheum 33*: 160–172, 1990.
60. Yunus M, Kalyan-Raman UP, Kalyan-Raman K: Primary fibromyalgia syndrome and myofascial pain syndrome: clinical features and muscle pathology. *Arch Phys Med Rehabil 69*:451–454, 1988.
61. Yunus M, Masi AT, Calabro JJ, Miller KA, Feigenbaum SL: Primary fibromyalgia (fibrositis): clinical study of 50 patients with matched normal controls. *Semin Arthritis Rheum 11*:151–171, 1981.

Appendix—Postexercise Muscle Soreness

Reviews of postexercise (delayed-onset) muscle soreness (not "charley horse," muscle strain or tear, cramps, or chronic leg pain) were published as early as 1902[31] and, more recently, in 1983,[19] in 1984,[2] and in 1986.[38] Hough[31] in 1902 had not yet recognized the important difference between concentric (shortening) and eccentric (lengthening) contractions. In many ways, the soreness of muscles following exercise is similar to a myofascial pain syndrome, but in other ways, it is different. Because postexercise muscle soreness has been so well studied, understanding the similarities and differences in the two conditions should help to better understand myofascial trigger points (TrPs). The features of delayed-onset muscle soreness are reviewed here and are related to TrPs as to features that are similar, those that are different, and those that have an equivocal relationship.

Similarities

Muscle Shortening

In two separate studies,[11,12] vigorous eccentric exercise produced significant shortening of the biceps brachii muscle on the day following, but not immediately following, the exercise. The muscle gradually returned close to its baseline length during the next 4 days. Reduced ability to shorten the muscle fully on a voluntary basis followed a similar time course.

Muscles with active or latent TrPs are also restricted in stretch length and in active shortening, but these restrictions remain as long as the TrPs are present.

Training Effect

Training with *mild slow* eccentric exercise prior to vigorous eccentric contractions protects against postexercise soreness. In addition, a vigorous bout of exercise performed a week after a first vigorous bout caused significantly less muscle shortening, less creatine kinase release into the blood, and less pain.[11] A similar reduced effect was also observed 2 weeks following a strenuous bout of eccentric exercise.[42] The same was true when a modest exposure to eccentric exercise preceded the strenuous test by 2 weeks.[12] Although mild daily eccentric exercise for 1 or 2 weeks prior to strenuous exercise provided protection, the same work expended as concentric exercise did not.[52] Another study found that training effect could still be seen 6 weeks following a single bout of exercise, and that the training effect is specific to eccentric exercise.[9]

Intensive progressive eccentric bicycle ergometry exercise for 8 weeks increased eccentric work capacity 375% with little change in maximal dynamic concentric muscle strength.[24] Biopsies taken before and immediately after a maximal eccentric exercise stint showed increased numbers of type 2C fibers and selective glycogen depletion of type 2B fibers. This indicates that type 2 fibers were selectively affected by the exercise. Ultramicroscopically, the fine structure was well preserved. An increased volume density of mitochondria was seen with no change in Z-band widths.[24]

Vigorous eccentric contractions performed at long muscle length caused markedly greater weakness of the muscle that lasted several times longer than the weakness caused by eccentric contractions performed at short muscle length. This occurred despite the fact that the contractions performed at short muscle length were stronger (produced more work) than those at long muscle length.[34,44]

Conditioning of muscles also makes them more resistant to activation of myofascial TrPs. Whether this protective effect against the development of TrPs is equally specific to training by eccentric exercise has not been tested experimentally.

Resting Electromyographic Activity

Careful quantification of electromyographic (EMG) activity in the medial and lateral heads of the gastrocnemius muscle at 24, 48, and 72 hours after strenuous eccentric exercise showed no increase in average EMG activity in the 11 subjects studied.[6] Similarly, the biceps brachii[32] and other muscles[33] were electrically silent at times when there was pain and restriction of elbow extension following eccentric exercise.[32]

This demonstrates that neither the shortening of the muscle, nor its painfulness, are caused by true muscle spasm. Similarly, tense muscles with myofascial TrPs show no increased resting EMG activity.[22,53]

Response to Treatment

Most (but not all) studies have shown that anti-inflammatory drugs provide little or no relief of postexercise muscle soreness, weakness, and shortening.[14,21,33,49] Because prostaglandin E_2 may be important in muscle repair, prostaglandin blockers, such as aspirin, may be not only useless, but actually detrimental to restoration of the contractile elements.[15] Similarly, aspirin has not been found useful in the relief of pain referred from myofascial TrPs.[59]

Vitamin E was ineffective in reducing the soreness, loss of range of motion, and weakness that resulted from exhausting eccentric exercise;[20] nor has it been found helpful, generally, in the management of myofascial pain syndromes except for some cases of nocturnal calf cramps associated with gastrocnemius TrPs.

Clinical experience has shown that postexercise stiffness may be prevented or markedly reduced by 500 mg or more of vitamin C (preferably timed release) taken so that it is available at the time of the exercise. To our knowledge, this has not been tested in controlled experiments (*see* Volume 1, page 139).[58]

Differences

The sharpest contrasts between postexercise muscle soreness and a myofascial pain syndrome are in the location of the pain and tenderness, and in the time course of symptoms. In addition, marked serum enzyme changes occur in association with postexercise muscle soreness but not as a rule in myofascial pain syndromes. The weakness of each apparently stems from different causes. Static stretching and warm-up exercises do not prevent the muscle soreness from exhaustive eccentric exercise,[30] but are helpful in relieving pain and stiffness associated with myofascial TrPs.

Location of Pain and Tenderness

During episodes of delayed-onset muscle soreness, pain and tenderness are often described as generalized throughout most of the muscle belly.[2] In other studies, the tenderness is described as localized at the region of the distal musculotendinous junction.[2,47]

In myofascial pain syndromes, the pain is primarily referred, often to areas well beyond the muscle that harbors the responsible TrPs. Often, the patient is unaware of the TrP in the muscle that is causing the pain. In myofascial syndromes, the local tenderness is most marked at the TrP and extends with reduced intensity along the taut band associated with the TrP. Tenderness may extend to and include the musculotendinous attachment of that band. Tenderness is also present in the pain reference zones of TrPs.

Time Course

Muscle soreness appears between 8 and 24 hours following eccentric exercise,[57] increases in intensity to reach a peak at 24–72 hours, and is usually gone in 5–7 days. Subjects often describe such exercised muscles as "stiff" and "tender."[2]

Soreness peaked at 24–48 hours following eccentric exercise depending on the age and training of the subjects and the exercise protocol used.[10,11,32,33,41,56,57] Vigorous exercise every 2 weeks produced soreness that peaked in 48 hours after the first bout and in 24 hours after subsequent bouts.[42] Soreness may not be gone until the fifth day,[41,42] the seventh day,[32] or until 2 weeks[47] after vigorous eccentric exercise.

The histological damage from a severe bout of eccentric exercise may take as long as 12 weeks for recovery.[15]

After sudden trauma, pain referred from acute myofascial TrPs appears immediately at the time of injury or within a few hours. In chronic myofascial pain syndromes due to repetitive overload and fatigue, the pain usually develops gradually over a period of days or weeks, sometimes months. After either type of onset, the myofascial pain may gradually resolve spontaneously or run a chronic course.

Response to Treatment

Two muscle-stretching techniques,[41] myofascial manipulation and a muscle-energy technique, had no effect on the muscle soreness, but stretch is effective for treatment of myofascial pain.

Blood Indices

Following vigorous eccentric exercise, some indicators of muscle damage peak in the blood much earlier than others.

The concentration of plasma interleukin-1 (IL-1),[16] total thiobarbituric acid-reactive substances,[37] lactic dehydrogenase (LDH),[25,37,57] serum creatine phosphokinase (CPK),[57] aspartate aminotransferase (AST),[37] and serum glutamic oxaloacetic acid transaminase (SGOT)[25,57] all peaked within the first 24 hours. However, plasma creatine kinase (CK) concentration[11,16,33,42,43] and muscle uptake of the radioisotope 99m technetium pyrophosphate[45] may not peak until 5 or 6 days after exercise. Blood lactic acid was unchanged following eccentric exercise.[51] Jones *et al.*[33] concluded that the pain is more likely to arise from stress on the connective tissues than from damage to the contractile elements.

No increase in serum enzymes has been found in association with chronic myofascial pain syndromes, unless the patient has some coincidental disease. Acute-onset myofascial pain syndromes have not been critically tested for these enzyme changes, partly because the effects of trauma frequently associated with activation of the TrPs would confuse the issue.

Weakness

The weakness caused by TrPs and that caused by postexercise muscle soreness appear to be caused by different mechanisms. Paavo and associates[47] found that 40 minutes of vigorous eccentric exercise reduced strength to 50% of baseline, whereas corresponding concentric exercise reduced it only to 80% of baseline. Sargeant and Dolan[50] reported that the reduction in maximum voluntary contraction persisted up to 96 hours after eccentric exercise. In a study of bouts of exercise repeated every 2 weeks,[42] it took 2 weeks for strength to recover after the initial bout, and only one week or less after subsequent bouts. The weakness is not primarily due to inhibition by pain because it is most marked immediately following the exercise, it is demonstrable by direct electrical stimulation, and some recovery from weakness may occur in 24 hours, prior to the time of maximum soreness.[42] The weakness of sustained maximum isometric contraction is not due to neuromuscular junction failure.[36] The weakness associated with postexercise soreness appears to stem from damage to the contractile apparatus of the muscle as evidenced by so many enzyme changes.

Both active and latent TrPs characteristically cause a modest degree of muscle weakness that is not due to conscious avoidance of pain. The weakness persists as long as the TrPs remain. This mild persistent weakness caused by TrPs is probably caused by reflex inhibition.

Relationship Unclear

Swelling

Swelling appeared clinically in sore muscles following strenuous eccentric exercise.[47] An increase of 11% and 17% in weight caused by edema was observed in rabbit triceps surae muscles 24 and 48 hours, respectively, following vigorous eccentric exercise, but not 6 days following exercise.[7] Biopsies of human anterior tibial muscles 48 hours after eccentric work showed a significantly higher water content than contralateral muscles following concentric work.[26] Volume plethysmography of the leg on the side of exercised triceps surae muscles showed significant increase in calf volume 24, 48, and 72 hours following exercise, compared to the non-exercised contralateral leg.[6] A comparison of tissue pressures and biopsy following eccentric exercise of one tibialis anterior muscle and after concentric exercise of the other[26] found muscle fiber swelling as a predominant feature only after eccentric exercise. A comparable study[56] and an intramuscular pressure study[33] of the forearm flexors found no significant difference between the control and exercised limbs. However, the forearm flexors are not prone to developing a compartment syndrome.

The question as to whether the region in the vicinity of myofascial TrPs is characterized by edema has not been clearly resolved. Two reports[4,8] of biopsies in fibrositis described the presence of interstitial fluid. Their descriptions of "fibrositis" suggest that the authors were studying persons with myofascial TrPs (rather than fibromyalgia as the latter is now perceived by rheumatologists).[5]

Histological Differences. The histological changes that appear after vigorous eccentric exercise indicate exposure of the muscle to the stress of that specific mechanical overload[39] rather than to metabolic distress. This is consistent with the much greater mechanical efficiency of eccentric, as compared to concentric, exercise.[13,35,46–48,50] The net mechanical efficiency of concentric and eccentric work was computed based on force-plate measurement of mechanical work and analysis of expired air for energy expenditure.[35] The mechanical efficiency of concentric work averaged 19.4%. The efficiency of eccentric work, in many instances, exceeded 100%; eccentric work was produced with much less metabolic cost.

Biopsies of human muscles exposed to exhausting eccentric exercise[27,28] showed no abnormality of fiber organization or regeneration at the cellular level. At the subcellular level, severe disorganization of the striation pattern was seen within an hour following the exercise and at 2 and 3 days thereafter. Immediately after exercise, nearly half of the myofibrillar Z bands (which join one sarcomere to the next) showed marked broadening, streaming (scattered broadening), and sometimes total disruption. Most remarkable was the observation that sarcomeres near the affected Z-bands were either supercontracted or disorganized and out of register with the Z-bands. Seven days after the exercise, much recovery had occurred. Supercontraction is characteristic of a contraction knot, and one was illustrated.[27]

Biopsies of the vastus lateralis muscle taken before, and up to 6 days following, strenuous eccentric exercise were observed for immunocytological changes. Only the 3-day specimens showed remarkable changes. Intermediate filament protein responded with microscopic immunofluorescence using an antibody specific to desmin. The authors[23] suggested that the abundant longitudinal "desmin" extensions and strongly autofluorescent granules represented an increased synthesis of desmin and reorganization of the cytoskeletal system in order to restructure the distorted myofibrillar elements.

Fridén and co-workers,[27,28] McCully,[38] and Armstrong[3] concluded that the primary lesion in delayed-onset muscle soreness was disruption of myofibrillar structure due to mechanical overload rather than to a metabolic disturbance.

A subsequent biopsy study of severe eccentric bicycle exercise[46] showed myofibrillar tearing and edema immediately after exercise. In this study, after 10 days, there was myofibrillar necrosis, inflammatory cell infiltration, and no evidence of myofibrillar regeneration. At that time, muscle glycogen was still depleted in both type 1 and type 2 fibers. These changes cannot be attributed simply to increased metabolic demand caused by muscular activity.

No biopsy studies of *acute* myofascial TrPs are known. However, most reports of fibrositis prior to 1977 fit the description of chronic myofascial TrP syndromes much better than they fit the current definition of fibromyalgia.[54] This terminology issue is clarified in Chapter 28 of this volume, under Fibromyalgia. Several studies of fibrositis (using the pre-1977 definition) have reported contraction knots,[29,40,55] and one describes disintegration of the actin filaments where they connect to the Z-bands.[17]

The acute activation of myofascial TrPs is strongly, but not exclusively, related to overload caused by vigorous lengthening contractions. Superimposed reflex contractions may contribute additional overload responsible for activating TrPs. In these acute situations, the myofascial TrP-inducing overload is an instantaneous one-time stress as compared to the cumulative stress effects of prolonged eccentric exercise.

A myofascial TrP may result from a more focal and severe mechanical disruption of the type described in muscle soreness, but one that establishes a self-sustaining feedback loop through the central nervous system.[53]

Magnetic Resonance Findings. Magnetic resonance imaging[18] of runners with post-exercise muscle soreness showed bright rims around both heads of the gastrocnemius muscle and the soleus muscle immediately after vigorous exercise. However, after 24–72 hours, when pain and rhabdomyolysis had developed, signal intensity was markedly increased only at the medial head of the gastrocnemius muscle. In trained athletes, imaging abnormalities tended to be located near the attachments of the muscles, in the region of myotendinous junctions. Magnetic resonance image abnormalities appeared preceding other evidence of injury, including pain and histochemical changes, and lasted as long as 2 weeks following resolution of other changes.

Spectra obtained by magnetic resonance spectroscopy before and immediately after eccentric exercise showed normal resting phosphorylated metabolite levels and normal intracellular pH.[1] However, 24 hours later, when muscle soreness was apparent, inorganic phosphate levels were increased an average of 42%. No significant changes occurred in other metabolites, including phosphocreatine and adenosine triphosphate (ATP). This result could be attributed to a defect in oxidative metabolism, to tissue necrosis associated with the ultramicroscopic lesions described previously, or to sarcolemmal damage that permitted influx of inorganic phosphate.[1]

No magnetic resonance imaging or spectroscopy studies of myofascial TrPs are known to us.

These observations on muscle soreness induced by vigorous eccentric exercise do not apply to the therapeutic value of a limited number of slow eccentric contractions used to inactivate myofascial TrPs, or to recondition muscles, as discussed under Sit-ups and Sit-backs in Volume 1 (*see* Fig. 49.11).[60]

References

1. Aldridge R, Cady EB, Jones DA, *et al.*: Muscle pain after exercise is linked with an inorganic phosphate increase as shown by ^{31}P NMR. *Biosci Rep* 6:663–667, 1986.
2. Armstrong RB: Mechanisms of exercise-induced delayed onset muscular soreness: a brief review. *Med Sci Sports Exerc 16*:529–538, 1984.
3. Armstrong RB: Muscle damage and endurance events. *Sports Med* 3:370–381, 1986.
4. Awad EA: Interstitial myofibrositis: hypothesis of the mechanism. *Arch Phys Med 54*:440–453, 1973.
5. Bennett RM, Goldenberg DL (editors): The fibromyalgia syndrome. *Rheum Dis Clin North Am 15*: 1–191, 1989.
6. Bobbert MF, Hollander AP, Huijing PA: Factors in delayed onset muscular soreness of man. *Med Sci Sports Exerc 18*:75–81, 1986.
7. Brendstrup P: Late edema after muscular exercise. *Arch Phys Med Rehabil 43*:401–405, 1962.
8. Brendstrup P, Jespersen K, Asboe-Hansen G: Morphological and chemical connective tissue changes in fibrositic muscles. *Ann Rheum Dis 16*: 438–440, 1957.
9. Byrnes WC, Clarkson PM: Delayed onset muscle soreness and training. *Clin Sports Med* 5:605–614, 1986.
10. Clarkson PM, Byrnes WC, McCormick KM, *et al.*: Muscle soreness and serum creatine kinase activity following isometric, eccentric, and concentric exercise. *Int J Sports Med 7*:152–155, 1986.
11. Clarkson PM, Dedrick ME: Exercise-induced muscle damage, repair, and adaptation in old and young subjects. *J Gerontol 43*:M91–M96, 1988.
12. Clarkson PM, Tremblay I: Exercise-induced muscle damage, repair, and adaptation in humans. *J Appl Physiol 65*:1–6, 1988.
13. Dick RW, Cavanagh PR: An explanation of the upward drift in oxygen uptake during prolonged

sub-maximal downhill running. *Med Sci Sports Exerc 19*:310–317, 1987.
14. Donnelly AE, McCormick K, Maughan RJ, *et al.*: Effects of a non-steroidal anti-inflammatory drug on delayed onset muscle soreness and indices of damage. *Br J Sports Med 22*:35–38, 1988.
15. Evans WJ: Exercise-induced skeletal muscle damage. *Phys Sportsmed 15*:89–100, 1987.
16. Evans WJ, Meredith CN, Cannon JG, *et al.*: Metabolic changes following eccentric exercise in trained and untrained men. *J Appl Physiol 61*: 1864–1868, 1986.
17. Fassbender HG: *Pathology of Rheumatic Diseases*. Springer-Verlag, New York, 1975 (Chapter 13, pp. 303–314).
18. Fleckenstein JL, Weatherall PT, Parkey RW, *et al.*: Sports-related muscle injuries: evaluation with MR imaging. *Radiology 172*:793–798, 1989.
19. Francis KT: Delayed muscle soreness: a review. *J Orthop Sport Phys Ther 5*:10–13, 1983.
20. Francis KT, Hoobler T: Failure of vitamin E and delayed muscle soreness. *Ala Med 55*:15–18, 1986.
21. Francis KT, Hoobler T: Effects of aspirin on delayed muscle soreness. *J Sports Med Phys Fitness 27*:333–337, 1987.
22. Fricton JR, Auvinen MD, Dykstra D, *et al.*: Myofascial pain syndrome: electromyographic changes associated with local twitch response. *Arch Phys Med Rehabil 66*:314–317, 1985.
23. Fridén J, Kjörell U, Thornell L-E: Delayed muscle soreness and cytoskeletal alterations: an immunocytological study in man. *Int J Sports Med 5*:15–18, 1984.
24. Fridén J, Seger J, Sjöström M, *et al.*: Adaptive response in human skeletal muscle subjected to prolonged eccentric training. *Int J Sports Med 4*: 177–183, 1983.
25. Fridén J, Sfakianos PN, Hargens AR: Blood indices of muscle injury associated with eccentric muscle contractions. *J Orthop Res 7*:142–145, 1989.
26. Fridén J, Sfakianos PN, Hargens AR, *et al.*: Residual muscular swelling after repetitive eccentric contractions. *J Orthop Res 6*:493–498, 1988.
27. Fridén J, Sjöström M, Ekblom B: A morphological study of delayed muscle soreness. *Experientia 37*:506–507, 1981.
28. Fridén J, Sjöström M, Ekblom B: Myofibrillar damage following intense eccentric exercise in man. *Int J Sports Med 4*:170–176, 1983.
29. Glogowski G, Wallraff J: Ein beitrag zur Klinik und Histologie der Muskelhärten (Myogelosen). *Z Orthop 80*:237–268, 1951.
30. High DM, Howley ET, Franks BD: The effects of static stretching and warm-up on prevention of delayed-onset muscle soreness. *Res Quart Exercise Sport 60*:357–361, 1989.
31. Hough T: Ergographic studies in muscle soreness. *Am J Physiol 7*:76–92, 1902.
32. Jones DA, Newham DJ, Clarkson PM: Skeletal muscle stiffness and pain following eccentric exercise of the elbow flexors. *Pain 30*:233–242, 1987.
33. Jones DA, Newham DJ, Obletter G, *et al.*: Nature of exercise-induced muscle pain. In *Advances in Pain Research and Therapy*. Vol. 10, edited by M. Tiengo *et al.* Raven Press, Ltd., New York, 1987 (pp. 207–218).
34. Jones DA, Newham DJ, Torgan C: Mechanical influences on long-lasting human muscle fatigue and delayed-onset pain. *J Physiol 412*:415–427, 1989.
35. Komi PV, Kaneko M, Aura O: EMG activity of the leg extensor muscles with special reference to mechanical efficiency in concentric and eccentric exercise. *Int J Sports Med (8 Suppl) 1*:22–29, (Mar) 1987.
36. Kukulka CG, Russell AG, Moore MA: Electrical and mechanical changes in human soleus muscle during sustained maximum isometric contractions. *Brain Res 362*:47–54, 1986.
37. Maughan RJ, Donnelly AE, Gleeson M, *et al.*: Delayed-onset muscle damage and lipid peroxidation in man after a downhill run. *Muscle Nerve 12*:332–336, 1989.
38. McCully KK: Exercise-induced injury to skeletal muscle. *Fed Proc 45*:2933–2936, 1986.
39. McCully KK, Faulkner JA: Injury to skeletal muscle fibers of mice following lengthening contractions. *J Appl Physiol 59*:119–126, 1985.
40. Miehlke K, Schulze G, Eger W: Klinische und experimentelle Untersuchungen zum Fibrositissyndrom. *Z Rheumaforsch 19*:310–330, 1960.
41. Molea D, Murcek B, Blanken C, *et al.*: Evaluation of two manipulative techniques in the treatment of postexercise muscle soreness. *J Am Osteopath Assoc 87*:477–483, 1987.
42. Newham DJ, Jones DA, Clarkson PM: Repeated high-force eccentric exercise: effects on muscle pain and damage. *J Appl Physiol 63*:1381–1386, 1987.
43. Newham DJ, Jones DA, Edwards RHT: Plasma creatine kinase changes after eccentric and concentric contractions. *Muscle Nerve 9*:59–63, 1986.
44. Newham DJ, Jones DA, Ghosh G, *et al.*: Muscle fatigue and pain after eccentric contractions at long and short length. *Clin Sci 74*:553–557, 1988.
45. Newham DJ, Jones DA, Tolfree SE, *et al.*: Skeletal muscle damage: a study of isotope uptake, enzyme efflux and pain after stepping. *Eur J Appl Physiol 55*:106–112, 1986.
46. O'Reilly KP, Warhol MJ, Fielding RA, *et al.*: Eccentric exercise-induced muscle damage impairs muscle glycogen repletion. *J Appl Physiol 63*:252–256, 1987.
47. Paavo V, Komi PV, Rusko H: Quantitative evaluation of mechanical and electrical changes during fatigue loading of eccentric and concentric work. *Scand J Rehabil Med (Suppl.) 3*:121–126, 1974.
48. Romano C, Schieppati M: Reflex excitability of human soleus motoneurones during voluntary shortening or lengthening contractions. *J Physiol 90*:271–281, 1987.
49. Salminen A, Kihlström M: Protective effect of indomethacin against exercise-induced injuries in mouse skeletal muscle fibers. *Int J Sports Med 8*:46–49, 1987.
50. Sargeant AJ, Dolan P: Human muscle function following prolonged eccentric exercise. *Eur J Appl Physiol 56*:704–711, 1987.
51. Schwane JA, Watrous BG, Johnson SR, *et al.*: Is lactic acid related to delayed-onset muscle soreness? *Phys Sportsmed 11*:124–131, 1983.

52. Schwane JA, Williams JS, Sloan JH: Effects of training on delayed muscle soreness and serum creatine kinase activity after running. *Med Sci Sports Exerc 19*:584–590, 1987.
53. Simons DG: Myofascial pain syndrome due to trigger points, Chapter 45. In *Rehabilitation Medicine*, edited by Joseph Goodgold. C.V. Mosby Co., St. Louis, 1988 (pp. 686–723).
54. Simons DG: Muscle pain syndromes, Chap. 1. In *Myofascial Pain and Fibromyalgia*, edited by J.R. Fricton and E.A. Awad. Raven Press, New York, 1990 (pp. 1–41).
55. Simons DG, Stolov WC: Microscopic features and transient contraction of palpable bands in canine muscle. *Am J Phys Med 55*:65–88, 1976.
56. Talag TS: Residual muscular soreness as influenced by concentric, eccentric, and static contractions. *Res Quart 44*:458–469, 1973.
57. Tiidus PM, Ianuzzo CD: Effects of intensity and duration of muscular exercise on delayed soreness and serum enzyme activities. *Med Sci Sports Exerc 15*:461–465, 1983.
58. Travell JG, Simons DG: *Myofascial Pain and Dysfunction: The Trigger Point Manual*. Williams & Wilkins, Baltimore, 1983.
59. *Ibid.* (pp. 91).
60. *Ibid.* (pp. 680–681, Fig. 49.11).

Index

Page numbers of definitive presentations are in boldface. Illustrations and tables are in italics.

INDEX TO VOLUME 1

INDEX TO VOLUME 1

INDEX TO VOLUME 1

VOLUME I

VOLUME 1

INDEX TO VOLUME 1

INDEX TO VOLUME 1

Index to Volume 2

With a few exceptions, an anatomical structure is listed according to the descriptive adjective that identifies it instead of collectively according to the noun category. Thus the iliopsoas muscle will be found under **I,** iliopsoas, not under **M,** muscle.

The page numbers of the definitive presentation on a topic are set in **bold face** type. A page number that refers to an illustration or table is *italicized.*

INDEX TO VOLUME 2

INDEX TO VOLUME 2

INDEX TO VOLUME 2

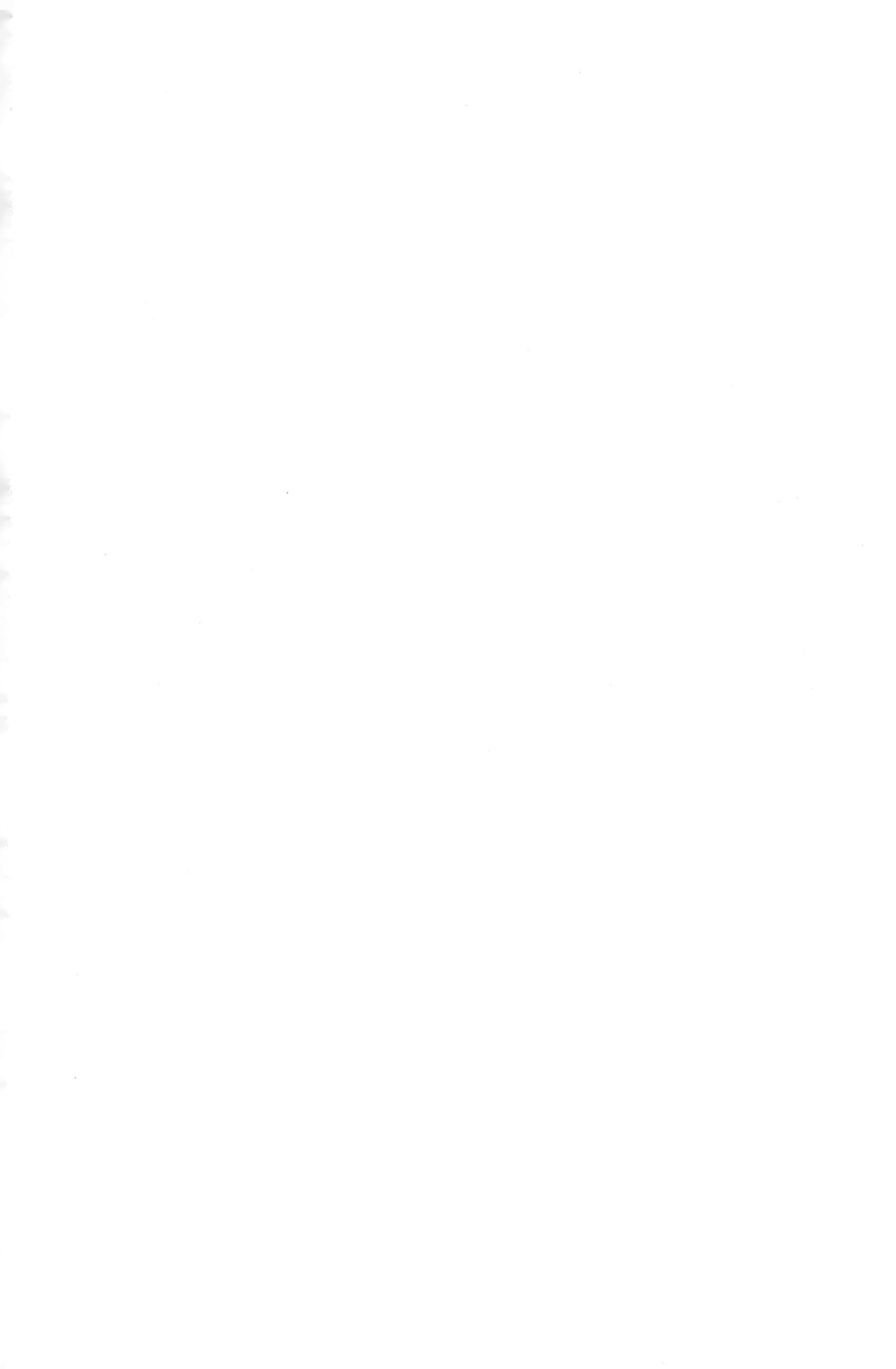

Pain Patterns